OXFORD TEXTBOOK OF
OPHTHALMOLOGY

OXFORD MEDICAL PUBLICATIONS

OXFORD TEXTBOOK OF
OPHTHALMOLOGY

VOLUME 1
Sections 1–2.10

Edited by

David L. Easty
Professor of Ophthalmology

and

John M. Sparrow
Consultant Senior Lecturer

University of Bristol

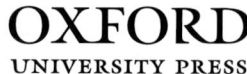

OXFORD
UNIVERSITY PRESS

OXFORD
UNIVERSITY PRESS

Great Clarendon Street, Oxford OX2 6DP

Oxford University Press is a department of the University of Oxford.
It furthers the University's objective of excellence in research, scholarship,
and education by publishing worldwide in

Oxford New York

Athens Auckland Bangkok Bogotá Buenos Aires Calcutta
Cape Town Chennai Dar es Salaam Delhi Florence Hong Kong Istanbul
Karachi Kuala Lumpur Madrid Melbourne Mexico City Mumbai
Nairobi Paris São Paulo Singapore Taipei Tokyo Toronto Warsaw
with associated companies in Berlin Ibadan

Oxford is a registered trade mark of Oxford University Press
in the UK and in certain other countries

Published in the United States
by Oxford University Press Inc., New York

Database right Oxford University Press (maker)

First published 1999

British Library Cataloguing in Publication Data
Data available

Library of Congress Cataloging in Publication Data
Data available

ISBN 0–19 262557 8 (2 volume set)
0–19 262995 6 (volume 1)
0–19 262998 0 (volume 2)
(Available only as a two volume set)

Typeset by Wyvern 21 Ltd, Bristol
Printed in Hong Kong

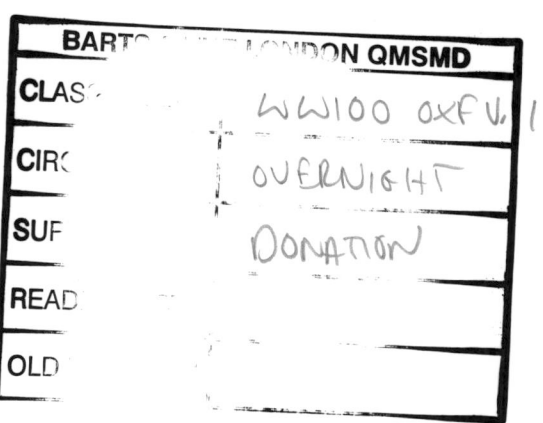

Preface

In producing the *Oxford Textbook of Ophthalmology* we have attempted to reconcile the conflicting demands presented by the need for a broad coverage with the need to discuss all topics at a depth sufficient to render the text useful to a wide readership. By including chapters written by experts from many parts of the world we have captured a breadth and depth of opinion which will provide stimulation and knowledge at many levels. For this we have relied most heavily on the contributing authors, but have also benefited a great deal from the opinions of our section advisers. If we have achieved our goal then this text will be of value to training and practising ophthalmologists in a diversity of situations. By far the greatest time and effort expended in producing the book has been generously given by the contributing authors, to whom we, as editors, are extremely grateful. Their reward will be derived from a readership which gains knowledge and translates this into safe and effective medical practice.

Section advisers

Bertil Damato, Liverpool
Peggy Frith, Oxford
Rodney Grey, Bristol
Richard Harrad, Bristol
Gordon Johnson, London
Wojciech Karwatowski, Leicester
William Lee, Glasgow
Philip Murray, Birmingham

Rachael North, Cardiff
Mike Potts, Bristol
Ralph Rosenthal, Rockville, USA
Mike Saunders, London
David Taylor, London
John Thompson, Leicester
Andrew Tullo, Manchester

We are grateful to Bethany Williams, Karen Bailey, Anne Hugh, Joan Smith and Anne Williams for secretarial support, Gill Bennerson for photographic assistance, Dr Irene Butcher for her excellent administration and team of copy-editors, and the staff of Oxford University Press for technical and other support.

D.L.E
J.M.S
March 1999

To Božana, Valerie, Marina, and Julia

David Easty

To Gemma and Victoria

John Sparrow

Contents

Volume 2

         A. Tufail and Gary N. Holland

2.11.11 Congenital and acquired periorbital skeletal
         anomalies   792
         Peter Ward-Booth

2.11.12 Congenital disease – inherited disorders of
         metabolism   801
         Charles A. Pennock

2.12 Neuro-ophthalmology

    2.12.1   Neuro-ophthalmic history and examination
             of the afferent visual system   813
             Clare Bailey

    2.12.2   Neuroradiology of the orbit and visual
             pathways   824
             Ivan Moseley

    2.12.3   Papilloedema, pseudopapilloedema, and local
             causes of optic disc swelling   830
             Michael A. Burdon and M.D. Sanders

    2.12.4   Retrobulbar optic nerve disease   839
             Paul Riordan-Eva

    2.12.5   Chiasmal disease and the visual system 843
             Shirley H. Wray

    2.12.6   Disorders of visual perception   857
             Christopher Kennard

    2.12.7   Disorders of higher visual function   859
             Gordon T. Plant

    2.12.8   Disorders of the pupil   862
             John Brazier and S.E. Smith

    2.12.9   Supranuclear eye movement abnormalities 866
             Elliot M. Frohman and David Zee

    2.12.10 Infranuclear disorders of eye movements aris-
             ing in the brainstem   871
             James F. Acheson

    2.12.11 Nystagmus   877
             Christopher J. Lyons

    2.12.12 Facial palsy and other disorders of the face 881
             Roger B. Ellingham and Katarzyna Ellingham

    2.12.13 Headache   886
             Thomas R. Hedges, Jr. and T.R. Hedges, III

    2.12.14 Vascular malformations   893
             William Westlake

    2.12.15 Multiple sclerosis   898
             Robert M. McFadzean

2.13 Intraocular tumours

    2.13.1   Uveal melanoma   907
             B. Damato

    2.13.2   Retinoblastoma   918
             Judith Kingston

    2.13.3   Other intraocular tumours   926
             B. Damato

2.14 Epidemiology

    2.14.1   Scientific method.

        2.14.1.1 Clinical measurement instruments:
                  reliability and scaling   933
                  *N. Andrew Frost and John M. Spar-
                  row*

        2.14.1.2 Scientific methods in epidemiology 936
                  John R. Thompson

    2.14.2   Epidemiology of ocular diseases

        2.14.2.1 Basic epidemiological concepts in
                  ophthalmology   948
                  Joanne Katz

        2.14.2.2 Global perspective on blindness 953
                  Gordon J. Johnson

        2.14.2.3 Screening for ocular disease   957
                  Richard Wormald and Scott Fraser

2.15 Tropical ophthalmology

    2.15.1   Ocular infections and infestations   961
             Hugh R. Taylor and Rasik B. Vajpayee

    2.15.2   Childhood blindness: vitamin A deficiency
             and measles infection in developing countries 973
             Clare Gilbert

    2.15.3   Ophthalmic service provision in the Third
             World   981
             David Yorston

2.16 Paediatric ophthalmology

    2.16.1   Embryology of the eye and orbit   985
             Garry N. Shuttleworth

    2.16.2   Postnatal growth and visual development 994
             Cathy Williams

    2.16.3   Developmental abnormalities

        2.16.3.1 Developmental abnormalities of the
                  posterior segment of the eye   998
                  Stephen B. Kaye and S. Siddiqui

        2.16.3.2 Developmental abnormalities of the
                  cornea and anterior segment   1006
                  Stephen B. Kaye and P. Rao

    2.16.4   Examination of the eye in children   1012
             Arvind Chandna and Rowena McNamara

    2.16.5   Paediatric orbital disease: developmental,
             neoplastic, and inflammatory   1030
             *Maria Portellos, Nicholas J. Volpe, and
             Katrinka Heher*

    2.16.6   Corneal and external eye disease in children 1035
             Douglas J. Coster and Li Lim

    2.16.7   Cataract in infancy and childhood: aetiology,
             treatment, and correction   1043
             Isabelle Russell-Eggitt

    2.16.8   Retinal disease and dystrophies   1050
             Richard Markham

    2.16.9   Retinopathy of prematurity   1063
             David Clark and Colin E. Willoughby

3 Principles of surgery and anaesthesia

Index [1]

Contributors

JAMES F. ACHESON
Consultant Ophthalmologist, National Hospital for Neurology and Neurosurgery, University College London Hospitals NHS Trust, UK
2.12.10 Infranuclear disorders of eye movements arising in the brainstem

ALFONSO ANTON-LOPEZ
Glaucoma Specialist, Hospital General (Segovia) and Instituto de Oftalmobiologia Aplicada IOBA (Valladolid), University of Valladolid, Spain
2.10.3 Glaucoma definition and classification

W.J. ARMITAGE
Senior Research Fellow, Division of Ophthalmology, University of Bristol, UK
2.6.1 Anatomy and physiology of the cornea
3.9 Eye banking

ANNETTE S. BACON
Consultant Ophthalmologist, Royal Berkshire Hospital, Reading, UK
3.5 Oculoplastic surgery

PAUL BADENOCH
Senior Medical Scientist and Senior Lecturer, Flinders Medical Centre and Flinders University of South Australia, Adelaide, South Australia
1.2.1 Bacteriology, virology, and mycology

CLARE BAILEY
Specialist Registrar in Ophthalmology, London, UK
2.12.1 Neuro-ophthalmic history and examination of the afferent visual system

JEREMY BARTLETT
General Manager – UK Operations, Sterile Services International Ltd., Cardiff, UK
3.2 Cleaning and sterilization of instruments

CAROLINE R. BAUMAL
Vitreoretinal Surgeon, New England Eye Center and Associate Professor, Tufts University School of Medicine, Boston, Massachusetts, USA
1.5.2 Physical and biological effects of lasers on ocular tissues

PARIMAL BHATTACHERJEE
Professor of Ophthalmology and Visual Sciences, University of Louisville Medical School, Kentucky, USA
1.4.4 Anti-inflammatory drugs

ALAN C. BIRD
Professor of Clinical Ophthalmology, Moorfields Eye Hospital, London, UK
2.9.5 Hereditary pigmentary retinal and macular dystrophies

GRAEME BLACK
Lecturer in Ophthalmology and Genetics, University of Manchester, UK
1.1.2 Molecular biology and molecular genetics: basic principles

P. BLAKE
Wilmer Eye Institute, Baltimore, Maryland, USA
2.1.4 The orbit in neuro-ophthalmology

J. BOULTON
Specialist Registrar, Bristol Eye Hospital, UK
1.4.5 Ocular lubricants and tear replacements

WILLIAM M. BOURNE
Professor of Ophthalmology, Mayo Medical School and Consultant in Ophthalmology, Mayo Clinic, Rochester, Minnesota, USA
1.6.3 Specular and confocal microscopy

JOHN BRAZIER
Consultant Ophthalmologist, University College Hospital, London, UK
2.12.8 Disorders of the pupil

NEIL M. BRESSLER
Professor of Ophthalmology, Wilmer Ophthalmological Institute, Johns Hopkins University School of Medicine, Baltimore, Maryland, USA
2.9.3 Age-related macular degeneration

S. BRESSLER
Wilmer Ophthalmological Institute, Johns Hopkins University School of Medicine, Baltimore, Maryland, USA
2.9.3 Age-related macular degeneration

FRANK V. BUFFAM
Clinical Professor, Department of Ophthalmology, University of British Columbia, Vancouver, Canada
2.1.6.2 Investigation of lacrimal disease
3.7 Treatment of lacrimal obstruction

MICHAEL A. BURDON
Consultant Ophthalmologist, Birmingham and Midland Eye Centre, City Hospital NHS Trust, Birmingham, UK
2.12.3 Papilloedema, pseudopapilloedema, and local causes of optic disc swelling

C.R. CANNING
Consultant Ophthalmologist, Southampton University Hospitals Trust, UK
3.2 Proliferative diabetic retinopathy

ARVIND CHANDNA
Consultant Paediatric Ophthalmologist and Lead Clinician, Royal Liverpool Children's Hospital, UK
2.2.3 Introduction to childhood strabismus
2.16.4 Examination of the eye in children

DEVRON H. CHAR
Professor of Ophthalmology, Radiation Oncology, and The Francis I. Proctor Foundation, University of California, San Francisco, USA
2.1.5 Orbital disease; overview

S. CHARLES
Charles Retina Institute, Memphis, Tennessee, USA
3.19 Pathogenesis and repair of retinal detachment

LEO T. CHYLACK
Professor and Vice-Chairman (Research), Harvard Medical School and Director of Research, Center for Ophthalmic Research, Brigham and Women's Hospital, Boston, Massachusetts, USA
2.7.9 Prospects for a medical treatment of age-related cataract

GEORGE A. CIOFFI
Director, Ocular Research Laboratory and Senior Scientist, Discoveries in Sight, Portland, Oregon, USA
2.10.2 Anatomy and circulation of the anterior optic nerve

DAVID CLARK
Consultant Ophthalmologist, Walton Hospital, Liverpool, UK
2.16.9 Retinopathy of prematurity

KEITH T. R. CLARK
Marketing Manager (Ophthalmology), Ethicon Ltd., Edinburgh, UK
3.3 Suture materials in ophthalmic surgery

MICHAEL COLE
Consultant Ophthalmologist, Torbay Hospital Eye Department, Torquay, Devon, UK
2.2.1 Anatomy of the extraocular muscles and associated cranial nerves

J.R.O. COLLIN
Consultant Opthalmic Surgeon, Moorfields Eye Hospital and Honorary Consultant Ophthalmic Surgeon, Hospital for Sick Children, Great Ormond Street, London, UK
3.5 Oculoplastic surgery

STUART D. COOK
Consultant Ophthalmologist, Bristol Eye Hospital, UK
2.4.1 External eye: anatomy and physiology, examination, and investigation

DOUGLAS J. COSTER
Professor of Ophthalmology, Flinders Medical Centre, Adelaide, South Australia
2.16.6 Corneal and external eye disease in children

B. DAMATO
Consultant Ophthalmologist, St Paul's Eye Unit, Royal Liverpool University Hospitals, UK
2.13.1 Uveal melanoma
2.13.3 Other intraocular tumours

JOHN K.G. DART
Consultant Ophthalmologist, Corneal and External Disease Service, Moorfields Eye Hospital, London, UK
2.3.4 Contact lenses in adults

GARRY DAVIS
Orbital Fellow, Moorfields Eye Hospital, London, UK
2.1.2 The investigation of orbital disease

JEREMY P. DIAMOND
Consultant Ophthalmologist, Bristol Eye Hospital, UK
1.4.3 Antibiotic, antiviral, and antifungal agents
3.24 Endophthalmitis

A. JANE DICKINSON
Consultant Ophthalmologist, Royal Victoria Infirmary, Newcastle upon Tyne, UK
2.5.1 Anatomy, physiology, and malformations of the eyelids

ROBERT M.L. DORAN
Consultant Ophthalmic Surgeon, General Infirmary, Leeds, UK
2.16.12 Non-accidental injuries in babies

RICHARD DOWNES
Consultant Ophthalmic Surgeon, Queen's Medical Centre, University Hospital, Nottingham, UK
2.5.2 Inflammatory lid diseases and degenerative processes of the lids

PAUL J. DRIVER
Associate Professor of Ophthalmology, The Eye Institute, Robert Wood Johnson School of Medicine, Camden, New Jersey, USA
2.11.4 Connective tissue disease

HARMINDER DUA
Chair and Professor of Ophthalmology, University Hospital, Queens Medical Centre, University of Nottingham, UK
2.8.3 Immunological aspects of uveitis

A.V. DURRANT
Senior Lecturer in Physics, Physics Department, The Open University, Milton Keynes, Buckinghamshire, UK
1.5.1 The physics of light and lasers

ELIZABETH EAGLING
Consultant Ophthalmic Surgeon, Birmingham and Midland Eye Hospital, UK
3.22 Lacerations and foreign bodies

DAVID L. EASTY
Professor of Ophthalmology, University of Bristol and Head, Division of Ophthalmology, Bristol Eye Hospital, UK
2.6.3 Corneal infectious disease
2.6.4 The cornea in immunological, degenerative, and metabolic disease
3.10 Corneal grafting
3.11 Corneal refractive surgery

ROGER B. ELLINGHAM
Registrar in Ophthalmology, Bristol Eye Hospital, UK
2.12.12 Facial palsy and other disorders of the face

KATARZYNA ELLINGHAM
Registrar in Radiology, Bristol Eye Hospital, UK
2.12.12 Facial palsy and other disorders of the face

DAVID B. ELLIOTT
Senior Lecturer, Department of Optometry, University of Bradford, UK
2.7.8 Effects of cataract on visual function

G.T. FAHY
Consultant Ophthalmologist, Leicester Royal Infirmary, UK
2.1.6.1 Lacrimal gland neoplasms

SHARON FEKRAT
Assistant Professor, Vitreoretinal Surgery, Duke Eye Center, Duke University Medical Center, Durham, North Carolina, USA
2.9.3 Age-related macular degeneration

PETER FELLS
Honorary Consulting Ophthalmic Surgeon, Moorfields Eye Hospital, London, UK
2.2.6 Mechanically restricted ocular movements and myopathies

F. FIGUEIREDO
Consultant Ophthalmologist, Director of Corneal, External
Disease and Refractive Surgery, Royal Victoria Infirmary,
Newcastle upon Tyne, UK
3.10 Corneal grafting
3.11 Corneal refractive surgery

F.W. FITZKE
Professor of Visual Optics and Psychophysics, Institute of
Ophthalmology, London, UK
1.6.10 Visual field analysis

C. STEPHEN FOSTER
Professor of Ophthalmology, Harvard Medical School and
Director, Immunology Service, Massachusetts Eye and Ear
Infirmary, Boston, USA
2.4.4 Scleritis and episcleritis
3.17 Cataract surgery in patients with uveitis

SCOTT FRASER
Glaucoma Fellow, The Glaucoma Unit, Moorfields Eye
Hospital, London, UK
2.14.2.3 Screening for ocular disease

F.T. FRAUNFELDER
Professor of Ophthalmology, Oregon Health Sciences
University, Portland, USA
*1.4.1 Pharmacological principles, delivery of topical ocular
medication, and drugs which affect the pupil*
1.4.6 Side-effects of topical ocular medication
2.11.8 Ocular toxicology

F.W. FRAUNFELDER
Oregon Health Sciences University, Portland, USA
1.4.6 Side-effects of topical ocular medication
2.11.8 Ocular toxicology

KENN A. FREEDMAN
Clinical Assistant Professor, Department of Surgery, Mercer
University School of Medicine, Macon, Georgia, USA
2.1.3 Inflammatory conditions of the orbit

P. FRITH
Consultant Ophthalmic Physician, Radcliffe Infirmary, Oxford
and University College London Hospitals, UK
2.11.5 Skin and mucous membrane disorders

ELLIOT M. FROHMAN
Assistant Professor of Neurology and Ophthalmology and
Director, Multiple Sclerosis Program, University of Texas
Southwestern Medical Center, Dallas, USA
2.12.9 Supranuclear eye movement abnormalities

N. ANDREW FROST
Research Fellow, University of Bristol, Bristol Eye Hospital,
UK
2.7.3 Physical aspects of lens clarity and image degradation
2.7.7 Optical effects of cataract
2.14.1.1 Clinical measurement instruments: reliability and scaling

ALEC GARNER
Emeritus Professor of Pathology, Institute of Ophthalmology,
University of London, UK
1.3 Inflammation, wound repair, degeneration, and neoplasia

RAF GHABRIAL
Consultant in Ophthalmic Plastic and Orbital Surgery,
Concord Hospital, Sydney, New South Wales, Australia
2.5.3 Tumours of the eyelid

CLARE GILBERT
Clinical Lecturer, Department of Preventive Ophthalmology,
Institute of Ophthalmology, London, UK
*2.15.2 Childhood blindness: vitamin A deficiency and measles
infection in developing countries*

JULIAN F. GILTROW-TYLER
Principal Optometrist, Bristol Eye Hospital, UK
2.3.7 Low vision aids

P.R. GODDARD
Directorate of Clinical Radiology, Bristol Royal Infirmary,
UK
1.6.6 Radiology in ophthalmology

ELIZABETH GRAHAM
Consultant Medical Ophthalmologist, St Thomas' Hospital
and National Hospital of Neurology and Neurosurgery,
London, UK
2.8.7 Uveitis associated with systemic disease

MICHAEL J. GREANEY
Specialist Registrar, Southampton Eye Unit, Southampton
General Hospital, UK
1.6.1.1 Loupe, slit lamp, and ophthalmoscopy

KEVIN-GREGORY EVANS
Senior Lecturer and Consultant Ophthalmologist, Imperial
College London, UK
2.9.5 Hereditary pigmentary retinal and macular dystrophies

RODNEY H.B. GREY
Consultant Ophthalmologist, Bristol Eye Hospital, UK
2.9.4 Vascular occlusive disease of the retina

NEIL D. GROSS
Resident, Department of Otolaryngology, Oregon Health
Sciences University, Portland, USA
*1.4.1 Pharmacological principles, delivery of topical ocular
medication, and drugs which affect the pupil*

JOHN J. HARDING
Professor of Ocular Biochemistry, Nuffield Laboratory of
Ophthalmology, University of Oxford, UK
2.7.2 Physiology and biochemistry

B. HARNEY
Consultant in Ophthalmology, Gloucester Royal Infirmary,
UK
1.6.7 Fluorescein angiography

RICHARD HARRAD
Consultant Ophthalmologist, Bristol Eye Hospital, UK
2.2.4 Sensory adaptations to strabismus
3.16 Strabismus surgery

JULIE M. HARRIS
Lecturer, Department of Psychology, University of Newcastle
upon Tyne, UK
2.2.2 Binocularity

T.R. HEDGES, III
Pennsylvania Hospital, Philadelphia, USA
2.12.13 Headache

THOMAS R. HEDGES, JR.
Professor of Ophthalmology, University of Pennsylvania,
Philadelphia, Pennsylvania, USA
2.12.13 Headache

KATRINKA HEHER
Assistant Professor of Ophthalmology, Children's Hospital of
Philadelphia, Pennsylvania, USA
*2.16.5 Paediatric orbital disease: developmental, neoplastic, and
inflammatory*

EUGENE M. HELVESTON
Professor of Ophthalmology and Chief, Section of Ophthalmology, Indiana University School of Medicine, Indianapolis, USA
2.2.5 Strabismus

EMER HENRY
Glaucoma Research Fellow, Princess Alexandra Eye Pavilion, Edinburgh, UK
1.4.2 Antiglaucoma medication

DAVID HENSON
Senior Lecturer (Clinical Visual Science), University Department of Ophthalmology, Royal Eye Hospital, Manchester, UK
1.6.2 Instruments: compound microscopes, illumination systems,diagnostic lenses, keratometers, and photokeratoscopes

R.A. HITCHINGS
Professor of Ophthalmology, University College London, UK
2.10.9 The secondary glaucomas

WILLIAM G. HODGE
Assistant Professor of Ophthalmology, University of Ottawa, Ontario, Canada
2.4.2 Infectious conjunctivitis – a clinical approach

GARY N. HOLLAND
Professor of Ophthalmology, UCLA School of Medicine and Jules Stein Eye Institute, Los Angeles, California, USA
2.8.5 Uveitis associated with infections
2.11.10 Immunodeficiency (AIDS)

DARREN W.A. HOOK
Research Scientist, Nuffield Laboratory of Ophthalmology, University of Oxford, UK
2.7.2 Physiology and biochemistry

CREIG S. HOYT
Professor of Ophthalmology and Pediatrics and Vice-Chairman, Department of Ophthalmology, University of California, San Francisco, USA
2.16.10 Neuro-ophthalmic disease in childhood

C.D. ILLINGWORTH
Specialist Registrar, Bristol Eye Hospital, UK
2.1.1 Anatomy of the orbit and lacrimal apparatus

JEFFREY J. JAY
Consultant Ophthalmologist, Tennent Institute of Ophthalmology, University of Glasgow, UK
2.10.6 The natural history of primary open-angle glaucoma

P. JEFFERIES
Ophthalmologist, Flinders Medical Centre, South Australia
2.9.1 Applied anatomy and physiology of the retina

GORDON J. JOHNSON
Rothes Professor of Preventive Ophthalmology, International Centre of Eye Health, Institute of Ophthalmology, London, UK
2.14.2.2 Global perspective on blindness

ROBERT W. JOHNSON
Consultant Anaesthetist, Bristol Eye Hospital and President, Ophthalmic Anaesthesia Society, UK
3.1 Anaesthesia in ophthalmology

J.E. KABALA
Consultant Radiologist, Bristol Royal Infirmary, UK
1.6.6 Radiology in ophthalmology

WOJCIECH S. KARWATOWSKI
Consultant Ophthalmologist, Leicester Royal Infirmary, UK

2.10.5.1 Intraocular pressure measurement and optic nerve examination

JOANNE KATZ
Professor of International Health, Ophthalmology, Biostatistics and Epidemiology, Johns Hopkins University, Baltimore, Maryland, USA
2.14.2.1 Basic epidemiological concepts in ophthalmology

STEPHEN B. KAYE
Consultant Ophthalmologist, Royal Liverpool Children's Hospital, UK
2.16.3.1 Developmental abnormalities of the posterior segment of the eye
2.16.3.2 Developmental abnormalities of the cornea and anterior segment

PETER R. KELLER
Corneal Research Fellow, Department of Ophthalmology, University of Dundee, UK and Associate Lecturer, Centre for Ophthalmology and Visual Science, University of Western Australia
1.6.4 Corneal topography

CHRISTOPHER KENNARD
Professor of Clinical Neurology, Imperial College School of Medicine, London, UK
2.12.6 Disorders of visual perception

MARSHALL P. KEYS
Attending Staff, Children's National Medical Center and Clinical Associate Professor, Department of Ophthalmology, Georgetown University, Washington, DC, USA
2.16.13 Dyslexia

PENG T. KHAW
Professor of Glaucoma Studies and Wound Healing, Consultant Ophthalmic Surgeon, and Director, Paediatric Glaucoma Clinic and Wound Healing Research Unit, Moorfields Eye Hospital and Institute of Ophthalmology, London, UK
2.16.11 Neonatal glaucomas
3.15 Glaucoma surgery

A. KIJLSTRA
Professor of Experimental Ophthalmology, University of Amsterdam, The Netherlands
1.1.1 Immunology and the eye

SIMON KILVINGTON
Honorary Research Fellow, Department of Microbiology and Immunology, University of Leicester School of Medicine, UK
1.2.2 Parasite infections of the eye

JUDITH KINGSTON
Consultant Paediatric Oncologist, St Bartholomew's Hospital, London, UK
2.13.2 Retinoblastoma

YOSHIAKI KITAZAWA
Professor and Chairman, Department of Ophthalmology, Gifu University School of Medicine, Japan
2.10.8 Primary angle closure glaucoma

GORDON K. KLINTWORTH
Professor of Pathology and Joseph A.C. Wadsworth Research Professor of Ophthalmology, Duke University, Durham, North Carolina, USA
2.6.2.1 Superficial corneal dystrophies
2.6.2.2 Predominantly stromal dystrophies
2.6.2.3 Posterior corneal dystrophies
2.6.2.4 Corneal ectasias

EVA M. KOHNER
Emeritus Professor of Medical Ophthalmology, St Thomas'
Hospital, London, UK
2.11.1 Diabetes and the eye

GREGORY B. KROHEL
Professor of Ophthalmology and Neurology, Albany Medical
Center Hospital, New York, USA
2.1.3 Inflammatory conditions of the orbit

THEODORE KRUPIN
Professor of Ophthalmology, Medical School, Northwestern
University, Chicago, Illinois, USA
2.10.1.2 Aqueous humour dynamics

PETER R. LAIBSON
Professor of Ophthalmology, Thomas Jefferson University
School of Medicine, and Director, Cornea Service, Wills Eye
Hospital, and Medical Director, Lions Eye Bank,
Philadelphia, Pennsylvania, USA
3.12 Excimer laser corneal surgery

D.F.P. LARKIN
Consultant Ophthalmic Surgeon, Moorfields Eye Hospital and
Honorary Research Fellow, Department of Pathology,
Institute of Ophthalmology, London, UK
*2.4.3 Immunological, neoplastic, and degenerative diseases of the
conjunctiva*

JOHN LEEMING
Clinical Scientist, Bristol Eye Hospital, UK
1.4.3 Antibiotic, antiviral, and antifungal agents

MICHAEL A. LEMP
Clinical Professor of Ophthalmology, Georgetown University,
Washington DC, USA
2.11.4 Connective tissue disease

LI LIM
Senior Registrar, Singapore National Eye Centre
2.16.6 Corneal and external eye disease in children

RICHARD D. LISMAN
Clinical Professor of Ophthalmology, New York University
School of Medicine; Clinic Chief, Division of Ophthalmic
Plastic Surgery, Manhattan Eye and Ear Hospital, New York,
USA
3.21 Fractures of the orbit

CHRISTOPHER LYONS
Assistant Professor, University of British Columbia and Head,
Department of Ophthalmology, British Columbia Children's
Hospital, Vancouver, Canada
2.12.11 Nystagmus

DAVID MABEY
Professor of Communicable Diseases, London School of
Hygiene and Tropical Medicine and Consultant Physician,
Hospital for Tropical Diseases, London, UK
1.2.3 Chlamydial agents

DENISE MABEY
Senior Registrar in Ophthalmology, St Thomas' Hospital,
London, UK
1.2.3 Chlamydial agents

RICHARD MARKHAM
Consultant Eye Surgeon, Bristol Eye Hospital, UK
2.16.8 Retinal disease and dystrophies
3.18 Peripheral retinal degeneration

GAVIN W. MARSH
Lecturer in Ophthalmology, Department of Ophthalmology,
University of Bristol, UK
2.6.3 Corneal infectious disease
*2.6.4 The cornea in immunological, degenerative, and metabolic
disease*

KRISTINA MAY
Senior House Officer in Ophthalmology, General Infirmary,
Leeds, UK
2.16.12 Non-accidental injuries in babies

ROBERT M. McFADZEAN
Consultant Neuro-Ophthalmologist, Institute of Neurological
Sciences, Glasgow, UK
2.12.15 Multiple sclerosis

CHARLES N.J. McGHEE
Professor of Ophthalmology, University of Dundee, UK
1.6.4 Corneal topography

SUZANNE P. McKEE
Associate Director, Smith-Kettlewell Eye Research Institute,
San Francisco, California, USA
2.2.2 Binocularity

ROWENA McNAMARA
Orthoptist, Eye Department, Hillingdon Hospital, Middlesex,
UK
2.2.3 Introduction to childhood strabismus
2.16.4 Examination of the eye in children

PAUL MEYER
Department of Ophthalmology, Addenbrooke's Hospital,
Cambridge, UK
1.6.8 Anterior segment vascular imaging

JAMES MILITE
Associate Adjunct Attending Surgeon, New York Eye and Ear
Infirmary, USA
3.21 Fractures of the orbit

NEIL R. MILLER
Professor of Ophthalmology, Neurology, and Neurosurgery
and Frank Walsh Professor of Neuro-Ophthalmology,
ohns Hopkins Medical Institutions, Baltimore, Maryland,
USA
2.1.4 The orbit in neuro-ophthalmology

JAMES E. MORGAN
Consultant Senior Lecturer, University of Wales College of
Medicine, Cardiff, UK
2.10.10 Genetics of glaucoma

IVAN MOSLEY
Director of Radiology, Moorfields Eye Hospital, London,
UK
2.12.2 Neuroradiology of the orbit and visual pathways

P.I. MURRAY
Professor of Ophthalmology, University of Birmingham, UK
2.8.6 Uveitis confined to the eye

C.S. NG
Specialist Registrar, Leicester Royal Infirmary, UK
2.8.2 Classification and epidemiology of uveitis
2.8.8 Principles of clinical management of uveitis

RACHEL V. NORTH
Lecturer, Department of Optometry and Vision Sciences,
Cardiff University, UK
2.3.1 Optical principles

COLM O'BRIEN
Consultant Ophthalmic Surgeon, Mater Hospital, Dublin, Ireland
1.4.2 Antiglaucoma medication
2.10.7 The management of glaucoma (medical, laser) and indications for surgery

STEPHEN J. OHLRICH
Consultant Ophthalmologist, Princess Alexandra Hospital, Brisbane, Australia
2.5.2 Inflammatory lid diseases and degenerative processes of the lids

JANE M. OLVER
Consultant Ophthalmologist and Oculoplastic Surgeon, Western Eye Hospital and Charing Cross Hospital, London, UK
2.8.1 Anatomy and physiology of the uveal tract

DEMETRIOS PAPAKOSTOPOULOS
Honorary Consultant and Scientific Director, Electrodiagnostic Department, Bristol Eye Hospital, UK
1.6.9 Visual electrodiagnosis (diagnostic psychophysiology)

BEN PARKIN
Specialist Registrar in Ophthalmology, Southampton General Hospital, Hampshire, UK
2.3.5 Optics of aphakia and pseudophakia

CARLOS E. PAVÉSIO
Consultant Ophthalmic Surgeon, Moorfields Eye Hospital, London, UK
2.8.4 Clinical features of uveitis

CHARLES A. PENNOCK
Consultant Paediatric Chemical Pathologist, Southmead Hospital NHS Trust and United Bristol Hospitals NHS Trust; Honorary Senior Lecturer in Child Health, University of Bristol, UK
2.11.12 Congenital disease – inherited disorders of metabolism

STEPHEN R. PERRY
Consultant Ophthalmologist, Kidderminster General Hospital, UK
2.11.7 Phacomotoses

ROSWELL R. PFISTER
Professor of Ophthalmology, University of Alabama, and Director, Eye Research Laboratories, Brookwood Medical Center, Birmingham, Alabama, USA
3.23 Mechanical and chemical injuries of the eye

NICHOLAS PHELPS BROWN
Director (retired), Clinical Cataract Research Unit, Oxford, UK
2.7.6 Classification and pathology of cataract
2.11.9 Systemic disorders associated with cataract

GORDON T. PLANT
Consultant Ophthalmologist, National Hospital for Neurology and Neurosurgery, Moorfields Eye Hospital and St Thomas' Hospital, London, UK
2.12.7 Disorders of higher visual function

MARIA PORTELLOS
Affiliate Staff Member, Children's Memorial Hospital, Chicago, Illinois, USA
2.16.5 Paediatric orbital disease: developmental, neoplastic, and inflammatory

M.J. POTTS
Consultant Ophthalmic Surgeon, Bristol Eye Hospital, UK
2.5.3 Tumours of the eyelid
2.11.2 Thyroid eye disease

CARMEN PULIAFITO
Vitreoretinal Surgeon, New England Eye Center and Professor of Ophthalmology, Tufts University School of Medicine, Boston, Massachusetts, USA
1.5.2 Physical and biological effects of lasers on ocular tissues

MAURICE F. RABB
Professor of Ophthalmology, University of Illinois at Chicago and Chairman, Department of Ophthalmology, Mercy Hospital and Medical Center, Chicago, Illinois, USA
2.11.3 Cardiovascular, renal, hypertensive, and haematological disorders

P. RAO
Royal Liverpool Children's NHS Trust, UK
2.16.3.2 Developmental abnormalities of the cornea and anterior segment

CHRISTOPHER RAPUANO
Associate Surgeon, Cornea Service and Co-Director, Refractive Surgery Department, Wills Eye Hospital; Associate Professor of Ophthalmology, Jefferson Medical College of Thomas Jefferson University, Philadelphia, Pennsylvania, USA
3.12 Excimer laser corneal surgery

MARIE RESTORI
Consultant Medical Physicist, Moorfields Eye Hospital, London, UK
1.6.5 Ultrasound in ophthalmic diagnosis

N.S.C. RICE
Consulting Ophthalmic Surgeon, Moorfields Eye Hospital, London, UK
2.16.11 Neonatal glaucomas

PAUL RIORDAN-EVA
Consultant Ophthalmologist, Farnborough Hospital, Orpington, Kent, UK
2.12.4 Retrobulbar optic nerve disease

ROBERT RITCH
Professor of Clinical Ophthalmology and Chief of the Glaucoma Service, New York Eye and Ear Infirmary, USA
2.10.1.1 Anatomy and physiology of the anterior chamber angle

ANA RIVERA
Consultant Ophthalmologist, Instituto Oftalmologico del Norte, Buenos Aires, Argentina
2.16.10 Neuro-ophthalmic disease in childhood

BIANCA ROJAS LOPEZ
Ophthalmic Research Institute, Madrid, Spain
3.17 Cataract surgery in patients with uveitis

JACK ROOTMAN
Professor and Head of Ophthalmology and Professor of Pathology, University of British Columbia and Vancouver General Hospital and Health Sciences Centre, Canada
3.8 Orbital surgery

A. RALPH ROSENTHAL
Director, Division of Ophthalmic Devices, Food and Drug Administration, Rockville and Visiting Professor of Ophthalmology, Wilmer Institute, Johns Hopkins University School of Medicine, Baltimore, Maryland, USA

1.1 Biological basic principles

1.1.1 Immunology and the eye

A. Kijlstra

The eye as an immune privileged site

Preservation of visual function is essential for the evolutionary success of many species including human beings. The high level of specialization of the human visual system does not allow irreversible damage caused by intense inflammation and it has therefore been hypothesized that active mechanisms should be available to the human eye to chose those immune effector functions that are minimally damaging to its delicate structures.

The ability of an organ to select certain arms of the immune response and actively suppress others is called 'immune privilege'. Basic scientists in the field of ocular immunology use the term 'immune privilege' to describe the observation that foreign tissues or cells enjoy prolonged survival when placed into the eye as compared to other sites of the body such as the skin. The phenomenon that antigens placed in the anterior chamber of the eye elicit a deviant immune response is currently named anterior chamber associated immune deviation.

Not only is the induction of systemic immunity to intraocularly placed antigens modified (afferent arm) but it also has been shown that the expression of the inflammatory response is altered (efferent arm). The immune privilege of the eye depends on a number of factors such as: (a) blood–ocular barriers and avascularity of various structures; (b) absence of lymphatic channels within the eye; (c) the presence of local antigen-presenting cells; and (d) the presence of factors creating an active immunosuppressive environment.

Blood–ocular barriers and avascularity of several structures in the eye play an important role in both afferent and efferent arms of the immune response. The avascularity of the vitreous, lens, and cornea impede the traffic of both antigens and cells. The absence of intraocular lymphatics implies that antigens and cells from the intraocular compartment mainly leave the eye directly via Schlemm's canal into the bloodstream. This has a number of consequences including a large dilution of antigens and cells and a main uptake by the spleen as a lymphoid organ. Apart from direct drainage into the bloodstream some intraocular antigens may leave the eye via the so-called uveoscleral outflow system and reach local lymph nodes via the orbital lymphatics.

The presence of immunocompetent cells within various structures of the eye has only recently been generally appreciated. It is now evident, however, that various tissues of the eye contain large networks of macrophages and professional antigen-presenting cells and that the distribution of these cells in, for instance, the uveal tissue is not largely different from that seen in other sites of the body. The intraocular microenvironment, however, dictates the functions and ultimate properties of these cells.

The immunosuppressive environment of the anterior chamber is now well established. Elegant experiments performed by Streilein and coworkers have shown that aqueous humour derived factors modify professional antigen-presenting cells in such a way that they are unable to generate a delayed-type hypersensitivity response against certain antigens. Characterization of the responsible factors in aqueous has identified transforming growth factor-β as one of the critical elements in mediating anterior chamber associated immune deviation. Factors in aqueous that have been identified as playing a role in the final inflammatory response include calcitonin-related peptide, vasoactive intestinal peptide, α-melanocyte stimulating hormone, and also transforming growth factor-β. These factors have been shown to interfere with T-lymphocyte activation. Immunosuppressive factors have not only been identified in the aqueous humour but have also been observed in extracts from the cornea, iris, and ciliary body; however, they seem to be lacking in the conjunctiva, sclera, and limbus.

The immune privilege of the eye is thus an important feature to prevent damage to the eye by intense inflammation. It is mediated by suppression of both afferent and efferent arms of the immune system through the action of local immunosuppressive factors on the function of both antigen-presenting cells and the effector T lymphocytes. It is believed that alterations in the immunosuppressive properties of the ocular microenvironment may play a role in the pathogenesis of ocular inflammation.

Immunology of ocular surface disorders

Innate and adaptive immune responses

The surface of the eye is continuously being bombarded by infectious micro-organisms from its environment. Under normal conditions nothing disastrous happens since the eye is equipped with a number of defence mechanisms whereby it prevents infection of its structures. Apart from various physical barriers such as the blink reflex and rapid tear flow, the human tear film contains a number of potent antimicrobial proteins. The antimicrobial defence can be divided into innate and adaptive defence mechanisms, whereby the innate defence (or non-adaptive) is represented by the proteins lactoferrin and lysozyme, whereas secretory immunoglobulin A is responsible for the adaptive immune response on the ocular surface.

Lysozyme

Lysozyme was first described by Fleming, who discovered its lytic action on bacterial cell-wall material, especially of *Micrococcus lysodeikticus* and denoted this protein as lysozyme. Lysozyme is an antibacterial enzyme; it acts as a muramidase by hydrolysing *N*-acetylmuramic (β1–4) *N*-acetylglucosamine linkages of the peptidoglycan constituting bacterial cell walls, causing ultimate lysis of these cells. Human tear fluid contains the highest concentration of lysozyme as compared to other body fluids. Reported levels in normal tears vary from 0.5 to 4.5 g/l and are not influenced by tear flow. The presence of lysozyme in tears is a reliable parameter for lacrimal gland function. In dry eye states like Sjögren's syndrome, lysozyme levels in tears are markedly reduced.

Lactoferrin

Lactoferrin is an iron-binding protein, belonging to the transferrin family. This protein is thought to act as a defence protein against bacterial invasion, owing to its bacteriostatic and bactericidal properties. Lactoferrin can interact with lipopolysaccharide and thereby alter the membrane of Gram-negative bacteria allowing subsequent lysis by lysozyme. Due to its iron-binding capacity it can prevent bacterial colonization of the external ocular structures by depriving the ocular mucosa of free iron, which is an essential factor for bacterial growth. Recently it was shown that lactoferrin can also inhibit the induction of keratitis by herpes simplex virus. Apart from this antimicrobial effect, this protein may also be involved in the regulation of inflammatory disorders. In human tears an anticomplementary effect was found to be associated with tear lactoferrin. On the ocular surface, tear lactoferrin may therefore have an anti-inflammatory function by dampening complement activation during inflammatory processes.

The iron-binding capacity of lactoferrin may implicate another function of this protein in the tear film with respect to reactive oxygen species. In biological systems, the production of the highly reactive hydroxyl radical is known to occur via the so-called Fenton type Haber–Weiss reaction, whereby iron is known to function as an effective catalyst. Owing to the iron-binding capacity of lactoferrin, this protein has been shown to influence OH· formation suggesting that it may protect the ocular mucosal surface against reactive OH· species, which can be formed during inflammatory conditions.

Lactoferrin levels in normal human tears have been measured and the concentration was shown to range between 1 and 2 g/l, representing about 25 per cent of total tear protein content. Levels in normal human tears were found to vary largely and tend to decrease with older age. Markedly decreased levels of tear lactoferrin have been reported in diseases affecting the lacrimal gland like Sjögren's syndrome.

Secretory immunoglobulin A

The adaptive ocular surface immune response is represented by secretory immunoglobulin A. Secretory immunoglobulin A is the predominant antibody in tears. Immunoglobulin A in external secretions is usually present in a dimeric form containing the additional polypeptides J (joining) chain and a glycoprotein called secretory component. Immunoglobulin A in secretions is therefore denoted as secretory immunoglobulin A and has a molecular weight of 385 kDa. This assembled secretory immunoglobulin A molecule is a product of two different cell types: immunoglobulin A with J chain is produced by plasma cells and secretory component by epithelial cells. External secretions contain about equal amounts of the immunoglobulin A1 and A2 subtypes.

The primary site of the secretory immune system of the eye is located in the lacrimal gland. Immunoglobulin A in tears is thought to be locally produced by interstitial plasma cells after homing to main and accessory lacrimal gland tissue. Intracellular transport of immunoglobulin A by acinar epithelial cells and secretion to the lacrimal lumen requires dimerization and combination of immunoglobulin A by J chain and subsequent coupling to secretory component. In the lacrimal glands, secretory component is synthesized by the acinar epithelial cells and acts as a membrane receptor for immunoglobulin A, picking up immunoglobulin A produced by plasma cells after which the complex is endocytosed and subsequently secreted into the lacrimal ducts. Apart from main and accessory lacrimal immunoglobulin A secretion, there may be additional sources for this protein in tears such as the conjunctiva.

Immunoglobulin A levels in tears are found to vary between 0.1 and 0.6 g/l and depend on the assay method used as well as the conditions during tear collection. There is a marked influence of tear flow rate on immunoglobulin A levels: being high in non-stimulated tears and dropping after stimulation of tear flow. Extremely high levels of secretory immunoglobulin A are detected on the ocular surface during closed eye conditions.

Selective immunoglobulin A deficiency is one of the most common immune deficiencies in humans with an incidence of approximately 1 in 500. In some individuals this immunodeficiency is compensated by the production and release of secretory immunoglobulin M on the ocular surface. The incidence of external ocular infectious or inflammatory disease in secretory immunoglobulin A deficiency has not yet been reported in the literature suggesting that it has either been overlooked until now or that it is not a significant problem.

Ocular surface disease

Autoimmune disease

Classical examples of autoimmune conjunctivitis include pemphigoid and pemphigus vulgaris. Cicatricial pemphigoid is characterized by ulceration of the conjunctiva followed by progressive fibrosis and symblepharon formation. The disease is considered to be caused by a reaction of circulating autoantibodies directed against the conjunctival basement membrane followed by complement activation and influx of polymorphonuclear granulocytes.

Pemphigus is an intradermal blistering disorder and does not affect the conjunctiva as seriously as pemphigoid. Pemphigus is mediated by a circulating autoantibody directed against the intercellular cement substance.

Autoimmune diseases of the cornea include peripheral ulcerative keratitis: Mooren's ulcer. This ulcerating disease of the cornea is also thought to be mediated by circulating autoantibodies directed against the cornea. Although a number of potential antigens have been mentioned, the identity of the causal antigen(s) has not yet been firmly proven.

Allergic conjunctivitis

The allergic response in the conjunctiva, whereby the immune system reacts to inoffensive foreign substances is an important cause of inflammation of the ocular surface. Epidemiological studies have indicated that the incidence of allergic conjunctivitis may reach values as high as 20 per cent in certain populations and age groups. In general, the milder forms commence in the first and second decade of life and may disappear spontaneously at a later age. Allergic conjunctivitis is a classical example of a type I hypersensitivity reaction. There are a number of clinical entities within this group such as seasonal allergic conjunctivitis, perennial allergic conjunctivitis, vernal conjunctivitis, and contact lens associated giant papillary conjunctivitis.

The mast cell plays a key role in the inflammatory process of allergic conjunctivitis. The conjunctiva contains an abundant amount of mast cells and in allergic individuals these cells have been sensitized with immunoglobulin E antibodies directed against innocuous antigens such as grass pollen, house dust mite, or animal dander. Interaction of the sensitized mast cell with these antigens leads to an immediate stimulation of the cell which subsequently releases its granules (Fig. 1). The mast cell granules contain a large number of mediators including histamine, platelet-activating factor, leukotrienes, and prostaglandin D. These mediators cause dilation of blood vessels, increased vascular permeability, stimulation of nerve endings, and stimulation of mucus secretion, which explain most of the symptoms observed such as redness, chemosis, and itching. Since most of these effects are mediated by histamine the pharmacological intervention in allergic conjunctivitis has mainly been directed to this mediator or to stabilizing the mast cell to prevent discharge of its granules containing histamine. Histamine has been shown to stimulate nitric oxide synthesis and it is possible that some of the effects ascribed to histamine are due to nitric oxide release.

A type I reaction typically has an early phase starting immediately after contact with the allergen and may be followed by a late phase after 6 to 12 h. In the early phase the mast cell is the key player whereas in the late phase other leucocytes

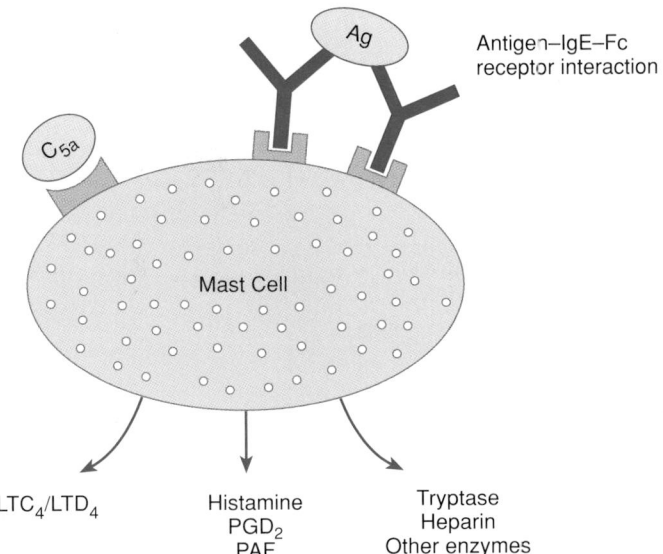

Fig. 1 Activation of mast cells and release of mediators.

(eosinophils, granulocytes, and lymphocytes) infiltrate the conjunctiva.

Why some individuals respond to inoffensive airborne substances such as plant pollen or animal dander by producing immunoglobulin E antibodies is not yet known. The allergic response involving immunoglobulin E antibodies has had an advantage during evolution in the combat of various species against parasites. Most individuals in the modern Western world are not bothered by parasites anymore and it has been hypothesized that this arm of the immune system is now free to react with various other substances such as grass pollen or the faeces of house dust mites.

It has recently become clear that the immunoglobulin E production by B lymphocytes is regulated by T-helper lymphocytes of the so-called T-helper type 2 (Th2). The division of T-helper lymphocyte subpopulations into Th1 and Th2 types is based upon the cytokines these cells produce (Fig. 2). Th2 cells produce the cytokine Il-4, which triggers immunoglobulin E synthesis by B lymphocytes. The Th1 response is characterized by an interferon-γ response leading to cellular immune reactions. Of interest is the fact that the cytokines produced by each T-helper subset inhibits the other subset. Immunotherapy is now aimed at shifting the Th2 response in 'allergy' predisposed individuals to a Th1 type of response.

Corneal immunology

The cornea has been shown to play an active role in regulating the local immunosuppressive environment. This statement is based on the fact that corneal extracts and supernatants of cultured corneal cells inhibit lymphocyte proliferation. Although transforming growth factor-β is expressed by the cornea and may be involved in the immunosuppressive activity, other as yet unidentified components may also contribute to the observed phenomena. Analysis of cytokine expression during experimental corneal transplantation showed that a surgical

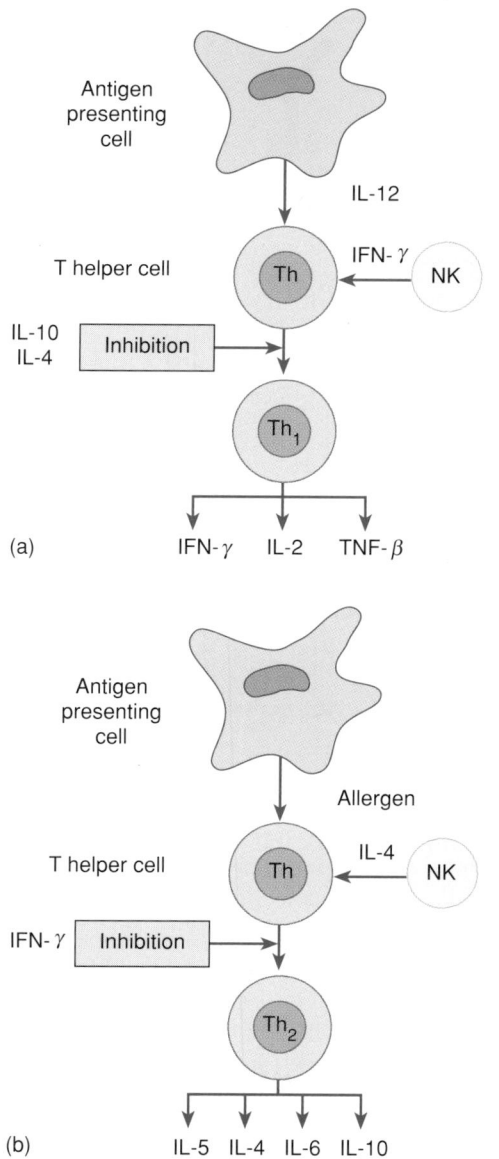

Fig. 2 Two types of helper T-cell clones were originally identified by their distinct cytokine secretion patterns. T-helper type 1 (Th1) and Th2 clones are reciprocally regulated *in vivo* by the cross-regulatory cytokines interferon-γ and interleukin 4 (IL-4). Th1 cells play a major role in cellular immunity, whereas Th2 cells are involved in the humoral immune response.

stimulus to the cornea readily induces expression of interleukin 10 (IL-10), a potent inhibitor of the Th1 arm of the immune response.

Evidence is now accumulating that the cornea also plays a key role in regulating inflammation at the ocular surface. It has been known for some time that the cornea is capable of producing IL-1. IL-1 is an extremely important cytokine with numerous functions including the ability to activate cells to produce cytokines that attract inflammatory cells. Corneal cells stimulated with IL-1 have been shown to produce IL-8 which is a chemoattractant for polymorphonuclear granulocytes. It has been hypothesized that induction of IL-8 production during anoxia may explain the massive influx of polymorphonuclear

granulocytes on the ocular surface during closed eye conditions (sleep).

The action of IL-1 is kept under strict control by a naturally occurring antagonist: the IL-1 receptor antagonist. The cornea has been shown to constitutively express this antagonist, indicating a continuous control of the proinflammatory action of IL-1.

Despite active immunoregulation and defence mechanisms on the ocular surface the cornea is susceptible to various infections. Reactivation of neurotropic herpes viruses is an important cause of corneal inflammation. Factors controlling latency and recrudescence of herpetic eye disease in humans are not well known at the present time and many animal models are currently being used to study the pathology of this infection.

Bacterial keratitis

The incidence of bacterial keratitis is increasing due to the growing popularity of contact lenses to correct refractive errors. Microbial ulcerative keratitis is the most devastating complication of contact lens wear and *Pseudomonas aeruginosa* is the organism most frequently isolated from these ulcers. The relative risk for and incidence of this disorder is dependent on the lens type (soft or rigid) and the lens-wearing modality (daily wear or extended wear). Several well-controlled studies have shown that overnight wear of contact lenses (including disposable lenses) is the most important risk factor for contact lens related ulcerative keratitis.

The pathogenesis of *P. aeruginosa* induced keratitis is thought to be multifactorial in origin. The first prerequisite is the contamination of the contact lens with the bacterium whereby the inoculum often arises from a contaminated contact lens case or a direct 'in eye' adhesion of the bacteria. The second factor of importance is the integrity of the corneal epithelium. Both *in vitro* and *in vivo* studies have demonstrated that binding of *P. aeruginosa* to the corneal epithelium depends on the condition of these cells, whereby corneal hypoxia and epithelial defects enhance binding of the micro-organisms to the cells. A third factor that has not received much attention until now involves the role of mucosal immunity in contact lens associated bacterial keratitis.

Experimental studies suggest a protective role for secretory immunoglobulin A in the pathogenesis of *P. aeruginosa* induced keratitis and the incidence of keratitis could be decreased by vaccinating the experimental animals. A similar approach has been followed in experimental models of acanthamoeba keratitis. Whether stimulation of the mucosal ocular immune response by vaccination may prevent infectious keratitis in contact lens wearers is a subject that deserves further investigation.

Cornea transplantation immunology

Transplantation of the cornea is the most frequently performed transplantation procedure in the world. In the United States approximately 40 000 corneal transplantations are being performed annually with success rates exceeding 90 per cent in the uncomplicated first-time operations.

The high success rate of corneal transplantation has been

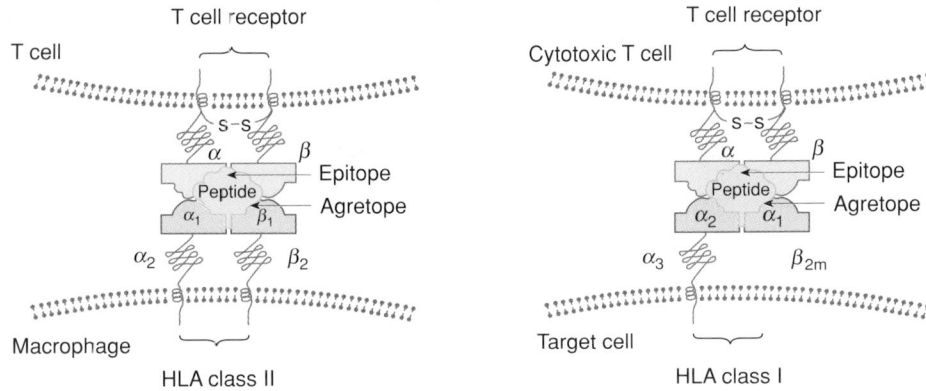

Fig. 3 The interaction of T cells is mediated by the interaction of the T-cell receptor with a peptide that is presented to the T cell in a pocket of an human leucocyte antigen (HLA) membrane protein. HLA class I molecules present antigenic peptides to T cells carrying the CD8 marker on their membrane (cytotoxic T cells), whereas HLA class II antigen presentation is directed towards T cell having the CD4 marker on their surface (helper T cells).

explained by assuming that the cornea was not able to sensitize the host. This hypothesis has now been refuted by numerous experiments. The cornea is capable of expressing human leucocyte antigens (HLA) such as HLA class I and II and graft failure has been ascribed with HLA class I incompatibilities. Another explanation for the success of corneal grafts was the possibility that donor corneal tissue was rapidly replaced by recipient cells. This hypothesis is also not valid since only the corneal epithelium is replaced but this is not the case for endothelium or stroma. The third explanation for acceptance of corneal grafts included the avascularity of the cornea. The avascularity of the cornea is indeed an important factor dictating the success of this type of graft and increased graft failures are associated with heavy neovascularization of the recipient tissue bordering the graft. Of the older theories only the avascularity of the cornea thus remained as a valid explanation for the success of penetrating keratoplasties and recently other mechanisms influencing graft acceptance have been put forward.

A deviant immune response against antigens placed in the anterior portion of the eye may account for the success of corneal grafting. As mentioned above this deviant immune response is characterized by the absence of a delayed-type hypersensitivity response and complement-fixing antibodies. The observation that the cornea can produce several immunosuppressive factors suggests that the tissue itself may play a prominent role in maintaining an immune privileged environment.

Despite the immune privileged nature of the cornea the major cause of graft failure is still due to immunological reactions. The sequence of events leading to an immunological rejection of a corneal graft can shortly be summarized as follows. Foreign antigens of the donor cornea are picked up by recipient Langerhans' cells located at the limbus adjacent to the graft. These antigen-presenting cells migrate to the local draining lymph nodes and present the antigen to T lymphocytes. Once activated the sensitized T cells circulate through the body until they encounter antigen that is locally presented

within or around the graft. The interaction of antigen on an antigen-presenting cell with a T cell requires presentation of peptide portions of the antigen via HLA molecules on the antigen-presenting cell to the T-cell receptor (Fig. 3). This local interaction leads to the release of various cytokines by the T cells including interferon-γ and also members of the chemokine family of cytokines. This leads to a massive influx of aspecific inflammatory cells such as monocytes and granulocytes. The local release of interferon-γ results in a further increase of HLA expression on resident corneal cells which may then also present antigen to sensitized T cells thereby enhancing the inflammatory response.

Intraocular inflammatory disorders

The immunology of intraocular disorders is mainly centred around the pathogenesis of uveitis. Uveitis is now used as a general term to describe any intraocular inflammation and is not only limited to the uvea but also includes the adjacent tissues such as the retina, vitreous, and optical nerve. Uveitis is considered to be caused by infectious and non-infectious mechanisms and is an important cause of visual impairment. The fact that uveitis is immune mediated stems from the observation that a number of uveitis entities show a strong association with certain HLA antigens such as HLA B27 in acute anterior uveitis, HLA A29 in birdshot chorioretinopathy, and HLA B51 in Middle Eastern and oriental patients with Behçet's disease. Other observations supporting an immune-mediated mechanism include the presence of activated lymphocytes in the ocular fluids of these patients as well as the favourable clinical response to a variety of immunosuppressive agents.

Immunogenetics and intraocular inflammation

Antigen presentation occurs in the context of cell membrane proteins of the major histocompatibility complex. There are a number of different loci encoding the genes for the major histocompatibility complex antigens. The major histocompatibility complex class I genes in humans are divided into HLA A, HLA B, and HLA C while those of the class II are known as HLA DR, HLA DP, and HLA DQ. These genes are located on chromosome 6 in humans and are highly polymorphic. To date there are nearly 75 class I alleles and about 30 different class II alleles, as detected by serological means. Analysis of the alleles by molecular biological approaches has resulted in a further subdivision of the HLA specificities.

All nucleated cells can virtually express the HLA membrane proteins, but there is a marked difference in expression between cell types and tissues. Professional antigen-presenting cells display a strong constitutive expression of the major histocompatibility complex proteins whereas most other cells show a weak presence or seem absent. Expression of the major histocompatibility complex proteins is markedly upregulated on the cell membrane following exposure to interferon-γ.

Antigen presentation to CD4-positive T cells occurs via HLA class II, whereas CD8 cells interact with antigen-presenting cells via HLA class I (see Fig. 3). Elimination of, for instance, virus-infected cells occurs via recognition of these cells by CD8-positive T cells in the context of HLA class I. Interaction of HLA class II with T cells is of importance in other types of cell-mediated immunity and in the stimulation of the differentiation of B lymphocytes to antibody-producing plasma cells.

There are a number of intraocular disorders that are associated with certain alleles of the HLA system. Numerous theories have been put forward to explain this association, but the most plausible is that the HLA system dictates the strength and type of immune response against a certain pathogen. Infection of the eye and the following inflammatory response is dictated by the genetic make-up of the individual, whereby the HLA antigens probably play a prominent role.

Animal models

Numerous animal models have been set up to study the pathogenesis of autoimmune uveitis. The antigens used for such studies include a number of retinal proteins such as: rhodopsin, phosducin, recoverin, S antigen, and interphotoreceptor retinoid binding protein.

These antigens are capable of inducing retinal autoimmune disease in a number of laboratory animals including mice, guinea pigs, rats, and primates. Autoimmune anterior uveitis can be induced in experimental animals by using melanin protein. The diseases induced by S antigen and interphotoreceptor retinoid binding protein are the most thoroughly investigated models described until now and have clarified the pathogenesis and treatment of uveitis in humans. As yet it is still a matter of debate whether any of these antigens (with the possible exception of recoverin) play a causative role in the clinical disease. The animal models have taught us that uveitis is a T-cell mediated disease which can be effectively treated by suppressing T-cell functions.

Another widely used animal model (rat, mouse) for uveitis involves the systemic (footpad) administration of endotoxin. Endotoxin-induced uveitis is characterized by iris hyperaemia, miosis, increased protein and fibrin in the anterior chamber, and massive cell infiltration in iris, ciliary body, retina, and choroid. This model has played a major role in our current understanding of the role of cytokines in the pathogenesis of intraocular inflammation.

Cancer-associated retinopathy

As mentioned above the only clinical autoimmune condition affecting the retina in which a causative antigen has now been identified, is the so-called 'cancer-associated retinopathy'. This is a rare form of retinal degeneration associated with certain forms of cancer, most notably small lung cell carcinoma. The tumour or its metastases have not infiltrated the eye and retinopathy may be apparent before the diagnosis of cancer is made.

Patients with this condition have been shown to have circulating autoantibodies directed against a 26 kDa calcium-binding protein in the retina named recoverin. Not all lung cancer cells express recoverin and only those patients in whom the cancerous cells express the recoverin develop autoantibodies against this protein. Furthermore, it has been shown that immunization of Lewis rats with recoverin leads to immune-mediated retinal destruction. This is therefore the first well-described example of an autoimmune disease of the retina in humans, whereby ectopic expression of recoverin on cancer cells induces an autoimmune response, cross-reacting with retinal protein, resulting in retinal degeneration.

Infectious uveitis

A number of frequently observed clinical uveitis entities are caused by infectious mechanisms. *Toxoplasma gondii* is a frequent cause of posterior uveitis and reactivation of the latent parasite in the retina with an ensuing immune response may lead to intense intraocular inflammation. Although it was initially thought that secondary autoimmune phenomena are involved in the pathogenesis of ocular toxoplasmosis recent investigations of the antigenic specificity of the intraocular inflammatory T cells indicate that these cells are directed against the parasite but not against retinal proteins. Other infections of the uvea in which immunological factors may play a prominent role include herpes simplex and varicella zoster virus induced uveitis.

Immunocompromised patients are especially prone to develop uveitis. Cytomegalovirus is an important cause of uveitis in patients with acquired immune deficiency syndrome (AIDS). Of the uveitis cases seen in patients with AIDS it has been estimated that approximately 90 per cent is due to cytomegalovirus. Of the patients with AIDS, up to 40 per cent may encounter cytomegalovirus retinitis in the later stages of their disease. In these patients the retinitis is most certainly due to a cytopathic effect of the virus instead of an immune-mediated inflammatory response. Herpes zoster retinitis in patient with AIDS may have a fulminant course leading to blindness in a matter of days. The rapid progress in the treatment of human immunodeficiency virus (HIV) infection may

Table 1 Cytokine families and examples of their members

Cytokine family	Members
Interleukin (IL)	IL-1α, IL-1β, IL-2, IL-3, IL-4, IL-5, IL-6, IL-7, IL-8, IL-9, IL-10, IL-11, IL-12, IL-13, IL-14, IL-15, IL-16, IL-17
Colony-stimulating factor (CSF)	G-CSF, GM-CSF, M-CSF, EPO
Interferon (IFN)	IFN-α, IFN-β, IFN-γ
Chemokine	GRO-α, GRO-β, GRO-μ, MIP-1α, MIP-1β, MCP-1, MCP-2, MCP-3, RANTES, IL-8
Growth factor (GF)	EGF, FGF, HGF, IGF, KGF, NGF, PDGF, TGF, VEGF

lead to a change in the occurrence of infectious uveitis in this patient group.

Cytokines as mediators of intraocular inflammation

Cytokines are low molecular weight proteins that play an important role in the communication between various cell types. They function through specific interaction with receptors on their target cells. Sometimes the target is present at a distance (endocrine), but in most cases cytokines work within tissues and interact with the same cell (autocrine), with neighbouring cells of the same tissue layer (intracrine), or with adjacent cellular layers (paracrine). After interaction with the target cell a cytokine can either induce proliferation, differentiation, secretion, or migration depending on the cell and cytokine involved.

The cytokine field has markedly benefited from recent developments in molecular biology and the development of immunochemical assays which are capable of detecting cytokines in cell culture supernatants or body fluids at the picogram level.

The cytokines have been subdivided into a number of families (Table 1), whereby the interleukin family represents the cytokines involved in immunoregulation which is also among the functions of some members of the interferon family. Colony-stimulating factors influence the generation of certain cell types in the bone marrow and thus play an important role in haematopoiesis. The chemokines represent a group of proteins involved in the attraction and activation of inflammatory cells such as macrophages and granulocytes. A large group of cytokines are involved in activities including wound healing and tissue repair and are listed above.

A number of cytokines play an essential role in dictating which types of cells or antibody classes will be involved in defence. Cytokines such as interferon-γ and IL-12 induce the formation of cellular immunity mediated by T-helper cells of the Th1 class, whereas the cytokine IL-4 is involved in the immediate-type hypersensitivity responses by stimulating Th2 lymphocytes that regulate immunoglobulin E production by B cells (see Fig. 2). Balance between the cytokines mentioned above is crucial in determining the outcome of the immune defence mechanisms employed to combat infectious disease. Since intraocular structures may suffer from bystander damage of the inflammatory response, it has been hypothesized that the immune defence within the eye should be deviated to a benign Th2-type response.

Cytokine research in ophthalmology has mainly been involved in analysing the role of cytokines during intraocular inflammation. Various cytokines have now been detected in clinical as well as experimental samples (Table 2). The observations made to date have clearly shown that various inflammatory cytokines can readily be detected in inflamed eyes. Another approach, to study the exact sequence of events during intraocular inflammation, comes from laboratory experiments whereby the effects of the intraocular administration of recombinant cytokines is being studied. To date all cytokines tested so far (IL-1, IL-8, IL-6, tumour necrosis factor) can induce uveitis, while IL-1 appears to be the most potent initiator of ocular inflammation.

Cytokines may also play a role in postsurgical inflammation after cataract removal and insertion of an intraocular lens. It has been shown that residual lens epithelial cells of the capsule are stimulated to produce IL-1 and prostaglandins following an interaction with plastic material. This in turn may stimulate fibroblasts to produce collagen resulting in postoperative cataract. The sequence of events delineated here have been obtained from *in vitro* experiments with human lens epithelial cells. *In vivo* experiments using a cataract extraction model in rabbits showing that IL-1 receptor antagonist could markedly block postsurgical inflammation supports this hypothesis.

An extension of these studies now involves the research on inhibition of the cytokine network via various inhibitors. At

Table 2 Cytokines detected in ocular material of patients with different forms of uveitis

Type of uveitis	Cytokine
Anterior	IL-8, interferon-γ
Intermediate	IL-8
Posterior	Tumour necrosis factor, IL-2, IL-6, IL-8, interferon-γ, leukotriene
Panuveitis	IL-6, IL-8
Undefined	Tumour necrosis factor, IL-1, IL-6

IL, interleukin.

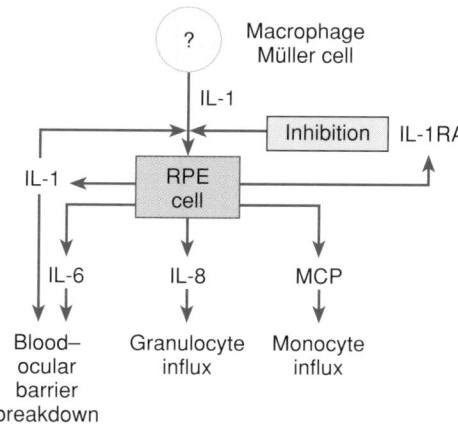

Fig. 4 The retinal pigment epithelial cell plays a key role in posterior segment inflammation. Interleukin 1 (IL-1) is the key trigger of the production of inflammatory cytokines such as IL-6, IL-8, and monocyte chemotactic protein and may be controlled by the IL-1 receptor antagonist.

present the general idea is that this area is extremely complex in view of the fact that some cytokines such as tumour necrosis factor may have different roles in inflammation depending upon the compartment under study. Experimental models, for instance, have clearly shown that blocking systemic tumour necrosis factor worsens the intraocular inflammation, whereas other experimental data suggest an important proinflammatory role for tumour necrosis factor within the eye during uveitis. In addition the actions of a number of the inflammatory cytokines are redundant. Interfering with the network will need to be performed by targeting various cytokines at the same time.

A new approach to understanding the role of cytokines involves the use of transgenic animals which express a cytokine gene under the control of an eye-specific protein. Examples include the expression of interferon-γ under the control of the rhodopsin gene or a lens crystallin gene. In both models the animals acquire serious intraocular inflammation.

The source of cytokines during intraocular inflammation may include infiltrating inflammatory cells but may also derive from resident cells within the eye. The retinal pigment epithelial cell has been shown to produce high levels of inflammatory cytokines such as IL-6 and IL-8, when appropriately stimulated (Fig. 4). This cell type is now being extensively studied *in vitro* to delineate mechanisms that may control intraocular cytokine release.

Immunology of the orbit

Inflammatory disorders of the orbit include lacrimal gland disease as seen in sarcoidosis or Sjögren's syndrome, pseudotumours, orbital muscle inflammation as observed in Graves' ophthalmopathy, and orbital myositis.

Sjögren's syndrome

Sjögren's syndrome is an autoimmune disease of the lacrimal and salivary glands resulting in a decreased tear production followed by keratoconjunctivitis. The lacrimal gland of these

patients is heavily infiltrated with T lymphocytes and later becomes atrophic. The disease is characterized by the presence of circulating autoantibodies designated as anti-Rho and anti-La. An antigen of the lacrimal gland to which the autoimmune response is directed has not yet been identified and a causative role for the circulating autoantibodies has not been proven. There is a strong debate as to whether or not infection with the Epstein–Barr virus is involved in the pathogenesis of this disease.

Graves' ophthalmopathy

Graves' ophthalmopathy is characterized by inflammation and swelling of orbital muscles resulting in proptosis and exophthalmos. Vision loss may occur due to an increased pressure within the orbit leading to compression of the optic nerve. Graves' ophthalmopathy is closely linked to Graves' disease of the thyroid. This latter disease is an autoimmune disease caused by circulating autoantibodies directed against the thyroid gland. A causal relationship between the autoimmune thyroid disease and the orbital disease has not yet been proven until now.

Tumour immunology of the eye

Immune surveillance

Although an immune attack against body constituents may cause serious inflammation of the organs or tissues involved there are situations in which such an autoimmune response may be beneficial to the host. This is especially the case in those situations whereby normal cells turn into cancerous cells. The continuous elimination of cancerous or even precancerous cells by the immune system is called 'immune surveillance'. Evidence for a continuous role of the immune system in fighting cancer stems from observations of an increased incidence of leukaemias, lymphomas, and other types of cancer in patients whose immune system is suppressed by drugs or viral infection (e.g. HIV).

Recognition of tumour cells is mediated via aberrant expression of certain proteins (tumour antigens) on these cells, whereby the antigens must be presented to the immune system via HLA molecules also residing on the tumour cell. Single recognition via HLA is not sufficient and additional cell surface interactions are necessary to activate the immune cells fully to kill the tumour cell. One such additional recognition system is comprised of the so-called 'B7' marker on the tumour cells which can interact with its 'CD28' counterpart on the cytotoxic T lymphocyte (Fig. 5). The ability of certain tumours to be eliminated by the immune system is thus highly dependent on the expression of these antigens on the tumour. Despite the presence of these antigens some tumours still escape immune surveillance possibly due to the active production of immunosuppressive factors such as transforming growth factor-β.

Cancer immunotherapy

Stimulation of the immune response against the tumour by devising cancer vaccines has shown dramatic responses in cer-

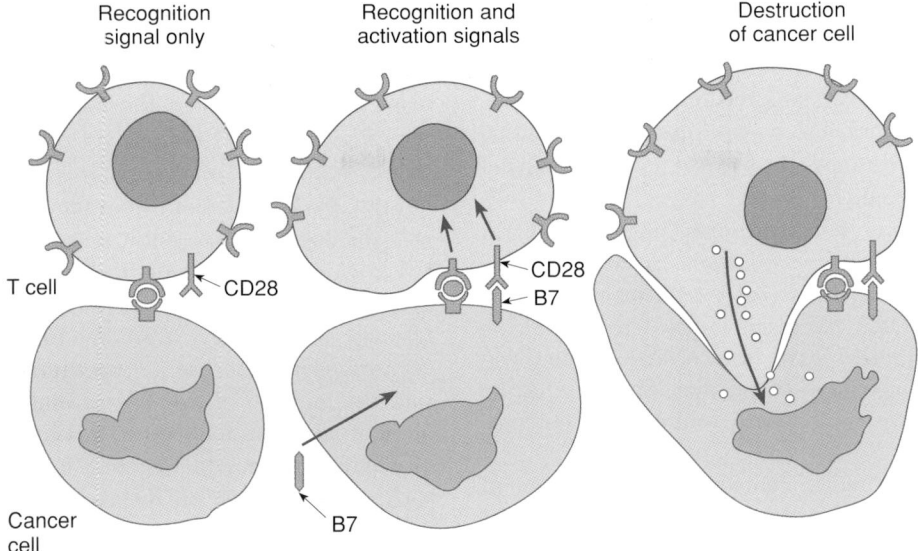

Fig. 5 Recognition of tumour cells by T cells is mediated via an interaction of the T-cell receptor with tumour antigens presented in the pockets of human leucocyte antigen (HLA) molecules residing on the tumour cell. Single recognition via HLA (as shown on the left side of the figure) is not sufficient and additional cell surface interactions, such as an interaction with the B7 protein on the tumour cell with the CD28 molecule on the T cell is necessary to activate the cytotoxic T cells fully to kill the tumour cell.

tain types of tumours but has failed in many others. Promising results are envisaged in the control of tumours induced by viruses. Vaccination against the papillomavirus is expected to play a prominent role in the treatment and prevention of, for instance, cervical carcinoma.

Other forms of immunotherapy include the *ex vivo* propagation of lymphocytes that have infiltrated the tumour and reinfusion of these cells into the patient and cytokine treatment of patients to either stimulate the immune system or enhance the expression of recognition markers (B7 or HLA molecules) on the cancer cells. Combinations of conventional therapy (surgery, radiation, and chemotherapy) which is expected to remove the large mass of tumour cells followed by immunotherapy to kill the few remaining cells may hopefully lead to complete eradication of certain types of tumours in the coming decades.

Tumour immunology of the eye

Many tumours can arise in the eye and adnexa. In view of its dramatic impact on both the clinician and patient this section focuses on the tumour immunology of the eye using uveal melanoma as an example.

Uveal melanoma is the most common intraocular tumour with an annual incidence of 6 per million in the Caucasian population. The high rate of metastasis and mortality of patients has stimulated a large body of research concerning various aspects of this tumour including possible immunological treatment modalities.

Both humoral and cellular immunity against melanoma antigens has been observed in patients with uveal melanoma, but no significant correlations have been found between the presence of these responses and patient survival. Active stimulation of the immune response by using a melanoma-derived cancer vaccine has shown a significant decrease in tumour mass in one patient with choroidal melanoma.

A number of genes encoding antigens that are expressed by melanoma cells and that can be recognized by T cells have now been identified and have been collectively named MAGE (melanoma antigen encoding gene) genes. As outlined above, the ability of a T cell to kill the melanoma cell is not only dependent on the production of tumour antigens but is only possible if the cell presents the intracellularly processed tumour antigen peptides in the context of HLA molecules. Uveal melanoma cells have been shown to express HLA molecules to a varying degree and current research is aimed at modulating the expression of HLA molecules on these cells by cytokines such as interferon. Clinical trials with interferon are not only being performed in view of the role of interferon in the upregulation of HLA expression but also as a result of this cytokine's antiproliferative effect on the tumour as well as immunostimulatory effects on certain T-lymphocyte subpopulations.

Future prospects in immunotherapy of inflammatory eye disease

The oldest form of immunotherapy is represented by the desensitization protocols to treat allergic conditions such as asthma. With our current knowledge of the Th1 and Th2 arms of the immune response the rationale for this treatment is now explained as a rerouting of the T-cell response from a Th2-driven immunoglobulin E type of response to a non-response or a Th1-type response. For autoimmune conditions such as uveitis it would be desirable to change a devastating Th1-mediated cellular immune response to a more benign Th2 response.

Immunotherapy can intervene in the initial phases of the immune response or can be directed at the effector mechanism of inflammation. Intervention in this later phase includes blocking of adhesion molecules, suppression of T-cell function, elimination of inflammatory T-cell populations, or inhibiting the mediators of inflammation such as cytokines or products of the arachidonic acid cascade.

Interferons are known to induce the expression of both HLA class I and II molecules and have also been described as being antiviral and antiangiogenic. Interferon treatment might counteract the inhibition of HLA expression induced by certain viral infections. Clinical responses have been observed using systemic therapy with interferon-α in, for example, ocular Behçet's disease but have not yet been confirmed in randomized clinical trials.

An important event during inflammation is the expression of cell adhesion molecules on both the vascular endothelium of blood vessels in the vicinity of the inflamed site as well as on the cells that are predisposed to leave the blood compartment. Experimental studies have shown that disruption of the leucocyte endothelial cell interaction by administration of antibodies directed against these cell molecules can lead to a considerable decrease in uveitic inflammation and may offer future therapeutic possibilities in the human situation.

Once inflammation is triggered it causes damage by releasing a wide variety of molecules, for example cytokines, prostaglandins, leukotrienes, and proteolytic enzymes. Manipulation of the cytokine network has shown a clinical response in rheumatoid arthritis. Administration of monoclonal antibodies against the cytokine tumour necrosis factor-α caused a considerable relief of symptoms in these patients. Application of anti-tumour necrosis factor-α antibodies in animals undergoing endotoxin-induced uveitis, however, paradoxically worsened the disease.

Since the immune response starts with an interaction between the T cell and an antigen-presenting cell this interaction may be a suitable target for therapeutic intervention. The interaction between the antigen-presenting cell and the T cell can be blocked using anti-T-cell receptor antibodies. Although this approach seems to work in animal models, it is not yet suitable for treatment in humans.

Administration of monoclonal antibodies against the CD4 or CD8 marker on T cells and thus depletion of these lymphocyte subpopulations has been tried in various experimental and clinical settings. Experimental corneal graft survival could be enhanced by treating rats with monoclonal anti-CD4 antibodies. In experimental uveitis, administration of these antibodies has been shown to prevent autoimmune disease. A similar approach has been used in patients with rheumatoid arthritis and vasculitis by administration of either Campath-1H (humanized monoclonal antibody against an antigen present on all lymphocytes) or anti-CD4 with reasonable success. As yet, only one patient with uveitis who was treated with a monoclonal anti-CD4 antibody has been reported.

Another mechanism of T-cell inhibition is the well-known action of cyclosporin A that inhibits IL-2 production which is essential for the proliferation of these cells. FK506, a newer drug, has a similar mechanism and has been shown to be effective in patients with non-infectious uveitis. Both drugs have systemic side-effects, with hypertension and nephrotoxicity being the major problem. Rapamycin, one of the newest immunosuppressants, was originally a macrolide antibiotic. Experimental studies have shown that it is not only effective in uveitis, but can also be used as an adjuvant in order to reduce considerably the doses of cyclosporin A.

Corticosteroids are still the most potent anti-inflammatory drugs known. They affect various facets of the immune response but also have a profound effect on the generation of the various mediators of inflammation. Their disadvantages are the large number of side-effects if given in an effective dose. Topical administration often leads to secondary cataract and glaucoma. Systemic therapy may lead to numerous side-effects such as hypertension and diabetes mellitus. If dosage is reduced it is often necessary to add other immunosuppressives, such as cyclosporin or azathioprine. New developments in this field include the 'soft' topical steroids such as loteprednol, which is metabolized much more rapidly than the traditional steroids and is therefore expected to induce glaucoma less frequently. It has an anti-inflammatory effect in animal uveitis models and its effectiveness in clinical settings is currently being evaluated.

Oral tolerance induction

Although it is still a matter of controversy many ophthalmologists still believe that autoimmune processes play an important role in the pathogenesis of clinical uveitis. Since autoimmunity may be defined as a state of loss of self tolerance the aim is to restore the state of tolerance again. One of the current strategies to induce tolerance to autoantigens involves the mucosal administration of antigen. Mucosal surfaces challenged include the intestinal, nasal, and also the conjunctival mucosa. Mucosal-induced tolerance has been shown to be effective in the treatment of experimental autoimmune uveitis. Although the exact mechanisms involved are not yet clear it has been suggested that the effect may be based on a shift from aggressive tissue damaging Th1 type of autoimmune response to a more benign Th2 response. Oral tolerance strategies have now also been performed in clinical settings. Patients with multiple sclerosis have been fed with myelin basic protein and in rheumatoid arthritis, studies are ongoing with collagen-containing capsules. Favourable clinical responses have been reported by Nussenblatt's group who fed uveitis patients with soluble retinal antigens.

Further reading

Gery, I. and Streilein, J.W. (1994). Autoimmunity in the eye and its regulation. *Current Opinion in Immunology*, **6**, 938–45.

McMenamin, P.G. (1994). Immunocompetent cells in the anterior chamber. *Progress in Retinal and Eye Research*, **13**, 555–85.

Nussenblatt, R.B., Whitcup, S.M., and Palestine, A.G. (1996). *Uveitis, fundamentals and practice*. Mosby, St Louis, USA.

Roitt, I., Brostoff, J., and Male, D. (1993). *Immunology*. Mosby, St Louis, USA.

1.1.2 Molecular biology and molecular genetics: basic principles

Graeme Black

The importance of inherited factors in human disease should not be underestimated. Around 50 per cent of conceptions abort spontaneously, the majority as a result of major chromosomal disorders, which also account for approximately 2.5 per cent of childhood deaths.

From the genetic standpoint, a huge number of diverse disorders—diabetes, cancer, coronary heart disease, and schizophrenia for example—have a substantial genetic contribution to their aetiology. Within ophthalmology, 'polygenic conditions'—those which have both genetic and environmental components such as cataract, age-related macular disease, glaucoma, and myopia—comprise an enormously important group in terms of both workload and morbidity.

The mendelian, or single gene, disorders are the easiest to characterize at the molecular level. Around 4000 autosomal dominant, recessive, and X-linked inheritance patterns have now been described and, with the technological revolution of the 'new genetics', more and more of the genes underlying these diseases are now being mapped and isolated.

Basic molecular genetics

Genetic material

The basic molecule of inheritance is DNA, deoxyribonucleic acid. This consists of a skeleton—an alternating sugar–phosphate backbone—along which the four nucleotides (adenine, cytosine, guanine, and thymine) are hung. Fundamental to the understanding of all genetic processes is the fact that the function of DNA, both as a store of information which encodes all proteins and as the molecule which controls their expression, is dependent on its sequence of bases. Thus the majority of proteins which bind to DNA do so by means of an interaction between their three-dimensional structure and specific DNA sequence sites, or motifs.

The vast majority of DNA within mammalian cells is situated in the nucleus. In addition, a small amount of DNA is found within the mitochondrion, which is unique as a mammalian cellular organelle with its own genome separate from the nucleus. The mitochondrial DNA is a closed circular molecule 16 569 base pairs (bp) in length, which encodes ribosomal RNAs, transfer RNAs, and polypeptides of the respiratory chain and energy-transducing system (NADH dehydrogenase, apocytochrome-b and subunits of both cytochrome oxidase and ATP synthase). Recently, certain diseases, such as Leber's hereditary optic neuropathy and Kearns–Sayre syndrome, have

been shown to be caused by mutations in mitochondrial DNA. Since the sperm contributes only nuclear material to the formation of the zygote, the cytoplasm and its contents are almost exclusively maternally derived. Therefore such mitochondrially inherited diseases pass only through the maternal line and often preferentially affect tissues, particularly those which are neural and muscular, with high metabolic requirements.

Structure and function of chromosomes

The DNA within the human nucleus is divided into 23 pairs of chromosomes (Fig. 1). There are 22 pairs of autosomes, which are numbered according to size. In addition there is one pair of sex chromosomes, X and Y, responsible for sex determination. Females have two X chromosomes (i.e. 46,XX), whilst males have one X and one Y chromosome. The Y chromosome carries little genetic information and is generally (apart from a short pairing region) non-homologous to the X chromosome.

The Y chromosome. It is the presence of the Y chromosome which determines maleness. Thus Turner's syndrome (45,XO) and triple X (47,XXX) individuals are female, but Klinefelter (47,XXY) individuals are male. Although relatively gene poor, with few genes unique to it, it is one of these Y chromosome genes, the testis-determining factor, which is responsible for the switch to maleness early in development.

The X chromosome. Mammals, like many other animals with a chromosomal mechanism of sex determination, require a system of dosage compensation to equalize the genetic contribution of the sex chromosomes in the two sexes. This is achieved by inactivation of one X chromosome in each somatic cell of the female, a process termed lyonization. The DNA of the inactive X is tightly coiled and highly methylated and thus inaccessible to the apparatus of transcription. It is seen as the a darkly staining (heterochomatic) mass under the light microscope, the Barr body. With the exception of a few genes along its length, the inactive X is untranscribed.

Inactivation occurs early in development so that approximately half of a female's cells will have each X chromosome inactivated. As the process is random, however, the ratio may differ between different individuals. Thus if carrier females of X-linked syndromes show a skewed X-inactivation pattern they may manifest the disease themselves.

At a purely biological level divisions of the DNA into chromosomes are arbitrary, but by definition they must be identical between members of the same species. Once in discrete packages, the DNA can function conveniently at all times within the cell cycle. This packaging of chromosomes changes at different times of the cell cycle; from highly relaxed and uncoiled during interphase to facilitate transcription, to tightly coiled during metaphase of cell division to enable movement of the chromosomes to the poles of the mitotic/meiotic spindle.

Each chromosome contains a single, uninterrupted DNA molecule with, at either end, a telomere. This is a hairpin-shaped structure important in maintaining the integrity of the chromosome and protecting it from enzymatic degradation. At

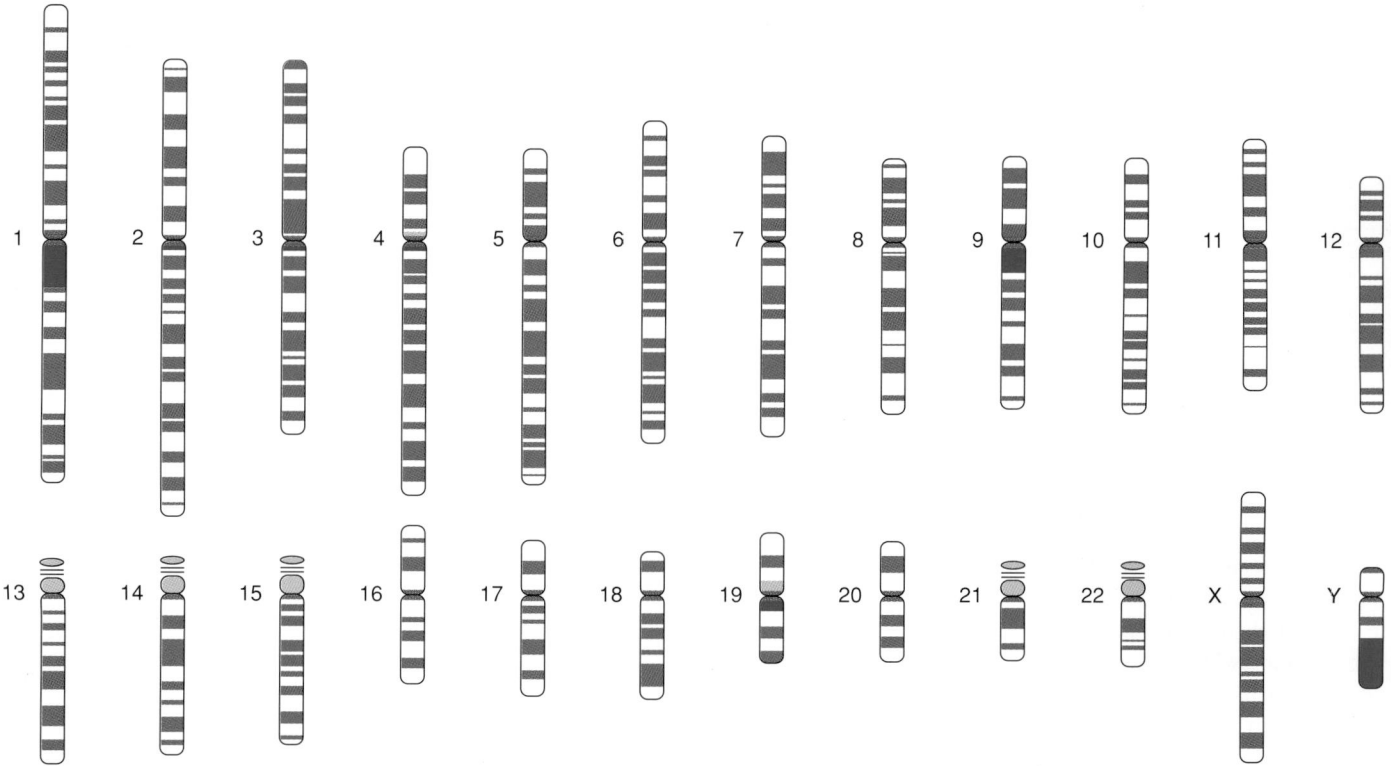

Fig. 1 Ideogram of the human chromosomes. This is a diagrammatic representation of human chromosomes as they would be seen after staining in order to differentiate one from another. A male has a pair of each of numbers 1 to 22, one X, and one Y.

some point along the chromosome's length is a single centromere, formed from an interaction of proteins with specific DNA sequences. These are of particular importance during cell division to ensure accurate partitioning of the chromosomes between daughter cells.

The remainder of each chromosome is not homogeneous. This can be inferred from analysis of Giemsa stains of metaphase chromosome spreads, which are used for karyotype analysis and detailed cytogenetic chromosome analysis. The chromosomes show characteristic banding patterns, with light and dark areas clearly distinguished. The light bands correspond approximately to gene-rich regions of the chromosome which replicate early in the cell cycle.

Packaging of DNA within the nucleus

In total the DNA content of each cell is approximately 10^9 bp, which if stretched out would be around 1 m long. In order to fit into the nucleus, therefore, the chromosomes are packaged in a highly organized fashion into chromatin, which comprises approximately one-third DNA, one-third histone proteins, and one-third non-histone proteins (Fig. 2).

The initial packaging of DNA is around the histone proteins. These are highly conserved, positively charged proteins (due to a high lysine and arginine content) which interact with the negatively charged DNA. The histones form an octomer around which the DNA (approximately 150 bp) is coiled twice, to form a nucleosome. This structure, a 10-nm fibre, resembles 'beads on a string'. This is in turn coiled into a solenoid structure, the 30-nm fibre.

Higher orders of packaging are then achieved by coiling this structure on a proteinaceous 'scaffold'. As the scaffold proteins—the numerous non-histone proteins—are also responsible for the functioning of the DNA (transcription, replication, coiling, and so on), the DNA is relatively mobile on this suprastructure, attached only at intervals along its length at scaffold attachment regions or SARs. Such a system allows different regions, or domains, of chromosomes to be separately bound by proteins and differentially coiled. Such domains include the genetic 'units' of replication and gene activity and are one means of achieving differential control of transcription, facilitating tissue, and cellular and temporal specificity of gene activity.

Coding potential of DNA

In order to search for genes amongst our DNA it is important first to comprehend the magnitude of such a task. Our 3×10^9 bp of DNA contains an estimated 50 000 to 100 000 genes. However, these comprise only a small fraction of the total DNA, probably less than 10 per cent. The greater part does not code for proteins and has no apparent biological function. This non-coding DNA comprises sequences which are often repeated many times within an individual, some as many as 10^5 to 10^6 times throughout the genome.

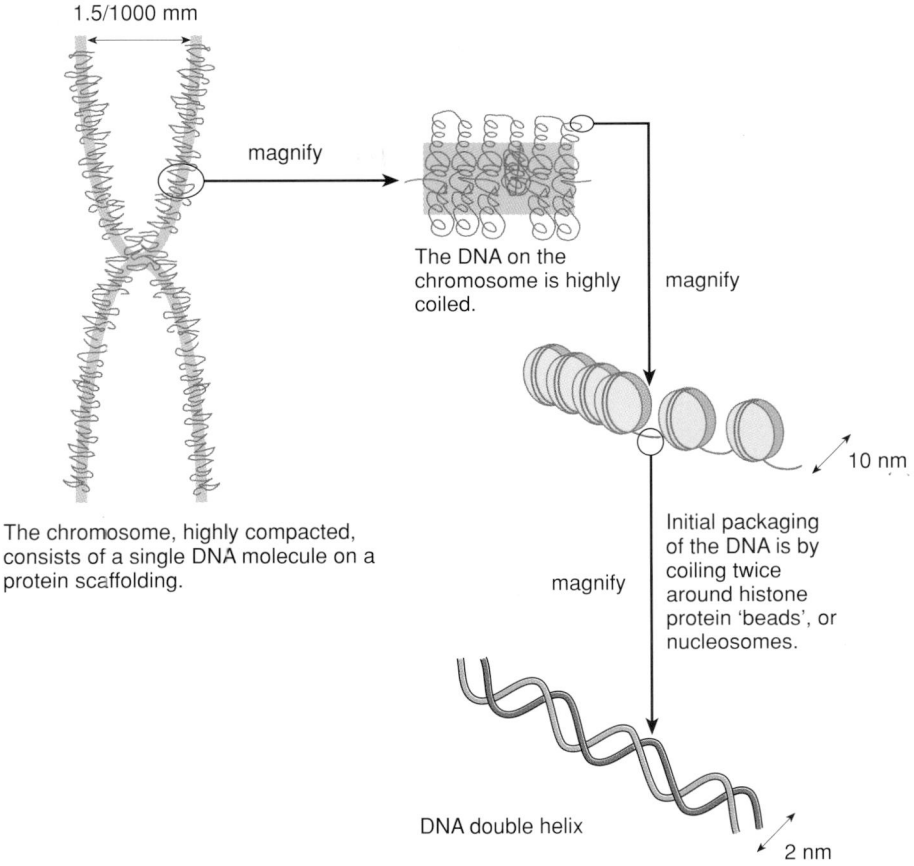

Fig. 2 Chromatin packaging in chromosomes.

Gene

At the DNA level, the 'unit of inheritance' is the gene, but what exactly *is* a gene? The information in DNA is transferred to RNA during the process of transcription, by means of the enzyme RNA polymerase. This exists in three forms—RNA polymerases I, II, and III—which oversee the transcription of class I genes (ribosomal RNA genes), class II genes (genes transcribed into messenger RNA), and class III genes (transfer RNA genes), respectively. It is the class II genes, those which are transcribed into messenger RNA, whose message, once modified, passes into the cytoplasm and is translated into polypeptides. Therefore it is these genes which, in medical terms at least, are of greater interest. These class II genes consist of more than simply an interrupted coding sequence.

Mosaic nature of genes

In higher eukaryotes, the class II genes are not a continuous stretch of DNA, but are normally interrupted, or mosaic (Fig. 3). Those sequences which interrupt the gene are termed introns, those which are ultimately responsible for expression, exons. At transcription, the gene is read from the 5′ ('5 prime') to the 3′ end, according to the convention of orientation of the base sequence with respect to the DNA backbone.

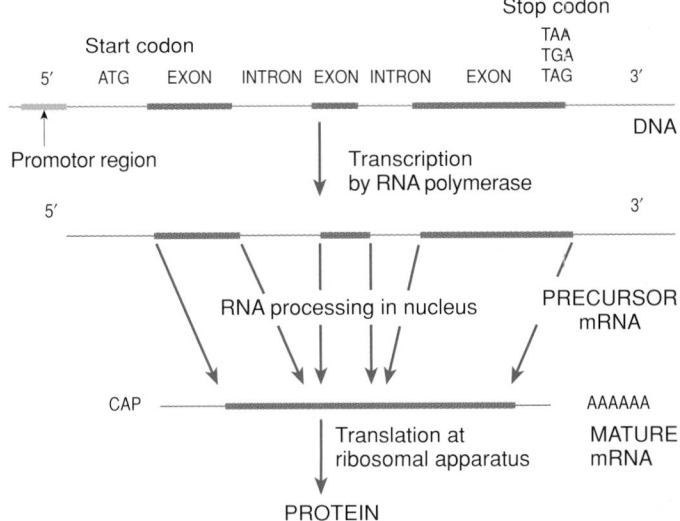

Fig. 3 The structure of the gene.

Control sequences

In order to recognize the beginning of any gene in a sea of DNA, the transcription apparatus must recognize certain DNA sequence motifs around the gene. Although not part of that

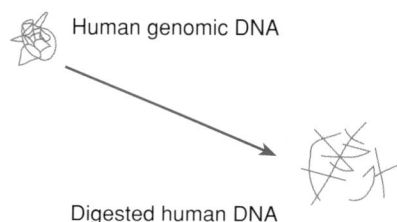

Human genomic DNA

Digested human DNA

Digestion of human DNA

Human genomic DNA is usually extracted from white blood cells although it can be extracted from any nucleated cell. Once extracted, it is kept in solution.

Restriction enzymes, found in bacteria, cut DNA at specific sequence sites along its length. Such sites are usually between 4 and 6 base pairs in length. (For example the enzyme EcoR1 cuts the sequence GAATTC). Given that an individual's DNA sequence varies from another's, so the positions of cutting sites may also vary between individuals.

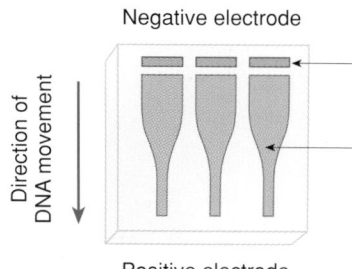

Negative electrode

Direction of DNA movement

Notch, or well into which is placed digested DNA

Digested DNA, after blue electrophoresis arranged by order of size

Positive electrode

Gel electrophoresis is a technique which arranges the cut DNA molecules according to size. A gel slab is placed in electrolytic buffer and the digested DNA is loaded into notches in the gel. A current is placed across the gel and the DNA (which is negatively charged due to the phosphate backbone) moves towards the positive terminal. The gel acts as a retarding medium, slowing the passage of the DNA, the larger molecules moving more slowly than the smaller ones. After electrophoresis the DNA fragments are arranged such that the larger molecules are near the starting point, the smallest farthest away from it.

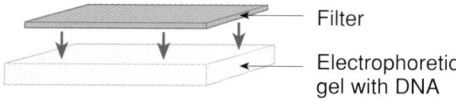

Filter

Electrophoretic gel with DNA

Southern blotting. The DNA is transferred to an adsorbant membrane, or filter, such that the relative positions of the molecules are exactly preserved.

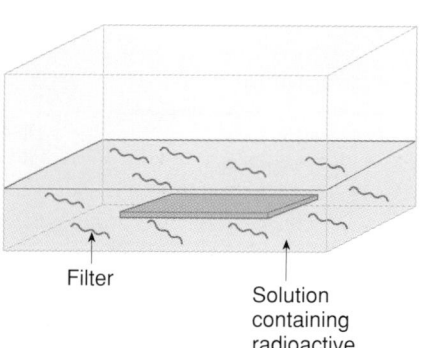

Filter

Solution containing radioactive probe

Hybridization with radiolabelled cloned probe.

A clone is a single, specific human DNA fragment which has been inserted into a host (for example a bacterium). When that host is grown in culture and DNA prepared from it, large amounts of the human DNA molecule may be prepared.

When a small amount of this molecule is radioactively labelled and used in experiments it is referred to as a **probe.**

If, in the correct experimental conditions, the filter is bathed in a solution containing the radiolabelled probe, the probe will bind to those DNA fragments on the filter, (and no other) to whose sequence it is identical (i.e, complementary). This technique is termed **hybridization.**

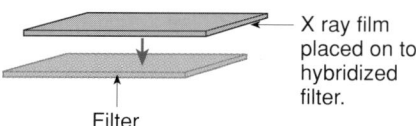

X ray film placed on to hybridized filter.

Filter

Autoradiography. The filter, to which the radioactive DNA is adherent, is placed against an X-ray film. The X-ray film is exposed wherever the radioactivity is situated.

(a)

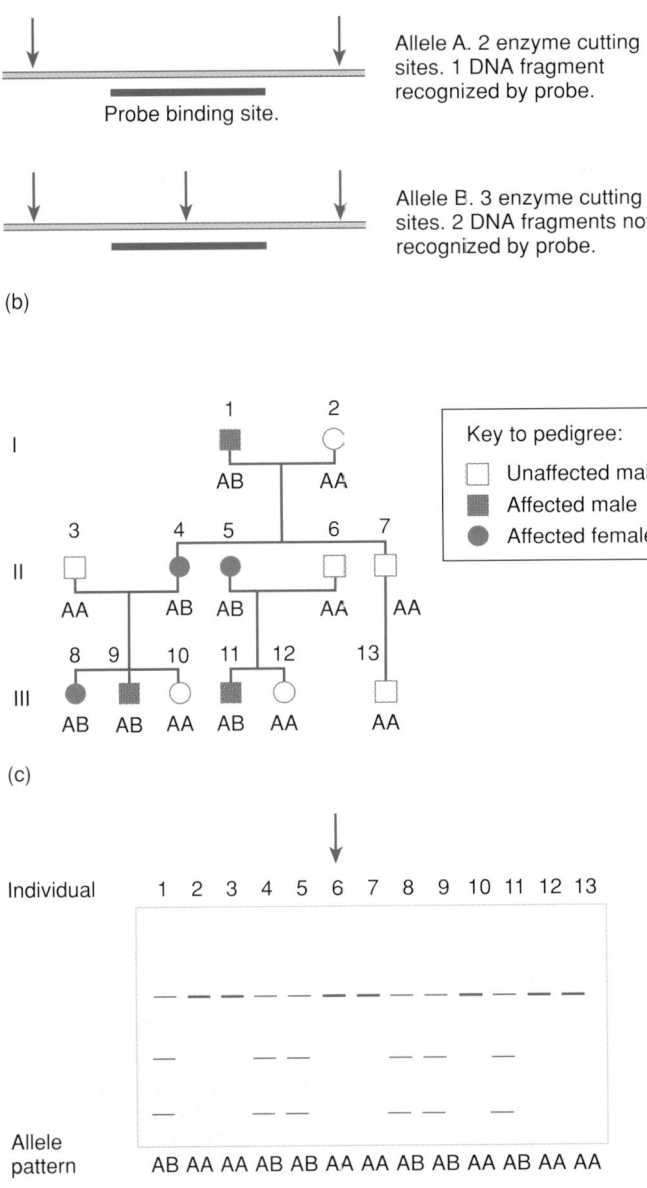

Allele A. 2 enzyme cutting sites. 1 DNA fragment recognized by probe.

Probe binding site.

Allele B. 3 enzyme cutting sites. 2 DNA fragments now recognized by probe.

(b)

Key to pedigree:

☐ Unaffected male
■ Affected male
● Affected female

(c)

Individual   1 2 3 4 5 6 7 8 9 10 11 12 13

Allele pattern   AB AA AA AB AB AA AA AB AB AA AB AA AA

(d)

Fig. 4 Restriction fragment length polymorphisms. (a) Techniques used for restriction fragment length polymorphism analysis. (b) Restriction enzyme pattern of different alleles. Every individual carries two alleles, one on each identical chromosome. (c) Autosomal dominant pedigree. Allele B is only seen in affected individuals, suggesting a possible association (linkage) between the disease gene and the restriction fragment length polymorphisms. (d) Result of analysis of pedigree with restriction fragment length polymorphisms. A allele shown as largest band, B allele as two smaller bands. Individual with two A alleles have a single, intense band.

unit which is transcribed, without these sequences the genes would not function.

1. Immediately prior to the point of origin of transcription at the beginning of the gene lie DNA sequences, termed promoters, to which transcription factors bind to form a three-dimensional complex which facilitates the binding of the RNA polymerase.

2. Tissue specificity is achieved by means of tissue-

specific or even gene-specific sequences (also found close to the 5′ end of the gene) to which bind further transcription factors.

3. The rate of transcription may be significantly boosted by 'enhancer' regions. These may lie considerably further from the gene at the 3′ or 5″ ends or even within an intron of the gene.

4. At the 5′ end of many mammalian genes is often found a region which contains a large number of the dinucleotide cysteine–guanine (5′–3′). This is termed a 'CpG island'. Such dinucleotides are relatively uncommon and may be enzymatically altered by a methylase which adds a methyl group to the cysteine residue of the pair. Methylated cysteine guanine regions help to regulate gene activity.

Untranslated sequences

Before passage into the cytoplasm, the messenger RNA molecule is processed. The introns are spliced out and both the 5′ and 3″ ends are modified—a 5′ cap and the 3′ polyadenine tail are added—to ensure stability of the messenger RNA following its exit from the nucleus. Employing the ribosomal apparatus, the messenger RNA is read from the 5′ end and translated, via the triplet code, into a polypeptide moving from amino to carboxy termini. Only a section of the mature messenger RNA is translated into the polypeptide; this is termed the 'open reading frame'. The remainder may be important in ensuring stability of the messenger RNA in its passage between the nucleus and the cytoplasm.

Basic techniques of molecular genetics

Family analysis

In any branch of medicine, it is impossible to make a statement about a disease without first accurately defining a disorder. Accurate characterization of families is essential for effective genetic analysis. Even then, it may not be possible to differentiate between genetic forms of the same disorder. For example, tuberous sclerosis, one of the phakomatoses, exists in two distinct genetic forms which are clinically indistinguishable. The two identical disorders are encoded by different, although perhaps related, genes on separate chromosomes (chromosomes 9 and 16). This is termed locus heterogeneity.

Genetic mapping

The main aim of genetic analysis is to demonstrate an association (linkage) between the disease phenotype and a previously mapped anonymous 'marker', or polymorphism, for the disease. At the level of the gene, such an association is the result of the disease gene and the anonymous marker lying close to one another on the same chromosome. Statistically the chance of 'crossing-over'—meiotic recombination—occurring between such closely linked DNA sequences is small, and they therefore follow one another through the generations.

Once such an association has been demonstrated and has been proven to be statistically significant, those that carry the 'at risk' form of the marker, be they born or unborn, can be identified. Appropriate family members can then be counselled as to their risk of either developing the disease themselves or of passing it on to their progeny.

Polymorphisms

A polymorphism is defined as a detectable difference between individuals, phenotypic or genotypic, caused by the existence of varying forms of a gene or DNA sequence and are present in the population at a frequency higher than that caused by mutation alone. Many different forms have been used as marker systems; formerly, major blood groups such as ABO and rhesus were useful, if laborious to use.

Polymorphisms may be detected at the protein level. Different individual proteins, although functionally almost identical, often vary in amino acid sequence; and electrophoresis (Fig. 4) can detect differences in around 30 per cent of different proteins. Although time-consuming and inefficient to use for genetic analysis, such electrophoresis is regularly used for the detection of haemoglobin variations.

Currently the most frequently used polymorphisms for genetic analysis are DNA polymorphisms. Two common types will be described here.

Restriction fragment length polymorphisms

Restriction fragment length polymorphisms are one of the most basic of the DNA polymorphisms and are described in detail in Fig. 4. Unfortunately certain features inherent to their nature reduce their efficacy as tools in molecular biology. First, many restriction fragment length polymorphisms rely on the presence or absence of a single restriction enzyme site. This means that there are only two possible alleles: they are dimorphic (see Fig. 4(b)). Since, for an autosome, there are four different chromosomes, two maternal and two paternal participating at meiosis, there is a limited ability to follow the one chromosome linked to the mutated gene using such a system. In addition, analysis takes several days and can require a large amount of DNA. Therefore other polymorphisms, or microsatellites, whose variation is based on different underlying mechanisms of change, are now beginning to be used.

Microsatellite polymorphisms (Fig. 5)

Scattered throughout the human genome are short regions where certain nucleotide pairs, for example AC, are repeated in tandem several times (i.e. ACACACACACACACAC). Such a region is termed a microsatellite repeat. Very occasionally during DNA replication, the DNA polymerase may misread the number of AC pairs in a tandem array, and produce an array that is slightly shorter or longer. It is such non-functional differences which can be detected and which provide the basis for the marker systems.

Such oligonucleotide repeats have many advantages as genetic tools.

1. They have far higher levels of variability between individuals, with more than two possible alleles

2. They are common throughout the human genome. It is estimated that there is one such microsatellite approximately every 50 to 100 000 bp and, because detection is based on the polymerase chain reaction (Fig. 6), small amounts of DNA can be used and analyses rapidly performed.

During genetic analysis, indications as to the location of the gene will be sought in order to direct the initial study to a particular chromosomal region and, by so doing, to decide upon which polymorphisms must be used. Such directions may come from a number of sources.

1. Inheritance pattern. In the case of sex-linked or maternally inherited disorders, the inheritance pattern alone may give some indication of where in the human genome to search for a gene. In the case of autosomal disorders other clues will have to be sought.

2. Examination of each of a patient's chromosomes and their exact banding patterns, known as karyotype analysis, particularly of those individuals with atypical forms of a disorder, may reveal localized chromosome abnormalities which may help in the localization of the disease gene within the genome.

Visible chromosome deletions helped in the localization of the retinoblastoma locus to chromosome 13 and of one of the loci involved in oculocutaneous albinism (tyrosinase positive) to chromosome 15.

Occasionally a deletion may cause the manifestation of a complex phenotype, due to the deletion of two or more genetic loci: this is termed a contiguous gene syndrome. Examples include: (a) a large deletion of the short arm of the X chromosome causing X-linked retinitis pigmentosa, Duchenne muscular dystrophy, and chronic granulomatous disease; (b) a deletion of chromosome 11 which causes the WAGR phenotype (Wilms' tumour, aniridia, genitourinary abnormalities, and mental retardation). In these cases, if the location of one of the loci is already known, the deletion need not be visible at the microscopic level to aid in the localization of a disease locus.

Chromosome translocations may also help to map a disease locus: those involving the X chromosome have been particularly helpful in localizing several of the genes involved in X-linked ocular diseases (e.g. choroideraemia, Norrie's disease).

3. The study of a variety of inherited disorders has shown that a remarkable overlap can exist in the phenotypic expression of similar genetic defects in different mammals (examples are given in Table 1). Controlled mating and pedigree analysis in animal models can pinpoint the map position of mendelian genetic disorders. Since many large segments of the linkage groups of, for example the mouse, are preserved in humans, a gene's approximate chromosomal location in humans can be inferred from the location of its homologue in the mouse.

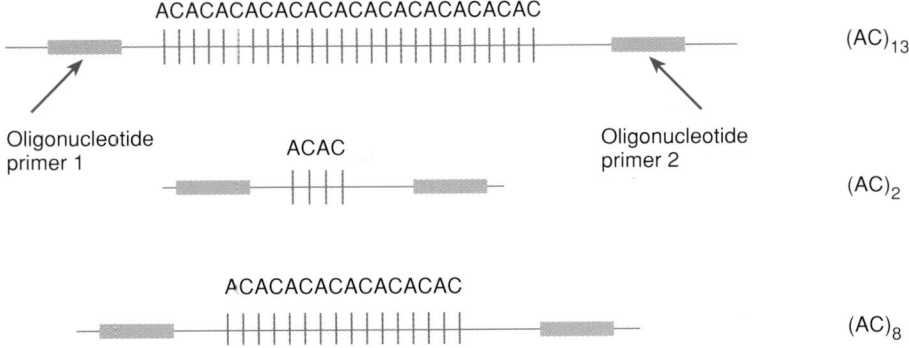

Fig. 5 Microsatellite polymorphism. In the case of a microsatellite marker, differences between alleles are detected on the basis of different size of a repeating sequence (here AC). The top allele and the middle allele therefore differ in length by 22 bp.

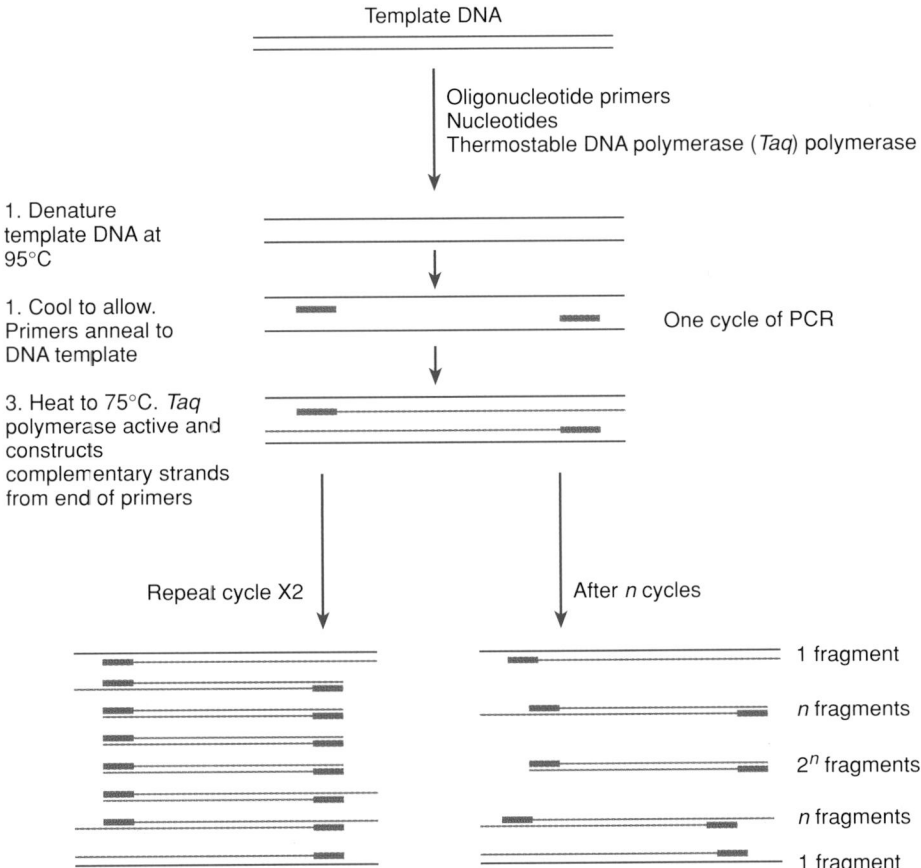

Fig. 6 Polymerase chain reaction is a technique for amplifying short regions of DNA (usually under 1000 bp), between regions of known sequence. Oligonucleotide primers complementary to these regions are added, along with nucleotides and the reaction enzyme, a thermostable DNA polymerase from the bacterium *Thermus aquaticus* (*Taq*). After *n* cycles, there is an exponential increase in the number of molecules whose ends correspond to the two primers (*box bottom right*). These are then demonstrated by electrophoresis.

Table 1 Mouse models for human ophthalmic diseases

	Mouse mutant	Gene locus	Human disorder
Albinism/defects in pigmentation	Himalayan	Tyrosinase	Tyrosinase-negative OCA
	Pink-eyed dilution	'P' locus	Tyrosinase-positive OCA
	Splotch	PAX3 gene	Waardenburg's syndrome
Aniridia	Small eye	PAX6 gene	Aniridia
Cataract	Eye lens obsolescence (Elo)	γ-crystallin	Autosomal dominant cataract
	Guinea-pig cataract	ζ-crystallin	—
	Philly mouse	β-crystallin	—
Pigmentary retinopathy	rds mouse	Peripherin/rds	Autosomal dominant retinitis pigmentosa
	rd mouse	β-Phosphodiesterase	Autosomal recessive retinitis pigmentosa
	Shaker-1 locus	Myosin gene	Usher's syndrome

rds, retinal degeneration slow; OCA, oculocutaneous albinism.

4. A feature of the mapping of an increasing number of inherited diseases has been the observation that disorders which are defined as clinically separate, but whose underlying biological pathogenic mechanism is similar, may be caused by mutations in the same gene. This is defined as allelic heterogeneity and examples amongst inherited ocular disease are given in Table 2. Such information may help to direct initial genetic analysis of unmapped disorders to specific genomic regions.

If a disorder is autosomal and there are no obvious factors which lead to its positioning within a particular genomic interval, a long, laborious search for the genetic needle through the genomic haystack must ensue. Any gene can follow another through a single mating and therefore, in order to estimate whether an association between two loci (for example, the disease gene and a marker) is significant statistically, a large number of meiotic divisions must be examined. This analysis is called linkage analysis. Analysis will be either of one large family or of several smaller families. If there is heterogeneity within the disorder then the latter approach is potentially flawed since it is extremely difficult to map simultaneously two

or more genes which cause a single heterogeneous disorder. It is this that has, until recently, hindered the progress in the genetic characterization of many forms of retinitis pigmentosa, which cannot be reliably distinguished.

Physical mapping
Once a gene has been assigned to a chromosomal location by genetic means, its location is usually localized to an interval of several million base pairs. This is therefore only the first step, albeit an important one, towards its isolation. Thereafter, physical means must be sought for dissecting and characterizing this region and, in general, two complementary approaches have been used to this end: the candidate gene approach and 'positional cloning'.

Candidate gene approach
Once a protein whose biological function is known has been isolated, its amino acid sequence can be determined. This in turn can be used to estimate the sequence of the gene which encodes it. With this knowledge short nucleotide sequences (oligonucleotides) can be constructed to isolate and map that

Table 2 Allelic heterogeneity amongst ophthalmic disorders

Chromosome	Locus	Disorder
Xp11	NDP	Norrie's disease; X-linked familial exudative vitreoretinopathy
6p	Peripherin/rds	Autosomal dominant retinitis pigmentosa; retinitis punctata albescens; macular dystrophy; vitelliform macular dystrophy; butterfly-shaped pigment dystrophy
3q	Rhodopsin	Autosomal dominant retinitis pigmentosa; autosomal recessive retinitis pigmentosa; congenital stationary night blindness; sectoral retinitis pigmentosa
5q	BIG–H3	Granular corneal dystrophy; lattice corneal dystrophy type I; Avellino's corneal dystrophy

rds, retinal degeneration slow.

gene. As a result the chromosomal localizations of the genes which encode many proteins are well documented.

In recent times there has been an exponential increase in the number of anonymous DNA segments which have been isolated, characterized, and sequenced throughout the human genome. As a number of these sequences are expressed (i.e. they are genes), a map of transcribed sequences has been constructed despite the fact that the function of the majority remains unknown.

Therefore the chromosomal localization of many genes is known; for some the corresponding protein is known; for others the only information available is tissue expression profile. Once a disease has been mapped to a given chromosomal location, those mapped genes which are expressed in the tissue of interest can be examined in affected individuals to hunt for mutations. Such a candidate gene approach has been particularly successful for many of those genes which have been defined as the cause of eye disease; for example, of those genes which are known to be responsible for retinitis pigmentosa both rhodopsin and peripherin were characterized by this method.

Positional cloning (Fig. 7)

For a significant number of disorders, once a chromosomal localization has been ascertained, there are no candidate genes in the region. (Such a situation will, in a very short time, cease to occur once all the genes of the genome have been successfully mapped.) In this case the laborious process of analysing the whole region must be undertaken. The basic aims of such an approach are as follows.

1. To clone every sequence from the interval. With intervals of several million base pairs in length, such

a strategy is laborious and time-consuming. However, recent developments which have allowed the insertion of large human DNA segments of around 10^6 bp into, for example, yeast cells (yeast artificial chromosomes) have greatly speeded up the process.

All the isolated segments can be used in an attempt to define submicroscopic deletions in patients with the disease. Such deletions, often under 100 000 bp in length, will shorten the interval of interest dramatically as they identify relatively large causative mutations. Many genes isolated by positional cloning have relied on the identification of such chromosomal rearrangements.

2. To isolate genes from the region. Once assembled, the DNA segments from the region of interest can be searched for potential gene sequences from a region, which include:

    (a) identification of sequences which show conservation between distantly related species. Since DNA sequences which have no function show little conservation through evolution, such conservation suggests that the sequence has a function (i.e. it is expressed);

    (b) identification of regions at the 5′ end of genes involved in control of gene expression ('CpG islands');

    (c) isolation of complementary DNA sequences. Messenger RNAs from a given tissue can be extracted and converted, using reverse transcriptase, into complementary DNA (cDNA) 'libraries'. There are now a variety of techniques for screening such libraries with cloned sequences from any interval and, by so doing, extracting genes which are expressed in the tissue of interest.

Following their isolation, candidate genes must be sequenced, their intron/exon boundaries and their patterns of expression defined. Once this has been carried out, the search for causative mutations in affected individuals will confirm the gene as that responsible for a given disorder.

Summary

Through the application of molecular genetics, much progress has been made in our understanding of specific ocular mendelian disorders. Characterization of ocular proteins has allowed the isolation of autosomal genes involved in retinal disorders (retinitis pigmentosa, stationary night-blindness, vitelliform macular dystrophy), whilst positional cloning approaches have been successful in the mapping and cloning of X-linked ocular genes (e.g. Norrie's disease, choroideraemia, and ocular albinism) and the aniridia gene (PAX6 locus). In addition animal models have proved a powerful complementary approach. Within ophthalmology enormous advances have been

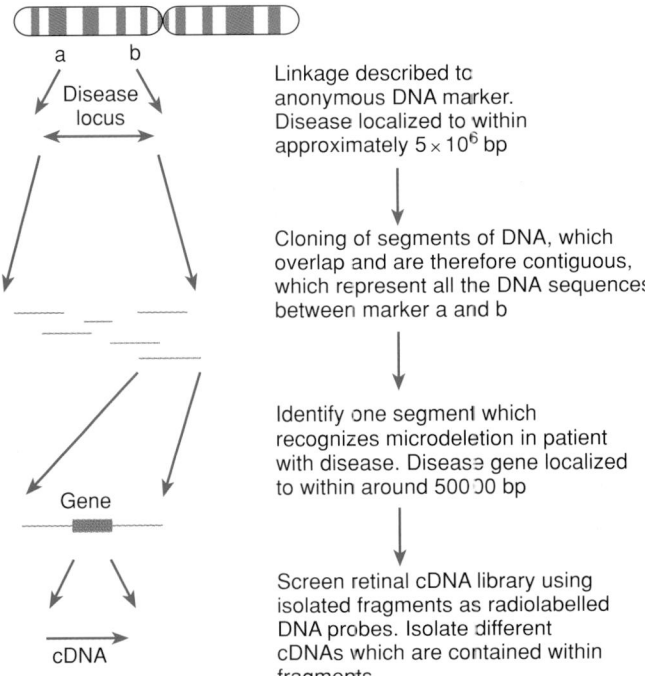

Fig. 7 Localization of a disease gene by positional cloning.

Linkage described to anonymous DNA marker. Disease localized to within approximately 5×10^6 bp

Cloning of segments of DNA, which overlap and are therefore contiguous, which represent all the DNA sequences between marker a and b

Identify one segment which recognizes microdeletion in patient with disease. Disease gene localized to within around 50000 bp

Screen retinal cDNA library using isolated fragments as radiolabelled DNA probes. Isolate different cDNAs which are contained within fragments seen in the field of the inherited retinal dystrophies, inherited cataract syndromes, and systemic disorders involving the eye.

Genetic analysis of complex inherited disorders (polygenic disorders) is hindered by problems of heterogeneity and, in many cases, by the late onset of symptoms. However, the analysis of related, albeit uncommon, disorders which segregate in a defined mendelian fashion is considerably simpler and has been successful for certain forms of the diseases, such as certain familial glaucomas, macular degenerations, and cataracts. Hopefully study of these will shed light on the genetic bases of such complex visual disorders.

With the rapid acceleration in the efficacy of molecular techniques it is likely that many more genes involved in the pathogenesis of eye diseases will be isolated and characterized in the near future, opening the door on a new era of understanding of the pathogenesis of disease and of biochemical and developmental processes. At the same time this will lead to improvements in diagnosis and assessment of prognosis and may in turn lead to progress in treatment, both by traditional and genetic means.

Further reading

McKusick, V.A. (1994). *Mendelian inheritance in man*, 11th edn. Johns Hopkins University Press, Baltimore, MD.

Singer, M. and Berg, P. (1991). *Genes and genomes*. University Science Books, Mill Way, CA.

Strachan, T. and Read, A.P. (1996). *Human molecular genetics*. Bios Scientific Publishers, Oxford.

1.2 Microbiological basic principles

1.2.1 Bacteriology, virology, and mycology

Paul Badenoch

A basic understanding of the micro-organisms that invade the eye is important for the proper diagnosis and treatment of ocular infections. This chapter provides a brief summary of the biology of bacteria, viruses, and fungi as a background to clinical sections later in the book. We begin with a few historical notes.

Discovery of microbiology

That certain diseases are due to microscopic organisms is a recent concept. It was long believed that illnesses, particularly epidemics, were sent as punishment by the gods. The idea of contagion being due to tiny creatures, however, can be found in classical writing. Lucretius, for example, wrote of 'the seeds of disease' in the first century BC. Such abstract thought would not re-emerge in Europe until the Renaissance. In a visionary expression of the germ theory, Girolamo Fracastoro wrote in 1546 of disease being due to minute seeds which could spread from person to person.

The discovery of the microbial world by Antony van Leeuwenhoek (1632–1723) marked the beginning of microbiology as a science. Leeuwenhoek was a highly skilled lens maker with an insatiable curiosity about nature. He described all the main types of unicellular organisms that we know today, including bacteria and yeasts. As no one could equal Leeuwenhoek's expertise at constructing simple microscopes, and the early compound microscopes suffered from major optical defects, there was little progress in the field for more than a century. From about 1820, significant improvements to the compound microscope rekindled interest in the study of microbial life.

Leeuwenhoek's work made scientists wonder about the origin of the 'little animals'. There were two main schools of thought: that the observed micro-organisms arose by spontaneous generation or from germs present in the air. The theory of spontaneous generation, held as self-evident for centuries, was not generally discarded until the latter half of the nine-teenth century as the weight of negative evidence accumulated. For example, Lazzaro Spallanzani had demonstrated that an organic infusion could be kept free of contamination if hermetically sealed and boiled, and that microbial growth would occur only when untreated air entered the flask. In addition, John Tyndall found that the regrowth of bacteria from dried hay after boiling, long taken as evidence for spontaneous generation, could be explained by the presence of thermoresistant forms (endospores).

An appreciation of the role of micro-organisms in the transformation of organic matter gradually developed. The theory that yeast was responsible for the fermentation of alcohol was proposed as early as 1837, but was not accepted until the work of Louis Pasteur several decades later. He showed that different fermentative processes occur in the presence of different micro-organisms. While studying the fermentation of butyrate, he observed that bacteria at the the edge of a drop became immotile when air was introduced and that the reaction would cease. He introduced the terms 'aerobic' and 'anaerobic' to designate life in the presence or absence of oxygen. Pasteur was the first to appreciate that some micro-organisms can use either of two energy-yielding mechanisms depending on the availability of oxygen: aerobic respiration and fermentation. The mechanisms were associated with different growth rates and different end products.

Pasteur suspected that micro-organisms could be agents of human infectious disease. It had already been demonstrated that particular fungi were responsible for disease in wheat, rye, potatoes, and silkworms. *Beauveria bassiana*, shown in Fig. 3, is celebrated as being the first micro-organism proven to cause a specific disease. Agostino Bassi showed it to be the agent of muscardine in silkworm larvae in 1835. Furthermore, Joseph Lister had reasoned that surgical sepsis resulted from contamination of exposed tissue and developed methods to prevent the access of micro-organisms to wounds. This approach was markedly successful and was important indirect evidence for the germ theory. The conclusive demonstration of bacteria as specific agents of disease was made by Robert Koch in 1876, working on anthrax. His experiments fulfilled criteria proposed by Friedrich Henle as necessary to establish a causal relationship between a micro-organism and a disease. These criteria were: (a) the organism must be present in every case of the disease; (b) the organism must be isolated from the host in pure culture; (c) the disease must be reproduced when the organism is inoculated into a healthy susceptible host; and (d) the organism must be recoverable once again from the experimentally infected host. The criteria are now known as Koch's postulates.

Diagnostic ocular microbiology as we know it began in 1879 when Theodor Leber cultured *Aspergillus* from a corneal ulcer and Albert Neisser observed diplococci in conjunctival exudates. These bacteria, *Neisseria gonorrhoeae,* were first cultured from the eye by Löffler and Leistikow in 1882. Koch was in Egypt at the time investigating a cholera outbreak. Although he did not confirm the agent of cholera until he went on to India, he isolated a bacterium responsible for epidemic conjunctivitis (the Koch–Weeks bacillus, *Haemophilus aegyptius*).

The anthrax work and a number of important technical advances at the time, such as the introduction of agar and the development of a differential staining method by Christian Gram, ushered in the golden age of medical bacteriology. By the turn of the century, most of the major bacterial agents of human disease had been discovered.

During this period, filters were used to test fluids for bacteria. In 1892 Dimitri Ivanovsky made the surprising observation that the infectious agent of tobacco mosaic disease could not be removed by filtration. It soon became apparent that many other plant and animal diseases were caused by submicroscopic, filter-passing agents. These agents became known as viruses, but their true nature remained obscure for the next 50 years.

Classification of bacteria

Living things can be divided into five kingdoms: bacteria, protozoa, plants, animals, and fungi. Essentially, a bacterium is a single-celled organism with a circular chromosome that is not enclosed within a nucleus. No microtubular spindle forms during DNA replication. The cell contains vacuoles, mesosomes, and 70S ribosomes but no complex, membrane-bound organelles. Several planetomycete species are exceptions in that they have a cell nucleus. Nutrients are taken up in molecular form. The ninth edition of *Bergey's Manual of determinative bacteriology* lists over 2000 species although, undoubtedly, many remain to be discovered. Only a small percentage inhabit humans and only a fraction of these are harmful. The classification of bacteria remains an evolving science, but microbiologists are optimistic that the current understanding is beginning to reflect natural relationships. However, one must keep in mind Bergey's tenet that 'bacterial classifications are devised for microbiologists, not for the entities being classified'.

The bacterial kingdom, Procaryotae, consists of eubacteria and archaeobacteria. This division is based on such fundamental differences as the chemistry of the cell wall and the composition of transfer RNA. The eubacteria are further divided into Gram positive or Gram negative, again based on the chemistry and structure of the cell wall. One group of eubacteria, the mycoplasmas, has no cell wall. In ophthalmology, the procaryotes of significance are all wall-possessing eubacteria. Archaeobacteria are often found in extreme environments or as symbionts in the digestive tract of animals.

Bacteria are either spheres (cocci) or straight, curved, or spiral rods (bacilli). Their size ranges from chlamydiae and mycoplasmas as small as 0.2 μm to amongst the largest cells known. *Epulopiscium fishelsoni,* a bacillus found in the gut of surgeonfish, measures 600 × 80 μm! Shape, Gram-stain characteristics and oxygen requirement are important features in classification (Table 1). The major groupings, particularly in medical bacteriology, are also determined by whether the cell is motile, forms an endospore, or requires a host cell for replication.

Bacterial cell wall

The bacterial protoplasm is enclosed by a unit membrane consisting of a bilayer of phospholipids and proteins. Many of the metabolic functions performed by organelles in eucaryotic cells are carried out by the cell membrane proteins in bacteria. The membrane is the major barrier to the passage of solutes between the cell and the environment. The movement of water across the membrane occurs by passive diffusion. 'Facilitated' diffusion is mediated by proteins that bind molecules on the outside of the membrane and expedite their entry into the cell. This mechanism is substrate-specific but, like passive diffusion, operates in the direction of the concentration gradient. To take up nutrients against a gradient, the proteins must be coupled to a supply of metabolic energy. This process is called active transport, as in the case of lactose uptake by *Escherichia coli.* Here, the binding affinity of lactose to the transporter protein on the internal surface of the membrane is reduced compared with that on the external surface.

The major strengthening component of the cell wall is the sac of peptidoglycan external to the cell membrane. Peptidoglycan is a polymer of the hexose sugars *N*-acetylglucosamine and *N*-acetylmuramic acid. Strands are cross-linked by short peptide chains. The layer of peptidoglycan is thick (20–80 nm) in Gram-positive bacteria but relatively thin ($\leq$ 10 nm) in Gram-negative bacteria (Fig. 1). Teichoic acids are found among the peptidoglycan of most Gram-positive bacteria. They are polymers of ribitol or glycerol, or complexes of these alcohols with sugars and amino acids, and constitute important surface antigens. Most are bound covalently to *N*-acetylmuramic acid, but some extend below the peptidoglycan and bind to glycolipids in the membrane. The functions of teichoic acids are uncertain, but they are believed to facilitate the passage of ions. The cell wall of some Gram-positive bacilli, namely the mycobacteria and some nocardia, contains waxes and glycolipids which render the surface hydrophobic. In the Ziehl–Neelsen stain, boiling carbol fuchsin penetrates the wall of these bacteria and resists extraction by acid. Hence, they are referred to as 'acid-fast' under conditions that decolorize other bacteria.

Gram-negative bacteria have a second membrane external to the peptidoglycan sac. The outer membrane is anchored to the peptidoglycan by lipoprotein bridges and consists of lipopolysaccharide, phospholipid, and a small number of proteins. The polysaccharide chains of lipopolysaccharide are important antigenic determinants (the 'O' antigens) and the membrane component, lipid A, is extremely toxic. Lipopolysaccharide is known as 'endotoxin' as it is only released on lysis of the bacterial cell. The uptake of essential polar molecules occurs through protein channels called porins. Tear lysozyme, which

Table 1 Description of bacteria associated with ocular disease

Bacteria	Culture conditions	Principal ocular diseases
Gram-positive cocci		
Enterococcus faecalis	Facultative anaerobe	Endophthalmitis
Staphylococci	Facultative anaerobes	Many
Streptococci	Facultative anaerobes	Many
Gram-positive bacilli		
Atypical mycobacteria	Aerobes	Keratitis
Bacillus cereus	Aerobe	Endophthalmitis
Clostridium perfringens	Anaerobe	Panophthalmitis
Mycobacterium leprae	Aerobe	Leprosy
Propionibacterium acnes	Anaerobe	Chronic postoperative endophthalmitis
Filamentous Gram positive		
Actinomyces israelii	Anaerobe	Canaliculitis
Nocardia asteroides	Aerobe	Scleritis
Gram-negative cocci		
Chlamydia trachomatis	Requires host cells	Trachoma, inclusion conjunctivitis
Neisseria gonorrhoeae	Aerobe	Ophthalmia neonatorum
Gram-negative bacilli		
Bartonella henselae	Aerobe	Cat-scratch disease
Eikenella corrodens	Facultative anaerobe	Dacryocystitis
Enterobacteriaceae	Facultative anaerobes	Conjunctivitis
Haemophilus influenzae	Aerobe	Conjunctivitis
Moraxella spp.	Aerobe	Keratitis
Pseudomonas aeruginosa	Aerobe	Many
Spiral Gram negative		
Borrelia burgdorferi	Complex; microaerophilic	Lyme disease
Treponema pallidum	Not culturable on artificial media; considered microaerophilic	Syphilis

hydrolyses the bond between N-acetylglucosamine and N-acetylmuramic acid, cannot access the peptidoglycan of Gram-negative bacteria without disruption of the outer membrane. This can occur in the presence of complement and specific antibody.

The region between the cell membrane and the outer membrane is known as the periplasmic space. It contains a number of proteins, such as digestive enzymes, that in Gram-positive bacteria are simply secreted into the surrounding medium. The function of many periplasmic enzymes is the removal of phosphate groups from nutrients to increase their membrane permeability. Other periplasmic proteins capture specific nutrients, for example amino acids, sugars, and ions, and direct them to active transport systems.

A number of features can be found on the surface of bacterial cells. For example, a coating of polysaccharide called the glycocalyx is common. The terms 'capsule' and 'slime layer' refer to the dense region adjacent to the wall and the more diffuse region extending outwards, respectively. The glycocalyx is important in adherence, in resisting dessication, and as camouflage against phagocytes. Many Gram-negative bacteria have fimbriae, hair-like structures that facilitate adherence to host cells. Fimbriae-mediated adherence of *Pseudomonas aeruginosa* to glycoproteins on corneal epithelial cells is important in the initiation of keratitis. While some authors use the terms 'fimbriae' and 'pili' interchangeably, others reserve 'pili' to describe a small number of longer filaments which include the sex pilus (see below). Fimbriae are also important in the adherence of some Gram-positive bacteria, although the structure of the filaments is quite different. Fimbriae of Gram-negative bacteria are composed of subunits of pilin protein. The fimbriae of *Streptococcus pyogenes*, the best characterized among Gram-positive bacteria, consist of two intertwined chains of M protein.

Many bacilli are motile. The most common mechanism of propulsion is by flagella, long helical filaments which anchor beneath the cell wall. Flagella are distributed in either a polar or peritrichous fashion and constitute the bacterial 'H' antigens. Some non-flagellated bacteria use an intriguing army tank-like mechanism to glide across surfaces. *Capnocytophaga ochracea*, occasionally isolated from serious eye infections, is an example of a glider.

Bacterial nutrition

When reduced to their elements, bacteria are made of hydrogen, oxygen, carbon, nitrogen, phosphorus, sulphur, potassium, sodium, and traces of about eight other metals. The complexity

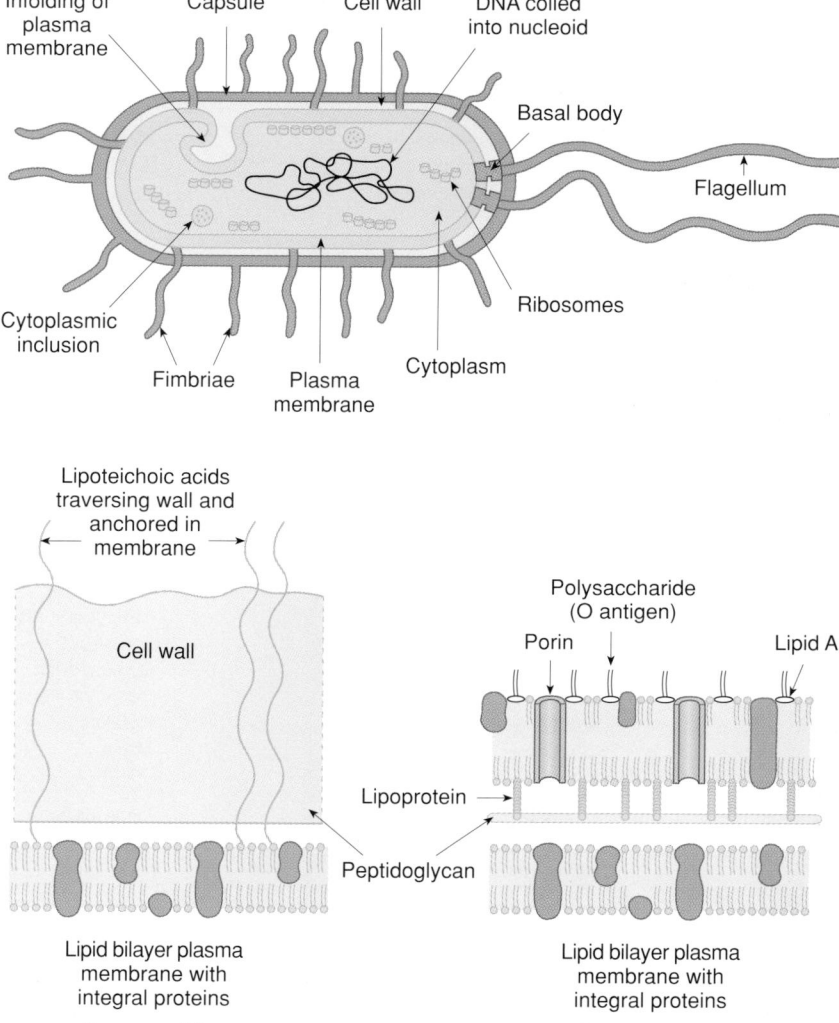

Fig. 1 The general structure of a bacterium and cross-sections through the Gram-positive and Gram-negative cell wall. (Reproduced from Mims *et al.* 1993 with permission.)

of bacterial nutrition lies in the chemical form in which four of these, namely carbon, nitrogen, sulphur, and oxygen, must be available. Bacteria of medical significance obtain carbon from organic nutrients, often from the same substrate used to produce energy. Most bacteria obtain nitrogen and sulphur from inorganic nitrates and sulphates, but some require these in reduced form as found in peptides. Oxygen is obtained from organic nutrients or water, or taken up as O_2. Molecular oxygen also plays an important role in the production of energy by many bacteria.

The major organic constituents of the cell are nucleic acids, proteins, polysaccharides, and complex lipids, all synthesized from about 70 different molecular building blocks. The energy required for biosynthesis is supplied principally as adenosine triphosphate. Adenosine triphosphate is produced by three basic mechanisms: photosynthesis, substrate-level phosphorylation (fermentation), and oxidative phosphorylation (respiration). The last two are relevant here. These reactions tumble down the thermodynamic gradient, resulting in products that have a lower free energy than the reactants. Some of the released energy is captured as the addition of a phosphate group to adenosine diphosphate via a high-energy bond.

In fermentation, organic molecules serve as both electron donors and electron acceptors. The oxidation level of the substrate is partitioned in products that are relatively reduced or oxidized, such as the fermentation of glucose into ethanol and CO_2. These reactions are mediated by coenzymes that can be reversibly oxidized or reduced, nicotinamide adenine dinucleotide being an example. In respiration, inorganic molecules serve as the ultimate electron acceptors. This is most commonly O_2 and the process is called aerobic respiration, but a few bacteria use nitrate, sulphate, or carbonate in a process called anaerobic respiration. Bacteria that use aerobic respiration only to generate energy are called obligate aerobes. Bacteria that use fermentation only and for which molecular oxygen is toxic are obligate anaerobes. Facultative anaerobes can switch between fermentation and respiration depending on the presence of O_2. A few facultative anaerobes use fermentation only but are not inhibited by O_2.

The components of the electron transport chain are the machinery of respiration. They are oriented across the cell membrane so that their oxidation creates a proton gradient. The re-entry of protons into the cell drives adenosine triphosphatase to generate adenosine triphosphate. The degradation of nutrients is more complete in respiration than in fermentation, and more energy per mole of substrate is produced.

Some bacteria require particular growth factors as precursors of constituents that they are unable to synthesize. Examples are the requirement for haemin and nicotinamide adenine dinucleotide by *Haemophilus influenzae* and for vitamin B_6 by *Abiotrophia* species, agents of crystalline keratopathy.

Bacterial growth

Most bacterial strains grow rapidly when nutrients are available, some having a doubling time as short as 20 min. Studies with *Escherichia coli* have shown that chromosome replication is coupled closely with cell division. Replication is initiated when helicases make a split in the double-stranded DNA, forming a 'bubble'. Short priming sequences of RNA are placed on each strand by RNA polymerase. DNA is then added to these sequences by DNA polymerase III using the parent strands as templates. This proceeds simultaneously in both directions around the chromosome, creating two replication 'forks'. The RNA is excised and replaced with DNA by DNA polymerase I and the segments of the new strands are joined by DNA ligase. The chromosome remains in contact with the cell membrane during replication, attached at the forks to an infolding called a mesosome. The process may be pictured as a loop of string being pulled through a knot and separating into two strands as it emerges. The mesosome is split by the synthesis of new membrane and wall, and the daughter chromosomes separate. A septum then forms, leading to cell division by binary fission.

A number of cellular features contribute to the speed of bacterial growth. The cytoplasm of rapidly growing cells teems with ribosomes and RNA. Genes for proteins with related functions are often linked on the chromosome, and are transcribed into one polygenic messenger RNA (mRNA). Coding sequences are not interrupted by introns as in eucaryotes, so that post-transcriptional modification of mRNA is unnecessary. New rounds of chromosomal replication and transcription can begin before the preceding rounds are completed. There being no nuclear membrane, the translation of a strand of mRNA can begin while it is still being transcribed.

Environmental factors that influence growth include temperature, acidity, osmotic pressure, ionic strength, and the availability of nutrients. Most pathogens grow well between 30 and 37°C and prefer a neutral pH. The presence of a particular substrate can induce enzymes involved in its metabolism. Conversely, the presence of an end product will inhibit enzyme synthesis. In either case, the control acts at the level of mRNA transcription. The substrate or product combine with a repressor protein and alter its activity. The repressor binds to an operator region on the chromosome which controls the transcription of a group of genes, known collectively as an operon. Another example of enzyme regulation is catabolite repression. For example, when glucose is available the production of enzymes necessary for the metabolism of other substrates is repressed.

The cells of certain Gram-positive species form endospores when faced with adverse conditions. Sporulation begins with the isolation of a daughter chromosome by inward growth of the cell membrane. An envelope consisting of peptidoglycan and protein is synthesized and the spore is liberated upon autolysis of the parent cell. Many of the cytoplasmic components sequestered within the spore are degraded and replaced. A gel of calcium dipicolinate forms, reducing the water content of the spore and contributing to its heat resistance. Spores survive for hours in boiling water, but are rapidly killed by autoclaving (121°C, 1.1 kg/cm^2). For germination, the envelope must first be cracked by sublethal exposure to heat, enzymes, or chemicals. A new vegetative cell then develops. *Bacillus cereus* and *Clostridium perfringens* are examples of sporulating species that can cause serious ocular infection.

Genetic change in bacteria

Bacteria have developed a number of strategies to bring about genomic change. This can be important in allowing the cell to take advantage of favourable circumstances or to survive adversity, such as when the environment contains pernicious substances such as antibiotics. Genetic change occurs by mutation or recombination. Mutations occur spontaneously or are induced by mutagens. Sometimes only a single nucleotide is affected; on other occasions a number of bases might be deleted, replaced, inserted, or inverted. Mutations are usually harmful to the cell, but some confer a selective advantage.

Genetic recombination can result from transformation, transduction, conjugation, or transposition. In transformation, DNA fragments from dead cells are taken up and integrated into the genome of recipient cells. The identification of the 'transforming principle' for capsule production in *Streptococcus pneumoniae* in the early 1940s was the first direct evidence that DNA was the conveyer of genetic information. In transduction, DNA is carried between cells by bacterial viruses (bacteriophages).

Conjugation is a common mechanism of gene transfer among Gram-negative bacilli. The process is controlled by small circular units of DNA called plasmids which replicate independently from the main chromosome. Many plasmids direct the formation of sex pili. The tip of a pilus binds to a recipient cell and the pilus retracts, pulling the cells together. A copy of the plasmid then passes through a cytoplasmic tunnel. Some plasmids integrate into the chromosome. If not interrupted, a copy of the entire chromosome including the plasmid can be transferred from these cells. Plasmid mobilization is known to occur rapidly within populations, spreading genes controlling new phenotypic characteristics. Most antibiotic resistance, such as that to tetracycline and chloramphenicol, is acquired from plasmids. Many toxins are also plasmid-encoded, an example being the haemolysin of *Escherichia coli*. Plasmids are used by molecular biologists to transfer genes between species and to make commercial quantities of important proteins.

Finally, genetic change is also effected by moveable segments of DNA called transposons. These elements have insertion sequences flanking their genes and can insert at homologous sites. Transposons on plasmids allow integration of plasmid DNA into the host chromosome. This can lead to rapid and extensive genetic recombination within a bacterial population.

Structure and classification of viruses

In the last years of the nineteenth century, Martinus Beijerinck turned his attention to tobacco mosaic disease. The infectious agent was unusual because it passed through filters that retarded all known bacteria. Beijerinck found that it diffused in agar and was seemingly unaffected by alcohol treatment. He concluded that the agent was not merely a small bacterium but rather a living molecule, a 'fluid infectious principle'. Such ultramicroscopic agents became known as viruses. Their composition remained obscure until 1935 when Wendell Stanley crystallized tobacco mosaic virus and deduced that it consisted largely of protein. Within 2 years, RNA had also been found and the true nature of viruses began to be appreciated.

Viruses infect bacteria, protozoa, fungi, plants, and animals. They alternate between intracellular and extracellular stages, existing in the latter as inert infectious particles called virions (Fig. 2). Virions consist of nucleic acid surrounded by a protein shell, the capsid. Some viruses have additional proteins within the capsid. Capsids consist of subunits called capsomers arranged in either a helical or icosahedral fashion. An icosahedron is a regular polyhedron having 12 corners, 30 edges, and 20 triangular faces, known to architects as a 'geodesic dome'. Icosahedral capsids contain two types of capsomers: pentamers at the corners and hexamers elsewhere. They are, in turn, composed of subunits and bind to five or six other capsomers, respectively. The size of a capsid is determined by the number and size of the capsomers. For example, the icosahedron of adenovirus is smaller than that of herpes simplex virus, despite having more capsomers. Adenovirus has 252 small capsomers (six along each edge giving 12 pentamers and 240 hexamers), while herpes has 162 large capsomers (5, 12, 150). The capsids of many human viruses are enveloped in a membrane derived from the host cell.

The viral genome is RNA or DNA, either single- or double-stranded, usually linear but in some cases circular. Most capsids contain only one nucleic acid segment, but the larger RNA viruses have up to 12. The viral genome is haploid except in retroviruses where it is diploid. The size of the genome ranges widely. Virions of molluscum contagiosum virus, for example, contain over 50 times more DNA than those of hepatitis B virus. However, one cannot assume a simple relationship between genome size and the number of proteins coded. This is affected by whether one or both DNA strands are transcribed, in one or both directions, and in how many reading frames. Repeated sequences or introns may be present. Also, a single RNA transcript can be rearranged to give several mRNAs that are translated into different proteins.

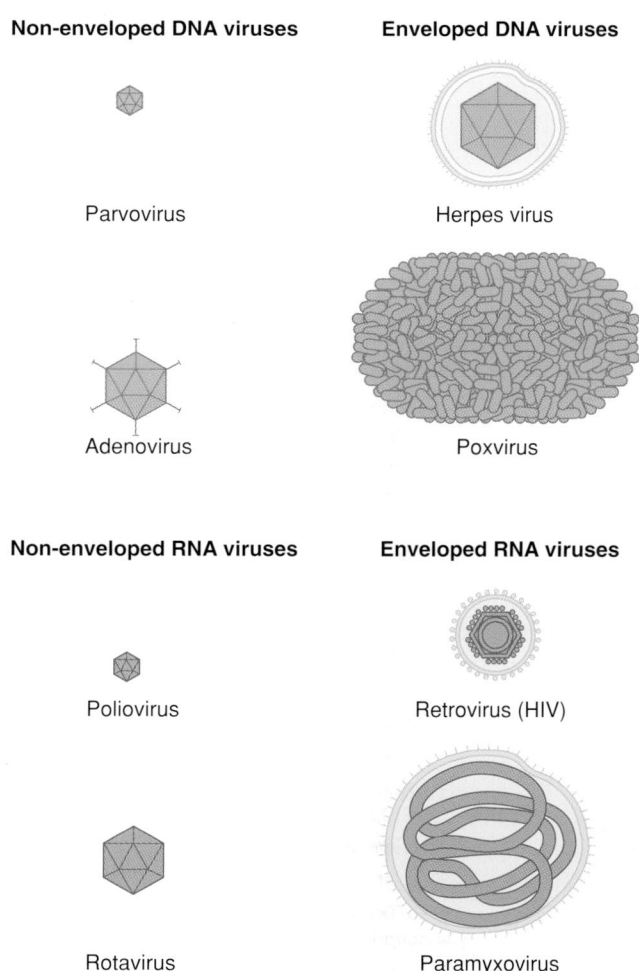

Fig. 2 Examples of virus morphology, variety, and size (scale: 1 cm = 100 nm). (Reproduced from Mims *et al*. 1993 with permission.)

A number of the features which determine the classification of viruses are given in Table 2. The primary criteria for the delineation of families are the morphology of the virion, the nature of the nucleic acid, and the strategy of replication. The family name may reflect these properties, for example Picornaviridae from the Italian *piccolo*, meaning small, and RNA. Viruses are often grouped informally according to their target organ or associated disease, such as the respiratory viruses and hepatitis viruses.

Viral replication

The important steps in viral replication are attachment to the host cell, penetration, uncoating, protein synthesis, nucleic acid replication, and virion assembly and release. Whereas bacterial and plant viruses require a mechanism to get through the cell wall, animal viruses bind directly to the cell membrane. To facilitate attachment, many virions have ligands on specific molecules on their surface. Adenovirus, for example, has a

Table 2 Features of viruses associated with ocular disease

Family	Virus	Genome	Capsid symmetry	Envelope	Principal ocular diseases
Adenoviridae	Human adenovirus	Linear dsDNA, 36–38 kbp	Icosahedral	–	Keratoconjunctivitis
Bunyaviridae	Rift Valley fever virus	Circular (–) ssRNA, 3 segments, total of 12–13 kb	Loosely helical	+	Conjunctivitis, uveitis, retinitis
Herpesviridae	Herpes simplex	Linear dsDNA, 152 kbp	Icosahedral	+	Many
	Herpes zoster	Linear dsDNA, 124–126 kbp	Icosahedral	+	Many
	Cytomegalovirus	Linear dsDNA, 230 kbp	icosahedral	+	Retinitis
	Epstein–Barr	Linear dsDNA, 172 kbp	Icosahedral	+	Many
Papovaviridae	Human papillomavirus	Circular dsDNA, 8 kbp	Icosahedral	–	Conjunctival papilloma
Paramyxoviridae	Measles virus	Linear (–) ssRNA, 16 kb	Helical	+	Cataract, retinitis
	Mumps virus	Linear (–) ssRNA, 15 kb	Helical	+	Many
	Newcastle disease virus	Linear (–) ssRNA, 15 kb	Helical	+	Acute follicular conjunctivitis
Picornaviridae	Enterovirus 70 and cocksackie virus A24	Linear (+) ssRNA, 7–8 kb	Icosahedral	–	Acute haemorrhagic conjunctivitis
Poxviridae	Molluscum contagiosum	Linear dsDNA, 179 kbp	Brick-like	+	Lid lesions
Retroviridae	Human immunodeficiency virus	Linear (+) ssRNA, diploid, 2 × 9 kb	Icosahedral	+	Chorioretinitis
	Human T-cell lymphotropic virus type 1	Linear (+) ssRNA, diploid, 2 × 9 kb	Icosahedral	+	Uveitis
Togaviridae	Rubella virus	Linear (+) ssRNA, 10 kb	Icosahedral	+	Cataract, retinitis

ss, single-stranded; ds, double-stranded; kb, kilobases; kbp, kilobase pairs; (+), positive sense; (–), negative sense.

ligand-bearing fibre extending from each pentameric capsomer. Virions make use of a variety of membrane glycoproteins as their receptors, such as permeases and hormone receptors. The human immunodeficiency virus (HIV) uses the CD4 glycoprotein present on some leucocytes. The specificity of the ligand–receptor interaction is an important factor in the host range and tissue tropism of viruses.

Ligand binding triggers receptor-mediated endocytosis. Once inside the cell, some viruses rely on their containing vesicle fusing with a lysosome, and the acidic conditions that ensue, to initiate capsomer dissociation. Enveloped viruses often fuse directly with the cell or vesicle membrane, releasing their capsid into the cytoplasm where it undergoes enzymatic degradation. Irrespective of the mechanism, the result is that the viral genome is usually fully uncoated.

Viruses have a number of strategies for pirating the protein-synthesizing machinery of the cell. In some single-stranded RNA viruses such as hepatitis C, the genome serves directly as mRNA. One of the proteins coded is an RNA-dependent RNA polymerase which transcribes viral RNA into complementary (negative-sense) copies. These act as templates for the synthesis of new genomes. Virions of other RNA viruses have a (–) sense genome and they need to pack an RNA polymerase to generate (+) sense mRNA. The HIV genome is (+) RNA but, instead of functioning as mRNA, it is transcribed by a viral RNA-dependent DNA polymerase (reverse transcriptase). This gives an RNA–DNA intermediate leading to double-stranded DNA which inserts into a chromosome. Full length (+) transcripts associate in pairs to form the diploid genomes of new virions. In DNA viruses such as adenovirus and the herpesviruses, the genome is transcribed in the nucleus by cellular DNA-dependent RNA polymerase. Molluscum contagiosum virus, a large poxvirus, carries its own RNA polymerase into the cell and can replicate in the cytoplasm.

Each family of DNA viruses has its own mechanism of DNA replication. In adenovirus, for example, the 5′ end of each DNA strand is a mirror image of the other and has a covalently bound protein primer. Replication proceeds from both ends, involving virally coded DNA polymerase. The herpesviruses encode most of the enzymes that are necessary to increase the pool of nucleotides and to copy DNA. This is important for replication in resting cells, such as in herpes simplex virus infection of neurones of the sensory ganglia. Herpes simplex virus can persist indefinitely in these cells. Latently infected neurones contain between 10 and 100 copies of the viral genome as circular concatenated molecules in the nucleus. Unusual (–) RNA transcripts known as LATS (latency-associated transcripts) inhibit mRNA production. Herpes simplex virus reactivation is poorly understood, but is associated with changes in immunological or hormonal status.

Viral proteins and nucleic acid accumulate in the cell and assemble into capsids. Genetic recombination may occur before or during packing. RNA molecules of poliovirus, for example, pair and crossover in a manner analogous to DNA recombination. The influenza A virus genome consists of eight RNA segments and reassortment can occur in cells infected with more than one strain. This may result in a subtype having a novel haemagglutinin and an antigenic shift. The appearance of such a strain in 1918 resulted in a pandemic and 21 million recorded deaths.

A common mechanism for the release of virions is extrusion through the cell membrane with the acquisition of an envelope. Other viruses escape through breaks in the membrane without envelopment. This usually follows cell death and is characterized by the sudden appearance of large numbers of free virions. In contrast, release by budding does not necessarily kill the cell and may continue for a long period. The envelope of herpesviruses is acquired by budding through the inner lamella of the nuclear membrane. The virions then pass along the cisternae of the endoplasmic reticulum to the exterior of the cell.

Some viruses have genes for proteins which combat host defences and help dissemination. Such proteins, known as virokines, might inhibit proteolytic enzymes, stimulate the proliferation of nearby uninfected cells or mimic the receptor of an antiviral cytokine. The glycoprotein E-glycoprotein I complex of herpes simplex virus, for example, is a virokine that binds to the Fc (fragment crystallizable) region of immunoglobulin G and inhibits complement-mediated cytolysis. Another example is the product of the UL18 gene of cytomegalovirus. This virokine is a homologue of the large peptide of the major histocompatibility complex class I molecule. It binds to the surface of infected cells and is believed to inhibit their recognition by cytotoxic cells.

Oncogenes

Oncogenes are genes that can transform normal cells into cancer cells. They were first discovered in retroviruses. Ellerman and Bang demonstrated in 1908 that leukaemia could be transmitted between chickens by the injection of cell-free filtrates and hypothesized that a virus was responsible. Further studies found that various cancers could be transmitted in rats, cats, turkeys, and other species. The development of cell culture techniques in the 1960s led to the identification of retroviruses as the causative agents. The genes responsible for transformation were called viral oncogenes.

Viral oncogenes were initially thought to be of viral origin and important in their lifecycle. However, when scientists examined cells from uninfected animals, genes similar to viral oncogenes were found. These 'proto-oncogenes' are now considered to be normal components of all vertebrate cells, and related genes have been found in insects and yeasts. Many have no known retroviral homologue. They code for proteins that are crucial in the control of cell growth and differentiation. It is assumed that proto-oncogenes have been incorporated into retroviruses during infections, and that having the ability to transform cells is of some advantage to the virus.

Retroviruses produce tumours either by integrating close to a proto-oncogene and corrupting its normal function or by coding for an oncoprotein. Retroviral oncoproteins act by interfering either with the transcriptional control of cellular genes or with signal transduction between the surface of a cell and its interior, thus resulting in loss of contact inhibition. For example, human T-cell lymphotropic virus type 1 encodes a transcriptional activator protein which increases the production of interleukin 2, a T-cell growth factor. This, and the effect of the activator on several proto-oncogenes, results in a lymphocytic leukaemia.

The term 'oncogene' now applies to any gene associated with transformation, including those of oncogenic viruses which do not have a cellular homologue. Other viruses strongly associated with human malignancies are papillomavirus (skin and genital carcinomas), Epstein–Barr virus (Burkitt's lymphoma, B-cell lymphomas, nasopharyngeal carcinoma), and hepatitis B and C (hepatocellular carcinoma).

Fungi

The concepts and language of mycology can be daunting to those outside the field. However, as fungi constitute one of the five kingdoms of the living world, a degree of complexity is to be expected. In any case, coming to terms with a small number of words and ideas is invaluable in understanding the interaction of fungi and the eye. A short glossary of common terms is given in Table 3.

Fungi are eukaryotic organisms. Although once considered to be plants, they lack chlorophyll. The fungal cell wall resembles that of plants architecturally but not chemically, consisting of chitin or cellulose in a matrix of proteins and lipids. The presence of a cell wall prevents fungi from engulfing other micro-organisms. Fungi feed by secreting enzymes which degrade organic matter. Substrates are then absorbed and used for energy production by respiration or fermentation. Most fungal species are free-living in soil where they function as recyclers of biological material. Some are parasitic on plants or animals. The great majority have no direct interaction with humans. A number are beneficial, even prized, such as brewers' yeast, cheese moulds, and truffles. Fewer than 100 species are pathogenic in otherwise healthy people, with perhaps 200 others capable of opportunist infection. A summary of fungi important in ophthalmology is given in Table 4.

Most fungi form a vegetative structure called a mycelium, a multinucleated mass of cytoplasm enclosed within a branched system of tubes. A mycelium arises when a spore germinates,

Table 3 Glossary of common terms in mycology, supplementary to the text

Blastoconidium	A conidium formed by budding along a hypha, pseudohypha or single cell, as in the yeasts
Conidiophore	A conidia-bearing branch of a mycelium
Dematiaceous	Having black or brown pigment
Dermatophyte	A fungus with the ability to infect skin, hair, or nails
Deuteromycete	In some classifications, a member of the imperfect fungi
Dimorphic	Having two forms
Floccose	Cottony or woolly, in tufts
Fusiform	Spindle-shaped
Geniculate	Bent, like a knee
Germ tube	The initial hypha from a germinating spore or yeast
Glabrous	Having a smooth, even surface
Hyphomycete	An imperfect mould, as distinct from an imperfect yeast
Macro/microconidia	Large and small forms of spores produced by a single fungus; macroconidia are frequently multicellular
Moniliform	Shaped like a necklace or a string of beads
Mould	A fungus that cause mouldiness and exists as a filamentous colony
Phialide	A cell with a terminal opening through which conidia are extruded
Pseudohypha	A chain of elongated cells intermediate between a chain of budding cells and a true hypha, marked by constrictions rather than septa at the junctions
Pseudomycelium	A mass of pseudohyphae
Saprobe	A fungus that feeds on dead or decaying organic matter (formerly *saprophyte*)
Septate	Having cross-walls
Spherule	A large, circular structure containing spores, characteristic of *Coccidioides immitis*
Thallus	The actively growing vegetative part of a fungus

putting out a long thread (hypha) which branches as it elongates. Cytoplasm normally streams towards the growing tips and disappears from the older, central parts of the mycelium. Mycelia are rarely seen in nature as they develop underground. Mushrooms, however, form fruiting bodies which project above the surface.

Yeasts have lost the mycelial form of growth and reproduce by budding. As the bud enlarges, the nucleus divides and a cross-wall forms. *Candida albicans*, a yeast involved in ocular infection, forms pseudohyphae under certain nutritional conditions. Most yeasts do not live in soil but have become adapted to environments with a high sugar content, such as flower nectar and rotting fruit. Some fungi can switch between a mycelial and a budding form depending on the temperature. *Histoplasma capsulatum*, for example, develops as a mycelium in soil but as a yeast at 37°C or in the course of an infection.

The morphology of a fungus can vary markedly during its lifecycle. The form that appears after sexual reproduction (the teleomorph) is often very distinct from that which appears after asexual division (the anamorph). Some fungi produce two kinds of sex cells on a single mycelium, but most require contact between two compatible mycelia for sexual reproduction. Most

fungal infections of the eye result from spores produced by anamorphs of opportunistic fungi. Since it is rare for more than one strain to be involved in an infection, only the anamorph is seen in stains and cultures. This is a relief for the non-mycologist, as the anamorph and teleomorph usually have different names. *Fusarium solani* and *Nectria brevicona*, for example, are the same organism. In addition, some fungi have more than one anamorph classified in different genera, and the teleomorphs of a genus of anamorphs can be multigeneric and vice versa.

Asexual spores form at the tips of hyphae and are of two general types, conidia and sporangiospores (Fig. 3). Conidia are naked spores seen in many saprobes and dermatophytes. Sporangiospores are spores produced within a sac-like structure, a sporangium. They are released by rupture of the sporangium and disperse in the breeze. The mechanism of formation of sexual spores is important in the classification of fungi.

Fungal classification

Various systems of classification have been devised for fungi. There is general agreement for a primary division into 'lower'

Table 4 Classification of fungi associated with ocular infection

Fungus	Principal ocular diseases	Description
Candida albicans	Keratitis, endophthalmitis	Yeast-like imperfect fungus of the class Blastomycetes, order Cryptococcales, family Cryptococcaceae
Cryptococcus neoformans	Endophthalmitis, chorioretinitis	Yeast-like anamorph also in the Cryptococcaceae family; the teleomorph is a basidiomycete, *Filobasidiella neoformans*
Acremonium potronii	Keratitis	Imperfect mould of the order Moniliales, family Moniliaceae
Sporothrix schenckii	Endophthalmitis	Imperfect, dimorphic fungus of the Moniliaceae family, growing as a yeast at 37°C and as a mycelium at lower temperatures
Coccidioides immitis	Conjunctivitis, lid infection	Another dimorphic fungus in the Moniliaceae family, growing as a mycelium with arthrospores in soil and as a spherule with endospores in tissue
Histoplasma capsulatum	Chorioretinitis (presumed ocular histoplasmosis syndrome)	An anamorph in the Moniliaceae family, growing as a yeast at 37°C and as a mycelium in soil. The teleomorph is the ascomycete *Ajellomyces capsulatus*
Blastomyces dermatitidis	Lid and orbit infection	As for *H. capsulatum*. The teleomorph is *Ajellomyces dermatitidis*
Aspergillus spp.	Keratitis, endophthalmitis	Anamorphs are in the Moniliaceae family, teleomorphs are ascomycetes of the order Eurotiales, family Trichocomaceae
Alternaria spp.	Keratitis	Imperfect mould of the order Moniliales, family Dematiaceae
Fusarium solani	Keratitis, endophthalmitis	An anamorph in the Moniliales order, family Tuberculariaceae. The teleomorph is an ascomycete, *Nectria brevicona*
Pseudallescheria boydii	Keratitis, endophthalmitis	Ascomycete of the order Microascales, family Microascaceae; the anamorph is *Scedosporium apiospermum*
Rhizopus and *Absidia* spp., *Mucor circinelloides*	Orbital cellulitis, orbital apex syndrome	Lower fungi of the order Mucorales.
Rhinosporidium seeberi	Oculosporidiosis	*Incertae sedis*; possibly a zygomycete

and 'higher' fungi. Lower fungi, the zygomycetes, form sporangiospores and have non-septate hyphae. Higher fungi, which include most of the species of medical importance, form conidia on the tips of septate hyphae. These organisms cannot be considered multicellular, however, as each septum has a pore through which cytoplasm and nuclei move freely.

A small number of zygomycetes are pathogenic. Several members of the order Mucorales, including *Rhizopus* and *Mucor* species, are agents of mucormycosis which may involve the orbit. Recent evidence suggests that *Pneumocystis carinii* and *Rhinosporidium seeberi* are also lower fungi. Zygomycetes are noted for the production of large 'zygospores' (see Fig. 3). When hyphae of two compatible strains meet, each produces a short branch which divides to form a cell called a gametangium. The gametangia then fuse to produce a thick-walled zygospore. The behaviour of the two fungi is identical; there is no 'female' or 'male'. Meiosis occurs when the zygospore germinates. The growing hypha produces a sporangium and its haploid spores develop into mycelia.

Higher fungi are subdivided into Ascomycotina and Basidiomycotina based on the mechanism of sexual reproduction. The ascomycetes are heterothallic, meaning that strains have distinct male or female structures. When strains of opposite sex come into contact, the structures fuse into a multinucleated zygote

called an ascogonium. The ascogonium sprouts a short hypha containing a nucleus from each parent. The nuclei fuse and genetic recombination occurs, followed by meiosis and mitosis. Spores are produced endogenously in the elongating hypha, now termed an ascus (see Fig. 3). The ascus ruptures, the spores are released and a new round of haploid growth commences. In basidiomycetes, fusion also occurs between mycelia of suitable mating types, but karyogamy is postponed. Therefore, most basidiomycetes exist in a heterokaryon state for most of their lifecycle. Eventually, a club-shaped structure called a basidium forms in which the nuclei fuse. Meiosis and mitosis lead to the production of four spores attached to the end of the basidium. A droplet of liquid appears at each point of attachment, hydrostatic pressure builds and the spores shoot off into the environment. The most conspicuous basidiomycetes are the mushrooms.

A sexual cycle has not been observed for many of the asexually reproducing fungi isolated in the laboratory. Most are assumed to be heterothallic ascomycetes that either have strict mating requirements or have lost the ability to produce sexual spores. Therefore, a provisional grouping called the conidial or 'imperfect' fungi has been devised from which strains are moved into Ascomycotina or Basidiomycotina on the discovery of a sexual stage. Useful classifications among imperfect fungi

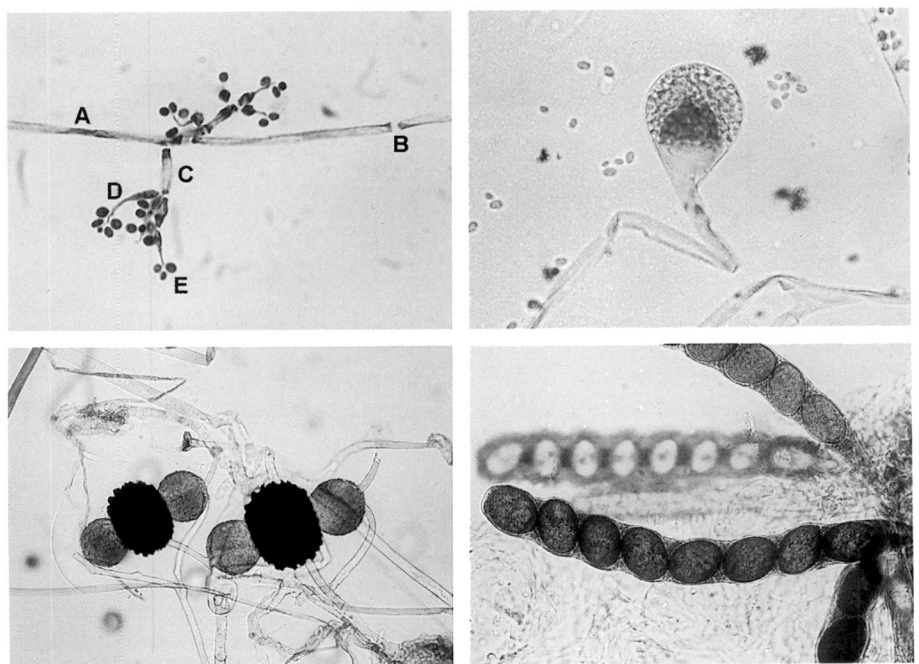

Fig. 3 Important features of fungi. (*Top left*) Culture of an imperfect fungus, *Beauveria bassiana*, from a corneal ulcer. A, hypha; B, septum; C, conidiophore; D, conidogenous cell; E, conidia. (*Top right*) A sporangium of the zygomycete *Absidia corymbifera,* an agent of mucormycosis. (*Bottom left*) A pair of black-staining zygospores with their suspensor cells. (*Bottom right*) An ascus containing eight ascospores. (The last three photomicrographs are from D.H. Ellis (ed.) (1987). *Kaminski's teaching slides on medical mycology,* by courtesy of Dr David Ellis of the Women's and Children's Hospital, Adelaide.)

are made on the basis of the morphology and ontogeny of the conidia and conidiogenous cells.

The term 'yeast' is not a formal taxon and these organisms are found in all three groups of higher fungi. *Cryptococcus neoformans,* for example, is a basidiomycete; *Saccharomyces cerevisiae* (brewers' yeast) is an ascomycete and *Candida albicans* is an imperfect fungus. The mechanism of sexual reproduction in *Cryptococcus neoformans* is similar to other basidiomycetes, but the organism is unusual in spending the majority of its lifecycle as a budding cell derived from a basidiospore. In most ascomycetous yeasts, the mating process involves haploid vegetative cells fusing into a zygote and transforming into an ascus. The germinating ascospores produce haploid vegetative progeny. However, the vegetative cells of *Saccharomyces cerevisiae* are diploid and transform into asci containing four haploid ascospores. Pairs of germinating ascospores, or the first vegetative cells derived from them, then fuse to form diploid vegetative cells.

Interaction of micro-organisms with the eye

We live in harmony with the great majority of microbial species, including those that reside on us as normal flora. Nevertheless, the body attempts to limit the number of microbes on the ocular surface by the action of the lacrimal system and eyelids. This makes it difficult for organisms to adhere to the corneal epithelium, a formidable barrier in its own right. Occa-

sionally, an organism will have the opportunity and the means to cause an infection. If the ocular surface is disturbed, for example by a foreign body or a block in the lacrimal drainage, potentially harmful bacteria can multiply and invade the adnexae or the eye itself.

Most of the bacteria that infect the eye live in the skin, nose, or mouth. Sometimes a pathogen will be introduced from the environment, perhaps by an animal bite or on a contact lens. Organisms can also spread to the eye from within the body, examples being herpes simplex virus emanating from the nerve supply and *Candida albicans* from the blood. An important risk factor for the latter is intravenous drug abuse, resulting in *Candida* endophthalmitis.

Bacteria have varying degrees of specificity for ocular tissues. For example, *Actinomyces* commonly infects the canaliculi but is rarely a problem at other sites, while *Bacillus cereus* infection is predominantly intraocular. Staphylococci, streptococci, and pseudomonads, however, can invade many ocular tissues. Relatively few viruses attack the eye, a consequence of both their host and tissue specificity. The small size of the viral genome limits their ability to thrive in a wide range of environments. Most fungal infections of the eye originate from airborne spores that gain a foothold as a result of a wound.

For an ophthalmologist reading the clinical sections later in the book, it might be helpful to consider infections from the micro-organism's point of view. That is, think of the pathogenic process as a sequence involving microbial attachment, penetration, feeding and multiplication, direct and indirect effects on tissue, combatting the host response, and escape. When dealing with a serious ocular infection, an understanding of the basic biology is important in making the best treatment decision.

Further reading

de Hoog, G.S. and Guarro, J. (ed.) (1995). *Atlas of clinical fungi*. Centraalbureau voor Schimmelcultures, Baarn, The Netherlands/Universitat Rovira i Virgili, Reus, Spain.

Holt, J.G., Krieg, N.R., Sneath, P.H.A., Staley, J.T., and Williams, S.T. (ed.) (1994). *Bergey's manual of determinative bacteriology*, 9th edn. Williams & Wilkins, Baltimore. [The major treatise on bacterial identification, in one volume.]

Mandell, G.L., Bennett, J.E., and Dolin, R. (ed.) (1995). *Principles and practice of infectious diseases*, 4th edn. Churchill Livingstone, New York.

Mathews, C.K. and van Holde, K.E. (1996). *Biochemistry*, 2nd edn. Benjamin/Cummings, Menlo Park, California. [A well-illustrated resource of bacterial structure and metabolism.]

Mims, C.A., Playfair, J.H.L., Roitt, I.M., Wakelin, D., and Williams, R. (1993). *Medical microbiology*. Mosby, St Louis.

Pepose, J.S., Holland, G.N., and Wilheimus, K.R. (ed.) (1996). *Ocular infection and immunity*. Mosby, St Louis. [A treasury of ocular microbiology.]

Rippon, J.W. (1988). *Medical mycology*, 3rd edn. Saunders, Philadelphia.

White, D.O. and Fenner, F.J. (1994). *Medical virology*, 4th edn. Academic Press, San Diego. [Recommended for every ophthalmologist's bookshelf.]

1.2.2 Parasite infections of the eye

Simon Kilvington

Parasite infections affect millions of people worldwide causing considerable suffering and economic hardship. Far from declining, many parasitic diseases are increasing throughout the world. Climatic changes from global warming has aided the spread of many parasite diseases, whilst starvation and the breakdown in sanitation that accompanies war has caused the re-emergence of others. The impact of human immunodeficiency virus (HIV) and acquired immune deficiency syndrome (AIDS) has also seen the emergence of 'new' opportunistic parasites as well as the increased prevalence of others.

Many human parasite infections have included descriptions of ocular involvement and it is beyond the scope of this chapter to detail them all. Attention will therefore focus on the more commonly described eye infections caused by *Toxoplasma*, *Acanthamoeba*, *Toxocara*, *Onchocerca*, and microsporidia. Other parasites that may be associated with ocular disease are included in Table 1.

Toxoplasmosis

Toxoplasma gondii is an obligate intracellular parasite causing the zoonotic disease of toxoplasmosis in humans. Members of

the cat family (*Felidae*) serve as the definitive host for the organism from which the parasite oocysts are excreted into the environment. The oocysts can then infect other animals, including humans, which act as secondary hosts. Toxoplasmosis occurs worldwide and the incidence varies depending on geographical location, eating habits, and climate. In the United States approximately 50 per cent of the population have been infected by the age of 40 years, whilst in some European countries the figure is over 90 per cent.

Biology

The lifecycle of *T. gondii* is complex, involving both sexual and asexual reproduction. Three main lifeforms of *T. gondii* occur: (a) the oocyst which is produced from the sexual cycle in the small intestine of the cat and contains sporozoites; (b) the tachyzoite of the asexual invasive form found in secondary hosts which are derived from pseudocysts; and (c) the tissue cyst that contains bradyzoites.

The oocysts are shed in cat faeces and are commonly ingested by rodents and other animals. The sporozoites are released and penetrate the gut to enter the blood stream where they are phagocytosed by macrophages. Resistant to phagocyte destruction, rapid binary fission occurs that eventually ruptures the macrophage to release the tachyzoite progeny that invade other cells. The tachyzoite measures 3×7 μm and is crescentric in shape. In response to the host T-cell immunity the tachyzoites are initially contained in a microcolony called a pseudocyst. Eventually a true tissue cyst is formed containing slowly dividing bradyzoites. The tissue cysts range from 10 to 100 μm and can occur in any organ but are most commonly found in the myocardium, skeletal muscle, and brain. The cysts may persist for life and can reactivate to release the bradyzoites when the immune system is compromised. Although humans can become infected directly from cat oocysts, the commonest route of infection is the consumption of bradyzoites from raw or undercooked meat.

Disease

In most cases, acquired infection in adult life is asymptomatic or causes only mild fatigue, sore throat, fever, or lymphadenopathy that resolves within a few months. In the immunocompromised patient, toxoplasmosis can be a severe and life-threatening condition. Central nervous system infection is one of the leading causes of death among patients with AIDS. Although rare, transplant acquired toxoplasmosis can be fatal as the recipients of donor organs are usually immunosuppressed for therapeutic reasons.

The most devastating effect of toxoplasmosis is seen in congenital infection when the parasite crosses the placenta from an infected mother to invade the fetus. Severe birth defects can result including hydrocephalus, encephalitis, blindness, and mental retardation. The severity of the infection is greatest when the disease is acquired during the early stages of pregnancy. In later pregnancy the baby may appear normal but symptoms can manifest themselves months or years later.

The most common sequela of congenitally acquired toxo-

Table 1 Other parasites for which ocular involvement has been described

Organism	Disease	Biology	Mode of transmission	Geographic distribution	Ocular symptons	Laboratory diagnosis	Treatment
Protozoa							
Entamoeba histolytica	Amoebiasis: infection of the gut and liver	Anaerobic amoeba: trophozoite and cyst stage	Faecally contaminated food and water	Worldwide	Papilloedema, retinal haemorrhage	Faecal microscopy, culture, serology	Metronidazole, emetine, chloroquine (hepatic amoebiasis)
Plasmodium spp.	Malaria: infection of the liver and blood cells due to P. falciparum, P. vivax, P. ovale, and P. malariae	Complex lifecycle involving mosquito (sporozoites) and humans (merozoites)	Anopheles mosquito	Africa, Asia, and Latin America	Retinal haemorrhage (from anaemia); retinopathy following chloroquine therapy	Blood microscopy, serology	Chloroquine and primaquine (liver stages). Drug resistance: quinine, mefloquine, sulphadoxine + pyrimethamine
Leishmania donovani	Visceral leishmaniasis (kala-azar): infection of liver, spleen, bone marrow, and other organs	Flagellate promastigotes (sandfly), amastigotes in macrophages	Phlebotomus sandfly	Mediterranean, Asia, Africa, and South America	Bilateral retinal haemorrhages	Microscopy, serology, culture	Antimony, amphotericin B, pentamidine
Leishmania tropica, and L. braziliensis	Cutaneous leishmaniasis (skin sores) and mucocutaneous leishmaniasis (nose, mouth, and palate destruction)	Flagellate: promastigotes (sandfly), amastigotes in macrophages	Phlebotomus sandfly	L. tropica: Mediterranean, Asia, Africa, Central and South America; L. braziliensis: Central and South America	Eyelid and corneal lesions, destructive loss of eye in mucocutaneous infection	Microscopy, serology, culture	Antimony, amphotericin B, pentamidine
Trypanosoma cruzi	American trypanosomiasis (Chaga's disease): chagoma (local swelling) at primary site of infection Acute infection: fever, malaise, lymphadonopathy, hepatosplenmegaly. Chronic infection: heart arrhythmias and dilation	Flagellate: trypomastigotes (triatomid bug), amastigotes (humans)	Triatomid bug	Mexico, Central and South America	Unilateral palpebral oedema: Romaña's sign (diagnostic)	Microscopy, serology, culture	Nifurimox, benznidazole
Nematodes							
Taenia solium	Cysticercosis: infection by pig tapeworm	Tapeworm, egg, ocosphere and cysticerci	Infected pig meat	Worldwide	Periorbital pain, diplopia, ptosis, blurring and loss of vision, retinal detachment	Ophthalmascopic examination of eye, microscopy of faeces, serology, computed tomography	Praziquartel, metrifonate, surgical removal
Loa loa	Loiasis ('eyeworm'): microfilarial worm	Adult worms (humans), microfilariae (flies)	Chrysops (mango flies)	Central and West Africa	Retinopathy, uveitis, migration of worm in eyelid and vitreous and anterior chamber	Blood microscopy	Diethylcarbamazine
Trichinella spiralis	Trichinosis: worm infection of muscle	Worm and cyst	Infected meat	Worldwide	Bilateral palpebral oedema, retinal haemorrhage	Microscopy of muscle biopsy	Thiabendazole, mebendazole
Echinococcus granulosus	Echinococcosis ('hydatid disease'): fluid-filled cysts in internal organs	Tapeworm (dog), eggs and cysts (herbivores), cysts (humans)	Ingestion of contaminated dog faeces	Worldwide	Proptosis, corneal ulcer	Serology (arc 5 antigen), radiology, microscopy of biopsy tissue	Surgical removal, mebendazole, albendazole
Schistosoma spp.	Schistosomiasis ('bilharzia'): fluke infection of rectum (S. mansoni, S. japonicum) or bladder (S. haematobium)	Worms and eggs (humans), sporocysts, and cercariae (snails)	Cercariae from infected water snails burrow into skin of humans	Far East, Middle East, Africa, and South America	Choroiditis, retinal haemorrhage, egg granulomas in conjunctiva	Microscopy of faeces and urine, serology	Praziquantel, metrifonate

plasmosis is the late manifestation of ocular infection as retino-choroiditis. Patients are usually asymptomatic until later in life, with a peak incidence of symptomatic disease occurring in the second and third decades. It has been estimated that retinochoroiditis will occur in about 80 per cent of congenitally infected people by 20 years of age. Approximately 100 people born in Britain annually may be affected by retinochoroiditis, about a fifth of the 500 to 600 congenitally infected births each year.

Ocular toxoplasmosis is thought to result from the rupture of dormant cysts and the release of bradyzoites. These invade and multiply in the surrounding tissue causing an inflammatory reaction in the retina and choroid. The disease is rarely bilateral, except in the severely immunocompromised host. Features that suggest toxoplasmosis on ophthalmic examination include bilateral macular involvement, and chorioretinal degeneration with a normal appearing retina surrounding typical punctate lesions. The active lesions are located deep in the retina and appear cream coloured with elevated patches and hazy margins. The retina is thickened and necrosis and oedema are present. Retinal vasculitis and occasionally haemorrhage may surround an active lesion. Fundoscopy may be difficult as the inflammatory reaction in the vitreous can produce a blurred picture that obscures the legions. On healing the lesions pale, atrophy, and develop black pigment (Figs 1 and 2).

When the lesion is peripheral then the prognosis for full recovery of visual acuity is excellent. However, if the lesion is located near the macula then the associated oedema can result in affected central acuity. This usually improves when the inflammation subsides although complete recovery of visual acuity may not occur. In the worst instance, permanent loss of central vision can occur if the macular is involved directly.

The retinal lesions in patients with AIDS are extensive and can cause severe or permanent visual impairment if left untreated. Full thickness retinal necrosis with retinal tears and detachment may develop. These features can be confused with cytomegalovirus retinopathy. However, a prominent anterior

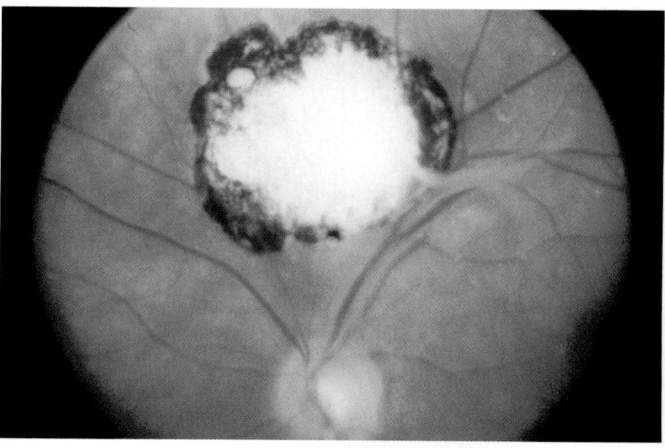

Fig. 2 Toxoplasmosis: fundus photograph showing well-defined yellow scar.

chamber and vitreous inflammatory reaction should alert the clinician to the possibility of toxoplasmosis.

Diagnosis

Active toxoplasmosis may be diagnosed by culture or histological detection of the organism from body fluids and tissue. However, these are not routinely available and the standard laboratory diagnostic test is the demonstration of rising antibody titre using indirect immunofluorescence, latex agglutination, Sabin–Feldmann dye test or enzyme-linked immunosorbent assay. Such is the prevalence of antibody to *T. gondii* in the population that serological tests alone cannot be used to diagnose active ocular infection. Diagnosis of *Toxoplasma* retinochoroiditis is therefore made on the basis of clinical findings on ophthalmic examination with serology serving to confirm the diagnosis. Such cases are often confusing because the antibody level may be only slight. Most authorities consider the presence of active typical retinal lesions and rising antibody titre to be diagnostic of ocular toxoplasmosis. The absence of serum antibody can be used to exclude a diagnosis of toxoplasmosis.

Treatment

In the immunocompetent person, ocular toxoplasmosis is a self-limiting disease and does not usually require treatment. Without intervention, the inflammation gradually subsides and the lesion usually heals in 6 to 8 weeks. Instances of when ocular toxoplasmosis treatment should be commenced are: (a) lesions in the papillomacular area that threaten visual acuity; (b) large retinal lesions greater than two disc diameters, with pronounced vitritis; and (c) all lesions in the immunocompromised host. The object of therapy is to stop the multiplication of the parasite during the active stage of the disease. The tachyzoites but not the tissue cysts of *T. gondii* are sensitive to pyrimethamine, sulphadiazine, trimethoprim, clindamycin, and spiramycin. Recent reports indicate that azithromycin and atovaquone may be cysticidal and are being evaluated for clinical use. Conventional treatment for ocular toxoplasmosis comprises a synergistic combination of pyrimethamine and sulphonamides with

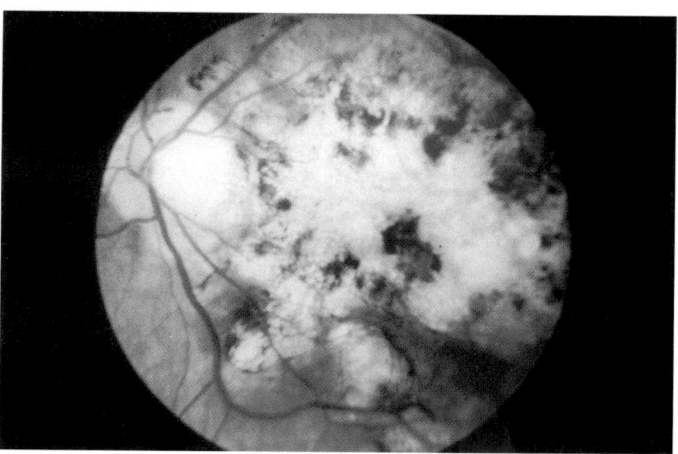

Fig. 1 Toxoplasmosis: fundus photograph showing large areas of retinochoroiditis.

the inclusion of corticosteroids. Pyrimethamine is toxic to humans as it is a folate antagonist. Folinic acid (leucovorin) is therefore given concomitantly to diminish host toxicity. Studies have shown that this treatment can reduce the size of the retinal inflammatory lesion in approximately 50 per cent of cases although treatment does not effect the duration of the inflammatory activity.

Acanthamoeba keratitis

Acanthamoeba is a genus of free-living amoeba found in most soil and aquatic environments. The organism causes two distinct forms of disease in humans, granulomatous amoebic encephalitis and *Acanthamoeba* keratitis. Granulomatous amoebic encephalitis is a rare and invariably fatal opportunistic infection of the central nervous system in the immunocompromised host. In contrast, *Acanthamoeba* keratitis affects previously healthy persons and occurs with far greater frequency. Since the disease was first described in the United States in 1975 several hundreds of cases have been reported worldwide. In the United Kingdom, the incidence of *Acanthamoeba* keratitis has risen steadily each year, with some 100 new cases diagnosed in 1996. Although *Acanthamoeba* keratitis can arise from accidental trauma to the cornea, contact lens wearers are most at risk from infection and account for 80 to 90 per cent of cases. Poor lens hygiene practices, notably the use of non-sterile saline rinsing solutions and defaulting on recommended cleaning and disinfection steps are recognized risk factors.

Biology

Acanthamoeba is characterized by a feeding and dividing trophozoite and dormant cyst stage. Several species have been attributed to causing keratitis but *A. castellanii* and *A. polyphaga* are most commonly identified. The trophozoites range from 25 to 40 μm in length, depending on the species, and show numerous needle-like projections termed 'acanthapodia' (Fig. 3). Cysts are formed from the trophozoites in response to adverse conditions. These are circular, double walled, and range from 15 to 28 μm. The intermittent joining of the inner and outer cyst walls creates a polygonal arrangement in most species (Fig. 3). The resistance of *Acanthamoeba* cysts to extremes of temperature, desiccation, and disinfection accounts for the almost ubiquitous distribution of the organism in the environment.

Acanthamoeba keratitis is characterized by acute pain with perineural and ring-shaped infiltrates in the corneal stroma (Fig. 4). In advanced cases, severe inflammation of neighbouring intraocular structures follows, with scleritis, iritis, and cataract. Corneal perforation may occur in endstage disease. In the early stages of the disease, the presence of a stromal haze within the cornea can lead to a misdiagnosis of herpes simplex keratitis. Although only one eye is usually affected, cases of bilateral infection have been reported.

Most human specimens on which histopathological descriptions are available originate from corneal transplantation and accordingly describe late stages of the disease, probably modified by drug therapy. Disruption and necrosis of stromal lamel-

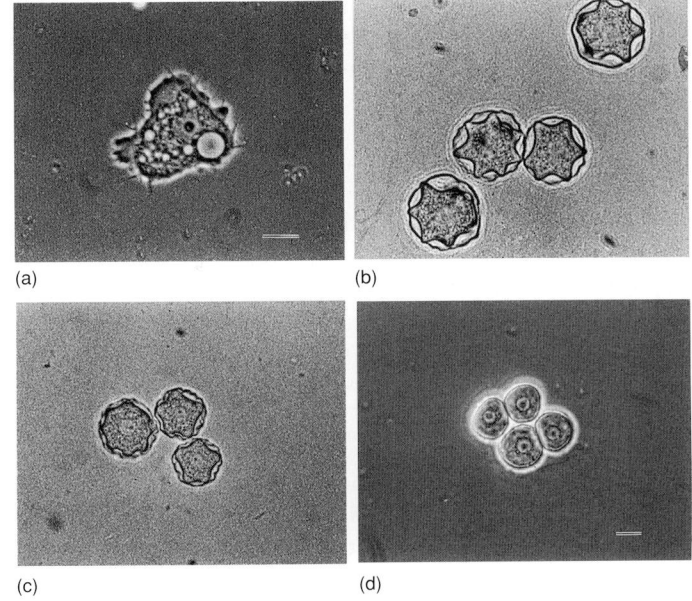

(a)   (b)

(c)   (d)

Fig. 3 Morphological characteristics of *Acanthamoeba*.

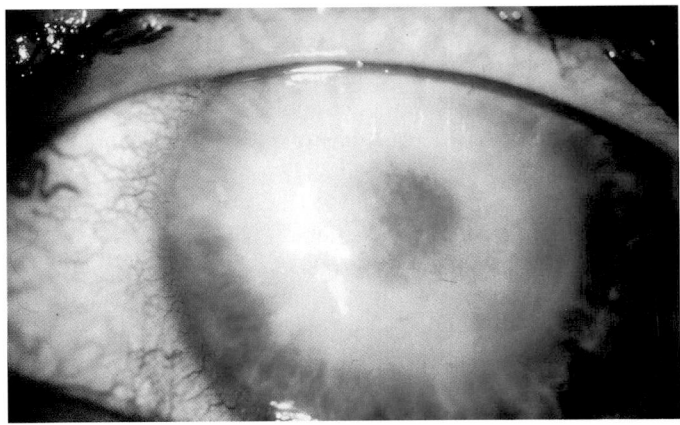

Fig. 4 *Acanthamoeba* keratitis: cornea photograph showing ring infiltrates.

lae and invasion of amoebae deep into the stroma to the Descemet's membrane are seen. Infiltrates of neutrophils and occasionally lymphocytes and plasma cells are also found in this region. However, *Acanthamoeba* can also be present in tissue relatively free of inflammation.

Diagnosis

Acanthamoeba keratitis should be suspected in any symptomatic patient who is a contact lens wearer or presents with a recent history of ocular trauma. Clinical findings such as intense pain and ring infiltrates in the cornea would also suggest *Acanthamoeba* keratitis. However, diagnosis can only be made through laboratory investigations. This is achieved by the culture or histological staining of corneal scrapings or biopsy material. Culture isolation is made by inoculating tissue on to nonnutrient agar (NNA) (1.5 per cent w/v in distilled water) spread with a dense suspension of the bacterium *Escherichia coli* (NNA–*E. coli*). The plates are sealed, incubated at 32 to 35°C for up to 7 days and examined microscopically for the presence of trophozoites migrating away from the inoculum site. If the patient is a contact lens wearer, fluid and biofilm from the storage case should also be cultured (after concentration by centrifugation) as this can often yield the organism when a corneal specimen proves negative. However, the results should be interpreted cautiously as approximately 10 per cent of health contact lens wearers can harbour *Acanthamoeba* in their storage cases.

Treatment

In the untreated state, *Acanthamoeba* keratitis can result in permanent blindness. The resistance of the cysts to most antimicrobial agents at concentrations tolerated by the cornea makes *Acanthamoeba* keratitis one of the most difficult ocular infections to manage successfully. This results in the need for prolonged medical treatment, often lasting a year or more, to eliminate the organism from the cornea. *Acanthamoeba* are sensitive to propamidine isethionate (Brolene 0.1 per cent), hexamidine di-isethionate (desomedine 0.1 per cent), chlorhexidine gluconate (0.02 per cent), and polyhexamethylene biguanide (PHMB 0.02 per cent). Of these, PHMB has proved the most successful. When combined with prompt diagnosis and intensive topical therapy PHMB has dramatically improved the prognosis in *Acanthamoeba* keratitis enabling many cases to be cured medically with restored normal vision. However, the compound is not licensed for patient use and is currently available at only a few centres in the United Kingdom.

The role of corticosteroids in the management of *Acanthamoeba* keratitis is controversial. Steroid treatment may allow the organism to penetrate the cornea more readily by immunosuppressing the host. However, this may be offset by tempering the host inflammatory response that is responsible for some of the tissue damage and severe pain. Contrary opinion considers the host inflammatory response to be an important factor in controlling the infection and some clinical evidence has suggested that steroid therapy is more likely to result in medical therapy failure necessitating surgical intervention.

When medical therapy fails in *Acanthamoeba* keratitis the only recourse is penetrating keratoplasty. Whilst this serves to remove the bulk of the infected corneal tissue, remaining viable organisms can result in graft reinfection in approximately 50 per cent of cases.

Prevention

Many cases of contact lens associated *Acanthamoeba* keratitis can be attributed to some form of negligence in recommended lens hygiene procedures. The presence of *Acanthamoeba* in sites such as natural water, bathing pools, and tap water represent a constant challenge to the contact lens wearer. Therefore, recommended lens cleaning and disinfecting methods should be strictly adhered to and only sterile commercial saline used for the rinsing and storing of lenses. In addition, lenses should never be rinsed or stored in tap water as *Acanthamoeba* have been isolated from domestic tap outlets.

Toxocariasis

Toxocara canis is a roundworm parasite of the dog causing toxocariasis in humans. Less frequently, the disease can be caused by the cat roundworm *Toxocara cati*. Infection results in a clinical syndrome in which the worm migrates in the host viscera producing the systemic condition known as visceral larva migrans. If the worm reaches the eye, ocular larva migrans occurs. Toxocariasis occurs worldwide and approximately 200 cases of ocular larva migrans have been reported in Great Britain and 500 in the United States.

Biology

The adult *T. canis* worm measures 10 to 15 mm in length and lives in the small intestine where large numbers of eggs (75 × 90 µm) are produced that pass with the faeces. In the soil, the larvae develop inside the eggs and can be ingested by other dogs. In young animals the eggs enter the small intestine where the larvae (350–450 µm) hatch, penetrate the mucosa, and are carried through the hepatic circulation to the heart and lungs. There they moult twice and escape from the capillaries into the alveoli. They again enter the stomach via the trachea and oesophagus by being coughed up and pass to the small intestine where they grow to adulthood to continue the lifecycle.

In older animals which have developed immunity the lifecycle fails to be completed. Instead the larvae penetrate the intestinal mucosa and wander through the host tissues for long periods. In a pregnant animal, the changes in hormone balance and possible depression of the host immune response, results in the larvae becoming reactivated. They enter the blood and are carried across the placenta to the fetal circulation before arriving at the fetal lungs where the developmental cycle is completed.

Disease

Humans can become infected with *Toxocara* eggs from their close association with pets or from faecally contaminated ground. The worm cannot complete its lifecycle in the human and becomes arrested in various tissues after penetrating the intestinal mucosa and entering the blood. This results in visceral larva migrans and is characterized by fever, malaise, leucocytosis with marked eosinophilia, hepatomegaly, cough, myalgias, and high titres of isohaemagglutinins. The disease is essentially benign and self-limiting. Although rare, myocarditis, encephalitis, and pneumonia can result with fatal consequences.

Ocular larva migrans is usually seen in older children and young adults. Eosinophilia is less common in ocular larva migrans and the severity of the symptoms can range from mild involvement through to serious ocular destruction. The most important differential diagnosis in ocular larva migrans is retinoblastoma because if misdiagnosed it can result in the enucleation of the affected eye.

Commonly encountered eye lesions are chronic endophthalmitis with retinal detachment, posterior pole granuloma

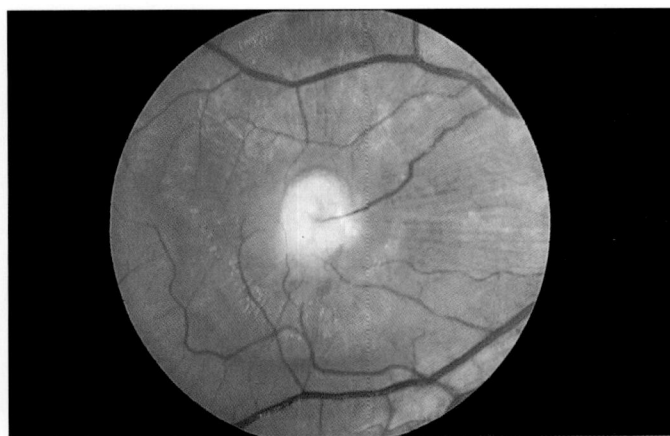

Fig. 5 Macular granuloma due to *Toxocara* infection. (By courtesy of Christopher Dean Hart, Bristol Eye Hospital.)

(Fig. 5), and peripheral granuloma. Initial signs are strabismus, esotropia, leukocoria (a white pupillary reflex), and decreased visual acuity or total loss of vision. The granulomatous lesion is usually unilateral, solitary, and painless and is generally located posteriorly, in close proximity to the optic nerve and disc. The retina is usually involved but lesions have been observed in the iris. The granulomatous lesion is usually solitary, raised, grey or yellow in colour, semispherical, and occasionally umbilicated.

Diagnosis

The importance of differentiating ocular larva migrans from retinoblastoma requires careful and thorough investigation. Definitive diagnosis relies on the detection of the larvae in tissue sections. However, the larvae are usually degenerate when granuloma formation has occurred and difficult to visualize. Diagnosis therefore depends on serological testing. Enzyme-linked immunosorbent assay is positive in 78 per cent of those with visceral larva migrans but only in 45 per cent of ocular larva migrans cases. Simultaneous antibody detection in vitreous humour and serum may provide a differential diagnosis, with a higher titre in the vitreous humour than the serum signifying ocular larva migrans.

Treatment

Therapy is not needed in a majority of visceral larva migrans and ocular larva migrans cases as clinical symptoms are mild and resolve after several weeks or months. However, in acute ocular toxocariasis periocular steroids may be required to control inflammation although the results are often conflicting. Diethylcarbamazine, thiabendazole, and mebendazole are active against the larvae in visceral larva migrans and ocular larva migrans although the timing of the treatment can greatly affect the therapeutic results. The destruction of the larvae may, however, cause an even greater destructive inflammatory response. Vitrectomy aids the repair of retinal detachments secondary to the larva granuloma.

Prevention

Children are most at risk from toxocariasis and are commonly infected when they ingest eggs either directly from infected puppy or kitten faeces or from contaminated soil and vegetation. Approximately 10 to 20 per cent of dogs and 90 per cent of puppies may be infected with *T. canis* in the United Kingdom. Regular worming of puppies and dogs and preventing animals from fouling public areas are effective control measures.

Onchocerciasis

Onchocerca volvulus is a filarial nematode causing onchocerciasis or river blindness in humans. The disease is transmitted by biting flies of the genus *Simulium*. The larvae and pupae of *Simulium* attach to submerged objects in fast-running, well-oxygenated water. As the flight range of the adult fly is limited, human infection is associated with areas bordering rivers and streams. The disease manifests itself as dermatitis, subcutaneous nodules, sclerosing lymphadenitis, and ocular lesions. Onchocerciasis occurs in equatorial Africa, the Sahara, Yemen, and limited areas of Central and South America. In Africa alone it is estimated that more than 30 million people are infected with the parasite resulting in blindness rates of 10 per cent of the adult population in some regions.

Biology

Microfilariae in the subepidermis of infected humans are taken up with blood when the *Simulium* bites. The larvae pass into the gut and then enter the flight muscles where they undergo two moults. Finally, the larvae migrate to the head and become long, thin, infective forms that enter the proboscis. These enter the skin of humans when the fly again feeds. Infective larvae mature into adults as they move through the subcutaneous tissues, with males and females mating and becoming encapsulated by fibrous tissue in prominent subcutaneous nodules. Within the nodules, the females produce microfilariae that migrate into the nearby subepidermal tissues, with those in the head region reaching the tissues of the eye. Female worms measure 30 to 80 cm in length and males 3 to 5 cm. They have a lifespan of 9 to 14 years. Microfilariae range from 250 to 300 μm in length.

Disease

Microfilariae in the eye can be seen by slit lamp examination. Microfilariae have been observed in the conjunctiva, cornea, anterior and posterior chambers, vitreous, uvea, inner retinal layers, posterior sclera, and optic nerve. The ocular lesions are mainly the result of microfilarial invasion, but allergic reaction to parasite antigen may also play a role. The opacity in keratitis is caused by the death of microfilariae within the cornea (Fig. 6). Blindness results from lesions producing sclerosing keratitis and, less commonly, active optic neuritis (Fig. 7). The sclerosing keratitis produces an opaque 'apron' spreading over the lower half of the cornea. Posterior lesions in the retina produce sclerosis of the choroidal vessels and total blindness.

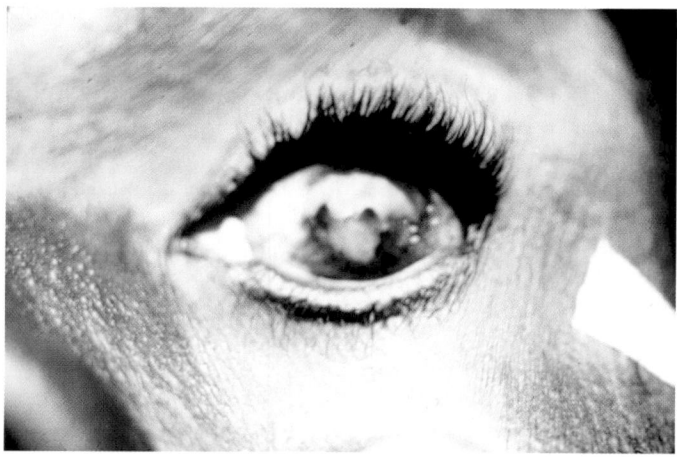

Fig. 6 Corneal scarring in a patient with a history of onchocerciasis. (By courtesy of C.D. Mackenzie.)

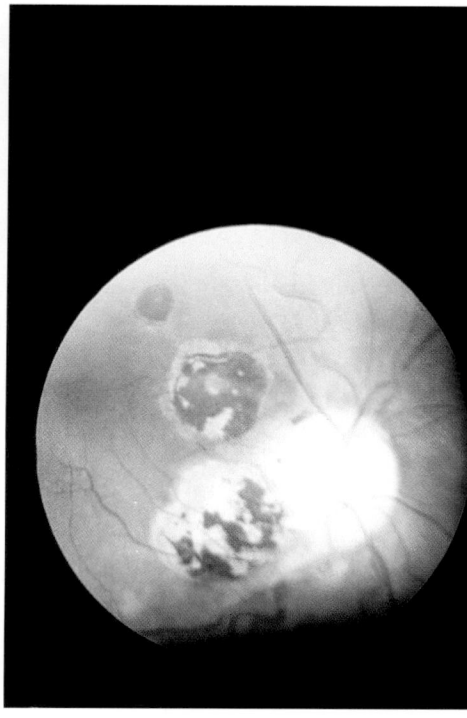

Fig. 7 Optic atrophy with inactive choroidoretinitis due to onchocerciasis. (By courtesy of C.D. Mackenzie.)

Dense vascular sheathing may extend along retinal vessels for a considerable distance beyond the optic nerve head. Partial or complete primary optic atrophy may also occur.

Diagnosis

Diagnosis is usually made by observing microfilariae in the eye and by histological biopsy examination of skin, subcutaneous nodules, or eyes. Aspirate from a nodule, or lymph expressed from a superficial skin incision, can be taken for microscopic detection of microfilariae. The parasite is rarely found in blood. When no microfilariae can be found, the patient can be given a single 50 mg oral dose of diethylcarbamazine. If severe itching and a skin rash develops within the next 24 h, a diagnosis of onchocerciasis is likely (Mazzotti test).

Treatment

Diethylcarbamazine has traditionally been the drug of choice for the treatment of onchocerciasis. However, therapy usually causes severe itching (Mazzotti reaction) which few patients can tolerate and diethylcarbamazine is now considered too toxic for use. Ivermectin is now recommended for the treatment of onchocerciasis at a dose of 150 µg/kg orally once, repeated every 6 to 12 months. The same dose is recommended for children but without the repetition of treatments. This reduces the microfilarial count to near zero within a week and eliminates those in the cornea and anterior chamber in 3 months.

Microsporidiosis

Microsporidia is a non-taxonomic designation used to describe the group of organisms belonging to the phylum *Microspora* contained within the subkingdom Protozoa. Microsporidia are obligate intracellular spore-forming parasites. Approximately 100 genera encompassing 1000 species have been described and these infect a variety of invertebrate and vertebrate hosts. It is only recently that certain species have been recognized as human pathogens. *Encephalitozoon hellem*, *Nosema corneum*, *N. ocularum*, *Microsporidium africanum*, and *M. ceylonensis* have been reported to cause keratitis or keratoconjunctivitis in HIV-positive and, occasionally, non-HIV-positive people.

Biology

The microsporidia have a lifecycle comprising merogenic (proliferative) and sporogenic (spore forming) stages. The spores are ovoid or piriform, 1.5 to 5.0 µm long, and comprise an exospore and endospore. The spore contains a coiled polar tube or filament connected with a complex extrusion apparatus and a nucleated, infective sporoplasm.

After ingestion by a suitable host, the physiological conditions of the digestive tract stimulate the spores to force the polar filament into the host cell membrane. The sporoplasm then migrates through the tube and enters the cytoplasm where asexual multiplication (merogony) and spore formation (sporogony) occur. Sporoplasms usually infect the gut epithelium where they develop or become transferred, probably by the action of phagocytic cells, to the circulation for infection of other organs. The spores, released to the environment from the intestinal or urinary tract, are ingested by a new host.

Disease

Ocular symptoms include conjunctival irritation, photophobia, foreign body sensation, and decreased visual acuity. Conjunctival hyperaemia, mixed follicular–papillary tarsal conjunctival reaction, and recalcitrant punctate epithelial keratopathy may be demonstrated by slit lamp examination. The keratitis may be severe but rarely results in corneal ulceration. Some patients may be only mildly symptomatic or intermittently asymptomatic. However, in deep stromal infections corneal ulceration, keratouveitis, and hyphaemia can result.

Where biopsy material has been examined, organisms have been observed on the inner side of the corneal stroma with necrosis and acute inflammation present at the centre. They have also been found anterior to the plane of Descemet's membrane. The corneal lamellae may also be necrotic and infiltrated by neutrophils and mononuclear cells.

Diagnosis

Detection of microsporidia is usually made by examination of conjunctival or corneal scrapings or biopsy. Urine and pulmonary specimens should also be examined in suspected ocular microsporidiosis. Spores within infected cells can be identified by routine stains such as Giemsa, Gram, or haematoxylin and eosin. Fluorochromes that stain the chitin in the spore wall (e.g. Uvitex 2B or Calcafluor White) may also be used. However, these are not specific for microsporidia spores as fungi and *Acanthamoeba* cysts will also stain with these compounds.

Microsporidia have also been isolated by cell culture but it is a difficult procedure that may not propagate all species. Polymerase chain reaction assays have been described for several species and will greatly aid the accurate diagnosis of infections.

Treatment

The medical treatment for ocular microsporidium infection is still experimental. Preliminary results suggest that albendazole may be effective and clinical trials are in progress.

Further reading

Kean, B.H., Tsieh, S., and Ellsworth, R.M. (1991). *Color atlas/text of ophthalmic parasitology*. Igaku-Shoin, New York.

Khaw, M. and Panosian, C.B. (1995). Human antiprotozoal therapy: past, present, and future. *Clinical Microbiology Reviews*, 8, 427–39.

Kilvington, S. and White, D.G. (1994). *Acanthamoeba*: biology, ecology and human disease. *Reviews in Medical Microbiology*, 5, 12–20.

Muller, R. and Baker, J.R. (1990). *Medical parasitology*. Gower Medical, London.

Peters, W. and Gilles, H.M. (1995). *Colour atlas of tropical medicine and parasitology*. Mosby-Wolfe, London.

Weber, R., Bryan, R.T., Schwartz, D.A., and Owen, R. (1994). Human microsporidial infections. *Clinical Microbiology Reviews*, 7, 426–61.

1.2.3 Chlamydial agents

David Mabey and Denise Mabey

History

The scarring sequelae of trachoma, entropion, and trichiasis, were well known to the ancient Egyptians, and were described in the Ebers Papyrus of 1900 BC, as well as in ancient Greek, Roman, and Arabic medical texts. The disease first became prominent in Europe after the Napoleonic campaigns in Egypt in 1798/99, when both the French and British armies were severely affected by 'military ophthalmia', and introduced the disease into Europe on their return. Although this was long before the 'germ theory' of disease causation was generally accepted, it was obvious to all careful observers that the disease was contagious, and many countries introduced compulsory isolation and quarantine laws against trachoma in the nineteenth century.

In 1907 Halberstaedter and von Prowazek, who were in Indonesia with Albert Neisser's expedition to study syphilis, observed intracellular inclusion bodies in scrapings taken from the conjunctiva of patients with follicular trachoma which they named 'Chlamydozoa', from the Greek word *chlamys*, meaning cloak, because of the characteristic way in which the inclusions were draped around the cell nucleus. They were able to infect orang utans with conjunctival scrapings from trachoma patients, and to find similar intracellular inclusions in infected animals. In 1909 Lindner observed similar intracellular inclusions in conjunctival scrapings from an infant with ophthalmia neonatorum in Germany, but it was not until 1957 that the causative agent, now called *Chlamydia trachomatis*, was isolated in pure culture, in embryonated hens' eggs, by T'ang and colleagues in Peking. Koch's postulates were fulfilled shortly afterwards by Jones and colleagues, when trachoma was induced in a blind volunteer following experimental inoculation.

Classification and structure

The genus *Chlamydia* belongs to the order Chlamydiales, which contains one family, the Chlamydiaceae. It consists of four species: *C. trachomatis*, *C. pneumoniae*, *C. psittaci*, and *C. pecorum*. *Chlamydia* are Gram-negative bacteria, but highly unusual in that they can only replicate inside eukaryotic host cells. *Chlamydia trachomatis* and *C. pneumoniae* are almost exclusively human pathogens, whereas *C. psittaci* affects a wide variety of wild and domesticated birds and animals, only occasionally affecting humans; and *C. pecorum* is an infection of ruminants. Unlike *C. pneumoniae* and *C. psittaci*, which commonly cause systemic illness in humans, *C. trachomatis* infection is usually confined to mucosal epithelial surfaces in the eye and genital tract, although it may cause pneumonitis in infants or in the immunocompromised.

Using an immunofluorescence test developed in the 1960s, Wang *et al.* identified 15 serotypes of *C. trachomatis*: types A, B, Ba, and C, which cause trachoma in endemic areas, types D–K, which cause genital tract and neonatal infections throughout the world, and types L1, L2, and L3 which belong to the more invasive LGV biovar, and cause the uncommon sexually transmitted disease lymphogranuloma venereum. No differences have been identified between the 'trachoma' and 'genital' serotypes which can explain their distinct epidemiology; volunteer experiments have shown that 'genital' strains are capable of causing typical trachoma.

As obligate intracellular parasites which have to transfer

from one cell to another in order to survive, *Chlamydia* have evolved a unique lifecycle, and exist in two forms: the spore-like, metabolically inert, infectious particle, adapted to extracellular survival, known as the elementary body; and the metabolically active reticulate body, which replicates by binary fission within an intracytoplasmic inclusion in the host cell.

The elementary body has a rigid cell wall although, unlike that of other Gram-negative bacteria, it does not contain peptidoglycan. It is about 0.3 μm in diameter. It contains a dense nucleus, eccentrically positioned, and the cytoplasm consists of moderately dense, amorphous material containing numerous ribosomes. Freeze-etching or scanning electron microscopy reveals projections on the elementary body surface, arranged hexagonally.

A cysteine-rich protein of approximately 40 kDa, known as the major outer membrane protein (**MOMP**), makes up some 60 per cent by mass of the cell wall; multiple disulphide cross-linkages within the MOMP are thought to confer rigidity to the elementary body. The MOMP gene, *omp1* has been sequenced from a number of strains of *C. trachomatis*, and has been shown to contain four variable and five conserved domains. The variable domains, at least three of which are surface exposed, contain species-specific epitopes which distinguish *C. trachomatis* from *C. pneumoniae* and *C. psittaci*, as well as serotype-specific epitopes identified in the immunofluorescence test of Wang. In addition to the MOMP, the cell wall contains another abundant cysteine-rich protein known as OMP2, and lipopolysaccharide with endotoxin activity, similar to that found in other Gram-negative bacteria.

Attachment, uptake, and intracellular replication

Chlamydia has a small genome of approximately 1000 kb, and appears to lack the capacity to synthesize many metabolites which are essential for growth. In particular, *Chlamydia* lacks enzymes of the cytochrome oxidase pathway, and is therefore unable to synthesize adenosine triphosphate, making it an 'energy parasite'.

Chlamydia is actively taken up by host cells, although these are not usually 'professional' phagocytes; in the case of *C. trachomatis*, the usual host is a columnar epithelial cell of the conjunctiva or genital tract. The mechanisms by which *Chlamydia* attaches to and enters host cells has not been clearly identified, in spite of considerable efforts in many laboratories. Several candidate 'adhesins' have been proposed on the elementary body surface, including and OMP2, on the basis of inhibition of attachment by treatment with monoclonal antibodies or trypsin digestion. A more recent theory, based on inhibition and reconstitution experiments, proposes that a glycosaminoglycan present at the chlamydial surface, containing heparin sulphate, mediates attachment, displacing host cell glycosaminoglycan by molecular mimicry. There is no clear consensus as to whether *Chlamydia* is taken up by host cells through the phagocytic pathway or by pinocytosis (receptor-mediated endocytosis). The determination of the precise mechanisms by which *Chlamydia* attaches to and is ingested by host cells will probably

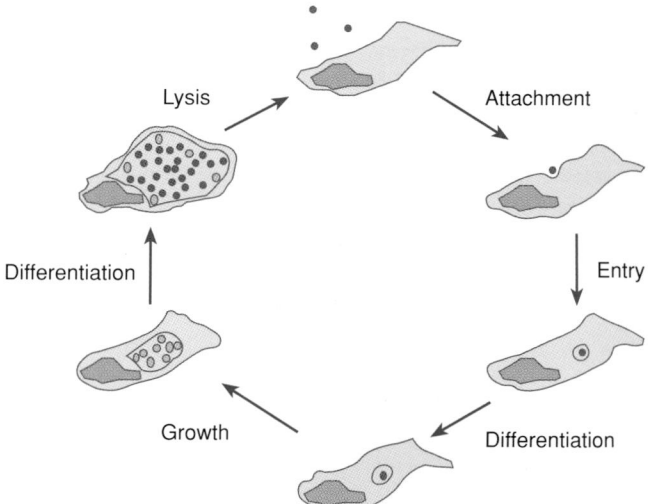

Fig. 1 Schematic representation of the chlamydial intracellular lifecycle. Completion of the cycle requires approximately 40 h.

have to await the development of a system for its genetic manipulation, although inspection of the total genomic sequence of *C. trachomatis* (published on the Internet in 1998) may provide clues through the identification of homologues of other bacterial adhesins.

Having been ingested, *Chlamydia* is able to survive by inhibiting the fusion of the intracytoplasmic endosomes in which it is contained with lysosomes, whose contents are acidic and bactericidal. Once again, the mechanism underlying this inhibition is not clear, although it can be mediated by purified outer membrane preparations in the absence of viable organisms.

Soon after internalization, the elementary body starts to differentiate into the larger, metabolically active reticulate body, with the cell wall losing its rigidity through dissociation of disulphide linkages in the cysteine-rich outer membrane proteins. Reticulate bodies grow and divide by binary fission until, 25 to 30 h after internalization, reticulate bodies start to differentiate back into elementary bodies. By 48 h postinfection, the chlamydial inclusion may contain more than 1000 chlamydiae, mostly elementary bodies, and the infected cell usually lyses, releasing these, by 72 h postinfection. The chlamydial lifecycle is shown in Fig. 1.

When cells infected with *C. psittaci* are grown in medium lacking certain amino acids, infection may become latent; non-replicating organisms persist within the cells, starting to replicate again when the medium is replenished. It has been suggested that such latent infections may occur with *C. trachomatis in vivo*, under the influence of host cytokines such as interferon-γ; but this has not been convincingly demonstrated.

Immunity and pathogenesis

Although repeated infections often occur, and play an important role in the pathogenesis of blinding trachoma, epidemiological considerations suggest that protective immunity follows ocular exposure to *C. trachomatis*; it is unusual to find active trachoma in, or to be able to isolate the organism from, adults in endemic communities. Encouraged by this observation, several groups conducted field trials of trachoma vaccines in the 1960s, as well as vaccine experiments in primates.

These trials showed that it was possible to stimulate protective immunity with whole cell vaccines, but that protection was short lived and serotype-specific. Moreover, in some cases, it appeared that vaccination led to more severe inflammatory disease on rechallenge. In the Taiwan monkey (*Macaca cyclops*), the hypersensitivity induced by vaccination was shown to be species-specific, and to persist longer that the protective response. The conclusion was that the immune response to chlamydial infection is a two-edged sword: it can lead to protection, but it also plays an important role in pathogenesis. Indeed, since *Chlamydia* produces no known toxin, it is possible that the pathogenesis of chlamydial infection is almost entirely mediated by the host immune response.

In recent years, attempts have been made to develop a subunit chlamydial vaccine. An important objective was to identify the chlamydial antigens and epitopes that were the targets of protective immune responses, which should be included in the vaccine, and those responsible for damaging hypersensitivity reactions, which should be excluded. Certain serotype-specific monoclonal antibodies, which recognized variable regions of MOMP, were shown to have neutralizing activity *in vitro*, and most vaccine candidates evaluated subsequently contained MOMP epitopes, the goal being to stimulate the production of antiMOMP antibody at the exposed mucosal surface. Unfortunately results have been disappointing, probably because insufficient efforts were made to stimulate cell-mediated immune responses (see below).

Experiments in monkeys and guinea pigs appeared to have identified a chlamydial antigen which stimulated hypersensitivity in previously exposed animals as a heat shock protein of 57 kDa, homologous to the GroEl protein of *Escherichia coli*, which is secreted by infected cells; but subsequent experiments have failed to confirm the initial findings. Several studies have found that antibodies to this protein are more common in subjects with severe sequelae of genital or ocular chlamydial infection, but the significance of this observation is not clear.

Histopathology

An acute inflammatory response, with a profuse purulent exudate, is characteristic of the early stages of primary infection with *C. trachomatis*. Polymorphs are attracted to the site of infection by cytokines (for example tumour necrosis factor-α) and chemokines (for example interleukin-8) released from macrophages or epithelial cells stimulated by chlamydial antigens, for example lipopolysaccharide. Polymorphs have powerful antichlamydial activity, releasing a variety of metabolites with chlamydiacidal activity, and after a few days the number of organisms is reduced and the acute inflammatory response subsides. In the absence of treatment, a chronic inflammatory response supervenes, characterized by the clinical and pathological hallmark of active trachoma—the subconjunctival lymphoid follicle. Follicles contain typical germinal centres, consisting pre-

dominantly of B lymphocytes, with T cells in the parafollicular region which have been shown in a primate model of trachoma to contain a majority of CD8$^+$ cells. Between follicles the inflammatory infiltrate contains plasma cells, dendritic cells, macrophages, and polymorphs in addition to T and B lymphocytes. Epithelial cells express major histocompatibility complex class II molecules at this stage of the infection, presumed to be induced by interferon-γ.

Clearance of infection

Being an intracellular pathogen, it would appear probable that cellular immune mechanisms, rather than antibody, play the major role in clearance of chlamydial infection; and there is considerable experimental evidence to support this 'common sense' hypothesis. The central importance of CD4$^+$ lymphocytes in chlamydial clearance has been recently confirmed in major histocompatibility complex class II gene knockout mice. These mice express no major histocompatibility complex class II (the molecule which presents foreign antigens to CD4$^+$ cells), and as a result are totally unable to resolve chlamydial infections of the genital tract. Mice deficient in antibody, however, through disruption of the gene for the μ-chain constant region, resolve infection normally, although they are somewhat more susceptible to reinfection than normal animals. β$_2$-Microglobulin gene knockout mice, which express no major histocompatibility complex class I, resolve infection normally, suggesting that, in the mouse, CD8$^+$ lymphocytes (which recognize antigen in the context of class I) play little role in clearance.

Such evidence as there is in humans also suggests that cell-mediated immune responses are more important than antibody in the clearance of ocular chlamydial infection, and that T-helper type 1 cells play a key role. These cells secrete a number of cytokines including interferon-γ, which has been shown both *in vitro* and in animal models to exert an inhibitory effect on the intracellular replication of *Chlamydia*. Gambian children who spontaneously cleared ocular chlamydial infection were found to have stronger lymphocyte proliferative responses to chlamydial antigens (whole organisms, MOMP, and the 57 kDa heat-shock protein) than persistently infected subjects. Moreover, subjects with moderate to severe conjunctival scarring due to trachoma were found to have relatively weaker responses to these antigens than age- and sex-matched controls with normal eyes from endemic areas. There were no differences in antibody levels between the groups. Cytotoxic T-cell responses to chlamydial antigens, mediated by CD8$^+$ cells, have been demonstrated in some subjects from trachoma-endemic communities, and there was a suggestion that these responses were protective.

Protection from infection

Animal models have given conflicting evidence concerning the relative contribution of antibody and cell-mediated immune responses to protection from infection. Passive transfer experiments have shown that antibody can protect from genital tract infection in the guinea pig, whereas in the mouse cell-mediated immune responses appear to play the major role. Ocular secretions from children with trachoma were shown to neutralize chlamydial infection in the monkey eye many years ago, and antichlamydial secretory immunoglobulin A levels were shown to be inversely correlated with the number of viable *Chlamydia* shed from the human cervix; but no evidence was found to support a protective role for antichlamydial antibody of the secretory immunoglobulin A or immunoglobulin G class in protection from ocular infection in a trachoma-endemic community.

Recently, the *omp1* gene (encoding MOMP) has been sequenced from a number of genital and ocular chlamydial isolates, and several strains have been identified which differ by one or more inferred amino acids from the prototype serotypic strain, suggesting that antigenic drift may occur in *C. trachomatis*, perhaps driven by the need to escape from neutralizing antibody responses at the site of infection. More variants were identified among genital isolates from a group of prostitutes in Nairobi than in ocular isolates from trachoma-endemic communities, suggesting that such an escape mechanism may be more important among genital than among ocular strains. Recent evidence suggests that recombination may also occur between strains of different serotype, providing another possible mechanism of antigenic variation.

Our own longitudinal studies of families with trachoma in The Gambia have shown that the incidence of ocular infection in adults is reduced by approximately 50 per cent compared to young children, whereas the duration of (untreated) infection is reduced from a mean of approximately 10 weeks in young children to less than 2 weeks in adults. This suggests that the acquired immune response affects the ability to clear infection to a greater extent than the ability to resist reinfection.

Pathogenesis

A variety of proinflammatory cytokines are expressed at the conjunctival surface in subjects with inflammatory trachoma, including tumour necrosis factor-α, interleukin-1β, interferon-γ, interleukin-12, and transforming growth factor-β1. *In vitro* studies have shown that the chemokine interleukin-8, which is strongly chemotactic for polymorphs, is secreted by epithelial cell lines following infection with *Chlamydia*. Moreover, chlamydial elementary bodies activate complement via the alternative pathway, generating further chemotactic molecules, an effect due at least in part to lipopolysaccharide. Studies in the guinea pig have shown that immunosuppressed animals with persistent infection mount a powerful and prolonged acute inflammatory response, with a high incidence of sequelae such as hydrosalpinx.

On the basis of experiments in mice, guinea pigs, and monkeys, Bavoil *et al.* have proposed a convincing model for the induction of the acute inflammatory response to *Chlamydia*, involving the stimulation of macrophages by chlamydial lipopolysaccharide to produce tumour necrosis factor-α and interleukin-12, the secretion of interferon-γ by natural killer and T-helper type 1 cells, an influx of polymorphs due to complement activation and interleukin-8 secretion, increased endothelial expression of cellular adhesion molecules such as intercellular adhesion molecule-1, and the secretion of transforming growth factor-β.

The serious sequelae of chlamydial infection, such as entropion, are due to fibrosis, which progresses over many years in those repeatedly exposed to reinfection or suffering from chronic infection. There is evidence that subjects with trachomatous scarring have relatively impaired cellular immune responses to chlamydial antigens, and that they clear infection less rapidly than exposed controls without scarring. The mechanism driving the scarring process is not well understood; it is presumably due to the continuing expression of fibrogenic cytokines such as transforming growth factor-β resulting from repeated or continuing inflammatory stimuli.

Genetic susceptibility

It is not clear why some subjects in trachoma-endemic areas develop conjunctival scarring while others, apparently similarly exposed, do not. The possibility of a genetic predisposition was suggested by the observation that in Tanzania, having a mother with trichiasis was an important risk factor for the condition. Case–control studies in The Gambia have found an association of the major histocompatibility complex class I type *A6802 with moderate to severe scarring; this allele was present in 18 per cent of cases, and 7 per cent of controls. Moreover, polymorphisms in the promoter region of the tumour necrosis factor-α gene, possibly associated with increased transcription and hence secretion of tumour necrosis factor-α, were also associated with scarring disease.

Further reading

Barron, A.L. (ed.) (1988). *Microbiology of Chlamydia*. CRC Press, Boca Raton, Florida.

Bavoil, P.M., Hsia, R.-C., and Rank, R.G. (1996). Prospects for a vaccine against *Chlamydia* genital disease 1. Microbiology and pathogenesis. *Bulletin de l' Institut Pasteur*, **94**, 5–54.

Bobo, L., Novak, N., Mkocha, H., *et al.* (1996). Evidence for a predominant proinflammatory conjunctival cytokine response in individuals with trachoma. *Infection and Immunity*, **64**, 3273–9.

Conway, D.J., Holland, M.J., Bailey, R.L., *et al.* (1997). Scarring trachoma is associated with polymorphism in the tumor necrosis factor alpha gene promoter and with elevated TNF-alpha levels in tear fluids. *Infection and Immunity*, **65**, 1003–6.

Jones, B.R. (1975). The prevention of blindness from trachoma. *Transactions of the Ophthalmological Society UK*, **95**, 16–33.

Mabey, D.C.W., Bailey, R.L., and Hutin, Y.J.F. (1992). The epidemiology and pathogenesis of trachoma. *Reviews in Medical Microbiology*, **3**, 112–19.

Morrison, R.P., Feilzer, K., and Tumas, D.B. (1995). Gene knockout mice establish a primary role for major histocompatibility complex class II-restricted responses in *Chlamydia trachomatis* genital tract infection. *Infection and Immunity*, **63**, 4661–8.

Rank, R.G. and Bavoil, P.M. (1996). Prospects for a vaccine against *Chlamydia* genital disease. II. Immunity and vaccine development. *Bulletin de l' Institut Pasteur*, **94**, 55–82.

Schachter, J. and Dawson, C.R. (1978). *Human chlamydial infections*. PSG Publishing, Littleton, Massachusetts.

1.3 Inflammation, wound repair, degeneration, and neoplasia

Alec Garner

Inflammation and wound repair

Flamma, the Latin word for flame, provides the clue to the early understanding of the inflammatory process. Celsus, in the first century AD, defined the four cardinal signs as *calor* (heat), *rubor* (redness), *tumor* (swelling), and *dolor* (pain), the first three of which draw attention to the vascular component. In recent years, however, it has become evident that, important as they are, vascular changes are not the key element and a working definition of inflammation might be that it is a process whereby cells and soluble plasma constituents collect around an injurious substance and tend to destroy it.

Tradition has also recognized two broad types of inflammation: acute, in which there is a non-specific response coming on within a matter of hours, usually resolving within days, and characterized clinically by conspicuously increased vascularity; and chronic, in which the vascular component is less evident and which takes much longer to both develop and resolve. This temporal distinction is commonly reflected histologically with evidence in the former of polymorphonuclear leucocyte accumulation, whereas lymphocyte and macrophage infiltration is typical of the latter. Unfortunately, these associations do not always hold as, for instance, in the predominantly macrophage and lymphoid cell infiltration present from the outset in viral infections, and, conversely, the continued outpouring of polymorphonuclear leucocytes in long-standing osteomyelitis. Consequently, given that the terms acute and chronic are firmly entrenched, most pathologists prefer to define them in terms of their histological features irrespective of the timings, and it is in that sense that they are used here.

Mediators of inflammation

The initiation, maintenance, and termination of inflammatory processes is subject to a vast number of influences, although not all are of equal significance. The reader should look elsewhere for a detailed discussion of what is an extremely complex topic. It is enough for present purposes to note the main categories of mediators and to draw attention to those considered to be of major relevance.

Soluble plasma-derived mediators

Kinin system

Kinins are small peptides cleaved from much larger protein molecules in the circulating plasma through the enzymatic action of kallikrein. The latter is itself activated when extravasated blood makes contact with negatively charged stromal structures such as collagen fibres or when the blood-clotting cascade is set in motion. One of the better characterized kinins is bradykinin which not only promotes arteriolar dilatation and plasma leakage but also may contribute to the subsequent healing process through a capacity to stimulate fibroblastic activity.

Complement system

The complement system is a cascade of plasma proteins which, when activated, can facilitate phagocytosis and proteolysis of the target tissue. It can be triggered by specific antigen–antibody interaction and as such is a factor in chronic inflammation. Alternatively a variety of non-specific agencies may be involved, including the effects of bacterial products, which means that it can also be involved in acute inflammation (in both temporal and histological senses).

Clotting cascade and fibrinolytic sequence

Fibrin, formed by activation of the clotting cascade early in the inflammatory process, and its subsequent breakdown products are chemotactic for phagocytic leucocytes.

Soluble tissue-derived mediators

Vasoactive amines

Histamine, prominent in basophils and mast cells, is a potent vasodilator substance involved in the initial stages of acute inflammation and immunoglobulin E-mediated hypersensitivity reactions.

Cytokines

These are peptides produced by inflammatory cells, fibroblasts, and vascular endothelium which help to regulate the activity of other inflammatory cells. They are of various kinds.

Interleukins   Essentially the product of macrophages, currently some 12 interleukins are recognized. Their main function is to regulate the immune system, although they may have other effects. Interleukin 1 (IL-1), for instance, helps to recruit polymorphonuclear leucocytes as well as being a major pyrogen.

Interferons   Originally so designated because of their antiviral properties, they can also enhance immunological activity.

Colony-stimulating factors   In the context of inflammation these stimulate macrophage and granulocyte proliferation. They are products of fibroblasts, lymphocytes, vascular endothelium, and macrophages themselves.

Tumour necrosis factors   Products of activated lymphocytes and macrophages and initially identified through their effects on tumour cells, such factors have been shown to interact with other cytokines to facilitate leucocyte adhesion to the vascular endothelium and to stimulate polymorphonuclear leucocyte activity. Tumour necrosis factor may also be involved in the caseation necrosis characteristic of tuberculosis.

Transforming growth factors   As their name implies, these cytokines, of which there are two, participate in the regulation of cell proliferation. With respect to inflammatory processes the more important is tumour necrosis factor-β which, derives from macrophages and platelets, is chemotactic for leucocytes and, through its action on fibroblasts, figures in wound repair.

Other leucocyte-derived substances
The granules of neutrophil polymorphonuclear leucocytes, eosinophils, and macrophages contain proteolytic enzymes which if exocytosed can produce extensive tissue damage.

A phospholipid product of leucocyte membrane lysis, known as platelet-activating factor, has an extremely wide range of functions: besides being a potent promoter of microvascular leakage it serves to recruit additional leucocytes and appears to enhance several other inflammatory responses.

Arachidonic acid derivatives
A normal component of all cell membranes, arachidonic acid can be broken down enzymatically as a result of tissue damage to produce two principal groups of inflammatory mediators. Those resulting from cyclo-oxygenase activity include prostaglandins and prostacyclin with vasodilator properties, and thromboxane with vasoconstrictor and platelet-aggregating activities. Concurrent lipoxygenase activity produces several potent vasoconstrictor substances known as leukotrienes.

Other factors
These include platelet-activating factor, free oxygen radicals, neuropeptides, and endothelium-derived factors.

Cellular (leucocyte) mediators

Polymorphonuclear leucocytes (neutrophils)
Variously referred to as polymorphonuclear leucocytes to indicate the segmented character of their nuclei, or neutrophils as a reflection of the amphophilic character of a cytoplasm replete with fine granules, these are numerically the predominant leucocyte type. They are motile, readily leaving the circulating blood and migrating through the tissues in a chemotactic fashion to reach the source of infection or other irritation. (It might be noted, however, that polymorphonuclear leucocytes do not readily leave the retinal circulation due to the characteristic encircling interendothelial cell junctions.) Once in the tissues they may influence the outcome in the following ways.

1. Phagocytosis of microbial or other foreign material, following which intracellular lysosomes (primary polymorphonuclear leucocyte granules) fuse with the endocytosed vesicle (phagosome). A cocktail of lytic enzymes is then released into the phagosome. Phagocytosis is promoted by a range of receptors on the polymorphonuclear leucocyte surface for bacterial products and soluble inflammatory mediators. Coating the offending particle with specific antibody or products of the third component of the complement system, an activity known as opsonization, greatly increases the effectiveness of the process.

2. Extracellular secretion of antimicrobial proteins, lysozyme, and other degradative enzymes.

3. Production of reactive oxygen metabolites ('free radicals') which, in addition to helping to kill or dispose of the phagocytosed material, are also responsible for much of the tissue damage associated with acute inflammation. The requisite burst of respiratory activity involves the uptake of large amounts of oxygen, with the corollary that polymorphonuclear leucocyte microbicidal action is markedly impaired under conditions of relative ischaemia.

Polymorphonuclear leucocytes are short-lived with an average half-life of 7 h after leaving the bone marrow and, correspondingly, invariably die at the inflammatory site to become pus cells.

Monocytes and macrophages
Monocytes are circulating leucocytes that arise from the same bone marrow progenitors as the granulocytes (neutrophils, eosinophils, and basophils) but which move less rapidly in response to chemotactic stimuli. Until they leave the circulation they are functionally inert but in the tissues they tend to acquire rather more cytoplasm and are transformed into macrophages able to engulf and digest irritant material. Macrophages have a much longer lifespan than other phagocytic leucocytes and they can even be a component of healthy tissues: such semipermanent or resident macrophages are sometimes called histiocytes. The process of activation is principally a response to the ingestion of foreign substances and interaction with a number of soluble mediators of inflammation as well as specific antibody. In contrast to polymorphonuclear leucocytes they usually survive the phagocytic process.

The products of activated macrophages are legion and include a range of lysosomal and other lytic enzymes, coagulation factors, complement components, cytokines, growth factors, extracellular matrix and other proteins, prostaglandins and related lipids, and reactive oxygen metabolites. Some macrophages subjugate their phagocytic potential to a predominantly secretory role and, in respect of an associated fairly abundant, pale-staining, cytoplasm filled with rough endoplasmic reticulum, are termed epithelioid cells.

Eosinophils

Eosinophils are phagocytic cells with bilobed nuclei and prominent eosinophilic cytoplasmic granules. Most are found in the tissues as opposed to the circulating blood and are particularly associated with immunoglobulin E-mediated allergic responses and helminthic infections. They respond to several chemotactic factors but of special interest is the effect of histamine and a complex eosinophil chemotactic factor A released by basophils and mast cells.

Activation results in degranulation, the specific granules responsible for the cytoplasmic eosinophilia containing a number of substances, with emphasis on a distinctive major basic protein, that have helminthotoxic and other degradative properties.

Basophils and mast cells

Both types of cell originate from precursors in the bone marrow but, whereas basophils are confined to the circulation, mast cells are limited to the tissues. They are the source of virtually all the body's histamine and are an integral element of immunoglobulin E-mediated hypersensitivity reactions, release of the vasoactive amine being triggered by interaction between specific immunoglobulin E and receptors for the crystallizable fragment (Fc) of the antibody on the basophil/mast cell surface. Other less specific mediators of inflammation may also be associated with basophil/mast cell activation.

Lymphocytes and plasma cells

Lymphocytes are the mediators of inflammatory responses specific to a given irritant and depend on stereochemical recognition of moieties peculiar to the irritant by receptor molecules on the lymphocyte surface. They are small cells with round nuclei and scanty cytoplasm that originated during embryogenesis from pluripotential stem cells in the bone marrow. There are three basic types that can be distinguished on the grounds of function and differentiation antigens on the cell surface (cluster of differentiation or CD antigens): T lymphocytes, B lymphocytes, and natural killer cells.

T lymphocytes   Such cells have been modified by passage of their progenitors through the fetal thymus gland. They have a primary role in the recognition of antigen and are usually required for the initiation of B-lymphocyte activity as well as direct cell-mediated immune responses. Two major subsets are recognized: CD4 and CD8.

Helper cells (CD4)   These either serve to induce or suppress (mainly the former) the activity of other T and B lymphocytes. The various activities are mirrored by the presence of additional distinctive CD antigens on the various helper cells.

Suppressor cells (CD8)   Cells in this group are also responsible for the cell-mediated cytotoxicity seen in virus infections and graft rejection, in addition to serving to terminate inappropriate immune responses.

B lymphocytes   These are lymphocytes capable of forming antibody and normally found in the follicular regions of regional lymph nodes. The response is antigen-specific and facilitated by helper T-cell activity. Activation involves a massive increase in protein synthesizing capacity and hence of endoplasmic reticulum and cytoplasmic volume. The result is a plasma cell which has a characteristic eccentric nucleus.

Natural killer cells   These are mononuclear cells that appear to be a part of the normal lymphocyte population but with markers for neither T nor B cells, although it may be that they are T-cell precursors. They are able to kill tumour and other cells without specific antigen recognition or the interaction of antibody. Modulation of immune responses may be another and more fundamental function.

Acute inflammation

Histopathology

The essential feature is the presence within the affected tissue of large numbers of polymorphonuclear leucocytes. In established lesions the neutrophils may be particularly concentrated in a relatively walled-off cavity to form an abscess, many of them necrotic with eosinophilic cytoplasm and barely recognizable nuclei (pus cells). Other liquefied, necrotic tissue residues are also seen. Prominent vascularity relating mostly to thin-walled venules and capillaries is usual, the dilated vessels being stuffed with erythrocytes (vascular congestion or hyperaemia). Moderate numbers of macrophages are also seen and at the time of biopsy, which is rarely within the first few hours, scattered lymphocytes (but not plasma cells) are common.

Pathophysiology

The first clinically identifiable event is increased redness due to vascular dilatation although experiments indicate that this is preceded by a transient arteriolar constriction. The dilatation incurs increased blood flow which raises the temperature of the affected part as well as making it red. An accompanying but separately mediated increase in vessel permeability promotes leakage of plasma and there is tissue swelling. The consequent accumulation of extravascular protein tips the osmotic balance in favour of yet more fluid extravasation until, eventually, the attendant increase in blood viscosity causes the flow to slow down such that the temperature falls and the initial bright redness becomes more dusky in colour. Pain is probably the result of raised pressure in the affected tissue secondary to oedematous swelling and increased firing of afferent sensory nerves. The transport of plasma across the vessel wall is in part an active transcellular event and in part due to the opening of intercellular junctions, the latter also facilitating the passage of leucocytes from the circulation. In respect of polymorphonuclear leucocytes and monocytes emigration is also a function of amoeboid cell activity and enzymatic digestion of the vascular basement membrane. Polymorphonuclear leucocytes are the cells initially involved and movement is maximal when the circulation has slowed and they are able to adhere to the venular wall under the influence of specific adhesion molecules, expression of which is enhanced in the presence of cytokines. They move towards the injurious stimulus through a gradient of chemotactic mediators. Proteolytic enzymes released by polymorphonuclear leucocytes and macrophages as they respond to the irritant are a principal factor in generating the associated tissue necrosis.

Chronic inflammation (diffuse)

Causes

Allowing that chronic inflammation is here arbitrarily defined on histological rather than temporal criteria, it is still appropriate to consider the circumstances in which it arises.

1. Persistence of an irritant originally provoking an acute reaction. In this case an intermediate state, sometimes referred to as subacute inflammation, may be seen.

2. Immune reactions wherein the primary response is lymphocytic. The exciting agent can be either exogenous, as in viral infection, or endogenous, as in the autoimmune diseases.

Histopathology

For reasons already elaborated the various types of inflammation are preferably described and identified on histological criteria. Accordingly, chronic inflammation is characterized by diffuse lymphoid cell infiltration with variable numbers of macrophages and variable vascularity. Focal necrosis is common but rarely so conspicuous as in acute inflammation. Where the chronicity is temporally related plump active fibroblasts may also be seen as part of an attempted reparative process. Plasma cells accompany the lymphocytic component in states that involve significant B-cell activation.

Pathophysiology

Immunological mechanisms, as indicated by the predominance of lymphocytes, play a much more important role in chronic inflammation than in the acute process. The presence of macrophages usually reflects a dual function: initial processing of antigen as a prerequisite for immunological activity and elimination of ingested irritants.

Chronic inflammation can, however, result from the presence of foreign material with little immunological potential, in which case macrophages may be the predominant cells. Chalazion provoked by leaked sebaceous secretion is an apposite example.

Chronic inflammation (granulomatous)

Causes

Here again there are two main categories, those conditions that are immunologically based and those that are not. Delayed hypersensitivity reactions are particularly associated with granulomatous inflammation and can be elicited by a variety of agents, including certain bacteria, such as the tubercle bacillus, and a number of helminths. Sarcoidosis is another disease state characterized by granulomatous inflammation, although in this condition immunological mechanisms other than delayed hypersensitivity appear to be involved. Essentially non-immune granulomas may form around indigestible particulate matter which may be exogenous, as in the response to inert materials such as talc, or endogenous, as in the reaction to the leaked sebaceous secretion of a chalazion or the haematogenous residues responsible for cholesterol granulomas.

Histopathology

The essential component of granulomatous inflammation is the presence of macrophages, grouped in sheets or nests, with a surrounding infiltrate of lymphoid cells and, possibly, of other leucocyte types (the presence of eosinophils may suggest a parasitic infection) (Fig. 1). The finding of epithelioid macrophages is particularly typical of immunologically based granulomas. Multinucleated giant cells, formed by fusion of epithelioid and, to a lesser extent, other macrophages are another frequent, though not inevitable, finding. Ingested exogenous material may be observed and it is then that the term foreign body granuloma is most appropriate. Fibrous tissue formation is usual and may be conspicuous, especially where the granuloma has an immunological basis.

Pathophysiology

The development of a granuloma is promoted by the protracted presence of particulate and poorly degradable material. Cytokines released by lymphocytes, especially T cells, appear to be involved in the maturation of monocytes into epithelioid macrophages in immunologically based granulomas. In turn, the epithelioid cells secrete fibroblast-activating factors and other cytokines that stimulate collagen synthesis.

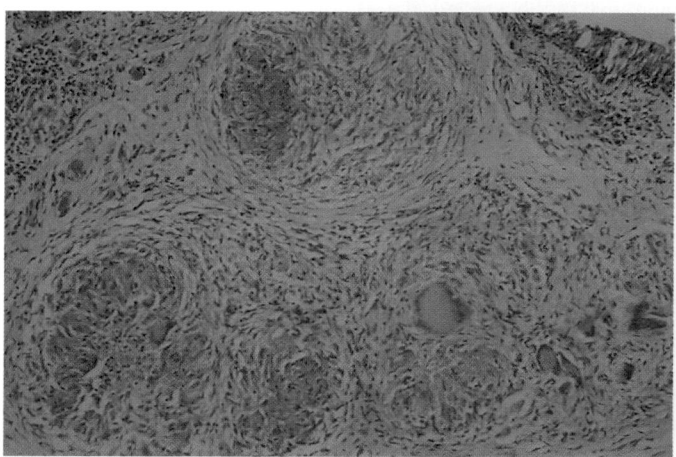

Fig. 1 Chronic granulomatous inflammation. Scattered within loose connective tissue clusters of pink-staining macrophages (one of them including a conspicuous multinucleated giant cell). The surrounding stroma is diffusely infiltrated with lymphocytes (haematoxylin and eosin, × 180).

Wound repair

Commensurate with the removal of necrotic products of the inflammatory process is reparative activity involving regeneration of damaged parenchyma or replacement by scar tissue.

Regeneration

The capacity for renewal of damaged tissue is related to:

- the extent to which the underlying structure or scaffolding of the original tissue persists

- the regenerative potential of the relevant cells. Corneal epithelium, for example, has a considerable potential for replication whereas corneal endothelium has very little.

The stimulus to regeneration is complex but of major importance are growth-modulating factors released from macrophages and other adjacent cells as well as both cell–matrix and cell–cell interactions.

Scarring

Where the extent of any necrosis or innate cellular behaviour precludes regeneration the deficiency is liable to be replaced by fibrous tissue. Three overlapping phases are recognizable:

- resolution, in which the products of necrosis are removed by host macrophages

- proliferation, when the injured tissue is invaded by new capillary blood vessels and fibroblasts to constitute granulation tissue (Fig. 2). The fibroblasts synthesize collagen precursors which aggregate and polymerize in the extracellular milieu (in neural tissues such as the retina, astrocytes substitute for fibroblasts, forming extensive fibrillary processes as opposed to extracellular collagen)

- remodelling, when the collagen polymers form yet

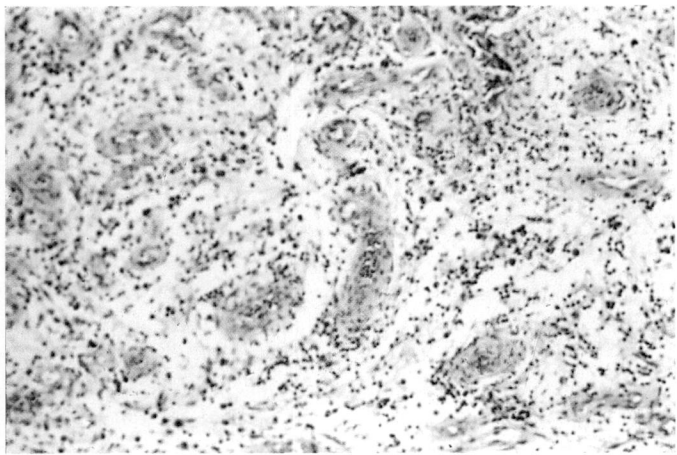

Fig. 2 Granulation tissue. Nascent capillary blood vessels characterized by plump endothelium are seen within a loose matrix diffusely infiltrated with leucocytes (haematoxylin and eosin).

more stable linkages. Even so the tensile strength rarely reaches that of the original tissue and the more extensive the scar the weaker it is likely to be. Reduction in the size of the scar (cicatrization) is primarily attributable to active contraction on the part of myofibroblasts but there is also some reduction through degradative enzymatic activity.

Contrary factors in the reparative process include glucocorticoid administration and deficiencies of protein or vitamin C. Local adverse influences include persistence of infection, residual unresolved necrotic areas, the presence of foreign material, and undue physical stresses. An adequate blood flow or other local source of nutrition is important if healing is to proceed.

Excessive scar tissue growth (keloid formation) rarely occurs, and then most often in black people, but the cause is unknown.

Excessive granulation tissue projecting from the surface of an open wound may prevent re-epithelialization of the surface and need to be removed surgically. (Such reddish, velvety tissue does not constitute a granuloma and should not be confused.)

Degenerations

The concept of degenerative disease covers a range of cellular and extracellular disorders in which there is detrimental modification of previously healthy tissue. As such the term might also include dystrophic conditions but convention generally limits the latter to situations attributable to a primary genetic abnormality such that the affected individual has a potential defect from conception albeit not expressed until later life. In which case degenerative disorders are probably best thought of as those in which non-genetic, acquired factors are fundamental.

The endpoint of all cellular degeneration, however it might be initiated, is cell death.

Cell death

There are two forms of cell death appropriate to living tissues: necrosis, which usually concerns multiple cells, and apoptosis, which is a process affecting single cells.

Necrosis

The term necrosis refers to the degradative changes that follow cell death. (The cells of biopsied tissue that is immediately immersed in histological fixative are dead but not necrotic.) The changes can develop through either the activation of lytic enzymes in the dead cell (autolysis) or the activity of similar enzymes derived from leucocytes attracted to the scene. The former produces increased eosinophilia of the cytoplasm in tissue sections stained with haematoxylin and eosin, as well as nuclear condensation (pyknosis) progressing to fragmentation (karyorrhexis) or lysis (karyolysis), and is known as coagulation necrosis. Associated inflammatory responses may add to the degradation with destruction of the entire cell to constitute liquefaction necrosis.

Pathogenesis

Necrosis can be caused in several ways, ischaemia, wherein it is preceded by potentially reversible biochemical events, being the most common. Of major importance in this circumstance is an inability to generate adenosine triphosphate in the absence of oxygen which leads to failure of the ionic pump mechanism essential for the maintenance of isotonicity. Accordingly there is an influx of calcium and sodium ions, the latter resulting in acute cellular oedema. Degeneration of organelle membranes may produce laminated whorls in the cytoplasm known as 'myelin figures' and there is mitochondrial swelling. In the presence of continued ischaemia there is further structural damage to cell membranes, both of organelles and the cell boundary. This is because of increased phospholipase activity in response to the massive influx of calcium from the extracellular compartment through deficiency of energy-dependent adenosine triphosphatase. Principal among the several consequences is the release of degradative lysosomal enzymes. The rise in calcium ions also further impairs mitochondrial function.

The leucocytic contribution to necrosis, in the form of polymorphonuclear leucocytes and macrophages, is a response to the leakage of cell constituents into the extracellular milieu.

Activated oxygen species (oxygen atoms with single unpaired electrons in an outer orbital) are also a potent cause of necrosis. They may arise spontaneously as a normal event but are prone to be increased where there is:

- excess oxygen (they are the agents likely to be responsible for retinal endothelial cell injury in the retinopathy of prematurity)

- inflammation (generated by phagocytic leucocytes during the burst of respiratory activity involved in creating the appropriate conditions for microbiocidal activity)

- reperfusion injury after ischaemia (when xanthine that has accumulated in the ischaemic phase is oxidized)

- chemical toxicity (products of catabolism)

- ionizing radiation tissue damage.

Occurring as superoxide (O_2^-), hydrogen peroxide (H_2O_2), and hydroxyl radicals (OH^-), such moieties are extremely reactive and will steal electrons from any available source, especially lipids. Consequently, they serve to damage the membranes of cytoplasmic organelles and the cell surface in addition to certain thiol-rich enzymes, such as adenosine triphosphatase, and nuclear DNA.

Calcification

A late sequel of necrosis in some situations is 'dystrophic' calcification. (The term dystrophic calcification, used to distinguish it from metastatic calcification wherein there is an underlying metabolic defect, is unhelpful since the process is not genetically determined: it is better seen as a degenerative state.) The mechanism is uncertain but appears to involve two phases.

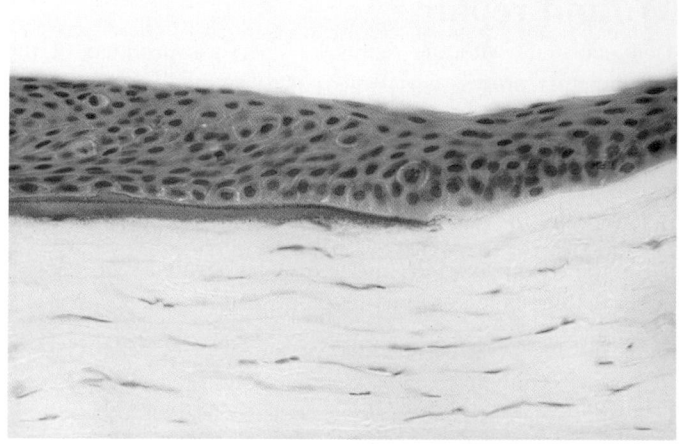

Fig. 3 Dystrophic calcification (cornea). Two-thirds of Bowman's layer sandwiched between the substantia propria and the overlying epithelium is stained a deep purple in contrast to the unstained remainder. The staining represents calcium salt deposition in a patient with band keratopathy (haematoxylin and eosin, × 320).

First is initiation, wherein calcium ions attach to acidic phospholipids present on the surfaces of membrane-bound vesicles derived from dead cells. Secondly, propagation follows the initial nucleation as a function of local calcium and phosphate concentrations to form hydroxyapatite crystals (Fig. 3).

Apoptosis

Apoptosis is a form of cell death that is primarily physiological, constituting a mechanism for the removal of redundant or effete cells. A literal meaning of the Greek is 'falling off' or 'drop-out'. It can be observed in both physiological and pathological states.

Morphogenesis

There are two underlying events: priming and triggering. Priming includes the accumulation of enzymes essential for the subsequent events, although the mechanism and nature of the stimulus is as yet unknown. Triggering involves activation of the accumulated enzymes and this can occur in two ways: physiological and pathological.

Physiological triggering This is important in the remodelling of embryonic tissues, the deletion of unwanted lymphocyte clones, the elimination of potential neoplastic cells, and many other activities. As an example, proliferation of neurones in the embryonic central nervous system invariably exceeds requirements and those that do not make contact with other neurones undergo apoptosis. In this instance it seems that inadequate formation of nerve growth or other trophic factors by the isolated cells is the trigger. Indeed, there seems to be a general rule that cells formed in excess of the body's capacity to sustain them are programmed to die through apoptosis. In which case genetic influences are likely to be of major importance in the apoptotic process and, conversely, there is evidence from study of animal tumours that some cancers are promoted by defects in the relevant genes. The triggering process involves an increase in calcium ions in the cytoplasm with attendant stimulation of specific messenger RNA activity and protein synthesis. The latter includes overexpression of an interleukin-1β converting enzyme which then activates specific proteases.

Pathological triggering Tissue injury insufficient to cause necrosis may, nevertheless, be enough to provoke death of isolated cells through apoptosis, possibly by allowing a rise in intracellular calcium. Radiation damage and minor ischaemia frequently achieve their effects in this way. Apoptotic cell loss is also a feature of most viral infections, and neurodegenerative and autoimmune disorders.

At a structural level the affected cells first lose contact with neighbouring cells and shrink, frequently with fragmentation, before being phagocytosed and forming residual lysosomal bodies. Phagocytosis can be a function of 'professional' macrophages or adjacent parenchymal cells. The initial changes reflect an influx of calcium ions which serve to activate accumulated enzymes able to degrade the cytoskeleton and nucleus. The process is short-lived, the events leading to nuclear condensation and cell fragmentation taking only a few minutes with the whole sequence, including phagocytic degradation taking only a few hours. Moreover, because the cellular changes do not involve the surface membrane, cell components are not released into the surrounding space and an inflammatory response, such as attends necrosis, does not occur.

Elastotic degeneration

The yellowish accumulations sometimes seen at the corneoscleral limbus and known as pingueculas probably represent degenerate elastic tissue. Histologically they present as thickened, convoluted fibres surrounded by a granular matrix and may include variably sized concretions (Fig. 4). Uptake of Verhoeff's stain for elastic is usual and immunoelectron microscopy demonstrates an affinity for antibodies to both the amorphous elastin and microfibrillar protein components of elastic tissue. Earlier doubts concerning the nature of pingueculas were based on negative responses to elastase digestion and certain other elastic tissue stains. Such discrepancies may be the outcome of conformational changes in the elastin molecule, although the precise nature of the degeneration is obscure. Undue exposure to ultraviolet light may be an aetiological factor.

Amyloidosis

The term amyloidosis embraces a heterogeneous collection of disorders characterized by the mainly extracellular deposition of proteins that, while varying in composition, share distinctive staining properties. Uptake of Congo red with green birefringence (dichroism) when tissue sections are viewed using crossed polarizing filters is a commonly applied criterion.

Although whole proteins may be involved, most amyloids are derived from fragments of specific precursor proteins that polymerize to form randomly oriented, interlacing fibrils with a constant 10 to 15 nm diameter. One of the more frequent

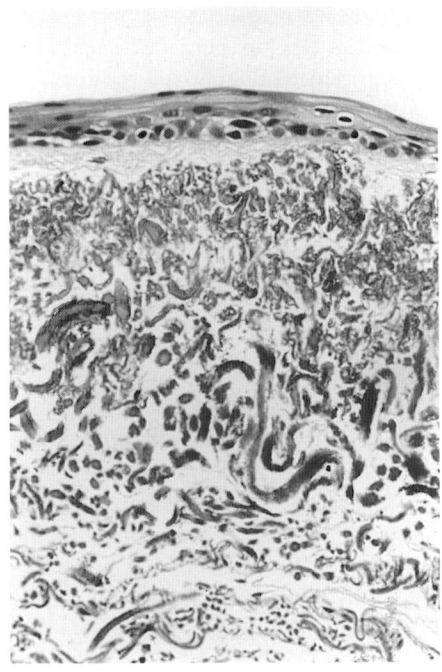

Fig. 4 Pinguecula. The stroma beneath the epithelium of the bulbar conjunctiva includes numerous coarse, folded fibres, some of them disintegrating to a more granular state (haematoxylin and eosin, × 320).

amyloids, arbitrarily named AA amyloid, is formed from part of an acute phase protein synthesized by the liver in acute inflammation. Monoclonal immunoglobulin light chain fragments can also polymerize to form amyloid (AL amyloid). Other identified sources include certain hormones, a protein thought to come from a cell surface receptor protein observed in Alzheimer's disease, a variant of a circulating prealbumin also known as transthyretin, and gelsolin which is an actin-binding serum protein.

There are several ocular and adnexal amyloid states. Some that are inherited, and consequently regarded as dystrophies, include the corneal lattice dystrophies and vitreal amyloidosis. The nature of the protein in the more common localized form of lattice dystrophy (type 1) is uncertain but there is evidence of a mutant form of gelsolin in the systemic form (type 2 or Meretoja's syndrome). A mutant transthyretin has been implicated in vitreal amyloidosis. Non-hereditary, localized amyloid deposits may occur in the cornea, conjunctiva, eyelids, or orbit and it is probably justifiable to describe them as degenerative states. A variety of amyloid types have been reported but it is interesting to speculate that, particularly with respect to the anterior situations, the amyloid sometimes may have originated from keratin as has been postulated in the context of cutaneous amyloidosis.

Lenticular degeneration

Cataract formation is discussed elsewhere and comment at this point will be confined to the observation that, irrespective of the cause, most cataracts are eventually characterized by degeneration of lenticular fibres. Commencing as increased hydration related to membrane abnormalities, the fibres suffer progressive breakdown of their intracellular organelles and eventually disintegrate to form rounded globules of residual denatured lens protein.

Neoplasia

Neither the terms tumour, which in theory could refer to any abnormal swelling, nor neoplasm, which taken literally means simply new growth, adequately covers the pathological state to which they conventionally refer. Essentially, the concept implied is that of excessive and persistent local cell proliferation unrelated to the needs of the host and not subject to normal controls.

It might be noted in passing that undue tissue proliferation can occur in childhood that is not strictly neoplastic. Mostly classified as hamartomas, such tumours present as circumscribed growth of defined tissue components ceasing at the end of the systemic growth process. Choristomas represent a comparable proliferation of tissue elements not normally found at the affected site, a common example in respect of the eye being an epibulbar dermoid. They have no potential for malignancy.

Morphology

Tumours are conveniently divided into two groups defined according to their anticipated behaviour which is generally, and conveniently from the standpoint of biopsy diagnosis, reflected in their histological appearances. There are exceptions, however, and prognostication based on morphology alone is not always reliable.

Benign

Benign tumours grow relatively slowly and expand so as to compress the adjacent extracellular connective tissue and form a capsule separating the proliferating mass from neighbouring structures (Fig. 5). There may also be some active capsule synthesis by nearby fibroblasts but the tumour does not directly contribute to the process. The proliferating cells are differentiated and resemble those of the parent tissue in respect of size and shape (Fig. 6). Mitotic figures are usually infrequent.

Malignant

Growth is invasive rather than expansile so that capsule formation is not a feature (Fig. 7). The cells of individual tumours vary from high levels of differentiation to total anaplasia with scant evidence of their origin (Fig. 8). Variation in cell size and shape (pleomorphism or atypia) is common and there is an enhanced ratio of nuclear to cytoplasmic volume. Increased intensity of nuclear staining with haematoxylin (hyperchromatism) is often seen and mitotic figures, some of them atypical, are increased as a measure of the rate of tumour growth. Markedly enlarged nuclei or multiple nuclei may be found and nucleoli are often conspicuous by virtue of their size and number.

Laboratory aids to prognosis and diagnosis

Unfortunately, prognostication based on histological differences is not infallible, especially where tumours of low grade

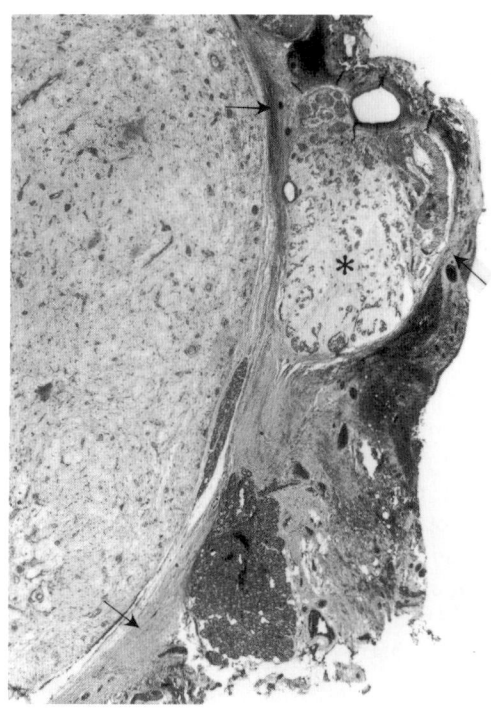

Fig. 5 Pleomorphic adenoma (lacrimal gland). The boundary of the tumour is smooth and defined by a fibrous tissue capsule (arrows). Sometimes, as here, nodules of tumour may expand into the capsule (asterisk) but not beyond it (haematoxylin and eosin, ×16).

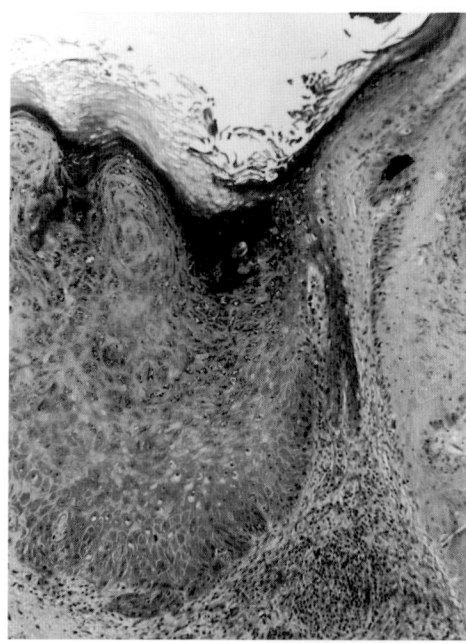

Fig. 6 Squamous cell papilloma. The benign neoplastic proliferation is wholly in terms of seemingly normal squamous epithelium with expected maturation through prickle and granular cell layers to surface keratin (haematoxylin and eosin, ×100).

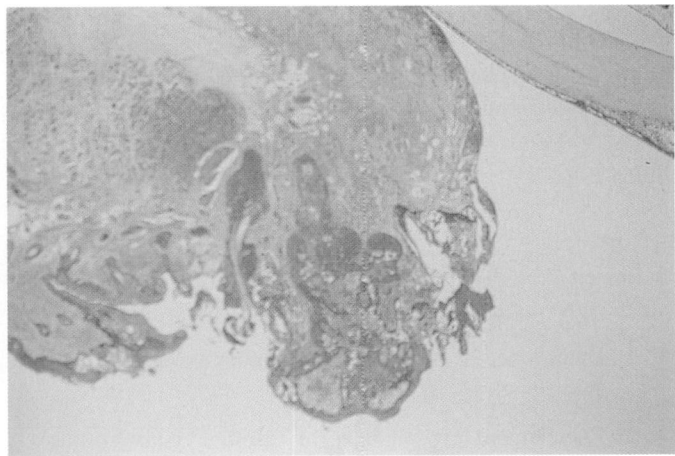

(a)

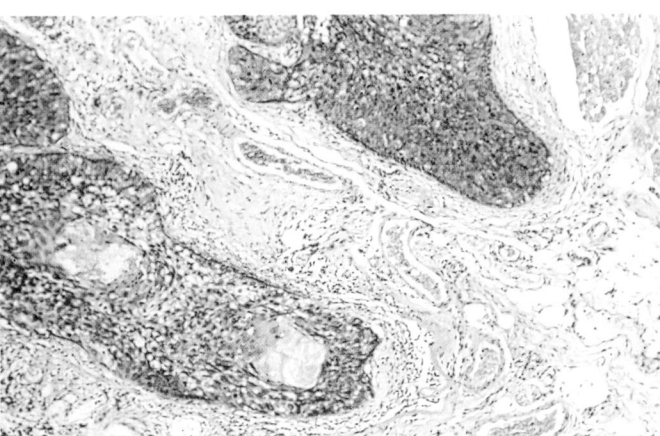

(b)

Fig. 7 Sebaceous carcinoma (meibomian gland). (a) The margin of the upper eyelid is destroyed and replaced by an irregular, non-encapsulated tumour (haematoxylin and eosin, × 20). (b) At higher magnification the infiltrative nature of the tumour is apparent, as well as limited differentiation in the form of some foamy, vacuolated cells (haematoxylin and eosin, × 100)

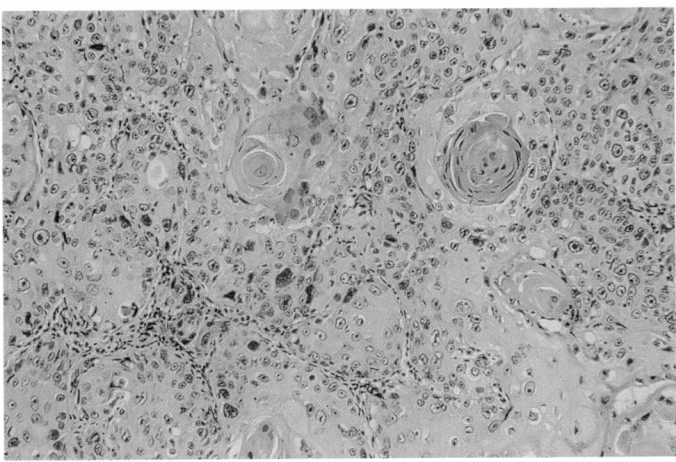

Fig. 8 Squamous cell carcinoma (conjunctiva). The tumour overall is only moderately differentiated, many cells having irregular, hyperchromatic nuclei. Squamous origin is evident, however, in the form of occasional pink-staining concentric keratin 'pearls' (haematoxylin and eosin, × 180).

malignancy are concerned. Consequently, other measures of tumour behaviour have been investigated.

DNA flow cytometry measures the DNA content of cells held in suspension both at an individual cell and overall sample levels. In this way, given that the DNA content is increased in cells subject to chromosomal reduplication (aneuploidy) in the neoplastic process, atypical cells may be identified. Furthermore, the percentage of proliferating cells can be assessed, this being generally higher in malignancy. Cells in the growth phase of some tumours can also be labelled using an antibody to the *Ki-ras* oncogene. Conversely, evidence of a reduction in a widespread tumour suppressor gene p53 can be sought by measuring levels of its protein products. The increased protein synthesis accompanying cell proliferation involves transcription of DNA to ribosomal RNA, an activity that is reflected morphologically in the emergence of nucleolar organizer regions. These are increased in number in some tumours, including melanomas, and can be demonstrated histologically with appropriate silver staining.

Nevertheless, all these additional techniques are restricted in their application because of limitations on the type of tissue that can be used (whether fixed or fresh, for example), inconstancy of the described features in tumours of differing histogenesis, and, not least, expense and availability.

Determination of tumour histogenesis can be helped by treating histological sections with antibodies to specific tissue elements. Labelling the antibodies with fluorescein or an enzyme such as horseradish peroxidase enables them to serve as markers for the corresponding antigen. Thus, tumours of neural crest derivation are commonly characterized by a specific protein (S-100), while actively growing melanotic tumours often stain with an antibody referred to as MB-45. Astrocytic tumours stain with antibody to glial fibrillary acidic protein, and so on. Here again, however, the finding that marker specificity is often far from absolute substantially reduces the use of immunohistochemical diagnosis.

Molecular basis

Fundamental to the neoplastic process is non-lethal genetic damage such that the affected cell clones are liberated from the constraints of genes designed to modulate proliferative activity. The evolution from normality to neoplasia is a multistep process, witness the progression through the various degrees of cell dysplasia seen in so-called Bowen's disease of the limbal conjunctiva (Fig. 9) to preinvasive disease (carcinoma *in situ*) and invasive squamous cell carcinoma. As in this example, progression to frank malignancy is far from inevitable and the transformation can stop at any stage. Benign tumours appear to develop somewhat differently in that dysplastic cells are not a usual feature and malignant transformation is uncommon. Squamous cell papillomas, for instance, do not give rise to carcinomas. There are exceptions, however, as in the case of pleomorphic adenomas of the lacrimal gland which do occasionally spawn a malignant tumour (usually after repeated recurrence of an incompletely excised lesion).

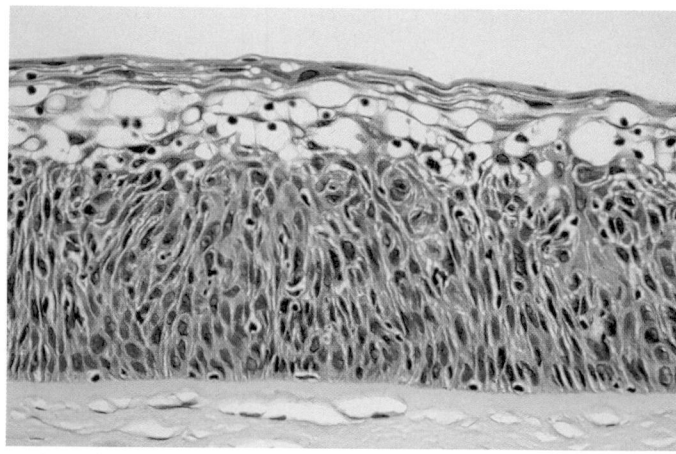

Fig. 9 Epithelial dysplasia (corneoconjunctival limbus). The corneal epithelium is thickened through abnormal proliferation of cells with irregular, hyperchromatic nuclei. The epithelial basement membrane and Bowman's layer are intact, however, so distinguishing the process from frank, invasive carcinoma (haematoxylin and eosin, × 240).

Several types of gene are involved in the evolution of neoplastic states.

Oncogenes

Derived from genes (proto-oncogenes) concerned with normal growth and differentiation as a result of either structural or regulatory changes, oncogenes promote defective control of cell proliferation. Changes can result from point mutations, chromosomal translocations or gene amplification. Alteration of just one of the paired genes is adequate for increased synthesis of the corresponding oncoprotein.

Tumour suppressor genes (antioncogenes)

Downregulation of cell proliferation is the function of a second class of genes. These are a normal cell component and neoplasia is promoted by their deletion or inactivation, usually as a result of gene mutation. But, because suppressor genes show recessive behaviour, deletion of both alleles is required before there is an effect. The genetic abnormality in retinoblastoma involves growth suppressor genes located on the long arm of chromosome 13 (13q14) and loss of both, that is two mutational events or 'hits' are necessary if a tumour is to develop. Because loss of a single suppressor gene has no effect, cells damaged in this way are viable and, should the deletion involve a germ cell, the abnormality can be passed on to succeeding generations. Affected individuals then need only one more hit for neoplasia to ensue and, correspondingly, tumours related to loss of suppressor gene function are often associated with a familial tendency. Retinoblastoma is a pertinent example but others include schwannomas in neurofibromatosis patients and Wilms' tumour of the kidney. By far the most common suppressor gene to show defective expression, however, is p53 located on chromosome 17 (17p13.1) and implicated in over 50 per cent of patients with carcinomas of the colon, breast, and lung.

Apoptosis genes

These are the genes responsible for programmed cell death as defined earlier. Deletion or inactivation has been demonstrated in respect of certain animal tumours and is almost certainly also a factor in human neoplasia.

Tumour development is also a function of the soil as well as of the seed. Blood flow and availability of metabolites, the status of the immune system and hormonal influences may also be important.

Metastasis

A capacity for distant metastasis is the ultimate expression of malignant neoplasia involving a cascade of events.

1. Emergence of a subclone of tumour cells with metastatic potential.

2. Detachment from adjacent tumour cells through downregulation of cadherin proteins involved in normal cellular cohesion.

3. Adhesion to and penetration of basement membrane promoted by increased expression of receptors for laminin, fibronectin, and other matrix proteins.

4. Invasion of the extracellular matrix through the agency of proteolytic enzymes derived from macrophages, fibroblasts, and the tumour cells themselves.

5. Penetration of blood or lymph vessel walls related to the secretion of an autocrine motility factor.

6. Interaction with circulating host lymphoid cells, especially natural killer cells, with the possibility of tumour cell death.

7. Formation of tumour cell emboli (enhanced by interaction with platelets).

8. Adhesion of tumour emboli to vascular basement membrane at the destination as a function of a range of adhesion molecules with specific affinities. Differences in affinity may account for the predilection of certain tumours to metastasize to particular tissues. (The association of uveal melanoma metastases with the liver is a probable example.)

9. Extravasation by mechanisms equivalent to those involved in the earlier intravasation.

Causation

This a complicated subject but an essential property of any carcinogen is the ability to disrupt the normal genetic control of cell proliferation. There are three major ways of achieving this.

1. Introduction of viral DNA into the genome may act as a promoter of oncogene activity. Oncogenic RNA viruses function by inducing the cell to produce a DNA copy under the influence of a reverse transcriptase which then acts similarly to activate proto-oncogenes.

2. Chemical substances may damage the DNA and, since the subsequent repair process is prone to error, there

is a risk that mutations will develop in the genes controlling cell proliferation.

3. Physical agencies, especially ultraviolet and ionizing radiations, can also serve to damage DNA resulting in mutation or translocation of relevant genes.

Individual predisposition is also involved, whether through genetic, immunological, or other mechanisms and carcinogenesis depends on interaction between these endogenous and exogenous factors.

Little is known about the specific causes of intraocular tumours although reverse transcriptase activity, consistent with a viral aetiology, has been reported in retinoblastoma. There is also evidence from a study of animal neoplasia that a protein induced by simian virus 40 can inactivate the retinoblastoma gene product. A slightly increased incidence of uveal melanoma in blue-eyed individuals and its marked rarity in black people could indicate an aetiological role for sunlight.

Further reading

Alison, M.R. (1992). Repair and regenerative processes. In *Oxford textbook of pathology*, Vol. 1: *Principles of pathology*, (ed. J.O'D. McGee, P.G. Isaacson, and N.A. Wright), pp. 365–89. Oxford University Press, Oxford.

Cotran, R.S., Kumar, V., and Robbins, S.L. (1994). *Robbins: pathologic basis of disease*, (5th edn). Saunders, Philadelphia. [A deservedly popular textbook covering both general and systemic pathology, distinguished by its clarity and authority.]

Garner, A. and Klintworth, G.K. (ed.) (1994a). *Pathobiology of ocular disease: a dynamic approach*, (2nd edn). Marcel Dekker, New York. [Helpful in relating general pathological principles to specific ocular and adnexal conditions.]

Garner, A., Sarks, S., and Sarks, J.P. (1994b). Degenerative and related disorders of the retina and choroid. In *Pathobiology of ocular disease, a dynamic approach*, (2nd edn), (ed. A. Garner and G.K. Klintworth), pp. 631–74. Marcel Dekker, New York.

Klintworth, G.K. (1994). Degenerations, depositions, and miscellaneous reactions of the ocular anterior segment. In *Pathobiology of ocular disease, a dynamic approach*, (2nd edn), (ed. A. Garner and G.K. Klintworth), pp. 743–94. Marcel Dekker, New York.

Lewis, J.G. (1994). Overview of oncogenesis. In *Pathobiology of ocular disease, a dynamic approach*, (2nd edn), (ed. A. Garner and G.K. Klintworth), pp. 1345–54. Marcel Dekker, New York.

McGee, J.O'D., Isaacson, P.G., and Wright, N.A. (ed.) (1992). *Oxford textbook of pathology*, Vol. 1: *Principles of pathology*. Oxford University Press, Oxford. [A comprehensive multiauthor textbook with especially excellent coverage of inflammatory and neoplastic processes.]

Norton, L. (1991). Clinical aspects of cell and tumor growth kinetics. In *Comprehensive textbook of oncology*, Vol. 1 (2nd edn), (ed. A.R. Moossa, S.C. Schimpli, and M.C. Robson), pp. 409–14. Williams & Wilkins, Baltimore.

Proia, A.D. (1994). Inflammation. In *Pathobiology of ocular disease, a dynamic approach*, (2nd edn), (ed. A. Garner and G.K. Klintworth), pp. 63–99. Marcel Dekker, New York.

Rudin, C.M. and Thompson, C.B. (1997). Apoptosis and disease: regulation and clinical relevance of programmed cell death. *Annual Reviews of Medicine*, **48**, 267–81.

Tarin, D. (1992). Tumour metastasis. In *Oxford textbook of pathology*, Vol. 1: *Principles of pathology*, (ed. J.O'D. McGee, P.G. Isaacson, and N.A. Wright), pp. 607–33. Oxford University Press, Oxford.

Turner, N.C. (1992). Acute inflammation. In *Oxford textbook of pathology*, Vol. 1: *Principles of pathology*, (ed. J.O'D. McGee, P.G. Isaacson, and N.A. Wright), pp. 351–65. Oxford University Press, Oxford.

Wyllie, A.H. and Duvall, E. (1992). Cell death. In *Oxford textbook of pathology*, Vol. 1: *Principles of pathology*, (ed. J.O'D. McGee, P.G. Isaacson, and N.A. Wright), pp. 141–57. Oxford University Press, Oxford.

1.4 Pharmacological basic principles

1.4.1 Pharmacological principles, delivery of topical ocular medication, and drugs which affect the pupil

*F.T. Fraunfelder and Neil D. Gross**

Topical ocular medications remain patient friendly, relatively inexpensive, non-invasive, convenient, and easy to apply. Topical ocular agents also hold distinct advantages over systemically delivered drugs. They allow focusing of pharmacological activity to the eye with the ultimate goal of increased drug efficacy. This method concomitantly limits general distribution and decreases the risk of side-effects. Topical application of ocular medicine reigns as the most common method of drug delivery to the eye.

Since most medications were initially designed for systemic use, the pharmacological properties of topical ocular agents are among the least publicized. Yet, this knowledge proves to be quintessential to the delivery of safe and effective patient eye care. Unlike medicines administered orally, topical eye medications that reach systemic circulation avoid first-pass metabolism. Topical ocular medication reaches systemic circulation via absorption from large mucosal surfaces (conjunctival and nasal mucosa), the effects of which resemble intramuscular or intravenous administration. These agents reach the target organ before reaching the liver where the drug is metabolized. Oral β-blockers first pass through the liver before reaching the target organ. This is why therapeutic blood levels of β-blockers can be reached with eyedrops alone in up to 6 to 8 per cent of patients. In addition, 1 per cent of Japanese or Chinese, 2.4 per cent of African-Americans, and 8 per cent of Caucasians do not have the P-450 enzyme CYP2D6 to metabolize the drug. Therefore, higher blood levels occur. Nelson *et al.* reported over 30 deaths associated with the use of timolol eyedrops between 1978 and 1985, and many other topical eye drugs have shown significant systemic side-effects. Paediatric patients are particularly vulnerable because instillation volumes are constant regardless of body size. The tailoring of medication to the individual patient's history, needs, and level of compliance is important in the assessment of the risk to benefit ratio essential to clinical practice.

Basic pharmacology of topical eye agents

Pharmacokinetics is the rate at which the body processes a drug, including absorption, distribution, metabolism, and elimination. Together, these elements determine the ultimate bioavailability of topical eye medication. The various factors that influence the degree to which a drug becomes available include age, body weight, sex, and pigmentation. Less intrinsic factors include the disease process, drug interactions, and instillation techniques. Most topically applied ocular medications miss their primary target, the eye, since only a small per cent of the eyedrop enters the eye. It becomes apparent, then, that the proper administration of ocular medication involves consideration of each of its pharmacokinetic properties.

Absorption

Topical ocular agents are not uniformly absorbed, if absorbed at all. Experiments in rabbit models demonstrate that less than 5 per cent of an administered topical agent is absorbed intraocularly, with estimates in humans ranging from 1 to 10 per cent. For the drugs that are absorbed into the eye, this occurs through two major routes: corneal and extracorneal. The individual properties of each compound ultimately define the path of absorption. In general, small lipophilic drugs are more easily absorbed across the cornea. Conversely, extracorneal pathways can more easily accommodate larger and less lipophilic agents. Regardless of the drug, however, absorption is governed by several related factors: (a) ocular contact times, (b) drug concentration, (c) tissue permeability, (d) the cornea, and (e) extracorneal sites.

Ocular contact time

The length of time that an agent contacts tissue directly affects its absorption into that tissue. For ocular medication, residence time at the absorption site is exceptionally short compared to other routes of administration. Most of an instilled drop will have disappeared from the conjunctival sac within 15 to 30 s of instillation, while complete elimination from the tear film occurs within 15 min. Ocular contact time is especially sensitive

*This study was supported, in part, by an unrestricted grant from Research to Prevent Blindness, New York, United States.

to extraocular fluid dynamics. Dynamic constituents such as tear volume, tear turnover, and blinking play critical roles in the ocular absorption of topical drugs. The average human tear volume in the cul-de-sac is 7 µl with only 1 µl in the precorneal tear film and with a short-term maximum cul-de-sac capacity of 25 to 30 µl. Roughly 10 µl transitory drug remains following instillation and blinking. The basal tear flow rate, which averages 1.2 µl/min (16 per cent) and decreases variably with age, nearly doubles upon instillation of medication. Reflex blinking displays great variability and reacts strongly to both physical and emotional stimulation. Paradoxically, it serves two opposing absorptive functions. While mixing the agent into the tear film solution, blinking simultaneously pumps excess drug away from the cul-de-sac and into the nasolacrimal duct at an average rate of 2 µl/min. The mixing allows increased intraocular absorption, while the pumping action decreases contact time.

Drug concentration

Solubility factors aside, ocular absorption follows first-order kinetics. The amount of a drug entering the eye is linearly related to tear film concentration. Dilution from lacrimation, such as psychophysical stimulation, tends to produce an exponential decay in drug concentration. Reflex tear rates vary significantly (3–400 µl/min), not only between patients, but also for the individual. Drug concentrations may decrease due to successive topical administration of different ocular agents. Therefore, a 3- to 5-minute interval between drops is recommended to prevent wash-out effects.

Tissue permeability

Most drugs cross the cornea via passive transport, with the concentration gradient as the driving force. This movement varies exponentially with time until the cell membrane becomes saturated with solute and diffusion approaches a plateau. However, therapeutic doses rarely reach saturation and generally abide by first-order kinetics. Tissue permeability is governed primarily by the physiochemical factors of passive transport. The most notable factors include: acid–base dissociation, partition coefficient, and drug molecular structure and solubility. Temperature, tissue surface area, and thickness also influence tissue permeability.

Cornea

The cornea is the primary site of intraocular absorption. It is directly proportional to temperature and inversely related to the square root of molecular weight. Since the cornea has a high lipid content, lipophilic drugs pass with the least difficulty. The cornea is a five-layer structure of which only three are significant barriers to absorption. The cornea resembles a sandwich with a hydrophilic stroma flanked by lipophilic epithelial and endothelial layers. The stroma and endothelium act in unison as a single hydrophilic layer. Although less porous, the epithelial layer maintains a lipid content 100 times greater than the highly collagenated stroma. Charged particles penetrate both layers poorly. The corneal epithelium and its release of drug to stroma determine the rate-limiting barrier to diffusion. Any drug intended to cross the cornea must strike a balance between

the lipophilicity required to enter and the hydrophilicity needed to leave. Only weak acids and bases are capable of adapting to such biphasic solubility requirements.

The dissociation constant of a particular agent also determines diffusion across the cornea, albeit strictly by indirect affiliation to lipid solubility. The ionized form of a drug is only minimally lipid soluble. Alkaloids, or weak bases, remain unionized at physiological pH and show greater lipid solubility at decreased pH. A modest decrease in pH translates to increased absorption. Weak acids (i.e. timolol) show the opposite properties. Depending upon the dissociation constant of a given drug, lacrimation can greatly enhance or diminish corneal absorption. Therefore, the drugs best suited to cross the cornea are small, moderately lipophilic, and partially unionized under physiological conditions.

Extracorneal

Topical eye agents are absorbed through the conjunctiva, sclera, and lacrimal apparatus. The conjunctiva has greater permeability, blood flow, and a surface area 17 times that of the cornea. To a lesser degree than the cornea, movement across the conjunctiva increases with lipophilicity and is relatively permeable to hydrophilic drugs. The conjunctiva shows greater permeability for some topical eye medications (e.g. β-blocking agents) and can significantly reduce ocular bioavailability by offering a competing absorptive route.

Drugs can cross the porous sclera much easier than the cornea, especially for hydrophilic agents. Hydrophilic agents can pass the sclera at a rate up to 80 times that of the cornea. Scleral absorption can be quite substantial and may prove to be a viable alternative to transcorneal therapy for drugs that target the retina, uvea, or ciliary body.

Greater than 80 per cent of topically applied ocular medication is lost to drainage in the lacrimal system. Lacrimal drainage is 100 times faster than the corneal absorption rate. The rate of lacrimal drainage for an ophthalmic solution is linearly related to the volume instilled and the amount the eye can hold. Eyedroppers deliver an average volume of 39 µl (ranging 25–56 µl), which exceeds the maximum cul-de-sac capacity. Overflow is inevitable from even a single drop. Brown et al. demonstrated that 2.5 per cent phenylephrine administered to neonates in 8 and 30 µl aliquots showed no difference in pupillary response, while plasma phenylephrine concentrations were double in patients who received the larger dose size. Therefore, a single instillation volume of 20 µl or less is considered ideal for ensuring adequate bioavailability and decreasing side-effects due to excess drug volume.

Intraocular distribution

Once a drug has been absorbed into the eye, it is rapidly, although not uniformly, portioned among various tissue components. Anatomical considerations play an important role in ultimately determining which compartments are exposed. For example, anteroposterior distribution is limited by the lens. Other physical barriers, such as the iris, ciliary body, and aqueous humour flow, also protect the posterior segment from drug exposure. Consequently, topical drugs that cross the cornea are distributed almost exclusively within the anterior segment. The iris and ciliary body, which together represent the biophase of most topical ocular agents, are of particular interest to the clinician. Concentrations in the ciliary body are often higher than in the aqueous humour. This comes as no surprise when one accounts for scleral absorption. Conversely, the iris relies much more heavily on corneal absorption and distribution from the aqueous humour. When isolated from the ciliary body, iris drug levels nearly equal those of the aqueous humour.

Other factors that influence drug distribution include tissue permeability, ion trapping, and drug–protein binding. Protein–drug binding is the primary force in the bioavailability of many topical medications. Mikkelson *et al.* found a 75 to 100 per cent decline in the amount of drug delivered to the target tissue due to protein binding. Protein–drug complexes can also act as substantial drug reservoirs, primarily from two sources—tear solution and the iris. The protein in tears is comprised of albumin, globulin, and lysozyme and accounts for less than 2.0 per cent of total tear volume. Under normal conditions, this amount of protein binding is nominal. However, in cases of severe irritation, disease, or chronic inflammation protein binding from tears can become significant. In contrast, the pigmented iris affects on pharmacological activity have been well documented in mydriatics, miotics, and ocular antihypertensive medications. These studies have repeatedly shown a slower onset of drug activity due to pigmented cell binding of lipoid soluble drugs with the result of decreased maximum effect and longer duration of drug action.

Intraocular metabolism and elimination

Topical ocular agents undergo metabolism by a host of esterases found in tears, the adnexa, and ocular tissues. Within the corneal epithelium, drugs are subject to metabolism by significant amounts of choline esterases. Metabolism is stereospecific for the laevo form of a drug, and since the inactive raceme will often exhibit toxic effects, most solutions are formulated as single isomers.

A decrease in aqueous drainage, as in patients on some forms of glaucoma medication, may lengthen the elimination half-life in patients taking multiple ocular medications. A β-blocking agent or carbonic anhydrase inhibitor could enhance the effect of other ocular medications by decreasing aqueous humour secretion and slowing elimination. A secondary route of intraocular elimination is the uveoscleral outflow pathway. Drug eliminated by this route avoids the trabecular meshwork and percolates through the ciliary muscle *en route* to the suprachoroidal space, where it can be either reabsorbed or enter the systemic circulation.

Prodrugs, preservatives, and other agents that affect delivery

Lipophilic prodrugs, drugs converted into active form during or after intraocular absorption, are designed to employ corneal esterases as a means of increasing intraocular absorption. They are often esterified to increase lipophilicity and selectively augment potency at the target tissue. Studies of timolol and phenylephrine prodrugs show significant increases in the ocular absorption ratio with no change in the delivery to ocular tissues, thereby increasing the therapeutic index.

Preservatives prolong the shelf-life of topical medications by their bacteriostatic or cidal qualities. Most preservatives have side-effects. Benzalkonium chloride, a preservative widely used because of its antimicrobial activity at a wide range of pH, can cause significant corneal and conjunctival irritation and epithelial erosions at or near clinical concentrations (0.01–0.04 per cent). Preservatives often increase corneal epithelial permeability, allowing for significant augmentation of drug bioavailability. These potential advantages must be weighed against their potential tissue toxicity. In the case of benzalkonium chloride, the use of low concentrations (> 0.01 per cent) appears to offer an acceptable balance between inhibiting microbial growth and limiting toxicity. Bioavailability of drugs is enhanced by viscous vehicles, especially at viscosities of 0.1 to 0.2 cm²/s. This increased viscosity can cause an increase in tear film saturation of up to 80 per cent due primarily to slower draining and prolonged corneal contact time. Tonicity can also affect bioavailability. Although hypertonic solutions can leach fluid out of the eye and increase drug dilution, solution tonicities are tolerated without changes in corneal permeability. Topical solutions with a tonicity between 270 and 620 mmol have been shown to minimize changes in tissue permeability, discomfort, and lacrimation.

Drug delivery vehicles

The ideal drug delivery system has a versatile vehicle that can maximize contact time and increase conveyance to target tissues with minimal discomfort and irritation. Differences do exist between the delivery devices.

Aqueous solutions

Solutions remain the most popular vehicle for delivery of topical eye medication. The definition of a solution necessitates that all ingredients be fully dissolved. Water is invariably the liquid medium of choice. It is easily applied, causes few visual symptoms, and complications are generally minimal. Solutions, however, exhibit the shortest ocular contact times and have relatively poor ocular absorption with limited bioavailability. Aqueous solutions are subject to degradation by hydrolysis and evaporation, both of which can result in significant changes in drug concentration. Nevertheless, aqueous solutions continue to be preferred due to their ease of application, ocular comfort, and few side-effects.

Suspensions

Suspensions are composed of an active ingredient in fine, particulate form suspended in a saturated solution of the same. Nearly all are water-based and have active agents with diminished water solubility. Upon application, the solution in the suspension is diluted by tears. Entrapped particles within the suspension are intended to dissolve and replenish the drug concentration in the tear film. This allows a more sustained delivery as well as a rapid initial deposit of dissolved drug. The rate of dissolution is inversely proportional to particle size, meaning theoretically that an optimal particle size exists for each drug. Suspensions tend to stay in the cul-de-sac longer than solutions and therefore have a more prolonged ocular contact time compared to solutions. The drug bioavailability from suspensions is greater than that of solutions. The most significant drawback of a suspension, however, is the precipitation of drug. All require vigorous shaking prior to each application. Foreign body sensation after application with the use of suspensions is not uncommon due to crystal formation of some drugs under certain conditions.

Ointments

Ointments rank as the third most common delivery vehicle. They consist of a semisolid lipoid preparation containing lipid soluble drugs. The most common base is petroleum with anhydrous lanolin in mineral oil. Petroleum is inert and not absorbed by the conjunctiva or cornea. Ointments are designed to liquify at body temperature and are dispersed by the shearing action of blinking. Ointment can also become entrapped in the cornea, fornices, or lashes, which are capable of acting like reservoirs (Fig. 1).

Ointments are also retained on the eye longer, since their passage through the lacrimal outflow system is slow. This results in a drug turnover rate that is low (0.5 per cent/min). Total bioavailability is substantially higher than from aqueous solutions or suspensions. Ointments require less frequent dosing. Ointments can undergo phase separation of emulsions or precipitation of lipid-insoluble particles depending upon environmental conditions and the specific formulation. They can be difficult to self administer in consistent doses, and by the nature of application, increase the risk of ocular injury. Furthermore, they can be uncomfortable and often interfere with vision. Patient compliance can be unreliable, especially for day use since cosmetically and visually they may be unacceptable to the patient.

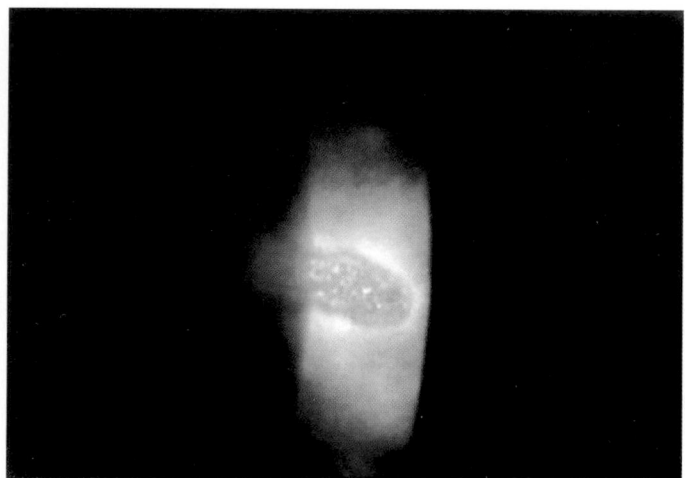

Fig. 1 Ointment entrapped in corneal depression after patching the eye. Once the patch is removed, the ointment globules are washed out within a few hours.

Solid delivery systems

Solid delivery systems attempt to avoid the pulsatile delivery with conventional vehicles. The ultimate goal is to provide a constant drug concentration at the target tissue by means of a sustained drug release that follows zero-order, rather than first-order, kinetics. Thus, solid delivery vehicles appear most effective for rapidly absorbed drugs that demonstrate marked fluctuations in target tissue concentration. This slower and more uniform delivery allows smaller doses to achieve local therapeutic levels with less frequent instillations, inherently reducing the risk of systemic side-effects. Other goals of solid vehicles include more accurate dosing, possible targeting of ocular tissues through non-corneal routes and increased shelf-life of medication. Most notably, these devices aim to increase patient compliance through safety and convenience.

When considering solid inserts, there are two main categories: soluble and insoluble. Soluble inserts release drug by either dilution or erosion, and occasionally both. Most soluble inserts are swelling controlled, meaning they swell upon hydration and release the active agent into the tear film. They do not follow zero-order kinetics. Neither do most erodable inserts, which are chemically controlled and release drug as a result of hydrolysis. Unfortunately, both forms of soluble inserts have increased potential side-effects from initial burst 'leaching' by tears. It is the insoluble insert, however, that promises better drug delivery control. These include drug-saturated hydrogel contact lenses and membrane-bound delivery units, such as the Ocusert therapeutic system. Contact lenses allow increased ocular contact time and absorption. Their effectiveness depends largely upon the specific medication, soaking time, lens thickness, drug concentration, and molecular weight. For example, drug molecules larger than 500 kDa are too large to manoeuvre into or out of the lens. If lenses are adequately soaked (e.g. 25 min), bioavailability is greatly augmented without concomitant delay in peak time. Although the soaking method is generally preferred for its better bioavailability, drugs can be applied while the lens is in place. Even so, these devices have yet to offer constant delivery, and like the soluble inserts, tend to release the drug in potentially damaging bursts. In the case of pilocarpine, 90 per cent of the drug is released in the first 20 min. Therefore, drug-saturated contact lenses appear useful for only a handful of clinical situations, particularly acute ocular inflammation or infection.

The only solid delivery devices to approach zero-order kinetics are the membrane-bound systems. These insoluble inserts, with the therapeutic agent sandwiched between two polymer layers, are currently the most consistent method of drug deployment. Such delivery heralds the possibility of increasing non-corneal absorption of hydrophilic agents and thus expanding the clinician's pharmacological options. The primary advantage of membrane-bound drug inserts is reduction in dosage necessary to achieve therapeutic effect. Studies with pilocarpine Ocusert in glaucoma patients showed an average drug delivery per day eight-fold less than drops, while achieving the same therapeutic goals. Thus, they can significantly reduce the risk of systemic absorption and side-effects. The slow, constant release is particularly desirable for long-term therapy, both in terms of efficacy and reduction of side-effects. They are also convenient, requiring less frequent instillation than other vehicles. The Ocusert delivery system is, however, expensive and causes a foreign body sensation in some patients. Enthusiasm for these devices has been further muted by occasional therapeutic failures and reluctance of both ophthalmologists and patients to abandon more conventional remedies. The use of other devices such as nanoparticles, gel strips, and liposomes are also currently under investigation as future delivery alternatives.

Drugs that affect the pupil

A discussion of the pharmacokinetics, delivery vehicles, and proper instillation techniques of topical ocular medication is somewhat esoteric without a relevant clinical context. Therefore, an elaboration upon commonly employed agents is worthwhile. We shall focus our discussion on the mydriatics and cycloplegics, as these are the mainstay of diagnostic ophthalmology. They are employed primarily as a means of examining intraocular anatomy and evaluating refractive function. Other uses include diagnosis of Horner's syndrome, preoperative and postoperative management of patients undergoing intraocular surgery, and therapy for conjunctival congestion, anterior uveitis, and secondary glaucoma.

Two main classes of drugs exist as mediators of mydriasis and cycloplegia: the anticholinergic and adrenergic agents. Anticholinergic drugs antagonize parasympathetic activity at both the iris constrictor muscle and longitudinal muscle fibres of the ciliary body, which are responsible for accommodation. Thus, they are applied topically to the eye to produce both cycloplegia and mydriasis. All cycloplegics produce mydriasis. Conversely, the adrenergic agents stimulate the iris dilator muscle. They are effective only as mydriatics and show no cycloplegic action. The anticholinergic and adrenergic agents are often used in combination as a means of maximizing a mydriatic effect.

Drugs used for refraction

Anticholinergic drugs, the only drugs to produce cycloplegia, have proven useful for estimating errors in refraction. More specifically, it is the short-acting cycloplegics (e.g. cyclopentolate hydrochloride and tropicamide) that are best suited for this purpose. Cyclopentolate has a rapid onset of action (20–45 min) and a relatively short duration (3–24 h). Tropicamide is a weaker cycloplegic, with an even quicker onset (15–30 min) and shorter duration of action (2–6 h). Thus, when using tropicamide, a cycloplegic refraction may be performed within 20–35 min. Few significant side-effects have been reported with these agents, and they are generally considered safe. They can be administered alone, together, or in conjunction with phenylephrine allowing the doctor to titrate the desired effect. Other anticholinergic agents available for refractive error estimation include atropine sulphate, homatropine hydrobromide, and scopolamine hydrobromide. These drugs typically show a slower onset and much longer duration of action; up to 18 days for atropine. They often result in prolonged blurred near vision

and can precipitate an attack of acute angle closure glaucoma in eyes with anatomically narrow angles. Thus, while they may be indicated for children up to 5 or 6 years, these long-acting anticholinergics are rarely employed in adults except to treat uveitis.

Anticholinergic and adrenergic drugs used for fundoscopic examination

Both anticholinergic and adrenergic agents are useful in facilitating ophthalmoscopic viewing of the fundus, as well as retinal photography. The pharmacological goal is wide pupillary dilation with relative sparing of accommodation. Given alone, 1 per cent tropicamide can rapidly induce adequate mydriasis with short-term cycloplegia, which makes it useful for routine fundoscopic screening in adults. As an adrenergic agent, phenylephrine causes mydriasis without cycloplegia. It demonstrates a rapid onset (45–60 min) and duration of only 2 to 3 h. Hydroxyamphetamine is a similar but less clinically recognized adrenergic agent. Although these agents show less residual blurring of vision, they are known to cause more frequent systemic side-effects. Therefore, they are typically administered in a low dose solution and often in combination with an anticholinergic. Other adrenergic mydriatics, such as epinephrine or its prodrug, dipivalyl epinephrine, produce less mydriasis than vasoconstriction and are rarely used for diagnostic purposes.

Application of topical eye medication

The authors' recommendation for application of topical ocular medication is the depot method, described nearly two decades ago. This technique is the same for both solutions and ointments, and if employed properly, should maximize ocular absorption and minimize systemic exposure. The best method is to have another person apply the medication (Figs 2, 3, and 4).

- Tilt the patient's head posteriorly so that the optical

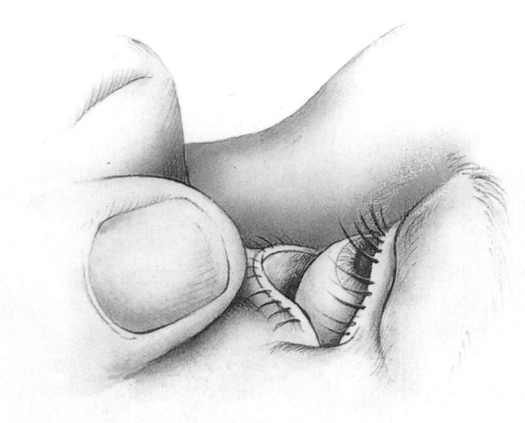

Fig. 2 Inserting topical medication: retract lower eyelid.

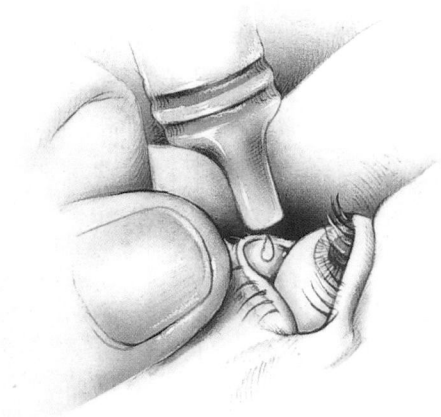

Fig. 3 Inserting topical medication: drop into lower fornix.

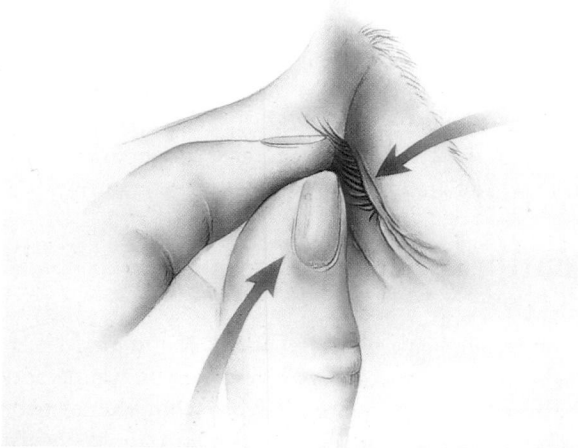

Fig. 4 Inserting topical medication: close the lids.

axis is vertical. With one hand resting on the cheek, grasp the lower eyelid below the eyelashes with the thumb and index finger. Lightly retract the eyelid at a right angle away from the globe, forming a small pocket out of the palpebral and bulbar conjunctiva.

- Hold the dropper as near the site of deposition as possible without touching the ocular or periocular tissues. Unsteadiness can most easily be eliminated by resting the hand with the dropper on the hand holding the eyelid.

- Instruct the patient to look upward. This prevents the drop of medicine from hitting the cornea, which stimulates tearing.

- Dispense a single drop of ophthalmic solution into the pocket formed by the lower conjunctival sac and hold the lid forward momentarily to allow the drop to collect in the lower cul-de-sac.

- Advise the patient to look downward, while the lower lid is pulled upward and returned to contact with the upper eyelid. This method maximizes the volume of the cul-de-sac.

- Release the lower lid and allow the eyelids to seal gently. The eyelids should remain closed for 3 min. Lid closure prevents activation of the lacrimal 'pump' pushing medication into the lacrimal outflow system. Each blink causes this 'pumping' action.

- Instruct the patient not to blink, flutter, or squeeze the eyelids as any of these will activate the lacrimal pump for approximately 3 min. Before the eyelids are opened, blot any excess medication away from the inner canthus. Wait 5 to 10 min between applications when applying more than one eye medication.

A patient can apply their own medication in the following way (Fig. 5):

- Tilt the head back, rest the hand on the cheek, and grasp the lower eyelid below the lashes. The lid is gently lifted away from the eye.

- Hold the dropper over and as near to the eye as is safe; the hand with the dropper is resting on the hand holding the lower eyelid.

- Looking up, apply 1 drop of medication into this 'pocket'.

- Keep the eyelids closed for more than 3 min, blotting away any excess medication before opening the eyes.

The clinical significance of lid closure has been well documented, revealing a dramatic increase in ocular contact time and decline in lacrimal drainage. For example, Zimmerman demonstrated that merely closing the eyelids for 3 min can decrease plasma concentrations of timolol by 65 per cent when measured 60 min after topical application. Likewise, the therapeutic benefits of nasolacrimal occlusion are substantial, par-

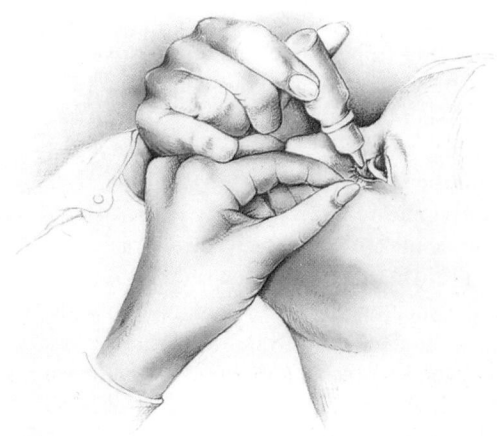

Fig. 5 Inserting topical medication: without assistance.

ticularly for drugs absorbed via non-conjunctival routes. Pressure over the lacrimal sac can allow for a decrease in both the frequency and dose of some topical ocular agents, including several antiglaucoma agents. However, it is difficult for patients to perform nasolacrimal occlusion routinely, so this technique is seldom used. Lid closure is as effective as properly applied pressure over the lacrimal outflow system, and far easier to do.

Further reading

Apt, L., Henrick, A., and Silverman, L.M. (1979). Patient compliance with use of topical ophthalmic corticosteroid suspensions. *American Journal of Ophthalmology*, **87**, 210–14.

Armaly, M.D. and Rao, K.R. (1973). The effect of pilocarpine Ocusert with different release rates on ocular pressure. *Investigative Ophthalmology and Visual Science*, **12**, 491–6.

Brown, R.H., Wood, T.S., *et al.* (1987). Improving the therapeutic index of topical phenylephrine by reducing drop volume. *Ophthalmology*, **94**, 847–50.

Edeki, T.I., Huabing, H., and Wood, A. (1995). Pharmacogenetic explanation for excessive β- blockade following timolol eye drops. Potential for oral-ophthalmic drug interaction. *Journal of the American Medical Association*, **274**, 1611–13.

Fraunfelder, F.T. (1976). Extraocular fluid dynamics: how best to apply topical ocular medication. *Transactions of the American Ophthalmological Society*, **74**, 457–87.

Fraunfelder, F.T. and Meyer, S.M. (1985). Possible cardiovascular effects secondary to topical ophthalmic 2.5 per cent phenylephrine. *American Journal of Ophthalmology*, **99**, 362–3.

Green, K. (1993). The effects of preservatives on corneal permeability of drugs. In *Biopharmaceutics of Ocular Drug Delivery*, (ed. P. Edman), p. 47. CRC Press, Boca Raton, Florida.

Harris, L.S. and Galin, M.A. (1971). Effect of ocular pigmentation on hypotensive response to pilocarpine. *American Journal of Ophthalmology*, **72**, 923–5.

Lederer, C.M. and Harold, R.E. (1986). Drop size of commercial glaucoma medications. *American Journal of Ophthalmology*, **101**, 691–4.

Lee, V.H.L. and Robinson, J.R. (1986). Topical ocular drug delivery: recent developments and future challenges. *Journal of Ocular Pharmacology*, **2**, 67–108.

Lynch, M.G., Brown, R.H., *et al.* (1987). Reduction of phenylephrine drop size in infants achieves equal dilation with decreased systemic absorption. *Archives of Ophthalmology*, **105**, 1364–5.

Massey, R.J., Hanna, C., Goodart, R., and Wallace, T. (1976). Effect of drug vehicle on human ocular retention of topically applied tetracycline. *American Journal of Ophthalmology*, **81**, 151–6.

Mikkelson, T.J., Chrai, S., and Robinson, J.R. (1973). Altered bioavailability of drugs in the eye due to drug protein interaction. *Journal of Pharmacology Science*, **62**, 1648–53.

Mishima, S. (1981). Clinical pharmacokinetics of the eye: Procter lecture. *Investigative Ophthalmology and Visual Sciences*, **21**, 504–41.

Nelson, W.L., Fraunfelder, F. T., Sills, J.M., *et al.* (1986). Adverse respiratory and cardiovascular events attributed to timolol ophthalmic solution, 1978–1985. *American Journal of Ophthalmology*, **102**, 606–11.

Ramselaar, J.A.M., Boot, J.M., *et al.* (1988). Corneal epithelial permeability after instillation of ophthalmic solutions containing local anesthetics and preservatives. *Current Eye Research*, **7**, 947.

Schoenwald, R.D. and Chien, D.S. (1987). Ocular absorption and disposition of phenylephrine and phenylephrine oxazilidine. *Biopharmaceutics and Drug Disposition*, **9**, 527–38.

Shell, J.W. (1982). Pharmacokinetics of topical applied drugs (therapeutic review). *Survey of Ophthalmology*, **26**, 207–18.

Sieg, J.W. and Robinson, J.R. (1975). Vehicle effects on ocular drug bioavailability. I. Evaluation of fluorometholone. *Journal of Pharmacology Science*, **64**, 931–6.

Urtti, A. (1985). Pilocarpine release from matrices of alkyl half-esters of poly (vinyl methyl ether/maleic anhydride). *International Journal of Pharmacology*, **26**, 45.

Urtti, A. and Saliminen, L. (1993). Minimizing systemic absorption of topical administered drugs (therapeutic review). *Survey of Ophthalmology*, **37**, 435–56.

Zimmerman, T.J., Kooner, K.S., Kandarakis, A.S., and Zeigler, L.P. (1984). Improving the therapeutic index of topically applied ocular drugs. *Archives of Ophthalmology*, **102**, 551–3.

Zimmerman, T.J., Sharir, M., Nardin, G.F., and Fuqua, M. (1992). Therapeutic index of epinephrine and dipivefrin with nasolacrimal occlusion. *American Journal of Ophthalmology*, **114**, 8–13.

1.4.2 Antiglaucoma medication

Colm O'Brien and Emer Henry

Despite the acknowledged multifactorial aetiology of glaucoma, present therapy is based on lowering intraocular pressure in an effort to halt the progression of optic disc damage and visual field loss. Intraocular pressure is determined by aqueous humour flow dynamics. Antiglaucoma agents exert their hypotensive effect by suppressing aqueous humour formation and/or facilitating aqueous outflow.

There is no mandatory level for an ideal intraocular pressure. A target pressure should be established for each patient, a level which is considered relatively safe and unlikely to cause further damage to the optic nerve. The peak intraocular pressure prior to treatment and the severity of optic disc damage and visual field loss should be considered, together with other factors such as age, race, family history of glaucoma, and the presence of other ocular or systemic disorders. In selecting a treatment regimen to achieve this target pressure, it is important to weigh the benefits of treatment against the potential side-effects, and the cost and inconvenience to the patient.

Currently, there are six main groups of antiglaucoma drugs:

- β-adrenergic antagonists
- miotics
- sympathomimetics
- carbonic anhydrase inhibitors
- prostaglandin analogues
- hypertonic agents.

Therapy is usually started with a single topical agent, such as a β-antagonist.

Assessment of the efficacy of the agent requires close monitoring of ocular pressure, the optic disc, and visual function. If the pressure is not lowered sufficiently, a further agent may be substituted for or added to the initial drug.

Patient co-operation is vital to successful medical control. It is essential to explain to each individual the nature of both the disease and treatment. Advice should be given on the possible local and systemic side-effects associated with each agent. Patients should be instructed on the correct method of instillation of their drops. Clinical trials also suggest that manually occluding the puncta or closing the eyes following instillation, limits nasolacrimal mucosal absorption and consequent systemic side-effects.

When patients are using several agents, they should be advised to leave an interval of at least 5 min between each agent to allow adequate ocular absorption. It may be wise to provide a timetable for drug instillation to maximize patient compliance. Finally, each patient must be reviewed frequently until a satisfactory treatment regimen has been established which appears to be halting the progression of visual loss.

β-Blockers

β-Blockers have been the mainstay of medical management of glaucoma for the past 15 to 20 years. They are potent hypotensive agents but systemic side-effects limit their use in a significant proportion of the glaucoma population.

Both β1 and β2 receptors are found in the eye, in the ciliary body, arterioles, and choroid. Antagonists may be non-selective in their action (timolol, levobunolol, and carteolol), or relatively β1 selective (betaxalol).

Mode of action

β-Blockers suppress aqueous humour secretion with minimal effect on outflow. The exact mechanism by which they achieve this is unclear and it is probable that blockade occurs at a number of sites including the non-pigmented ciliary epithelium and by induction of vasoconstriction in the arterioles supplying the ciliary processes. Comparative studies have shown that non-selective agents are marginally better in lowering intraocular pressure than β1-selective antagonists but their effectiveness may diminish with long-term use due to drug modulation of ocular receptors.

Indications

β-Blockers are useful in all forms of glaucoma and are first-line agents in primary open angle glaucoma and ocular hypertension. They have a significant synergy with miotics and carbonic anhydrase inhibitors but have minimal additive effects when used with sympathomimetics.

Local side-effects

These are relatively uncommon, usually mild and include conjunctival irritation, allergic blepharoconjunctivitis, corneal anaesthesia, and punctate keratitis. Preservative-free preparations of timolol and levobunolol are available for sensitized patients.

Systemic side-effects

These may be severe and represent the major restriction to the more widespread use of β-blockers. They gain access to the systemic circulation by absorption through the conjunctiva, and the mucosa of the nasolacrimal system and nasal cavity. Therefore, punctal occlusion by gentle finger pressure for 2 to 3 min following instillation should be recommended to minimize systemic side-effects.

Respiratory

Bronchospasm may be induced by blockade at bronchiolar β2 receptors and this is a particular risk in patients with already established reversible airways disease. Non-selective agents are contraindicated in these patients and the cardioselective betaxolol may be used but with great caution. If in doubt, the advice of a respiratory specialist should be sought before commencing therapy. In elderly patients, long-term treatment with non-selective antagonists causes deterioration in respiratory function, resulting in diminished exercise tolerance and reduced forced expiratory volume on spirometry.

Cardiovascular

Beta-1 blockade may result in bradycardia, heart block, and systemic hypotension. Cardiac side-effects have also been implicated in the increased risk of falls in elderly glaucoma patients. Prior to starting treatment, heart rate should be measured by the ophthalmologist. If the rate is less than 60 beats/min, then β-blockers should not be prescribed. If there is doubt about potential cardiac problems, an electrocardiogram should be carried out and the patient referred for a cardiology opinion.

Metabolic

Glucose intolerance may be exacerbated in insulin-dependent diabetes mellitus and the symptoms of hypoglycaemia may be masked. Elevation of serum lipoproteins has been reported.

General

Lethargy, dizziness, headaches, depression, and hallucinations have all been reported, especially in the elderly population. Other problems include gastrointestinal upset, impotence, decreased libido, and exacerbation of myasthenia gravis.

Preparations

1. Timolol is a non-selective antagonist, causing β1- and β2-receptor blockade and is available in 0.25 and 0.5 per cent aqueous solutions. It is effective within 30 min, peaks at 2 h, and may persist for up to 24 h. It is usually administered twice daily and at the lowest concentration which will achieve an adequate hypotensive effect. Timolol LA is a long-acting gel preparation with a lower side-effect profile which may be administered once daily.

2. Levobunolol is also non-selective and prepared in a 0.5 per cent solution. It has equal potency to timolol and has peak effect at 2 to 6 h. It has a longer duration of effect and may therefore be given once daily.

3. Carteolol is a non-selective agent with intrinsic sympathomimetic activity. This may have the added benefit of increasing optic nerve head perfusion and

reducing the likelihood of systemic complications. It is available in 1 and 2 per cent concentrations and administered twice a day.

4. Betaxolol is the only selective β1 antagonist currently available. It is relatively cardioselective and is therefore safer in patients with respiratory disease where, however, it should still be used with caution. It is prepared in a 0.5 per cent solution and is prescribed twice a day.

Miotics

Parasympathomimetics have been used in glaucoma treatment since the nineteenth century. Indirect cholinergics which inhibit cholinesterase are no longer in clinical use due to the unacceptable level of side-effects. Direct acting agents such as pilocarpine continue to form an important part of antiglaucoma therapy.

Mode of action

Cholinergics increase aqueous humour outflow. Muscarinic receptor stimulation causes the longitudinal fibres of the ciliary muscle to contract and this in turn pulls on the scleral spur to open up the trabecular meshwork. In addition, sphincter pupillae contraction causes miosis and this is of benefit in situations of angle closure.

Indications

Pilocarpine is widely used as a second-line agent in primary open angle glaucoma and is one of the main therapeutic options in angle closure glaucoma. It has good additive effect when used with both β-blockers and sympathomimetics. It is contraindicated in malignant and uveitic glaucoma.

Local side-effects

Parasympathomimetics induce miosis and ciliary spasm.

1. Miosis decreases night vision and visual acuity in those with axial lens opacities. It further constricts an already compromised visual field, resulting in diffuse depression of the hill of vision.

2. Sustained ciliary spasm gives rise to brow ache which may wane with time. It also causes varying myopia which is troublesome and particularly poorly tolerated by younger patients.

3. Stronger concentrations of pilocarpine may induce forward movement of the lens–iris diaphragm, causing shallowing of the anterior chamber and paradoxical angle closure.

Older indirect acting anticholinesterase drugs are associated with a higher incidence of ocular side-effects.

1. External problems include contact dermatitis, chronic conjunctival injection, and more rarely ocular pemphigoid.

2. Breakdown of the blood–aqueous barrier results in variable iritis. Posterior synechiae may arise from the combination of the latter and chronic miosis. Iris cysts occur at the pupillary margin and resolve on discontinuation of use.

3. Other reported problems include a cataractogenic effect and an increased risk of retinal tears and detachments.

Systemic side-effects

These are rarely reported in patients using direct acting miotics. Cholinergic toxicity may present with gastrointestinal disturbance such as diarrhoea, abdominal cramps, and increased salivation. Bradycardia and bronchospasm also occur.

Preparations

1. Pilocarpine in drop form is available in 0.5, 1, 2, 3, and 4 per cent concentrations. It is effective within 20 min, peaks at 2 h, and lasts 4 to 6 h. It therefore requires frequent instillation, usually four times a day, which has an adverse effect on compliance. It may be used less often if given in combination with β-blockers. Pilocarpine is also available in a viscous acrylic gel, prepared in a 4 per cent concentration. This has prolonged contact time reducing the required frequency of administration to once daily, usually at night and there appears to be a lower frequency of side-effects and better patient compliance. A pilocarpine insert (Ocusert) is a continuous delivery device which is placed into the fornix once weekly. It induces less intense miosis and less variability of myopia, making it more acceptable to younger patients.

2. Carbachol 0.75 to 3 per cent has both direct and indirect actions and has a longer duration of action than pilocarpine. Its use is usually limited to cases resistant to pilocarpine.

Sympathomimetics

Adrenergic agonists were once a major part of glaucoma management for many years but with the advent of more effective agents with fewer side-effects, they have been consigned to a secondary role.

Mode of action

The mechanism is not fully understood. Alpha-receptor stimulation reduces aqueous humour secretion and increases trabecular outflow. Beta-receptor stimulation increases uveoscleral outflow but also acts to increase aqueous secretion. The overall effect, however, is to decrease intraocular pressure.

Indications

Adrenergic agonists have been used in primary open angle glaucoma as an adjunct to either β-blockers or miotics. They are less effective in lowering intraocular pressure than either pilocarpine or β-blockers. They have minimal synergy with non-selective β-blockers but appear to have greater effect when used in combination with either betaxolol or pilocarpine.

Local side-effects

The frequency of local side-effects is the major drawback of sympathomimetics and has made these agents unpopular with both patient and practitioner.

1. Conjunctiva: many patients develop conjunctival irritation on injection. Up to 20 per cent develop allergic blepharoconjunctivitis. Long-term use of epinephrine is associated with adrenochrome deposits in the conjunctiva, cornea, and lacrimal system. Sympathomimetics stimulate conjunctival cellular activity, in particular inflammatory cells and fibroblasts. This can be of significance in patients who undergo filtration surgery, as prior treatment with adrenergic agonists can have a deleterious effect on surgical outcome, carrying an increased risk of bleb scarring and failure.

2. Mydriasis may precipitate angle closure.

3. Cystoid macular oedema has been reported in aphakic and pseudophakic individuals. This may resolve on cessation of treatment.

Systemic side-effects

1. Cardiovascular side-effects may be significant and include hypertension, tachycardia, and arrhythmias. Patients with established cardiovascular and cerebrovascular disease and those with diabetes and hyperthyroidism should be closely monitored for complications. Orthostatic hypotension has been reported with apraclonidine use.

2. Central nervous system problems include headache, nervousness, and sleep disturbance.

3. Gastrointestinal upset may involve abdominal pain, diarrhoea, and nausea and vomiting.

Preparations

1. Adrenaline is available in 0.5, 1, and 2 per cent concentrations. It is effective within 1 h of administration and lasts up to 24 h. It is usually given twice a day.

2. Dipivefrin 0.1 per cent is a prodrug which is converted to adrenaline on absorption into the eye. At a concentration of 0.1 per cent it has equal potency to adrenaline 1 per cent and is associated with a lower incidence of ocular side-effects.

3. Apraclonidine, an α_2-agonist, is a synthetic clonidine analogue. It is a powerful suppressant of aqueous formation and is effective within 1 h of administra-

tion. It is generally used for short-term prevention of surgical- or laser-induced pressure spikes, for example following laser iridotomy, trabeculoplasty, and capsulotomy. Long-term use with twice or three times daily instigation is restricted by the high incidence of allergic blepharoconjunctivitis, systemic side-effects, and the reduced hypotensive effect that occurs with chronic use.

4. Brimonidine is a new, highly selective α_2-agonist which has recently become available. It is a potent ocular hypotensive and appears to have a better safety profile and none of the tachyphylaxis associated with long-term apraclonidine use. It is administered twice daily in a 0.2 per cent concentration.

Carbonic anhydrase inhibitors

Mode of action

The enzyme carbonic anhydrase has a significant role in the production of aqueous humour. It catalyses the formation of bicarbonate from carbonic acid in the non-pigmented ciliary epithelial cells and this is linked to the passage of sodium from plasma to aqueous. Carbonic anhydrase inhibitors are sulphonamide derivatives which can lower the intraocular pressure by up to 65 per cent. A secondary hypotensive effect may be mediated by the induction of acidosis.

Indications

The systemically administered inhibitor, acetazolamide, has a highly potent hypotensive effect and is of particular use in conditions of acute, severe intraocular pressure rise, such as angle closure glaucoma. Long-term use in the treatment of primary open angle glaucoma has been restricted by the frequency and severity of systemic side-effects with full dose therapy. Dichlorphenamide has a longer duration of action and may be given less often. Dorzolamide is a topical preparation which has recently become available. It is becoming increasingly popular as a second-line agent in primary open angle glaucoma. Carbonic anhydrase inhibitors have a good additive effect with β-blockers and miotics. They should be used with caution in patients with a history of renal impairment.

Local side-effects

Many patients complain of burning, stinging and tearing, and a metallic taste following the instillation of dorzolamide. About 10 per cent develop evidence of allergic blepharoconjunctivitis.

Systemic side-effects

A large proportion of patients develop systemic problems when treated with full dose, oral carbonic anhydrase inhibitors.

1. General side-effects are common and include malaise and lethargy.

2. Gastrointestinal upset such as anorexia, heartburn,

nausea, taste disturbance, abdominal discomfort, and diarrhoea occur frequently.

3. Paraesthesia of the peripheries is common and may diminish with time.

4. Renal and metabolic: hypokalaemia is not uncommon with long-term therapy and patients require regular monitoring of electrolytes and oral potassium supplementation if indicated. Metabolic acidosis and urinary frequency may also occur. Renal calculi form in up to 5 per cent of those on long-term treatment. This is thought to be related to decreased urinary citrate with consequent reduction in the chelation and solubilization of urinary calcium.

5. Rare complications include bone marrow suppression causing agranulocytosis, thrombocytopenia, and rarely aplastic anaemia. Stevens–Johnson syndrome has also been documented.

Preparations

1. Acetazolamide in oral form is available in 250 and 500 mg tablets. The onset of action is within 1 h, peaking at 4 h, and lasting up to 12 h. A slow-release 250-mg tablet is available. Parenteral acetazolamide is administered in intravenous bolus of 500 mg and has an immediate effect which lasts up to 4 h.

2. Dichlorphenamide is administered in a starting dose of 100 to 200 mg followed by 100 mg twice daily maintenance dose.

3. Dorzolamide 2 per cent is a topical carbonic anhydrase inhibitor which can reduce aqueous humour secretion by up to 25 per cent. It does not appear to have any of the severe systemic side-effects associated with oral carbonic anhydrase inhibitors. It is administered three times daily if given alone but can be reduced to twice daily when used in combination with a β-blocker.

Prostaglandin analogues

Prostaglandin analogues are highly effective hypotensive drugs which appear to have minimal systemic side-effects.

Mode of action

Synthetic analogues of prostaglandin $F_{2\alpha}$, such as latanoprost, facilitate uveoscleral outflow and can lower the intraocular pressure by up to 30 per cent.

Indications

Latanoprost has been used on patients with primary open angle glaucoma and ocular hypertension where it appears to be as potent as timolol. It has a good additive effect with aqueous humour suppressants such as β-blockers.

Local side-effects

Conjunctival irritation and hyperaemia have been reported in up to 30 per cent of patients. Increased iris pigmentation is also a recognized effect, particularly in green–brown coloured irides.

Systemic side-effects

Latanoprost has not been associated with significant cardiovascular or respiratory complications.

Preparations

Latanoprost in a 0.006 per cent solution is administered once daily in the evening.

Hyperosmotic agents

Mode of action

Systemically administered hyperosmotic agents increase blood osmolality and create an osmotic gradient between the blood and intraocular fluids. This draws water out of the eye leading to a reduction in intraocular volume and pressure.

Indications

Hyperosmotic agents are used for rapid reduction of intraocular pressure, in situations of acute and severe pressure rise which are refractory to other treatment options.

Side-effects

1. Nausea and vomiting commonly occur following administration of sweet compounds such as glycerol.

2. Cardiovascular problems arise due to a sudden increase in the cardiac preload. Congestive heart failure and myocardial infarction are recognized complications especially in patients with already compromised cardiac function.

3. Neurological effects include headache, vertigo, and confusion. There are also reports of subdural and subarachnoid haemorrhage following treatment with hyperosmotic agents.

4. Renal and metabolic: diuresis resulting from hyperosmotic therapy may precipitate urinary retention, especially in elderly men with prostatic hypertrophy. Glucose-based compounds may precipitate hyperglycaemia and even ketoacidosis in diabetics.

5. Anaphylaxis has been reported in association with mannitol.

Preparations

1. Oral forms include glycerol and isosorbide. The recommended dose is 1 to 2 g per kilogram of body

weight. Peak hypotensive effect is achieved at 1 h and may last for up to 4 to 6 h.

2. Intravenous mannitol is administered in a dose of 1 to 2 g per kilogram of body weight. It is infused over 30 min and reaches peak activity at 30 min. Its effects may last for up to 6 h.

The future

There are an ever increasing number of antiglaucoma drugs becoming available, as present agents are revised and refined, and newer agents are developed.

Future treatment may focus on manipulating other factors involved in the pathogenesis of glaucomatous optic neuropathy. The challenge now is to develop agents which have a neuroprotective effect on retinal ganglion cells and enhance blood supply to the optic nerve head.

Further reading

Allen, R.C., Hertzmark, E., Walker, A.M., and Epstein, D.L. (1986). A double-masked comparison of betaxolol versus timolol in the treatment of open angle glaucoma. *American Journal of Ophthalmology*, **101**, 535–41.

Alm, A. and Stjernschantz, J. (1995). Effects on intraocular pressure and side-effects of 0.005 per cent latanaprost applied once daily, evening or morning. *Ophthalmology*, **102**, 1743–52.

Beasley, H. and Fraunfelder, F. (1979). Retinal detachments and topical ocular miotics. *Ophthalmology*, **86**, 95.

Bene, D.J. and Zimmennan, T.J. (1994). Perspectives in the drug treatment of glaucoma. *Current Opinion in Ophthalmology*, **5**, 99–104.

British Medical Association and Royal Pharmaceutical Society of Great Britain (1996). *British National Formulary*, March, Number 31.

Broadway, D.C., Grierson, I., O'Brien, C., and Hitchings, R. (1994). Adverse effects of topical anti-glaucoma medication 11. The outcome of filtration surgery. *Archives of Ophthalmology*, **112**, 1446.

Camras, C.B., Alm, A., Watson, P., *et al.* (1996). Latanaprost, a prostaglandin analogue for glaucoma therapy: efficacy and safety after 1 year of treatment in 198 patients. *Ophthalmology*, **103**, 1916–24.

Chacko, D.M. and Camras, C.B. (1994). The potential of alpha-2 adrenergic agonists in the medical treatment of glaucoma. *Current Opinion in Ophthalmology*, **5**, 76–84.

Coakes, R.L. and Brubaker, R.F. (1973). The mechanism of timolol in lowering intraocular pressure. *Archives of Ophthalmology*, **96**, 2045–52.

Diggory, P., Cassels-Brown, A., Vall, A., Abbey, L., and Hillman, J. (1995). Avoiding unsuspected respiratory side-effects of topical timolol by using cardioselective or sympathetic agents. *Lancet*, **345**, 1604–6.

Diggory, P. and Franks, W. (1996). Medical treatment of glaucoma—a reappraisal of the risks. *British Journal of Ophthalmology*, **80**, 85–9.

Lippa, E.A., *et al.* (1992). Dose response and duration of action of dorzolamide, a topical carbonic anhydrase inhibitor. *Archives of Ophthalmology*, **110**, 495.

Lowis, R.A. (1989). Medical management of glaucoma. In *Duane's clinical ophthalmology*, Vol. 3 (ed. W. Tasman and E.A. Jaeger). Lippincott, Philadelphia.

Nagasubramanian, S., Hitchings, R., Demailly, P., *et al.* (1993). Comparison of apraclonidine and timolol in chronic open angle glaucoma—a three month study. *Ophthalmology*, **100**, 1318.

Nordland, J.R., Pasquale, L, Robin, A., *et al.* (1995). The cardiovascular, pulmonary and ocular hypotensive effects of 0.2 per cent brimonidine. *Archives of Ophthalmology*, **113**, 77–83.

Pavan-Langston, D. (1996). *Handbook of ocular drug therapy and ocular side effects of systemic drugs*, (4th edn) pp. 235–42. Little, Brown, London.

Salminen, L. (1990). Systemic absorption of topically applied ocular drugs in humans. *Journal of Ocular Pharmacology*, **6**, 243–9.

Schuman, J.S. (1996). Clinical experience with brimonidine 0.2 per cent and timolol 0.5 per cent in glaucoma and ocular hypertension. *Survey of Ophthalmology*, **41** (suppl 1), S27–37.

Schumar, R.A. and Podos, S.M. (1993). Medical treatment of newly diagnosed open angle glaucoma. *Journal of Glaucoma*, **2**, 211–22.

Serle, J.B. (1996). A comparison of the safety and efficacy of twice daily brimonidine 0.2 per cent versus betaxolol 0.25 per cent in subjects with elevated intraocular pressure. *Survey of Ophthalmology*, **41** (suppl 1), S39–47.

Sherwood, M., Migdal, C., Hitchings, R., *et al.* (1993). Initial treatment of glaucoma: surgery or medications. *Survey of Ophthalmology*, **37**, 293–305.

Strahlman, E.R., *et al.* (1996). The use of dorzolamide and pilocarpine as adjunctive therapy in patients with elevated intraocular pressure. *Ophthalmology*, **103**, 1283–93.

Urtti, A. and Salminen, L. (1993). Minimizing systemic absorption of topically administered ophthalmic drugs. *Survey of Ophthalmology*, **37**, 435–56.

Watson, P., Stjernschantz, J., Beck, L., *et al.* A six-month randomized, double-masked study comparing latanaprost with timolol in open-angle glaucoma and ocular hypertension. *Ophthalmology*, **103**, 126–37.

1.4.3 Antibacterial, antiviral, and antifungal agents

Jeremy Diamond and John Leeming

Infections of the eye and its adnexae are common causes of ocular disease. They range from self-limiting inflammation of the external eye to sight-threatening endophthalmitis.

The choice of agent for treatment of microbial disease is dependent upon the susceptibility of known or suspected causative organisms, the site and severity of infection, possible side-effects, patient compliance with treatment regimens, and cost. The route of application is dependent upon the ability of the chosen agent to penetrate to the site of infection at a concentration likely to be effective against the causative organisms. Options include topical drops and ointments; subconjunctival, subtenon, intracameral, or intravitreal injections; and systemic administration. Finally, the frequency of drug application is determined by the half-life of the drug at the site of infection.

Favoured treatment regimens for serious ocular infections are frequently unlicensed. Inclusion of a regimen in this chapter does not indicate approval by any regulatory body, but is a reflection of common ophthalmic practice.

Antibacterial agents

External ocular infection

External ocular bacterial infections can usually be treated effectively using topical antibacterial preparations. Acute bacterial conjunctivitis is a self-limiting condition but there is evidence that the course of infection can be shortened by antibiotics. Blepharitis is usually a chronic condition with no single cause; antibiotics can be helpful in a proportion of cases.

Very high peak concentrations of antibiotic are achieved at the site of infection by topical application, but dilution by tears rapidly reduces the concentrations of most eye-drop formulations necessitating frequent dosing to maintain drug levels above minimum inhibitory concentrations. This is a particularly important consideration in invasive infections (bacterial keratitis and ulcers). Ointments persist longer than drops but are less comfortable for patients and blur vision. Collagen shields soaked in antibiotic, which have been shown to increase both peak drug levels and prolong drug elution time, can be used in severe infection. Penetration of the corneal stroma is a consideration in invasive infection; this is aided by disruption of the tight junctions of the corneal epithelium as a consequence of epithelial or stromal infection.

Most of the commercially available ophthalmic antibiotic preparations are satisfactory for the treatment of bacterial conjunctivitis, blepharitis, and mild keratoconjunctivitis, which are normally treated empirically. However, for bacterial ulcers more attention must be given to factors such as the spectrum of activity of the agent and whether it is bactericidal or merely bacteristatic. Where possible choice of antibiotic should be guided by laboratory data. Combination therapy is usually employed to provide the required broad-spectrum cover when the causative organism has not been identified.

Ophthalmia neonatorum requires systemic antibiotic treatment (again guided by microbiology results) in order to minimize the incidence of serious sequelae.

Chloramphenicol

Chloramphenicol is available as both 0.5 per cent drops and 1 per cent ointments. It was developed in the 1940s and for much of the period since has been a popular choice in the treatment of non-invasive external eye disease. The advantages of chloramphenicol are that it has a broad spectrum of activity, being effective against the majority of ocular pathogens (but not *Pseudomonas aeruginosa* or *Chlamydia trachomatis*), it is inexpensive, is available in unpreserved preparations, and it has a low incidence of local sensitivity reactions. The major problem with chloramphenicol is its association with bone marrow toxicity. This may take the form of a reversible, dose-related suppression, or irreversible, idiosyncratic aplastic anaemia. The latter is less common but more serious, being associated with a mortality in the order of 50 per cent. The incidence of serious aplastic anaemia is around 1 in 30 000 oral courses but is much rarer following the administration of eye-drops. There have been over 38 million prescriptions for topical chloramphenicol in England alone since 1980, but only eight cases of bone marrow suppression associated with topical chloramphenicol have been reported for the United Kingdom since 1966. There have been at least 23 further cases of marrow suppression documented worldwide though these mainly followed prolonged courses of weeks or months and several cases were also exposed to other risk factors. However, as a result of these reports American authorities have recommended that chloramphenicol eye-drops are used only in cases where bacterial isolates are resistant to all other available agents and a family history of drug-related haemopoietic toxicity has been excluded, advice

which effectively precludes use of this drug in the United States. While chloramphenicol remains a popular first-line topical agent in Europe and Australia, its use should be restricted to short courses.

Fusidic acid

Fusidic acid is available as 1 per cent viscous drops which liquefy in contact with the eye. This preparation has proved popular, largely because of the persistence of fusidic acid after application, which facilitates reduced frequency of application compared to most other formulations (one drop twice daily recommended). Fusidic acid has a narrow spectrum of activity and in other infective processes is used mainly as an antistaphylococcal agent, usually in combination with another agent to combat the tendency of bacteria to acquire resistance rapidly (noted *in vitro* but not often reported *in vivo*). However, at the high concentrations achieved in the eye, fusidic acid may have useful activity against some other ocular pathogens including streptococci and *Haemophilus* spp., and there are trial data demonstrating outcomes comparable with chloramphenicol in conjunctivitis. *Pseudomonas aeruginosa* and most other Gram-negative bacteria are resistant to fusidic acid, precluding its use as a first-line agent in the treatment of keratitis.

Polymyxin-based combinations

Polymyxin B sulphate is a bactericidal antibiotic available in combination with bacitracin (ointment), trimethoprim (drops and ointment), and neomycin plus gramicidin (drops). The rationale behind these products is that the combination of complementary narrow-spectrum agents can produce preparations active against a wide range of bacteria. Polymyxin is active against most Gram-negative ocular pathogens, including *Pseudomonas aeruginosa*, bacitracin is active against staphylococci, streptococci, and *Neisseria* spp.; trimethoprim is active against many Gram-positive and Gram-negative bacteria, but not *Pseudomonas aeruginosa*; neomycin has a similar spectrum of activity to trimethoprim but is inactive against streptococci. With the exception of neomycin (see below), these agents are of low toxicity (used topically) and in trials clinical results compared favourably with chloramphenicol and gentamicin in the treatment of conjunctivitis. However, some organisms causing bacterial keratitis (e.g. *Serratia* spp.) are inherently resistant, acquired resistance rates among ocular pathogens are relatively high, and the preparations are not reliably bactericidal. These factors limit their usefulness in invasive infections.

Tetracyclines

Tetracycline and chlortetracycline are both available in topical ophthalmic preparations. The indications for use of these bacteristatic agents is limited by the inherent resistance of many Gram-negative bacteria and the acquired resistance of some staphylococci. Their most important use is for the treatment of chlamydial infections.

Aminoglycosides

The aminoglycosides are bactericidal antibiotics which act by inhibiting bacterial protein synthesis. The aminoglycosides available for ophthalmic use can, for convenience, be divided into those active against *Pseudomonas aeruginosa* (gentamicin and tobramycin) and those that are not (neomycin and framycetin). With this exception they have similar spectra of activity, being effective against most Gram-negative bacteria and staphylococci but considerably less so against streptococci. However, gentamicin and tobramycin are effective at lower concentrations and a much lower proportion of clinical isolates have acquired resistance to these agents. Furthermore, in addition to their systemic toxicity, neomycin and framycetin are often irritant when topically applied and can cause sensitization after prolonged application. For these reasons neomycin and framycetin have limited application in ophthalmic practice. The rapid bactericidal action of gentamicin and tobramycin and their activity against *Pseudomonas aeruginosa* make them useful agents in the treatment of bacterial keratitis, but they do not penetrate the cornea well. Locally prepared fortified solutions (typically gentamicin at 15 g/l) are therefore generally used until the condition improves. At such concentrations marked corneal epithelial toxicity may arise, especially after prolonged use. Simultaneous instillation of a β-lactam agent is necessary for empirical therapy to cover streptococcal infection and improve activity against staphylococci.

β-Lactams

The β-lactam based agents (penicillins and cephalosporins) are relatively unstable in aqueous solution and so are not commercially available as eye-drops. However, solutions suitable for topical therapy of bacterial keratitis can be formulated locally from intravenous preparations. Penicillin G has a narrow spectrum of activity but can be used (at 0.1–0.5 MU/ml) for the treatment of keratitis known to be caused by sensitive *Streptococcus pneumoniae* (note that β-lactam resistance is now a problem in many centres). Cephalosporins (e.g. cephazolin and cefuroxime, 50 mg/ml) are resistant to staphylococcal β-lactamases and are used in combination with aminoglycosides in the empirical treatment of keratitis. Methicillin-resistant staphylococci are not susceptible to cephalosporins.

Fluoroquinolones

Ciprofloxacin and ofloxacin have been formulated for topical ophthalmic use (0.3 per cent preparations). These are synthetic broad-spectrum bactericidal agents, particularly active against the majority of Gram-negative pathogens, including *Haemophilus* spp., *Neisseria gonorrhoeae*, *Chlamydia trachomatis*, and Enterobacteriaceae. Both ofloxacin (versus chloramphenicol or aminoglycosides for conjunctivitis, blepharitis, blepharoconjunctivitis, and keratoconjunctivitis) and ciprofloxacin (versus tobramycin or placebo for conjunctivitis) have proved successful in the treatment of superficial eye disease. No serious side-effects of fluoroquinolone application were reported in any of these trials.

For the treatment of bacterial keratitis fluoroquinolones have the advantage that they penetrate the cornea well. Ciprofloxacin has greater activity against *Pseudomonas aeruginosa* than ofloxacin, while ofloxacin is more soluble than ciprofloxacin at physiological pH and exhibits better penetration into the

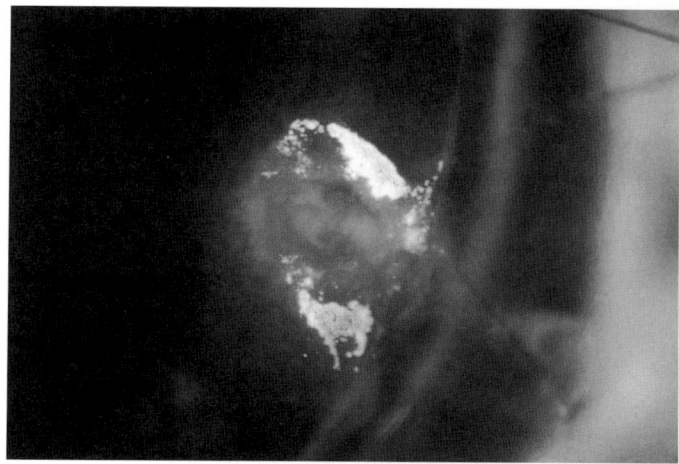

Fig. 1 Ciprofloxacin precipitate in a bacterial corneal ulcer. (By courtesy of Mathew Wade, Royal Perth Hospital.)

cornea. The reduced solubility of ciprofloxacin has resulted in precipitation after prolonged and frequent application to corneal ulcers (Fig. 1). Both ciprofloxacin and ofloxacin have been the subject of large multicentre comparison with more conventional treatment (mainly fortified combinations of cephazolin with gentamicin or tobramycin) for the treatment of bacterial keratitis of various aetiologies. Results were encouraging and suggested that monotherapy with either ciprofloxacin or ofloxacin eye-drops could reasonably be substituted for multiple-drug regimens. A note of caution must be sounded before this option is adopted widely because treatment failures have occurred in cases of streptococcal keratitis. Furthermore, fluoroquinolone resistance has been noted particularly among isolates of *Pseudomonas aeruginosa* and staphylococci in areas where fluoroquinolones are used extensively. The isolation of resistant strains from bacterial keratitis not responding to topical ciprofloxacin has also been reported. Close monitoring of the local prevalence of such strains will be important where quinolones are adopted as empirical treatment for keratitis, particularly in hospital-acquired cases.

Vancomycin

Vancomycin (3.3 per cent) can be prepared for topical application and may be useful in the treatment of methicillin-resistant *Staphylococcus aureus* or *Staphylococcus epidermidis* keratitis. Its value in serious infection should preclude its use as an empirical agent in the treatment of infections caused by more susceptible organisms.

Intraocular infection

Endophthalmitis is one of the most devastating eye diseases, and prevention of subsequent blindness presents a major therapeutic challenge.

Achieving therapeutic levels of antimicrobial agents in the anterior chamber and vitreous is difficult for a number of reasons. Access of topically applied drugs is limited by the corneal epithelium and endothelium, which inhibit transfer of fat

Table 1 Intravitreal anti-infective agents. Drugs made up to a volume of 0.1 ml for injection

Agent	Dose	Toxicity
Aminoglycosides		
gentamicin	0.1 mg	Retinal toxicity
amikacin	C.4 mg	Less toxic than gentamicin
Cephalosporins		
ceftazidime	2.0 mg	Minimal
ceftriaxone	3.0 mg	Minimal
Miscellaneous		
vancomycin	1.0 mg	Minimal
clindamycin	1.0 mg	
dexamethasone sodium phosphate	0.4 mg	
Antiviral drugs		
foscarnet	1200–2400 µg	
ganciclovir	200–400 µg	
cidofovir*	20 µg	
Antifungal drugs		
amphotericin B	5–10 µg	Retinal toxicity
miconazole	25–50 µg	

*Experimental data

insoluble agents into the anterior chamber. Once in the eye, drug diffusion posteriorly is against the anteriorly directed flow of aqueous humour and is impeded by the lens/iris diaphragm. Penetration of systemically administered drugs to the vitreous cavity is restricted by the impermeable retinal capillary bed. Many drugs are actively transported out of the vitreous cavity, further reducing achievable intraocular concentrations. Although these barriers are compromised by inflammation allowing increased penetration of fat insoluble compounds, intravitreal antibiotic injections are usually required to achieve adequate drug concentrations in the vitreous. Selected agents are generally made up to a volume of 0.1 ml and given via separate syringes to avoid risk of precipitation. Administration often follows diagnostic or therapeutic vitrectomy, and may be repeated if necessary after 2 to 4 days, especially where clinical signs suggest a persistence, or increase in inflammation. Despite the difficulties with absorption, intravitreous antibiotic injections are often supplemented by drugs administered systemically (Table 1).

The selection of intravitreal antibiotic treatment for endophthalmitis remains controversial because of the difficulties encountered in evaluating treatment outcomes in an objective manner. Some antibiotics, notably the aminoglycosides, have proven toxic to the retina when administered into the vitreous cavity. Retinal damage may also arise despite sterilization of the vitreous, probably as a consequence of toxins released from dead or dying organisms and white cells. Consequently some clinicians employ intravitreal injections of a steroid given concurrently with an antibiotic in an attempt to reduce inflammation.

Aminoglycosides

The activities of gentamicin and tobramycin are discussed above; amikacin, which is not available as an eye-drop, has similar characteristics but is active against some bacterial isolates with acquired resistance to gentamicin and tobramycin. Gentamicin (100–200 µg), tobramycin (200 µg), and amikacin (400 µg) may be injected intravitreally in the treatment of Gram-negative endophthalmitis. In the treatment of Gram-positive endophthalmitis aminoglycosides are useful components of combination regimens as they act synergistically with vancomycin and β-lactams against many isolates of enterococci, streptococci, and staphylococci, and with clindamycin against *Bacillus cereus*. Aminoglycosides have the theoretical advantage over anti-Gram-negative β-lactams such as ceftazidime of demonstrating 'concentration-dependent killing' (their bactericidal effect increases with increased concentration above minimum inhibitory concentrations) and of exhibiting reduced susceptibility to 'inoculum effects' (their activity is not greatly diminished at high concentrations of bacteria). They also exhibit a marked postantibiotic effect (activity against exposed susceptible cells persists after concentrations have fallen below minimum inhibitory concentrations).

Intravitreous injections of gentamicin at a dose as low as 400 µg have been associated with macular infarction. Rabbit studies have suggested that amikacin is less toxic than gentamicin but retinal infarction has also been reported with this agent.

Although often employed as an adjunct to intravitreal therapy, systemically administered gentamicin does not appear to penetrate the vitreous cavity well, even in the presence of scleral trauma.

Cephalosporins

The cephalosporins offer an alternative to the aminoglycosides for covering Gram-negative endophthalmitis and although clinical experience is rather limited they have been employed successfully for this purpose. Intraocular cephalosporins have a considerably reduced incidence of retinal toxicity compared with aminoglycosides. The current favoured agent is ceftazidime (2 mg), a third-generation agent with good antipseudomonal activity. Ceftazidime has poor activity against most Gram-positive bacteria and so should be combined with an agent such as vancomycin for broad-spectrum cover.

Although most systemic cephalosporins do not penetrate the intact vitreous cavity well, scleral lacerations improve vitreous drug levels considerably. Systemic ceftazidime has been shown to penetrate inflamed vitrectomized eyes, giving intraocular concentrations above the minimum inhibitory concentration for many Gram-negative organisms.

Vancomycin

Vancomycin is a bactericidal antibiotic which inhibits cell wall synthesis in Gram-positive bacteria. Gram-negative bacteria are inherently resistant. Although its use was limited following development of semi-synthetic β-lactams, it has re-emerged as the prime agent for treatment of methicillin-resistant *Staphylococcus aureus*. The great majority of both aerobic and anaerobic Gram-positive species are susceptible to vancomycin but resistance has recently emerged among strains of enterococci. These are an increasing problem in many regions of the developed world. In addition to intravitreal injection (1 mg), it may be given intravenously (1 g 12 hourly) in the treatment of endophthalmitis, though its ocular penetration by this route is poor.

Fluoroquinolones

The fluoroquinolones are well absorbed through the gastrointestinal tract, and ciprofloxacin (oral and intravenous) has been shown to penetrate the vitreous cavity relatively well. Moreover, vitreous drug levels have been shown to increase in the presence of scleral perforations. The fluoroquinolones have a broad spectrum of activity as outlined previously. For these reasons fluoroquinolones are a reasonable choice where systemic treatment is given to augment intravitreal injections for intraocular infection.

Carbapenems

Imipenem and meropenem are the first widely available members of this new class of β-lactams. They are β-lactamase resistant and have very broad spectra of activity encompassing most Gram-positive cocci, Gram-negative organisms including *Pseudomonas aeruginosa*, and anaerobic bacteria, but not methicillin-resistant staphylococci. They are relatively small molecules with low protein binding ratios and penetrate well into closed body tissues including the eye. Despite their apparent suitability for systemic treatment of intraocular infection, experience with these agents in ophthalmic practice is currently limited.

Clindamycin

Clindamycin inhibits bacterial protein synthesis and is active against many Gram-positive bacteria and against anaerobic, but not aerobic, Gram-negative bacteria. Its spectrum includes *Staphylococcus aureus* and *Streptococcus pneumoniae* and the α-haemolytic streptococci. This drug is well absorbed orally and some success has been reported in the systemic treatment of Gram-positive intraocular infection. Intraocular clindamycin (1 mg) has proved effective against *Propionobacterium acnes* and *Bacillus cereus* endophthalmitis but less so for coagulase-negative staphylococcal endophthalmitis.

Antivirals

The development of antiviral agents has been restricted because viruses are obligate intracellular parasites which depend upon the biochemical machinery of the host cells for most of their metabolic activities. Hence, development of antiviral agents which affect only virus particles or virus-infected host cells has proved difficult. Potential sites of action of antiviral agents include attachment and penetration of the virus to the host cell, certain aspects of viral replication (such as virus-encoded thymidine kinase and reverse transcriptase of viral RNA genomes), and assembly and release of new particles. Antiviral agents are generally active only against a narrow spectrum of viruses because of the specificity of their targets. None of the currently available antiviral agents are active against non-replicating or latent virus. Most are moderately toxic and must be used with caution; the side-effects and contraindications are not comprehensively covered in this chapter.

Viruses are primarily classified according to the type of nucleic acid (DNA or RNA) they contain, whether the virus has an envelope, and their host range. Subdivisions are made serologically. Ophthalmologically important DNA viruses fall mainly into two groups: the herpes viruses (herpes simplex types 1 and 2, varicella zoster, and cytomegalovirus) and adenoviruses (various distinct serotypes causing follicular conjunctivitis, pharyngoconjunctival fever, and epidemic keratoconjunctivitis). Important RNA viruses include the picornaviruses enterovirus 70 and coxsackievirus A24 (agents of acute haemorrhagic conjunctivitis), and the retroviruses (human immunodeficiency virus, HIV, types 1 and 2).

Idoxuridine

Idoxuridine is a nucleoside analogue of thymidine which is incorporated into replicating viral nucleic acid (primarily herpes viruses), rendering those particles non-infective. Although it is active upon replicating host cells it is preferentially taken up by virus-infected cells. Idoxuridine has been shown to be active against herpes simplex keratitis and is available as a 0.1 per cent solution or a 0.5 per cent ointment. This agent can induce local sensitivity reactions including punctal stenosis.

Vidarabine

Vidarabine (adenine arabinoside) is a substituted purine nucleoside which probably acts by interfering with viral DNA synthesis. Vidarabine is active against herpes viruses and, like idoxuridine, can effect host cells as well as infected cells. It is available as a 3 per cent ophthalmic ointment administered five times daily. Topical vidarabine appears less toxic than idoxuridine.

Trifluridine

Trifluridine (trifluorothymidine, F_3T) is a fluorinated analogue of thymidine which blocks viral DNA synthesis via inhibition of thymidylate synthase. A 1 per cent solution applied topically every 2 to 4 h is active against herpes simplex virus infection. It is water soluble and appears more active against herpes virus keratitis than either idoxuridine or vidarabine.

Acyclovir

Acyclovir is a purine nucleoside analogue which differs from guanine by having an acyclic side chain. It becomes active against herpes-infected cells following conversion to acyclovir monophosphate by virus-encoded thymidine kinase. Thereafter it is phosphorylated to acyclovir triphosphate which competitively inhibits viral DNA polymerase and, once incorporated into DNA, causes termination of DNA synthesis.

Acyclovir is primarily active against herpes simplex viruses, though it also exhibits activity against varicella zoster and, to a lesser extent, cytomegalovirus. It is available as a 3 per cent ophthalmic ointment, administered five times daily in the treatment of herpes simplex keratitis. Its efficacy against herpes simplex stromal keratitis and keratitis associated with first division zoster is less clear.

Oral acyclovir (800 mg, five times daily for 7 days) is useful in the treatment of herpes zoster while intravenous acyclovir (30 mg/kg/day) is used for serious herpes infections, for example acute retinal necrosis and encephalitis. Acyclovir is also available as a 5 per cent ointment for skin lesions.

Valaciclovir

Valaciclovir is a recently launched prodrug (valyl ester) of acyclovir. Acyclovir is released by hydrolysis after systemic absorption. Activity, and probably side-effects, are similar to acyclovir but bioavailability is improved allowing reduced dosage frequency (1 g orally, three times daily for 7 days recommended for herpes zoster). It is currently only available in tablet form.

Famciclovir

Famciclovir is a new orally administered antiviral prodrug, with properties similar to valaciclovir. After hydrolysis to penciclovir it is converted into penciclovir triphosphate (by the action of virus-specific thymidine kinase) which inhibits viral DNA polymerase by competing with deoxyguanosine triphosphate for incorporation into the DNA chain. Famciclovir has a similar spectrum of activity to acyclovir but has a 10 to 20 times longer half-life, allowing more convenient dosage schedules: 250 mg three times daily (for 7 days in the treatment of shingles and 5 days for genital herpes simplex).

Ganciclovir

Ganciclovir is a purine nucleoside analogue of guanine, closely related to acyclovir. It seems to act by competing with deoxyguanosine for incorporation into DNA, resulting in termination of DNA synthesis. In contrast to acyclovir, ganciclovir is phosphorylated to its active form by cytomegalovirus as well as herpes simplex virus kinases. It is also phosphorylated by cellular enzymes, but concentrations of the active metabolite are much higher in infected than in non-infected cells and viral polymerases are more susceptible than the human equivalent.

Ganciclovir is used primarily in the treatment of cytomegalovirus retinitis in acquired immune deficiency syndrome (AIDS). It is given in an induction dose (10 mg/kg/day, for 2–3 weeks), followed by long-term maintenance treatment (5 mg/kg/day). Side-effects of intravenous ganciclovir include severe myelotoxicity, requiring reduction or cessation of treatment in about one-third of patients. Ganciclovir should not be administered systemically to patients receiving zidovudine because of the high risk of neutropenia. Intravitreous administration avoids the problems associated with systemic use, but

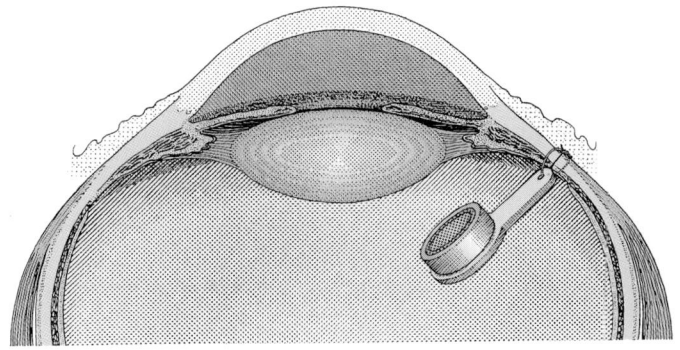

Fig. 2 Ganciclovir implant in the vitreous cavity in the treatment of cytomegalovirus retinitis. Ethylene vinyl acetate covers the ganciclovir pellet on all but its top surface, which is coated with polyvinyl alcohol. (Reproduced from Sanborn *et al.* 1992 with permission. Copyright American Medical Association.)

must be given repeatedly and has the disadvantage of not affecting extraocular cytomegalovirus infection, or infection of the fellow eye. The development of ganciclovir implants has improved long-term control of cytomegalovirus retinitis (Fig. 2), being effective for up to 8 months. Intravitreal injections of liposome-encapsulated ganciclovir has also been used to prolong the effect of this drug. The introduction of an oral preparation of ganciclovir (100 mg three times daily) may facilitate long-term systemic treatment.

Foscarnet

Foscarnet, an inorganic pyrophosphate analogue which acts by inhibiting viral DNA polymerases, has activity against cytomegalovirus. The drug can be administered intravenously (120–180 mg/kg/day induction dose followed by 120 mg/kg/day maintenance therapy), or via intravitreous injection. Systemically administered foscarnet causes nausea, vomiting, headache, and nephrotoxicity in up to 50 per cent of patients. Foscarnet and ganciclovir have been given in combination against cytomegalovirus retinitis, but because of the high incidence of side-effects foscarnet is normally reserved for patients for whom ganciclovir cannot be given or is not effective.

Cidofovir

Cidofovir is an experimental acyclic nucleoside analogue with broad-spectrum anti-DNA virus activity via competitive inhibition of viral DNA polymerase. Its activity against cytomegalovirus is 10 times that of ganciclovir and 200 times that of foscarnet. Early data suggests that a single 20 μg intravitreous dose will induce prolonged arrest of cytomegalovirus retinitis. Trials also suggest that topical application may prove to be of value in the management of adenovirus keratoconjunctivitis, for which there is currently no effective treatment.

Antifungal agents

The indolent nature of fungal infection combined with poor ocular penetration of antifungal agents (in part due to elevated tissue-binding) means that antifungal chemotherapy is often required over a prolonged period. Furthermore, laboratory determination of antifungal sensitivities is difficult because results are greatly affected by laboratory variables such as growth media employed, pH, temperature, inoculum size, and atmosphere. Correlation between *in vitro* susceptibility data and clinical response is uncertain for many drug/fungus combinations. Thus, close clinical observation of the effect of therapy is required thoughout a course of treatment. Three main classes of antifungal drugs are available.

Polyenes

The polyene antibiotics induce an increase in fungal cell envelope permeability and cell lysis mediated by their interaction with ergosterol, a lipid occurring only in fungal cell membranes. The polyenes used in ophthalmic fungal infection are amphotericin B, natamycin, and nystatin.

Amphotericin B is widely used in ophthalmology. In the treatment of anterior segment fungal infections it is administered topically at a concentration of 2.5 to 10 mg/ml. Higher concentrations cause corneal epithelial toxicity, particularly when used over long periods. Treatment is usually initiated every 30 to 60 min and extended over 4 to 6 weeks. It has long been considered the agent of choice for the treatment of fungal endophthalmitis because of its broad spectrum of activity, but note that *Fusarium* isolates are often not susceptible. Amphotericin B is less toxic than other polyenes when administered systemically, but is poorly absorbed into the eye. Intravenous treatment (0.5–1.0 mg/kg/day) is therefore usually augmented with intravitreous injection (5–10 μg in 0.1 ml).

Natamycin is too toxic to be administered intravitreously or intravenously but is less irritant than amphotericin B when administered topically (5 per cent suspension or a 1 per cent ointment). Nystatin has also been used topically in the treatment of fungal keratitis.

Azoles

These broad-spectrum antimycotic agents have several modes of action. At low concentration they inhibit synthesis of ergosterol, a component of fungal cell membranes, while at high concentration they cause direct cell membrane damage. The most widely used azoles are listed in Table 2.

Miconazole is relatively well tolerated and can be used topically (1 per cent solution), intravitreally (25–50 μg in 0.1 ml), or intravenously (200–3600 mg/day). Ketoconazole is also applicable topically (1–5 per cent solution) and is well absorbed after oral administration (200–400 mg daily). Clotrimazole is given topically (1 per cent solution) or orally (60–150 mg/kg/day). Fluconazole is given topically (2 per cent solution) and orally or intravenously (400 mg/day). These agents (particularly fluconazole) have been shown to penetrate the eye after systemic administration and there have been reports of success-

Table 2 Antifungal antibiotics

Polyenes	Azoles	Pyrimidines
Amphotericin B	Miconazole	Flucytosine
Natamycin	Ketoconazole	
Nystatin	Clotrimazole	
	Fluconazole	
	Itraconazole	
	Econazole	

ful treatment of candidal endophthalmitis using systemic fluconazole alone.

Pyrimidines

These agents are cytotoxic drugs with antimycotic activity. Flucytosine, the most important pyrimidine, is converted within the fungal cell into 5-fluorouracil which is subsequently incorporated into RNA. It may be used both topically (1 per cent solution) and orally (50–150 mg/kg/day). It is often used in combination with amphotericin B.

Further reading

Cantrill, H.L., Henry, K., Melroe, H., Knobloch, W.H., Ramsay, R.C., and Balfour, H.H. (1989). Treatment of cytomegalovirus retinitis with intravitreal ganciclovir. Long-term results. *Ophthalmology*, **96**, 367–74.

Carlson, A.N., Foulks, G.N., Perfect, J.R., and Kim, J.H. (1991). Fungal scleritis after cataract surgery. Successful outcome using itraconazole. *Cornea*, **11**, 151–4.

Diaz-Llopis, M., Espana, E., Munoz, G., *et al* (1994). High dose intravitreal foscarnet in the treatment of cytomegalovirus retinitis in AIDS. *British Journal of Ophthalmology*, **78**, 120–4.

Fraunfelder, F.T. and Bagby, G.C. (1983). Ocular chloramphenicol and aplastic anemia. *New England Journal of Medicine*, **308**, 1536.

Gigliotti, F., Hendley, J.O., Morgan, J., Michaels, R., Dickens, M., and Lohr, J. (1984). Efficacy of topical antibiotic therapy in acute conjunctivitis in children. *Journal of Pediatrics*, **104**, 623–6.

Gordon, Y.J., Romanowski, E.G., and Araullo-Cruz, T. (1994). Topical HPMPC inhibits adenovirus type 5 in the New Zealand rabbit ocular replication model. *Investigative Ophthalmology and Visual Science*, **35**, 4135–43.

Kirsch, L.S., Arevalo, J.F., Chavez de la Paz, E., Munguia, D., de Clercq, E., and Freeman, W.R. (1995). Intravitreal ciclofovir (HPMPC) treatment of cytomegalovirus retinitis in patients with aquired immune deficiency syndrome. *Ophthalmology*, **102**, 533–43.

Lambert, H.P. and O'Grady, F.W. (1992). *Antibiotics and chemotherapy*, (6th edn). Churchill Livingstone, Edinburgh.

Leibowitz, H.M. (1991). Antimicrobial effectiveness of ciprofloxacin 0.3 per cent ophthalmic solution in the treatment of bacterial conjunctivitis. *American Journal of Ophthalmology*, **112**, 29S–33S.

Luttrull, J.K., Lee Wan, W., Kubak, B.M., Smith, M.D., and Oster, H.A. (1994). Treatment of ocular fungal infections with oral fluconazole. *American Journal of Ophthalmology*, **119**, 477–81.

McCulley, J.P., Binder, P.S., Kaufman, H.E., O'Day, D., and Poitier, R.H. (1982). A double-blind, multicenter clinical trial of acyclovir vs idoxuridine for treatment of epithelial herpes simplex keratitis. *Ophthalmology*, **89**, 1195–200.

McDermott, M.L., Tran, T.D., Cowden, J.W., and Buggé, C.J.L. (1993). Corneal stromal penetration of topical ciprofloxacin in humans. *Ophthalmology*, **100**, 197–200.

Mandell, G.L., Bennett, J.E., and Dolin, R. (ed.) (1995). *Principles and practice of infectious diseases*, (4th edn). Churchill Livingstone, New York.

O'Brien, T., Maguire, M.G., Fink, N.E., Alfonso, E., McDonnell, P., and the Bacterial Keratitis Study Research Group (1995). Efficacy of ofloxacin vs cefazolin in the therapy for bacterial keratitis: report from the bacterial keratitis study research group. *Archives of Ophthalmology*, 113, 1257–65.

Parks, D.J., Abrams, D.A., Sarfarazi, F.A., and Katz, H.R. (1993). Comparison of topical ciprofloxacin to conventional antibiotic therapy in the treatment of ulcerative keratitis. *American Journal of Ophthalmology*, 115, 471–7.

Sanborn, G.E., Anand, R., Torti, R.E., *et al.* (1992). Sustained-release ganciclovir therapy for treatment of cytomegalovirus retinitis. *Archives of Ophthalmology*, 110, 188–95.

Sinclair, N.M. (1988). A comparison of fusidic acid viscous eye drops and chloramphenicol eye ointment in acute conjunctivitis. *Current Therapeutic Research*, 44, 468–74.

Snyder, M.E. and Katz, H.R. (1992). Ciprofloxacin-resistant bacterial keratitis. *American Journal of Ophthalmology*, 114, 336–8.

Weinberg, D.V., Murphy, R., and Naughton, K. (1994). Combined daily therapy with intravenous ganciclovir and foscarnet for patients with recurrent cytomegalovirus retinitis. *American Journal of Ophthalmology*, 117, 776–82.

Whitley, R.J. and Gnann, J.W. (1992). Acyclovir: a decade later. *New England Journal of Medicine*, 327, 782–9.

1.4.4 Anti-inflammatory drugs

Parimal Bhattacherjee and Mordechai Sharir

Anti-inflammatory drugs consist of heterogeneous groups of compounds differing in chemical structure, biology, and mode of action and can be broadly classified as steroidal and non-steroidal. Although the principal mechanism of anti-inflammatory action of each group is different, there is some degree of overlap between the classes. Pharmacology of non-steroidal and steroidal drugs is described in the following section.

Non-steroidal anti-inflammatory drugs

For almost 2000 years, willow bark extracts have been used in medical practice for treating arthritis and other inflammatory conditions. The active ingredients in the willow bark extract were identified as salicin and salicylic acid in the nineteenth century, and subsequently acetylsalicylic acid, now commonly known as aspirin, was synthesized. In 1972, Vane's group in England discovered that aspirin and indomethacin inhibit the synthesis of prostaglandins and suggested that such an inhibition is the basis of antipyretic and anti-inflammatory actions of aspirin and aspirin-like drugs. The non-steroidal anti-inflammatory drugs represent a diverse group of compounds with common mechanisms of action.

Pharmacology

Arachidonic acid present in the cell membrane phospholipid moiety, released by phospholipase A_2, is metabolized by prosta-glandin synthases (cyclo-oxygenases) to prostaglandins, thromboxane, and prostacyclin (Fig. 1) in response to biological stimuli. Prostaglandins and thromboxane mediate vasodilation, increased vascular permeability, leucocyte infiltration, and platelet aggregation. These products are formed *de novo* and released during inflammatory reactions in various animal and human tissues including ocular tissues. Numerous pharmacological studies have established that the anti-inflammatory effects of all non-steroidal anti-inflammatory drugs are due to the inhibition of prostaglandin synthases.

Non-steroidal anti-inflammatory drugs in the treatment of ocular inflammation

There are a large number of non-steroidal anti-inflammatory drugs of varying anti-inflammatory potency. For the treatment of ocular inflammation, a topical or intraocular mode of administration is preferred to systemic administration, because of severe gastrointestinal problems that accompany long-term treatment. Almost all non-steroidal anti-inflammatory drugs used clinically for the treatment of pain and inflammation of internal organs are administered orally. However, for the treatment of ocular inflammation, only those compounds with proven bioavailability and efficacy are used; these compounds are discussed below.

Flurbiprofen and suprofen

Both drugs are propionate derivatives that have been approved in the United States for the inhibition of intraoperative miosis. The 0.03 per cent flurbiprofen and 1.0 per cent suprofen ophthalmic solutions penetrate the cornea in sufficient concentrations to inhibit the synthesis of various prostaglandins. Evidence shows that when used in conjunction with tropicamide or cyclopentolate, flurbiprofen and suprofen significantly increased the mean pupil size as compared to placebo. But other reports indicated that the effect was marginal and influenced by the surgical technique, iris colour, presence of diabetes, and patient age. Few studies suggest some benefit with the use of 0.03 per cent flurbiprofen, but none with 1.0 per cent suprofen, in reducing cystoid macular oedema and suppression of the breakdown of the blood–aqueous barrier during the early postoperative period. The effect of 0.03 per cent flurbiprofen on post-laser uveitis has been disappointing; but unlike topical corticosteroids, it does not tend to increase the intraocular pressure, especially in steroid-responders.

A multicentre study suggested that 1.0 per cent suprofen may have some benefit in alleviating the discomfort and pain associated with contact lens induced giant papillary conjunctivitis, shortening the duration of symptoms.

Ketorolac tromethamine

In 0.5 per cent concentration, ketorolac was as efficacious as 0.1 per cent dexamethasone phosphate in reducing the adnexal and intraocular inflammatory response following cataract surgery, as judged by slit lamp biomicroscopy and fluorophoto-

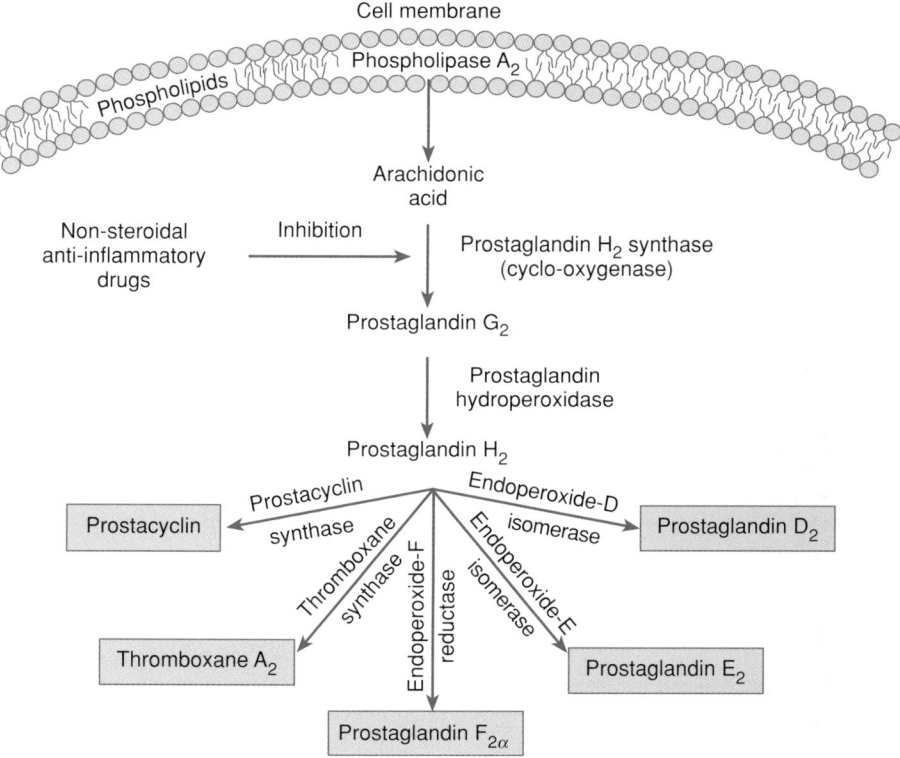

Fig. 1 Biosynthetic pathways of prostaglandins and the site of actions of non-steroidal anti-inflammatory agents.

metric studies. This acetate derivative could also be useful in the reduction of angiographic cystoid macular oedema, acute postoperative or chronic, but vision was not improved unless steroids were also added. Despite its anti-inflammatory properties, ketorolac does not significantly delay corneal wound healing.

Diclofenac sodium

Diclofenac sodium is a phenylacetic derivative, and is available as 0.1 per cent sterile ophthalmic solution (Voltaren Ophtha). Diclofenac appears to inhibit the prostaglandin synthase pathway, and therefore significantly reduce the bioavailability of prostaglandins. At high concentrations of diclofenac, the production of leukotrienes is indirectly lowered due to the shunting of arachidonic acid into triglyceride formation. Specifically, the concentrations of prostaglandin E_2 are reduced following photorefractive surgery in the rabbit, although there is no decrease in the inflammatory reaction, as judged by histological preparations. Thus, some studies have suggested alternative mechanisms by which diclofenac exerts its anti-inflammatory and analgesic effects, possibly via other arachidonic acid metabolites.

Evaluation of the ability of diclofenac to decrease postoperative inflammation has demonstrated some benefit in patients who underwent extracapsular cataract surgery with the implantation of posterior chamber intraocular lens. While the

ciliary injection and anterior chamber response were reduced, the intraocular pressure was not significantly changed when compared to a vehicle alone or to steroids. Other studies showed that diclofenac can effectively inhibit the immediate inflammatory response after laser trabeculoplasty and can be as effective as flurbiprofen in sustaining intraoperative pupil dilation.

Diclofenac might slow early corneal epithelial wound healing following abrasions, but appears to have lesser or no effect on the stroma where deep wounds or contact lens trauma are concerned.

Side-effects of non-steroidal anti-inflammatory drugs

All non-steroidal anti-inflammatory drugs are local irritants. The spectrum of complaints associated with their use ranges from transient conjunctival hyperaemia, stinging, burning, excessive tearing, and fogged vision to severe reactions of allergy, idiosyncrasy, and other types of hypersensitivity that necessitate their discontinuation. Ketorolac is formulated as a tromethamine salt, and caffeine is added to suprofen to alleviate pain and decrease local irritation.

With the exception of flurbiprofen, all other non-steroidal anti-inflammatory drugs are preserved in benzalkonium chloride which may augment local discomfort, and special caution must be employed in contact lens wearers, where some advocate abandoning the use of non-steroidal anti-inflammatory drugs altogether due to burning and pain. As mentioned earlier, non-steroidal anti-inflammatory drugs could delay wound healing and worsen punctate keratitis.

Contraindications

Due to the fact that non-steroidal anti-inflammatory drugs have aspirin-like properties, these compounds are contraindicated in patients with known allergy to aspirin. Caution should be employed in patients with bleeding problems and blood dyscrasia. Due to the fact that aspirin could worsen bronchospasm, special attention should be given when non-steroidal anti-inflammatory drugs are given to patients with bronchial asthma, hay fever, vasomotor rhinitis, nasal polyposis, and sinusitis.

Steroidal anti-inflammatory drugs

Glucocorticoids are potent anti-inflammatory agents with diverse mechanisms of actions and are most widely used in treating a variety of inflammatory diseases of various organs, including the eye. Anti-inflammatory and immunosuppressive actions of glucocorticoids were demonstrated as early as 1948. Since then, these compounds have proved extremely effective in treating immunoproliferative and connective tissue disorders, systemic lupus erythematosus, necrotizing vasculitis, allergy, and many other diseases. In ocular inflammatory diseases, acute or chronic, glucocorticoids given topically in small concentrations are the primary choice of treatment. The natural glucocorticoids such as cortisone and its metabolite, hydrocortisone, are effective only at high doses, which elicit undesirable side-effects. The derivatives of glucocorticoids, such as prednisolone and dexamethasone (Fig. 2), synthesized in the 1960s, are extremely potent with reduced side-effects. In this section, basic pharmacology and mechanisms of anti-inflammatory actions of glucocorticoids are described.

Anti-inflammatory activities

In general, inflammation of tissues are manifested inter- and intracellularly by increased vascular permeability and plasma protein exudation, leucocyte infiltration, and degradation of connective tissues. The presence of some or all of these responses depend on whether the inflammation is immunogenic or non-immunogenic and its severity. These inflammatory events are mediated by chemical mediators and factors elaborated by tissues and leucocytes during the course of inflammatory reactions. Actions that underlie anti-inflammatory activities of glucocorticoids are the inhibition of (a) biosynthesis of inflammatory mediators by neutrophils, basophils, fibroblasts, vascular smooth muscles, and endothelial cells; and (b) generation of immunoregulatory and proinflammatory factors (interferon-γ, interleukins, tumour necrosis factor-α) by macrophages and lymphocytes. The molecular mechanisms of anti-inflammatory actions of glucocorticoids are discussed below. For a detailed understanding

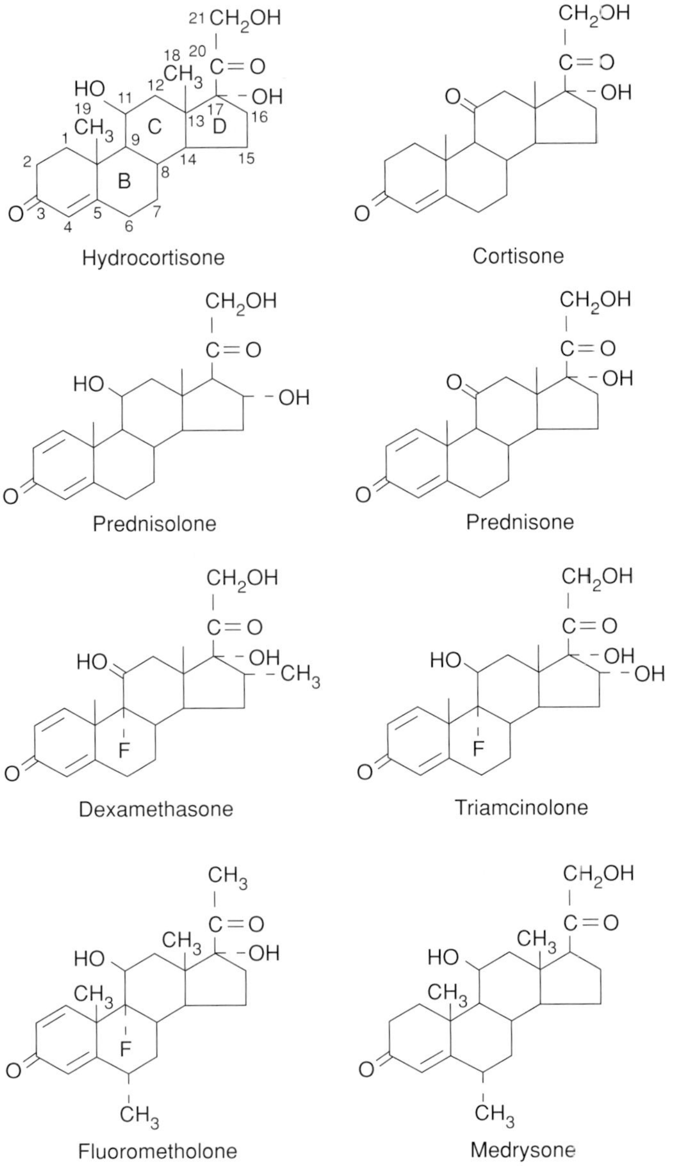

Fig. 2 Chemical structures of anti-inflammatory steroids used to treat ocular inflammatory diseases.

of glucocorticoid actions, see the review by Barnes and Adcock (1993).

Inhibition of synthesis of mediators

Eicosanoids

Arachidonic acid is converted to prostaglandins and leukotrienes and other hydroxy products by prostaglandin synthase 1 and 2 and lipoxygenases. Under normal physiology, prostaglandin synthase 1 is constitutive and during inflammation, prostaglandin synthase 2 is induced. Glucocorticoids share some of the anti-inflammatory actions of non-steroidal compounds discussed above. The principal differences of mode of action on prostaglandin synthesis between the two classes of compounds are that (a) the non-steroidal agents are direct inhibitors of prostaglandin synthase 1 and 2, and (b) glucocorticoids inhibit prostaglandin synthase 2 and the liberation of membrane arachidonic acid by phospholipase A_2, thus preventing the release of arachidonic acid, the substrate for prostaglandin synthase. The action of glucocorticoids on phospholipase A_2 is mediated by a small protein molecule, lipocortin 1 also known as calpactin 1. Lipocortins (1 and 2) are formed following occupation of cytoplasmic receptors by glucocorticoids and subsequent interaction of the receptor complex with DNA and relevant messenger RNA (mRNA) expression. Recombinant lipocortin 1 has a number of biological and anti-inflammatory activities and has potential for use in clinical practice as an anti-inflammatory agent.

Cytokines

A number of members of this family consisting of interleukins (IL), tumour necrosis factor-α, and granulocyte–macrophage colony-stimulating factor, are critical in the initiation and sustenance of chronic and immunological inflammation. Glucocorticoids inhibit the expression and actions of interleukins (1–6 and 8), tumour necrosis factor-α, and granulocyte–macrophage colony-stimulating factor at molecular levels. The molecular mechanisms are highly complex; their detailed discussion is beyond the scope of this section. To inhibit the formation of cytokines, glucocorticoids initially bind to the intracellular receptors. The glucocorticoid receptor complex then acts as a nuclear transcriptional regulator, a typical function of the steroid receptor superfamily, by binding to specific DNA sequences known as glucocorticoid response elements, resulting in the repression of gene transcription. In addition to the inhibitory effects on cytokine formation, glucocorticoids block the effects of some of the cytokines. The transcription factors, activator protein 1 and nuclear factor $_\kappa$B, mediate cellular effects of some of the cytokines such as tumour necrosis factor-α and of stimulated T lymphocytes by activating or repressing target genes such as IL-2 and IL-2 receptors. The activation of these factors during inflammation is inhibited by glucocorticoids. Cytokines also express intercellular adhesion molecule 1, probably mediated by nuclear factor $_\kappa$B; expression of this adhesion molecule which plays a mandatory role in recruiting leucocytes to inflamed tissue are downregulated by glucocorticoids.

The cellular and molecular mechanisms of anti-inflammatory activities of glucocorticoids in ocular inflammatory diseases are not different from other inflamed tissues. The treatment of ocular inflammatory diseases with glucocorticoids will remain in the forefront for the foreseeable future. It is possible that rapidly developing molecular technology will exploit glucocorticoid response elements and activator protein 1 to design highly targeted anti-inflammatory agents.

Glucocorticoid therapy in ocular inflammation

Glucocorticoid therapy is highly effective in the treatment of a variety of ocular inflammations. Ocular inflammatory diseases

that are commonly treated with glucocorticoids include allergic and vernal conjunctivitis, corneal diseases, iritis, anterior and posterior uveitis, sympathetic ophthalmia, and other ocular autoimmune diseases. The most widely used glucocorticoids are dexamethasone, betamethasone, prednisolone, cortisone, hydrocortisone, and fluorometholone. These drugs are administered topically in the form of ointment, suspension, or solution in concentrations ranging from 0.1 to 1.0 per cent. Systemic administration is restricted to the treatment of inflammation of the posterior segment or in connective tissue disorders.

Side-effects

Systemic glucocorticoid therapy causes a large number of undesirable side-effects, most important of which are pituitary–adrenal suppression, fluid and electrolyte disturbances, increased susceptibility to infections and posterior subcapsular cataracts; the latter two complications are common to ocular topical therapy. In addition to the last two complications of systemic administration, the most frequently encountered side-effects of ocular treatment are delayed wound healing and increased intraocular pressure, which is reversible on cessation of the treatment.

Further reading

Barnes, P.J. and Adcock, I. (1993). Anti-inflammatory actions of steroids: molecular mechanisms. *Trends in Pharmacological Sciences*, **14**, 436–41.

Ferreira, S.H. and Vane, J.R. (1979). Mode of action of anti-inflammatory agents which are prostaglandin synthetase inhibitors. In *Anti-inflammatory drugs*, (ed. J.R. Vane and S.H. Ferreira), pp. 348–83. Springer-Verlag, Berlin.

Flach, A.J. (1992). Cyclo-oxygenase inhibitors in ophthalmology. *Survey of Ophthalmology*, **36**, 259–84.

Flach, A.J. (1993). Non-steroidal anti-inflammatory drugs in ophthalmology. *International Ophthalmology Clinics*, **33**, 1–7.

Flower, R.J. (1989). Glucocorticoids and the inhibition of phospholipase A_2. In *Anti-inflammatory steroid action basic and clinical aspects*, (ed. R.P. Schleimer, H.N. Claman, and A.L. Oronsky), pp. 48–66. Academic Press, London.

Goldstein, I.M. (1988). Agents that interfere with arachidonic acid metabolism. In *Inflammation: basic principles and clinical correlates*, (ed. J.I. Gallin, I.M. Goldstein, and R. Snyderman), pp. 935–46. Raven Press, Philadelphia.

Hirata, F. (1989). The role of lipocortins in cellular function as a second messenger of glucocorticoids. In *Anti-inflammatory steroid action basic and clinical aspects*, (ed. R.P. Schleimer, H.N. Claman, and A.L. Oronsky), pp. 67–95. Academic Press, London.

Jaanus, S.D. and Lesher, G.A. (1995). Anti-inflammatory drugs. In *Clinical ocular pharmacology*, 3rd edn, (ed. J.D. Barlett and S.D. Jaanus), pp. 303–35. Butterworth-Heinemann, Boston.

Kulkarni, P.S. and Srinivasan, B.D. (1987). Non-steroidal anti-inflammatory drugs in ocular inflammatory conditions. In *Nonsteroidal anti-inflammatory drugs*, (ed. A.S. Lewis and D.E. Frust), pp. 107–25. Marcel Dekker, Basel.

Opremcak, E.M. (1994). Anti-inflammatory agents. In *Havener's ocular pharmacology*, (ed. T.H. Mauger and E.L. Craig), pp. 350–28. Mosby, New York.

Smith, W.L. (1989). The eicosanoids and their biochemical mechanisms of action. *Biochemical Journal*, **259**, 315–24.

1.4.5 Ocular lubricants and tear replacements

J. Boulton

Dry eye syndromes, though heterogeneous in aetiology, share many clinical features. They are common conditions; while severe dry eye has a prevalence of approximately 8 per 10 000 population, up to 200 per 10 000 use tear replacements. Current commercial preparations vary in composition; tonicity, electrolyte composition, viscosity agents, and preservatives. While significantly improving patient comfort, they elicit no significant improvement in the objective clinical dry eye parameters. Future products will incorporate our expanding knowledge of tear film structure, enzymology, and immunology, and should objectively improve epithelial health.

Historical perspective

The ancient Greeks used egg white and goose fat. Herbal tonics were thought to improve the production of tears by the brain in the eighteenth century. By the nineteenth century, oils and glycerins with added gelatin were being instilled. Some balanced electrolyte solutions were developed. These early attempts to mimic natural tears were frustrated by problems of sterility, stability, and biocompatibility. Subsequent research and commercial drive focused on the use of a less physiological but practical single active agent such as methyl cellulose. Clinically, however, these initially formed unsatisfactory sticky coatings on the lid margins.

Key issues in designing tear substitutes

Active ingredient

Commercial tear products contain one or more of the following:

- polyvinyl alcohol (1.4–3 per cent)
- polyvinyl pyrrolidone
- celluloses
- mineral oil
- petrolatum.

Electrolytes and osmolality

The tear film has an electrolyte balance that differs from that of serum and aqueous humour. Physiological concentrations of sodium, potassium, calcium, magnesium, and zinc are important in the maintenance of corneal health. Most tear substitutes use sodium chloride to achieve a suitable tonicity. Relative hypertonicity has been found in the tears of patients with dry

Table 1 Electrolyte composition of tears in normal subjects and patients with keratoconjunctivitis sicca (KCS)

	Normal subjects	KCS patients
Osmolarity	304.4 ± 0.4 molOsm/l	↑ by 3.5%
Electrolytes		
Sodium	133.2 ± 0.2 mmol/l	↑ by 6.5%
Potassium	24.0 ± 0.2 mmol/l	↑ by 3.5%
Calcium	0.80 ± 0.04 mmol/l	↑ by 3.5%
Magnesium	0.61 ± 0.03 mmol/l	↑ by 3.5%
Bicarbonate	32.8 ± 0.2 mmol/l	↑ by 3.5%

Source: Gilbard, J.P. and Rossi, R.R. (1994). *Advances in Experimental Medicine and Biology*, **340**.

eyes (Table 1). Many manufacturers have responded with a reduction of 10 per cent in the tonicity of their preparations. It is doubtful that this is of benefit.

Viscosity

Commercial products often incorporate agents such as celluloses and sodium hyaluronate to increase viscosity. When considering the flow properties of tear replacements, two contrasting states must be recognized; the open eye and the blink. When the eye is open, dry eye therapy aims for maximal retention of the tear film, lost through drainage and evaporation. This retention time is thought by some authors to be best increased with a high viscosity agent. No evidence exists, however, that viscosity is related to retention time. During the high shear conditions of the blink, low viscosity is clearly indicated to prevent damaging dragging forces on the epithelial surface.

Both natural and artificial tears are dilute polymer solutions. In fluid dynamic terms, these are of two types. In Newtonian solutions, the viscosity remains constant as shear rate increases. In non-Newtonian solutions, the viscosity decreases. Interestingly, most commercial preparations are in the former group, while in the latter group are natural tears and high molecular weight sodium hyaluronate.

Buffering

In natural tears, bicarbonate provides buffering. Tear replacements are buffered to pH 7.7 to 7.8 by one of many systems; bicarbonate, citrate, phosphate, or borate. Bicarbonate at a concentration of 12 mmol/l has been shown to restore epithelial health in damaged corneas.

Other ingredients

A number of proteins have been identified in natural tears. Their importance in defence and epithelial maintenance is well established, but they have not yet been incorporated into commercially available preparations. Antibacterial properties are provided by lysosyme and lactoferrin, whose concentration falls in dry eye. Epidermal growth factor has a role in the maintenance and healing of the corneal epithelium. Although it is detected in tears, more significant quantities are supplied from the corneal stroma. RGD peptide consists of three amino acids forming the binding site for fibronectin. It probably contributes to epithelial cell migration, tear stability, and bacteriostasis.

Vitamin A is supplied to the cornea in tears. Retinyl palmitate incorporated into an aqueous product was found to be significantly more efficacious than a leading commercial tear product in patients with Sjögren's syndrome and moderately severe sicca syndrome. Vitamin B_{12} improved healing three-fold in an experimental rabbit model in which epithelium was first denuded up to and including the limbus. Tear proteins bind vitamin B_{12} with more avidity than plasma proteins, while dietary absorption falls off in elderly people. This suggests that topical application may have theoretical advantages over oral administration. Supplementation in tear replacements has yet to prove efficacious in clinical trials.

Modulation of the immune response may be beneficial in conditions such as Sjögren's syndrome; the role of cyclosporin A and interferon-α have yet to be confirmed in clinical practice.

Preservatives

The commonly used preservatives include benzalkonium chloride, sorbic acid, chlorbutanol, parabens, thiomersal, and polyquad. Several authors have demonstrated the adverse effect of benzalkonium chloride on epithelial health as assessed by fluorophotometry. Recent attempts to minimize sensitivity problems by excluding preservatives have included disposable single dose preparations. These have shown significantly better performance at reducing rose bengal staining compared with a variety of commercially available preparations containing the preservatives listed above. Expense has limited their appeal.

Oncotic pressure

The addition of low viscosity polymers increases the oncotic pressure of the tear replacement. This has been shown experimentally to reverse epitheliopathy.

Administration

Drops

Patients should be made aware that symptoms vary with activity; the blink rate for example has been measured at 22 ± 9 per min under relaxed conditions, 10 ± 6 per min when reading a book at table level, and 7 ± 7 per min when viewing a VDU. In severe dry eye, relief of symptoms may necessitate the instillation of drops several times per hour. This still represents a flooding of the fornix followed by a relatively dry period. The logical response is to develop more physiological augmentation of the tear film.

Solid polymers

The placement in the inferior fornix of a solid water-soluble agent such as hydroxymethylpropylcellulose may provide continuous supplementation of polymer. In a small series of patients with moderate to severe rheumatoid arthritis, inserts

improved epithelial staining and were successfully manipulated by those with deforming arthropathy. However, the requirement for water is the major limiting factor in their effectiveness in severe dry eyes.

Continuous administration

In an effort to overcome the inconvenience of regular drop administration, techniques of continuous perfusion have been developed. Examples include:

- a peristaltic pump firing 5 μl droplets every 5 min
- a tunnelled subcutaneous tube delivering drops directly on to the cornea from a reservoir and ooze pump
- a micropump from a computer printer continuously saturating the eye with 22-picolitre droplets at 100 droplets per second, yielding 10–15 million drops per day.

Further reading

Advances in Experimental Medicine and Biology, 1994, **340**. [Entire volume devoted to new developments in tear physiology and substitutes.]
Holly, F.J. (1993). Diagnostic methods and treatment modalities of dry eye conditions. International Ophthalmology, **17**, 113–25.
Tsubota, K. (1994). New approaches to dry-eye therapy. International Ophthalmology Clinics, **34**, 115–28.

1.4.6 Side-effects of topical ocular medication

F.T. Fraunfelder and F.W. Fraunfelder

The adverse effects from topical ocular medication may be local, such as pseudo-ocular pemphigoid secondary to long-term glaucoma medication, or systemic, such as status asthmaticus secondary to a topical ocular β-blocker. Local adverse ocular drug reactions are often easier to recognize than systemic side-effects from an 'eyedrop'. A cause-and-effect relationship between a drug and an adverse event may be difficult to prove. This is compounded by incomplete information, polypharmacy, the rarity of an event, reluctance to rechallenge the patient with the drug, and so on. A comprehensive history is vital, with attention to over-the-counter and prescription agents, systemic or local disease, occupation, and multiple variables which may also cause health problems. The relationship between onset of symptoms and administration of the drug is important,

This study was supported, in part, by an unrestricted grant from Research to Prevent Blindness, New York, United States.

especially if the reaction does not fit the parameters of the expected signs and symptoms of the disease. Adverse drug reactions of all types are most frequent in patients who have a history of drug-related side-effects. The most important factor, however, is the health-care provider's awareness of possible adverse ocular effects attributable to the drug(s) in question. The absolute proof of a drug-induced effect is challenge/ rechallenge testing in a number of patients, which may be difficult to accomplish.

The human eye is relatively susceptible to toxic substances due to its rich blood supply and small mass. The eye and adnexae are composed of many types of tissue: muscles, tendons, secretion organs, permeable and semipermeable membranes, pigment cells, and so on. Because of these individual tissue and cell characteristics, and their varied metabolic reactions, each may show specific affinities and storage characteristics to various drugs and toxic substances. The number of types of drug-related adverse ocular reactions is, therefore, greater than most other areas of the body. Since the eye is a sensory organ, the patient may perceive adverse drug events sooner than with other non-sensory organ systems. Damage to the liver or kidney, the two most common organs adversely affected by drugs, may be as high as 80 per cent before an abnormality can be detected via clinical testing. However, only a fraction of 1 per cent of the eye may be involved and profound abnormalities noted, both by the patient and through clinical testing. Since most areas of the eye can be visualized by the ophthalmologist, he or she can more easily diagnose and help rule in or out a toxic response.

Adverse events attributable to drugs have been studied and classified as 'definite', 'probable', 'possible', and 'doubtful'. 'Definite' reactions usually occur within a reasonable interval following administration of a drug, follow a known pattern of response to the suspected drug, and are confirmed by improvement upon removal of the drug and by reappearance on rechallenge that cannot be explained by the known characteristics of the patient's disease. 'Probable' reactions occur within a reasonable interval after the drug is administered, follow a known response pattern, are confirmed on a suspicion of the drug but not on rechallenge, and cannot be explained by the known characteristics of the patient's disease or unknown factors. 'Possible' reactions occur within a reasonable interval, may or may not follow a known response pattern, but could be explained by the known characteristics of the patient's disease or unknown factors. 'Doubtful' reactions are more likely related to other factors than the suspected drug.

This chapter will discuss local and systemic side-effects from topical ocular medications, emphasizing the most common agents affecting the visual system. The National Registry of Drug-induced Ocular Side-effects is a clearing house for spontaneous reports of possible adverse ocular side-effects sent to the Food and Drug Administration, World Health Organization, and the National Registry. We will share these data upon request. Physicians suspecting adverse ocular drug reactions are encouraged to report their suspicions or cases to the National Registry of Drug-induced Ocular Side-effects (c/o the Casey Eye Institute, Oregon Health Sciences University, 3375 SW Terwilliger Boulevard, Portland, Oregon 97201–4197, fax 503 494–6864).

Local side-effects from topical ocular medication

Local side-effects may be due to the drug, vehicle, preservative, and/or metabolite. Toxic metabolites can be formed in the eye itself (i.e. iris–ciliary body, corneal epithelium, retinal pigment epithelial cells, and so on), or elsewhere in the body (i.e. liver). If the concentration of the offending drug in the tear film is high, the potential for adverse effects is accentuated. The concentration of a drug in the ocular tissues depends on a combination of factors: (a) the dosage of medication; (b) drug dilution secondary to factors such as lacrimation; (c) the rate of cul-de-sac drainage; and (d) the rate of drug absorption.

Factors which influence drugs to cause local adverse side-effects include:

- the inherent nature of the drug (some local anaesthetics may cause cell death by dehydration or chemical alteration of cellular proteins as they are protoplasmic poisons)

- the solubility of drugs can cause precipitate (topical ocular steroids and band keratopathy), or be secreted in the tear film via the lacrimal gland (isotretinoin and many antimetabolites)

- the pH of a drug is not compatible with patient comfort or causes tissue damage. This is especially true in agents with high pH.

Multiple-drug therapy can increase the incidence of adverse drug effects.

Local adverse ocular drug reactions usually occur within the first 7 to 10 days after onset of therapy, and most are reversible once the drug is discontinued. Typical signs and symptoms of local adverse ocular drug reactions include erythema, tearing, itching, burning, discharge, irritation, foreign body sensation, photophobia, and haloes around lights. Irreversible changes are unusual and primarily occur with long-term topical ocular treatment.

Toxic or irritative reactions from topical ocular medications are the most common adverse events seen in ocular toxicology. Blepharitis, conjunctivitis, and corneal disturbances are not uncommon. If the drug is discontinued, these events are seldom serious. However, if they go unrecognized and the medication is continued, blepharokeratoconjunctivitis medicamentosa can be serious. Corneal perforation with endophthalmitis can easily occur in a matter of weeks, including loss of the eye from the frequent use of topical ocular local anaesthetics. Long-term medications can cause an additional set of problems. For example, in sicca patients taking topical ocular medications frequently, the cornea and conjunctiva may not tolerate the toxic effects of the preservatives. Chemosis, erythema, and major disturbances of the cornea can occur. The same problems, however, to a much lesser extent, can be seen with long-term exposure to topical ocular medication, as with glaucoma

Table 1 Some of the medications commonly prescribed by ophthalmologists, and their side-effects

Class	Drug	Ocular side-effects	Comments
Aminoglycoside(s)	Gentamicin	Hyperaemia, mucopurulent discharge, chemosis, ulceration–necrosis, mild papillary hypertrophy, decreased healing, pallor, allergic reaction, blepharoconjunctivitis	One of the most common drugs to cause periocular allergic contact dermatitis
	Neomycin	Hyperaemia, ocular pain, oedema, burning sensation, allergic reaction, erythema, blepharoconjunctivitis, urticaria, punctate keratitis, overgrowth of non-susceptible organisms	Topical ocular application has been reported to cause allergic conjunctival lid reactions in 4% of patients
Antivirals	Idoxuridine, vidarabine	*Irritation*: lacrimation, hyperaemia, photophobia, ocular pain, oedema, ptosis, anterior segment ischemia; *cornea*: superficial punctate keratitis, oedema, filaments, wound healing, erosions, stromal opacities, superficial vascularization, epithelial dysplasia; *conjunctiva*: allergic reaction, hyperaemia, blepharitis, conjunctivitis, oedema; *lacrimal system*: canaliculitis, stenosis, occlusion	Idoxuridine has the highest degree of local irritation and toxicity. Not all side-effects are reversible after discontinuation of the drug
Sulphonamide	Sulphacetamide	Irritation, photosensitivity, ocular complications of Stevens–Johnson syndrome, lupoid syndrome, optic neuritis, transient myopia, periorbital oedema, overgrowth of non-susceptible organisms, allergic reaction	Skin sensitization may occur in medical personnel who handle this drug, i.e. dermatitis
Antimuscarinic (mydriatic)	Atropine	Decreased vision, decreased accommodation, mydriasis, irritation, hyperaemia, photophobia, ocular pain, oedema, increased intraocular pressure, allergic reaction, blepharoconjunctivitis, micropsia, decreased lacrimation, visual hallucinations	Topical ocular atropine may increase intraocular pressure in eyes with open angle glaucoma
Steroid(s)	Dexamethasone	Increased intraocular pressure, decreased resistance to infection, delayed healing, mydriasis, ptosis, posterior subcapsular cataracts, decreased vision, decreased accommodation, scotomas, constriction of visual field, colour vision defect, allergic reaction, conjunctival erythema, telangiectasia, punctate keratitis, lacrimation, photophobia, ocular pain, burning sensation, anterior uveitis, toxic amblyopia, optic atrophy	Glaucoma from the stronger steroids occurs in one-third of patients after 6 weeks of four times a day usage, and in most patients after 1 year of use
Miscellaneous	Polymixin	Irritation, ocular pain, allergic reaction, ptosis, paralysis of extraocular muscles, overgrowth of non-susceptible organisms	Topical ocular irritative and allergic reactions are common
	Bacitracin	Irritation, allergic reaction, oedema, urticaria, keratitis, delayed wound healing—toxic states, overgrowth of non-susceptible organisms	Allergic reactions are rare but quite irritating in high concentrations
	Chloramphenicol	Irritation, allergic reaction, non-specific conjunctivitis, depigmentation, keratitis, overgrowth of non-susceptible organisms	May cause latent hypersensitivity. Ocular side-effects most common in children. Aplastic anaemia rare

patients. Damage to the lining of the anterior surface of the eye can occur from the preservatives or as a direct effect of any one of a number of drugs or chemicals in various vehicles. These can cause chronic erythema, chemosis, and/or irritation, but can also have a significant effect on the tear film, which may aggravate ocular sicca. Superficial punctate keratopathy in a whorl pattern is suggestive of a toxic response from long-term topical ocular medication. This can be due to the drug or its preservative. Direct damage to the epithelium and underlying tissue can cause pseudo-ocular pemphigoid.

Allergic reactions can be acute (type I immunoglobulin E mediated hypersensitivity reactions) with anaphylactoid reactions occurring within minutes after instillation of the medica-tion (allergen), or they can occur more indolently (type IV delayed, hypersensitivity reaction) with adverse effects appearing within 24 to 72 h. Type I hypersensitivity reactions have occurred after instillation of essentially all topical ocular drugs used in ophthalmology. Contact blepharoconjunctivitis, a type IV hypersensitivity reaction, is associated with atropine, homatropine, aminoglycosides, antiviral agents, thimerosal, and ethylenediamine tetra-acetic acid.

If used frequently enough, all topical ocular medication can cause adverse reactions, even methylcellulose or artificial tears without preservatives. While many ointments do not contain preservatives, this vehicle can keep the medication in contact with the anterior surface of the eye for longer periods of time.

Table 2 Some frequently prescribed topical drugs and their side-effects

Class	Drug	Systemic side-effects	Comments
α-Antagonist	Apraclonicine	Dry nose and mouth, taste perversion, headache, asthenia, transient light-headedness	Systemic side-effects from topical ocular application rarely a cause to discontinue
β-Blocker	Timolol, carteolol, metipranolol	Asthma, bradycardia, dyspnoea, depression, arrhythmia, headache, congestive heart failure, asthenia, dizziness, cerebrovascular accident, hypotension, syncope, nausea, impotence, rhinitis, increased high density lipoprotein, hyperkalaemia, alopecia, confusion, psoriasis, nail pigmentation, skin disease, palpitation, hypoglycaemia, cerebral ischaemia	After topical ocular administration, peak systemic blood level is between 30 and 90 min after dosing. Effects can be seen immediately, or months to a year after therapy is started
Decongestant	Naphazoline	Headache, hypertension, nervousness, nausea, dizziness, asthenia, somnolence, arrhythmia, hyperglycaemia, hypothermia	Major systemic adverse reactions following use of ocular decongestants are rare and occur primarily when used more often than recommended by manufacturer
	10% neosynephrine	Hypertension, myocardial infarct, tachycardia, subarachnoid haemorrhage, arrhythmia, headache, syncope	Data suggests that 10% solutions should be used with caution in patients with cardiac disease, hypertension, aneurysms, or arteriosclerosis
Miotic	Acetylcholine	Bradycardia, hypotension, vasodilation, diaphoresis	Bradycardia and hypotension have been seen following irrigation of anterior chamber with acetylcholine
	Pilocarpine	Headache, diaphoresis, nausea, diarrhoea, salivation, tremor, bradycardia, hypotension, bronchospasm, confusion, depression, epistaxis, rhinorrhoea, tenesmus	Mothers on topical ocular pilocarpine may have infants with signs mimicking meningitis. Paediatricians should be aware of this and avoid unnecessary tests
Mydriatic	Cyclopentolate	Personality disorder, psychosis, ataxia, speech disorder, agitation, hallucinations, confusion, convulsion, tachycardia, fever, vasodilation, urinary retention, dry mouth	Systemic side-effects are not rare, especially in children
Antibacterial	Chloramphenicol	Aplastic anaemia, various blood dyscrasias	In some physicians' opinion, the only indication for topical ocular use is if the organism is resistant to all other antibiotics

Some of the most severe drug-induced lid reactions are associated with antibiotics in ointments. Table 1 lists the ocular side-effects caused by a few of the medications commonly prescribed by ophthalmologists.

Systemic side-effects from topical ocular medication

After instilling 1 drop of topical ocular medication in the eye, 60 to 80 per cent is absorbed systemically through the nasolacrimal system from beneath the inferior turbinate via the nasal mucosa. The remaining 20 to 40 per cent is absorbed through the conjunctiva and cornea. The contact of a drug over a large mucosal surface is essentially the same as giving the drug intramuscularly. As a result, some drugs administered to the eye can have substantial effects elsewhere in the body, for instance β-blockers or phenylephrine. Following oral administration of a drug, the active form of the drug is markedly decreased by the first order pass effect. The drug first passes through the gastrointestinal system with its pH and enzyme effects, and then reaches the liver before entering the bloodstream and travelling to the target organs. This first order pass has significant influence in decreasing the amount of drug that reaches the bloodstream to affect target organs. Conversely, topical ocular medication is absorbed systemically via the 'benign' corneal, conjunctival, and nasal mucosa, which are then channelled into the right ventricle and pumped to the lungs before reaching the left ventricle. After leaving the left ventricle, some passes

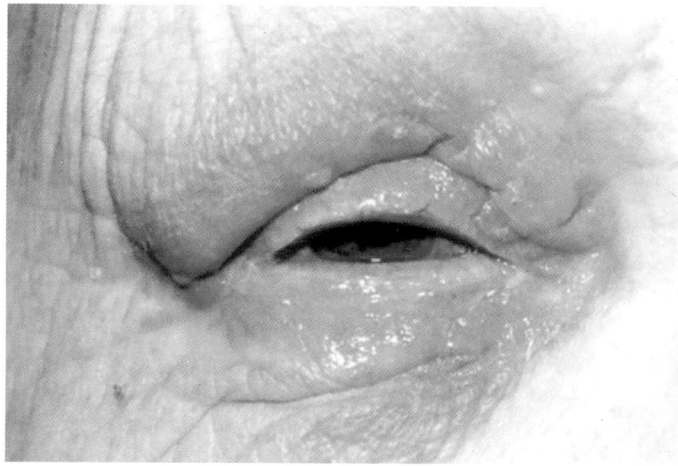

Fig. 1 A 74-year-old female who had previous exposures to topical ocular neomycin. Several days after repeat exposure, she showed the classic periorbital skin reaction secondary to a topical ocular medication.

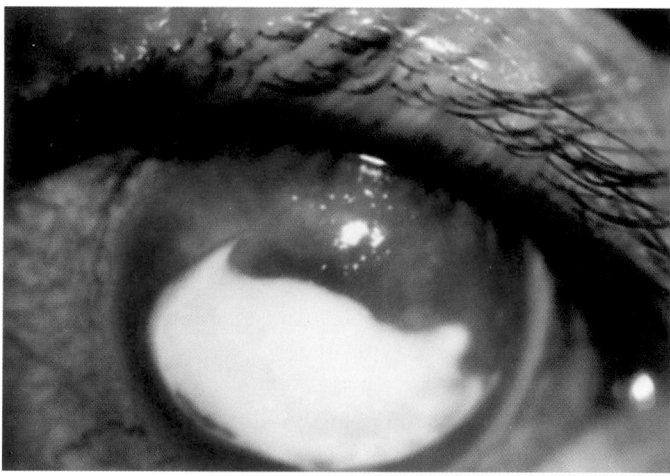

Fig. 4 A 60-year-old female developed a white opacity in her cornea following a penetrating keratoplasty. Snow-white crystalline opacity mimics a drug reaction, however, it was infectious crystalline keratopathy.

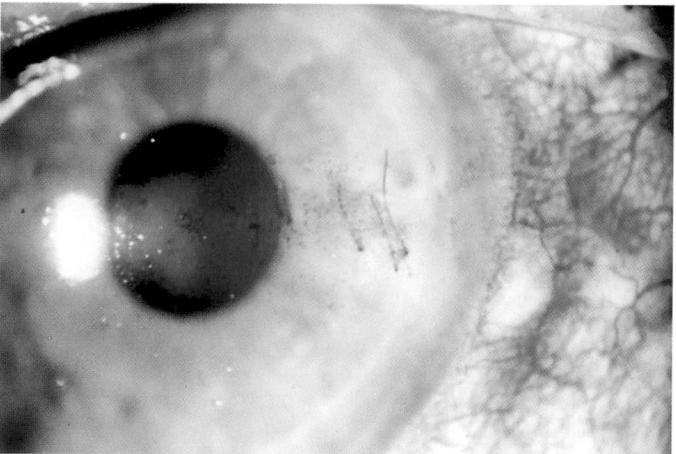

Fig. 2 A 56-year-old male using multiple drops of non-preservative-free articial tears developed filamentary keratitis with rose bengal.

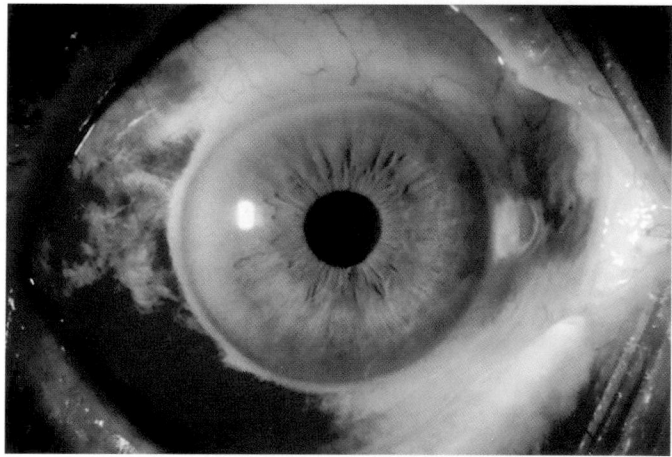

Fig. 5 A 23-year-old male taking sodium chloride ointment for corneal oedema developed subconjunctival haemorrhages. This was confirmed on rechallenge. It is well known that topical ocular hypertonic salt solutions or ointments can cause subconjunctival haemorrhages as well as nosebleeds.

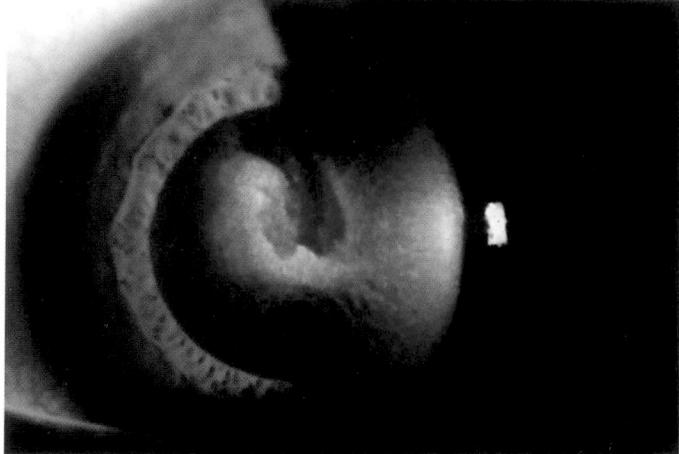

Fig. 3 A 16-year-old black male with severe, bilateral sicca developed a calcific band-like keratopathy from the use of topical steroid phosphate preparations applied six times daily.

through the liver and kidney, the sites of primary drug breakdown and where blood levels are decreased. Each drop (50 μl) of a 1 per cent solution contains 0.5 mg of the drug, which in some cases can cause systemic therapeutic blood levels of the drug, especially with bilateral application in elderly patients with lax eyelids (holds more drug). For example, a topical ocular β–blocker can cause therapeutic blood levels from 30 to 90 min after application to the eye because after its first pass through the heart, the drug is not metabolized to decrease its serum concentration.

Since many drugs applied topically to the eye can cause systemic effects, a comprehensive list is not practical. However, a partial list of the most frequently prescribed drugs and examples of their side–effects is presented in Table 2.

Conclusion

The clinician should maintain an awareness of the systemic side-effects of commonly used ophthalmic medications, especially those used in the management of glaucoma. Clinical data is often incomplete, and the doctor must use his or her scientific knowledge and clinical experience to evaluate a potential cause-and-effect relationship between an adverse event and a medication. Ocular and systemic side-effects from topical ocular medication are usually reversible, but some can be vision-threatening, such as chronic macular oedema in the aphakic eye secondary to epinephrine preparations for glaucoma, or life-threatening, such as severe hypertension from topical ocular 10 per cent phenylephrine used as a mydriatic. Therefore, the potential therapeutic value of a drug must be weighed against the potential adverse side-effects. With this in mind, the doctor must maintain a high index of suspicion that a new symptom or sign may be drug-related.

Figures 1 to 5 show drug-related ocular side-effects or suspected drug side-effects.

Further reading

Basu, P.K. (1983–4). Toxic effects of drugs on the corneal epithelium—a review. *Journal of Toxicology—Cutaneous and Ocular Toxicology*, **2**, 205.

Berdy, G.J., Abelson, M.B., Smith, L.M., and George, M.A. (1992). Preservative-free artificial tear preparations: assessment of corneal epithelial toxic effects. *Archives of Ophthalmology*, **110**, 528–32.

Bryant, J. (1969). Local and topical anesthetics in ophthalmology. *Survey of Ophthalmology*, **13**, 263.

Fiore, P.M., Jacobs, I.H., and Goldberg. D.B. (1987). Drug-induced pemphigoid spectrum of diseases. *Archives of Ophthalmology*, **105**, 1650–63.

Fraunfelder, F.T. (1986). Ocular β-blockers and systemic effects. *Archives of Internal Medicine*, **146**, 1073–4.

Fraunfelder, F.T. and Meyer, S.M. (1989). Systemic adverse reactions to glaucoma medications. *International Ophthalmology Clinics*, **29**, 143–6.

Fraunfelder, F.T. and Grove, J. (ed.) (1996). *Drug-induced ocular side effects*, (4th edn). Williams & Wilkins, Philadelphia.

Fraunfelder, F.T., Morgan, R.L., and Yunis, A.A. (1993). Blood dyscrasias and topical ophthalmic chloramphenicol. *American Journal of Ophthalmology*, **115**, 812–13.

Gerber, S.L., Cantor, L.B., and Brater, D.C. (1990). Systemic drug interactions with topical glaucoma medications. *Survey of Ophthalmology*, **35**, 205–18.

Hockwin, U.J. (1987). The human eye: initial and manifestation organ of drug-induced side effects. In *Drug-induced ocular side effects and ocular toxicology*, (ed. O. Hockwin), pp. 15–20. Karger, Basel.

Hughes, F.C., LeJeunne, C., and Munera, Y. (1992). Systemic effects of topical antiglaucomatous drugs. *Glaucoma*, **14**, 100–4.

Jenvert, G.I., Cohen, E.J., Donnenfeld, E.D., *et al.* (1985). Erythema multiforme after use of topical sulfacetamide. *American Journal of Ophthalmology*, **99**, 465–8.

Koneru, P., Lien, E., and Koda, R. (1986). Review—oculotoxicities of systemically administered drugs. *Journal of Ocular Pharmacology*, **2**, 385.

MacKool, R.J., Muldoon, T., Fortier, A., and Nelson, D. (1977). Epinephrine induced cystoid macular edema in aphakic eyes. *Archives of Ophthalmology*, **95**, 791–3.

Samples, J.R. and Meyer, S.M. (1988). Use of ophthalmic medications in pregnant and nursing women. *American Journal of Ophthalmology*, **106**, 616–23.

Schwab, I.R., Linberg, J.V., Gioia, V.M., *et al.* (1992). Foreshortening of the inferior conjunctival fornix associated with chronic glaucoma medications. *Ophthalmology*, **99**, 197–202.

Shell, J. (1982). Pharmacokinetics of topically applied ophthalmic drugs. *Survey of Ophthalmology*, **26**, 207–18.

Smith, R.E. (1990). Irritative conjunctivitis (toxic conjunctivitis). In *Current ocular therapy* (ed. F. Fraunfelder and F. Roy), pp. 413–14. W.B Saunders, Philadelphia.

1.5 Principles of the physics of light and lasers

1.5.1 The physics of light and lasers

T.B. Smith and A.V. Durrant

Light and coherence

Nature of light

Light is electromagnetic radiation. When propagating through space or transparent media light behaves as a wave. When interacting with electrons and atoms light is best thought of as a stream of particles, called photons, which carry energy and momentum. This duality is known as the wave–particle duality of light. Both aspects of electromagnetic radiation enter into a satisfactory explanation of the working of optical devices such as imaging systems, lasers, light detectors, and so on.

Light waves

Light of a precise colour is said to be monochromatic. A monochromatic light wave has precisely defined frequency, f, and corresponding wavelength, λ. The same is true of any monochromatic electromagnetic wave. Frequency is usually given in cycles per second, now called hertz (Hz). Wavelengths may be given in metres (m), nanometres (nm), ångstroms (Å), microns (μm), or any other convenient unit of length. It may be necessary to convert from one unit to another. For example 1 nm is 10^{-9} m, 10 Å, or 10^{-3} μm. Traditionally, light visible to humans covers a range of wavelengths from about 400 nm (4000 Å) for violet light to about 750 nm (7500 Å) for red light. At reduced sensitivity, however, visibility extends somewhat beyond this range. In any case visible light covers just a tiny portion of the full spectrum of electromagnetic waves which ranges from very short wavelengths of 0.1 nm or less for X-rays and gamma rays to many kilometres for radio waves (Fig. 1).

A familiar example of visible light is the strong yellow light emitted by a sodium lamp which has a wavelength of about 589 nm (5890 Å). This length is small compared to everyday macroscopic dimensions but actually large on the scale of most

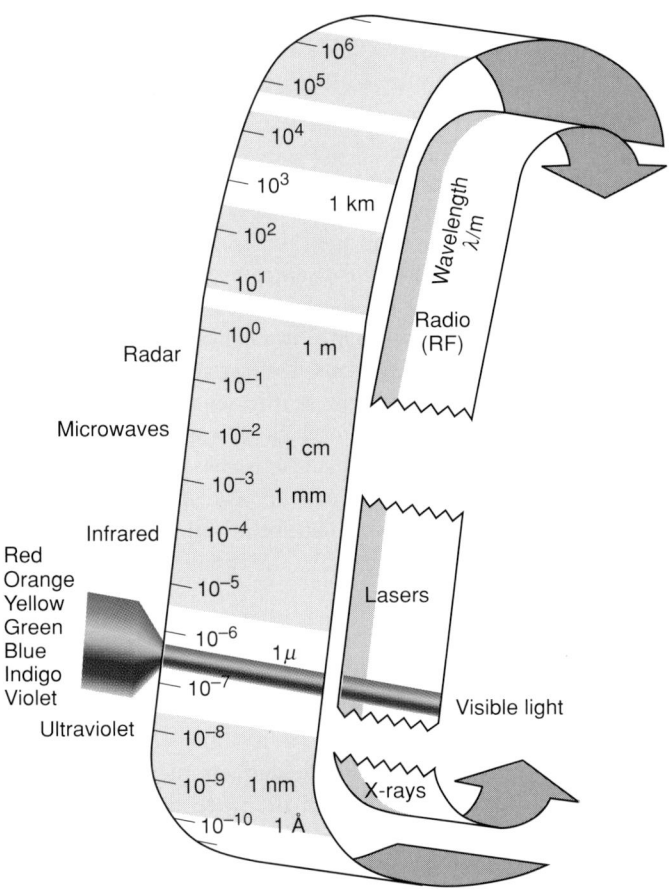

Fig. 1 Visible light covers a small part of the electromagnetic spectrum. The range of lasers as a group extends from ultraviolet to microwaves.

molecules. Consider for instance that the size of a water droplet is about 1 mm, but the size of a water molecule is a few ångstroms.

The frequency and wavelength of a monochromatic wave are not independent of each other, but are related by the equation $f\lambda = c$ where c is the speed of propagation. For waves in a vacuum or in air the speed of light is, to two decimal places, $c = 3.00 \times 10^8$ m/s.

The wave nature of light can be used to explain a variety of interference phenomena such as the colours of a thin oil film on water, the purple bloom seen on antireflection coated lenses,

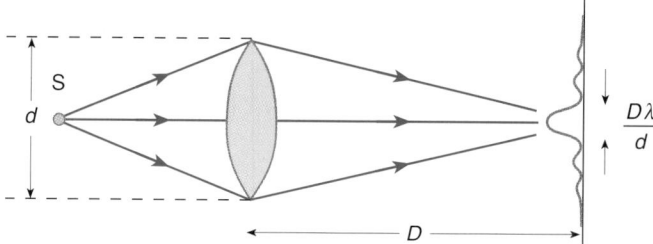

Fig. 2 The wave nature of light causes the image of an ideal point source to appear as a spot of finite width, shown here in exaggerated form.

and the speckle pattern sometimes produced by laser light. Another important example, known as diffraction, sets a fundamental limit on our ability to focus light to a small spot. The lens in Fig. 2 focuses monochromatic light (wavelength λ) from an ideal point source of light S on to a screen. Even if a perfectly made lens is used the focused image is not a point but a small blurred area surrounded by weak interference fringes. Most of the light is concentrated in a small region with a size of order $D\lambda/d$, where D is the distance from lens to screen and d is the diameter of the focusing lens. Should source S be very far from the lens, or equivalently if a collimating lens is used, then the light falling on the lens is effectively parallel. In this case D equals the focal length of the lens. For a lens with focal length 10 cm and diameter 1 cm this expression gives an approximate image size of 10 λ. For visible light this is a few microns, which is roughly the size of a small dust particle or red blood cell. Thus the wave nature of light imposes fundamental limits. For example it limits the resolution of a perfectly made optical microscope.

Photons

When light falls on a material surface some of it is reflected, some of it is transmitted, and some is absorbed. The relative proportions of these processes depend on the details of the chemical and physical make-up of the material and the wavelength of the light. Absorption mechanisms can best be understood by considering the particle aspects of light.

Light interacts with matter as if it were a stream of particles called light quanta or photons. Each photon carries a definite amount of energy. This is given up as an indivisible whole to a single atom, molecule, or ion if the photon is absorbed. Only if the photon carries sufficient energy can its absorption result in, for example, the rupture of a molecular bond. The energy of a single photon is given by the famous Einstein–Planck relation $E = hf$ where f is the frequency and h is a universal constant called Planck's constant which has the value of 6.626×10^{-34} J s. The Einstein–Planck relation relates the energy of photons to their frequency and thereby makes a connection between the particle and wave aspects of light. Since frequency, f, and wavelength, λ, are related by $f = c/\lambda$, the relation can also be written $E = hc/\lambda$, where c is the speed of light in a vacuum.

Using this formula we find that a photon of blue light with wavelength 450 nm carries an energy 6.626×10^{-34} J s $\times$ 3.00

$\times 10^8$ m/s $\div 450 \times 10^{-9}$ m $= 4.42 \times 10^{-19}$ J. Although this is a very small energy in everyday life, it is not small compared to energies associated with single atoms or molecules. In analysing the absorption of light by atoms and molecules, however, it is just these energies that one often needs to consider. The customary unit of energy for these processes is the electron volt (eV). One electron volt equals 1.6×10^{-19} J, to one decimal place. In these units the energy of a 450-nm photon is 4.42×10^{-19} J$/1.6 \times 10^{-19}$ J/eV $= 2.76$ eV. Thus for example blue light might rupture a molecular bond if the molecular binding energy is less than 2.76 eV but even large amounts of blue light would be almost ineffective in rupturing a bond when the binding energy exceeds 2.76 eV because it is very unlikely for a molecule to absorb more than one photon.

The fact that photons of higher frequency (shorter wavelength) carry more energy than photons of lower frequency (longer wavelength) explains why the ultraviolet component of sunlight can cause skin damage by rupturing molecular bonds in cells. But when this component is screened out, even long exposures to sunlight cause little damage since the photons in the screened light lack sufficient energy.

Coherence of light

There is a fundamental difference in coherence between laser light and light from traditional sources like the sun, sodium vapour lamps, tungsten filament bulbs, and candles. There are two types of coherence: temporal coherence and spatial coherence.

The temporal coherence of a light beam is a measure of its spectral purity. Light with perfect temporal coherence has a well-defined frequency and is therefore monochromatic. It also, therefore, has a corresponding well-defined wavelength. In reality all light comprises a spread (or bandwidth) of frequencies. Light from ordinary sources is spread over a wide band of frequencies, but laser light has a very narrow frequency spread and a corresponding high degree of temporal coherence.

The spatial coherence of a light beam describes the degree to which it can be focused to a point by a lens. Light from an ideal point source has a high degree of spatial coherence, for it can be collimated and focused to a point, limited only by diffraction effects (see Fig. 2). Laser light also has good spatial coherence, but light from conventional sources does not.

An ordinary incandescent filament lamp is a good example of a source with low spatial coherence. Figure 3 shows a heated filament and its image formed by a lens. Each small part of the filament emits light independently of all other parts and so can

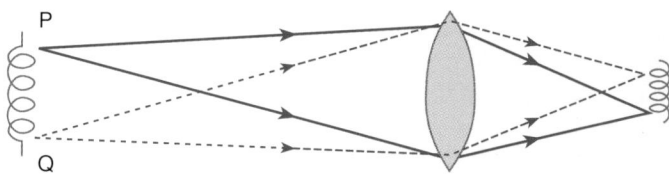

Fig. 3 Light from an incandescent filament is spatially incoherent. It can be focused to an image of itself, but not to a (diffraction blurred) point.

be considered an independent point source. Rays from a point P near one end of the filament are focused to a diffraction broadened spot on the screen. Similarly rays from any other point Q are focused to a different spot on the screen. Thus the lens forms an image of the filament. This image must be blurred very slightly by diffraction, but imperfections in design and manufacture of the lens may also cause distortion. To summarize: light from a conventional light source cannot be focused to a compact (diffraction broadened) spot, although it can be used to form an image of the source on a screen. Spatial coherence from such a source can be greatly improved by placing in front of the filament an opaque screen with a small pinhole, thereby reducing the effective size of the source. If the pinhole is small a spatially coherent beam of light is produced that can be focused to a diffraction broadened point. A heavy price is paid however, because the pinhole transmits only a tiny fraction of the light emitted by the filament.

In an analogous way the temporal coherence (spectral purity) of a light beam can be improved simply by passing it through a colour filter, again at the cost of reducing the transmitted intensity. Only a laser can produce intense beams of spatially and temporally coherent light.

The importance of spatial coherence

When one wants to deliver a beam of high power to a small well-defined region it is important to use a spatially coherent source, in effect a laser.

The maximum rate at which radiation energy is delivered to unit area of a target is commonly called the intensity of the radiation. (We note here that specialists use a range of terms when dealing with radiative power and energy.) Intensity is given in joules per second per square metre, that is watts per square metre (W/m^2). When the sun is directly overhead on a clear day it delivers to the surface of the earth about 10^3 W/m^2, that is 1 kW/m^2. Of course, less power per unit area is delivered when the sun is not directly overhead (Fig. 4).

It is possible to increase the intensity of the sun's light by means of a lens. However, the intensity we can achieve in this way is limited because the sun, although a powerful source, produces spatially incoherent light, since each point on the sun's surface radiates independently. Thus the lens actually produces an image of the sun, not a small diffraction broadened spot. For example, if the lens has a focal length of 10 cm, the diameter of this image is about 1 mm (10^{-3} m). And if the lens has a diameter of 1 cm it intercepts about 0.1 W of the sun's power to produce an intensity in the image of about 10^2 kW/m^2.

Light produced by lasers is coherent spatially (and temporally) and so can be used to produce very intense beams. A modest example is the 10 mW (10^{-2} W) beam of coherent light emitted in a 1-mm diameter collimated beam by an inexpensive helium–neon laser. A lens of focal length 10 cm will focus this beam to a diffraction broadened spot of size about 0. 1 mm (10^{-4} m) thus delivering a power density of roughly 10^3 kW/m^2 at the spot. Thus a very ordinary laser can produce a beam 'brighter than the sun'. In particular it is dangerous to look into a laser beam, for the eye's lens focuses the beam on to the retina producing extremely high intensities.

Absorption and emission of light

Electrons in matter can occupy only certain energy levels. In non-metallic matter these levels are often discrete. An electron can be caused to make a jump from one level to another by a photon of the correct frequency. Such jumps are called transitions. Consider two levels of energy, E_1 and E_2, where E_2 is the higher of the two. Photons in an incident beam of light of frequency, f, carry energy hf, where h is Planck's constant. These photons will be resonant with transitions between the two levels if $hf = E_2 - E_1$.

If initially an electron is in the lower energy level then resonant light can induce an upward transition to level E_2 (Fig. 5(a)). In a gas or solid there will be many such electrons, perhaps one for each atom. In that case many photons are absorbed from the beam causing its attenuation. It is true that electrons raised to the higher level by the absorption of photons will after a short delay fall back down in a random process called spontaneous decay (analogous to radioactive decay). But the photons released in this process do not restore the light beam, for they are radiated in all directions and not just the forward direction of the beam. Also their coherence is random; the waves are not in step with those of the incident beam. This is the mechanism by which fluorescence occurs.

If on the other hand, an electron is initially in the upper level then a resonant photon can, without itself being absorbed, induce a downward transition with the emission of a photon by the material (Fig. 5(b)). This process is called stimulated emission. Photons emitted by this process have the same frequency and direction as the incident photons and are locked to move in step with them. In other words these induced photons are coherent with the incident beam, and increase its strength. Stimulated emission is competed with by spontaneous decay, which removes electrons from the upper energy level within a

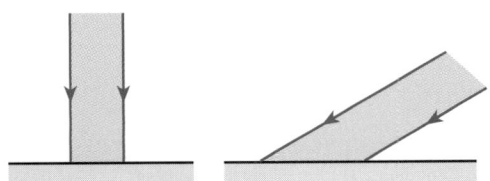

Fig. 4 Incident radiation delivers maximum power per unit area when it comes in at right angle to the surface.

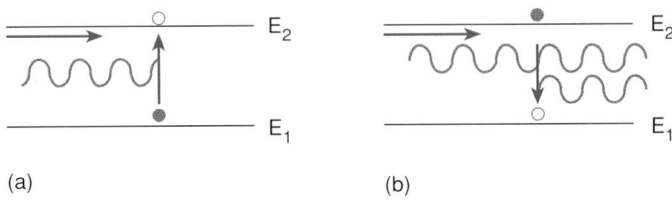

(a)   (b)

Fig. 5 (a) A resonant photon is lost in raising the energy of an electron. (b) But an electron in the upper energy level can be stimulated by a resonant photon to fall down and contribute an extra coherent photon.

short period of time called the lifetime of the level. Different energy levels have different associated lifetimes, generally varying from nanoseconds to milliseconds.

Laser physics

Light amplification by stimulated emission

The normal condition in any material is for all the electrons to be in the lowest available energy level. In that case resonant photons from the incident beam will be absorbed, resulting in attenuation of the beam. However, in some materials a physical mechanism can be found to raise or 'pump' electrons to an upper energy level. When the number of electrons in an upper energy level exceeds the number in a lower energy level there is said to be a population inversion between these two levels. A beam of light that is resonant with a downward transition of the inverted (pumped) material will be amplified by the stimulated emission of coherent photons. Stimulated emission, like absorption, occurs at a rate proportional to the intensity of the beam so that an incident light beam will be amplified. This is one principle behind the operation of the laser.

A laser is not simply a light amplifier; it is a device for generating intense coherent light. For laser action to occur two things are necessary. First, a population inversion must be achieved so that stimulated emission rather than absorption can occur. Second, a high light intensity must be established in the inverted (pumped) material so that stimulated emission dominates over spontaneous emission. In practice this involves the design of a suitable pumping mechanism for maintaining electrons in an excited state, and the use of an optical cavity in which the light intensity can build up to large values.

Pumping mechanisms

One way of pumping electrons into high energy levels is to produce an electrical discharge by passing a strong electric current through a gas. Collisions between the electrons in the current and the gas atoms produce a mix of excited ionized atoms and excited neutral atoms. The population of any particular excited energy level in an atom or ion depends on the competing processes of pumping by collisional excitation and loss from the level by spontaneous decay and possibly other mechanisms. Under favourable conditions one or more population inversions can be established and maintained by the electrical discharge. The population inversions in gas lasers such as the argon–ion laser and the helium–neon laser are produced in this way.

Population inversions of electrons in certain semiconductors can be produced by passing an electric current through junctions between two different semiconducting materials (p-n junctions). Diode lasers operating on this principle are used in compact disc players.

Another way of producing a population inversion is to use short-wavelength (i.e. energetic) photons from a 'pump laser' to pump electrons into high energy levels. In a dye laser, for example, a population inversion in a liquid dye can be produced by a 337 nm (ultraviolet) pumping beam from a nitrogen laser.

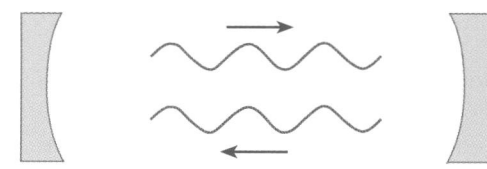

Fig. 6 Owing to its geometry the optical cavity stores standing waves along one axis at a certain frequency, thereby producing highly coherent light.

Optical cavity

A laser generates a high degree of temporal and spatial coherence by having the (pumped) amplifying medium inside an optical cavity. In its simplest form an optical cavity consists of two mirrors facing one another so that any light generated in the cavity can be continuously amplified as it bounces backwards and forwards between the mirrors (Fig. 6). Eventually a steady state is reached where the amplification is balanced by losses owing to light escaping from the cavity and the small amounts of light absorbed by even the best quality mirrors. Light in the cavity propagating in other directions will miss the mirrors and will thus experience less amplification and more losses.

Thus a laser cavity produces a high degree of spatial coherence by virtue of its directional selectivity. Initially light is produced in the cavity by spontaneous emissions in random directions. The cavity picks out the propagation directions normal to the mirrors for amplification into a strong spatially coherent beam. One of the mirrors, the output mirror, is partially transmitting and so allows a small fraction of the amplified light to escape to form the laser output beam.

The cavity also enhances the temporal coherence of the beam by virtue of its strong spectral selectivity. The two counter-propagating waves are equivalent to a standing wave, like the vibrations of a violin string, with an integral number of half wavelengths fitting between the mirror surfaces. As a result, the cavity will accept only particular discrete wavelengths. Again, there is competition between acceptable waves of different wavelengths, and only those that are very near to resonance with the inverted medium are amplified.

In summary, the spatial and temporal coherence of laser light is produced or enhanced by the directional and wavelength selectivity of the laser cavity, while the high powers are achieved by stimulated emission in the population-inverted medium inside the cavity. Different kinds of lasers put these principles into operation in different ways.

Types of lasers

There are hundreds of types of lasers. Some important characteristics of a given laser are as follows:

- whether its output is continuous or pulsed

- whether its output is limited to discrete wavelengths or is tuneable over a restricted range

- the location of its output in the electromagnetic spectrum

- the magnitude of its output power

- its efficiency (optical output power divided by input power)

- its cost.

There is a brief discussion of a selection of important lasers though more details will be found in the literature.

Gas lasers

Gas lasers have the common basic design illustrated in Fig. 7. The gas is contained in a discharge tube a metre or so long with a bore a millimetre or so across. Usually the gas inside is under a fairly low pressure. Population inversions are created by a variety of collision processes in an electrical discharge through the gas. The mirrors forming the cavity can be mounted internally in the gas chamber but it is often convenient to mount them externally. For high power lasers this is usually necessary for practical reasons of heat dissipation, and so on. One mirror is partially transmitting to allow a small fraction of the light to escape as the output beam.

The first gas laser was the helium–neon laser demonstrated by Ali Javin and coworkers in 1961. The helium–neon laser is an inexpensive low power continuous wave gas laser in which the population inversion is produced in neon by collisions with excited helium atoms in a discharge current of a few milliamps. The efficiency of these lasers is low, typically less than 0.1 per cent. Power outputs are limited to a few tens of milliwatts partly by the fact that excited energy levels in atomic gases typically have short lifetimes against spontaneous decay. The helium–neon laser can be made to operate on any one of a large number of neon transitions, thus offering a choice of discrete output frequencies. The most commonly used transition is, perhaps, that with a wavelength of 633 nm. This is the familiar red beam seen, for example at supermarket checkout counters.

Much higher continuous wave output power is obtained with noble gas ion lasers. The argon–ion laser is the most common of these. Like the helium–neon laser this is pumped by an electrical discharge, but the population inversion is between energy levels in ionized argon and is produced by a discharge of some tens of amperes. Although capable of producing high powers the argon ion laser operates at low efficiency (usually

less than 0.2 per cent), and thus the discharge unavoidably produces considerable heat which must be eliminated, usually by water cooling. The tube must be carefully designed to cope with the complicated dynamics of argon, ionized argon, and free electrons in the discharge, and it must withstand the high temperatures produced. Optical output power of several watts is possible at one of several different wavelengths. The usual choice is between the blue line at 488 nm and the green line at 514.5 nm. The krypton–ion laser is similar to the argon–ion laser, but gives a greater choice of lines in the visible spectrum, though with a weaker output. Argon–ion and krypton–ion lasers are extremely expensive, costing perhaps a thousand times as much as an ordinary helium–neon laser.

High output powers and efficiencies can be obtained more easily from gas molecular lasers. Molecules have a more complicated structure than atoms. They can vibrate and rotate in a large variety of different ways. The laws of quantum mechanics limit the rotational and vibrational energies of these motions to discrete values. The energy separations between adjacent rotational and vibrational levels are, however, much smaller than those between electronic energy levels in atoms. Consequently, the energy levels of a molecule appear as quasi-continuous bands. The very large number of energy levels in molecules and the long lifetimes of many of these levels provides great scope for laser action. The carbon dioxide laser operates at an efficiency of up to 20 per cent and can produce continuous wave outputs from less than 1 W to many kilowatts in a range of available infrared wavelengths between 9 and 11 μm. This is enough, when focused, to burn through metal plates. Not surprisingly carbon dioxide lasers have many industrial applications. Because wavelengths around 10 μm are strongly absorbed by water, carbon dioxide lasers are used in surgery. Furthermore, the wavelength of around 10 μm falls in a transparency window in the earth's atmosphere and so carbon dioxide lasers have found application in the communications industry.

Pulsed lasers can produce outputs in the ultraviolet region of the electromagnetic spectrum where it is difficult to achieve continuous laser action, due in part to the short lifetimes of the relevant energy levels. In the nitrogen laser the upper, pumped, level actually has a lifetime shorter than that of the lower level. Very rapid discharge (a few nanoseconds) of a high voltage capacitor through nitrogen gas excites the upper laser level and produces a population inversion. The subsequent laser action is self limiting as the stimulated and spontaneous emissions transfer electrons to the longer-lived lower level, thereby destroying the inversion. The pulsed laser output is at the ultraviolet wavelength of 337.1 nm and lasts for about 10 ns. Although the peak instantaneous output power of a nitrogen laser is phenomenal, its efficiency is low (a fraction of 1 per cent) and its time averaged power is modest. Typically the output can rise to 100 kW or higher at the peak of the pulse, but with a (typical) pulse repetition rate of about 50 Hz the time-averaged output power is just a few milliwatts. The ultraviolet photons from a nitrogen laser carry energy sufficient to study the photo-dissociation of molecules. Nitrogen lasers are moderately expensive.

Another important pulsed laser is the excimer laser which

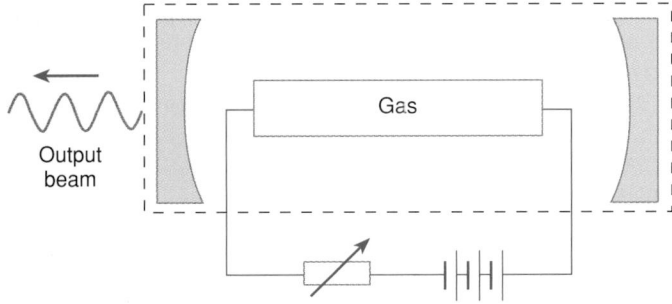

Fig. 7 Pumping by a direct current discharge. The left mirror is slightly imperfectly silvered to 'tap' the output beam from the radiation stored in the cavity.

Gas

Output beam

also has pulsed outputs in the ultraviolet region of the spectrum (Fig. 1). The word excimer is short for excited-state dimer. Noble gas atoms in the ground state do not form diatomic molecules (dimers) but the excited atoms can form long-lived excited-state dimers. Dissociation of the excited dimer into two ground state atoms with the emission of an ultraviolet photon is a basis for laser action. Excimer lasers are more efficient than nitrogen lasers and the power outputs and repetition rates are higher. The output wavelength is typically between 150 and 350 nm, depending on the noble gas used. Excimer lasers cost more than nitrogen lasers.

There are commercially available far-infrared gas molecular lasers which provide continuous wave or pulsed outputs at discrete wavelengths from about 30 μm to a few millimetres, thus extending the range of lasers to microwaves.

Solid state and semiconductor lasers

In solid state lasers the active medium consists of a small concentration of ions embedded in a crystalline or glass host material. Some of the excited energy levels of the ions are broadened into bands of very closely lying energy levels by interactions between the ions and the host material. As a result the ions have broad absorption bands and can be optically pumped by conventional light sources such as flash lamps and arc lamps, as well as by pump lasers. The host is usually in the form of a solid rod a few centimetres long and a few millimetres in diameter with polished and coated end faces which provide the cavity mirrors.

The first ever laser was a ruby laser demonstrated in 1960 by Dr T.H. Maiman. Ruby consists of an aluminium oxide crystal with a concentration of less than 1 per cent of impurity chromium ions which provide the active medium and give ruby its characteristic red colour. The chromium ions are pumped into a band of excited energy levels with a population inversion with respect to the ground state energy level by a pulse of white light from a flash lamp. The output is a pulse of red light of wavelength 694 mn and of relatively long duration (about a millisecond). Pulse repetition rates are limited to a few hertz due to the need to dissipate heat from the rod.

Other more efficient solid state pulsed lasers have been developed. In the neodymium–yttrium-aluminium-garnet (Nd–YAG) laser, neodymium impurity ions are introduced ('doped') into a crystal of yttrium-aluminium-garnet. YAG lasers are usually pumped by flash lamps or by diode lasers to give infrared output pulses at or near a wavelength of 1.06 μm. The pulse duration is typically a few hundred nanoseconds with pulse repetition rates as high as thousands of hertz. The peak power of about 100 kW is similar to that of the nitrogen laser, but because the pulse duration is much longer the energy conveyed by each pulse is much larger, typically 10 J per pulse. The efficiency of these lasers depends upon the light source used for pumping and can reach 10 per cent. YAG lasers, like carbon dioxide lasers, are used in surgery. The 1.06 μm output can be carried by optical fibres and focused to provide a fine cutting tool. Visible and ultraviolet beams can be obtained by passing a powerful 1.06 μm output from a YAG laser through

certain crystals to produce harmonics. For example a (visible) frequency doubled output can be obtained at 530 μm.

An increasingly important class of lasers employ semiconductor materials such as gallium aluminium arsenide manufactured as diodes in the shape of small rectangular blocks of side lengths less than 1 mm. The active medium is a semiconductor junction pumped by a steady (DC) electrical current. At the junction, electrons in the conduction band can recombine with holes in the valence band accompanied by the release of photons. When the electric current through the diode is small this recombination occurs spontaneously and the device operates as an incoherent light-emitting diode. Light-emitting diodes of various colours find many uses as indicators and panel lights in modern electronics. When the current is increased a population inversion of electrons over holes is achieved and the device can become a diode laser with the end faces of the diode forming the cavity mirrors. Outputs from diode lasers are typically in the infrared and red, and they can be pulsed or continuous wave. Diode lasers are easily mass produced, are quite cheap, and have many familiar applications, for example in compact disc players.

Tuneable lasers

Many dye molecules have broad bands of energy levels accessible from the ground energy level by optical excitation. Dye molecules in liquid solvents can be efficiently pumped by other lasers, such as the argon ion laser, nitrogen laser, or excimer laser, to produce a high density of inverted molecules. The dye solution is contained in a small transparent cell between the two mirrors that form the optical cavity. The output of dye lasers can be continuous wave or pulsed depending on the pumping laser. Because the bands of energy levels in a dye are so broad dye lasers can easily be tuned through a bandwidth of about 50 nm. This is done by placing a wavelength-selective component such as a prism or diffraction grating in the optical cavity, or by replacing one of the mirrors by a reflecting diffraction grating on a rotatable mount. Many different dyes are commercially available. By choosing from a dozen or so different dyes one can operate a dye laser in any region of the optical spectrum and slightly beyond, although only wavelengths longer than the pump laser are available since the pump photons must have higher energy than the dye laser photons. The efficiency of conversion from pump input power to dye laser output power is of the order of 10 per cent. Dye lasers are often constructed in the laboratory from separately purchased components. Ready built they cost about as much as nitrogen lasers.

Recently, tuneable solid state lasers have started to become commercially available. Like dye lasers these lasers are pumped by other lasers. Typical of these is the titanium–sapphire laser which can be tuned from the red into the infrared. Other visible and even ultraviolet light can be produced by harmonic generation with a crystal.

Safety

The most obvious hazard associated with lasers is the damage that a laser beam can do to living tissue. The eye in particular is at risk since the beam can be focused by the eye lens on to the retina. This hazard depends on the output characteristics of the laser beam, and can be reduced by standard safety measures such as confinement of the beams and the wearing of suitable goggles. Particular attention should be paid to the possibility of unexpected reflections. Then too it should be remembered that the eye's natural protective reflexes may not be triggered by invisible infrared and ultraviolet beams. All laser users should be aware of the hazard classification of their laser and the recommended safety measures. A less obvious danger of using lasers are the very high voltage and current capabilities of the laser's power supply. Also, capacitors in the power supply may retain lethal charges long after the laser is switched off, especially if there is a fault in the circuitry.

Further reading

Davis, C.C. (1996). *Lasers and electro-optics fundamentals and engineering*. Cambridge University Press, Cambridge, UK. [A survey of lasers and their operation, together with their use in modern optical methods.]

Hecht, E. (1998). *Optics*, (3rd edn). Addison-Wesley, Reading, MA. [A treatment of most aspects of optics at undergraduate level including some mention of lasers.]

Hecht, J. (1992). *The laser guidebook*, (2nd edn). McGraw-Hill. [A very informative description of most types and properties of lasers.]

Lipson, *et al.* (1995). *Optical physics*, (3rd edn). Cambridge University Press. [A discussion of optical principles to graduate level, including some discussion of lasers.]

Ohanian, H.C. (1985). *Physics*. W.W. Norton & Co., New York. [A general survey of physics at the undergraduate level.]

Pedrotti, L.S. and Pedrotti, F.L. (1998). *Optics and vision*. Prentice Hall, Upper Saddle River, New Jersey. [Discusses optics and vision with a minimum of mathematics.]

Smith, G. and Atchison, D.A. (1997). *The eye and visual optical instruments*. Cambridge University Press, Cambridge, UK. [Contains little on lasers, but gives good discussions of the optics of the eye and instruments used with and for the eye.]

Zare, R.N., Spencer, B.H., Springer, D.S., and Jacobson, M.P. (1995). *Laser experiments for beginners*. University Science Books, Sausolito, California. [A basic experimental introduction to lasers.]

1.5.2 Physical and biological effects of lasers on ocular tissues

Caroline R. Baumal and Carmen Puliafito

Ophthalmologists have been at the forefront of technology with regard to diagnostic and therapeutic laser applications. In 1956, Meyer-Schwickerath pioneered the use of the xenon arc to produce retinal photocoagulation. In 1963, the ruby laser became the first commercial laser available for ophthalmological use. The argon, krypton, dye, and diode lasers are presently used for ocular photocoagulation. Photodisruption and photoablation have joined photocoagulation as established ophthalmic procedures. Lasers permit efficient and precise delivery of energy to a target tissue, with minimal damage to adjacent areas. Therapeutic lasers are often capable of cutting, shaping, or coagulating tissue. Diagnostic lasers obtain information about the state of tissue using low powered lasers in combination with sensitive detectors or imaging devices to probe tissue optical properties such as reflectance, scattering, and fluorescence. The unique properties of laser light and the optical properties of the eye make lasers particularly suitable for ophthalmological use.

Laser fundamentals

Laser is the acronym for Light Amplification by Stimulated Emission of Radiation. Stimulated emission was described by Einstein in 1917. When an excited atom is struck by an incoming photon possessing energy equal to the difference between the atom's higher and lower energy levels, the atom returns to its ground state by releasing a photon. The newly emitted photon has the same energy, direction, and phase as the incoming photon that triggered its release. Thus, stimulated emission results in the production of two identical photons with respect to wavelength, direction, and frequency. Lasers selectively amplify the energy transitions produced by stimulated emission to create a cascade of photons with identical properties.

Three components are present in ophthalmic lasers: (a) an active medium that emits coherent radiation; (b) a mechanism for energy input known as 'pumping'; and (c) a resonant cavity for oscillation, amplification, and release of photons produced by stimulated emission.

The active medium supports the process of stimulated emission by allowing a large number of atoms to exist in their energized state. The wavelength emitted is a function of the laser cavity's active medium which may be a gas (argon, krypton, carbon dioxide, helium with neon), liquid (organic dye), solid (an active element supported by a crystal such as neodymium supported by yttrium–aluminum–garnet, Nd–YAG), or a semiconductor (diode). Lasers are often named for their active medium. An energy input is required to permit most atoms of the active medium to exist in a higher energy state than ground state. This is known as population inversion, because it is opposite to the usual condition in which the majority of atoms are in their lowest energy state. The energy input to create population inversion is known as pumping and can be produced by an electric current (in gas lasers), a flash lamp (in solid crystal lasers), or by other lasers such as an argon source (in dye lasers). When population inversion occurs in the active medium, its atoms (or molecules) are primed for stimulated emission, whereby atoms relaxing from the excited state stimulate adjacent atoms to emit their energy as photons. Mirrors at the ends of the resonant cavity allow the photons to oscillate through the active medium which the pumping mechanism maintains in a state of population inversion. One of the mirrors is partially reflecting, allowing some of the photons to escape and form the laser beam. A prism or filter in the cavity is used to deviate photons with any wavelength other than that desired.

Lasers have mode structures produced by the optical fields

inside the cavities. Longitudinal or axial modes are the frequencies at which the laser cavity is resonant. Transverse modes are perpendicular to the direction of beam propagation and are related to the intensity distribution across the laser beam. The transverse mode determines the spatial distribution of laser light and the focusing property of the laser. The lowest mode (noted as the fundamental mode or TEM_{00}) has the lowest beam divergence, permitting focusing to a fine spot size which minimizes laser exposure to structures anterior and posterior to the focal point. Higher order modes have a less uniform beam profile. The fundamental mode is often used due to its focusing characteristics, but may not be desirable when very high energy levels are required as it represents only a small portion of the laser output.

The laser output can be continuous mode or pulsed, with pulse durations in the microsecond ($1\ \mu s = 10^{-6}\ s$) to femtosecond ($1\ fs = 10^{-15}\ s$) range. Gas lasers such as argon or krypton run only in the continuous mode, while solid and liquid lasers may be pulsed. The continuous laser beam is controlled by an external shutter and has a uniform power. In the pulse mode, energy is concentrated and delivered over a short duration resulting in average and peak powers. The rate of energy delivery, known as the radiant power, is equal to the energy measured in joules divided by the pulse duration in seconds. An increase in power can be achieved by increasing the energy, or more practically, by shortening the pulse duration. Q-switching and mode-locking are methods to reduce the period over which the energy is delivered. The Q-switch is an intracavitary shutter that allows rapid release of the energy as a short high power pulse. When the Q-switch shutter is closed, one of the mirrors in the resonant cavity is optically removed from the system, to prevent photon oscillations as the active medium is pumped. When maximal population inversion occurs, the Q-switch shutter is opened to expose the mirror, allowing photon oscillations, stimulated emission and light amplification to occur suddenly. The 'Q' refers to the quality factor of the laser cavity, which is the ratio of the energy stored in the cavity to the energy lost per cycle. Mode-locking produces ultrashort pulses in the picosecond ($1\ ps = 10^{-12}\ s$) to femtosecond range by synchronizing the phase relationships within the laser cavity utilizing a shutter near one of the cavity mirrors. Mode-locking in ophthalmic lasers is often accomplished by a saturable dye that absorbs low power radiation pulses, but becomes transparent on exposure to high power pulses. A typical mode-locked laser output consist of 7 to 10 pulses spaced over a total of 35 to 50 ns ($1\ ns = 10^{-9}\ s$), with a typical pulse width of 30 ps. The Q-switched laser output is a single pulse ranging from 2 to 30 ns. Maximum outputs for most Q-switched and mode-locked ophthalmic lasers are 10 to 30 mJ and 4.5 mJ, respectively.

Laser properties

Laser light has several unique properties that allow precise and efficient delivery of laser energy of a specific wavelength to a target with minimal adjacent tissue damage. These properties are monochromaticity, directionality, coherence, polarization, and intensity.

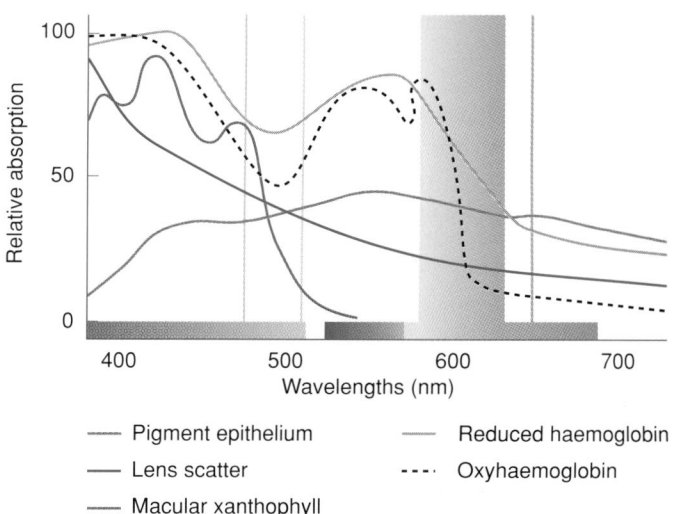

Fig. 1 Relative absorption versus wavelength for various ocular chromophores.

Monochromaticity refers to the discrete wavelength(s) emitted by the laser. This is due to a limited number of efficient electron transitions from the excited state to lower lying energy levels. Monochromaticity permits selection of a laser wavelength to enhance absorption or transmission by the target tissue with a certain absorption spectrum. The wavelength specificity of a laser typically exceeds the absorption specificity of pigments in the target tissue. The electromagnetic spectrum is composed of a broad range of radiation extending from short cosmic waves to long radio waves (Fig. 1). Current laser outputs include ultraviolet, visible, and infrared radiation (Table 1).

Directionality means that the laser beam is highly collimated (low divergence), allowing laser light to travel for considerable distances without widening. The degree of coherence describes the spatial and temporal synchronicity of the photons in the laser cavity. Polarization allows maximum energy transmission through the laser medium without loss due to reflection. Intensity is the power in a beam of a given angular size and brightness is the intensity per unit area. In ophthalmological lasers, the spot size is the diameter of the focused beam and its area is calculated by πr^2. Radiant energy is measured in joules ($1\ J = 1\ W \times 1\ s$) and radiant power is measured in watts ($1\ W = 1\ J/1\ s$). Laser irradiance is the power incident per unit area (W/cm^2), while radiant energy density is the energy per unit area (J/cm^2).

Tissue–photon interactions

Photons encountering a tissue surface can be reflected, scattered, transmitted, or absorbed. The energy of each photon is related to its wavelength and frequency by

$$E = h\nu = hc/\lambda$$

where h = Planck's constant (6.626×10^{-34} J s), ν = frequency, c = speed of light (3.0×10^8 m/s), and λ = wavelength. The frequency and energy of the photons decrease as the wavelength increases.

Table 1 Ophthalmic lasers and their wavelengths

Laser active medium	Wavelength	Colour
Argon	488.0 and 514.5 nm	Blue–green
	514.5 nm	Green
Carbon dioxide	10.6 μm	Infrared
Diode	810 nm (range 780–850 nm)	Infrared
Dye (tunable)	575 nm	Yellow
	590–600 nm	Orange
	630 nm	Red
Erbium	Erbium–YAG (2.94 μm)	Infrared
Excimer		
argon fluoride	193 nm	Ultraviolet
krypton chloride	222 nm	Ultraviolet
krypton fluoride	248 nm	Ultraviolet
xenon chloride	308 nm	Ultraviolet
xenon fluoride	351 nm	Ultraviolet
Helium–neon	632.6 nm	Red
Holmium	2.1 μm	Infrared
Krypton	647.1 nm	Red
	568.2 nm	Yellow
Nd–YAG	1064.0 nm	Infrared
Double frequency Nd–YAG	532.0 nm	Green
Ruby	694 nm	Red

Nd, neodymium; YAG, yttrium–aluminium–garnet.

The ability of a target to absorb radiation is measured by the attenuation of incident radiation after a certain length of the material has been traversed. The absorbance (A) is defined by

$$A(d) = \log[I_o / I(d)] = \varepsilon c d$$

where I_o = initial intensity, $I(d)$ = intensity at a distance d, ε = absorptivity of the material, and c = molarity of the material. Transmission is the portion of incident energy that is not absorbed after traversing a particular target thickness, and is defined by $T(d)$ where

$$T(d) = 10^{-A(d)} = e^{-\alpha d}$$

where $\alpha d = 2.3A$ defines the absorption coefficient α; α describes the fraction of incident energy that is absorbed per unit length of target material and is given in units of cm^{-1}. The thermal susceptibility of the irradiated tissue is denoted by the thermal relaxation time, τ, which represents the time required for the irradiated target tissue to carry away heat energy by conduction and is proportional to $1/4\alpha^2\kappa$ (where κ represents tissue diffusivity in cm^2/s).

The absorption maximum of a compound is the wavelength that has the highest probability of absorption. A plot of absorption versus wavelength produces an absorption spectrum that is characteristic of the chemical composition of a compound. Quantum yield measures the efficiency with which absorbed radiation produces chemical changes. The differences in spec-

tral absorption of different molecules allow selective damage to specific components of the target tissue. A chromophore is a molecule or a portion of it that absorbs photons of particular energy. Only the photons with wavelengths that match the absorption bands of the tissue chromophores are absorbed. A chromophore can undergo bond-breaking, ionization, or other types of molecular excitation depending on the energy of the absorbed photon.

When laser light reaches the target, its effect is dependent primarily upon its absorption. Sclera has a white appearance because it scatters almost all photons in the visible spectrum (400 to 700 nm) with little absorption. The cornea does not absorb photons in the visible range. Most photons are refracted and transmitted through the cornea with very little scattering (a small percentage are reflected at the air–cornea interface). Wavelengths shorter than 380 nm are limited by the ultraviolet-absorbing properties of the lens and cornea, and wavelengths longer than 1400 nm are restricted by water absorption. For retinal therapy, the laser must be able to penetrate the ocular media to interact with the target tissue. There is approximately 75 to 90 per cent transmission of electromagnetic radiation with a wavelength of 400 to 1064 nm through the ocular media. Scattering affects the distribution of photons in the target tissue. Scattering by the ocular media depends on the wavelength of incident light, and the size and refractive index of the scattering particle. In general, shorter wavelengths are scattered more than longer wavelengths for small particles.

Tissue effects of laser

The effect of laser light depends on both the properties of the target tissue and the laser. Laser wavelength, tissue absorbance, target diameter, exposure duration, energy, and power delivery to the target influence laser–tissue interaction. The most significant energy exchange with tissue occurs when photons are absorbed. The tissue effects of laser may be classified as photochemical, ionizing, or thermal depending on the parameters of laser wavelength, irradiance, and duration of exposure. More than one of these processes may be responsible for the clinical effects observed at intermediate values of irradiance and exposure.

Photochemical reactions primarily occur with low to moderate irradiances below coagulation thresholds and a laser wavelength below 320 nm. Absorption of a photon by the outer electrons provides an excited molecular state to drive a chemical reaction. This mechanism is most likely responsible for photoablation as produced by the excimer laser. In some instances, visible light can induce photochemical changes in photosensitized tissues, as with photodynamic therapy. Ionization requires high laser irradiances produced by a short exposure time in the nanosecond or picosecond range. The resultant energy strips the electrons from atoms and molecules, producing ionization and disintegration of target tissue into plasma. An example of ionization is photodisruption produced by the Nd–YAG laser, which delivers a near infrared wavelength to target tissues. Thermal effects occur primarily at a moderate irradiance, an exposure duration greater than 1 μs and a laser wavelength longer than used for photochemical effects. Both photocoagulation and photovaporization are produced by thermal mechanisms. Photocoagulation occurs when photon absorption or molecular vibrations produce a critical temperature rise sufficient to denature biomolecules, resulting in thermally induced structural changes in target tissues. For photovaporization, laser energy raises the tissue temperature in excess of 100°C (the boiling point of water) to produce tissue disruption. Clinically, this is used for incision and removal of tissue with haemostasis of adjacent blood vessels.

Photocoagulation

Photocoagulation is the commonest therapeutic application for laser of the retina, and its effect results from focal heating of tissue. Laser-induced thermal damage is proportional to the magnitude and duration of tissue temperature increase. The temperature rise is proportional to the light absorption in the target tissues, which is determined by how effectively its molecules absorb photons of a given wavelength. A moderate increase in retinal temperature under 100°C is associated with disruption of hydrogen bonds and van der Waal forces which stabilize molecular conformation. These conformational changes may manifest as loss of biological activity (enzyme inactivation) or structural integrity (alterations in cell membranes), resulting in cell necrosis, haemostasis, and coagulation. Water vaporization and gas bubble formation may occur with greater temperature increases. Photocoagulation lesions are immediately visible due to cellular necrosis and mechanical disruption of the normally transparent adjacent neurosensory retina. Delayed effects may result from inflammation and repair processes such as cellular proliferation, migration, and scar formation.

The photocoagulation burn for a given power is influenced by the amount of energy conducted by a specific wavelength, the duration of exposure, light scattering during transmission through the eye, and the optical and thermal properties of the absorbing tissue. For a burn of given intensity, decreasing the temperature rise increases the duration of exposure required. A higher temperature rise immediately produces a burn, while a lower temperature rise may result in a delayed appearance. The temperature elevation at the periphery of a burn may be lower than in its centre due to factors such as laser light scattering, heat conduction, and eye movements. This may account for the phenomenon of delayed expansion of a burn at its margin. The tissue temperature rise is proportional to the laser irradiance (which is the power incident per unit area). Smaller spots are more affected by heat dissipation to surrounding tissues and a higher irradiance is required to achieve the same central effect as for larger spots. Cooling of the centre of a large spot is less effective because immediately adjoining areas are also hot. For an increase in the spot size by two, less than four times as much power is required to reach the same temperature centrally.

Photocoagulation of the retina is often performed at durations of 100 to 200 ms, increasing up to 500 ms when an ocular media opacity is present. For a given amount of power,

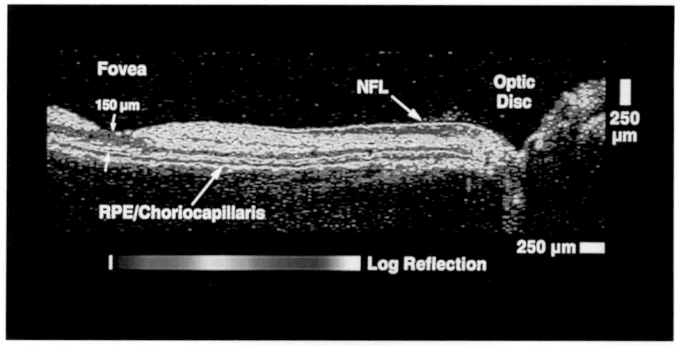

Fig. 2 Optical coherence tomography false colour image of a normal eye. The vitreous, fovea, optic disc, retinal nerve fibre layer, photoreceptors, and retinal pigment epithelium/choriocapillaris layer are identified. The central foveal thickness measures 150 μm.

decreasing the duration over which it is delivered increases the risk of tissue rupture and haemorrhage. Several hundred milliwatts are usually sufficient, although up to 1.0 W may be required. Spot sizes as small as 50 μm diameter are used to target individual vessels, whereas 100 to 500 μm are generally used for photocoagulation of the macula and retina, respectively.

Selection of a laser whose wavelength of emission matches the absorption characteristics of the target tissue in principle maximizes the therapeutic effect and minimizes side-effects. Most lasers for photocoagulation emit radiation in the visible portion of the electromagnetic spectrum, with the exception of the diode and long pulsed Nd–YAG lasers. The important chromophores in this range include melanin in the retinal pigment epithelium, choroidal melanocytes, iris pigment epithelium, and trabecular meshwork, haemoglobin in blood vessels, and xanthophyll in the inner and outer plexiform layers in the macula, as well as in some cataracts. Photoreceptor pigments and lipofuscin in elderly eyes are other potential chromophores. The three primary absorbers for retinal photocoagulation are melanin, xanthophyll, and haemoglobin (Fig. 2). Melanin absorption is maximal from 400 to 700 nm, absorbing blue, green, yellow, and red wavelengths in decreasing order. Melanin absorption decreases at longer wavelengths, resulting in deeper retinal burns. The argon green wavelength is absorbed at the level of the retinal pigment epithelium, krypton red produces a deeper burn, and Nd–YAG produces choroidal and even scleral effects. A deeper burn is less prominent clinically and often more painful. Haemoglobin in the inner retinal and choroidal vessels may be targeted to destroy or occlude leaky vessels. Haemoglobin absorbs blue, green, and yellow wavelengths well, with poor absorption of red and infrared wavelengths. The absorption spectrum of haemoglobin varies with its oxygen saturation and oxyhaemoglobin has poorer absorption of red than reduced haemoglobin. The two absorption maxima for oxyhaemoglobin are at 542 nm (green) and 577 nm (yellow), while reduced haemoglobin absorbs maximally at 555 nm (yellow). Blue, green, and yellow wavelengths can produce vasospasm in haemoglobin-containing structures. Longer wavelengths may produce vasospasm by absorption of laser light in the underlying retinal pigment epithelium with subsequent transfer of heat to adjacent retinal vessels. Yellow xanthophyll pigment absorbs wavelengths below 500 nm, absorbing blue strongly, green minimally, and yellow and red light negligibly. The blue wavelength from the argon blue–green laser is absorbed by the retinal xanthophyll pigment, while longer wavelength lasers avoid this effect.

Lasers for photocoagulation

The xenon arc photocoagulator emits monochromatic white light with wavelengths from 400 to 1600 nm, producing a full thickness retinal burn. Disadvantages include inability for selective targeting of ocular tissue, a long exposure duration of several seconds, and retrobulbar anaesthesia is required. Although rarely used in North America, the xenon arc is used in other areas of the world where lasers are unavailable. The ruby crystal laser was the first commercially available laser, although it was soon replaced by the argon laser. The ruby laser has an increased risk of subretinal haemorrhage due to its short pulse duration and is not useful for direct vascular treatment.

The argon laser can emit blue–green (488 and 514.5 nm) or green (514.5 nm) wavelengths. The standard argon blue–green laser produces 60 to 70 per cent blue light. Due to the potential hazards of the blue wavelength, it is no longer recommended for the treatment of macular disorders. Blue light is scattered more by media opacities and may be absorbed by inner retinal xanthophyll, producing undesirable neurosensory retinal damage. The white inner retinal burn that is produced may induce light scattering, preventing deeper laser penetration to the retinal pigment epithelium with repeated laser applications and obscuring post-treatment fluorescein angiographic imaging. Prolonged use of blue light may decrease colour discrimination in a tritan colour-confusion axis in ophthalmologists. The argon green wavelength is well absorbed by haemoglobin and melanin, with minimal xanthophyll absorption. This permits direct coagulation of retinal vessels, but does not allow treatment through haemorrhage.

The krypton laser emits either red (647.1 nm) or yellow (568.2 nm) wavelengths. Krypton red has no haemoglobin absorption and negligible xanthophyll absorption, with deeper penetration than argon green. Krypton red is used primarily for treatment of the retinal pigment epithelium and choroid. Closure of choroidal neovascularization by krypton red is secondary to laser light absorption by the retinal pigment epithelium and choroidal melanin and transfer of heat to adjacent blood vessels. Krypton red has better penetration than shorter wavelengths through nuclear sclerotic cataracts and mild vitreous or shallow subretinal haemorrhage. Due to deeper laser penetration, there is an increased risk of choroidal haemorrhage and disruption of Bruch's membrane. If an inadvertent haemorrhage occurs, the red wavelength is unable to coagulate vessels directly. Krypton yellow causes less retinal pigment epithelium damage than krypton red, but may cause inner retinal damage in the form of nerve fibre layer and ganglion cell oedema.

The tunable dye laser produces a range of monochromatic wavelengths including yellow (575 nm), orange (590–600 nm), and red (630 nm), in addition to blue (488 nm) and green (514 nm) produced by the argon laser used to pump the dye. Dye yellow (577 nm) absorption is negligible for xanthophyll, moderate for melanin (41 per cent absorption), and maximal for oxyhaemoglobin (70 per cent absorption) and deoxyhaemoglobin (82 per cent absorption), permitting direct therapy of abnormal retinal or choroidal vessels. Dye orange has not been as widely used, as high intensity juxtafoveal burns produced with 600 nm orange light produced inner retinal damage in the primate retina.

The Nd–YAG laser at 1064 nm is poorly absorbed by melanin, resulting in deep choroidal penetration. A crystal of potassium–titanium–phosphate can double the frequency of the Nd–YAG laser and decrease the wavelength in half to 532 nm (green). The double frequency Nd–YAG output is more highly absorbed by the retinal pigment epithelium and haemoglobin than argon green and is close to the absorption peaks of oxyhaemoglobin and deoxyhaemoglobin permitting effective vascular occlusion.

Most ophthalmic semiconductor diode lasers emit in the infrared region at 810 nm, and produce outer retina and choroidal damage while sparing the inner retina. Benefits of the diode laser include excellent penetration through serous fluid or retinal oedema and minimal absorption by intraocular media opacities. The diode laser requires greater power and a longer exposure duration to create clinical photocoagulation when compared to argon green.

Factors to be consider when selecting a laser wavelength for retinal photocoagulation are effective transmission through the ocular media, low absorption by macular xanthophyll to limit inner retinal damage, and effective penetration through haemorrhage or fluid anterior to the target tissue. For closure of retinal or choroidal blood vessels, direct haemoglobin absorption by the shorter wavelengths may be desirable. Dye yellow has minimal absorption by cataracts or xanthophyll with moderate melanin and maximal haemoglobin absorption. Argon green is useful for therapy of choroidal neovascularization in a poorly pigmented fundus and for treating large calibre vessels. Longer wavelengths such as krypton red and diode are favoured in the presence of a vitreous or retinal haemorrhage or lens opacity, as they are absorbed poorly by haemoglobin and are scattered less than shorter wavelengths.

While the histopathological effect of the various laser wavelengths used for photocoagulation has been studied in animals and humans, the clinical significance of these studies is uncertain. Therapy is often performed in eyes with concurrent ocular pathology that may interfere with laser effect. It is notable that heavy photocoagulation with any laser wavelength can produce varying degrees of a full thickness retinal burn due to heat conduction to the inner retina. Few studies have compared the clinical effect of different laser wavelengths and further evaluation is required.

Clinical applications

Laser photocoagulation is used to treat ocular disorders including diabetic retinopathy, macular oedema, choroidal neovascularization as well as to form an adhesion around retinal breaks and detachments. Retinal neovascularization may occur in proliferative diabetic retinopathy, sickle cell retinopathy, retinopathy of prematurity, and after retinal vein occlusion. Panretinal photocoagulation indirectly improves proliferative diabetic retinopathy by reducing the stimulus for neovascularization. This follows from the destruction of hypoxic retina, especially photoreceptors with their high oxygen requirement, creating tighter adhesions to the choriocapillaris and resulting in decreased vasoproliferative tendencies with better oxygen perfusion to the remaining viable retina. Retinal pigment epithelium cells may produce a substance to inhibit neovascularization, and thus may be released secondary to retinal photocoagulation.

Laser photocoagulation has proven beneficial for treatment of diabetic macular oedema and after branch retinal vein occlusion in selected patients. In diabetes, localized and diffuse forms of macular oedema are treated with focal and grid laser application, respectively. Focal treatment may reduce oedema by preventing fluid passage from the subretinal space through the retinal pigment epithelium and directly sealing leaking microaneurysms or capillaries. Damage by grid photocoagulation occurs primarily in the retinal pigment epithelium, with some effect on the photoreceptors and the underlying choriocapillaris. The mechanism of effect is unclear, but possibilities include reduction in blood flow, increased inner retinal oxygen, replacement of coagulated retinal pigment epithelium cells with new ones, and proliferation of endothelial cells in capillaries and venules overlying the lesions, capable of reinforcing the outer and inner blood–retinal barriers, respectively. The inner retinal effects are believed to result indirectly from targeting of the outer retina.

The mechanism of laser therapy for choroidal neovascularization involves thrombus formation and collagen shrinkage in vascular walls and surrounding connective tissue induced by laser-generated heat. As with diabetic neovascularization, laser treatment may cause the release of angiogenesis-inhibiting factors, cauterize vessels in the choriocapillaris, and seal breaks in Bruch's membrane that may engender choroidal neovascularization.

Laser iridectomy for angle closure glaucoma has been performed with argon and diode lasers. Argon iridectomy permits simultaneous coagulation of any haemorrhaging vessels, but may require numerous exposures, especially in lightly pigmented irises, and the Q-switched Nd–YAG laser is often preferred. Damage to the ciliary body (cyclodestruction) has been performed successfully with a contact diode laser. Argon or diode laser trabeculoplasty may control elevated intraocular pressure in selected forms of glaucoma. Initial theories of the mechanism of laser trabeculoplasty focused on its mechanical effects to shrink the superficial collagen of the corneoscleral meshwork to prevent closure of Schlemm's canal, while more recent theories focus on the biochemical effects of laser trabeculoplasty.

Photodisruption

Photodisruption uses high peaked power laser pulses to damage target tissue. When laser energy is concentrated in space and time to achieve high irradiance or density of power, optical breakdown or ionization of the target occurs. Optical breakdown is a sudden event, noted visibly as a spark and accompanied by an audible snap with target disruption. When focused to a small spot (usually less than 50 μm), short pulsed Q-switch and mode-locked Nd–YAG lasers can produce adequate irradiance to create optical breakdown and dissociate electrons from their atoms to produce plasma. Light energy can create plasma when high irradiance in the range of 10^{10} to 10^{12} W/cm^2 is produced. Q-switch pulses produce ionization mainly by focal target heating in a process called thermionic emission, whereas mode-locked pulses rely on multiphoton absorption. In either case, once the initial free electrons have been generated, plasma expands via electron avalanche or cascade if the irradiance is adequate to cause rapid ionization. Plasma absorbs and scatters incident radiation, thus shielding underlying structures that are in the beam path. The Nd–YAG photodisruptor utilizes energies significantly above retinal damage thresholds. Beam divergence after the focal point and plasma formation and shielding are mechanisms to reduce the radiant energy from reaching the retina and prevent adjacent damage.

The mechanism of Nd–YAG-induced tissue damage involves focal thermal effects and pressure waves. The microplasma temperature reaches up to 15 000°C focally. The high energy density is sufficient to create a microexplosion with vaporization and melting of liquids and solids in a small volume near the focal point. This occurs in the absence of absorption of energy by the targets and can occur in transparent targets. As the pulse duration is short, heat does not diffuse to surrounding regions. In biological systems, thermal denaturation of protein and nucleic acids is calculated as confined to a radius of 0.1 mm for a 1 mJ pulse. Although high local temperatures exist briefly, the total heat energy is low and clinical photocoagulation is not an important factor.

Several mechanisms generate pressure waves radiating from the zone of optical breakdown, such as rapid plasma expansion and stimulated Brillouin scattering, in which the laser light generates the pressure wave that scatters it. The focal heating may lead to vaporization, melting, and thermal expansion, generating acoustic waves. The shock wave begins immediately with plasma formation, and expands at a hypersonic velocity of 4 km/s, falling to sonic velocity within 200 μm. The acoustic transient lasts 50 ns at a distance of 300 μm from the focal point, while the pressure falls from a maximum of 101 000 to 10 100 kPa (1000 to 100 atm) within a distance of 1 mm. The shock wave is followed by cavitation, or vapour bubble formation which begins within 50 to 150 ns after breakdown in water. Cavity propagation velocity is approximately 20 m/s at 300 μm from the breakdown. The size of the damage zone depends on the irradiance and total energy, the plasma's duration, and the mechanical properties of the target tissue.

Clinical applications

The Nd–YAG output at 1064 nm is the only commercially used ophthalmic photodisruptor. Most Nd–YAG lasers employ the fundamental TEM$_{00}$ mode, so the spot size, and consequently the energy required for optical breakdown, can be minimized. Beam divergence typically ranges from 0.5 to 3.0 mrad. Most ophthalmic applications can be performed with a pulse energy of 5 mJ or less. Higher energies may be required in the presence of opaque ocular media. Due to greater control and relative safety of the Q-switch, mode-locking Nd–YAG lasers have fallen out of favour. A continuous wave helium–neon laser produces a 632.8 nm output aiming beam coaxial with the invisible Nd–YAG output.

Most cataract surgery is performed leaving the posterior lens capsule in place. This decreases the incidence of postoperative vitreoretinal complications and provides support for posterior chamber intraocular lenses. The posterior capsule may opacify with time and can be opened with Nd–YAG pulses of 1 to 2 mJ. Opacities in the anterior capsule and pupillary or anterior vitreous membranes may be sectioned by the Nd–YAG.

Intraocular lenses may be made of polymethylmethacrylate, silicone, acrylic, or glass. Nd–YAG laser damage to the intraocular lens during posterior capsulotomy may take the form of microcracks, melted voids, and large pulverized regions. Optical breakdown in polymethylmethacrylate and glass may be associated with self-focusing and self-trapping with both nanosecond and picosecond pulses. The damage threshold for glass is approximately 100 times greater than that for polymethylmethacrylate, but once glass damage occurs, it is often more extensive. Damage tends to be cumulative and intraocular lenses may be damaged more by a burst than by single laser pulses. Intraocular lenses designed to increase the separation between the intraocular lens and the posterior lens capsule may decrease damage from laser capsulotomy.

The Nd–YAG laser is useful for creating iridectomies as photodisruption does not depend on target pigmentation. Small, self-limited haemorrhages occasionally occur, and the Nd–YAG is unable to coagulate any significant bleeding. Openings are often achieved with a single Nd–YAG laser shot of 4 to 8 mJ. Nd–YAG laser cyclodestruction is effective to control intraocular pressure in selected patients.

Nd–YAG photodisruption may prove useful for posterior segment pathology. Experimental vitreous membranes in rabbits have been sectioned with 4 mJ pulses as close as 4 mm to the retina, without retinal injury. The risk of retinal or choroidal haemorrhage rises with proximity to the retina, and a lens (crystalline or intraocular lens) may be damaged if laser energy is deposited too close to its posterior surface.

Photoablation

Photoablation produced by the excimer laser utilizes short pulses of ultraviolet radiation to perform lamellar corneal surgery without thermal damage to adjacent tissue. Clinical use of excimer laser technology was approved in 1995 by the United States Food and Drug Administration for treatment of low to moderate myopia and a number of anterior corneal pathologies.

Excimers, or excited dimers, are molecules with bound upper states and weakly bound ground states, such as the rare gas excimers fluoride (F_2) and xenon (Xe_2), which emit radiation at 157 and 170 nm, respectively. These lasers are not practical clinically as oxygen absorption below 190 nm precludes working in room air. The best excimer laser performance has been demonstrated by the reaction of an excited rare gas atom with a halogen molecule. Several combinations have been investigated as the laser active medium (see Table 1). These rare gas monohalides emit energetic ultraviolet photons as they decay from the bound upper state to the rapidly dissociating ground state. The released photons possess enough energy not only to break molecular bonds, but to expel molecular fragments from the corneal surface. The process of controlled removal of material, in which molecules on the irradiated surface are broken into small volatile fragments by the excimer, has been termed 'ablative photodecomposition'. Ablative photodecomposition is likely caused by a combination of the high absorption for ultraviolet radiation possessed by organic polymers, which limits the depth of the radiation's penetration, and the high quantum yield for bond breaking, which results in the formation of numerous fragments in a small volume near the surface. Ablation is thought to result from the intense pressure build-up within this volume. With respect to the relative photochemical and thermal contributions to excimer ablation, there appears to be an increasing thermal effect at longer wavelengths.

Two ultraviolet excimer wavelengths, 193 and 248 nm, have been most extensively studied for cornea surgery. Corneal absorption rapidly increases below 300 nm. As water does not significantly absorb radiation between 193 and 293 nm, it must be the solid components of the cornea which are responsible for absorption in this region. The majority of corneal solids are proteins, particularly collagen which comprises about 70 per cent of the stromal dry weight. Protein absorption maxima around 190 nm have been associated with absorption by the C–N peptide bond.

Nucleic acids, primarily in the corneal epithelium, absorb at both 193 and 248 nm. The different types of glycosaminoglycans demonstrate absorption peaks around 190 nm and no significant absorption at 248 nm.

In 1983, Trokel and associates demonstrated that the 193 nm excimer laser was capable of precisely etching the cornea and laser damage was localized to the zone of ablation. Puliafito and colleagues compared the 193 and 248 nm excimer laser in human and bovine corneas. The lowest per pulse fluences at which human corneal ablation was observed were 46 mJ/cm^2 at 193 nm and 58 mJ/cm^2 at 248 nm. Corneal ablations with 193 nm were either trough- or slit-like depending on the width of exposure. Transmission electron microscopy revealed a zone of damaged stroma approximately 0.1 to 0.3 μm thick at the lesion edges which was interpreted as a thin band of thermal denaturation or photoablated material which was not completely ejected and adhered to the wall of the incision. Ablation with 248 nm produced incisions with a wider zone adjacent stromal damage at least 2.5 μm wide and more marked disruption.

The lowest radiant exposure for corneal ablation has been achieved with the 193 nm argon fluoride laser. Removal of corneal tissue with the lowest amount of energy may minimize damage secondary to excess heat build-up, shock waves, or photochemical damage to untreated tissues. A number of factors may account for the precise corneal ablation and minimal adjacent tissue damage observed with the 193 nm excimer. The absorption length of 193 nm radiation is only 3.7 μm, so that incident energy is deposited in a relatively small volume of tissue. The incident laser radiation is short pulsed (10 to 20 ns), minimizing heat diffusion beyond the irradiated area. At 193 nm, the energy per photon is high at 6.4 eV, which is sufficient to cleave peptide bonds (3.0 eV) or the adjacent carbon–carbon bonds (3.5 eV) of the polypeptide chains, especially as in collagen. The high quantum yield for peptide bond cleavage at 193 nm and the high absorption of stroma glycosaminoglycans may be responsible for the superior tissue removal and lower fluence requirement associated with 193 nm ablation. Radiation at 193 nm has yielded smoother surfaces than 248 nm, thus promoting more normal corneal re-epithelialization. A linear relationship exists between number of pulses and ablation depth. Ablation depth with each pulse can be reproduced to ± 2000 Å in most materials, accounting for the excimer lasers high level of reliability and reproducibility.

Clinical applications

Some refractive errors can be corrected by recontouring the cornea. Surgical procedures such as radial keratotomy, keratomileusis, keratophakia, and epikeratophakia can alter corneal curvature; however, these methods may lack reproducible incision depths or accuracy. During photorefractive keratectomy with the 193 nm excimer, the stroma is lathed to alter the corneal curvature *in situ* in a precise and reproducible manner. The optical axis is treated with disruption of Bowman's membrane. For correction of myopia, a circular beam of uniform irradiance is passed through a slowly enlarging or shrinking diaphragmatic opening to permit preferential ablation of the central cornea. Alternatively, a scanning slit that is wider in the centre may translate over the corneal surface.

The central ablation depth and diameter required to achieve a specified myopic correction has been calculated, assuming that the epithelium will regrow with a uniform thickness and produce a new corneal curvature determined by the new stromal curvature. Corneal flattening is determined by the equation:

$$\text{Ablation depth} = \frac{-S^2 D}{8(n-1)}$$

where $D = (n-1)/(1/R2 - 1/R1)$, n is the corneal index of refraction, $R1$ and $R2$ are the initial and final corneal radii of curvature, respectively, and S is the diameter of the ablation zone in mm. This formula has been approximated as:

$$\text{Ablation depth} = \frac{DS^2}{3}$$

where D is the intended dioptric correction and S is the diameter of the intended ablation zone. This reveals that an increase in the ablation zone diameter will result in a deeper ablation depth for a given myopic correction. This is important clinically as eyes treated with deeper ablations may experience more regression of the refractive effect.

The excimer is being evaluated for treatment of hyperopia and astigmatism. Hyperopic correction is achieved by sparing the visual axis and removing peripheral cornea tissue. Laser *in situ* keratomileusis combines the advantages of corneal lamellar surgery with the precision of excimer laser surgery. In this technique, a superficial flap in a cornea is temporarily separated, the stroma is shaped with the excimer, and the flap is replaced.

Phototherapeutic keratectomy is the removal of anterior corneal pathology with excimer laser. It is indicated in eyes with mild to moderate visually significant anterior corneal pathology that is not severe enough to warrant more invasive partial thickness or total keratectomy. It has been used to treat corneal scars and corneal dystrophies (such as granular, lattice, Reis–Buckler, crystalline, and anterior basement membrane dystrophy). There is an increased chance of significant refractive error changes with phototherapeutic keratectomy for cornea pathology deeper than 100 μm. Modification of the beam diameter, pulse repetition rate and depth of ablation per pulse according to extent of pathology. While the cornea is presently the most common target for excimer ablation, the laser is being investigated for non-corneal ophthalmic applications.

Carbon dioxide laser

The carbon dioxide laser efficiently emits radiation in the mid-infrared wavelength of 10.6 μm. This wavelength is strongly absorbed by water, making the carbon dioxide laser useful in any water-containing tissue. Heat diffusion away from the target area coagulates adjacent vessels for haemostasis. The carbon dioxide laser has been employed to treat ophthalmic pathology from the eyelids and adnexa to the vitreous. Disadvantages of the carbon dioxide laser are the degree of tissue shrinkage and vaporization. The rate of energy delivery determines the peak energy rise, which if controlled will minimize the area of undesired coagulation of surrounding tissue. The use of a pulsed carbon dioxide laser reduces thermal damage to surrounding tissue by allowing less time for heat conduction.

New developments in ophthalmic lasers

In order to increase the specificity and effectiveness of laser therapy, several new techniques have been investigated including selective photothermolysis, short pulse lasers, dye enhancement, and photodynamic therapy. The rationale is to target specific ocular structures with decreased energy requirements and to minimize damage to adjacent tissues. Lasers can be used to image ocular tissues as with the recently developed optical coherence tomography.

Selective photothermolysis

At the duration of exposure presently used for retinal photocoagulation, the neurosensory retina is thermally damaged due to its position adjacent to the retinal pigment epithelium, and this may adversely affect the final visual outcome. Selective photothermolysis describes thermally confined injury of pigmented target tissue caused by selective absorption of brief pulses of radiation. Selective thermal injury is produced by the unique properties of the target tissue, rather than precise aiming of the laser beam. After laser exposure, the target begins to dissipate heat by conduction to adjacent tissues. Selective target heating may be achieved when the energy is deposited at a rate faster than the rate of cooling. In order to achieve this effect, the pulse duration must be equal to or less than the target's thermal relaxation time. The length of exposure is determined by the target size. Other requirements include a wavelength that reaches and is preferentially absorbed by the target structure and a fluence sufficient to cause thermal damage. This method has successfully produced selective damage to blood vessels (3.0×10^{-7} s, 577 nm) and melanocytes (2.0×10^{-8} s, 351 nm).

Short pulse lasers

Repetitive exposure to short laser pulses can confine damage to absorbing structures at pulse energies below the threshold energy for single pulse damage. The heat flux out of the retinal pigment epithelium is negligible if very short pulse durations are used. However, higher temperatures are required with short pulses to produce thermal effects similar to long pulses. To avoid thermal damage, multiple subthreshold pulses are used to compensate for the lower pulse energy. Selective retinal pigment epithelium destruction with minimal damage to adjacent neural retina and choroid was produced in the rabbit retina by multiple subthreshold short laser exposures (514 nm, 5 μs, 1 to 500 pulses at 500 Hz, 2 to 10 μJ pulse energy). Ultrashort pulses in the picosecond to femtosecond range produce extremely high peak laser intensity with minimal pulse energy. Femtosecond pulsed lasers have been evaluated in rabbits (single 80 fs pulse, 625 nm) and energy deposition and retinal damage was found to be non-linear and produced fewer non-specific thermal effects.

Drug-enhanced laser absorption

Dye enhancement

Dye enhancement relies on the administration of an exogenous dye that concentrates in the target tissue. Localization of the laser effect is based on the similar wavelength of absorption for the exogenous agent and the emission from the laser. This may permit treatment with lower energy requirements with less adjacent tissue damage. Fluorescein dye absorbs in the blue region wavelength emitted from the argon blue–green laser and has been used to enhance argon laser therapy of retinal angiomas outside the macular region. Indocyanine green is a water soluble tricarbocyanine intravenous dye that is used as an angiographic agent to enhance visualization of the choroidal circulation and to characterize occult choroidal neovascularization and other choroidal disorders. As the wavelength of indocyanine green absorption at 805 nm is similar to that of diode laser emission (810 nm), intravenous indocyanine green administration immediately prior to diode treatment may permit selective photocoagulation of indocyanine green-filled choroidal neovascularization with lower energy requirements and decrease laser damage to adjacent normal retina. In animal models, indocyanine green-enhanced diode photocoagulation closed choroidal neovascularization with lower energy requirements than for diode laser alone.

Photodynamic therapy

Photodynamic therapy utilizes low intensity light of an appropriate wavelength to activate an exogenous photochemical agent. A photochemical interaction between the agent and light leads to *in situ* production of singlet oxygen and superoxide anions which interact with various cellular components (lipid membranes, proteins, and nucleic acids). This results in vascular thrombosis and cellular damage in the target tissue. Selective tissue targeting occurs as the photochemical agent preferentially concentrates in hyperproliferating and neoplastic tissues. Thermal damage to adjacent retina is minimized by direct application of low intensity light.

In ophthalmology, photodynamic therapy with the photosensitizer haematoporphyrin derivative has been used to treat intraocular melanoma and retinoblastoma with variable results. As vascular injury plays a role in photodynamic therapy-induced tissue destruction, it is being investigated for therapy of choroidal neovascularization. Photodynamic therapy with new second-generation photosensitizers including chloroaluminum sulphonated phthalocyanine, benzoporphyrin derivative monoacid ring A, and tin etiopurpurin (activated by 675, 692, and 664 nm wavelength light, respectively) have induced short-term closure of experimental choroidal neovascularization in animals.

Liposome drug delivery

Systemic administration of a liposome-encapsulated medication, followed by a controlled mechanism for local release, may provide a high drug concentration to specific intraocular structures. External low level irradiation with argon blue–green, dye yellow, and microwave irradiation have been used to produce targeted release of temperature-sensitive liposome content. Release of liposome-encapsulated dye and drug (carboxyfluorescein and cytosine arabinoside, respectively) in the anterior chamber of rabbits has been produced by external microwave-induced hyperthermia.

Optical coherence tomography

Optical coherence tomography is a new modality that produces high resolution, cross-sectional images of ocular structures *in vivo* and *in vitro*. Developed by researchers from Tufts University and the Massachusetts Institute of Technology, optical coherence tomography produces images with a longitudinal resolution of up to 10 μm. This is superior to B-scan ultrasound and the scanning laser ophthalmoscopy resolution of 150 and 300 μm, respectively. Ultrasound biomicroscopy produces image resolution up to 20 μm with a 100-MHz high frequency transducer, but depth of penetration is limited to 4 mm, preventing posterior segment applications.

Optical coherence tomography is similar to B-mode ultrasound, but uses reflection of light waves from different struc-

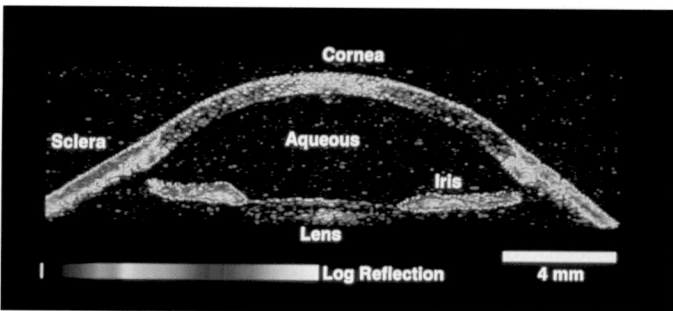

Fig. 3 Optical coherence tomography image of the anterior segment of the human eye.

tures in the eye rather than sound. Distance information is extracted from the time–of–flight delay of light reflected from different structures within the eye using low coherence interferometry. Low coherence light is produced by a continuous wave superluminescent diode source, coupled to a fibreoptic Michelson interferometer. Interference fringes appear at a detector only when the path length of light reflected from the eye matches a reference path length to within the coherence length of the light source. Microstructural features are determined by measuring the 'echo' time it takes for the light to reflect from the different structures at varying distances, analogous to ultrasound A-scan. The optical coherence tomography image of optical reflectivity is displayed in false colour. Bright colours such as red and white represent regions of high optical reflectivity and dark colours such as blue and black represent regions of minimal optical reflectivity. Figure 3 shows an optical coherence tomography image obtained by scanning through the centre of the fovea and optic disc in a normal eye. The cross-sectional anatomy and the layered structure of the retina are apparent. A highly reflective red layer corresponds to the retinal pigment epithelium and choriocapillaris. The contrast between this red layer and the neural retina forms a reproducible boundary for measurement of retinal thickness. The dark layer immediately anterior to this probably represents photoreceptor outer segments. The nerve fibre layer corresponds to the bright red reflective layer at the inner retinal margin.

Optical coherence tomography is useful to evaluate retinal architecture and has been used to characterize macular holes, vitreomacular traction, epiretinal membranes, and choroidal neovascularization. Quantification of retinal elevation in macular oedema and pigment epithelial detachments is possible. Visualization of anterior chamber structures and measurement of the peripapillary nerve fibre layer thickness may play a role in the evaluation of glaucoma.

A variety of lasers are presently available for ocular diagnosis and therapy. New developments in laser technology may further improve the resolution for ocular imaging and increase the specificity of tissue effects.

Further reading

Anderson, R.R. and Parrish, J.A. (1983). Selective photothermolysis: precise microsurgery by selective absorption of pulsed radiation. *Science*, **220**, 5247.

Hee, M.R., Baumal, C.R., Puliafito, C.A., *et al.* (1996). Optical coherence tomography of age-related macular degeneration. *Ophthalmology*, **103**, 1260–70.

Krauss, J.M. and Puliafito, C.A. (1995). Lasers in ophthalmology. *Lasers in Surgery and Medicine*, 17, 102–59.

L'Esperance, F.A. Jr. (1985). New laser systems and their potential clinical usefulness. In *Transactions of the New Orleans Academy of Ophthalmology. Symposium on the laser in ophthalmology and glaucoma update*, pp.192–209. Mosby, St Louis.

Lin C. (1993). Laser tissue interactions. Basic principles. *Ophthalmology Clinics of North America*, **6**, 381–91.

Mainster, M.A. (1985). Ophthalmic laser surgery: principles, technology and technique. In *Transactions of the New Orleans Academy of Ophthalmology. Symposium on the laser in ophthalmology and glaucoma update*, pp.81–101. Mosby, St Louis.

March, W.F., ed. (1990). *Ophthalmic lasers. A second generation.* Slack International, New Jersey.

Parrish, J.A. and Deutsch, T.F. (1984). Laser photomedicine. *IEEE Journal of Quantum Electronics*, **QE-20**, 1386–96.

Puliafito, C.A., Steinert, R.F., Deutsch, T.F., Hillenkamp, F., Dehm, E.J., and Adler, C.M. (1985). Excimer laser ablation of the cornea and lens. Experimental studies. *Ophthalmology*, **92**, 741–8.

Puliafito, C.A., Wong, K., and Steinert, R.F. (1987). Quantitative and ultrastructural studies of excimer laser ablation of the cornea at 193 and 248 nanometers. *Lasers in Surgery and Medicine*, **7**, 155–9.

Roider, J., Hillenkamp, F., Flotte, T., and Birngruber, R. (1993). Microphotocoagulation: selective effects of repetitive short laser pulses. *Proceedings of the National Academy of Sciences (USA)*, **90**, 8643–7.

Romanelli, J.F. and Puliafito, C.A. (1990). Metabolic studies of dye laser retinal photocoagulation. *International Ophthalmology Clinics*, **30**, 95–101.

Sliney, D.H., and Trokel, S.L. (1993). *Medical lasers and their safe use.* Springer-Verlag, New York.

Steinert, R.F., and Puliafito, C.A. (1985). *The Nd-YAG laser in ophthalmology. Principles and clinical applications of photodisruption.* W.B. Saunders, Philadelphia.

Trokel, S.L., Srinivasan, R., and Braren, B. (1983). Excimer laser surgery of the cornea. *American Journal of Ophthalmology*, **96**, 710–15.

1.6 Ophthalmic clinical examination

1.6.1 Methods of clinical examination

1.6.1.1 Loupe, slit lamp, and ophthalmoscopy

Michael J. Greaney

Meticulous ophthalmic examination requires an understanding of the techniques for using optical instruments as well as their features and limitations.

Loupe

It is impossible to measure the ratio of object to image dimensions if the image is virtual and located at infinity. The magnification produced by an optical system therefore refers to angular rather than linear magnification—the ratio of the angle at the eye subtended by the object when viewed through the optical system to that when it is viewed unaided at a standardized viewing distance of 0.25 m.

The magnified image produced by a loupe facilitates external ocular examination. In its simplest form it is a hand-held plus lens. When an object at the first principal focus of such a lens is viewed at d metres, the magnification (M) of the virtual image is the product of the dioptric power (D) and distance: $M = D \times d$. For example, a 32-dioptre lens produces 8× magnification of an object 0.25 m from the observer.

A binocular loupe consists of either a plus lens of high power or a Galilean telescope mounted in front of each eye on spectacles or a headband. Galilean telescopes allow a more practical working distance and magnifications from 2× to 6× are available, with a larger field of view in the lower range. In a Galilean telescope the second focal point of a positive lens coincides with the first focal point of a negtive lens to form an image at infinity. The resulting magnification (M) is the absolute value of the focal length of the objective lens (fo) divided by the focal length of the eye lens (fe): $M = (fo/fe)$. A combination of a +10 dioptre and a –20 dioptre lens will therefore magnify 2× or 0.5× depending on telescope orientation.

Direct ophthalmoscopy

A hand-held direct ophthalmoscope may be used to examine the anterior segment but is more useful for the posterior segment. The field of view is approximately 8° and for fundus examination, is limited by the most oblique light ray leaving the subject's pupil which enters the observer's pupil. It is therefore maximized by using a larger illumination aperture stop and by dilating the pupils of both the subject and observer and bringing them closer; dilating the observer's pupil is not expedient. Axial illumination allows maximum overlap of the observed and illuminated fields but if slightly offset vertically, specular reflection from the corneal surface is deflected from the line of vision. The image is virtual, erect, and magnified. The image of an emmetropic fundus is magnified 15×, whereas in a –10 dioptre myope it increases to 19× and in a +10 dioptre hypermetrope it reduces to 13×. In eccentric gaze the pupil becomes effectively elliptical, therefore when viewing the superior or inferior fundus periphery the ophthalmoscope should be rotated so that the offset fields of view and illumin-azntion fit within it (Fig. 1).

Dial-mounted neutralizing lenses alter the plane of focus and compensate for refractive errors in both the subject and obser-

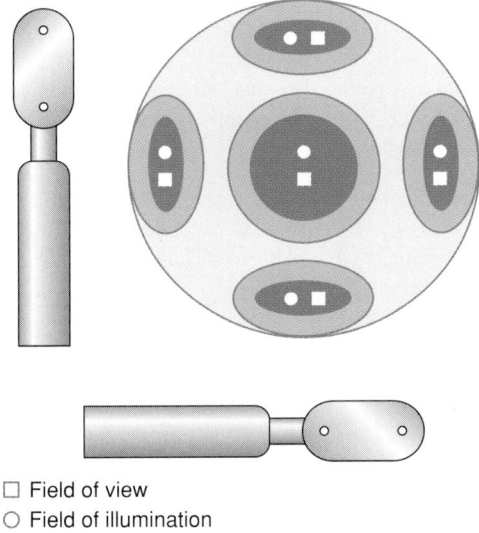

□ Field of view
○ Field of illumination

Fig. 1 When viewing the fundus periphery the pupil will become effectively elliptical. Because the fields of view and illumination are vertically offset, the direct ophthalmoscope must be orientated to fit both.

ver. They range in power from +20 to –20 dioptre (up to +44 to –45 dioptre in some models) and may permit a rough estimate of the subject's refractive error. A high degree of astigmatism prevents adequate fundus examination.

Many direct ophthalmoscopes have additional features: the contour of structures in the anterior segment and fundus and anterior chamber depth may be shown if illuminated obliquely by a slit beam. This is difficult for fundus lesions because of vertical alignment of illumination and observation but easier for the anterior segment if illuminated from the side and observed directly. Projection of a star, cross, or graticule on to the retina may establish eccentric fixation if it does not fall on the foveola when the subject looks directly at it. A green (red free) filter accentuates vascular structures, retinal nerve fibre changes, and retinal holes. Cobalt blue and yellow filters, respectively, highlight fluorescein and eliminate retinotoxic blue and ultraviolet wavelengths. The density of opacities in the ocular media can be assessed against the red reflex and in such eyes, illumination may be insufficiently bright to see fundus detail clearly.

Indirect ophthalmoscopy

The fundus is illuminated by a light mounted on spectacles or a headband (an indirect ophthalmoscope) or by a slit lamp (biomicroscope). The observer sees a real image of the fundus situated between him and an interposed condensing lens. Compared to direct ophthalmoscopy indirect ophthalmoscopy allows a larger field of view, is stereoscopic, overcomes refractive error and its more powerful illumination is more likely to penetrate unclear ocular media.

The field of view is wider than with a direct ophthalmoscope and is determined by lens diameter and distance from the eye. A higher power lens has a shorter focal length and working distance and therefore a wider field (Table 1). A real inverted aerial image is formed; magnification is the dioptric power of the eye (60 dioptres) divided by the dioptric power of the lens, for example a 20 dioptre general diagnostic lens magnifies 3×.

Gas filling the posterior segment of a phakic eye creates a large myopic shift by increasing the refractive power of the posterior lens surface. In this situation and in some high myopes, 'indirect' ophthalmoscopy can be performed without a condensing lens.

Indirect ophthalmoscope

A head-mounted light source is combined with eyepieces comprising a 2 dioptre positive lens in order that accommodation is not required to view the aerial image of the fundus. The arrangement of the fields of view and illumination is slightly elongated horizontally so that when the pupil appears elliptical in eccentric gaze, it is easier to examine the fundus periphery with the subject looking up or down than to the side. Moving around a recumbent subject to examine the peripheral fundus permits a horizontally elongated pupil for all sectors.

A variety of coloured filters and aperture stops can be placed in front of the light source. A flip-down teaching attachment comprises two transparent plates at 90° to each other but at 45° to the line of view. By deflecting light rays from the fundus to a second observer on either side, it reduces the brightness of the image seen by the principal observer. An argon laser delivery system can be incorporated to perform retinal photocoagulation.

Scleral indentation brings the peripheral retinal into view and allows a dynamic assessment which may reveal retinal holes by opening them. The globe may be indented directly but with conscious patients it is more comfortable if performed over the eyelid (Fig. 2).

Biomicroscopic indirect ophthalmoscopy

The slit lamp has a fixed plane of focus about 10 cm in front of the objective lens. The fundus image of an emmetropic eye is at infinity and can be seen only by interposing a negative lens to move the focus of the slit lamp to infinity, by moving the image to within the focusing range of the slit lamp using a positive non-contact lens, or by neutralizing the power of the cornea with a contact lens. The Hruby (–58.6 dioptre plano-concave) lens may be coupled to the biomicroscope and produces a narrow field, virtual, erect image. The Superfield, 90 dioptre, 78 dioptre, and the superceded El Bayadi 58.6 dioptre positive lenses produce a wide angle, real, inverted, aerial image. A 16× slit lamp eyepiece lens contains two positive lenses and can be employed as an astronomical telescope to

Table 1 Lenses used for indirect ophthalmoscopy (the second four are biomicroscopy lenses)

Lens	Diameter (mm)	Angular magnification	Field of view (°)	Working distance from cornea (mm)	Angular laser spot magnification
15 D	52	3.92	40	60	0.26
20 D	50	2.97	46	43.1	0.34
28 D	41	2.16	55	29	0.46
Panretinal	52	2.56	56	34.1	0.39
78 D	31	0.87	73	7.0	1.15
90 D	21.5	0.72	69	6.5	1.39
Superfield	27	0.72	120	6.5	1.39
Superpupil	16	0.43	120	2.4	

D, dioptre.

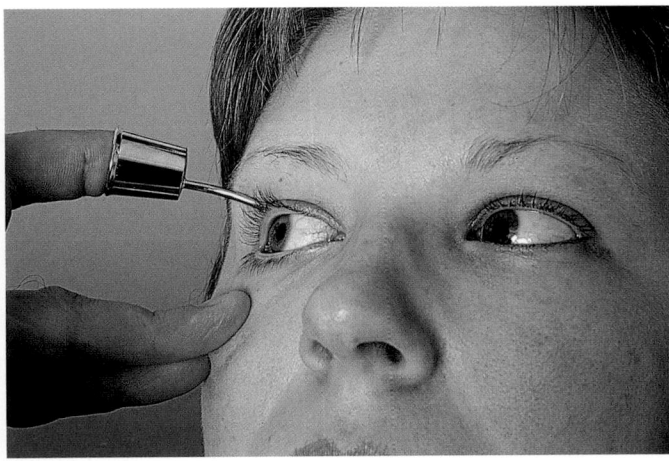

Fig. 2 A T-bar attached to a thimble worn on the index finger is used to indent sclera and retina. With the patient looking forward, the bar is placed just back from the eyelid margin over the sector of retina to be examined. As the patient then looks towards the area of interest, the eyelid is rolled back and pressed by the indenter while the other is retracted by the fingers or thumb of the same hand. This leaves the second hand free to hold a fundus-viewing lens.

produce an image similar to a 90-dioptre lens, if used in the same way but held in reverse. Optical power or mirrors can be incorporated into contact lenses to alter the field of view.

To use a non-contact fundus viewing lens, the slit lamp focused on the centre of the cornea, the lens is interposed at its correct working distance (perpendicular to the illuminating beam) and the biomicroscope is withdrawn until the red reflex becomes a clear fundus image (Fig. 3). Coaxial illumination facilitates lens alignment and fundus image detection, especially if the pupil is small. Reflections from the lens surface can be deflected by tilting the lens slightly vertically or by altering the angle of illumination. Observation of more peripheral retina requires eccentric patient gaze and lens repositioning; lens decentration to exploit the prismatic effect of the lens periphery

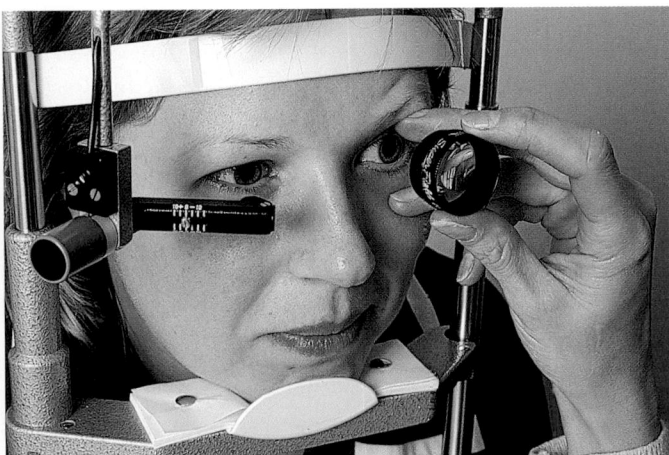

Fig. 3 Holding an indirect biomicroscopy lens between index finger and thumb allows use of the middle and ring fingers of the same hand to retract the eyelids. A movable fixation target in front of the fellow eye steadies gaze position and can be focused to compensate for refractive errors between +10 and −15 dioptre or for accommodation.

may also help. If the image seen is monocular, the lens is incorrectly centred with respect to the cornea.

Indirect ophthalmoscopy lenses

Aspheric lenses maintain image magnification across the field of view. The more convex surface should face the observer but with double-aspheric lenses, orientation is irrelevant. Glare and ghost images caused by reflection of light from each lens surface are reduced by multilayered lens coatings. Argon or diode laser transmission can be improved by wavelength-specific lens coating. Many lens sizes are available in solid yellow glass or with detachable yellow filters to eliminate retinotoxic blue and ultraviolet wavelengths. Detachable contact and non-contact adapters can be fitted to certain lenses to alter the field of view and magnification. Indirect ophthalmoscopy through a small pupil or in children is facilitated by using a higher power lens with a shorter working distance and wider field of view, for example a 28- or 30-dioptre lens rather than a standard 20-dioptre lens. These are features of the Superpupil lens, designed specifically for small pupil biomicroscopy. A monocular indirect ophthalmoscope may allow a better view through a small pupil than a binocular one (see Table 1).

Lenses can be disinfected using alcohol or glutaraldehyde and sterilized using ethylene oxide but should not be autoclaved.

Slit lamp

The slit lamp biomicroscope is used for direct observation of the anterior segment or for indirect ophthalmoscopy of the posterior segment. Features common to all slit lamps are a biomicroscope, an illumination system, and their mechanical supporting system.

The biomicroscope is a compound microscope which uses two or more lenses to increase magnification and reduce aberration. The objective lens forms a real inverted image which the eye lens magnifies and reimages at a comfortable working distance (usually infinity). Resolution of the biomicroscope may be improved by using shorter wavelengths of light to illuminate the object (e.g. when examining for flare in the anterior chamber) and by a shorter lens-to-object working distance (90 to 120 mm is the normal working distance to allow room for manipulations between the biomicroscope and the subject's eye).

Depth of field is limited by the optics of the slit lamp as demonstrated by slit lamp photography where it seems surprisingly shallow. It is increased by the observer's range of accommodation. Resolution is improved by object illumination with shorter light wavelengths (when examining for flare) and by a shorter lens to object working distance −90 to −120 mm is the norm to allow room for ocular manipulation.

In many slit lamp models the total magnification of the microscope is altered by flipping a lever below the eyepieces to change the revolving objective lenses (Fig. 4). This allows a choice of 10× and 16× magnification for the low power eyepieces and 16× and 25× for the high power. A different mechanism to change magnification involves turning a drum con-

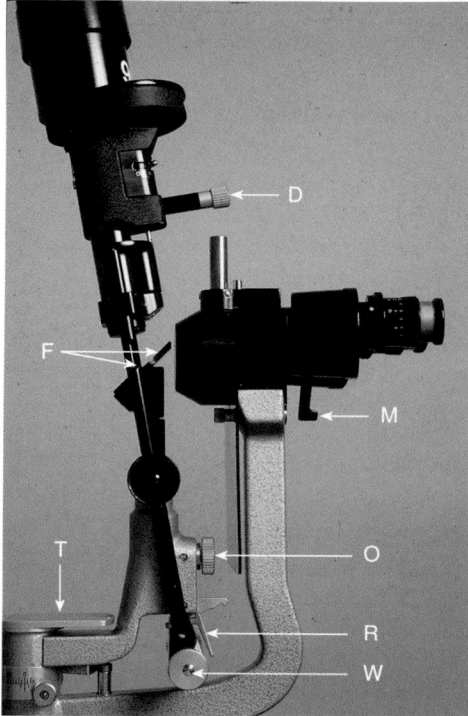

Fig. 4 The slit lamp illumination assembly may be tilted as much as 20° in 5° steps by releasing the ratchet (R). Full length mirror (F); beam diameter variator (D); beam width variator (W); 1.0×/1.6× objective magnification changer (M); dial to allow beam off-centration (O), tonometer footplate (T).

taining three Galilean telescopes of differing power (Fig. 5). Each can be rotated about a common axis, into line between the objective and eyepiece lenses and depending on telescope orientation, magnifications of 6.3×, 10×, 16×, 25×, and 40× are possible. With such a range there is no need to alter magnification further by changing the eyepieces and these are fixed at

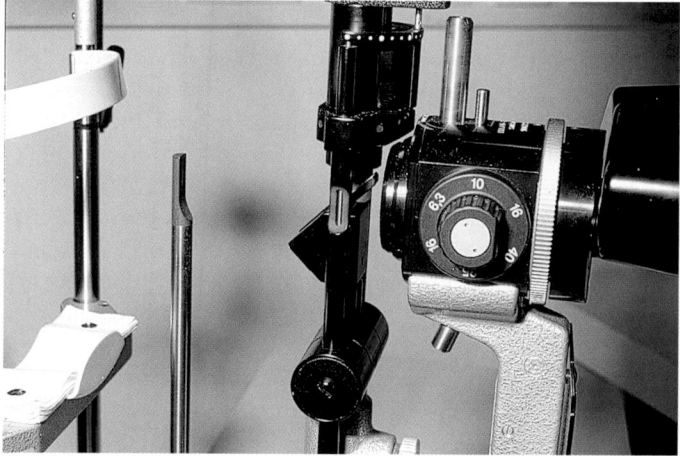

Fig. 5 Eyepieces can be set to compensate for observer refractive error by focusing each on a slit beam projected on to the flat non-reflective surface of the focusing rod (left). Magnification is indicated by the uppermost number on the rotating drum containing three Galilean telescopes.

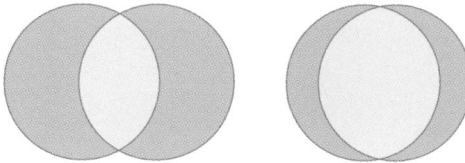

Fig. 6 When the stereovariator is disengaged the stereoscopic viewing angle is greater and the binocular field of view is small (left); when interposed, the angle is reduced and the binocular field of view is large (right)

12.5×. Zoom lens systems offer a third alternative for changing magnification.

A 13° angle of convergence between the oculars of the biomicroscope allows optimal stereoscopic viewing of an optical section. Binocular visual acuity is superior to monocular; however, when observing surfaces which are perpendicular to the line of observation, the physical features of the observed eye or the slit lamp may prevent binocular observation. By reducing the angle of stereoscopic observation to 4.5° (at the cost of stereopsis), the overlap between monocular fields (the binocular field) and therefore the visual acuity are improved (Fig. 6). This is accomplished with a stereo-variator incorporated into the optics of the biomicroscope between the objective lens and the magnification changer. It is useful when examining corneal endothelium, the posterior lens surface, anterior parts of the fundus when using a three-mirror lens, and in myopic fundus examination where the binocular field is smaller. Stereopsis may also be increased by increasing the magnification of the optical system.

For satisfactory binocular and stereoscopic examination, the biomicroscope eyepieces should be set to the interpupillary distance and setting the focus by adjusting for the uncorrected refractive error of the examiner. When the tonometer guide plate is replaced by the focusing rod, the focal plane of the slit beam corresponds with the black surface of the rod on to which it projects (see Fig. 5). Each eyepiece is then focused on the slit beam. This is done separately for the 10× and the 16× eyepieces. The dioptric correction for the 10× eyepiece is indicated by the numerals close to the scale on the eyepiece and must be tested separately from the correction for the 16× eyepiece which is indicated just above it (Fig. 7). Adjusting this setting by −1 to −2 dioptre will compensate for accommodation induced in younger examiners by the converging binocular tubes. If calibration is accurate, an oblique slit beam intersects the plane of focus in the centre of the field of view. If the planes of focus and illumination do not correspond, the central area may be illuminated but out of focus or the area which is illuminated and in focus may be off-centre.

Illumination system

The bulb used in modern slit lamps has a coiled tungsten filament. Increasing the voltage passing through the filament increases its temperature and shifts the spectral composition of emitted light towards shorter wavelengths. During use tungsten atoms evaporate from the hot filament to the cooler inner bulb surface. In bulbs filled with a halogen vapour, tungsten atoms

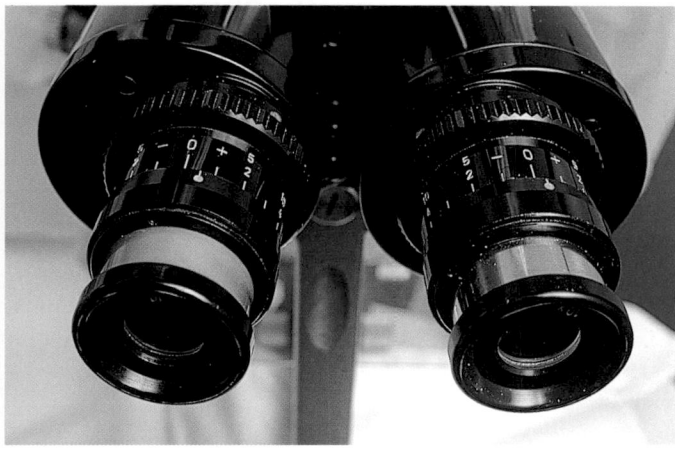

Fig. 7 When using the 10× eyepiece (shown here) the refractive error of the observer is set using the numerals close to the scale on the eyepiece and must be tested separately from the correction for the 16× eyepiece indicated just above.

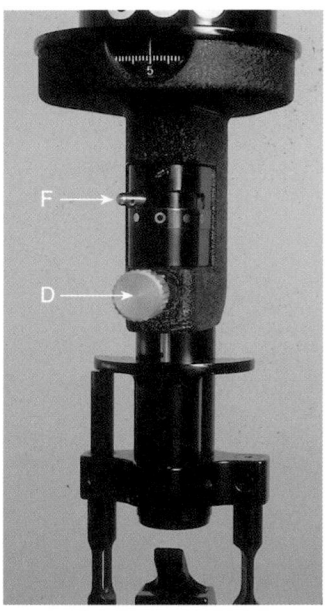

Fig. 8 A disc containing a wedge aperture (set at 5 mm in figure) and fixed-diameter apertures is housed in the illumination assembly and rotated by dial D. A second disc rotated by switch F has apertures which are empty, hold heat, 90 per cent grey, and red-free filters, and a spare aperture for a filter to be inserted.

combine with halogen atoms at the bulb surface and are returned to the filament. Conservation of the filament in this way extends its life and reduces the neutral density filter effect of tungsten deposited on the bulb. Light intensity is controlled by voltage regulation or by interposing neutral density filters (which do not affect the colour temperature).

The illumination unit and microscope are set back from the common axis around which they rotate. The light source is located above or below the microscope oculars and lights through a condensing and projection system to ensure a uniformly bright beam. A disc located in the path of the beam has both fixed diameter and wedge apertures, a blue filter, and a fixation star, while a second disc contains heat-absorbing, 10 per cent grey, and red-free filters (Fig. 8). The heat-absorbing filter should be used when the full beam is used at maximum voltage. A shutter controls beam width before the modified beam is deflected forward by a mirror or prism (see Fig. 4).

Fundus examination requires illumination from between the microscope oculars. A wider beam enables easier examination of the adnexa, whereas a narrow one is more useful for the cornea and anterior chamber. The slit beam can be rotated 90° to either side of vertical or tilted by as much as 20° to optimize the angle of optical section for gonioscopy and three-mirror lens examination. Tilting is achieved by an inclining mirror or prism, or by inclining the entire illumination assembly (see Fig. 4).

In certain positions, the upper part of the illumination mirror may obstruct the microscope, therefore for angles of 3 to 10° between the illumination unit and microscope, the short mirror should be used. In addition, the illumination unit should be inclined by 10° in order that all of the beam is reflected. Similarly, with the stereovariator set at 4.5°, the illumination unit should be displaced 10° to the left or right, or the short mirror can be used between the oculars at 0° and the unit inclined by 10°.

A fixation target for the eye which is not being examined comprises either a light or a concentric ring target behind a moveable lens (see Fig. 3). The latter allows subjects with refractive errors of between plus and minus 15 dioptres to see the target clearly and is less likely to stimulate accommodative convergence.

Methods of illumination

Using more than one technique to illuminate an ocular structure may reveal features which are not otherwise visible. With direct illumination, the centres of the fields of illumination and observation correspond; however, lateral displacement of the beam is required for viewing by retroillumination, scleral scatter, and specular reflection (Fig. 9).

Opaque objects are visible by direct illumination because of light reflected from their surface. Relatively transparent media are made visible against a dark backround because of light scattered by small particles within their structure. Where particle size is smaller than one-tenth of the wavelength of light (e.g. protein molecules of aqueous flare), it is best seen at right angles to an intense beam of shorter wavelengths because these are scattered more. Light scattering by larger particles becomes progressively less dependent on wavelength, e.g. cells in the anterior chamber or particles in the cornea.

Retroillumination uses a reflecting surface (such as the iris or retina) as a secondary source of illumination to highlight opacities, localized changes in refractive index, or pigment defects in more anterior structures. The iris is best retroilluminated through a small pupil (avoiding direct illumination); lens changes are best seen with the pupil dilated.

Laterally displaced light incident at the limbus is internally

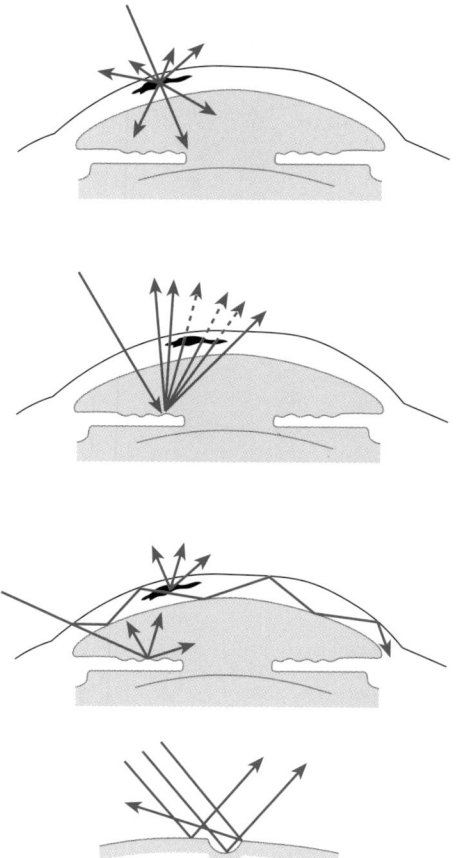

Fig. 9 Light pathways in slit ocular examination by (a) direct illumination, (b) retroillumination, (c) scleral scatter, and (d) specular reflection.

reflected across the cornea. Subtle corneal irregularities interrupt the passage of light and become visible because of scleral scatter. The effect is most useful when examining for corneal oedema.

Specular reflection highlights irregularities in a smooth reflecting surface occurring at the boundary of structures with different refractive indices because they reflect light at a different angle. The angle between the lines of illumination and observation is critical and the effect is therefore only seen monocularly. The effect is more pronounced for larger differences in refractive index, for example corneal endothelial cell soma and intercellular material. It is also used to examine corneal and lens epithelium and zones of discontinuity within the lens. Specular reflection is seen by focusing on the area of interest and changing the angle of illumination until the effect is observed or by fixing the angle between the biomicroscope and illumination units and scanning the area.

Further reading

Mainster, M.A., Crossman, J.L., *et al.* Retinal laser lenses: magnification, spot size and field of view. *British Journal of Ophthalmology*, **74**, 177–9.

Snead, M.P., Rubinstein, M.P. and Jacobs, P.M. (1992). The optics of fundus examination. *Survey of Ophthalmology*, **36**, 439–45.

Paul Spry

Visual acuity

Quantification of the visual system's ability to discriminate between points in visual space may be termed visual acuity. Clinical assessment of visual acuity is an integral but simple part of the ophthalmological examination. The aim of assessment is two-fold:

- to examine foveal visual function

- to permit determination of optimum optical correction.

Measurement ease with conventional letter charts masks the complex physiological and cognitive processes interacting to produce the result.

Terminology

Visual acuity may be defined as the reciprocal of the limit of ocular resolution at the eye's nodal point. The limit of resolution equals the angle subtended by two points seen to be just separated, in minutes of arc. Strictly, this threshold angle determines minimum separable acuity.

Care should be taken when using the terms limit of resolution and those of clinical visual acuity measurement. Whilst it is possible experimentally to quantify the former using experimental methods, such as gratings or point sources, clinically measured visual acuity relates to the smallest readable letter chart line or minimum legible acuity. This distinction is important because of the cognitive factors involved. Furthermore, clinical visual acuity is used to denote vision attained when refractive error is optimally corrected. Without correction, the term unaided vision (or simply vision) should be used.

Factors limiting visual resolution

The purpose of an optical system is the transfer of incident information from an object on to a receptive medium. Output resolution is dependent upon optical quality and detective ability of the receptive medium. For example, in a camera, the quality of the negative produced is determined by the lens optics and film grain size. This is analogous to the eye in which the resolution attained is determined by its optical system and neural processing capability. These two limiting factors will be examined in turn.

Optical system

The optics of the eye are not perfect. Three important factors serve to degrade the retinal image:

- refractive error

- ocular aberrations

- diffraction.

Providing the eye exhibits no refractive error, the two remaining factors determine resolution. Aberratic blur, resulting from chromatic and spherical aberrations, increases with greater pupil size.

In optical systems, shining light through a reducing circular aperture will produce a decreasing image size. However, at a certain point the image will no longer decrease but will start to grow steadily with further aperture reduction. This is due to bending of light by the edge of the aperture, termed diffraction, and produces distinctive image patterns. With circular apertures, the image formed consists of a central bright area surrounded by concentric alternating bright and dark rings. The central bright area is named the Airy disc in which 84 per cent of emergent light energy is contained. Point objects therefore do not produce point images, but small blur circles, the size of which is dependent upon the wavelength of light passing through the system, λ, and the aperture diameter, d. Equation 1 allows us to calculate the angular subtense of the Airy disc, θ, and its radius, R, from equation 2 where f is the focal length of the system. 1.22 is a constant for circular apertures.

$$\theta = \frac{1.22\lambda}{d} \qquad (1)$$

$$R = f \times \theta \qquad (2)$$

If Airy discs are too close together, they will merge, summating to appear as a single brighter point. Diffractive blur therefore limits resolution. Two diffractive blur patterns may first be resolved when the centre of one Airy disc (maximal intensity) falls upon the first dark circle (minimal intensity) of the other, that is they are separated by one disc radius. This degree of separation is referred to as the Rayleigh criterion and produces a depression between the Airy disc peaks equal to 74 per cent of their height, sufficient to permit resolution.

For the eye, minimum separable acuity by the Rayleigh criterion allows a theoretical minimum angle of resolution, θ_{min}, at the nodal point of the eye to be calculated using equation 3.

$$\theta_{min} = \frac{1.22\lambda}{d} \text{ radians} \qquad (3)$$

Example 1 Assuming a 3 mm pupil size and wavelength of 555 nm

$$\theta_{min} = \frac{1.22 \times 555 \text{ nm}}{3 \text{ mm}} = 2.26 \times 10^{-4} \text{ radians} = 47 \text{ seconds of arc.}$$

It can be seen that θ_{min} is inversely proportional to pupil size, so larger pupil sizes should optimize minimum separable acuity.

Pupil size thus plays an essential role in optimizing visual acuity, balancing aberrations, and diffractive effects. Providing the eye is in focus, minimum separable acuity is usually attained with pupil sizes between 2 and 3 mm.

Retinal anatomy

A significant correlation exists between clinically measured visual acuity and photoreceptor density. Visual acuity varies with eccentricity and is maximal foveally. In this region photoreceptor and ganglion cell populations are virtually equal. The absence of convergence of photoreceptors on single ganglion cells permits small receptive field size at the fovea.

Foveal cones are hexagonal in section, allowing dense packing to form the distinctive retinal mosaic. The cell population is approximately 147 000 cones/mm^2, average foveal cone size being approximately 2.0 μm with intercell distances of about 0.3 μm. Cone centre separation is therefore approximately 2.3 μm.

If two Airy discs are narrowly separated and fall upon a single or two neighbouring cones they will go unresolved. However, if Airy disc centres fall upon cones separated by a single cone, stimulated to a significantly lower level, resolution may occur.

Using equation 2, it is possible calculate the theoretical resolution limit by photoreceptor theory. Assuming the distance between two cone centres separated by a third to be 4.6 μm and the nodal point of the eye to be 17 mm in front of the retina:

$$\theta = \frac{R}{f} = \frac{0.0000046}{0.00017} = 0.000271 \text{ radians} = 56 \text{ seconds of arc.}$$

It can be seen that minimum separable acuity defined by both optical and retinal characteristics are closely matched. It is assumed that 'normal' ocular minimum angle of resolution is 1 minute of arc. However, it is not unusual for the limit of resolution to be smaller than this. Theories underlying increased visual acuity include contrast enhancement of diffractive patterns by complex retinal and greater foveolar photoreceptor density. With the distance separating three cone centres as low as 30 μm, the theoretical resolution limit is 36 s.

Clinical assessment

Snellen type charts

Since their publication in 1862, Snellen-based letters have become the standard of visual acuity assessment. The optotypes described are based upon the assumed minimum angle of resolution for high contrast objects, 1 minute of arc. Although supposedly minimum separable acuity, the actual measurement is of minimum legible acuity.

Test distances

In the United Kingdom and Western Europe the standard test distance is 6 m, although in some countries 5 m is used. In the United States, 20 ft is specified. These test distances are preferred because accommodation stimulated is less than 0.25 dioptre, the smallest unit of refractive error commonly prescribed.

Test symbols

Snellen's optotypes consisted of serif script constructed within a 5 × 5 or 5 × 6 grid. Modern chart design now uses non-serif letters on a 5 × 4 or 5 × 5 grid. Each grid unit subtends 1 minute of arc at a specified distance and letters are constructed such that gaps between letter limbs are a single unit width. Letter size is specified by the distance at which a single unit on the grid on which they are based subtends 1 minute of arc, for example each size 9 letter grid unit subtends 1 minute at 9 m.

Use of letters is problematical as the relative acuity required for perception of certain letters may differ from others of identical specified size. This is mainly due to the construction of letters within the grid, those letters with more limbs, such as E and B being more difficult to read than U and C whose interlimb spaces may exceed 1 minute of arc. Potential for confusion between letters may also play a part. Attempts to overcome this problem have included modified letter design and inclusion of letters calculated of 'equal legibility'. The most recent British Standard specified that the letters used should be of 5 × 4 non-serif construction and from the selection of equally legible letters D, E, F, H, N, P, R, U, V, and Z.

The truest clinical test of minimum separable acuity is use of symbols requiring only resolution and not recognition, such as the Llandolt C, with which gap orientation is the test criterion. The disadvantage of such a test is prolonged testing time and increased potential for confusion and error when used with a mirror.

Notation

Two options are available for expressing visual acuity:

- an absolute threshold visual angle

- a relative value, representing the acuity achieved referenced to a standard.

The Snellen fraction, an example of relative value, has been used almost exclusively since its publication.

$$\text{Visual acuity} = \frac{\text{test distance}}{\text{distance at which grid unit subtends 1 minute of arc}}$$

Visual acuity obtained at different test distances may be compared using decimal V, a direct decimal conversion of the Snellen fraction. However, it is unwise to use such notation routinely, test distance specification being a useful adjunct.

Chart layout

Progression of symbol size

Differences in letter size between lines influences the sensitivity and repeatability of a chart, whilst also affecting test speed. Virtually all charts are designed with geometric progressions. The British Standard, applied to many presently used Snellen-type charts, uses a progression close to a multiplication factor of √2.

Letter distribution and spacing

The rectangular layout of the Snellen type chart, with long axis vertical, permits greater numbers of smaller optotypes. The only British Standard design recommendation for layout is that letters within a row should be equally spaced and that the row separation should be at least 20 mm. This design presents a number of flaws:

1. It does not provide an accurate assessment in patients with reduced visual acuity.

2. It does not control the crowding phenomenon (the interaction of target contour with increasing proximity) which is known to be reduced in amblyopic patients.

LogMAR charts

Departing from many of the traditions associated with Snellen-type charts, logMAR charts represent a considerable reappraisal of visual acuity testing (Fig. 1). The generic name is an abbreviation for logarithm of the minimum angle of resolution, in minutes of arc. An eye that is capable of resolving 1 minute of arc has a logMAR score of 0, whilst resolution reduced to a level of 10 minutes scores 1.

LogMAR chart design addresses many of the problems inherent to Snellen chart layout and scoring:

1. These charts possess an equal number of letters per line, each separated by one letter width. Letters used are restricted to those of equal legibility as specified in the British Standard.

2. The distance between rows is equal to the letter height of the lower row.

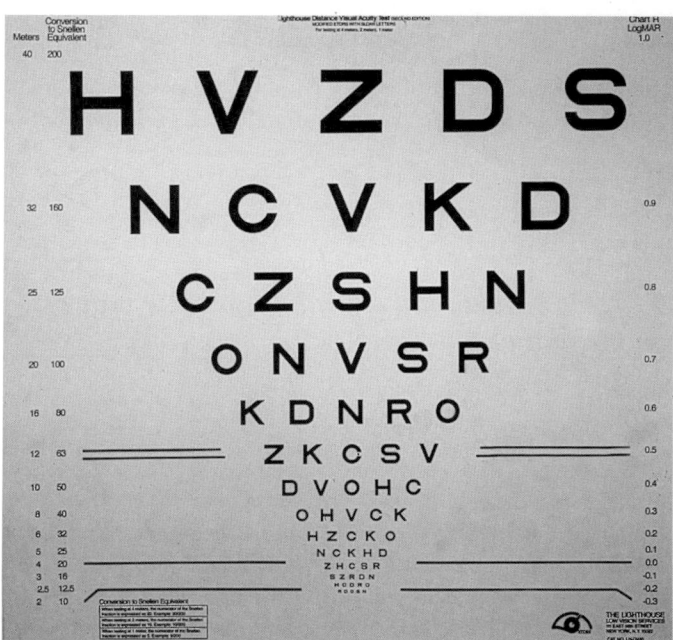

Fig. 1 LogMAR chart. (By courtesy of Mrs G. Bennerson.)

3. Progression of letter size is geometric, with a uniform logarithmic scaling factor of 0.1 log unit ($10\sqrt{10}$). The 14-line range subtends letters from 10 to 0.5 minute of arc (Snellen equivalent sizes 6/60 to 6/3). Scale truncation is avoided for better acuities and use of reduced testing distances permits low vision quantification, down to 6/480 equivalent at 0.5 m.

4. Each letter correctly identified may be scored. Due to equal difference of 0.1 logMAR unit between lines, each letter is worth 0.02 units. This permits increased accuracy regardless of visual acuity level. Additionally, it overcomes the problem of relative acuity inherent to use of letters.

LogMAR charts have long been of recognized value in research requiring accurate visual acuity measurement, due to increased sensitivity and the statistical advantages of the scoring system. However, these advantages appear to be outweighed by increased test time when speed is required during refraction. For this reason, Snellen-based chart designs remain more popular for routine refractive work.

Contrast sensitivity

As a high contrast task, visual acuity does not represent completely the visual requirements of everyday life, during which the majority of visual tasks are of medium to low contrast. Clinically, it is relatively common for a patient to present with symptoms describing visual disability not detectable by visual acuity assessment alone. For example, a patient with a degree of cataract may present with symptoms of reduced or even 'misty' vision, despite normal visual acuity. Quantification of the contrast sensitivity function provides supplementary information on visual function and may reveal such defects.

Visual acuity measures the reciprocal of threshold visual angle subtended by two high contrast points. Contrast sensitivity meaures the reciprocal of the threshold contrast at a specified visual angle. If an analogy with hearing is drawn, visual acuity is represented by the highest frequency audible tone at high volume, whereas contrast sensitivity is represented by the minimum volume audible at a given frequency (Fig. 2).

Contrast sensitivity testing

Sine wave gratings are the target of choice in contrast sensitivity function assessment as any degradation of the wave produces a reduction only in amplitude and form remains unchanged. Also, sine waves can be considered an essential element from which any pattern may be formed by their summation. This is important as visual system spatial processing may be characterized by the presence of a number of 'pathways', each of which are responsible for handling a small range of spatial frequencies.

A grating consists of repetitive sine waves and may be described using three parameters: orientation, spatial frequency, and contrast.

Spatial frequency relates to the light and dark bandwidth. Each dark and light band pair represents a single wavelength,

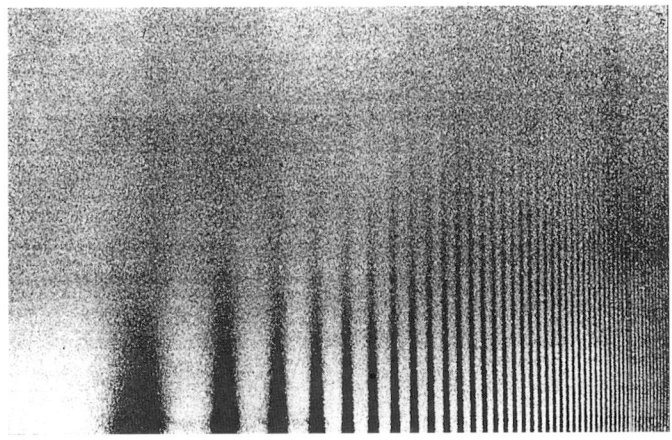

Fig. 2 Variable contrast and spatial frequency grating. This chart demonstrates increasing spatial frequency from left to right, with decreasing contrast from bottom to top. The limits of grating detection define the contrast sensitivity function. (By courtesy of Spalton *et al.* 1994.)

or cycle. Spatial frequency is specified in number of cycles/degree. So, thinner bandwidths represent a greater number of cycles/degree thus higher spatial frequency and vice versa. This method of notation allows contrast sensitivity function construction independent of test distance.

Contrast, C, may be defined as the difference between the light band luminance (L_{max}) and dark band luminance (L_{min}) as in eqn 4. If L_{max} is decreased or L_{min} increased, grating contrast is reduced.

$$C = \frac{L_{max} - L_{min}}{L_{max} - L_{min}} \qquad (4)$$

For a grating of a specified spatial frequency the contrast required for its detection is the contrast threshold, usually expressed as a percentage. In contrast sensitivity function assessment, its reciprocal, contrast sensitivity, is used. For example, at a spatial frequency of 20 cycles per degree a subject may just be able to perceive a grating with light band luminance of 55 units and dark band luminance of 45 units. Their contrast sensitivity would be:

$$\text{Contrast threshold, } C = \frac{55 - 45}{55 + 45} = \frac{10}{100} = 0.1 \text{ per cent}$$

$$\text{Contrast sensitivity, } = \frac{1}{C} = \frac{1}{0.1} = 10.$$

A graph of the variation of contrast sensitivity with spatial frequency is referred to as the contrast sensitivity function (Fig. 3). The contrast sensitivity function can be seen as a bell-shaped function with a negative skew. Contrast sensitivity is moderate at low spatial frequencies (< 2 cycles/degree) and becomes maximal over the intermediate spatial frequency range by physiological enhancement. Receptive field size, retinal on–off systems and lateral inhibition produce levels of sensitivity corresponding to contrasts of approximately 1 per cent in this 2 to 6 cycles/degree region. At higher spatial frequencies (> 6 cycles/degree) contrast sensitivity drops to where maximal

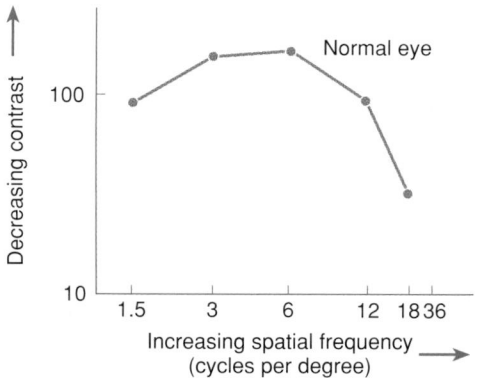

Fig. 3 Schematic contrast sensitivity function, normal eye. Maximum contrast sensitivity, around 1 per cent, can be seen to be in the medium spatial frequency range. Attenuation of the curve occurs at both low and high spatial frequencies. (Redrawn from Spalton *et al.* 1994, with permission.)

contrast defines the highest resolvable spatial frequency, limited by diffraction and aberrations and is equivalent to visual acuity. Stimuli with contrast levels within the contrast sensitivity function are detectable.

Physiological contrast sensitivity function variation

The more comprehensive description of the visual performance provided by contrast sensitivity function is subject to normal physiological variation. Contrast sensitivity declines with age, although the degree of change is highly variable between individuals. It is dependent upon both optical and neural components. Comparison of contrast sensitivity function assessment for the entire visual system with neural components alone indicates that this reduction is primarily due to retinal and neural cell loss and degenerative change, resulting in loss of ability to enhance contrast. Age-related optical changes, such as increased lenticular absorption, intraocular scatter, and senile pupillary miosis, only play a small role at higher spatial frequencies. The contrast sensitivity function is also reduced with decreased illumination.

Spatial processing

Fourier theory states that any waveform may be written as the sum of sine waves of defined spatial frequencies, amplitudes, phases, and orientations. The visual system may code information in this manner. Retinal level image processing breaks down an object into its component sine waves (Fourier transformation). These codes are transmitted to the visual cortex by a number of different cell routes or 'channels', each representing a narrow range of spatial frequencies. Cortical synthesis (Fourier analysis) of this coded spatial information allows interpretation to form a percept of the object.

Clinical assessment

Experimental psychometric methods, using computer-controlled sine wave gratings, do not lend themselves to clinical use due to complexity, prolonged testing times, and expense.

Accuracy and repeatability are also variable, depending on the psychophysical method.

Clinical tests should be swift, relatively inexpensive, and simple to perform. Ideally, measurement intervals should be sensitive to the smallest level of clinically important change and should be repeatable. Current instrumentation may be divided into two groups: those assessing single and those assessing multiple spatial frequencies.

Tests assessing multiple spatial frequencies

Arden test gratings

The Arden test gratings are a series of photographically produced plates. Each plate represents a single spatial frequency with contrast varying along its length. Seven plates cover a spatial frequency range from 0.2 to 6.4 cycles/degree at the specified viewing distance, 57 cm. The test is performed by withdrawal of the plate from a sheath exposing the gradually increasing contrast grating. The patient must subjectively report the time of grating detection. Each plate features a score continually changing along its length which is noted at the point of grating detection. The total score for all plates may be compared with normative data accompanying the test. The sinusoidal nature of the gratings permits use at different test distances so increasing the range of available spatial frequencies. Unfortunately, no information regarding plate contrast is provided, making localization of contrast sensitivity detriment impossible and normative data is not age-matched.

Vistech contrast sensitivity test system

Each chart in the Vistech system features circular targets organized into five rows and nine columns. The targets on individual rows are of the same spatial frequency with contrast decreasing in discrete $1/\sqrt{2}$ intervals. The five rows cover a range of spatial frequencies from 1.5 to 18 cycles/degree. Each target is a sinusoidal grating and is orientated vertically or tilted to the right or left. The test is objective, although not forced choice, since the patient is asked to identify target orientation or blank response. Charts are available at 3 m and 45 cm. Three different charts are obtainable for each test distance for repeated measurement. The last plate correctly identified is plotted on supplied graphical templates of contrast versus spatial frequency, enabling construction of a complete contrast sensitivity function which may be compared with normative data.

Major disadvantages of this test system are the relatively large contrast intervals present and only one target per chart for each spatial frequency/contrast combination. With no age-matched normative data, this combination of factors serves to reduce the sensitivity and repeatability of the test.

Tests assessing single spatial frequencies

The basis of such tests is that although determination of the complete contrast sensitivity function is ideal, this is unlikely to be achieved satisfactorily in clinical situations. Detailed accurate and repeatable assessment of a single spatial frequency is more beneficial than incomplete assessment of many. Spatial frequencies chosen are intermediate, close to contrast sensitivity function peak, argued as the most important contrast sensitivity function feature for predicting performance in everyday tasks.

Such tests represent the next evolutionary step from multiple spatial frequency tests, and have demonstrably increased repeatability due to concentration upon single spatial frequencies and adoption of criterion-free psychophysical procedures.

Cambridge low contrast gratings

This test utilizes square wave gratings of dot matrix construction. The test is designed for use at 6 m at which the spatial frequency is 4 cycles/degree. Assessment of lower spatial frequencies may be carried out at reduced test distances, the minimum of which should be 3 m due to visualization of the individual dots by subjects with normal visual acuity.

The test consists of a spiral bound A4 size book presented two pages at a time. Only one of the pair of pages contains a grating, the other being luminance matched. The patient makes a forced choice as to which page the grating is on. Contrast sensitivity is assessed four times according to a fixed protocol and a contrast threshold is obtained.

Pelli–Robson low contrast letter chart

The use of letters within this chart make it familiar to both patient and clinician, and thus easier to perform. This test is described as variable contrast letter chart as letter size remains constant throughout the chart but there is a gradual decrease in contrast. The chart consists of 16 groups of three capital letters, contrast being the same for letters within a given triplet, the difference in contrast between successive triplets being $1/\sqrt{2}$. The chart is read conventionally, from top right to bottom left. Contrast range within the chart is 100 to 0.9 per cent. The test distance may be varied, but is commonly used at 1 m, each letter subtending 3°. As letter structure consists of a complex and variable limb organization, it may be regarded as a selection of square wave targets of between 1 and 2 cycles/degree, so is not strictly a single spatial frequency target, although does assess contrast sensitivity function close to its peak.

The patient is asked to read down the chart until they make two or more errors within a triplet. The test is conducted by forced choice. The criterion used for threshold assessment makes this test highly repeatable, the influence of chance misreporting single letters not influencing the result.

Contrast sensitivity function and the detection of disease

Spatial frequency processing channels may be selectively affected by a pathology, causing reduced visual function undetectable by visual acuity.

Contrast sensitivity function testing has been useful in a variety of pathologies, for example optic neuropathies (including toxic varieties), diabetic retinopathy, cataract-induced glare disability (with addition of a glare source), and amblyopia. In such diseases there is potential for detection of subclinical damage in the form of reduced sensitivity to low and intermediate spatial frequencies.

Due to age-related variability, use of contrast sensitivity function alone as a screening technique is limited since results become physiologically less reliable in the elderly population in whom incidence of disease is highest. Any detectable abnormality will always require additional tests to establish a diagnosis. Contrast sensitivity function may be suitable for monitoring progressive change within individuals.

Tonometry

Lack of ocular structural rigidity requires a pressure within the eye which exceeds the surrounding tissues and atmospheric pressure. This maintains both corneal curvature and appropriate positioning of the posterior wall of the eye. Intraocular pressure depends on aqueous humour formation and outflow equilibrium and is influenced by factors affecting either of these two variables. Methods of intraocular pressure assessment fall broadly into three groups: manometry, indentation, and applanation. Manometry measures intraocular pressure directly and requires insertion of a small needle into the eye attached to a mercury or water manometer. Whilst useful for laboratory studies it is clearly unsuitable for clinical use.

Tonometry is the term applied to indirect intraocular pressure measurement. Ocular impressibility, such as by indentation or applanation, is used to estimate intraocular pressure.

Clinical measurement of intraocular pressure

Tonometry quantifies, as a pressure index, ocular resistance to an applied force. Although attempts have been made to measure intraocular pressure through the sclera, its structural irregularity and thickness of adjacent conjunctiva and ciliary body produces inaccuracy. Uniform corneal structure produces relatively constant corneal rigidity between individuals and this reduced source of error promotes it as the surface of choice for tonometry.

Indentation tonometry

The commonest indentation tonometer encountered is the Schiotz, designed in 1905. The principle of this technique is based upon the assumption that indentation is proportional to intraocular pressure.

The cornea of a supine patient is anaesthetized. A mobile plunger of known weight is allowed to indent the cornea, the amount of indentation being referenced to a surrounding concave footplate resting gently upon the cornea. Indentation produced may be read off on a 20-point scale, each point representing 1/20 mm of indentation. Intraocular pressure is determined from an accompanying calibration chart. A number of measurement errors are encountered with this method:

1. Instrument errors. Despite manufacturing standards, it is not unusual to find differences in measured pressures upon the same eye of up to 3 mmHg.

2. Reading errors. The space present between the pointer and scale permits parallactic error. Additionally, the cyclic fluctuation characteristic of the ocular pulse is a source of error if the required endpoint is not correctly identified.

3. Indentation principle errors. Indentation tonometers place a considerable weight upon the cornea, and consequently raise intraocular pressure. This factor is taken into account in the calibration data. However, indentation also displaces about 20 µl of aqueous. This is forced to exit the anterior chamber either via the trabecular meshwork, or, for the majority of displaced fluid, into the posterior chamber where it produces a variable degree of distension depending on ocular rigidity. Ocular coat rigidity therefore greatly influences measured intraocular pressure. The reaction to displaced aqueous is a compensatory increase in outflow and decreased intraocular pressure. This 'massaging effect' will continue with procedure duration, hence rapid testing using minimum number of readings to obtain maximum accuracy is essential.

Attempts to overcome this were made by Freidenwald. Using the facility to vary plunger weight, a nomogram was devised allowing intraocular pressure extrapolation from two measurements made with different plunger weights so negating the effect of ocular rigidity. Although preferable to single measurements, the nomogram result is affected significantly by errors in either reading. Use of more readings to reduce error is not advocated due to the massaging effect.

Although indentation is not the tonometric method of choice, it is useful where other techniques are unavailable or cannot be used clinically, for example when a patient is supine or severe corneal scarring is present.

Applanation tonometry

Theory

Applanation tonometry uses a small force to flatten the cornea. It is unaffected by ocular rigidity as only small areas of applanation are used and so negligible amounts of aqueous are displaced (approximately 0.5 µl). This method is based upon the Imbert–Fick law, which states that the pressure in a sphere filled with liquid and surrounded by an infinitely thin membrane can be measured by the counterpressure necessary to flatten this membrane to a plane. However, the eye does not fulfil these theoretical criteria. Notably, corneal rigidity resists flattening and surface tension of the tears attract the applanating body. However, Goldmann showed that when applanation diameters are close to 3 mm in diameter, these two forces cancel out. Also, at applanation diameter 3.06 mm, the relationship between applied force and intraocular pressure is arithmetically simple, 1 g of applied force being directly proportional to 10 mmHg.

Fixed area–variable force tonometers

Tonometers based upon Goldmann's principle exist in two forms: slit lamp mounted and hand-held . The applanating head design is common to both instruments and ensures correct applanation diameter (Fig. 4).

Measurement is achieved by anaesthetizing the cornea and instilling a small quantity of fluorescein. The applanating head

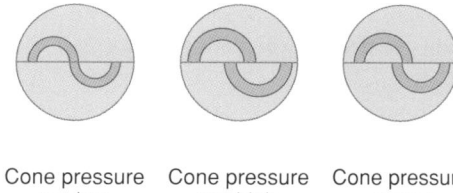

Cone pressure too low   Cone pressure too high   Cone pressure correct

Fig. 4 Schematic view through applanation tonometer head. The shaded areas represent the tear menisci defining the boundary of the area of applanation. (Redrawn from Henson 1983, with permission.)

is brought gently into contact with the cornea. Viewing through the head, it is possible to see the boundary of the applanated area by the presence of the fluorescein in the tear meniscus. The head contains two prisms with opposing bases that split the circular image into two semicircles by 3.06 mm. The inner edges should be aligned by adjustment of the applanating force. At this point it is possible to read intraocular pressure directly from the force adjustment dial (Fig. 5).

It is possible to view the ocular pulse through the tonometer head. It is preferable to chose systole as the measurement endpoint as it is less observer dependent than midpoint estimation and represents worst case scenario.

Non-contact tonometers

Frequently referred to as 'air puff' tonometers, such instrumentation was developed as a response to a need for topical anaesthetic-free tonometry. Instruments are based around a pneumatic system to briefly applanate the cornea. The required degree of applanation is ensured by collimated light emission and detection optical system, identifying maximal corneal reflectance at the point at which it is made flat. These instruments fall broadly into two groups depending upon how intraocular pressure measurement is calculated:

- measurement of time taken to point of required

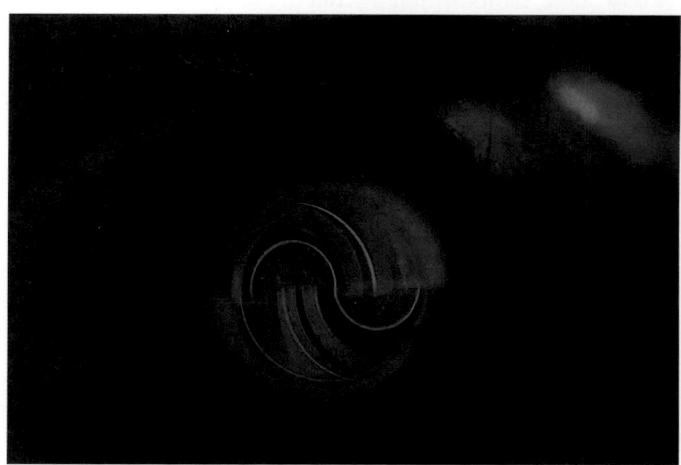

Fig. 5 View through Goldmann tonometer head. The semicircular tear menisci are made visible by installation of fluorescein and illustration with cobalt blue light.

applanation using a linearly increasing incident air pressure

● measurement of pneumatic system air pressure necessary to achieve required applanation.

Whilst having the advantages of applanation tonometers, the major drawback of such instruments is that they sample intraocular pressure over a very brief period of time and the mean of four readings is recommended to account for the arterial cycle.

Microprocessor-controlled tonometers

Applanation theory based tonometers have evolved to allow computer-controlled intraocular pressure determination. This is valuable due to the objective nature of measurements obtained.

Mackay–Marg based instruments

Modern examples based upon the principle first employed in the Mackay–Marg tonometer include the Tonopen and ProTon. These self-contained instruments are hand-held and used to applanate the cornea through a single use sterile polymer sheath. Each successful applanation, signalled by an audible bleep, generates an electronic signal which is converted by the internal microprocessor to mmHg and stored. Repeat measures are required in order to generate a mean reading with an associated reliability index, both of which are displayed.

Pneumotonometer-based instruments

This group of instruments utilize a pneumatic sensor placed upon the cornea. Gas flow into the sensor is increased until internal sensor pressure equals intraocular pressure, at which point a positive feedback loop is set up between the sensor and its base unit, the base unit sampling internal sensor pressure almost continually using an electronic transducer. Measurements are converted to mmHg, stored, and displayed as an intraocular pressure waveform, often referred to as the ocular pulse.

Instruments using this technology, such as the ocular blood flow tonograph, use this intraocular pressure pulse to estimate the pulsatile component of ocular blood flow.

Good test practice

Tonometric results may be subject to errors which are not directly test-related. Careful attention to positioning and instructing the patient, ensuring they are at ease with the procedure, will yield more representative results.

1. Target choice. Steady fixation throughout tonometry is required. Distant target use is preferable as accommodative effort reduces intraocular pressure by up to 2 mmHg. Necessity for fixation outweighs this, provided accommodative effects are borne in mind.

2. Eye and lid position. Contraction of the extraocular muscles alone can raise intraocular pressure dramatically, by up to 10 mmHg. If eyelids are squeezed, this increase may be as great as 30 mmHg. Involuntary

palpebral fissure widening, may also put pressure upon the globe and can elevate intraocular pressure by approximately 2 mmHg.

3. Patient position. If on a slit lamp, the patient should be comfortable, have a loosely fitting collar and without an outstretched neck as head position may affect venous drainage and so elevate intraocular pressure.

Further reading

Arden, G.B. (1988). Testing contrast sensitivity in clinical practice. *Clinical Visual Science*, **2**, 213–24.

Bailey, I.L. and Lovie, J.E. (1976). New design principles for visual acuity letter charts. *American Journal of Optometry and Physiological Optics*, **53**, 740–5.

Bennett, A.G. (1965). Ophthalmic test types; a review of previous work and discussions on some controversial questions. *British Journal of Physiological Optics*, **22**, 238–71.

Bennett, A.G. and Rabbetts, R.B. (1989). *Clinical visual optics*, (2nd edn). pp. 23–72. Butterworths, London.

Edwards, K. and Llewellyn, R. (1988). *Optometry*. Butterworths, London.

Elliott, D.B. (1987). Contrast sensitivity decline with ageing: a neural or optical phenomenon. *Ophthalmic and Physiological Optics*, **7**, 415–19.

Elliott, D.B., Sanderson, K., and Conket, A. (1990). The reliability of the Pelli–Robson contrast sensitivity contrast chart. *Ophthalmic and Physiological Optics*, **10**, 21–4.

Ferris, F.L., Kassoff, A., Bresnick, G.H., and Bailey, I. (1982). New visual acuity charts for clinical research. *American Journal of Ophthalmology*, **94**, 91–6.

Freidenwald, J.S. (1957). Tonometer calibration. *Transactions of the American Academy of Ophthalmology and Otology*, **61**, 108.

Henson, D.B. (1983). *Optometric instrumentation*, (2nd edn). Butterworths, London.

Katz, M. (1997). The human eye as an optical system. In *Duane's Clinical Ophthalmology*, Vol. 1 (ed. M. Tasman and E.A. Jaeger). Lippincott–Raven, Philadelphia.

Pelli, D.G., Robson, J.G., and Wilkins, A.J. (1988). The design of a new letter chart for measuring contrast sensitivity. *Clinical Visual Science*, **2**, 187–99.

Perkins, E.S. (1965). Hand held applanation tonometry. *British Journal of Ophthalmology*, **49**, 469.

Rubin, G.S. (1988). Reliability and sensitivity of clinical contrast sensitivity tests. *Clinical Visual Science*, **2**, 169–77.

Spalton, D.J., Hitchings, R.A., and Hunter, P.A. (1994). *Atlas of clinical ophthalmology*, (2nd edn). Mosby-Year Book, London.

Woodhouse, J.M. (1983). Practical applications of the contrast sensitivity function. *Ophthalmic and Physiological Optics*, **3**, 311–14.

Woodhouse, J.M. (1987). Contrast sensitivity measurement. *Optician*, **193**, 19–26.

Woods, R.L. and Thompson, W.D. (1993). A comparison of psychometric methods for measuring the contrast sensitivity of experienced observers. *Clinical Visual Science*, **8**, 401–15.

1.6.2 Instruments: compound microscopes, illumination systems, diagnostic lenses, keratometers, and photokeratoscopes

David Henson

Compound microscope

The range of magnifications and the large working distance (distance between the microscope objective and the eye) needed for both slit lamps and operating microscopes necessitates the use of compound rather than simple microscopes. In their most basic form, compound microscopes are composed of two optical elements, an objective and an eyepiece. A diagram of the optical arrangement of these two elements is given in Fig. 1(a). While they are shown in this figure as two simple positive lenses, in reality the eyepiece and occasionally the objective are composed of a series of lenses in order to reduce aberrations.

One of the problems of compound microscopes is that the final image is inverted with respect to the object. To overcome this, slit lamp microscopes and operating microscopes use a prism (see Fig. 1(b)) between the objective and the eyepiece to reinvert the image. The eyepieces and prism can usually be rotated around the optical axis of the microscope such that the instrument can be adjusted for practitioners with different interpupillary distances. This arrangement, which is the same as that found in a prism binocular, also has the advantage of shortening the length of the microscope.

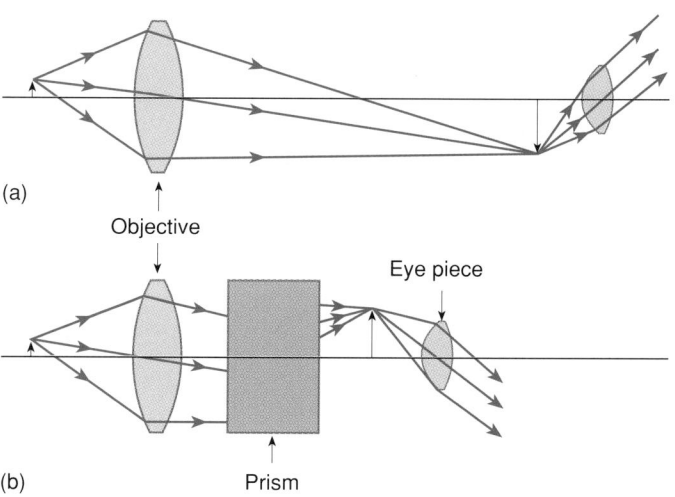

(a)

Objective

Eye piece

(b)   Prism

Fig. 1 (a) Optical arrangement of the objective and eyepiece in a compound microscope. (b) In the slit lamp microscope a prism is used to reinvert the image.

The resolution limit of a microscope can be specified in terms of its numerical aperture (NA) where the numerical aperture is defined as:

$$NA = n * \sin (a)$$

where *n* equals the refractive index of the medium between the objective and the eye (this would normally be air with a refractive index of 1.00) and *a* is the half angle subtended by the objective at the microscope's focal plane. The numerical aperture of a microscope, and hence its resolution limit, is dependent upon both the working distance and the diameter of the objective lens.

The working distance of slit lamp microscopes is normally kept fairly large in order to give plenty of room for attachments such as tonometers and to give room for the clinician to manipulate accessories such as fundus viewing lenses. The diameter of the objective lens is also kept fairly small in order to keep the depth of focus of the microscope as large as possible. This means that the numerical aperture of a slit lamp microscope is fairly small as is its resolving power and maximum useful magnification.

Longhurst states that for normal observers the maximum magnification should fall between 300 and 600 times the numerical aperture. Magnification beyond 600 times the numerical aperture is often called empty magnification which means that while the image is larger it is not possible to see any more detail. A typical slit lamp numerical aperture would be around 0.085 which would give an ideal maximum magnification of 25.5 to 50 times which is very close to the maximum magnification found on most slit lamp microscopes.

Compound microscopes usually provide a range of magnifications produced via either one or a combination of the following four techniques:

1. the use of different objectives
2. the use of different eyepieces
3. the Littmann–Galilean telescope principle
4. zoom optics.

Use of different objectives

This is one of the oldest and possibly still the most frequently used technique for obtaining different magnifications in slit lamps. The different objectives are usually placed on a turret that allows them to be fairly rapidly changed during an examination. The system is usually limited to two sets of objective lenses due to the confinements of space.

Use of different eyepieces

This technique is usually used to augment the range of magnifications provided by other techniques. It is not a very convenient technique as it requires the practitioner to pull out the current eyepieces and replace them with new ones. It is unusual for more than two pairs of eyepieces to be provided and hence this technique alone provides a very limited range of magnifications. In combination with two sets of objectives, it can provide four different magnifications, which is sufficient for most types of slit lamp examination.

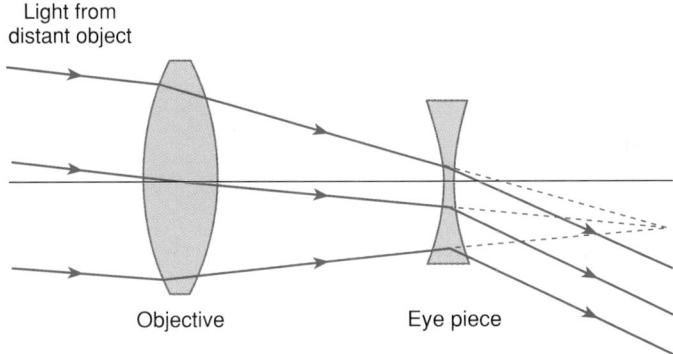

Fig. 2 Galilean telescope.

Littmann–Galilean telescope principle

The Galilean magnification changer, as developed by Littmann, is frequently found in some of the better slit lamps. It is a completely separate optical system that sits neatly between the objective and eyepiece lenses, and does not require either of them to change. It provides a larger number of magnifications than the previously mentioned techniques, typically five. It is called a Galilean system because it utilizes Galilean telescopes to alter the magnification.

Galilean telescopes have two optical components, a positive and a negative lens arranged in the manner shown in Fig. 2. Parallel light both enters and leaves the system and undergoes some degree of magnification which is dependent upon the power and separation of the two lenses. The Galilean telescope fits within the standard slit lamp microscope along with a relay lens in the manner shown in Fig. 3.

By reversing the order of the lenses in the telescope, a different magnification can be achieved (this time a minification) without altering any other optical elements. Thus, with the provision of two Galilean telescopes, both of which are reversible, four different microscope magnifications are available. Typically, slit lamps using this system also allow both telescopes to be removed from the optical path of the microscope, thereby increasing the range of magnifications to five.

Zoom optics

Rather than have a series of discrete magnifications most operating microscopes and some slit lamps have been produced with zoom systems. The optics of zoom systems is always a com-

promise between the ability to vary the magnification and aberrations continuously.

Illumination systems

The objective of the slit lamp illumination system is to produce a bright, evenly illuminated, finely focused, adjustable slit of light at the eye. To this end, virtually all slit lamp manufacturers have adopted the Koeller illumination system. It is optically identical to that of a 35 mm slide projector with the exception that a variable aperture slit takes the place of the slide and the projector lens has a much shorter focal length. Reflectors are occasionally positioned behind the lamp in order to increase the amount of light that passes through the condensers. The centre of curvature of any reflector is made to coincide with the filament of the bulb so as to reimage the filament back on itself. This arrangement ensures that there are no additional unwanted images of the filament.

In the Koeller illumination system, the filament of the bulb is imaged by the condenser lenses at or close to the projection lens (Fig. 4). The projection lens forms an image of the slit at the eye. The diameter of the projection lens is usually fairly small. This has two advantages: first, it keeps the aberrations of the lens down, which results in a better quality image; second, it increases the depth of focus of the slit and thereby produces a better optical section of the eye. While the optics of the condenser are not as critical as that of the other elements of the slit lamp, care must be taken in their design so as not to introduce too much chromatic aberration, which will tend to cause fringes at the slit image. A reduction of this aberration is normally achieved by using two or more lenses in the condenser system.

The width of the slit is controlled, usually in a continuous manner, via a mechanical arrangement. Its height is adjusted either in discrete steps with a series of apertures placed in front of the slit or continuously with a screw arrangement (Fig. 5). Different filters can be inserted into the illumination beam either to reduce the illumination when a wide slit aperture is used or to excite fluorescence in the eye when fluorescence has been used. In addition to this, rotation of the slit away from the vertical meridian is often available and an ability to tilt the projection system about a horizontal axis. These two additional degrees of freedom are included to assist in the examination of the fundus and the angle of the anterior chamber.

The light source used in virtually all slit lamp illumination systems is a tungsten filament bulb. For safety reasons, they are run on relatively low voltages. Some slit lamps can now be obtained with halogen-filled bulbs which have a considerably

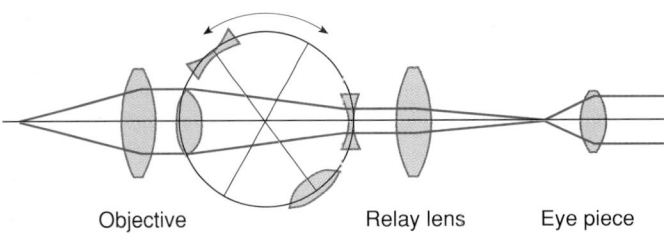

Fig. 3 Galilean telescope magnification changer.

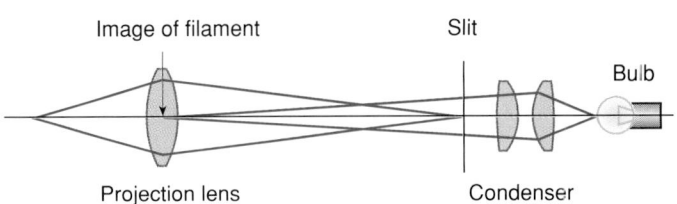

Fig. 4 The Koeller illumination system.

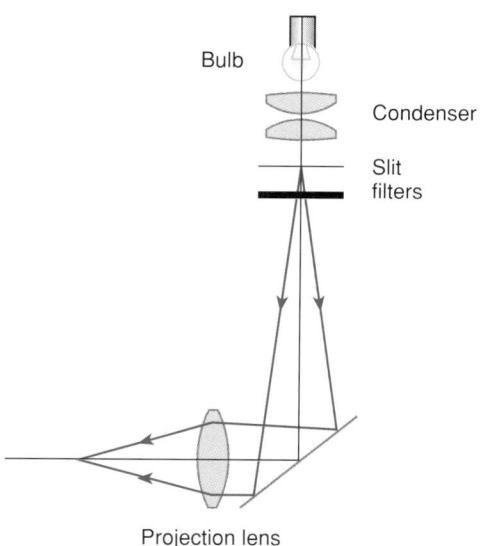

Fig. 5 Typical slit lamp illumination system.

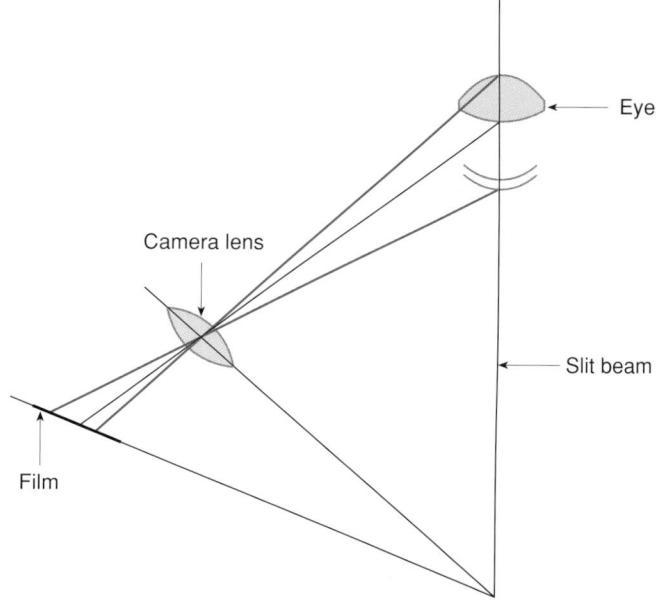

Fig. 6 Arrangement of camera lens and film for an in-focus slit section of the whole anterior segment, Scheimpflug's principle.

higher light output. These bulbs are useful in slit lamp photography and in instances where special techniques, such as pachometry, are practised.

Measurement of anterior eye using Scheimpflug's principle

The small depth of focus of conventional slit lamps puts considerable constraints on the use of the slit lamp for the measurement of thickness, optical radii, and the scattering properties of different optical elements. A solution to this problem was put forward by Scheimpflug in 1906. Scheimpflug was able to show that the whole optical section could be kept in focus if either the plane of the camera objective lens was tilted, the film plane tilted, or a combination of both (Fig. 6).

With a Scheimpflug camera it is also necessary to increase the depth of focus of the slit beam. This is normally achieved by placing a slit aperture over the illumination systems projection lens. This aperture, while reducing the amount of incident light, acts as a stenopeic slit on the illuminating beam.

Dragomirescu *et al.* helped develop a commercial slit lamp system (Topcon) which in addition to incorporating Scheimpflug's principle was capable of taking a series of photographs along different meridians. With this system it was possible to obtain a whole series of different sections which could then be combined to give a three-dimensional image.

One particular area of research where Scheimpflug photography has found wide application is in the monitoring of cataracts. The scattering properties of the lens are analysed, over time, from Scheimpflug images and from images of the lens taken with a retroillumination camera (Fig. 7).

Indirect ophthalmoscopy with slit lamp biomicroscope

Over the last few years an increasing number of ophthalmologists have opted to perform indirect ophthalmoscopy with a slit

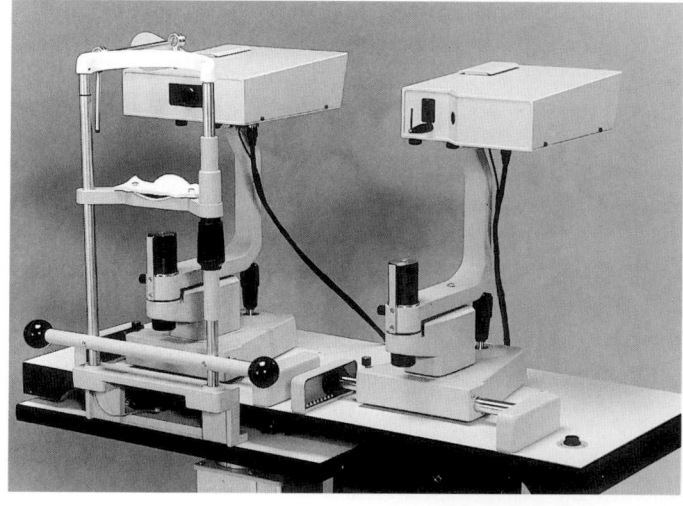

Fig. 7 Scheimpflug and retroillumination cameras. (By courtesy of Marcher Diagnostics.)

lamp biomicroscope and auxiliary fundus lens. Strictly speaking it is only the positive powered fundus lenses which form an intermediate image of the fundus between the ophthalmoscope lens and the observer, and hence can be described as indirect ophthalmoscopes. The advantages of such a system include stereoimaging of the fundus, adjustable magnification, a very flexible illumination system, and, with certain designs of fundus lenses, a very large field of view.

Slit lamp biomicroscopes cannot normally be focused any deeper into the eye than the anterior vitreous due to the refracting power of the cornea and lens. This problem can be overcome by one of two techniques. The first is to neutralize

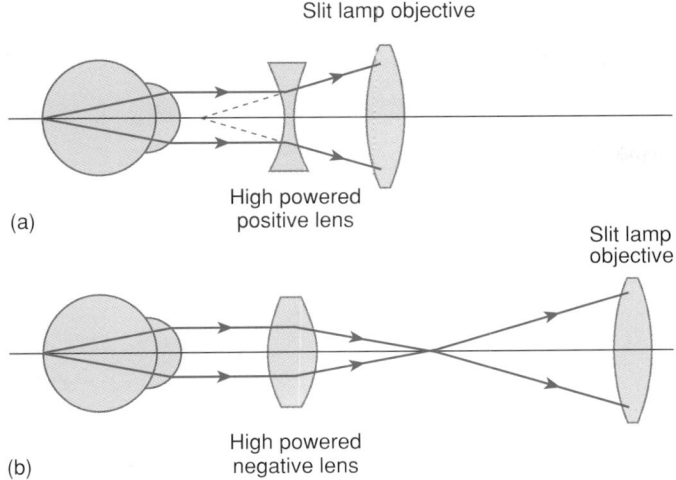

Fig. 8 Fundus examination: (a) with the aid of a negatively powered lens; (b) with the aid of a positively powered lens.

the power of the cornea with a high power negative lens (Fig. 8(a)), while the second is to use a high power positive lens to form an intermediate image of the fundus at the focal plane of the microscope (Fig. 8(b)). Both techniques can be used either with the auxiliary lens placed just in front of the eye or with the auxiliary lens in contact with the cornea.

Non-contacting lenses for viewing the fundus

One of the earliest non-contacting fundus lenses was developed by Hruby. This negative (–55 dioptre) lens was designed to neutralize the corneal power. It is easy to set up and provides a virtual erect image of the fundus. Its major limitation is the size of its field of view. The field of view of all negative fundus lenses is restricted by the pupil diameter and in the case of the Hruby lens can be as small as 5 to 8°, that is one disc diameter.

The problem of field size was overcome by El Bayadi who developed a +60 dioptre auxiliary lens which formed an inverted image of the fundus between the lens and the slit lamp microscope. The viewing system's optics is exactly the same as conventional indirect ophthalmoscope with the microscope being used to give both a stereo image of the fundus and variable magnification. The system is not reflex free although in practice this is not a major handicap as the clinician can move the ophthalmoscope lens and source around in order to displace the reflex away from any area of interest.

While the field of view of the El Bayadi lens was good, typically in the order of 40°, the overall image quality was poor. Subsequent developments of this lens led ultimately to the double aspheric Volk lens which is now available with a variety of powers including 90, 78, and 60 dioptre. The field of view of these three Volk lenses is approximately 70° although the area of observation is limited by the illuminator. Volk have recently produced a new double aspheric lens called the Superfield NC which has been specifically designed to give a large field of view (120°). The lens is 26 mm in diameter and has a working distance similar to that of the 90 dioptre lens of 6.0 to 6.5 mm with a magnification of 0.71. The final magni-

fication of the image is the product of this value and the slit lamp magnification.

Contacting lenses for viewing the fundus

One of the most widely used contacting fundus lenses is the one developed by Goldmann. This lens has a negative power of –64 dioptre with a field of view of approximately 30 to 40°. Again the field of view is restricted by the pupil which acts as the aperture stop in negative lens systems.

The Goldmann lens, like nearly all contacting fundus lenses, has a cone-like extension from its edge which stops the patient from blinking and reducing the optical quality of the lenses' front surface.

This lens normally incorporates a series of three mirrors which are set at slightly different angles such that, by successively viewing through each of them, the total retina can be examined (Fig. 9). The lens is rotated while on the eye in order to direct the illumination and viewing axes towards the region of the retina the clinician wishes to examine.

The Goldmann lens is most often used where high magnification is more important than large field of view such as a detailed inspection of the optic disc and macular. It is also used for retinal photocoagulation. This lens is less appropriate for general examination where the need to view through successive mirrors to see the whole of the fundus make examination times long and increases the potential for missing details.

Positive powered contact lenses have been designed by Rodenstock (the panfundoscope lens), Mainster, and Volk (the Volk quadraspheric) (Fig. 10). All these lenses give very large fields of view ranging from approximately 90° with the Mainster and panfundoscope lenses to 130° for the quadraspheric.

The panfundoscope was developed from the El Bayadi lens and has a power of +50 dioptre. It was one of the first large field auxiliary lenses and produces an intermediate image within the lens. While this is not a problem with regard to examining the fundus it may lead to damage of the lens when high energy lasers are used. The image quality of the panfundoscope also suffers from a large curvature of field, a problem that has been overcome in some of the alternate designs.

The Mainster lens uses aspheric surfaces on its anterior element in order to improve image quality. Its intermediate image

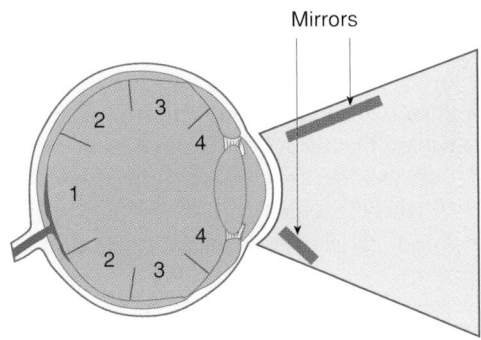

Fig. 9 The Goldmann three mirror lens showing the four regions of the retina visible through (1) the centre, and the three mirrors (2, 3, and 4).

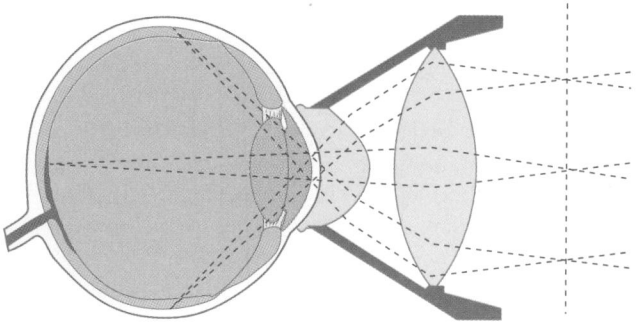

Fig. 10 The Volk quadraspheric lens.

is formed in front of the lens as it is in the quadraspheric lens which uses aspherical surfaces on both elements.

These lenses are used when very large field of view are required (quadraspheric field of view is 125° although the direct field of illumination is approximately one-third of the viewable area) and are especially useful for panretinal photocoagulation. The minification of the image (the quadraspheric magnification is 0.5) means that they are less suitable for detailed examination.

Photography through these lenses is very difficult due to the reflections from the different surfaces and the problems associated with keeping the illuminating beam separate from the viewing path through all the different elements. It is, however, interesting to note that the field of view of these lenses is relatively independent of the pupil size, large fields of view being obtained with only moderate dilation (4 mm).

Keratometers

Principles and theory of keratometry

Keratometers (also known as ophthalmometers) are instruments used to measure the radius of curvature of the anterior corneal surface (Fig. 11). This measurement is utilized in the fitting of contact lenses and to monitor corneal changes produced by contact lenses and ocular surgery. Keratometers are also occasionally used to assist in the recognition of certain corneal abnormalities and to check the radii of curvature of both hard and soft contact lenses.

Keratometers utilize the reflective properties of the cornea in order to measure its radius of curvature. By measuring the size of an image, formed by reflection from the cornea, of an object of known size and position, a measurement of the radius can be calculated. The theory of keratometry is depicted in Fig. 12, where it can be seen that the magnification of the image is equal to h'/h where h' equals the size of the image and h the size of the object. By similar triangles, it can be seen that

$$h'/h = f'/x = -r/2x \qquad (1)$$

where f' = the focal length of the corneal mirror, r = the radius of the cornea, and x = the distance between the object mire and focal point of the corneal mirror.

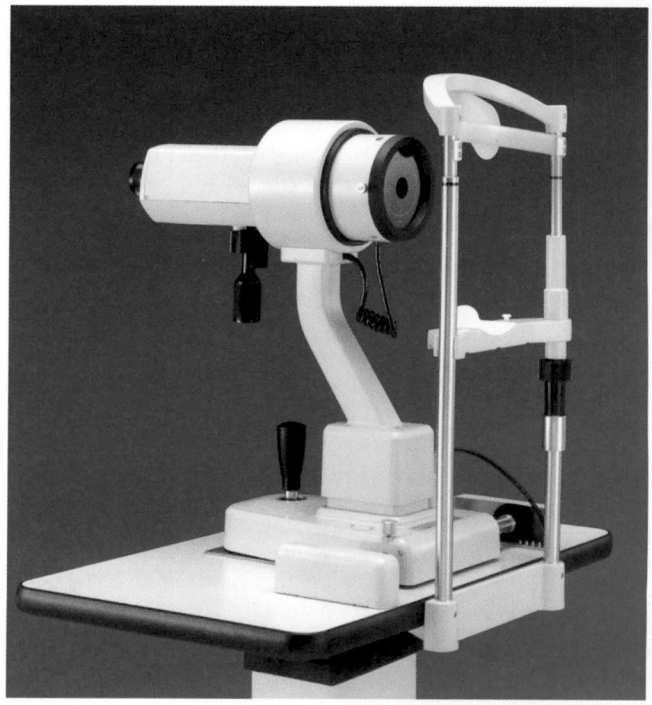

Fig. 11 Topcon keratometer. (By courtesy of Tinsley Medical Instruments.)

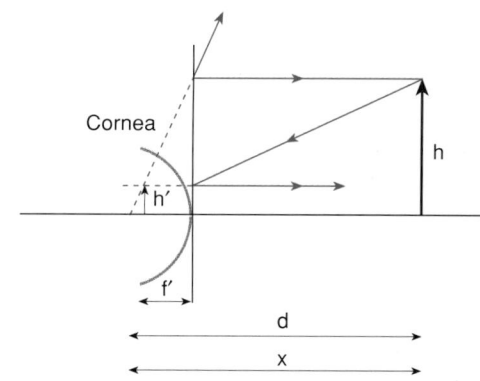

Fig. 12 The optical principles of the keratometer.

Transposing equation 1, we find that the radius of the cornea is

$$r = 2mx \qquad (2)$$

where m = the magnification of the image.

The magnification of the corneal image is of the order of 0.03 for a keratometer mire (test object) positioned approximately 15 cm from the eye. This magnification, or rather minification, makes the mire image so small that a compound microscope has to be used in order to measure its size accurately (Fig. 13). Because the object of known size (or mire) of the keratometer is invariably attached to the objective of this compound microscope, its image will only be seen in focus through the microscope when the mire is a given distance, d, from its image. If this distance is large, then the position of the mire image will

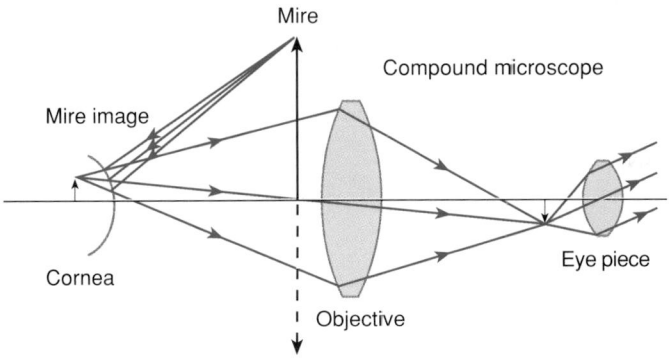

Fig. 13 The basic optical components of a keratometer.

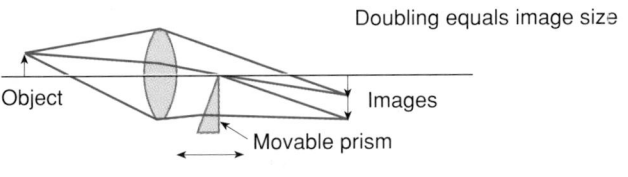

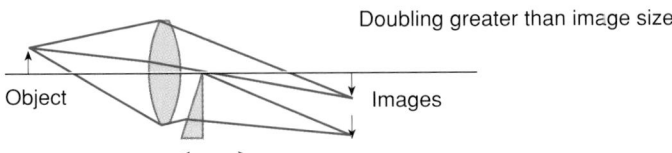

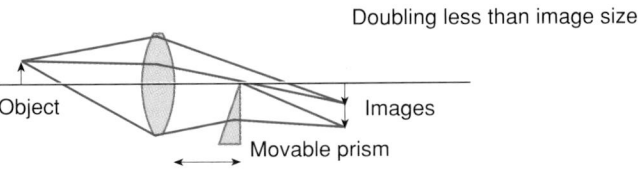

Fig. 14 The amount of doubling produced by a prism, placed between the objective of the keratometer and its image, is dependent upon the position of the prism.

be very close to the focal point of the corneal mirror, that is d will be approximately equal to x, in which case equation 2 can be rewritten as equation 3:

$$r = 2md \qquad (3)$$

Equation 3 is known as the approximate keratometer equation, while equation 2 is known as the exact keratometer equation. Since d is a constant for any particular instrument, the radius of the cornea is proportional to the magnification.

In theory, the size of the mire image could be measured by simply placing a measuring graticule within the microscope. However, a problem arises in keratometry due to the continual movement of the patient's eye. Every time the eye moves, the mire image moves, which makes it exceedingly difficult to measure with a fixed scale.

This problem has been successfully overcome by the use of a doubling system. The principles of one type of doubling system, a prism, are depicted in Fig. 14. Here it can be seen that the amount of doubling produced by the prism is dependent upon the position of the prism with respect to the objective lens. If this distance is reduced, the extent of doubling increases and if it is increased, the extent of doubling decreases.

By varying the position of the prism, the amount of doubling can be made to equal the size of the image. By then recording the position of the prism, the exact size of the image can be calculated. This technique overcomes the problem of eye movements because the two images stay in alignment when the eye moves.

Astigmatism

The centre of the average cornea is not spherical, but toric and in order to be fully specified it is necessary to have a radius of curvature measure along both its principle meridians. To align the mire images correctly the keratometer has to be rotated around its anteroposterior axis until the mires are aligned with one of the cornea's principal meridians. A measurement along the second principle meridian is obtained by rotating the keratometer through 90°.

One- and two-position keratometers

Because the axes of a toric surface are always at 90° to each other, some instrument manufacturers have designed kerato-

meters that incorporate two separate doubling systems which operate in mutually perpendicular meridians. Although these instruments still have to be rotated about their anterior and posterior axes in order to find one of the principal meridians, once this position has been found no further rotation of the instrument is necessary in order to obtain a radius measurement along the second principal meridian. This type of keratometer is known as a one-position instrument, while keratometers that require rotation through 90° in order to measure the second principal meridian are known as two-position instruments.

While the principal meridians of a toric lens are always at 90° to each other, those of the cornea need not be. This is because the corneal surface more closely approximates a toric ellipse and when an off-axis measurement is taken of a toric ellipse the principal meridians need not necessarily be at 90° to each other.

Area of cornea used during keratometry

It can be seen from Fig. 15 that the light reflected from the cornea comes not from its centre, but from two small areas on either side of the instrument axis. The size of these areas is dependent upon the effective aperture of the keratometer's objective. The principles upon which keratometry are based assume that a spherical surface exists between these two areas. This need not be the case. It is, in fact, well known that the normal cornea is not spherical, but flattens off towards its periphery. Because of this and because different keratometers reflect their mires from different regions of the cornea, two readings of the same cornea with two different keratometers may not give the same radius.

The fact that keratometers only record from two small areas

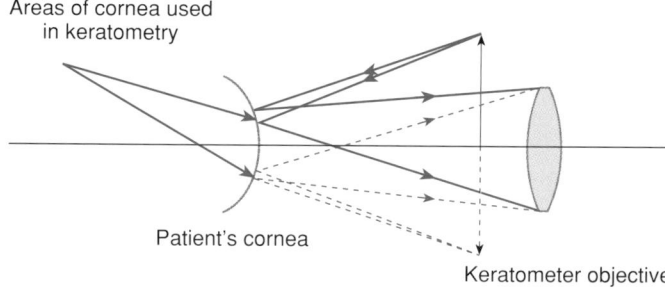

Areas of cornea used
in keratometry

Patient's cornea

Keratometer objective

Fig. 15 The two regions of the cornea from which the mire images are reflected.

of the cornea must make the clinician wary of relying on keratometer readings as the sole indicator of corneal distortion. It is theoretically feasible to have a small area of corneal irregularity that lies between the two areas measured with the keratometer. In this situation, the keratometry readings would be normal while the cornea itself was distorted. Similarly, it is possible to have corneal irregularities beyond the area of cornea measured with a keratometer.

Dioptric scales on keratometers

In addition to giving a measurement of the cornea's anterior radius of curvature, all currently produced keratometers also give an estimate of the total corneal power, that is the combined power of the front and back surfaces. To do this, keratometer manufacturers have had to assume certain values for the cornea's back surface. The majority of them have accepted the values adopted by Listing and Helmholtz who, in the production of a schematic eye, stated that the total corneal power could be reduced to a single curved surface with a refractive index equal to 1.3375. It should be recalled that the true refractive index of the cornea is 1.376.

The main value of these dioptric scales is to allow the contact lens practitioner to calculate the amount of residual astigmatism, this being defined as the amount of astigmatism that exists after a patient has been fitted with a hard spherical contact lens. Because the refractive index of the tears is very close to that used by keratometers to calculate total corneal power, the amount of astigmatism measured with the keratometer will be very close to that neutralized with a hard spherical contact lens. Thus, by comparing the amount of astigmatism measured with the keratometer with the ocular refraction, the practitioner can rapidly assess the extent of any residual astigmatism.

Calibration of keratometers

When the theory of keratometers was described at the beginning of this chapter, two equations were derived; the exact keratometer equation (2) and the approximate keratometer equation (3). Both of these equations are based on paraxial theory. Bennett has questioned whether the utilization of paraxial theory is valid in keratometry where the radii of the surfaces being measured are so very small. He takes a hypothetical instrument, which approximates a Bausch and Lomb keratometer, and calculates the angle, for a whole series of both

convex and concave radii, subtended by the mire image at the entrance pupil of the keratometer's microscope using:

1. The approximate keratometer equation
2. The exact keratometer equation
3. A ray tracing technique.

He finds that while all three conditions give an approximately linear relationship between corneal radius and angle subtended at the microscope objective, the use of paraxial theory results in an error of about 4 to 5 per cent. This means that a cornea of true radius 8.0 mm would be recorded as having a radius of curvature of 7.7 mm. The manufacturers of keratometers overcome this problem by calibrating their instruments on a series of known radii similar to those of the cornea. By doing this they reduce the errors induced by the use of paraxial theory to an insignificant level for any particular form of surface. If, however, a keratometer calibrated on convex surfaces is used to measure the radius of curvature of a concave surface, a large error will be introduced. While this is obviously not a problem when it comes to measuring the radius of curvature of the cornea, it is a problem when the keratometer is used to check the radii of curvature of contact lenses.

Eyepiece focusing errors in keratometry

In order for the majority of keratometers to give an accurate reading of the corneal curvature, it is essential that the eyepiece of the instrument be correctly focused. To facilitate this a graticule is invariably placed within the instrument upon which the eyepiece should be focused prior to making a radius measurement. The types of errors induced by incorrect focusing of the eyepiece can be reduced or eliminated by careful design of the keratometer's optics. Zeiss and Rodenstock have both designed keratometers without eyepiece focusing errors.

Measurement of the crystalline lens

The same theory as that used for the measurement of the corneal radius can be applied to a measurement of the front and back surfaces of the crystalline lens, a technique known as phakometry.

The most widely practised technique of phakometry is to photograph the reflected images from either the front or back surface of the lens, of an object of known size, and then to use the keratometer equation to calculate the radius of the equivalent mirror, that is a mirror which combines the refractive effects of the cornea (and lens when measuring the back surface of the lens) and the reflective properties of the crystalline lens surface. The calculation of the crystalline lenses' radii requires knowledge of the corneal radius of curvature and the distances between the different surfaces.

Types of optical systems incorporated in keratometers

Most of the currently produced keratometers fall into one of the following three categories:

1. Fixed doubling, variable mires

2. Variable doubling, fixed mires

3. Telecentric.

Three instruments are described here, one from each category mentioned above. Practically all modern keratometers have similar, if not identical, optical designs. This section ends with a brief description of an autokeratometer, which is capable of measuring the corneal radius without the clinician having to align a set of mires. Autokeratometers are bases upon the same principles as the other keratometers, that is it measures the size of the mire image.

Javal–Schiotz type keratometers

The Javal–Schiotz keratometer is a fixed doubling, variable mire, two-position instrument. The mires are attached to the front of small light boxes which, via a gearing arrangement, are made to move equally in opposite directions along a circular arc, the centre of curvature of which corresponds to the patient's eye. Doubling is achieved with a Wollaston prism placed behind the objective lens (Fig. 16). The whole instrument can rotate about its optical axis to enable measurement along any meridian.

The original mire pattern of the Javal–Schiotz keratometer is shown in Fig. 17. The stepped mire has a green filter over it while the square one is covered by a red filter. These filters help the practitioner to recognize when the mires overlap as any area of superimposition appears yellow. The appearance of the mire images as seen through the doubling system of the microscope is shown in Fig. 17.

Bausch and Lomb keratometer

The Bausch and Lomb instrument is a one-position, variable doubling keratometer. Two independently adjustable prisms, situated behind a special aperture stop, double the mire image along two mutually perpendicular meridians (Fig. 18).

When the instrument is correctly aligned, the operator sees three images of the instrument's mires (Fig. 19). The first is produced by light passing through aperture C and the vertically

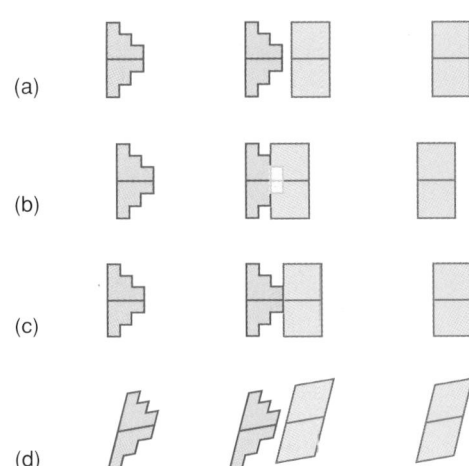

(a)

(b)

(c)

(d)

Fig. 17 The appearance of the Javal–Sciotz mires when (a) the mire separation is too large; (b) the mire separation is too small; (c) the mire separation is correct; (d) the mires are reflected off an astigmatic cornea, the axes of which do not coincide with those of the keratometer.

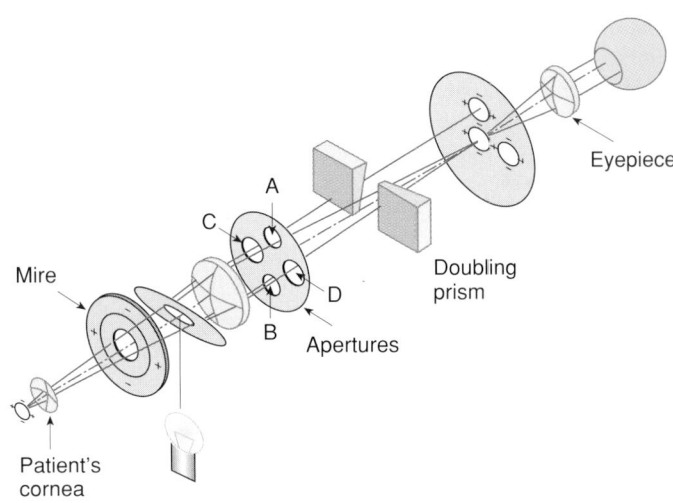

Fig. 18 Optics of the Bausch and Lomb keratometer. (Reproduced from Henson 1996, with permission.)

displacing prism. The second is produced by light passing through aperture D and the horizontally displacing prism, and the third by light passing through apertures A and B. Back and forth movement of the vertically doubling prism results in movement of the vertically displaced image, while movement of the horizontally doubling prism results in movement of the horizontally displaced image. The central image formed by the light passing through A and B is unaffected by movement of either prism. The apertures A and B act like a Schiener disc and double the central image of the mire when the intermediate image, produced by the objective lens, does not coincide with the focal point of the eyepiece lens. This system is designed to assist the operator in judging when the microscope is out of focus. Focusing errors still exist with this instrument when the eyepiece is incorrectly set.

In cases of high corneal astigmatism, it is impossible to keep

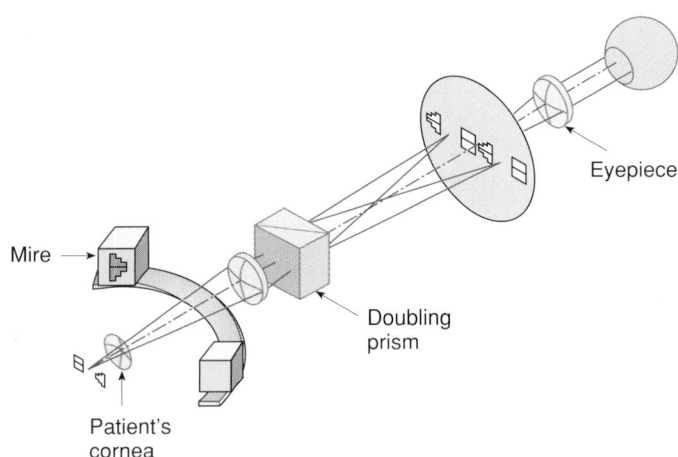

Fig. 16 Optics of the Javal–Sciotz keratometer. (Reproduced from Henson 1996, with permission.)

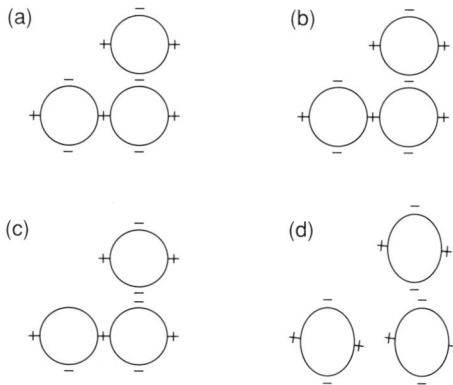

Fig. 19 Appearance of the Bausch and Lomb keratometer mires when (a) the vertical doubling is correct and the horizontal doubling is insufficient; (b) the vertical doubling is too great and the horizontal doubling is correct; (c) the vertical and horizontal degrees of doubling are correct; (d) the mires are viewed after reflection by an astigmatic cornea, the axes of which do not coincide with that of the keratometer.

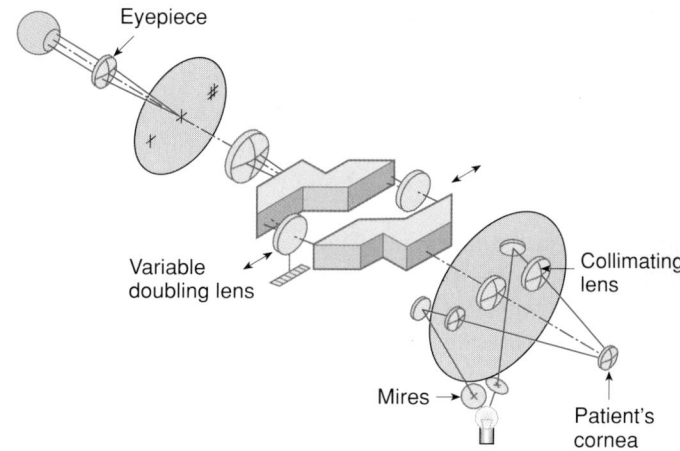

Fig. 20 Optics of the Zeiss keratometer. (Reproduced from Henson 1996, with permission.)

the central mire single along both astigmatic meridians. In this situation, the instrument needs to be focused for each meridian prior to a measurement in that meridian. One-position instruments assume that the two astigmatic axes are at 90° to each other. Because of the geometry of the cornea, this is not always the case.

Zeiss ophthalmometer

The Zeiss ophthalmometer is a variable doubling, two-position keratometer. The optics of the instrument have been designed so as to eliminate errors due to poor focusing. This has been achieved by:

1. placing the mires behind positive lenses which image them at infinity (collimated mires)

2. placing the doubling system at the focal point of the objective lens (telecentric principle).

The previously described variable doubling system, that of a prism moving along the axis of the instrument, is incompatible with the telecentric principle, which requires that the doubling system remains at the focal point of the objective lens. Zeiss have, therefore, developed a new type of doubling system which is composed of two cylindrical lenses that move in opposition to each other and move perpendicularly to the optical axis of the instrument (Fig. 20). The amount of doubling produced by these lenses, that is their prismatic effect, is proportional to the amount they are displaced from the optical axis.

The Zeiss ophthalmometer has a rather unusual recording system. The instrument has two scales: one records the radius of curvature and dioptral power of the front surface of the cornea, while the other reads the amount of front surface astigmatism. In use, the astigmatism scale should first be zeroed and a reading along one of the principle meridians made by rotating the knob that alters the radius of curvature scale. The instrument should then be rotated through 90° and the mires brought back into alignment by turning a second knob that alters the

qastigmatism scale. The operator can then read off from the two scales a prescription for the cornea, in dioptre. For optometrists and ophthalmologists in the United Kingdom who normally record in millimetres of radius, it is essential that the astigmatic scale remains at zero for both readings.

Optically, the instrument is a joy to use. The collimated mires have a much brighter image than those of many other instruments, which makes alignment easier. The freedom from focusing errors means that movements of the patient are less troublesome, for although they may result in a blurring of the images, they do not affect alignment. This freedom from focusing errors is also valuable when it comes to assessing the fit of soft contact lenses.

The mires of the Zeiss ophthalmometer are shown in Fig. 21. The appearances of the mire images through the doubling system of the microscope are shown in Fig. 21.

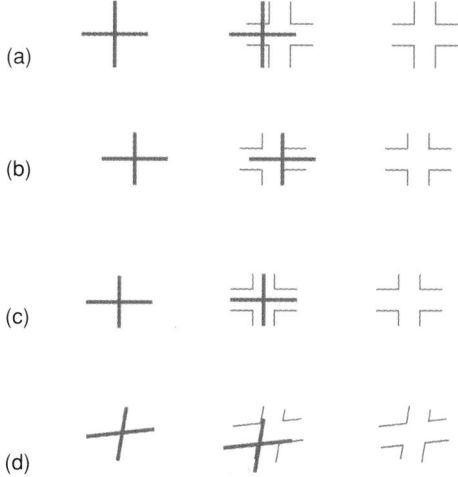

Fig. 21 Appearance of the Zeiss keratometer mires when (a) the amount of doubling is too large; (b) the amount of doubling is too small; (c) the amount of doubling is correct; (d) the mires are viewed after reflection by an astigmatic cornea, the axes of which do not coincide with that of the keratometer.

Humphrey autokeratometer

The Humphrey autokeratometer is designed to measure objectively the anterior corneal surface using the same basic theory as that of the standard keratometer.

The Humphrey autokeratometer does not require the optometrist to align any mire images. Once correctly positioned, the keratometer measures the cornea automatically. The mire of the Humphrey instrument is composed of three infrared emitting diodes arranged in a triangular shape whose image separation is approximately 2.6 mm at the surface of the cornea. In place of the observer it uses a solid state detector that records the exact position of each diode image after reflection from the cornea. From this it calculates the size of the mire image and the radius of curvature of the cornea. The speed with which these detectors operate is so fast that eye movements do not create a problem for the measurement system. The instrument does not, therefore, contain a doubling system.

In addition to measuring the central radius of curvature the Humphrey autokeratometer also measures the corneal radius at two additional peripheral locations along the horizontal meridian. The central measurements are taken with the patient looking straight into the instrument, while the peripheral ones are made with the patient looking 13.5° nasally and 13.5° temporally. The autokeratometer converts the peripheral readings into a measurement of the corneal shape factor (the degree to which it flattens off in the periphery) and an estimate of the vault height. It also calculates the position of the corneal apex and gives a conformance factor. The conformance factor indicates how well the measured cornea matches a theoretical cornea, the parameters of which are stored in the instrument. If the measured cornea conforms very badly with the theoretical one then this indicates an irregularly shaped cornea.

This instrument is a very good example of how electronics can overcome some of the optical problems encountered in the design of ophthalmic instruments. Similar autokeratometers are made by Canon and Topcon and it is now possible to get instruments which combine the functions of an autorefractometer with an autokeratometer.

Other techniques of corneal measurement

The keratometer in its basic form only gives information about the central radius of curvature. It does not measure the extent to which the cornea flattens towards its periphery or the exact location of the corneal apex (point of shortest radius).

In an attempt to overcome this problem, several keratometers were marketed with an optional attachment that allowed off-axis measurements. The attachment to the Bausch and Lomb keratometer (Topogometer) consisted of an illuminated fixation light that could be moved along two axes, both of which were perpendicular to the axis of the keratometer. Scales were attached to the Topogometer which indicated, in millimetres, the amount of decentration of the visual axis from the optical axis of the keratometer at the corneal surface.

A problem with such a system of peripheral assessment is that the mires of the keratometer reflect from just two areas of

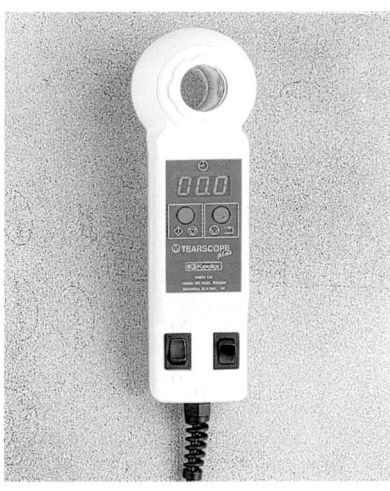

Fig. 22 Keeler tearscope, a modern, internally illuminated keratoscope. (By courtesy of Keeler Instruments.)

the cornea which, in the Bausch and Lomb instrument, are approximately 3 mm apart. When the patient is viewing eccentrically one mire will be reflected from a peripheral region 1.5 mm beyond that indicated on the scale while the other will be reflected from a region 1.5 mm closer to the apex. The resultant measurement will, therefore, not be a true measure of the radius of curvature at the indicated eccentricity.

An attempted solution to this problem was produced by Guilbert Routit with their topographic keratometer. They realized that the separation of the reflecting areas was a product of the mire size. The smaller the mires, the smaller the separation. The topographic keratometer had the facility for using just one of the mires, the other mire being turned off. The task of the clinician was to double the image by the size of the single mire. This effectively came from a very small region of the cornea and allowed the clinician to achieve a more accurate representation of the way in which the corneal curvature changed towards the periphery. Unfortunately, the accuracy of keratometer measurements reduces with the size of the mire, Douthwaite, so while these instruments were able to give clinicians a better understanding of peripheral corneal shape their accuracy on single measurements is below that of the larger mired keratometers.

The quest to gain more information on corneal topography, which has been boosted by the upsurge in refractive surgery, has largely been fulfilled via developments in photokeratoscopes.

The origins of the photokeratoscope date back to the nineteenth century with a simple device known as Placido's disc. This disc is essentially a flat black round plate upon which are attached a series of concentric white rings (Fig. 22). In the centre of the plate is a peephole and positive lens. Images of the concentric rings (mires) are viewed after reflection from the cornea through the positive lens. Any irregularities in the cornea display themselves as irregularities in the mire images. In its basic form, Placido's disc is only sensitive to gross irregularities of the corneal surface, such as may occur in certain pathologies. Gullstrand modified Placido's disc by attaching a camera to it that was capable of photographing the mire images. His instrument was called a photokeratoscope. By carefully measuring the size and shape of the mire images, Gullstrand was able to calculate the topography of the cornea. The theory and assumptions behind these calculations being exactly the same as that for a keratometer.

Ludlam and Wittenberg describe many of the shortcomings of Gullstrand's photokeratoscope. One of these is curvature of the image plane. With a large aperture system, such as that found in the photokeratoscope, the image becomes curved and it becomes impossible to obtain all the rings in focus at the film plane. This problem can be overcome by curving the object, that is by placing the rings on the inside of a bowl rather than on a flat plate.

A second problem is alignment of the patient's cornea with the photokeratoscope. Most measurements of corneal curvature are taken along the line of sight which is assumed to coincide with the corneal apex. It has, however, already been shown by Mandell and St Helen that the corneal apex does not necessarily coincide with the line of sight or any other common reference point. The third and final problem that Ludlam and Wittenberg mention relates to the analysis of the data. They found that the quality of the image produced was such that accurate measurement was not always possible.

Wesley-Jessen produced a photokeratoscope, known as the PEK (Photo Electronic Keratoscope), that resolved many of the problems outlined by Ludlam and Wittenberg. The mires of this instrument were placed on the inside of an elliptical bowl so that, for the average cornea, a flat image was produced in the film plane. In addition to this, Townsley developed a new mathematical treatment of the photokeratogram that does not require it to be taken symmetrically about the apex of the cornea.

Recently, several new photokeratoscopes and videokeratoscopes (instruments which use a video camera rather than conventional film) have taken advantage of the developments in computer technology to give rapid, on-line analysis of keratograms.

Unfortunately, there is no exact technique for the calculation of local corneal power from keratograms. All of the techniques used make certain assumptions which may or may not have important implications when it comes to obtaining absolute values of local corneal radius and power. One of the first groups to attempt a solution to this problem were Doss et al. whose techniques were further developed by Klyce. With this technique the average radius of the first ring's image is used to calculate the central radius of curvature a calculation which assumes a spherical cap. The radius and power measurements for peripheral regions of the cornea are then obtained via a series of smoothing and curve fitting equations which operate over small regions of the cornea starting at the centre and working towards the periphery.

Papers describing the operation of commercially produced instruments usually cite the papers of Doss et al. and Klyce but for proprietary reasons do not give details on how they calculate the local power or what assumptions they make. This means that their accuracy and reproducibility can only be evaluated by laboratory and clinical trials. Significant improvements to the analytical techniques have been described by both Wang et al. and Van Saarloos and Constable. These improvements are primarily in the calculation of peripheral radii and powers for both spherical and non-spherical surfaces.

One of the most widely used instruments is the corneal modelling system (CMS) made by Computed Anatomy. It uses a 32-ring videokeratoscope which covers almost the whole of the corneal surface (approximately 95 per cent). Results are presented in a variety of ways including the now frequently encountered topographic maps (Fig. 23).

The accuracy of its algorithms has been tested on a series of spheres by Hannush et al. and on a group of normal human eyes by Hannush et al. While its accuracy on spheres was found to be within the stated value (0.25 dioptres) its performance on real corneas highlighted a number of problems. Although the instrument has 32 rings quantitative data is only available for rings 1 to 27 (72 per cent of the corneal surface). Consistency of results was found to be dependent upon eccentricity, while 84 per cent of readings from rings 3 to 9 were within 0.50 dioptres, only 54 per cent of those from rings 1 to 27 were within 0.50 dioptres. The deterioration in accuracy with eccentricity is believed to result from mathematical assumptions underlying the methods of measurement. An analysis of reliability and accuracy on an asymmetric surface has been conducted by Heath et al. They found that the instrument was very sensitive to small alignment errors and for asymmetric surfaces had an error of more than 0.5 dioptres on 60 per cent of the measurement points.

The CMS technology is currently available in the topographic modelling system, TMS-1. This system has been evaluated for both accuracy and precision (repeatability of measurements) on calibrated spherical surfaces and normal human corneas by Wilson et al. The results of this evaluation concluded that it was sufficiently accurate for clinical applications where an accuracy of between 0.25 and 0.50 dioptres was needed. This study was not able to report on the instrument's accuracy on non-spherical or irregular surfaces due to problems of calibrating such surfaces and did not numerically quantify the results from the human subjects as did Hannush et al.

Another popular system is produced by Eye-Sys Laboratories (the corneal analysis system) (Fig. 24). This system again uses a videokeratoscope although this time there are only eight rings. Data is again presented in a variety of different forms which includes the colour-coded topographic maps. This system has also been evaluated on spherical surfaces by Wilson et al. who again concluded that it was sufficiently accurate for clinical applications.

An important parameter in the design of both photokeratoscopes and videokeratoscopes is the system they use to ensure that they are the correct distance from the cornea. The precision of this setting is a major determinant in the accuracy and precision of the instrument. The TMS-1 system uses the superimposition of scanning laser slits at the centre of the cornea while the Eye-Sys system uses the focusing of a cross-shaped target on the fourth ring's image. Wilson et al. have

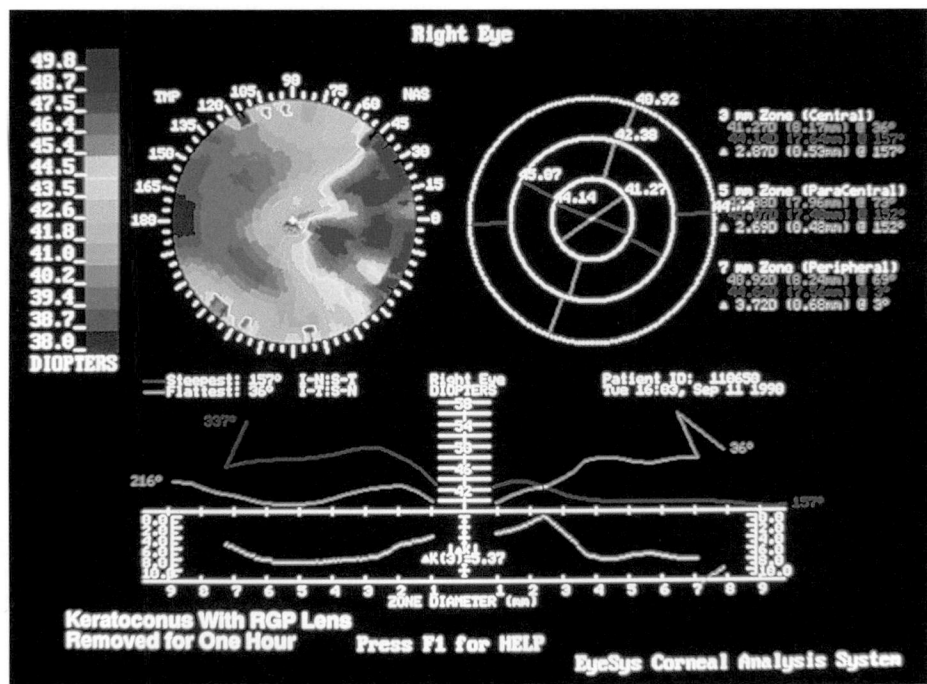

Fig. 23 Topographic map from Eye-Sys corneal analysis system. These images use colour to code the dioptric power of different corneal regions. (By courtesy of Keeler Instruments.)

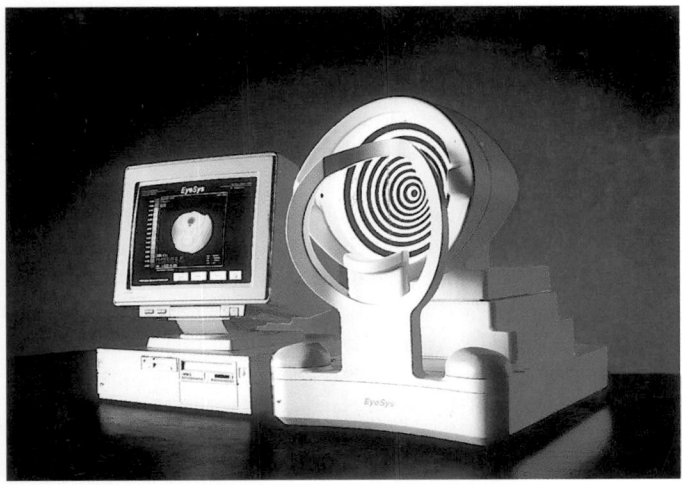

Fig. 24 Eye-Sys corneal analysis system. (By courtesy of Tinsley Medical Instruments.)

reported that while both systems are simple to use the TMS-1 system is not affected by peripheral distortions that may occur as a result of surgery.

The topographic information produced by videokeratography has led to new descriptive classifications of corneal shape that extend far beyond that developed for the earlier photokeratoscopes. The complex nature of the topographic plots has also led to the development of parametric descriptors of corneal topography which quantify the surface asymmetry and regularity. The TMS-1 incorporates three computerized algorithms,

simulated keratometry value, surface regularity index, and surface asymmetry index.

There are several other techniques for measuring the corneal surface which have yet to leave the research clinic. De Cunha and Woodward have developed a technique which projects vertical planes of light on to the cornea and then analyses the sections in order to derive topographical maps. This system, which is similar to that described by Thall *et al.*, overcomes a number of the problems outlined above with reference to photokeratograms such as (a) alignment with the cornea, (b) distorted and out of focus images, and (c) assumptions concerning the nature of the surface. Bonnet and LeGrand described a technique based upon stereo photography which has recently been further developed by Arffa *et al.*

Further reading

Arffa, R.C., Warnicki, J.W., and Rehkopf, P.G. (1989). Corneal topography using rasterstereography. *Refractive and Corneal Surgery*, **5**, 414.

Barker, F.M. (1990). Auxiliary lenses in fundus biomicroscopy— a comparison of field of view. *Journal of the American Optometric Association*, **61**, 544.

Barker, F.M. and Wing, J.T. (1990). Ultra wide field fundus biomicroscopy with the Volk quadraspheric lens. *Journal of the American Optometric Association*, **61**, 573.

Bennett, A.G. (1966). The calibration of keratometers. *Optician*, **151**, 317.

Bogan, S.J., Waring, G.O., Ibrahim, O., Drews, C., and Curtis, L. (1990). Classification of normal corneal topography based on computer assisted videokeratography. *Archives of Ophthalmology*, **108**, 945.

Bonnet, R. and Cochet, D (1962). New method of topographical ophthalmometry—its theoretical and clinical applications. *American Journal of Optometry*, **39**, 227.

Brown, N. (1973). The change in shape and internal form of the lens of the eye on accommodation. *Experimental Eye Research*, **15**, 441.

Brown, N. (1974). The change in lens curvature with age. *Experimental Eye Research*, 19, 175.

Brown, N. (1979). Photographic investigation of the human lens and cataract. *Survey of Ophthalmology*, 23, 307.

De Cunha, D.A. and Woodward, E.G. (1993). Measurement of corneal topography in keratoconus. *Ophthalmic and Physiological Optics*, 13, 377.

Douthwaite, W.A. (1987*a*). A new keratometer. *American Journal of Optometry and Physiological Optics*, 64, 711.

Douthwaite, W.A. (1987*b*). Corneal topography. *Contact Lens Journal*, 15, 7.

Doss, J.D., Hutson, R.L., Rowsey, J.J., and Brown, R. (1981). Method for the evaluation of corneal profile and power distribution. *Archives of Ophthalmology*, 99, 1261.

Dragomirescu, V., Hockwin, O., Koch, H.R., and Sasaki, K. (1978). Development of new equipment for rotating slit image photography according to Scheimpflug's principle. *Interdisciplinary Topics on Gerontology*, 13, 1.

El Bayadi, G. (1953). New method of slit lamp micro-ophthalmoscopy. *British Journal of Ophthalmoscopy*, 37, 625.

Emsley, H.H. (1963). *Visual optics*, Vol. 1, (5th edn). Hatton Press, London.

Gormley, D.J., Gersten, M., Koplin, R.S., and Lubkin, V. (1988). Corneal modelling. *Cornea*, 7, 30.

Hannush, S.B., Crawford, S.L., Waring, G.O., Gemmill, M.C., Lynn, M.J., and Nizam, A. (1989). Accuracy and precision of keratometry, photokeratoscopy, and corneal modelling on calibrated steel balls. *Archives of Ophthalmology*, 107, 1235.

Hannush, S.B., Crawford, S.L., Waring, G.O., Gemmill, M.C., Lynn, M.J., and Nizam, A. (1990). Reproducibility of normal corneal power measurements with a keratometer, photokeratoscope, and video imaging system. *Archives Ophthalmology*, 108, 539.

Heath, G.G., Gerstman, D.R., Wheeler, W.H., Soni, P.S., and Horner, D.G. (1991). Reliability and validity of videokeratoscopic measurements. *Optometry and Vision Science*, 68, 946.

Henson, D.B. (1996). *Optometric instrumentation*. (2nd edn). Butterworth-Heinemann, Oxford.

Klyce, S.D. (1984). Computer-assisted corneal topography: high-resolution graphic presentation and analysis of keratoscopy. *Investigative Ophthalmology and Vision Science*, 25, 1426.

Littmann, H. (1950). A new slit lamp apparatus. *American Journal of Ophthalmology*, 33, 1863.

Longhurst, R.S. (1967). *Geometrical and physical optics*, (2nd edn). Longman, London.

Ludlam, W.M. and Kaye, M. (1966). Optometry and the metrology. *American Journal of Optometry and Physiological Optics*, 43, 525.

Ludlam, W.M. and Wittenberg, S. (1966). The effect of measuring corneal toroidicity with reference to the line of sight. *British Journal of Physiological Optics*, 23, 178.

Mainster, M.A., Crossman, J.L., Erickson, P.J., and Heacock, G.L. (1990). Retinal laser lenses: magnification, spot size, and field of view. *British Journal of Ophthalmology*, 74, 177.

Mandell, R.B. (1965). *Contact lens practice: basic and advanced*. Thomas, Springfield, Illinois.

Mandell, R.B. (1966). Corneal curvature measurements by the aid of Moiré fringes. *Journal of the American Optometric Association*, 37, 219.

Mandell, R.B. and St Helen, R. (1971). Mathematical model of the corneal contour. *British Journal of Physiological Optics*, 26, 183.

Stone, J. (1962). The variability of some existing methods of measuring corneal contour compared with suggested new methods. *British Journal of Physiological Optics*, 19, 205.

Stone, J. and Francis, J. (1980). Practical optics of contact lenses and aspects of contact lens design. In *Contact lenses*, Vol. 1, (ed. J. Stone and A.J. Phillips), p. 91. Butterworths, London.

Thall, E.H., Lange, S.R. *et al.* (1993). Preliminary results of a new intraoperative corneal topography technique. *Journal of Cataract and Refractive Surgery*, 19, 193.

Townsley, M.G. (1967). New equipment and methods for determining the contour of the human cornea. *Contacto*, 11, 72.

Townsley, M.G. (1970). New knowledge of the corneal contour. *Contacto*, 14, 38.

Van Saarloos, P.P. and Constable, I.J. (1991). Improved method for calculation of corneal topography for any photokeratoscope geometry. *Optometry and Vision Science*, 68, 960.

Van Veen, H.G. and Goss, D.A. (1988). Simplified system of Purkinje image photography for phakometry. *American Journal of Optometry and Physiological Optics*, 11, 905.

Wang, J., Rice, D.A., and Klyce, S.D. (1989). A new reconstruction algorithm for improvement of corneal topographic analysis. *Refractive Corneal Surgery*, 5, 379.

Wilson, S.E. and Klyce, S.D. (1991). Advances in the analysis of corneal topography. *Survey Ophthalmology*, 35, 269.

Wilson, S.E., Verity, S.M., and Congert, D.L. (1992). Accuracy and precision of the corneal analysis system and the topographic modelling system. *Cornea*, 11, 28.

1.6.3 Specular and confocal microscopy

Steven J. Wiffen and William M. Bourne

Specular microscopy

Principles

David Maurice designed an instrument to examine and photograph the corneal endothelium of enucleated eyes and coined the term 'specular microscopy' in 1968. The specular microscope takes advantage of specular reflection of light from optical interfaces to image the endothelium. Light incident upon a surface may be transmitted, absorbed, or reflected. Reflection may be specular (mirror-like) from smooth surfaces, diffuse from rough surfaces, or a combination of these. The cornea serves its visual function by transmitting almost all incident light, but it is possible to see structures in the cornea because of the small proportion of light reflected and/or scattered from its interfaces. A greater proportion of incident light is reflected from interfaces of greater difference in refractive index. It has been estimated that 0.02 per cent of incident light is reflected from the posterior corneal–aqueous interface, whereas 0.4 per cent of incident light is reflected from the glass–tear interface when a contact objective lens is used. The reflectance of interfaces other than at the endothelium and epithelium is too low to allow them to be seen by specular microscopy. The orientation of cell borders perpendicular to the plane of the endothelial cell monolayer causes light to be scattered or reflected away from the observer, thus producing the visible dark outlines of the cells in the characteristic mosaic pattern (Fig. 1).

The slit lamp can be used to view the corneal endothelium using the principle of specular reflection, but the visible area of specular reflection is small due to the curvature of the cornea, there are many unwanted light reflexes, and magnification is limited to about 40 times. Scanning over a large area of

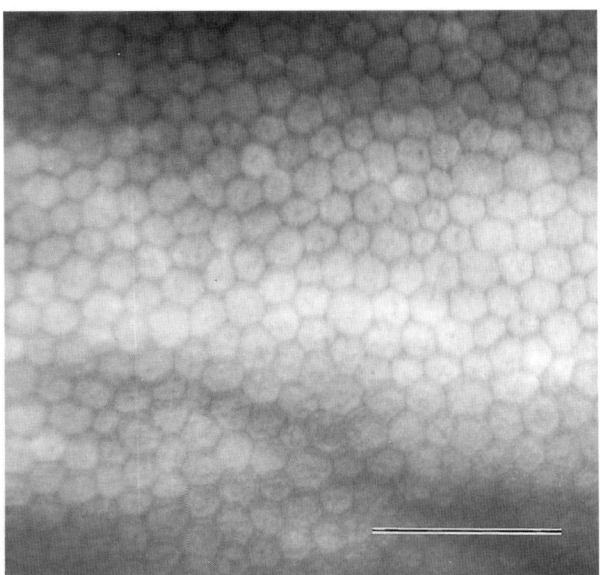

Fig. 1 Specular microscope photograph of normal human corneal endothelium. Endothelial cell density 3226 cells/mm², coefficient of variation 0.20, 90 per cent six-sided cells (bar = 100 μm).

endothelium requires constant repositioning of slit illumination and eyepieces, and eye movements are a problem. In the contact specular microscope the illuminating and image forming light rays pass through the same objective lens, thereby minimizing the angle of incidence and decreasing distortion and unwanted reflections. Light from the illuminating source is directed through part of the objective lens to the cornea and those rays that are specularly reflected pass back through a different portion of the objective. A dipping cone lens is used to applanate the cornea, eliminating the air–tear interface, reducing distortion due to corneal curvature, and dampening eye movements.

Overlap of the reflections from the tear film and the endothelium and scattering of light from the overlying stroma degrade the endothelial image. A narrow illumination beam decreases these effects, producing better contrast, but results in a narrow field of view. Modifications of the instrument have been made to increase the field without degrading image quality, leading to the development of 'wide-field' specular microscopes, which make observation and scanning of the endothelium easier and quantitative analysis of images more reliable. The disturbing effect of the tear interface reflection can be reduced by stepping down the refractive index of the dipping cone lens using a tip of fluorite coated with magnesium fluoride, thus reducing the difference in refractive index at the lens–tear interface. Use of a high-water content soft contact lens with a refractive index close to that of tears further reduces reflection from this interface. Scanning slit instruments, in which very narrow slit illumination is used at a small angle of incidence to scan an area of endothelium rapidly, can create optical sections of the cornea. The narrow slit effectively removes reflections from outside the focal plane and a high scanning frequency produces a continuous image. Such confocal instruments have the theor-

etical advantage of giving an image in the presence of some corneal oedema, but a relatively clear cornea is required in order to view the endothelium with any specular microscope.

Applanation of the cornea by the dipping cone lens of contact specular microscopes is the cause of artefacts called posterior corneal rings. These are dark lines with bright centres occurring in fixed positions concentric to the corneal centre. Applanation presumably produces shallow folds of the posterior corneal surface and the sides of these folds reflect light away from the observer, thus appearing dark in the specular image. As these rings occur in fixed positions for a given cornea they can be used to relocate specific areas of endothelium on repeated examination. Under certain circumstances in contact specular microscopy, the posterior corneal surface becomes visible in what has been called the relief mode. A relief image replaces a portion of the specular image and excrescences such as guttae in Descemet's membrane, or cells on the posterior endothelial surface, appear to be elevated towards the observer. This provides useful qualitative information for interpretation of abnormalities of the specular image.

With appropriate calculation of the magnification of the microscope (typically about 200×), endothelial cell density can be computed from the images obtained. Quantitative morphometric analysis of the endothelial cell monolayer was initially performed by fixed frame counting of the number of cells in a grid of known size, or by projecting images of the endothelium and tracing cell outlines with a digitizer. Proprietary computer software is now available for morphometric analysis of digitized specular microscopic images. Endothelial cell area can be estimated either by manual digitization of the positions of the cell apices, or by estimating the centre of each cell. The software typically computes mean endothelial cell density (cells/mm²), coefficient of variation of cell size (standard deviation/mean), and percentages of five-, six-, and seven-sided cells. Fully automated analysis of cells by computer software has still to be realized because of the difficulties involved in the determination of cell borders. Modern non-contact instruments with built-in cell analysis software provide rapid determination of endothelial cell density and morphology, but it is not possible to scan the endothelial mosaic with them in the same way as with contact microscopes. The rationale for morphometric analysis is that the human endothelium heals not by undergoing cell division, but by spreading of remaining cells. Changes in endothelial cell density or morphology may then reflect past trauma or indicate changes in function.

Uses of specular microscopy

The specular microscope has been used as a tool for examination of the corneal endothelium in the clinic and in the research setting, as well as for assessment of donor corneal endothelium in the eye bank prior to transplantation. Clinical specular microscopy can guide decision-making prior to anterior segment surgery when there is some concern about the state of the endothelium, for instance prior to secondary intraocular lens implantation. One of the most valuable uses of specular microscopy has been in the assessment of the response of the

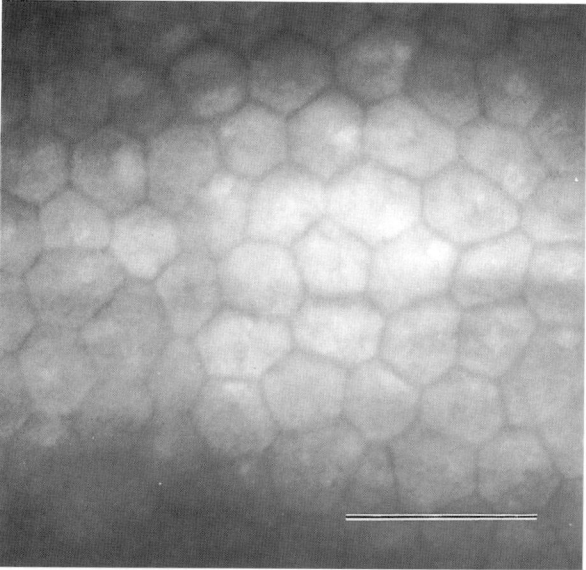

Fig. 2 Endothelium of a corneal transplant. Endothelial cell density 678 cells/mm², coefficient of variation 0.15, 68 per cent six-sided cells (bar = 100 μm).

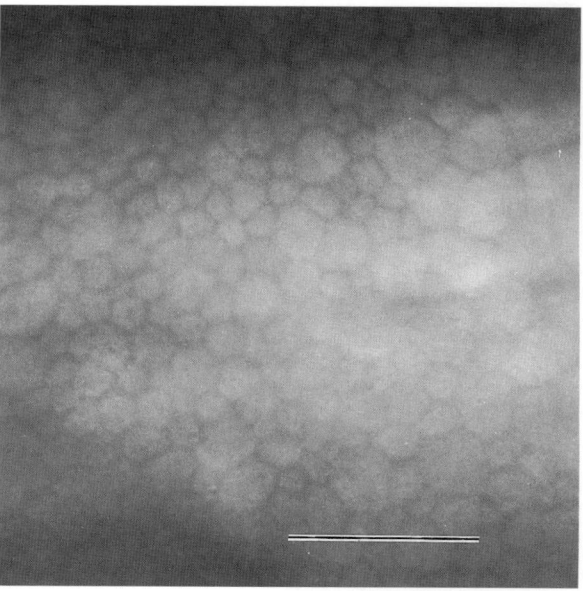

Fig. 3 Endothelium after long-term contact lens wear. Endothelial cell density 2114 cells/mm², coefficient of variation 0.75, 44 per cent six-sided cells. Marked polymegethism and pleomorphism (bar = 100 μm).

endothelium to various surgical procedures (Fig. 2). The effects of cataract surgery and intraocular lenses on the endothelium were not recognized until specular microscopy was used to examine the endothelium postoperatively. Responses of the endothelium to various insults, such as drugs, ocular irrigating solutions, and different forms of trauma, have been investigated by specular microscopy. Recently, specular microscopy has been employed in the assessment of the safety of keratorefractive procedures, such as excimer laser photorefractive keratectomy.

Changes in the specular microscopic appearance of the endothelium occur after both short- and long-term contact lens wear. Transient blebs appear in the endothelium after just 10 min of contact lens wear and with long-term wear there is increased variation of both endothelial cell area (polymegethism) and cell shape (pleomorphism) (Fig. 3). The significance of these changes is not known because the relationship between cell morphology and function is poorly understood. Diagnosis of some endothelial disorders is aided by specular microscopy. Conditions such as posterior polymorphous dystrophy and the iridocorneal endothelial syndrome (Fig. 4) have characteristic specular microscopic appearances. Specular microscopy is of limited use, however, in the presence of severe endothelial dysfunction with corneal oedema.

Specular microscopy has been used to examine the corneal epithelial surface. Newly emerged epithelial cells are small and are thought to enlarge with time before they are shed. Dry eye patients have smaller surface epithelial cells, whereas wearers of extended wear contact lenses have larger cells than normal, suggesting that epithelial turnover is slower in contact lens wear. Epithelial cell surface variations can be demonstrated by colour photography due to interference effects with differing thickness of the tear film.

Use of the specular microscope for the assessment of donor

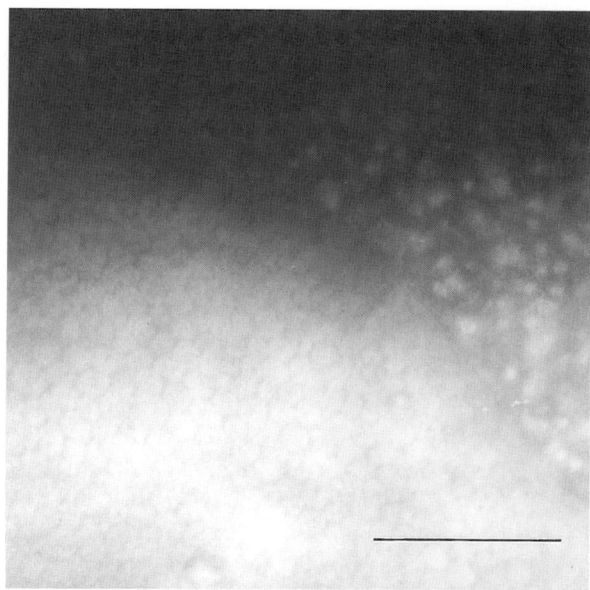

Fig. 4 Junction of ICE cells and endothelium in iridocorneal endothelial (ICE) syndrome (bar = 100 μm).

corneas in the eye bank allows for confirmation of findings of slit lamp examination and for the detection of subtle endothelial abnormalities, which may otherwise be missed. Specular microscopy is potentially valuable in the assessment of corneas which may otherwise be arbitrarily excluded on the basis of age and, in the absence of adequate tests of endothelial function, it provides the best assessment of donor endothelial quality. Knowledge of preoperative endothelial cell counts and morphology is essential for comparison with postoperative clinical measurements in the assessment of the effect of corneal transplantation on the endothelium, and for comparison of different methods of corneal preservation.

Confocal microscopy

Principles

Slit lamp images of the cornea have low contrast and low resolution because of the inherent low contrast of the tissue and the effects of light scattered from above and below the plane of focus. Resolution and contrast can be improved by reducing the field of view, thus reducing the effects of light scattered from the surrounding tissue. Taken to the extreme, one can use a point source of illumination and a point detection system. In this case, the illumination and detection systems need to be focused at the same point and hence are called confocal. Confocal systems using point or slit illumination and detection have to scan the object of interest to generate an image. Since the image is generated from a scanned light source, with little effect from scattered light above and below the plane of focus, confocal microscopes can produce high contrast optical sections with high lateral and axial resolution, even of thick, partially opaque tissue.

Several types of confocal microscope have been applied to ophthalmology. The tandem scanning confocal microscope uses a spinning Nipkow disc, which has two sets of pinholes arranged in continuous spirals, that scan across the surface to be examined as the disc rotates. Pairs of holes provide conjugate point illumination and detection and the pinhole apertures prevent light from outside the plane of focus from entering the system. The light throughput of the disc is low, so that objective lenses of high numerical aperture are required and, even then, with present low light level video technology, adequate resolution relies heavily on digital image processing. Confocal systems using scanning slit illumination, although having lower lateral and axial resolution than the Nipkow disc-based instrument, have greater light throughput, and with the use of high numerical aperture lenses can produce high contrast images without extensive image processing. Contact objective lenses and a coupling fluid are generally used with these instruments, but the cornea is not applanated. For clinical use, real-time scanning is necessary and video recording systems are generally used. The arc lamp light sources used for clinical applications are filtered to the visible spectrum and are within maximal permissible retinal exposure limits for examination times of several minutes. Laser confocal microscopes are used extensively for research purposes, but the scan rates of commercially available systems are too slow for real-time clinical application with video recording. The ability to examine structures within the eye depends on the working distance of the objective lens. It is presently feasible to examine the whole thickness of the cornea and, as lenses of longer working distance are developed, it will be possible to examine other parts of the eye *in vivo*.

Uses of confocal microscopy

The high resolution of the confocal microscope allows for examination of tissues at the cellular level *in vivo* and the

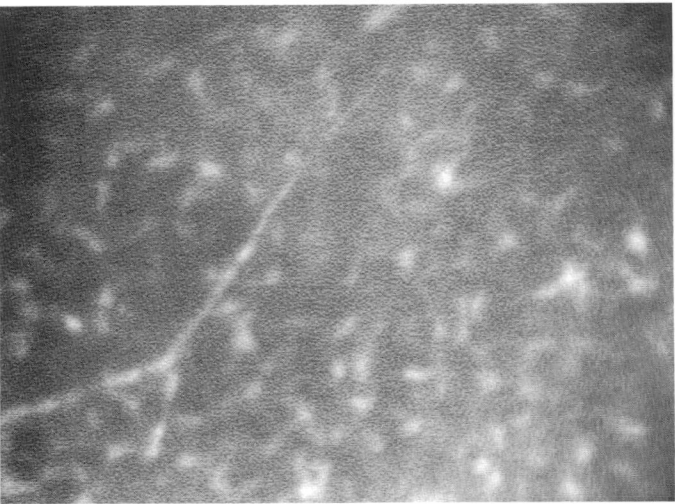

Fig. 5 Confocal microscope image of anterior stroma of human cornea, showing a corneal nerve and keratocyte nuclei (bar = 100 μm).

optical sectioning capability, with Z-axis reconstruction, provides the basis for three-dimensional analysis of tissue structure. These features have many potential applications in ophthalmology but have so far been applied mainly to the cornea. Whereas the specular microscope can only give adequate images of the endothelium and the epithelial surface, confocal microscopes can image cells within the epithelium and within the stroma (Fig. 5). The three-dimensional arrangement of keratocytes in the corneal stroma has been investigated, showing greater keratocyte density anteriorly. Quantification of keratocyte responses to injury and the ability to follow these types of cellular responses *in vivo* over time has direct application to corneal and keratorefractive surgery. It will be possible to investigate cellular reactions of the living cornea in conditions such as graft rejection and keratitis, or with contact lens wear, where this was not previously possible. Confocal microscopy has already been applied to the diagnosis of infectious keratitis. The presence of bacteria, fungi, and *Acanthamoeba* cysts and trophozoites can be established without the need for corneal biopsy. Confocal microscopy is also used for imaging the posterior segment and this aspect is covered elsewhere in this text.

Further reading

Jester, J.V., Cavanagh, H.D., and Lemp, M.A. (1990). Confocal microscopic imaging of the living eye with tandem scanning confocal microscopy. In *Noninvasive diagnostic techniques in ophthalmology*, (ed. B.R. Masters), pp. 172–88. Springer-Verlag, New York.

Koester, C.J. and Roberts, C.W. (1990). Wide-field specular microscopy. In *Noninvasive diagnostic techniques in ophthalmology*, (ed. B.R. Masters), pp. 99–121. Springer-Verlag, New York.

Leibowitz, H.M. and Laing, R.A. (1984). Specular microscopy. In: *Corneal disorders: clinical diagnosis and management*, (ed. H.M. Leibowitz), pp. 123–63. Saunders, Philadelphia.

Lemp, M.A. and Mathers, W.D. (1990). Color specular microscopy. In *Noninvasive diagnostic techniques in ophthalmology*, (ed. B.R. Masters), pp. 142–51. Springer-Verlag, New York.

Masters, B.R. and Kino, G.S. (1990). Confocal microscopy of the eye. In *Noninvasive diagnostic techniques in ophthalmology*, (ed. B.R. Masters), pp. 152–71. Springer-Verlag, New York.

Masters, B.R. and Thaer, A.A. (1994). Real-time scanning slit confocal microscopy of the *in vivo* human cornea. *Applied Optics*, 33, 695–701.

Maurice, D.M. (1968). Cellular membrane activity in the corneal endothelium of the living eye. *Experientia*, 24, 1094–5.

Sherrard, E.S. (1978). Characterization of changes observed in the corneal endothelium with the specular microscope. *Investigative Ophthalmology and Visual Sciences*, 17, 322–6.

Sherrard, E.S. and Buckley, R.J. (1982). The relief mode. New application of the corneal specular microscope. *Archives of Ophthalmology*, 100, 296–300.

Wilson, T. and Sheppard, C.J.R. (1984). *Theory and practice of scanning optical microscopy*. Academic Press, London.

Yee, R.W. (1994). Widefield specular microscopy and computerized morphometric analysis. In *External diseases: cornea, conjunctiva, sclera, eyelids, lacrimal system*, (ed. J.W. Chandler, J. Sugar, and H.F. Edelhauser), pp. 7.1–7.12. Mosby, London.

1.6.4 Corneal topography

Charles N.J. McGhee and Peter R. Keller

The cornea is the main refractive element of the human eye and contributes over two-thirds of its total optical power. The corneal contribution to optical performance can be described in terms of shape, regularity, and clarity. Measurement of the anterior corneal surface shape has evolved from qualitative to quantitative methods and is now known as the technique of corneal topography. Derived from the Greek *topos* meaning place and *graphien* meaning to write, the definition of corneal topography has been extended by common use from a description of surface shape to include the concept of optical power.

Corneal topography can be measured using a variety of techniques separated into two main categories, those based on (a) catoptric imaging, or (b) direct imaging. The first Purkinje–Sanson image, formed by the anterior corneal surface acting as a partial convex mirror, provides the optical basis of qualitative keratoscopy, keratometry, and quantitative photokeratoscopy. This erect, diminished, virtual image lies approximately 3 to 4 mm behind the anterior corneal surface slightly anterior to the entrance pupil plane. Its size varies proportionally with the radius of curvature of the reflecting surface such that by measurement of its height (knowing the object size and distance from the cornea), the radius of curvature can be calculated.

The keratometer is largely unchanged from the modification by Javal and Schiotz (1881) of von Helmholtz's ophthalmometer (1856). As an instrument for the measurement of corneal topography, the keratometer suffers from several important limitations and inherent assumptions which have been exposed by the demands of contact lens practice and keratorefractive surgery. Paramount in these limitations is the presumption that the cornea is spherical (whereas it is typically aspheric) and that the keratometer only measures two paracentral points separated by between 3 and 4 mm in two orthogonal principal meridia. Standard keratometry therefore does not allow assessment of either the very central, or mid to far peripheral zones of the cornea.

Keratoscopy overcomes the measurement area limitations of keratometry by the projection of a large disc of alternating black and white circles on to the corneal surface. The reflected image is viewed through a central aperture and evaluated qualitatively, comparing the relative size and compression of the ring images. A century after the first use of this target design, the Placido disc remains the basic mire target in photokeratoscopy and computed videokeratography. Keratoscopy has remained qualitative despite the introduction by Gullstrand of equations to quantify keratoscope photographs; a technique which proved to be labour intensive, error prone, and accordingly unpopular.

Computed videokeratography

Although several attempts have been made at quantifying keratoscopic data in the twentieth century, until recently the technique remained essentially qualitative. Instruments such as the Nidek photokeratoscope have been used with some success in the assessment of corneal disease processes and the management of postkeratoplasty astigmatism but lack objectivity (Fig. 1). Two important advances—the digital video camera and the advent of relatively inexpensive personal computer technology for quick accurate data analysis—have led to the rapid technical advances in corneal topography during the last decade. Computers can now drive the digitization of placido images and, through complex iterative mathematics, determine the shape of the reflecting surface under investigation. This is the essence of computed videokeratography.

Computed videokeratography can be conveniently broken down into three functional steps: (a) image capture, (b) surface reconstruction, and (c) data output.

- In image capture, an illuminated mire target is projected on to the cornea (Figs 2, 3), and the resultant virtual image formed by reflection is captured by video camera. Single frames are then isolated by computer 'frame grabber' and digitized.

- Next, the position and size of the digitized ring

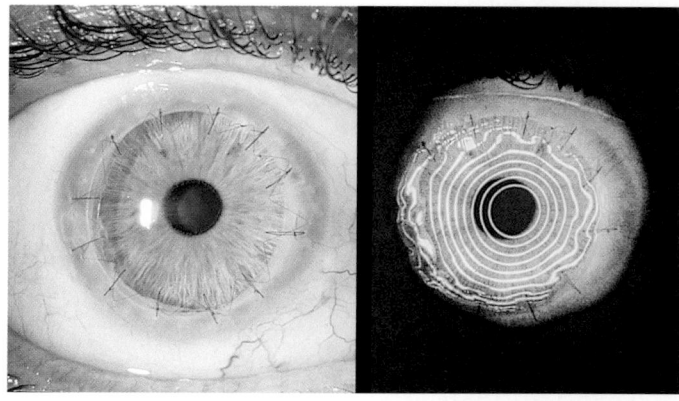

Fig. 1 A corneal graft with 1.5 dioptres of corneal astigmatism appears relatively spherical using the qualitative technique of photokeratoscopy.

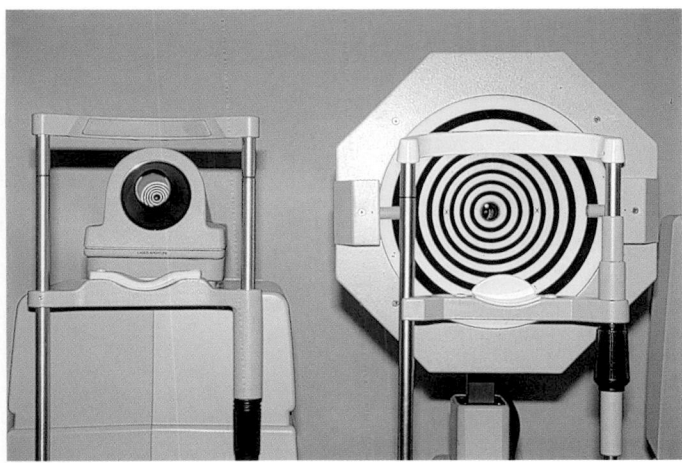

Fig. 2 The majority of computed video keratography systems continue to utilize a modified placido projection system. Targets vary in size and illumination (Tomey TMS-1 system left, Eyesys system right).

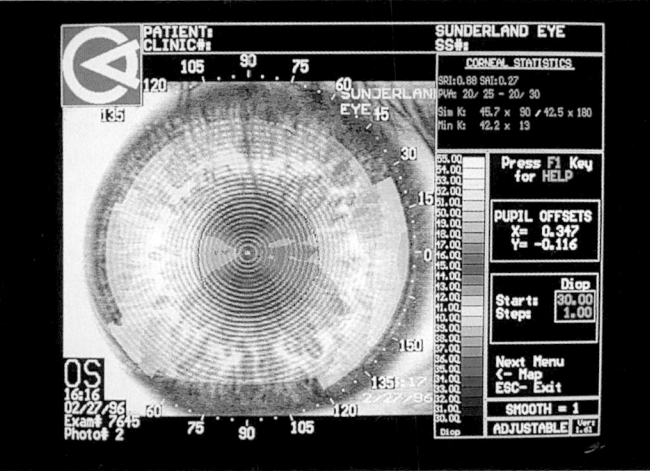

Fig. 3 The virtual image of the computed videokeratography mire pattern is captured and digitized to produce the topographic map, which can be displayed as either a colour or numerical map of corneal power. Note the scale, in dioptres, to the right of the corneal image.

images are determined by edge detection software which then feeds into proprietary algorithms which reconstruct the corneal surface by iteration. This process is repeated along each hemimeridian in turn, producing an array of surface co-ordinates. New and improved algorithms have accelerated such calculations without an increased sensitivity to noise.

- The very fact that computed videokeratography generate such a vast array of data has lead to the development of new display types capable of presenting the data in a readily assimilated format. Output of the many thousands of output data can be in the form of qualitative keratoscopic images; data tables; pseudo-three-dimensional wire mesh models; or the now familiar colour-coded curvature and power maps.

Feature recognition plays a significant role in the clinical utility of corneal power maps, the current standard display format. Colour coding is an integral component of this format which provides for rapid identification and assimilation of clinically important information from a complex data set, but introduces the choice of colour assignment and scale. As a general rule, warmer colours like oranges, reds, and pinks are associated with shorter radii and higher power (steeper) values, whilst cooler colours such as blues and greens are used for longer radii and lower (flatter) powers. For most applications the 'absolute' scale is adequate, wherein identical colours represent the same corneal power in all maps created with this scale. Such standardized scales allow easy comparison across individuals or time with the benefit of identical colours representing the same corneal power within each map. Alternatively, a 'normalized' scale can be applied to maps employing a standard set of colours of various incremental values to maximize visual impact and provide greater apparent detail. Chronological maps are less easily compared using the normalized scale since the same colour in each map may not necessarily represent the same power and dissimilar incremental steps may have been employed. Thus, the use of normalized colour coding necessitates constant reference to the individual scales on each map.

One of the main unresolved issues in corneal topography is the use of different forms of power to describe corneal shape. Although dioptric power and shape are intimately related and the concept of optical power has clinical meaning, it is strictly a misnomer to describe corneal shape in terms of power. A variety of different powers can be derived from the same corneal surface co-ordinates. The current standard, 'axial' power, is calculated using the distance from the surface point along its normal to the system reference axis. It is axis dependent and is considered the best representation of the optical performance of the cornea treated as a single refracting surface. Axial power is more robust to noise than the alternative 'instantaneous' (or local) power which is a more accurate representation of local curvature changes. Both axial and instantaneous power are paraxial approximations unlike the third alternative 'refractive' power which is calculated using ray-tracing techniques, Snell's law, and knowledge of the surface tangent. Although capable of accurately describing non-paraxial optics, further assumptions regarding the crystalline lens render this version of power unpopular in corneal topography.

Quantitative indices

Although rapid pattern recognition has been one of the breakthroughs of corneal topography output formats, the amount of quantitative data generated lends itself to the application of a number of simple mathematical techniques and the formulation of several useful numerical indices. Examples include simulated keratometry, surface asymmetry index, surface regularity index, and potential visual acuity. Several advanced mathematical techniques can be applied in the assessment of irregular astigmatism using corneal topography data, for example Fourier transformations, Taylor series expansions of wave aberration polynomials, and wave front approximation with Zernike polynomials.

The above discussions have been limited to keratoscope-based corneal topography systems. Of the range of other measurement techniques, only rasterstereography has progressed from research to clinical environments. It remains to be seen whether other techniques approach the level of clinical acceptance of computed videokeratography.

A multitude of commercial computed videokeratography units are now available, all sharing common basic principles, but varying substantially in the size, construction, and coverage provided by the Placido source and the method of presenting the analysed images. The accuracy of any particular corneal topography system is determined by a combination of instrument hardware and software and has been demonstrated to be about 0.25 dioptre for spherical test surfaces. The hardware of most systems incorporate sophisticated fixation and focusing devices, and by the combination of target size and working distance, enable coverage of almost the entire cornea, ranging from as little as 0.3 mm centrally to an 11 mm diameter peripherally. The great advantage of computed videokeratography systems over earlier methods of analysing corneal topography is the ability to measure in detail both the optically important central cornea and the mid-periphery, presenting the data in easily assimilated and interpreted display formats.

Computed videokeratography in clinical practice

Computed videokeratography has proved most useful as a research tool, but in addition has increasingly established its value in clinical ophthalmology and is essential in keratorefractive practice. The main clinical uses of computed videokeratography can be broadly divided into five categories:

1. classification of normal topography

2. identification of abnormal topography

3. pre- and postoperative assessment in keratorefractive surgery

4. management of astigmatism following intraocular surgery

5. planning contact lens fit.

Normal cornea

The normal cornea is characterized by a smooth regular surface which has been modelled with conic sections of increasing complexity and is now best described by a general ellipsoid. The average corneal apical radii are 7.87 ± 0.25 mm in the flat meridian, and 7.70 ± 0.27 mm in the steep meridian with an average range of flattening (p) of 0.83 ± 0.13 in the flat and 0.81 ± 0.16 in the steep meridia. This equates to an average central power of approximately 43.25 dioptres. The range of power found in the normal human cornea is from 39.00 to 48.00 dioptres, although a very small percentage of emmetropic subjects with normal corneas may have a central power of 50.00 dioptres or more. Interestingly an individual's corneas are often

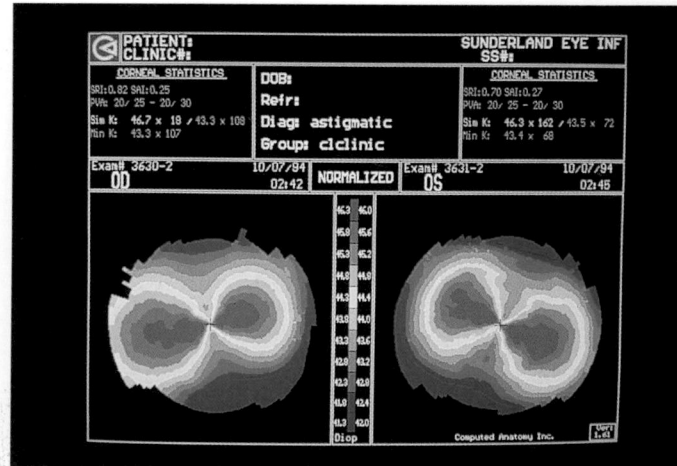

Fig. 4 Oblique astigmatism in an individual subject demonstrating mirror image enantiomorphism.

non-superimposable mirror images of each other (enantiomorphism) and knowledge of this symmetry can be useful in deciding whether a cornea is normal or not by comparison with topography of the contralateral eye (Fig. 4).

The exact morphology and topography of a given individual is unique; it is, however, important to establish the boundaries of normality. The first widely recognized classification of computed corneal topography illustrating the variation in a normal population was proposed by Bogan *et al.* (Bogan *et al.* 1990) which described five subgroups: (a) round, (b) oval, (c) symmetric bow-tie, (d) asymmetric bow-tie, and (e) irregular (Figs 5, 6). The majority of corneas are toroidal aspheres and therefore it is not surprising that the most common patterns identified are symmetric and asymmetric bow-ties, and that the prevalence of astigmatism increases with increasing ametropia.

Abnormal cornea

An appreciation of the topographical appearance of the normal cornea forms the basis for diagnosis in corneal abnormality. Gross abnormality rarely requires the introduction of subtle investigative techniques, but it is in the preclinical and subclinical stages of corneal disease and disorder that computed videokeratography proves invaluable.

Most contemporary computed videokeratography systems allow comparison of topographic maps of the same eye such that chronological changes can easily be identified. This information can be employed assessing (a) resolution of corneal warpage, (b) comparing preoperative and postoperative topography, (c) following myopic regression, (d) establishing keratorefractive ablation zone centration, and (e) differentiating between focal undertreatment, focal regression, and decentration in keratorefractive procedures.

Irregular astigmatism

Irregular astigmatism occurs both in the normal population as well as in those with pathologically abnormal corneas. Bogan *et al.* (1990) found a prevalence of irregular astigmatism in the

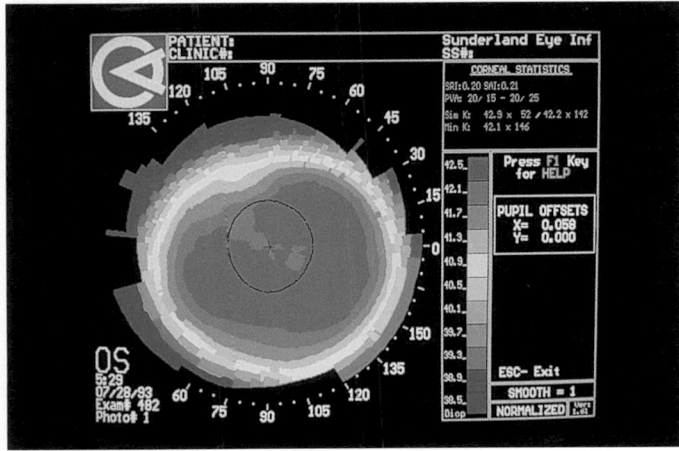

(a)

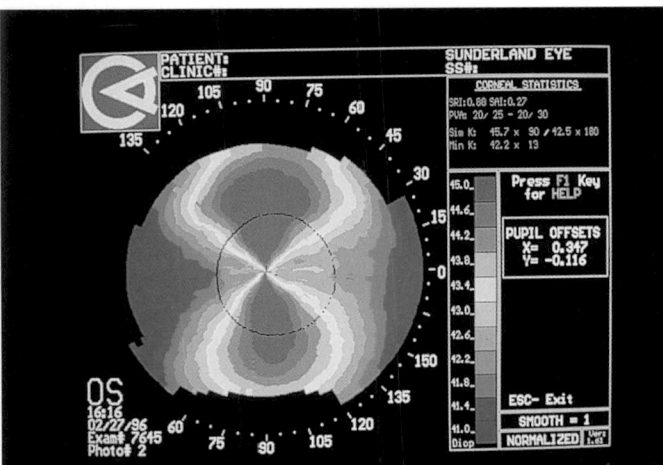

(b)

Fig. 5 (a) Round corneal topography; (b) symmetric bow-tie corneal topography.

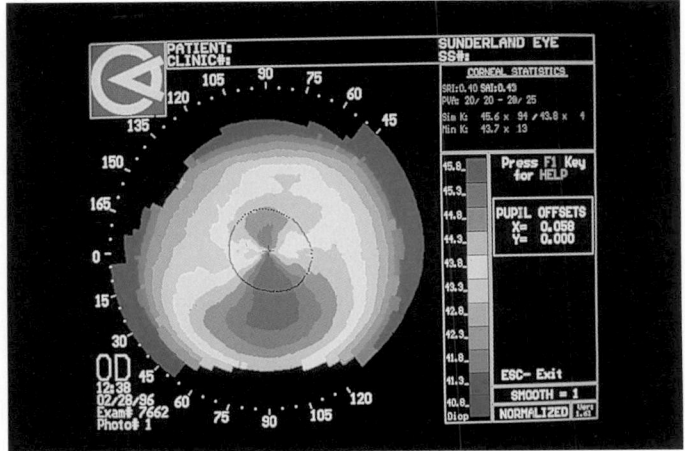

(a)

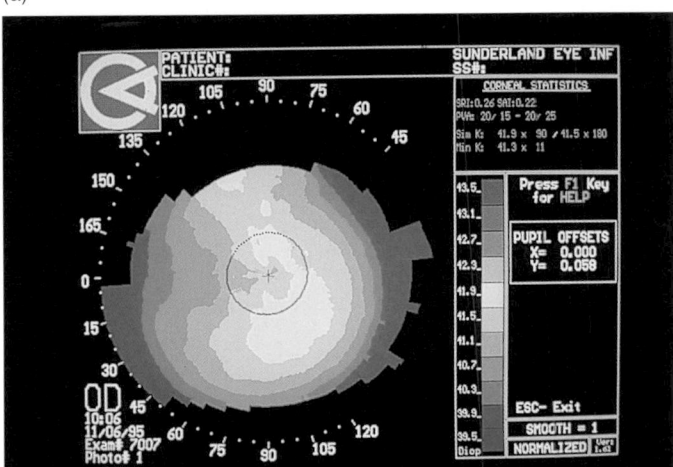

(b)

Fig. 6 (a) Asymmetric bow-tie corneal topography; (b) unclassifiable or anarchic corneal topography.

normal population of 7 per cent in the presence of normal spectacle corrected visual acuity and normal slit lamp appearance. Regular astigmatism, where the refractive power changes by uniform increments from one meridian to the next, can be distinguished from irregular astigmatism, where the irregularities in the curvature of the meridia conform to no geometrical pattern. It is only with the development of computed video-keratography to measure the curvature of thousands of different loci on the corneal surface accurately and rapidly, that the precise analysis of corneal astigmatic patterns, both regular and irregular, can be performed.

The clinician should be aware of the potential for significantly altered topography, not only after keratorefractive procedures, but also following keratitis, minor corneal trauma, and corneal epithelial disturbances. Pathological or abnormal irregular astigmatism has a number of diverse aetiologies which can broadly be categorized as follows:

1. Corneal dystrophies which disrupt the smooth regular corneal structure with keratoconus exhibiting the most common and a most spectacular form of irregular astigmatism

2. Inflammatory and infective agents causing architectural distortion of the cornea and subsequent irregular astigmatism, for example chemical injury, severe bacterial keratitis, or herpes simplex stromal keratitis

3. Trauma that distorts or disrupts the normal or pathological/weak cornea causing an irregular topographical appearance

4. Neoplastic lesions of the cornea, adjacent components of the globe, or neighbouring structures such as the lids, may induce corneal distortion. Pterygium formation is known to cause flattening of the cornea central to the leading apex resulting in irregular astigmatism.

Keratoconus

The presence of visual symptoms or clinical signs (including retinoscopy and biomicroscopic examination) can be quite variable in this relatively common condition and in early cases may frequently be absent. Therefore the only means for correct diagnosis of subclinical cases is by computed videokeratography.

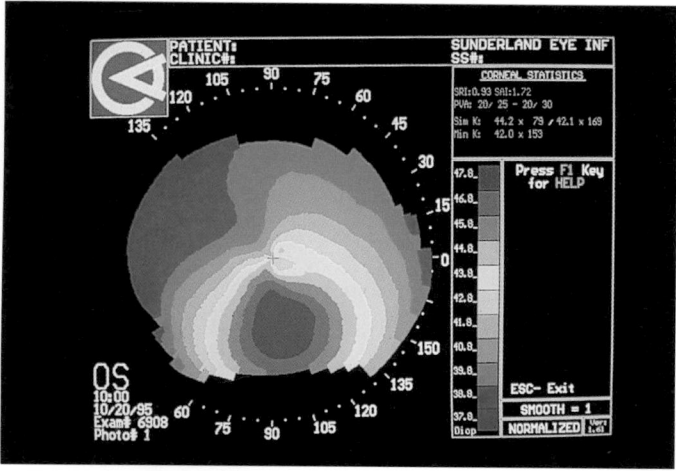

Fig. 7 Inferior 'oval' topographic appearance in early keratoconus.

The prevalence of keratoconus is 0.03 to 0.05 per cent, but may be as high as 6 to 12 per cent in those presenting for refractive surgery. Topographical subtypes have been proposed which include;

- oval—with cone involving only one to two quadrants, usually inferiorly, with fairly normal appearance outside this area (Fig. 7)

- globus—in which the cone involves most of the cornea (Fig. 8)

- nipple—with the cone involving less than 50 per cent of the central cornea, surrounded by a flatter normal cornea through 360°

- astigmatic—where the cornea is characterized by exaggerated bow-tie astigmatism, often steeper above, involving less than 50 per cent of the cornea but supported by clinical signs of keratoconus.

Artificial neural networks based upon various topographic indices have been applied to detection programmes for the screening and diagnosis of keratoconus and may benefit inexperienced observers. Subclinical topographic changes in central corneal power, differences in central corneal power between fellow eyes, and inferior–superior corneal asymmetry, have been found to be significantly different in keratoconics compared to normal controls.

Topographic lagoons

Corneal topographic lagoons are a recently described association of epithelial trauma and recurrent corneal erosion syndrome, and can be defined as reproducible areas of reduced dioptric power (3.00 dioptres or more) which are focal, small (approximately 1 mm diameter) and may occur in the absence of biomicroscopic evidence of corneal erosion syndrome. These anomalies are also noted to occur, but much more infrequently, in the normal population.

Computed videokeratography in keratorefractive surgery

The development of corneal topography systems has paralleled the technological advances in keratorefractive surgery. The clinical application of corneal topography measurement techniques is indispensable both in preoperative screening of candidates and in postoperative assessment of the procedure. It is important to identify by computed videokeratography and counsel patients with abnormal corneae and thus avoid suboptimal surgical outcomes.

Corneal topography is vital in documenting the postoperative course of refractive surgery and provides myriad detail in comparison to the clinical brevity of refraction and unaided visual acuity as benchmarks of success or failure. Decentration of greater than 1 mm may be associated with troublesome scotopic symptoms of glare and halo in younger subjects with large pupils, particularly with small ablation zones, and can only be identified by corneal topography (Fig. 9). High quality repro-

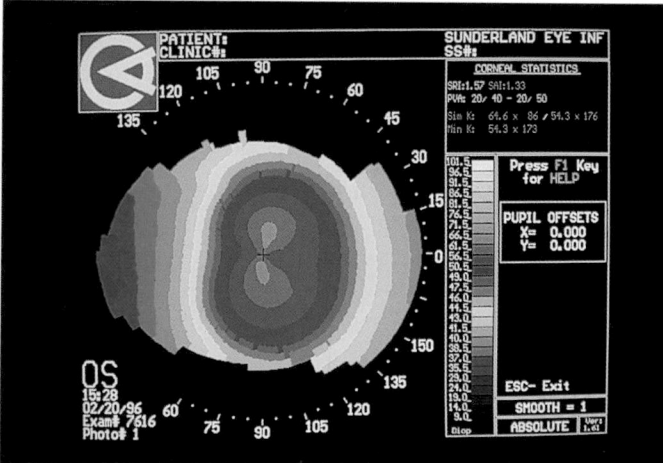

Fig. 8 A 'globus' topographic appearance in advanced keratoconus with the area of abnormally increased corneal power occupying more than 50 per cent of the central cornea.

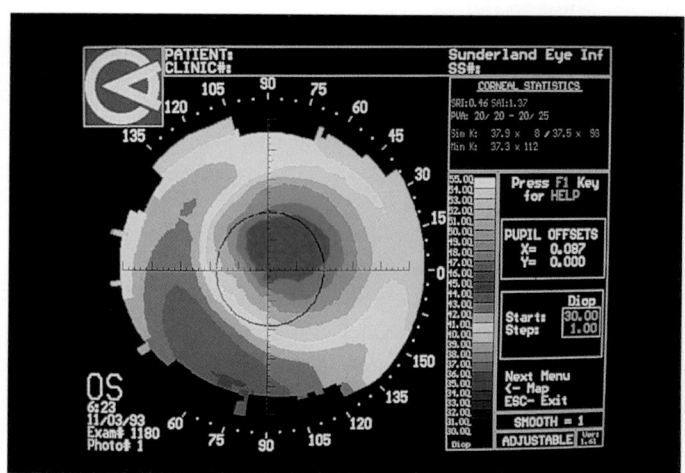

Fig. 9 Superotemporal decentration of an excimer laser PRK zone. Black outline circle represents the patient's pupil.

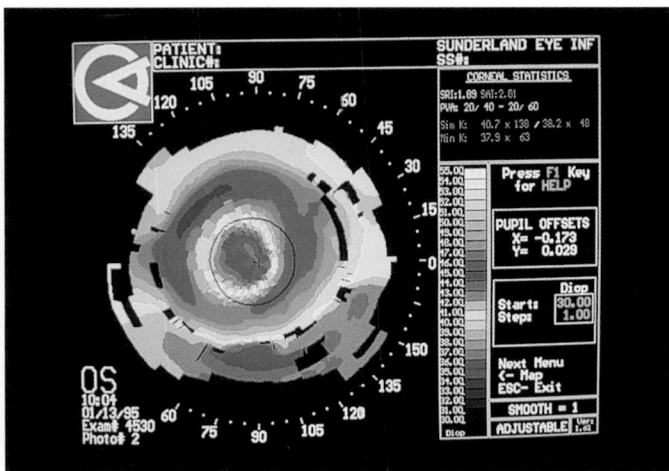

Fig. 10 A central topographic island is a round or oval central area of relatively greater dioptric power (more than 3.0 dioptre) within an excimer laser ablation zone. Fortunately the majority of islands resolve spontaneously.

ducible images should be obtained from all eyes by 1 month post-treatment and, presuming no topographic abnormalities are identified, further images at 3, 6, and 12 months represents routine topographic assessment. Topographic images are a powerful educational tool and preoperative and postoperative features, such as astigmatism, can be more readily explained to the patient when a graphical image is utilized.

Topographic central islands

In photorefractive keratectomy (PRK) and photoastigmatic refractive keratectomy (PARK) topographical irregularities are not uncommon, and it is important to differentiate transient from more permanent types. A 'central island' may be defined as a well-circumscribed, usually central, circular, or oval area of relatively greater corneal topographic power (>3.00 dioptres) within the region of reduced corneal topographic power created by excimer laser (PRK or PARK) (Fig. 10). These central islands may delay visual rehabilitation and cause visual symptoms such as monocular diplopia and decreased best corrected visual acuity. In the early postoperative period central islands are commonly encountered with up to 67 per cent of eyes demonstrating some degree of increased central power.

Management of astigmatism following intraocular surgery

Induced astigmatism following extracapsular cataract extraction and phacoemulsification cataract extraction can now be accurately quantified and studied with corneal topography analysis. The impact on both the central and peripheral cornea of the various incision placement techniques and different suturing methods can be analysed by computed videokeratography. It is not always obvious from subjective refraction and keratometric techniques which suture or sutures are overly tight (inducing a plus cylindrical error usually in the axis of the tight suture), and therefore warrant removal.

It is in the manipulation of corneal astigmatism following

penetrating keratoplasty that computed videokeratography analysis proves to be invaluable. Excessive astigmatism can be associated with poor uncorrected or best corrected visual acuity, tear film abnormalities, difficult contact lens fitting, and aesthenopic symptoms. Factors that may contribute to astigmatism include mismatch between donor and host tissues, irregular wound healing, and variations in suture placement, tension, and technique. Successful postoperative visual rehabilitation depends in part on accurate identification of the interrupted suture or sutures whose removal, or adjustment, would most effectively reduce astigmatism. Computed videokeratography can be a very useful adjunct to refraction and keratometry which are limited to describing one steep and one flat corneal meridian and hence may give an unrealistically simplified impression since complex asymmetric and irregular astigmatism may frequently occur following penetrating keratoplasty.

Contact lens practice

Many corneal topography systems now offer contact lens fitting modules which simulate fluorescein patterns providing a means for lens parameter alterations on screen. Although beneficial as a guide in contact lens base curve selection for the abnormal cornea, it is no substitute for trial lens fitting *in situ*.

Contact lens induced corneal warpage

This has been defined as contact lens induced changes in corneal topography, reversible or permanent, that are not associated with corneal oedema (to distinguish it from other pathologies) (Fig. 11). Mechanical and/or metabolic factors are thought to be responsible. Warpage is more likely to occur in rigid (polymethylmethacrylate) lens wearers rather than rigid gas permeable lens wearers and clinically significant warpage is rare in soft contact lens wearers. Rigid lens decentration is a known risk factor while total duration of wear is also related with a minimum reported wearing time being 3 months. Stable topography following discontinuation of lens wear may take as

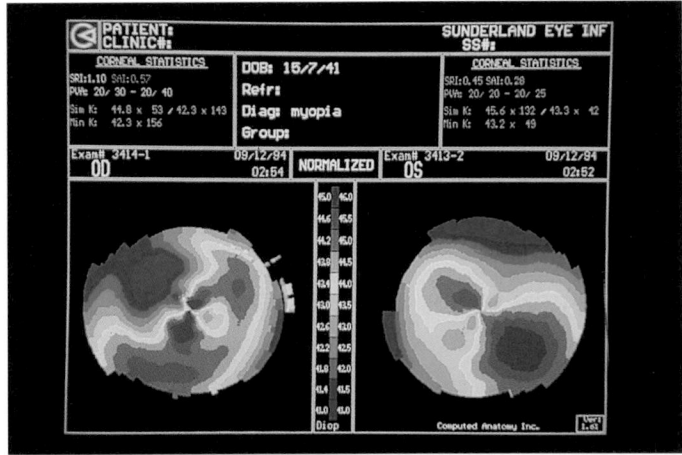

Fig. 11 Contact lens related corneal warpage following prolonged polymethylmethacrylate lens wear in the right eye demonstrates loss of the asymmetric bow-tie pattern, highlighted in the contralateral eye, and relative reduction in corneal power (flattening) in the superotemporal cornea.

long as 8 months. The importance of computed videokeratography screening to ensure stable corneal morphology prior to refractive procedures is obvious and the observation of a spherical refraction and reasonable corrected visual acuity (6/6–6/12) should not be interpreted as indicative of normality.

Further reading

Anastas, C.N., McGhee, C.N.J., and Bryce, I.G. (1996). Disciform keratitis causing severe irregular astigmatism. *Australian and New Zealand Journal of Ophthalmology*, 24, 69–70.

Binder, P.S. (1988). The effect of suture removal on post-keratoplasty astigmatism. *American Journal of Ophthalmology*, 105, 637.

Bogan, S.J., Waring, G.O., Ibrahim, O., Drews, C., and Curtis, L. (1990). Classification of normal corneal topography based on computer-assisted videokeratography. *Archives of Ophthalmology*, 108, 945–9.

Bryce, I.G., Morgan, S.J., McGhee, C.N.J., and Anastas, C.N. (1995). A classification of keratoconus by computed videokeratography. In *Proceedings of the 27th Annual Scientific Congress of the Australian College of Ophthalmologists*, 120 (abstract).

Burek, H. and Douthwaite, W.A. (1993). Mathematical models of the general corneal surface. *Ophthalmic and Physiological Optics*, 13, 68–72.

Cavanaugh, T.B., Durrie, D.S., Riedel, S.M., et al. (1993a). Topographical analysis of the centration of excimer laser photorefractive keratectomy. *Journal of Cataract and Refractive Surgery*, 19, 136–43.

Cavanaugh, T.B., Durrie, D.S., Riedel, S.M., et al. (1993b). Centration of excimer laser photorefractive keratectomy relative to the pupil. *Journal of Cataract and Refractive Surgery*, 19 (suppl), 144–8.

Cohen, K.L., Tripoli, N.K., Holmgren, D.E., and Coggins, J.M. (1995). Assessment of the power and height of radial aspheres reported by a computer-assisted keratoscope. *American Journal of Ophthalmology*, 119, 723–32.

Corbett, M.C., O'Brart, D.P.S., Saunders, D.C., and Rosen, E.S. (1994). The assessment of corneal topography. *European Journal of Implant and Refractive Surgery*, 6, 98–105.

Dingeldein, S.A. and Klyce, S.D. (1989). The topography of normal corneas. *Archives of Ophthalmology*, 107, 512–18.

Dingledein, S.A., Klyce, S.A., and Wilson, S.E. (1989). Quantitative descriptors of corneal shape derived from computer assisted analysis of photokeratographs. *Refractive and Corneal Surgery*, 5, 372–8.

Donders, F. (1897). *On the anomalies of accommodation and refraction of the eye*. London.

Guillon, M., Lyndon, D.P., and Wilson, C. (1986). Corneal topography: a clinical model. *Ophthalmic and Physiological Optics*, 6, 47–56.

Hannush, S.B., Crawford, S.L., Waring, G.O., Gemmill, M.C., Lynn, M.J., and Nizam, A. (1989). Accuracy and precision of keratometry, photokeratoscopy and corneal modelling on calibrated steel balls. *Archives of Ophthalmology*, 107, 1235–9.

Hannush, S.B., Crawford, S.L., Waring, G.O., Gemmill, M.C., Lynn, M.J., and Nizam, A. (1990). Reproducibility of normal corneal power measurements with a keratometer, photokeratoscope and video imaging system. *Archives of Ophthalmology*, 108, 539–44.

Harris, D.J., Waring, G.O., and Burk, L.L. (1989). Keratography as a guide to selective suture removal for the reduction of astigmatism after penetrating keratoplasty. *Ophthalmology*, 96, 1597.

Kennedy, R.H., Bourne, W.M., and Dyer, J.A. (1989). A 48-year clinical and epidemiological study of keratoconus. *American Journal of Ophthalmology*, 101, 107–12.

Kraff, C.R. and Robin, J.B. (1991). Topography of corneal disease processes. In *Corneal topography: measuring and modifying the cornea*, (ed. D.J. Schanzlin and J.B. Robin) pp. 39–46. Springer-Verlag, New York.

Levenson, D.S. and Berry, C.V. (1983). Findings on follow-up of corneal warpage patients. *Contact Lens Association of Ophthalmologists*, 9, 126–9.

Levin, S., Carson, C., Garret, S.K., and Taylor, H.R. (1995). Prevalence of central islands after excimer laser refractive surgery. *Journal of Cataract and Refractive Surgery*, 21, 21–6.

Lin, D.T.C. (1994). Corneal topographic analysis after excimer photorefractive keratectomy. *Ophthalmology*, 101, 1432–9.

McGhee, C.N.J. and Bryce, I.G. (1996). Natural history of central topographic islands following excimer laser photorefractive keratectomy. *Journal of Cataract and Refractive Surgery*, 22, 1151–8.

McGhee, C.N.J. and Weed, K.H. (1997). Computed videokeratography in clinical practice. In *Excimer lasers in ophthalmology: principles and practice*, (ed. C.N.J. McGhee, H.R. Taylor, D.S. Gartry and S.L.Trokel), pp. 97–125. Dunitz, London.

McGhee, C.N.J., Bryce, I.G., Anastas, C.N., et al. (1996). Corneal topographic lagoons a potential new marker for post-traumatic recurrent corneal erosion syndrome. *Australian and New Zealand Journal of Ophthalmology*, 24, 27–31.

Maloney, R.K. (1990). Corneal topography and optical zone location in photorefractive keratectomy. *Refractive Corneal Surgery*, 6, 363–71.

Morgan, J.F. (1975). Induced corneal astigmatism and hydrophillic lenses. *Canadian Journal of Ophthalmology*, 10, 207–13.

O'Brart, D.P.S., Saunders, D.C., Corbett, M.C., and Rosen, E.S. (1994). The topography of keratoconus. *European Journal of Implant and Refractive Surgery*, 7, 20–30.

Ruiz Montenegro, J., Mafra, C.H., Wilson, S.E., Jumper, J.M., Klyce, S.D., and Mendelson, E.N. (1993). Corneal topographic alterations in normal contact lens wearers. *Ophthalmology*, 100, 128–34.

van Saarloos, P.P. and Constable, I.J. (1991). Improved method for calculation of corneal topography for any keratoscope geometry. *Optometry and Visual Science*, 68, 960–5.

Walland, M.J., Stevens, J.D., and Steele, A.D.M. (1994). The effect of recurrent pterygium on corneal topography. *Cornea*, 13, 463–4.

Webber, S.K., McGhee, C.N.J., and Bryce, I.G. (1996). Decentration of photorefractive keratectomy ablation zones after excimer laser surgery for myopia. *Journal of Cataract and Refractive Surgery*, 22, 299–303.

Wilson, S.E. and Klyce, S.D. (1991a). Advances in the analysis of corneal topography. *Survey of Ophthalmology*, 35, 269–77.

Wilson, S.E. and Klyce, S.D. (1991b). Quantitative descriptors of corneal topography. A clinical study. *Archives of Ophthalmology*, 109, 349–53.

Wilson, S.E., Lin, D.T.C., Klyce, S.D., Reidy, J.J., and Insler, M.S. (1990a). Rigid contact lens decentration: a risk factor for corneal warpage. *Contact Lens Association of Ophthalmologists*, 16, 177–82.

Wilson, S.E., Lin, D.T.C., Klyce, S.D., Reidy, J.J., and Insler, M.S. (1990b). Topographic changes in contact lens-induced corneal warpage. *Ophthalmology*, 97, 734–44.

Wilson, S.E., Klyce, S.D., McDonald, M.B., et al. (1991a). Changes in corneal topography after excimer laser photorefractive keratectomy for myopia. *Ophthalmology*, 98, 1338–47.

Wilson, S.E., Klyce, S.D., McDonald, M.B., et al. (1991b). Changes in corneal topography after excimer laser photorefractive keratectomy for myopia. *Ophthalmology*, 98, 1338–47.

Wilson, S.E., Lin, D.T.C., and Klyce, S.D. (1991c). Corneal topography of keratoconus. *Cornea*, 10, 2–8.

Wilson, S.E., Wang, J.Y., and Klyce, S.D. (1991d). Quantification and mathematical analysis of photokeratoscopic images. In *Corneal topography: measuring and modifying the cornea*, (ed. D.J. Schanzlin and J.B. Robin) pp. 1–9. Springer-Verlag, New York.

1.6.5 Ultrasound in ophthalmic diagnosis

Marie Restori

Ultrasound is a vibrational form of energy with frequencies above 20 kHz: these frequencies lie beyond the audible frequency range of humans. Pulses of ultrasonic energy with nominal frequencies around 10 MHz are used for most diagnostic imaging.

Imaging techniques

To interpret the images formed using ultrasonic pulses an appreciation of imaging techniques and an understanding of the interactions of ultrasound with tissue are required.

Coupling of ultrasound to eye

Modern imaging systems provide adequate spatial resolution of the eye structures and sufficient sensitivity, to permit scanning through a closed eyelid. The exclusion of air between the probe face and the eye is achieved by smearing the face of the probe with a liquid coupling gel prior to application. Coupling to an open eye is only required in very high frequency (50 MHz) imaging of the anterior globe. Following eyelid surgery or in cases of severe trauma involving the eyelid, disposable sterile solid gel pads (3-mm thick) which mould to the shape of the closed eye can be interposed between the eyelid and the probe for comfort. Sterile probe covers are available for use in cases of human immunodeficiency virus (HIV) or other infections.

B-mode technique

The probe consists of an array of transducer elements and is selected on the basis of both frequency and footprint size. The transducer elements emit short pulses of high frequency ultrasound, in consecutive overlapping clusters to simulate a single moving transducer. Dedicated eye scanners often employ a single transducer mechanically rocked within an enclosed column of liquid. In the time intervals between the emission of ultrasonic pulses, echoes from underlying tissues are collected by the transducer elements. These echoes are converted to electrical signals and plotted on a screen as dots which are brightness modulated according to echo amplitude. Based on the arrival times of echoes at the face of the probe, devices can calculate the co-ordinates from which the echoes originate and display them accordingly. An average velocity in tissue of 1540 m/s is assumed when plotting the image. Eye scanners assume an average velocity of 1550 m/s in tissues. For each probe position on the eyelid, a cross-sectional B-mode image of the eye and orbit is produced (Fig. 1(a)) which is refreshed about 25 times per second, allowing good temporal resolution. B-mode images are usually displayed in shades of grey but occasionally other colours are selected. Sector probes or linear probes can be selected and produce trapezoidal and rectangular format images, respectively. Sector probes have smaller footprints which allow better access to the globe and provide a wider angle view of the posterior globe. Lateral resolution on sector format images decreases with depth but can be improved, at the expense of temporal resolution. Most images shown here were taken with a miniature 7 MHz sector probe on the Acuson 128XP system.

Serial B-scan sections of the eye in transverse, longitudinal, and oblique planes allow a three-dimensional mental impression of pathology to be obtained. The study of movements of echoes induced by and following voluntary eye movements is essential in ophthalmic diagnosis.

Colour flow mapping

This technique is used for imaging blood flow. A portion of the B-mode image (Fig. 1(b–h)) is selected and any displacement of echoes over short time intervals within this region is tracked by the system. Such displacements are converted into velocity data, colour encoded, and superimposed on to the B-mode image in 'real-time'. The convention is to display blood flowing towards the probe in red hues and away from the probe in blue hues. Pulsatile blood flow towards the probe such as that in the ophthalmic artery (Fig. 1(e)) is seen to flash at the heart rate in red. If the velocity scale on the colour flow map is set too low an 'aliasing' artefact may occur. This takes the form of a colour 'wrap-around' and blue hues appear in the red hues although, the flow within the ophthalmic artery is solely in the forwards direction towards the probe. To distinguish this artefact from true reverse flow (Fig. 1(g, h)) in the ophthalmic artery, an appropriate selection of velocity scale for the vessel under consideration is needed. Spectral Doppler techniques (see below) should always be used in conjunction with colour flow mapping when diagnosing true reverse flow. Many vessels can be imaged on the colour flow map such as the bundles of short posterior ciliary arteries (Fig. 1(b)), the retinal artery and vein (Fig. 1(c,d)), the ophthalmic artery (Fig. 1(e, f)), and blood vessels within tumours, detached retinae, and detached choroid. Although the short posterior ciliary artery bundles can be imaged as blocks of colour (Fig. 1(b)), the spatial colour flow map resolution is presently inadequate to display separately tiny adjacent vessels. Measurement of velocities in the posterior ciliary arteries is presently, unreliable.

Spectral Doppler techniques

A small sample volume ('gate') of the located blood vessel, typically 1.5 mm deep, is selected on the image. The 'gate' is displayed as two horizontal white lines (Fig. 1(d)) on the colour flow map. A graph of velocity of blood flow within the gated region versus time, known as the spectrogram/spectrograph (Fig. 1(d, f–h)) is plotted. The brightness of the graphical display at any point is a non-quantifiable indicator of the number of red blood cells moving with a particular velocity. For pulsatile vessels the trace will be repeated for each cardiac cycle. The convention is to display blood flow towards the probe above

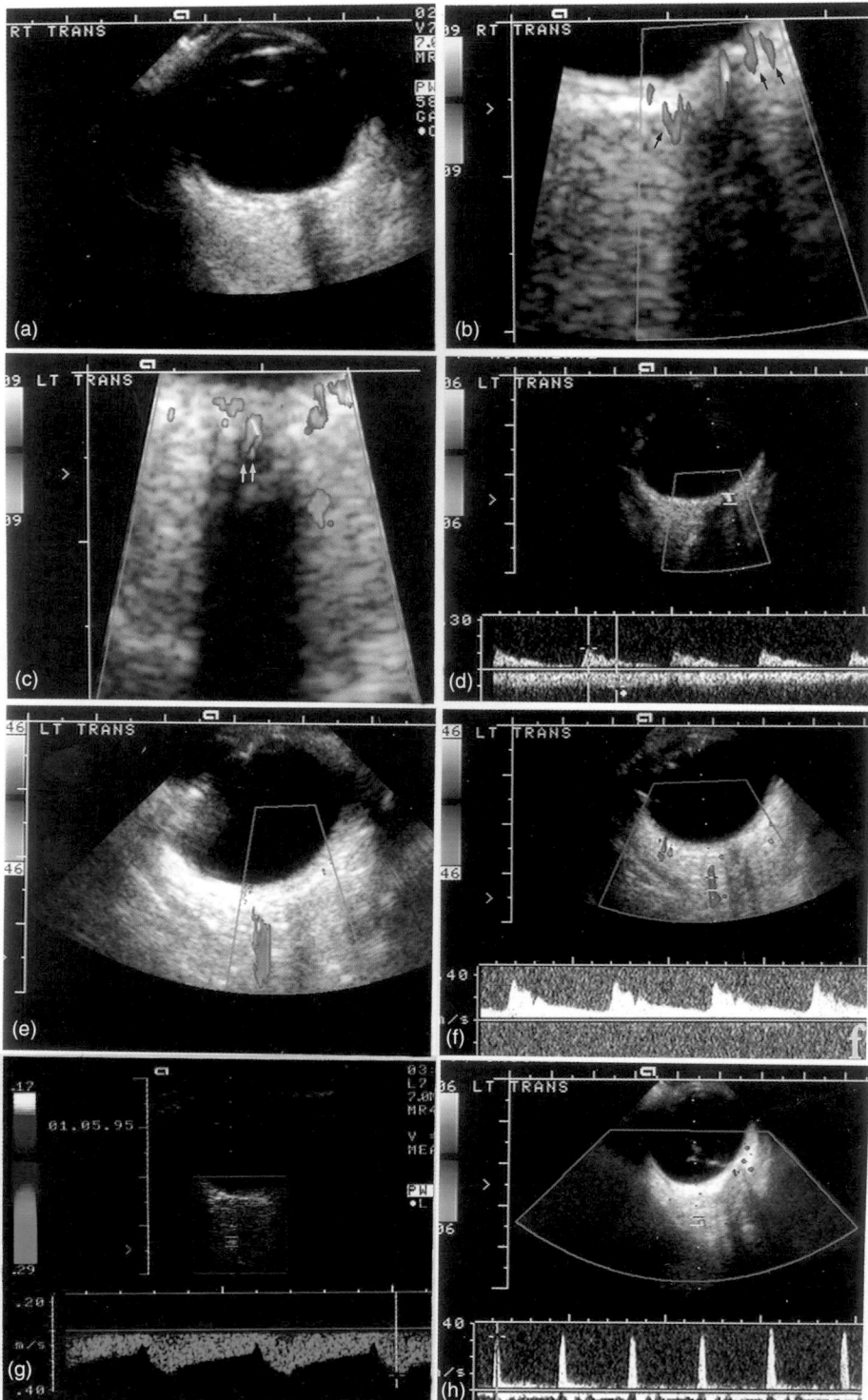

Fig. 1 B-mode images, colour flow maps in systole and spectrograms. (a) Normal eye; central section. (b) Colour flow map; expanded image: normal optic nerve and adjacent fat; posterior ciliary artery bundles (arrows). (c) Colour flow map; normal central retinal artery (red-arrow) and vein (blue-arrow). (d) Colour flow map and spectrogram; retinal artery (peak systolic velocity 12 cm/s) and retinal vein (peak velocity -10 cm/s); retinal vein is less pulsatile than retinal artery and is slightly out of phase with it. (e) Colour flow map; normal ophthalmic artery adjacent to nerve in superonasal quadrant. (f) Colour flow map and spectrogram; normal ophthalmic artery; peak systolic velocity 35 cm/s. (g) Colour flow map and spectrogram; reverse flow in ophthalmic artery; 100 per cent internal carotid artery occlusion. (h) Colour flow map and spectrogram; forward flow in ophthalmic artery during systole and reverse flow during diastole.

the X-axis and away from the probe below the X-axis. An audible output of the Doppler shift frequency allows optimization of the spectrogram by minor probe angulation; the audible output should have a maximum volume and frequency. Ideally, the incoming ultrasound pulses should travel along the lumen of the vessel; if this is not possible an angle correction is required. The direction of the interrogated pulses is indicated on the colour flow map by a dotted white line (Fig. 1(d)). At angles greater than 60° between the directions of the incoming pulses and the blood flow, velocity measurements become unreliable. Combined colour flow mapping and spectral Doppler techniques usually work by time-sharing of the transducer elements and therefore, whilst the spectral data is displayed, the colour flow map is static. Loss of the trace usually indicates movement of the eye, the probe, or both. Once the trace is located on the spectral Doppler display, it must be optimized by increasing the velocity scales until the peak systolic velocities are clearly visible. Aliasing is seen on the spectrogram as a wrap-around of data, the higher forward velocities being displayed below the baseline, that is, artefactually displayed as a reverse velocity. It is vital that no aliasing should be present on the spectrogram, if reverse flow in the ophthalmic artery (Fig. 1(g, h)) is to be diagnosed correctly. Reverse flow in the ophthalmic artery throughout the cardiac cycle is seen in 80 to 90 per cent diameter stenosis of the internal carotid artery and in its occlusions. Flow is seen to revert to forward flow post-endarterectomy. Power output settings for both colour flow mapping and spectral Doppler techniques should be set to a minimum value.

Colour Doppler energy/power maps

These images are similar to colour flow maps but indicate only where blood is flowing. No distinction is made between forward and reverse flow or velocities of flow. The image represents a vascular volume map and may prove useful in looking at tissue perfusion. The technique lends itself to low volume flow and low velocity situations. The loss of direction of flow information and splodges of colour on the images associated with small eye movements, however, make interpretation difficult in ophthalmology.

Echo-enhancing agents

Clinical trials into the use of echo-enhancing agents, such as stable micro-bubbles of a few microns in diameter, are on-going. Small quantities of these agents are introduced by intravenous injection, and allow very low volume blood flow to be highlighted on the colour flow or energy maps. Certain agents also resonate at harmonics of the interrogating ultrasound and harmonic imaging of blood flow may have a role in ophthalmic diagnosis.

Interactions of ultrasound in tissue

Conversion of the vibrational energy of the pulse to other energy forms, such as heat is known to occur in ocular tissues although the mechanisms of absorption are not fully understood. Higher frequencies are preferentially absorbed in tissue thereby reducing their penetration into tissue and restricting the frequencies that can be used in imaging. Specular reflection of some of the incident energy of an ultrasonic pulse may occur if the pulse strikes a large smooth boundary between two tissues that differs in acoustical impedance (approximately equal to the product of density and velocity of sound within a medium). The energy in the reflected pulse is dependent on the difference in acoustical impedance between the two tissues and the angle of incidence of the pulse with the boundary. If the boundary is approached obliquely by the ultrasonic pulse then the reflected pulse energy will be reduced and the forward transmitted pulse will be refracted, in accordance with Snell's law. Scattering of ultrasound occurs both at rough interfaces between different tissues and at any small discontinuities of density or elasticity within a tissue which are of similar size or less than a wavelength. The ultrasonic pulse energy is redirected into a continuum of directions with no energy loss. Scattering is frequency dependent and is of major importance in ultrasound imaging as it provides most of the signals used in diagnosis.

Normal eye

The appearances of the normal eye and orbit in central transverse B-mode sections are shown in Fig. 1. Most images are labelled RT for right eye or LT for left eye. Transverse sections are usually labelled 'trans' and longitudinal sections 'long'. In longitudinal sections the symbol 'a' on the top left of the image corresponds to the superior globe. In transverse sections, the symbol 'a' corresponds to the temporal right globe and the nasal left globe.

In the normal eye the vitreous cavity appears echolucent (acoustically empty). The coats of the eye and the orbital fat are strong scatterers of sound. The optic nerve is seen as a dark band within the echogenic region of the orbital fat. The ocular muscles are imaged as dark strips bounding the fat. Colour flow maps showing the normal appearance of the ophthalmic artery, the retinal artery and vein, and the bundles of short posterior ciliary arteries are shown in Fig. 1. Diagnosis using ultrasound imaging techniques is based on pattern recognition of echo topography, amplitudes, induced echo movements following voluntary ocular deviations, and blood flow characteristics within echogenic regions.

Diagnosis

Indications for ultrasound examination

Ultrasound examination is indicated when biomicroscopical examination of the eye is inadequate and in the diagnosis and monitoring of tumours.

Lens

The absence of the posterior lens interface echo in association with an ellipsoidal group of echoes in the vitreous cavity is suggestive of lens dislocation. Posterior lens capsule rupture is associated with a disruption of the posterior lens interface echo;

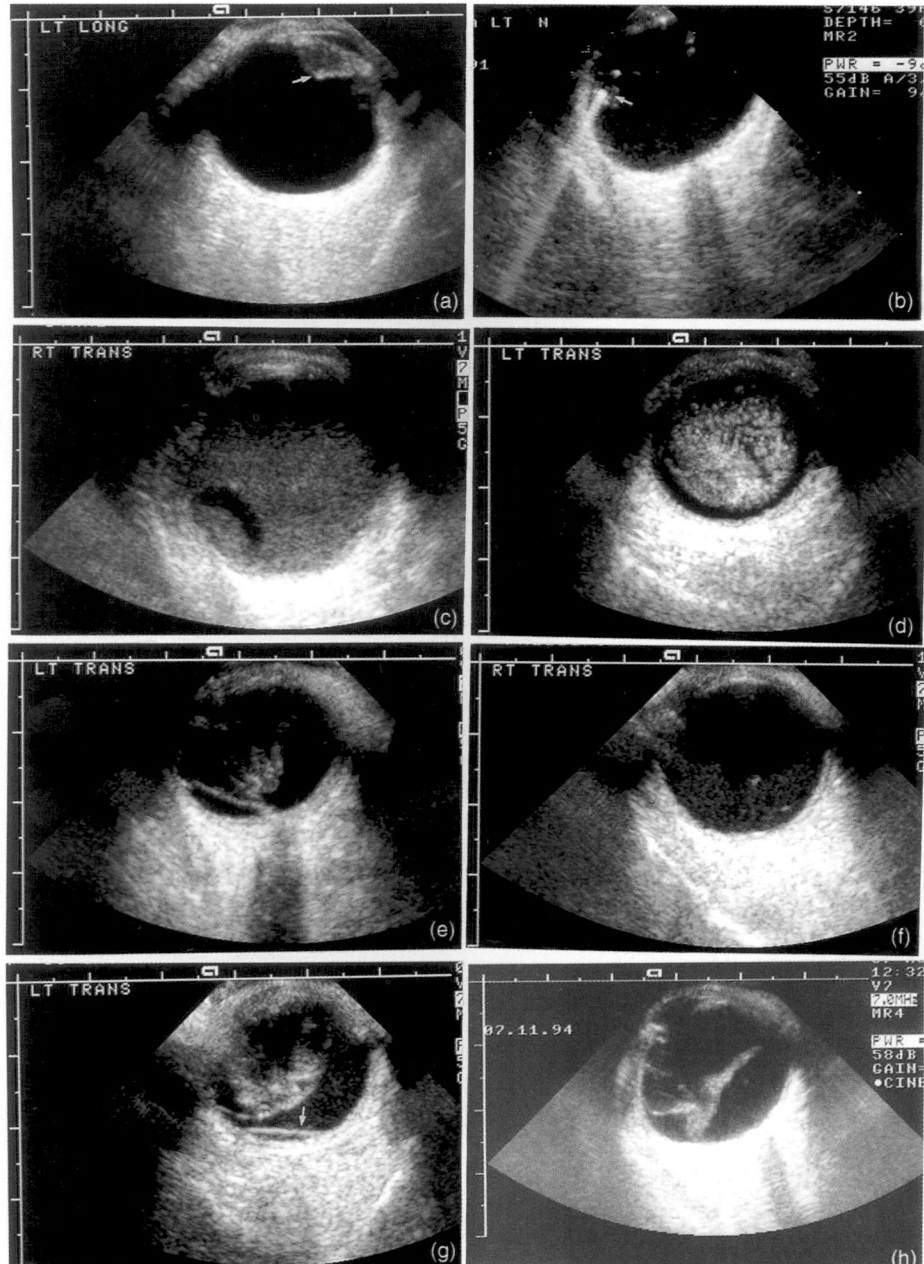

Fig. 2 B-mode images. (a) Ruptured posterior lens capsule (*arrow*). (b) Transverse section; foreign body (*arrow*); 'ringing' artefact. (c) Large eye; vitreous haemorrhage; large lacuna. (d) intragel asteroid hyalosis. (e) Posterior vitreous detachment attaching to disc; intragel haemorrhage. (f) Posterior vitreous detachment; retrohyaloid haemorrhage. (g) Posterior vitreous detachment; intragel and retrohyaloid haemorrhage; fluid level (*arrow*) in retrohyaloid space. (h) Right eye; transverse section; trauma; posterior vitreous detachment incarcerated into posterior temporal retina; intragel haemorrhage.

on occasions echoes are seen within the lens which extrude (Fig. 2(a)) into the vitreous cavity.

Vitreous

Foreign bodies appear as discrete highly echogenic opacities which depending upon size, shape, and orientation may give rise to a reverberation artefact ('ringing'; Fig. 2(b)) and/or may attenuate the sound sufficiently to cast a shadow. Head posi-

tioning during scanning permits the differentiation of foreign bodies and small gas/air bubbles. Dispersed echoes within the vitreous cavity associated with haemorrhage (Fig. 2(c)) and inflammatory cells are indistinguishable on ultrasound examination. In contrast, asteroid hyalosis (Fig. 2(d)) is more echogenic than even dense haemorrhage and has a more sluggish response following ocular deviations. The presence of lacunae (Fig. 2(c)) may suggest that posterior vitreous detachment is imminent.

Posterior vitreous detachment

Posterior vitreous detachment in an eye with clear vitreous is indicated by faint echoes arising from portions of the posterior hyaloid interface which form a continuous line during ocular movements. A Weiss ring, if detected, is seen as a small, faint circular group of echoes within the vitreous cavity. The patterns of posterior vitreous detachment associated with vitreous opacities are, however, varied. One or other of the intragel or retrohyaloid compartments may be clear (Fig. 2(d–f)) and one or both may be partly or wholly filled with echoes. If both compartments contain echoes, it may be the difference in echogenicity between the compartments (Fig. 2(g)) which outline the posterior hyaloid face. Intragel echoes may lie along the posterior hyaloid interface. Retrohyaloid opacities tend to have a more uniform distribution of echoes both in terms of echogenicity and spacing (Fig. 2(f)) as does postvitrectomy haemorrhage. On occasions fibrin sheets are seen in the retrohyaloid space as fine sheets of high amplitude echoes that shimmer with small unintentional eye movements. Similar in appearance to fibrin, fluid levels (Fig. 2(g)) may form on sustained gaze, which are distinguishable from fibrin as they disintegrate with eye movement. Incarceration of the gel anteriorly or posteriorly (Fig. 2(h)) may be indicated by an asymmetrical suspension of the gel in a stationary eye. A detached vitreous gel often demonstrates violent movements which continue for approximately 1 s following deviations of gaze, the retrohyaloid fluid remaining apposed throughout. Residual adhesions of the gel to the retina (Fig. 2(h)) or attachment of the gel to the optic disc (Fig. 2(e)) are best demonstrated during eye movements, particularly if the adhesions are tenuous. Vitreoretinal adhesions may indicate sites of neovascularization following branch vein occlusion, vitreous incarceration into the retina following trauma (Fig. 2(h)), or vitreous incarceration into fibrovascular membranes. The gel assumes reversed 'mirror image' positions at each extreme of ocular deviation. On occasions, a sheet of high amplitude echoes, arising from blood or fibrous tissue, may lie along the posterior hyaloid interface. An associated developmental adhesion to the disc may lead the posterior hyaloid interface to mimic retinal detachment in both echogenicity and topography, on a static B-mode image. Posterior hyaloid interface echo movements reflect the weight of the gel being thrown against the ocular wall in response to deviations of gaze. In contrast a fresh retinal detachment is bounded by fluid on either side and 'undulates' in response to ocular deviations. If doubt still persists, colour flow mapping will indicate the absence or presence of blood flow within the membrane.

Retina

Tractional retinal detachment

A detached vitreous gel may insert into the apex of a tractional retinal detachment seen as a tented, highly reflective membrane projecting pagoda-like into the vitreous cavity (Fig. 3(a)). The detached retina is continuous with the attached retina. Posterior to the tractional retinal detachment, there is a drop in the positional level of the echoes, accounted for by the absence of the

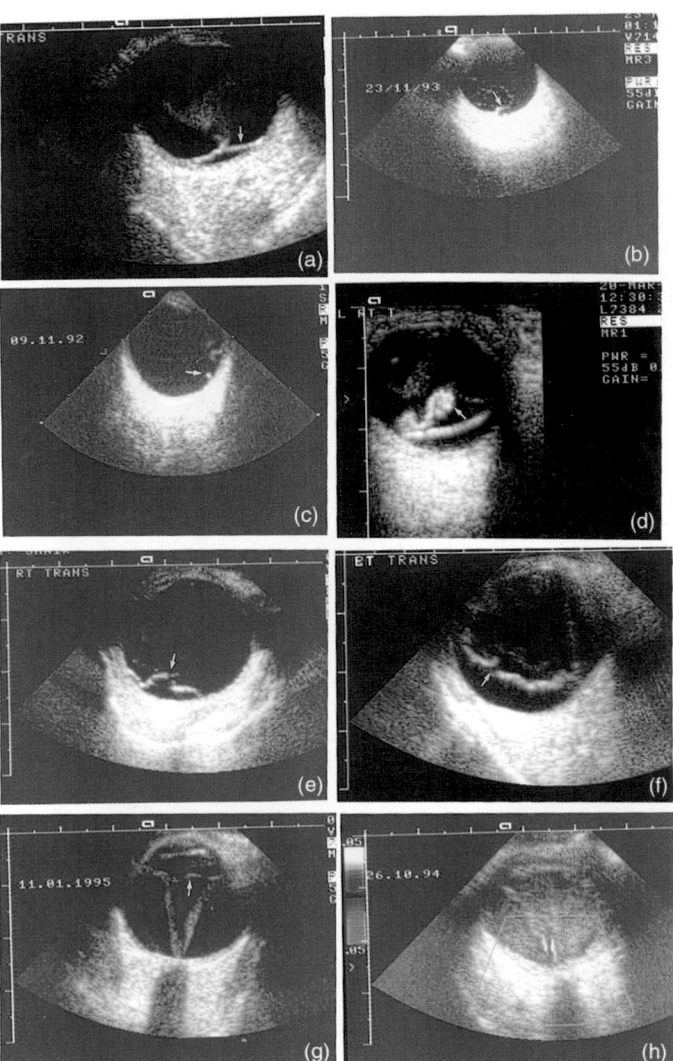

Fig. 3 Transverse B-mode images and colour flow maps in systole. (a) Posterior vitreous detachment; intragel opacities; tractional retinal detachment (arrow). (b) Right eye; posterior vitreous detachment; retinal tear (arrow, anterior edge). (c) Right eye; colour B-mode; large retinal tear (arrow, poster or edge) (d) Posterior vitreous detachment; retinal detachment with curled over giant retinal tear (arrow). (e) Posterior vitreous detachment; retinal detachment; retinal tear (arrow). (f) Posterior vitreous detachment; retinal detachment; retinal tear (arrow). (g) Right eye; detached retracted vitreous gel (arrow); total retinal detachment. (h) Colour flow map; total retinal detachment with blood flow shown (red); vitreous and subretinal haemorrhage.

retina in this region. In 'table-top' tractional retinal detachment the gel can be seen to have a wider area of adhesion to the detached retina. Generally, tractional retinal detachments do not demonstrate after-movements following ocular movements unless a retinal tear develops.

Retinal tears and rhegmatogenous retinal detachment

Retinal tears are displayed as two bright adjacent echo tags (Fig. 3(b, c)) continuous with the retinal surface. The combined length of these tags corresponds to the arc from which

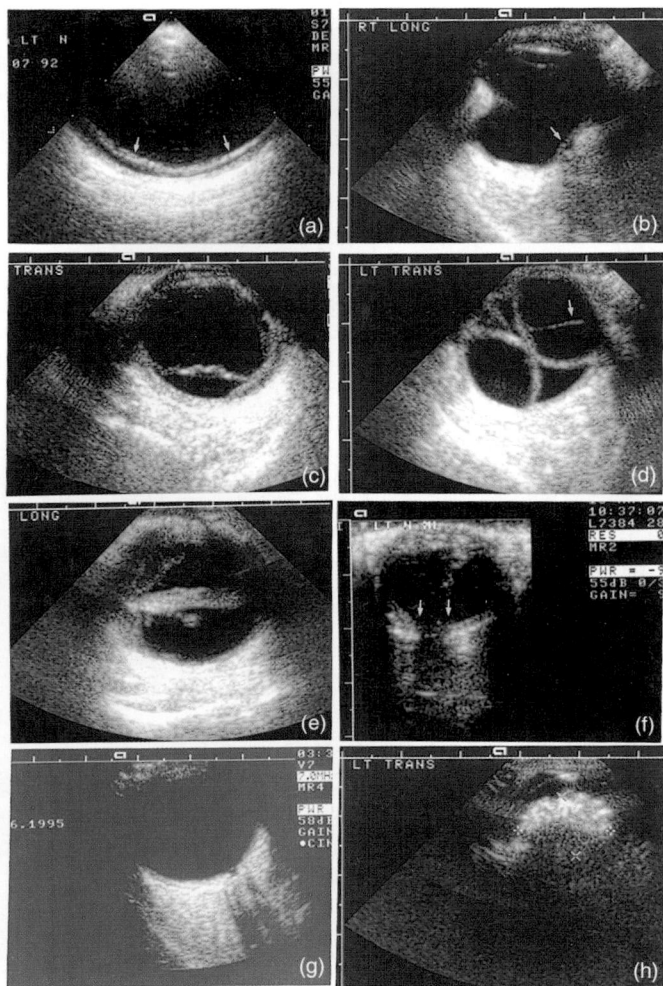

Fig. 4 B-mode images. (a) Transverse; silicone oil in vitreous; extensive retinal detachment (arrows). (b) Plombs; shallow retinal detachment lying posterior to inferior plomb (arrow). (c) Left eye; deviated temporal gaze; serous retinal detachment; anterior and posterior scleritis. (d) Deviated gaze; 'kissing' choroidal detachment; attachment to vortex ampullae of vortex vein (arrow). (e) Penetrating injury; transverse gel track of haemorrhage leading to superior scleral rupture; superior suprachoroidal haemorrhage. (f) Penetrating injury; transverse gel track of haemorrhage; large posterior scleral rupture (arrows). (g) Left eye; transverse; disc cupping. (h) Large retinoblastoma; heavy calcification casts shadow.

they were derived. In contrast, in an avulsed retinal vessel a single echo tag is defined. Attachment of the detached gel to the anterior edge of the tear can be delineated and this edge of the tear responds to gel movement whilst the posterior edge of the tear moves independently of the gel.

Retinal detachments give rise to a sheet of high amplitude echoes (Figs 3(d–h), 4(a–c)) and, if total, attachments to the ora serrata and optic disc (Fig. 3(g)) can be detected. Generally, there is associated posterior vitreous detachment. Recent retinal detachment gives rise to characteristic undulating after-movements. In massive preretinal retraction, these undulating after-movements become dampened or absent and the retinal leaves become shortened (Fig. 3(g)) and thickened by epiretinal fibrosis, sometimes producing a fixed folding and retinal 'cysts'.

Retinal tears associated with retinal detachment can be identified in some instances (Fig. 3(e, f)) but may be masked by retinal folding. A giant retinal dialysis or tear (Fig. 3(d)) will cause the retinal detachment to curl over and flap back and forth into and out of the plane of view, in response to deviations of the globe. Colour flow mapping may be required to aid in the diagnosis of retinal detachment, for example, when retro-hyaloid and subretinal opacities (Fig. 3(h)) make delineation of the retinal detachment echoes difficult. Pulsatile blood flow, typically 6 cm/s is detected in both recent and long-standing rhegmatogenous retinal detachment. Caution should be exercised in differentiating retinal detachment and posterior hyaloid membranes with fibrovascular stalk adhesions to the disc, in both of which blood flow can be detected. Subretinal cholesterol deposits characteristically swirl and stream for several seconds following eye movement. Silicone oil (Fig. 4(a)) and heavy liquid have velocities of sound considerably lower than in tissues (silicone oil velocity 982 m/s). On B-scan, eyes with silicone oil in the vitreous cavity appear elongated. Refraction of sound pulses at the interfaces between the oil and other ocular tissues produce many artefacts which are more pronounced with a sector B-scan format, owing to the varying angles of incidence of the incoming pulses. Plombs (Fig. 4(b)) are seen as echogenic clusters indenting the globe.

Serous retinal detachment

Serous retinal detachment may be associated with disciform lesions or scleritis (Fig. 4(c)). Disciform lesions are imaged as heterogeneous, echogenic lesions having an irregular anterior surface. Dispersed subretinal haemorrhage of variable amplitude may surround the disciform, and highly reflective drusen may be detected. Low velocity, low volume blood flow can be detected with the higher sensitivity systems (typically 5 cm/s) although when actively bleeding higher velocities (up to 20 cm/s) may be detected.

Choroid

Choroidal detachment when extensive and bullous, appear as highly echogenic convex lines on B-mode images. Attachment of the detached choroid to the vortex ampullae of the vortex veins (Fig. 4(d)) is pathognomonic of detached choroid and proves a useful feature in the differentiation of retinal and choroidal detachment. Shallow ciliochoroidal detachment can be detected by examining with a deviated gaze. Suprachoroidal haemorrhage (Fig. 4(e)) is echogenic and acoustically heterogeneous. The attachment to the vortex ampullae of the vortex vein can sometimes be detected amidst the haemorrhage. In contrast, the suprachoroidal space in choroidal effusion (Fig. 4(d)) is acoustically empty. In the presence of retinal detachment and choroidal detachment, blood flow can be imaged separately in both membranes. Typically, blood flow velocity in choroidal detachment is 8 to 10 cm/s compared to 6 to 8 cm/s in non-solid retinal detachment.

Sclera

A reduction of echogenicity and thickening of the posterior coats of the eye to greater than 2 mm (or 1.9 mm on a dedic-

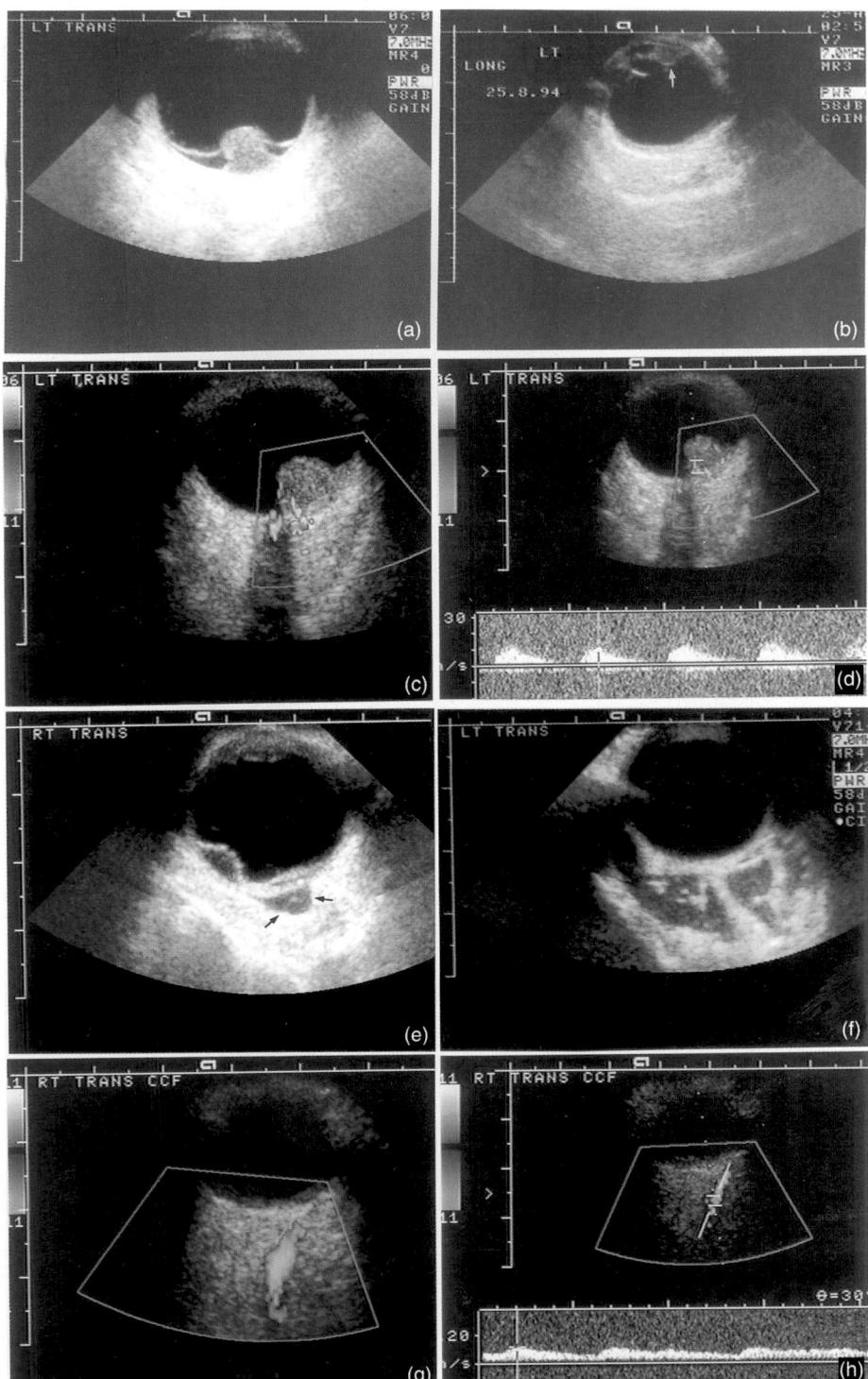

Fig. 5 B-mode, colour flow maps in systole and spectrograms. (a) 'Collar-stud' malignant melanoma; overlying retinal detachment. (b) Inferior iris malignant melanoma (arrow). (c) Colour flow map; posterior pole malignant melanoma; internal blood vessel (red). (d) Colour flow map and spectrogram; peak systolic blood flow velocity in malignant melanoma 10 cm/s. (e) Malignant melanoma; extrascleral spread (arrows). (f) Large orbital varices (child 4 years of age). (g) Colour flow map; caroticocavernous fistula; grossly dilated superior ophthalmic vein (red) with reversed blood flow direction. (h) Colour flow map and spectrogram; caroticocavernous fistula; reversed and pulsatile flow in dilated superior ophthalmic vein; peak systolic velocity 12 cm/s.

ated eye scanner) is consistent with posterior scleritis (Fig. 4(c)) in the non-nanophthalmic eye. This is sometimes accompanied by fluid in Tenon's capsule and the optic nerve sheath. Scleral rupture may be suggested by incarceration of vitreous gel (Fig. 4(e)) into the sclera or by a disruption in the continuity of the scleral echoes (Fig. 4(f)).

Intraocular tumours

Ultrasound is used in the diagnosis and monitoring of intraocular tumours. Retinoblastoma (Fig. 4(h)) are often calcified. Calcium is easily identifiable on B-mode having both the highest reflectivity and most marked attenuating properties of any naturally occurring substance in the eye, thus producing strong echoes and, if present in sufficiently wide deposits, it casts a shadow on more posterior structures. Low velocity blood flow can be detected within retinoblastoma (typically < 10 cm/s). Lesions are measured in two orthogonal planes to determine the base and maximum elevation dimensions. Lens-sparing radiotherapy also requires a measurement of the distance of the anterior cornea to posterior lens using ultrasound.

Malignant melanoma generally, gives rise to a group of acoustically heterogeneous echoes with a well-defined border, which connect to the uvea (Fig. 5(a, b)), and move with the coats of the eye. Internal blood flow (typically 10 cm/s) is usually identified in lesions (Fig. 5 (c, d)) measuring more than 2 mm in elevation. Replacement of the strongly scattered echoes of normal choroid by weaker echoes generated by the melanoma can produce an excavated appearance to the affected choroidal layer.

Serous retinal detachments overlying large tumours often exhibit higher velocity flow (typically 30 cm/s) than rhegmatogenous retinal detachment, presumably because the retinal vessels are stretched and their diameters reduced whilst volume blood flow is maintained. Caution must be exercised, therefore, when looking at tumour blood flow. Only vessels within a tumour rather than superficial vessels, which could be retinal in origin, should be sampled to avoid artificially high velocity flows being detected. Extraocular spread (Fig. 5(e)) can also be identified using B-mode imaging. The weaker echoes from tumour replace those of the more strongly scattering fat, producing a moth-eaten appearance of the fat in areas of spread. Optic nerve spread of melanoma causes the optic nerve to become echogenic. Choroidal haemangiomas generally have a higher reflectivity than melanoma and are acoustically homogeneous. Choroidal haemangioma generally give rise to easily detectable (high volume), high velocity flow (typically 20 cm/s). Secondary deposits are usually acoustically heterogeneous, with irregular anterior and posterior borders. Blood flow within secondary deposits tends to reflect blood flow patterns in the primary tumour.

Orbital lesions

Ultrasound is a useful adjunct to computed tomography and magnetic resonance imaging in the orbit. Capillary haemangioma demonstrate high volume, very high velocity internal blood flow (typically 50–150 cm/s). Orbital varices (Fig. 5(f)) can be seen to swell during a valsalva manoeuvre on the B-mode display. Dilation of the superior ophthalmic vein and reversal of blood flow direction within it (Fig. 5(g, h)) are easily detectable, though ultrasound examination is only occasionally needed when the clinical diagnosis is in doubt. The location, shape, acoustic texture, and internal blood flow of lesions all aid in determining their likely nature.

The future

Digital workstations will allow flexibility of image and data management. Three-dimensional visualization will aid in the interpretation of complex vascular relationships. New technology is leading to improvements in both spatial and temporal imaging resolution, permitting smaller detail to be defined and faster tissue movements to be recognized. An increase in imaging sensitivity in B-mode, colour flow and colour energy mapping will aid in detecting lower volume and lower velocity blood flow, allowing more accurate measurements of blood velocity. These improvements will permit more subtle tissue texture differences to be discriminated and will lead to increased confidence in diagnosis, in addition to the ability to make new diagnoses.

Further reading

Hedrick, W.R., Hykes, D.L., and Starchman, D.E. (1995). *Ultrasound physics and instrumentation*, (3rd edn). Mosby, St Louis.

McLeod, D. and Restori, M. (1979). Ultrasound examination in severe diabetic eye disease. *British Journal of Ophthalmology*, **63**, 533–8.

Pavlin, C.J. and Foster, F.S. (1995). *Ultrasound biomicroscopy of the eye.* Springer-Verlag, Berlin.

1.6.6 Radiology in ophthalmology

P. R. Goddard and J. E. Kabala

Imaging of the orbit has advanced considerably in recent years. The introduction of rapid microprocessing has permitted the use of techniques such as ultrasonography, computed tomography (**CT**), and magnetic resonance imaging (**MRI**), which provide much more soft-tissue detail than was available with plain films and conventional tomography. Contrast investigations (dacrocystography, angiography, and venography) have declined in importance (especially the last two) with the increased use of MRI and CT.

Plain film

Plain radiographs are produced by interposing the subject between a source of ionizing radiation (the X-ray tube) and a sheet of photographic film. The image obtained depends on the pattern of attenuation of the X-ray beam by the subject. Attenuation of the beam is complex and depends on a number of factors including its original energy and the composition of the attenuating tissue. Several tissue characteristics contribute to the overall effect, but the most important are atomic number and density; the higher either becomes the more the radiation is attenuated and the less the underlying photographic film is exposed. Areas of bone (high density and containing calcium of relatively high atomic number) therefore appear white, soft tissue of all sorts (largely water) is intermediate density, and air (for example in sinuses or in soft tissue after open injuries) virtually non-attenuating and therefore appears black. These principles explain the traditional weakness of plain films (very poor soft-tissue contrast and exposure of the patient to ionizing radiation) as well as its strength (good detail from bone and areas of calcification). Conventional tomography is done by rotating both the X-ray source and the film around a point at a predetermined level within the patient. This produces a plane that is in focus, while blurring out the image from points above and below the level of interest. It is now obsolete in the eye.

A wide range of traditional plain films of the skull and specific ophthalmological views (for example, optic foramina) is available, but it is worth noting that the information they offer (with some exceptions described below) is almost invariably indirect (for example, the demonstration of bone destruction due to adjacent tumour), and therefore these views are infrequently used in modern practice. A simple orbital view is useful to confirm or exclude a radio-opaque foreign body. If doubt persists about presence or location, CT or (with appropriate care) MRI or ultrasound may be used. Patients with suspected facial fractures are assessed with a series of plain films, for example occipitomental (**OM**), overtilted OM, and lateral. If, however, it is known that the patient will be assessed with CT, the plain films may be omitted; this protocol is particularly suited to the investigation of isolated fractures of the orbital floor. With a clinical diagnosis of orbital cellulitis or tumour, further investigation with CT or MRI is probably indicated and plain films are superfluous. Assessment of primary bone abnormalities (for example, fibrous dysplasia) with plain films may have some value.

Utrasound

This is an important tool for the assessment of lesions within the eyeball itself. Its usefulness may be limited where there is considerable retinal/vitreous haemorrhage and in the evaluation of retrobulbar lesions. Its specific role is discussed in a separate chapter.

Dacrocystography

Conventional dacrocystography is done by cannulating the inferior canaliculus with a fine cannula (metal or plastic) and

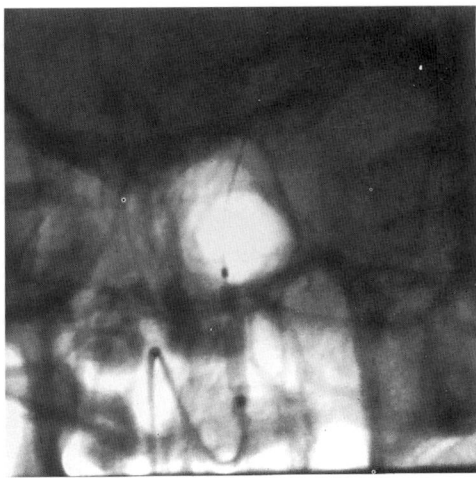

Fig. 1 Dilatation of nasolacrimal duct. Angioplasty balloon inflated in the left duct. Guide wire running into the inferior canaliculus, through the nasolacrimal duct and out of the nasal cavity, having emerged through the middle meatus.

injecting iodine-based contrast medium. Standard frontal (modified OM) and lateral radiographs may be obtained before and after the administration of contrast medium or the procedure may be done on a screening table with a digital-subtraction facility, which allows direct observation of the contrast flow and potentially a reduction in radiation exposure. The procedure demonstrates the anatomy and patency of the nasolacrimal ducts, and the level of any obstruction or stenosis. It is part of the investigation of epiphora, generally after flushing of the system has failed to resolve the problem. If a stricture is demonstrated, some centres have described success with radiologically controlled dilatation with an angioplasty-type, inflatable balloon introduced along a guide wire threaded down the nasolacrimal duct (Fig. 1). Manipulation of the guide wire from the inferior canaliculus through the sac into the duct may be difficult, and retrieval of the distal end from beneath the middle turbinate in the nasal cavity is easiest done with the cooperation of an ear, nose, and throat surgeon.

Functional assessment of the nasolacrimal duct may alternatively be done by the introduction of a drop of radionuclide, 4 MBq pertechnetate, into the medial angle of each eye, and then imaging with a γ-camera. This has the advantage of not requiring cannulation of the inferior cannaliculus and the possibility of demonstrating functional abnormalities of the duct. The anatomical detail is, however, inferior.

Computed tomography

CT is done by rotating a tightly collimated X-ray beam around a patient. The attenuated beam falls on a number of detectors. Calculations from the absorption profiles in multiple projections allow the reconstruction of a single plane within the patient. Sequential planes are imaged through the area of interest. Resolution is related to the thickness of the plane, 2-mm slice thickness usually being chosen for the orbits. It is generally easiest to scan in a transverse plane but the orbital floor

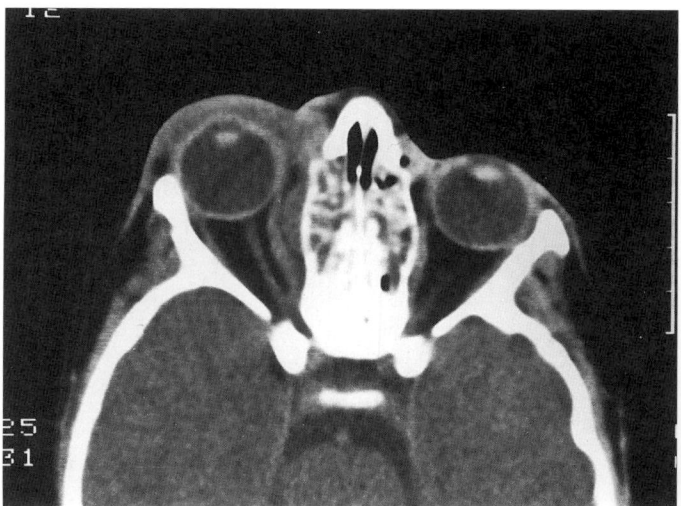

Fig. 2 Transverse CT scan through the orbits of an 8-year-old boy with orbital cellulitis. Inflammatory changes are shown in the ethmoid air cells and there is considerable oedema of the eyelids. The eye is proptosed and there is a subperiosteal abscess against the medial wall of the orbit, displacing the medial rectus.

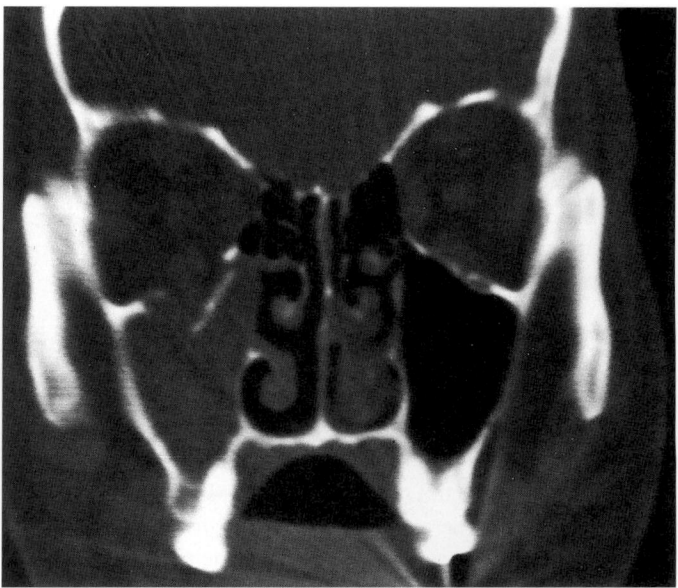

Fig. 3 Coronal CT scan showing a fracture of the floor of the left orbit with marked inferior displacement of a large bone fragment (classical blow-out fracture). There is herniation of orbital fat into the maxillary antrum, which is largely blood-filled. The inferior rectus also shows some downward displacement.

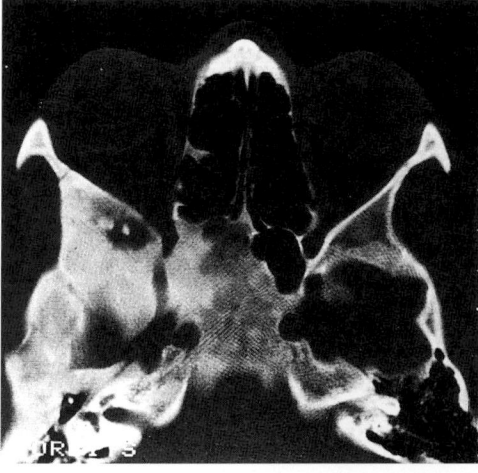

Fig. 4 Transverse CT scan through the orbits showing extensive predominantly right-sided skull base fibrous dysplasia with narrowing of the right optic nerve canal.

can only be properly assessed in the coronal plane. Images are displayed by manipulating an arbitrary grey scale so that different structures are emphasized. Bone windows (wide grey scale) reduce contrast; soft-tissue windows (narrow grey scale) increase contrast.

The advantage of CT is the marked increase in available contrast compared with plain films. It differentiates normal and abnormal soft-tissue structures from the lower-density orbital fat and the surrounding high-density bone. It has become the standard method for imaging tumours and inflammatory disease in and around the orbit (Fig. 2), for the assessment of bone configuration in the investigation and follow-up of fractures (Fig. 3), for subtle areas of calcification (drusen of the optic-nerve head), and for the assessment of primary bone disease (Fig. 4). CT has, however, a number of disadvantages. The patient receives a relatively high dose of radiation, particularly to radiosensitive organs such as the lens and the thyroid. Scanning in multiple planes is difficult, although the newer, reconstructive programmes and spiral CT may overcome some of the problems. Although soft-tissue contrast is good, differentiation of recurrent tumour from fibrosis and inflammatory lesions is not easy and may be impossible. Intracranial invasion is difficult to assess, especially when involving the meninges alone. Assessing the entire optic pathway adequately is also difficult and may be time-consuming.

Magnetic resonance

For this investigation the patient is placed in a powerful magnetic field, which causes the spinning protons of the subject's hydrogen nuclei to adopt a predominant alignment along the axis of the field. Radiofrequency pulses alter this alignment for short periods. The MR signal arises as the protons alter their alignment and different magnetic properties can predominate,

for example as they return to their original alignment or dephase with respect to each other. Different sequences of radiofrequency pulses have been developed to alter the imaging characteristics of the signal; they include T_1-weighted and T_2-weighted, and fat-suppression (for example short tau inversion recovery (STIR)), fast-scanning, and angiographic sequences.

The information obtained can be presented as a series of cross-sectional images in any plane (including oblique views) without altering the subject's position. MRI produces high soft-tissue contrast, providing excellent anatomical detail and

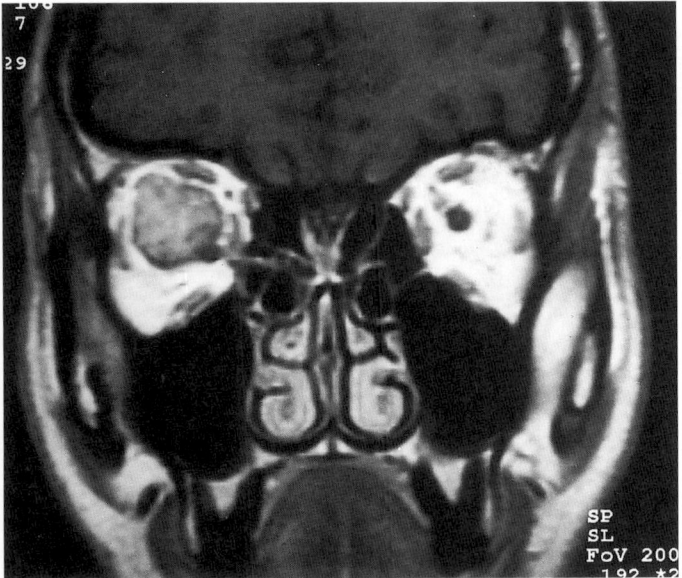

(a)

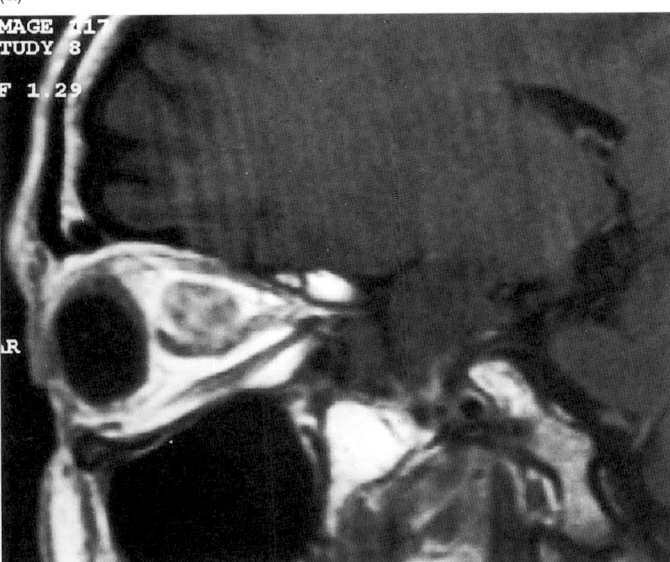

(b)

Fig. 5 Coronal (a) and sagittal (b) postgadolinium, T_1-weighted images showing a meningioma of the right optic nerve with inferomedial displacement of the nerve.

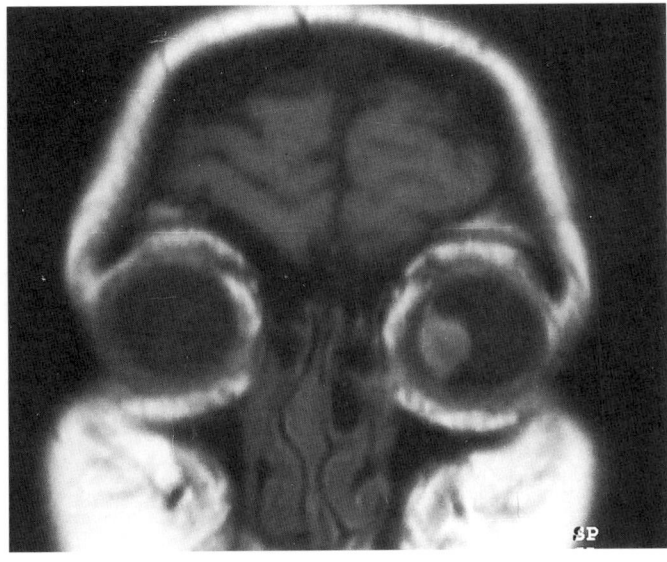

(a)

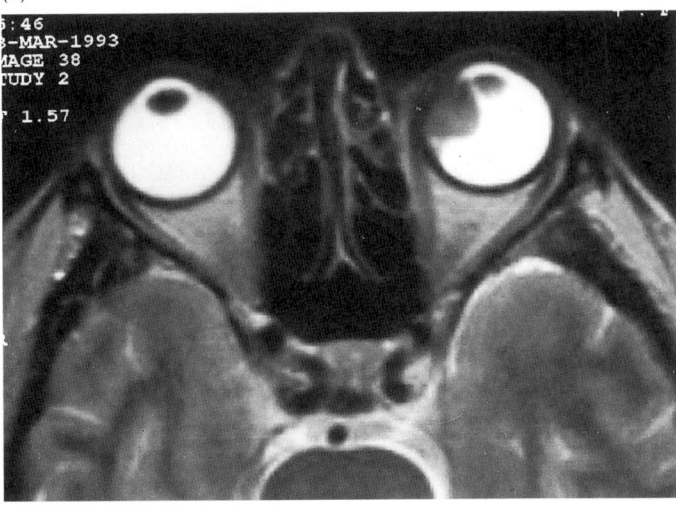

(b)

Fig. 6 Coronal T_1-weighted (a) and transverse T_2-weighted (b) images showing a large nasal malignant melanoma invading the adjacent ciliary body. It shows the classical appearance of low signal on T_2-weighted and high signal on T_1-weighted images due to the presence of melanin.

differentiation between diseased and normal tissue to a greater extent than CT. The signal void from flowing blood also offers generally good demonstration of the vasculature. MRI is therefore ideal for the assessment of tumours within the orbit (Fig. 5), including within the globe (Fig. 6), and in the surrounding region. Intracranial invasion, and involvement of cranial nerves and meninges, are best demonstrated with MRI, particularly with the use of intravenous gadolinium, which enhances (increases the signal on T_1-weighted scans) areas of involvement (Fig. 7).

MRI is very sensitive to the changes induced in tissue by inflammation from any cause, especially when using fat-suppression techniques. Orbital cellulitis is well demonstrated

and, although unproven, MRI is probably as sensitive as CT, if not more so, for the demonstration of intraorbital abscesses. MRI is excellent for the demonstration of thyroid eye disease and there is evidence to suggest some correlation between the intensity of the inflammatory changes demonstrated and the activity of the disease (Fig. 8). Episcleritis, lacrimal adenitis, and orbital myositis also appear to be well visualized on MRI. Optic neuritis will often be identified as high signal within the optic nerve on fat-suppression, T_2-weighted sequences.

Although the effects of trauma are well demonstrated on MRI, other methods compete well. In particular, CT, with its availability and excellent demonstration of bone and high-density foreign bodies, is the standard technique. MRI should, however, be considered where the soft-tissue lesion (damage to globe, nerve, or muscle) is of particular interest.

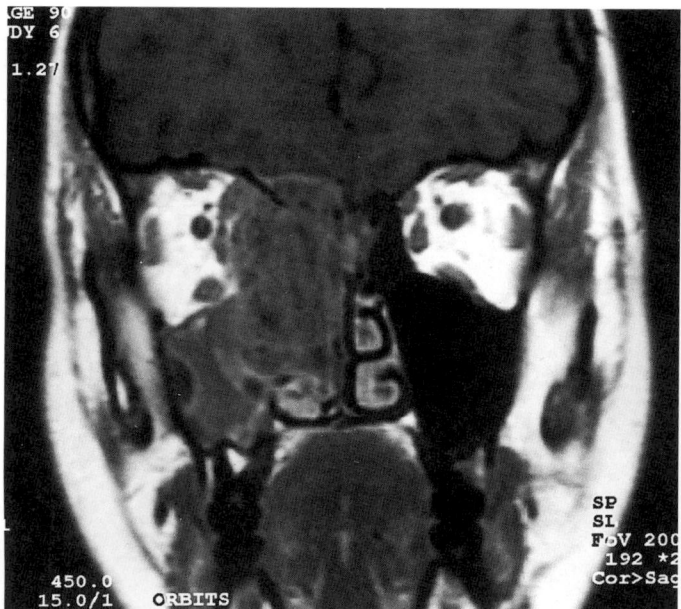

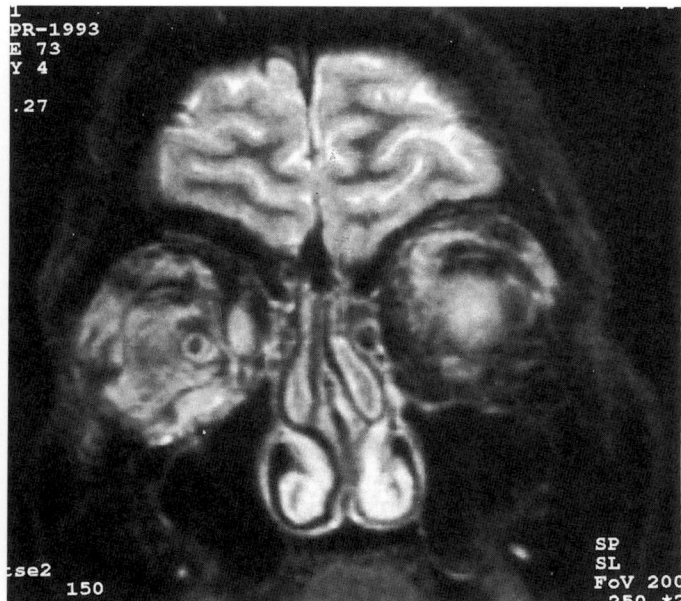

(a)

Fig. 7 Coronal, postgadolinium, T_1-weighted image of a 16-year-old female presenting with proptosis. There is a large rhabdomyosarcoma in the upper right nasal cavity extending into the orbit, displacing the medial rectus, ethmoid air cells, anterior cranial fossa (associated with meningeal invasion), and right maxilliary antrum (impeding sinus drainage, which has therefore filled up with secretions).

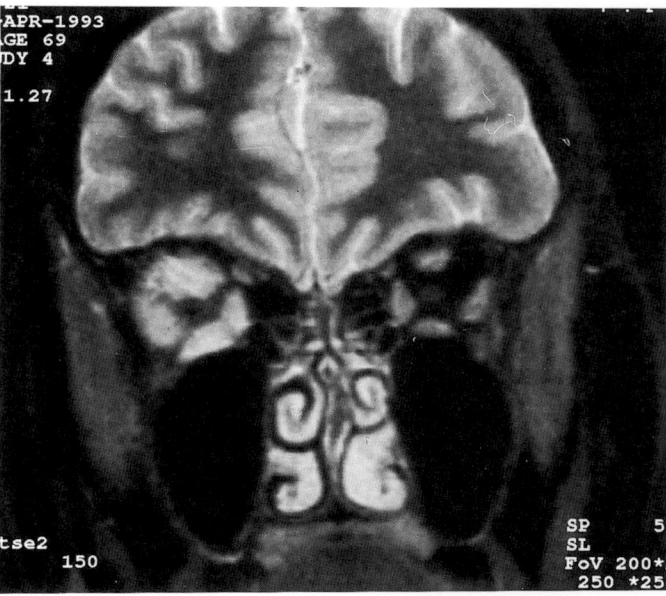

(b)

Fig. 8 Coronal STIR sequence through the orbits just posterior to the globes (a) and close to the orbital apex (b). There is severe active thyroid eye disease showing enlargement of the recti (grossly on the right) and increase in signal intensity from the muscles and the fat.

Problems with ocular movements due to innervation deficits are also best assessed with MRI. When an aneurysm of the circle of Willis is suspected, magnetic resonance angiography should also be used (classically in the painful IIIrd nerve palsy). With care it is claimed that this will diagnose all clinically important aneurysms.

The sensitivity of MRI for intracranial lesions and the ease of demonstration of the entire optic tract is an advantage in the investigation of visual-field problems of uncertain origin. MRI is the investigation of choice for suspected pituitary, cavernous sinus, brainstem, and occipital cortical lesions (Fig. 9).

MRI fails to show fine bone detail, cortical bone appearing essentially as a signal void. This is, however, an advantage in certain circumstances, particularly in the assessment of tumour invasion around the skull base, when MRI is untroubled by problems of density artefact from adjacent bone and the extent of the tumour is easily seen.

A few patients will be unsuitable for MRI. Ferromagnetic foreign bodies in sensitive sites (intracranial aneurysm clips, for example) and some medical implants (pacemakers, some otological implants) represent a hazard. Claustrophobia is occasionally prohibitive.

Angiography and venography

These procedures, particularly venography, are much less frequently used than in the past, largely due to the advent of MRI and CT. Angiography has a role in the assessment of arteriovenous malformations and intracranial aneurysms. It has no place in the routine assessment of tumours. Embolization,

either of an arteriovenous malformation or a large vascular tumour (classically preoperatively, for example with a juvenile angiofibroma invasive into the orbit), is a useful procedure, albeit not without hazard.

Future developments

Rapid scanning with MRI offers the potential to demonstrate the intraorbital structures during eye movements in normal individuals and patients with problems of ocular motility. The evaluation of more complex MRI sequences may allow the

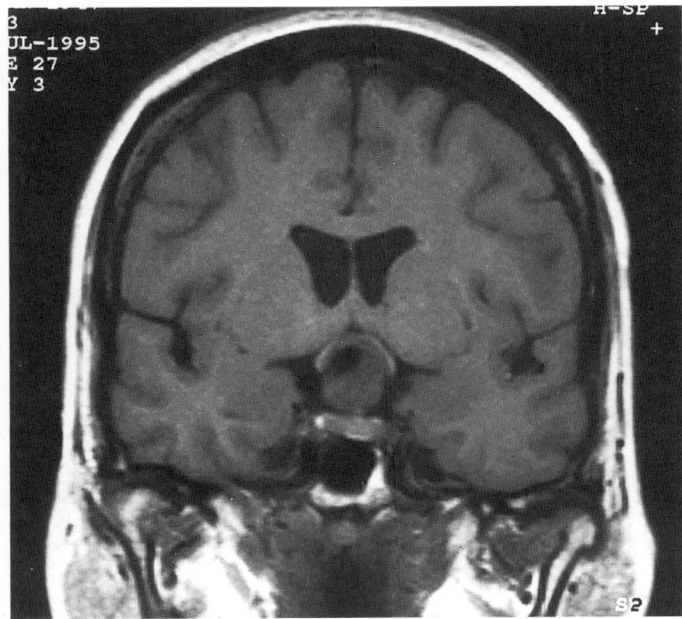

(a)

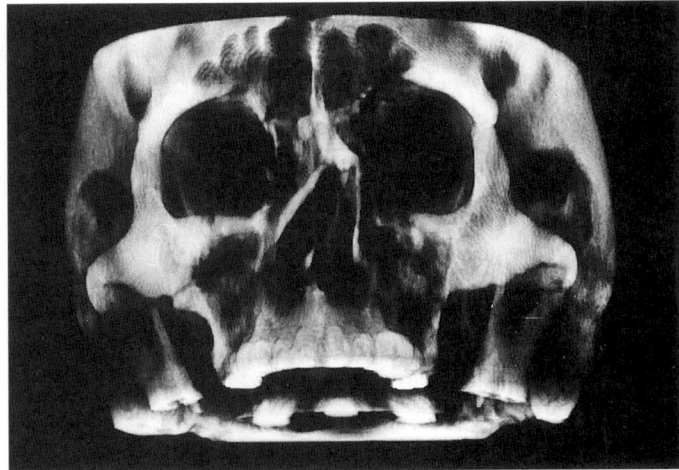

Fig. 10 Three-dimensional reconstruction of a CT scan of the facial bones demonstrating Le Fort II type fractures.

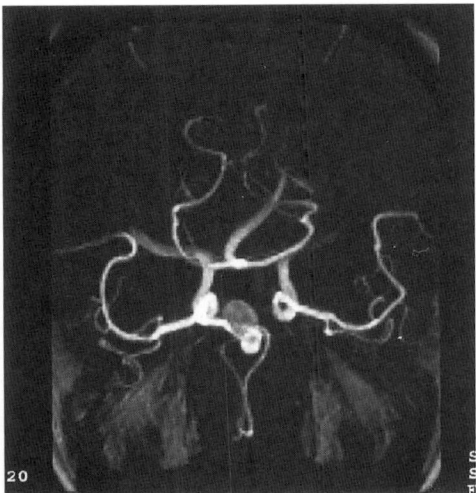

(b)

Fig. 9 Coronal T_1-weighted image (a) showing a large suprasellar mass elevating and compressing the optice chiasm. Magnetic resonance angiography confirmed the presence of an aneurysm of the anterior communicating artery (b). Both anterior cerebral arteries are seen to take origin from the right internal carotid artery.

delineation of the optic pathway distinct from the rest of the brain. MR spectroscopy and advanced radionuclide studies (positron-emission tomography) may allow functional imaging of the occipital cortex during visual stimulation.

Spiral CT scanners, in which a volume of a patient (for example the entire skull base and relevant vasculature) is scanned in a matter of seconds, rather than in a sequence of individual slices, offer the possibility of reconstructing high-quality images in any plane.

Three-dimensional reconstruction (Fig. 10) is already possible with current scanners (MRI and CT, conventional and spiral), given appropriate software, and is currently being refined. This may have particular importance in vascular and bone imaging or be linked with appropriate hardware to guide the surgeon within the orbit and cranium to reach tissue in potentially hazardous areas.

Further reading

Atlas, Scott W. (1992). Orbits. In *Magnetic resonance imaging* (2nd edn) (eds. D. D. Stark and W. G. Bradley Jr), pp. 988–1028. Mosley–Year Book Inc, St Louis.

Bloom, P. A., Ferris, J. D., Laidlaw, D. A. H., and Goddard, P. R. (1992). Magnetic resonance imaging. Diverse apperances of uveal malignant melanomas. *Archives of Ophthalmology*, **110**, 1105–11.

Jewell, F. M. *et al.* (1995). Video loop MRI of ocular motility disorders. *Journal of Computer Assisted Tomography*, **19**, 39–43.

Laitt, R. D. *et al.* (1994). The value of the short tau inversion recovery sequence in magnetic resonance imaging of thyroid eye disease. *British Journal of Radiology*, **67**, 244–7.

Mafee, M. F. (1995). Imaging of the orbit and imaging of the globe. In *Imaging of the head and neck* (eds. G.E. Valvassori, M. F. Mafee, and B. L. Carter), pp. 158–247. Thieme Medical, New York.

Moseley, I., Lloyd, G. A. S., and Sutherland, G.R. (1993). The orbit and eye. In *A textbook of radiology and imaging* (ed. D. Sutton), pp. 1287–310. Churchill Livingstone, Edinburgh.

Schwartz, R. B. (1995). Helical (spiral) CT in neurologic diagnosis. *Radiologic Clinics of North America*, **33**, 981–6.

Sheppard, S. (1995). Neurovascular Imaging. *Radiologic Clinics of North America*, **33**, 115–66.

1.6.7 Fluorescein angiography

B. Harney

Fluorescein angiography was introduced over 30 years ago and has stood the test of time. It has contributed to the understanding of many ocular diseases and remains an essential investigation in the management of disorders of the fundus. Although there have been considerable technical advances and although indications have changed, the fundamentals of technique and interpretation have altered little.

The dye

Fluorescein sodium is an orange-brown crystalline substance that belongs to the group of triphenylmethane dyes. It is a small molecule (376 mol. wt), but 80 to 90 per cent of the circulating dye is bound to plasma proteins. It diffuses freely out of all body capillaries apart from those of the central nervous system, of which the retina is a part, but does not enter the intracellular compartment in concentrations high enough to be visualized. It is relatively inert pharmacologically and is excreted by the liver and kidneys.

Fluorescent substances are stimulated to release energy in the form of light. Unlike phosphorescent substances, which continue to emit light after the stimulus ceases, fluorescence is only present while the substance is exposed to the exciting radiation. Absorption of a specific wavelength of radiation raises electrons to a higher energy level or excited state. As they spontaneously return to a lower energy level, they emit radiation, which may be less or equal to the absorbed energy but never greater. There is therefore a shift to longer wavelengths. When excited by a blue light (465–490 nm), sodium fluorescein in solution emits a yellow-green light (520–530 nm).

The camera

A number of techniques have been developed to record the transit of dye. The most commonly used involves serial photography on to a black-and-white film.

The camera produces a bright flash from a xenon light source. Before reaching the eye, the light passes through a blue filter called the excitor filter. The incident blue light stimulates fluorescence by the circulating fluorescein dye, and both the emitted green light and blue light, which is reflected back from the retina, then pass through a barrier filter. Because the wavelengths of blue and green light are relatively close in the electromagnetic spectrum, and because there is some overlap between the range of wavelengths transmitted by the excitor and barrier filters, some reflected blue light is allowed through to cause pseudofluorescence. Since the early days of angiography, filters have become much more efficient and pseudofluorescence has become less of a problem.

The film can be examined in negative or positive form. Stereo views produced by using a suitable attachment, or simply by moving the camera a little way from side to side between exposures, give useful information about differences in retinal thickness and the level of retinal abnormalities.

Newer techniques include videoangiography, digital imaging and storage techniques, and the scanning laser ophthalmoscope. No doubt the standard fundus camera will eventually be superseded, but the resolution obtained on a conventional negative has yet to be equalled.

The technique

The patient's pupils are dilated with tropicamide and phenylephrine. The patient is seated comfortably at the camera with his or her head on a head-rest. A large vein, if possible in the antecubital fossa, is cannulated. This technique is preferable to direct injection from a needle and syringe as it allows the patient to assume a more relaxed position, permits better timing of the injection and coordination with the photographer, and provides an initial route for medication and hydration should a serious reaction occur. Colour or red-free pictures are taken first. The dye is then injected rapidly, room lights extinguished, and photography started immediately to ensure that the earliest appearance of the dye is recorded. Approximately 20 pictures are taken at intervals of 1 to 2 s to follow the transit of the dye through the retinal and choroidal vasculature, and after a rest of a few minutes, late or residual pictures are taken.

Dosage

The dye is injected in an aqueous solution at a concentration of 10 to 25 per cent. We use 5 ml of a 20 per cent solution. There is no evidence that lower concentrations are associated with a lower incidence of adverse effects.

Oral fluorescein

Fluorescein can be administered orally to patients, for example children, who cannot tolerate injections. The pictures obtained do not allow analysis of the early phases of passage of dye through the circulation and give information only on the residual phases. This limits the usefulness of the technique and in practice oral fluorescein is rarely used. There is no evidence that oral administration reduces the incidence of serious side-effects, although the less severe reactions may be less frequent.

Adverse effects and precautions

Mild adverse effects are common. As the capillaries of the skin are permeable to fluorescein, all patients develop a yellowish tinge to the skin that fades after a day or so. The patient must also be warned that the urine will become bright yellow. Approximately 1/10 of patients will experience nausea. This usually occurs towards the end of the first sequence of photographs and lasts for only a few minutes. Very occasionally there may be vomiting.

Extravasation of fluorescein into surrounding tissues through a poorly positioned cannula should be avoided as it causes severe pain and, if little of the dye passes into the circulation, the procedure may have to be repeated. There have been reports of overlying skin necrosis requiring eventual grafting, although this is very rare.

Serious adverse reactions are fortunately rare, with an incidence of 2 to 5/1000 angiograms. Fatal reactions have been reported but with an incidence of less than 1/50 000 angiograms.

Reactions suggesting a hypersensitivity to the dye include urticaria, bronchospasm, angioedema, and anaphylactic shock.

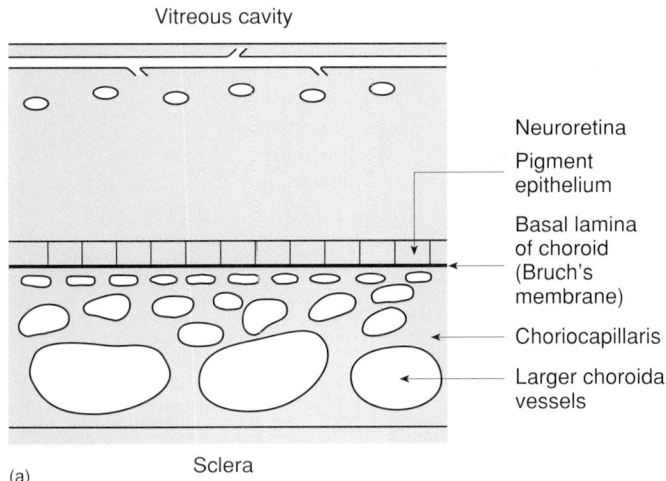

Fig. 1 Diagrams to demonstrate the passage of fluorescein dye through the blood vessels of the retina and choroid: (a) normal anatomy; (b) sequence showing fluorescein circulation.

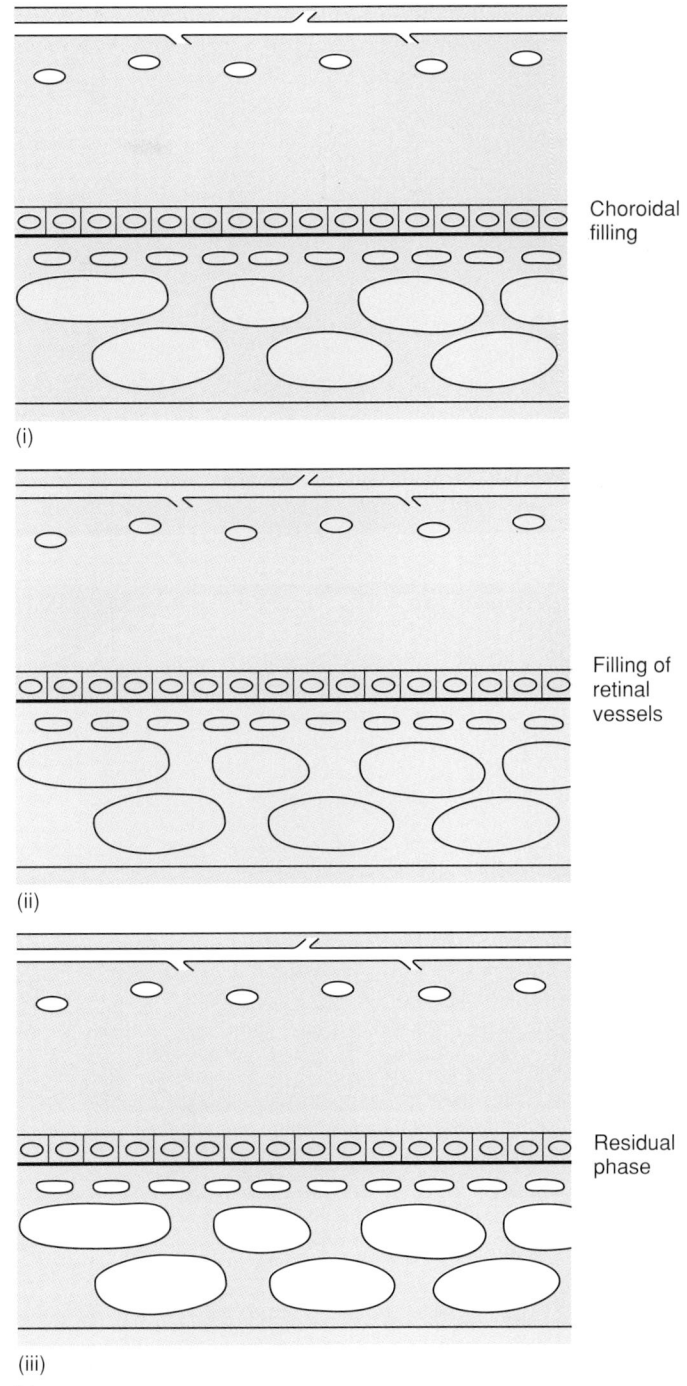

Urticaria develops from a few minutes to several hours after the injection and is treated with antihistamines. If urticaria develops soon after the injection, the patient should be monitored in case a more serious allergic reaction occurs. The more serious manifestations may develop within a few minutes of the injection and must be treated urgently.

A wide variety of cardiovascular complications have been reported, ranging from simple syncope to pulmonary oedema and myocardial infarction. The cause of these reactions is unknown. Some may be allergic phenomena, some may be simply a result of the stress associated with the investigation, and a proportion may be due to a direct effect of the dye.

Staff should be competent in cardiopulmonary resuscitation, and the equipment and medication required for the treatment of cardiovascular and emergencies and acute anaphylaxis should be at hand.

Contraindications to fluorescein injection are relative. The only absolute contraindication is a previous severe reaction. It would be wise to avoid fluorescein angiography unless strictly necessary if there is a history of recent myocardial infarction, increasing angina, or poorly controlled, severe asthma. There is no evidence that fluorescein is harmful to the fetus or neonate, but angiography is not recommended during pregnancy or lactation unless absolutely necessary. Renal failure is not a contraindication, but it will take longer for the fluorescein to be cleared from the circulation and a smaller dose can be given.

Interference with laboratory tests has been reported, particularly those where a colorimetric method is used. If tests of blood or urine are required, samples should be taken before rather than after fluorescein injection.

Interpretation of the angiogram

Negatives and transparencies are examined on a light box through magnifying glasses or a 20-D lens, or projected on to a screen. Stereo pairs can be examined in stereo viewers or with +10 D glasses. The examination is incomplete unless the angiogram is compared with colour pictures or, ideally, the patient re-examined with the angiogram at hand.

Passage of the dye (Figs 1 and 2)

The dye reaches the ocular circulation within a few seconds of injection, but the delay is variable depending on factors such as circulation time and compression of the arm.. Dye first appears in the eye as the choroid begins to fill via the short ciliary arteries 10 to 15 s after injection. The early pattern is

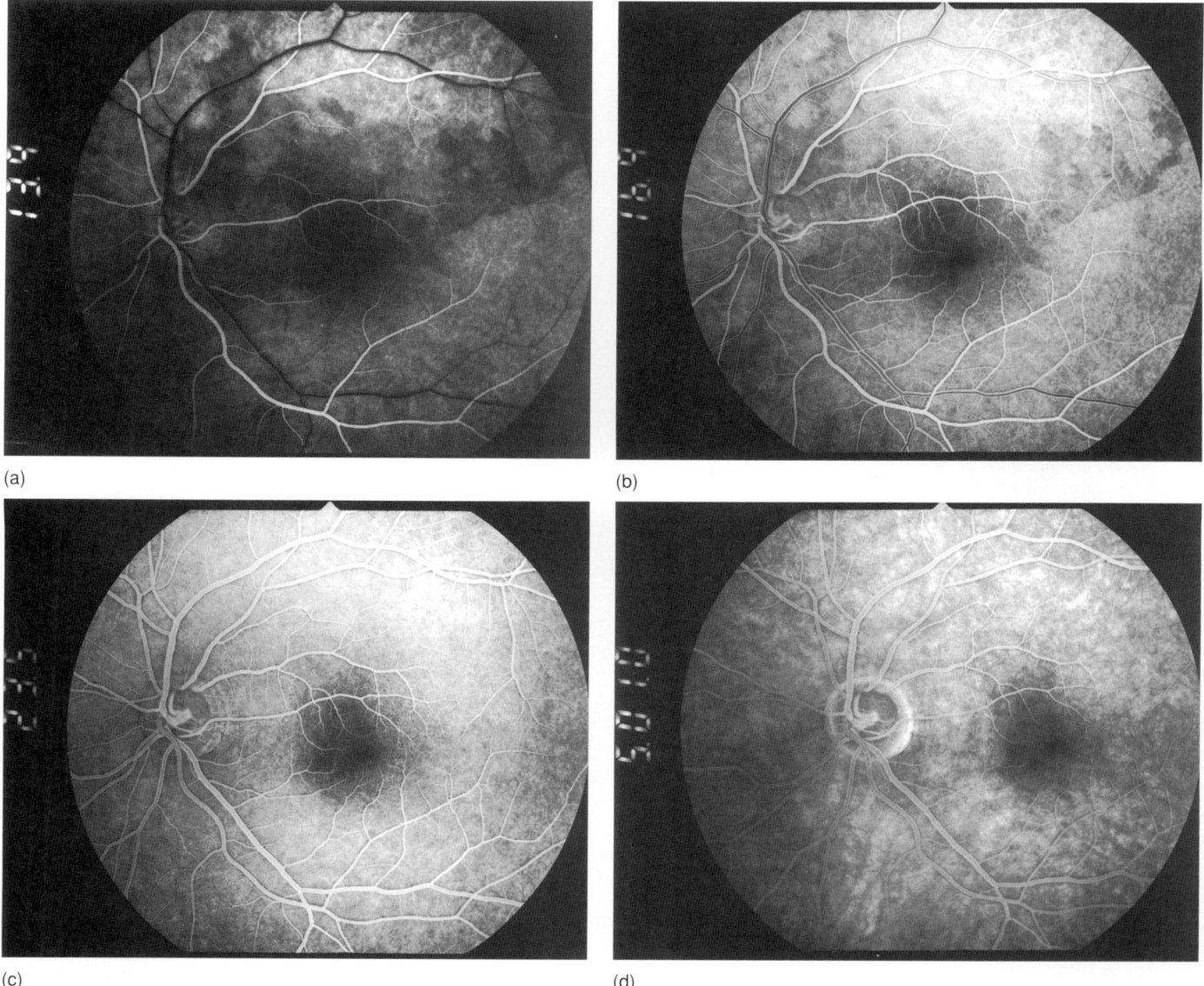

Fig. 2 Normal fluorescein angiogram. (a) Fluorescein angiogram 14 s after injection of dye showing patchy choroidal filling and dye within the retinal arterioles. (b) 17 s after injection showing dye within retinal arterioles and laminar fill of retinal veins. (c) 23 s after injection: full fluorescence with detailed view of macular capillaries. (d) 5 min after injection: dilute fluorescein within retinal vessels; residual staining of sclera.

one of patchy hyperfluorescence that becomes more uniform during the course of the transit. Details of the choroidal circulation are not demonstrated, as dye rapidly diffuses into the extravascular space from the fenestrated choriocapillaris and is taken up by Bruch's membrane. In the healthy eye, fluorescein is prevented from passing through the pigment epithelium (the outer blood–retinal barrier). The pigment epithelium thus provides not only a physiological barrier to the passage of dye, but also an optical barrier that reduces the level of fluorescence transmitted from the choroid. The mottled appearance of the choroidal fluorescence is the result of the masking effect of the pigment epithelium and the level of fluorescence will depend on such factors as age and race, which affect the degree of pigmentation within the retinal pigment epithelium. Choroidal fluorescence is reduced in the macular region because of the

greater density of pigment in the retinal pigment epithelium and the presence of yellow pigment in the outer retinal layers.

The capillaries of the optic nerve, and the cilioretinal artery if present, begin to fill at the same time as the choroid.

Dye reaches the retinal arterioles in less than a second after it first appears in the choroid. It then returns via the veins, filling them in a laminar fashion as tributaries empty into the main venules. There is no leakage from retinal capillaries (the inner blood–retinal barrier) in health, and a distinct picture of the retinal capillaries at the macula is obtained against the background glow of the choroid.

Eventually, as it recirculates, the dye becomes more dilute and the fluorescence within vessels fades. In the residual or late phase, dye remains only in those structures that have retained it. Normal sclera and lamina cribrosa take up dye and remain fluorescent after dye is no longer present in the circulation. Dye may also remain in fluid-filled compartments and other pathological structures. Normal blood-vessel walls do not take up dye and fluorescence within blood vessels in the residual phase is due to recirculation.

Abnormalities of angiograms

Abnormal flow rate

There is great variation in the time taken for the dye to reach the eye in the normal individual, but marked delay may be significant. Delay in venous filling is commonly seen in retinal venous occlusions.

Abnormalities of vascular architecture

Most abnormalities of the retinal vasculature are obvious clinically and fluorescein angiography merely confirms them. However, certain abnormalities such as long-standing capillary nonperfusion, which can be difficult to detect clinically, are easily assessed using fluorescein angiography.

Abnormal permeability of the inner or outer blood-retinal barriers

Fluorescein leaks from damaged retinal vessels or through the pigment epithelium, and persists in fluid-filled spaces.

Abnormalities in transmission of fluorescein (see below)

Traditionally, the interpretation of fluorescein angiograms has been assisted by classifying abnormalities as areas of hyperfluorescence and hypofluorescence.

Hyperfluorescence (Table 1)

Autofluorescence Some structures, for example superficial drusen of the head of the optic nerve, may be autofluorescent and will appear on a preinjection photograph taken with the excitor and barrier filters.

Pseudofluorescence (see above)

Leakage Fluorescence outside the normal pattern occurs where there is breakdown of either inner or outer blood-retinal barriers. For example, damaged retinal capillaries may leak (Fig. 3), and new vessels leak profusely. Leakage from the disc from dilated prepapillary capillaries occurs in papilloedema or papillitis. Leakage is characterized by a spread of hyperfluorescence from the abnormal structures during the course of the angiogram, giving rise to a persistent fluorescence with a 'fuzzy' outline.

Pooling Abnormal patterns of fluorescence occur when dye accumulates in fluid-filled spaces. Dye accumulates in the space beneath the pigment epithelium in pigment epithelial detachments. Different patterns of filling occur, but essentially the area of the detachment gradually becomes more hyperfluorescent, retaining a well-defined boundary (Fig. 4). In central serous retinopathy, dye appears between the neuroretina and pigment epithelium. A small, central, hyperfluorescent spot

Table 1 The interpretation of hyperfluorescence in the fluorescein angiogram

Accumulation of dye (hyperpermeability)
Leakage across blood–retinal barrier

Inner:
    microaneurysms
    retinal new vessels

Outer:
    Choroidal new vessels

Pooling in fluid-filled spaces
    central serous retinopathy
    pigment epithelial detachment
    cystoid macular oedema

Staining
Normal:
    disc
    sclera

Abnormal:
    drusen
    vessel walls in ischaemia
    scar tissue

Increased transmission
Normal:
    hypopigmentation of retinal
    pigment epithelium

Abnormal:
    retinal pigment epithelial atrophy

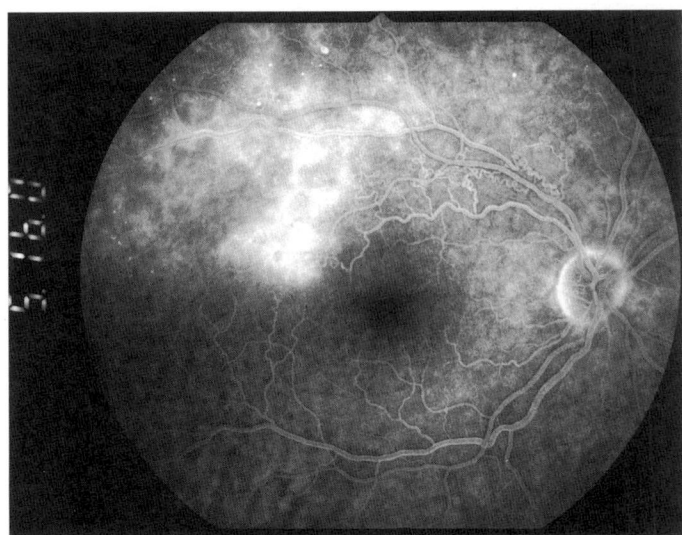

Fig. 3 Late picture of a branch retinal-vein occlusion to show hyperfluorescence caused by leakage of dye from the damaged retinal vascular bed.

enlarges concentrically as fluorescein fills the subretinal space. Occasionally, the pathognomonic 'smoke-stack' appearance is seen in the late pictures (Fig. 5). Dye pooling within cystoid spaces in the neuroretina gives a characteristic petalloid pattern (Fig. 6).

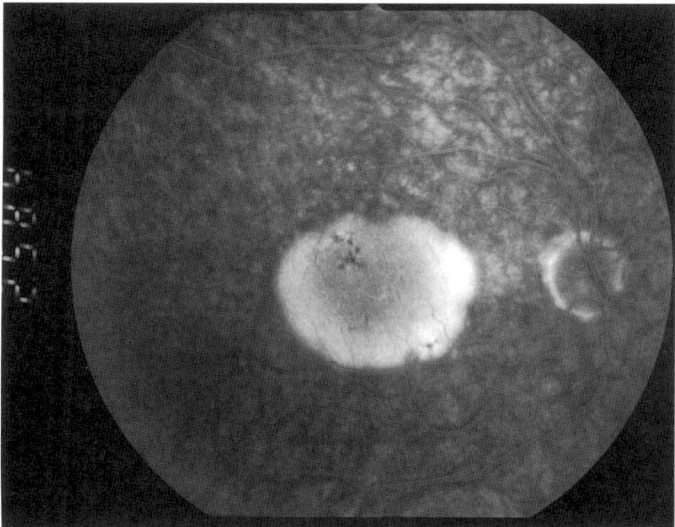

Fig. 4 Pooling of dye in a pigment epithelial detachment.

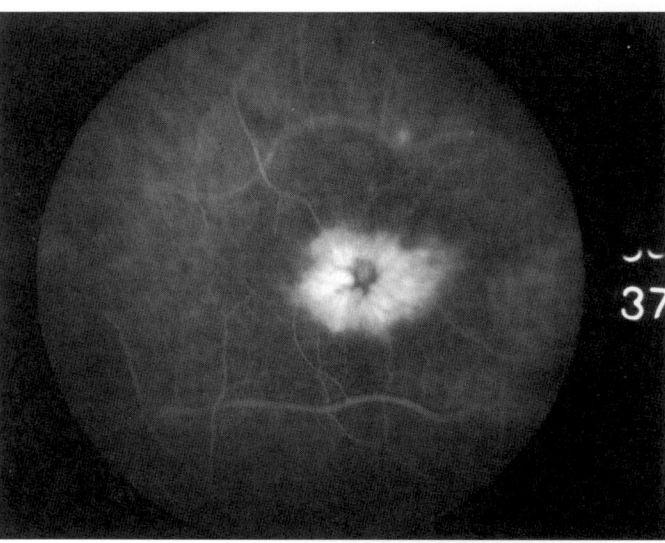

Fig. 6 Late picture showing typical petalloid appearance of hyperfluorescence in cystoid macular oedema.

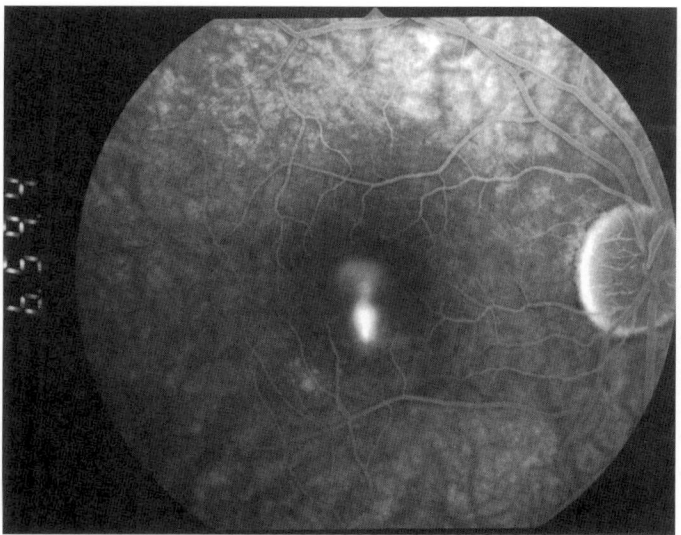

Fig. 5 Late picture showing smoke-stack appearance in central serous chorioretinopathy.

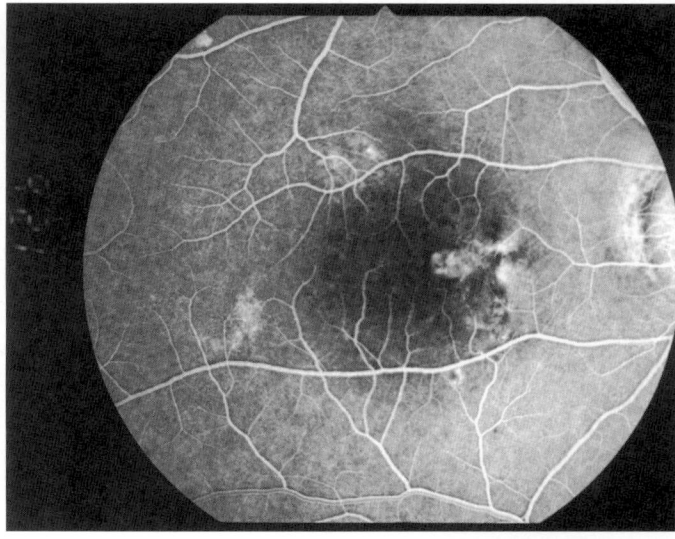

Fig. 7 Patches of hyperfluorescence corresponding to retinal pigment epithelial atrophy following attacks of central serous chorioretinopathy.

Window defect Abnormal patterns of hyperfluorescence are seen when disease processes reduce the pigmentation of the pigment epithelial without affecting its physiological barrier function. The shape of the fluorescent patch characteristically corresponds to the area of pigment epithelial atrophy seen as pallor clinically and, although it may increase in fluorescence as the angiogram progresses, the shape of the area remains constant (Fig. 7). If the disease process has also caused atrophy of the underlying choriocapillaris, larger choroidal vessels may be visible (Fig. 8). The staining of the underlying sclera means that the defect remains fluorescent after dye has left the circulation.

Staining

Staining describes the property of structures that absorb and retain dye and thus remain hyperfluorescent after dye is no longer visible in the circulation. Normal sclera and lamina cribrosa stain, as do structures, such as drusen and scar tissue, that are present in pathological states.

Hypofluorescence (Table 2)

Non-perfusion Reduced fluorescence is seen when dye does not reach parts of the circulation. Choroidal filling defects are often difficult to interpret because of the permeability of the choroidal circulation, which allows fluorescein to diffuse

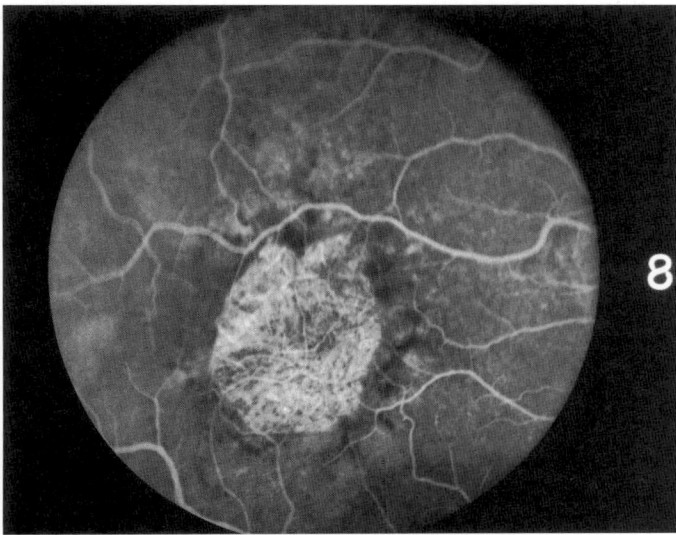

Fig. 8 Geographic atrophic age-related maculopathy.

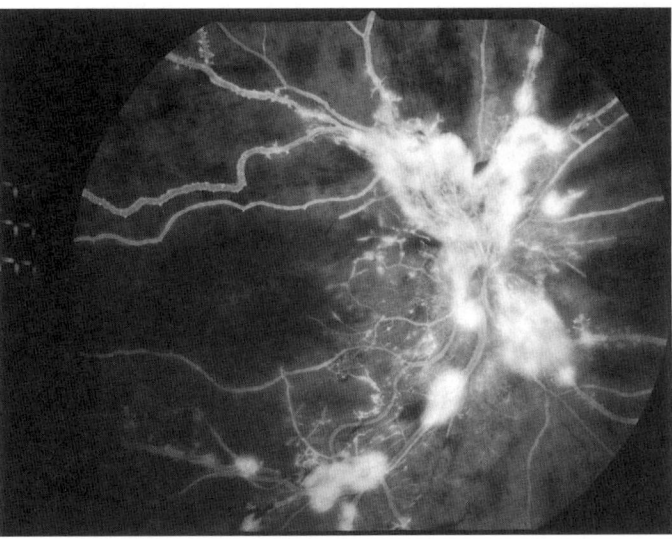

Fig. 9 Ischaemic occlusion of the central retinal vein showing widespread filling defect of the retinal capillary bed. The darkest areas of hyperfluorescence against the greyish background of non- perfused retina represent masking due to haemorrhage. There is intense hyperfluorescence due to leakage from new vessels arising from the disc.

Table 2 The interpretation of hypofluorescence in the fluorescein angiogram

Masking of normal dye transit
Media opacities
   vitreous haemorrhage
   lens/corneal opacities

Pigment
   blood
   melanin

Other
   exudates, oedema, fluid (rarely)

Failure of dye circulation
Retinal vessel closure
   large vessel
   capillary

Choroidal vessel closure
   segmental (large vessel)
   microinfarcts
   optic nerve ischaemia

rapidly throughout the extravascular space. Retinal filling defects can be seen in conditions such as diabetic retinopathy and retinal venous occlusion (Fig. 9). The affected area has a grey, featureless appearance and fluorescence is reduced though not absent. Vessel walls adjacent to non-perfused areas of retina often show increased fluorescence due to staining or leakage.

Masking or blockage Profound hypofluorescence is caused by materials that block the transmission of light. The most frequent cause is the accumulation of melanin pigment and haemorrhage. Lipofuscin deposits in the retinal pigment epithelium are responsible for blockage of choroidal fluores-

cence in some macular dystrophies. Large amounts of turbid fluid can cause a slight degree of hypofluorescence, but this is unusual and even rather extensive and thick-looking exudates often have little effect on underlying fluorescence.

Indications for fluorescein angiography

Indications for fluorescein angiography change with time. It has been a very important investigation in developing an understanding of various fundus conditions. Where the angiographic correlates of certain fundus appearances are known, fluorescein angiography is often no longer necessary and a decision can be made on the basis of clinical examination. An example would be proliferative diabetic retinopathy, where it is known that disc and retinal neovascularization indicate widespread retinal non-perfusion and laser treatment is planned without the need for further investigation.

Fluorescein angiography is rarely helpful in making a diagnosis, and it is often the case that where the diagnosis is equivocal on clinical examination it is also equivocal on angiography. Examples where the early promise of fluorescein angiography have not been fulfilled include the diagnosis of choroidal tumours and the differential diagnosis of disc swelling. To avoid unnecessary angiograms it is therefore important to know what question is being asked and whether fluorescein angiography is the best investigation to give the answer.

Main clinical uses

Investigation of retinal vascular disease

The main functions of fluorescein angiography are to determine the cause of visual loss, and to plan and monitor

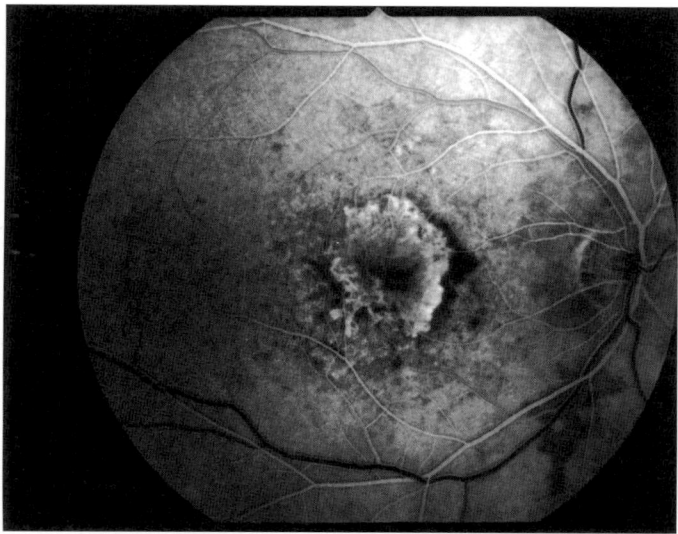

Fig. 10 Exudative age-related maculopathy with fluorescein delineating a large, subfoveal, neovascular network.

treatment. Angiography, although, as outlined above, no longer always necessary in the management of diabetic retinopathy, remains useful particularly in the investigation of diffuse macular oedema and in explaining visual loss. In the management of retinal venous occlusion, angiography is used to determine the extent of retinal non-perfusion and thus predict the risk of neovascular complications, and to determine the pattern of leakage from retinal capillaries responsible for sight-threatening oedema and exudate. The information is valuable for deciding on the frequency of review and planning laser therapy.

Management of macular disorders

Angiography has a very important use in the management of macular disorders. It is of particular value in the management of exudative maculopathy associated with choroidal neovascularization, most commonly encountered in age-related maculopathy. It is essential for defining a neovascular network that might be amenable to treatment and in monitoring progression or treatment (Fig. 10).

Angiography is used in the management of central serous chorioretinopathy, both in confirming the diagnosis where this is in doubt and in determining the position of the 'hot spot' should treatment be contemplated.

Angiography can help to differentiate between different patterns of macular dystrophy and may demonstrate changes where none is visible clinically.

Management of retinal inflammatory disease

Angiography is useful in determining the cause of visual loss and is particularly useful where vitreous haze obscures detail of the macula. Cystoid macular oedema may often be demonstrated by fluorescence angiography where it was not obvious clinically. Patterns of retinal perfusion and vessel involvement can help in diagnosis.

Management of choroidal tumours

Angiography has been used in the past to help distinguish between elevated choroidal tumours that were difficult to define clinically, for example melanomas, secondaries, and haemangiomas. In practice the diagnosis is usually made clinically and angiography rarely allows an unequivocal confirmation.

Investigation of disc disorders

Angiography has been used to differentiate between pathological disc swelling and pseudopapilloedema. The pathologically swollen disc shows leakage from dilated prepapillary capillaries. In practice, where there is doubt clinically, the fluorescein angiogram is often equivocal and cannot reliably be used to exclude or confirm raised intracranial pressure. Clinical considerations, including history and additional signs and symptoms, are more important.

Indocyanine-green angiography

Indocyanine green was first used for fundus angiography in the early 1970s, but its low level of fluorescence meant that good-quality images were difficult to achieve. More recently, developments in videoangiography, digital angiography with computing systems, and the scanning laser ophthalmoscope have led to considerable improvements in picture quality and indocyanine green is fast becoming an important adjunct to fluorescein angiography in the investigation of certain fundus disorders.

Properties of indocyanine green

Indocyanine green is a water-soluble tricarbocyanine dye. It absorbs and emits light in the near infrared with peak absorption at 805 nm and fluorescence at 835 nm. The longer wavelengths permit better penetration through overlying pigments such as haemoglobin, melanin, and xanthophyll, allowing better visualization of the choroid. The molecule is large and is 98 per cent bound to plasma proteins. Unlike fluorescein, therefore, indocyanine green leaks only slowly through fenestrated, normal, and abnormal choroidal vessels.

Indocyanine green is not metabolized *in vivo* and is excreted into the bile after passage through the liver. It has a low incidence of adverse effects.

Dosage and administration

Concentrations of 10 to 25 mg/ml have been used to give a dose of 1 to 5 mg/kg. The dye is injected into an arm vein.

Adverse effects

Indocyanine green has been used for some time in the study of liver function and cardiac circulation. The incidence of adverse effects is low, ranging from approx. 0.1 to 0.3 per cent, and of these the majority are minor. The concentration of dye has generally been higher in ophthalmology, but a survey of complications in Japan showed only 13 adverse reactions in 3774 angiograms (0.34 per cent), of which only three were classed as serious and required treatment. Hypotension is quoted as the most frequent serious adverse reaction but the mechanism is uncertain. The incidence of serious reactions is similar to that observed with fluorescein. Although extremely rare, deaths have been reported, and appropriate precautions therefore have to be taken.

Cameras

Because of the low level of fluorescence, high-quality images have only recently become available with advances in video-angiography and computerized digital-imaging systems. Standard fundus cameras can be used with modifications, but scanning laser ophthalmoscopes detect lower levels of fluorescence and have advantages over conventional systems.

Uses of indocyanine angiography

Indocyanine green is considered as an adjunct to, rather than a replacement for, fluorescein angiography. The two most significant properties of indocyanine green are its fluorescence in the infrared spectrum, thus allowing penetration through pigment, and the low level of leakage of the dye from choroidal capillaries. This allows better visualization of the choroidal vascular architecture, which is obscured in fluorescein angiography by the retinal pigment epithelium and by the profuse early leakage of fluorescein from the choriocapillaris.

Investigation of subretinal neovascular membranes

So far, the most important clinical application of indocyanine green angiography has been in the investigation of neovascular membranes, which are ill-defined on angiography, either because of rapid early leakage of dye or because of masking by blood or pigment. In occult choroidal neovascularization, a significant proportion of well-defined extrafoveal networks are detected and treatment has shown promising results. However, indocyanine green fails to delineate fully up to 20 per cent of networks that are well-defined with fluorescein and the two investigations are often used together to glean the maximum information.

The diode laser also functions in the infrared, and indocyanine green-enhanced, diode-laser treatment of poorly defined choroidal neovascular membranes has been successful in some cases.

Other uses

Indocyanine green is being increasingly applied to a wide range of fundus conditions and is shedding new light on disease mechanisms, although it is only in the field of exudative age-related maculopathy that it has had an impact on clinical management.

Studies of choroidal ischaemia are limited by the size of the molecule and its protein binding, which restricts its circulation into parts of the choroidal capillary bed. In the study of choroidal tumours, interesting observations have been made, but so far indocyanine green has not proved useful clinically in differential diagnosis. Indocyanine-green videoangiography has provided insights into the mechanisms of central serous chorio-

retinopathy, where a widespread choroidal vascular permeability is demonstrated. Fluorescein angiography is still the preferred clinical investigation, however, as it is better able to demonstrate active leak. Choroidal inflammatory disorders are currently being studied using the technique.

At present we do not yet know the full potential of indocyanine-green angiography or what its place will be in the day-to-day management of eye disease.

Further reading

[Books: the recommended books contain many references to important original articles not mentioned below.]

Gass, J. D. M. (1987). *Stereoscopic atlas of macular diseases*. Mosby, St Louis. [An established reference with many fluorescein angiograms to illustrate a detailed text.]

Harney B. A., Dean Hart, C. J. D., and Grey, R. H. B. (1994). *Atlas of fluorescein angiography*. [An introduction to the technique with illustrations to demonstrate the fundamentals of interpretation and examples of angiograms in a range of clinical disorders.]

Ryan, S. J. et al. (1994). *Retina* (2nd edn). Mosby, St Louis. [A comprehensive three-volume work covering all aspects of vitreoretinal disease. Volume 2 contains a chapter dedicated to fluorescein angiography, but angiographic findings are also described where relevant to specific disease processes elsewhere in the text.]

[Articles]

Bartsch, D-U., Weinreb, R. N., Zinser, G., and Freeman, W. R. (1995). Confocal scanning infrared laser ophthalmoscopy for indocyanine green angiography. *American Journal of Ophthalmology*, **120**, 642–51.

Branch Vein Occlusion Study Group (1984). Argon laser photocoagulation for macular oedema in branch vein occlusion. *American Journal of Ophthalmology*, **98**, 271–82.

Branch Vein Occlusion Study Group (1986). Argon scatter photocoagulation for prevention of neovascularisation and vitreous haemorrhage in branch vein occlusion. *Archives of Ophthalmology*, **104**, 34–41.

Cartlidge, N. E. F., Ng, R. C. Y., and Tilley, P. J. B. (1977). Dilemma of the swollen optic disc: a fluorescein retinal angiography study. *British Journal of Ophthalmology*, **61**, 385–9.

Central Vein Occlusion Study Group (1995). A randomised clinical trial of early panretinal photocoagulation for ischemic central vein occlusion. *Ophthalmology*, **102**, 1434–44.

Chahal, P. S., Neal, M. J., and Kohner, E. M. (1985). Metabolism of fluorescein after intravenous administration. *Investigative Ophthalmology and Visual Science*, **26**, 764–8

Davis, D. L. and Robertson, D. M. (1973). Fluorescein angiography of metastatic choroidal tumours. *Archives of Ophthalmology*, **89**, 97–9.

Haining, W. M. (1981). Video funduscopy and fluoroscopy. *British Journal of Ophthalmology*, **65**, 702–6.

Hayreh, S. S. (1974). Recent advances in fluorescein fundus angiography. *British Journal of Ophthalmology*, **58**, 391–412.

Kohner, E. M. and Dollery, C. T. (1970). Fluorescein angiography of the fundus in diabetic retinopathy. *British Medical Bulletin*, **26**, 166–70

Macular Photocoagulation Study Group (1989). The use of fundus photographs and fluorescein angiograms in the identification and treatment of choroidal neovascularisation in the macular photocoagulation study. *Ophthalmology*, **96**, 1526–34.

Maumenee, A. E. (1968). Fluorescein angiography in the diagnosis and treatment of lesions of the ocular fundus. *Transactions of the Ophthalmological Societies of the United Kingdom*, **88**, 529–56.

Novotny, R. and Alvis, D. L. (1961). A method of photographing fluorescence in circulating blood in the human retina. *Circulation*, **24**, 82–6.

Olk R. J. and Lee C. M. (1993). Indications for fluorescein angiography in the managment of diabetic retinopathy. In *Diabetic retinopathy: practical management* (ed. R. J. Olk and C. M. Lee), pp. 129–39. Lippincott, Philadelphia.

Pettit, T. H., Barton, A., Foos, R. Y., and Christensen, R. E. (1970). Fluorescein angiography of choroidal melanomas. *Archives of Ophthalmology*, **83**, 27–38.

Romanchuk, K. G. (1982). Fluorescein. Physicochemical factors affecting its fluorescence. *Survey of Ophthalmology*, **26**, 269–83.

Sanborne, G. E., Magargal, L. E., and Jaeger, E. A. (1987).Venous occlusive disease of the retina. In *Clinical ophthalmology* Vol. 3, Ch. 15 (ed. T. D. Duane). Harper and Row, New York.

Sanders, M. D. and Ffytche, T. J. (1967). Fluorescein angiography in the diagnosis of drusen of the disc. *Transactions of the Ophthalmological Societies of the United Kingdom*, **87**, 457–68.

Woon, W. H. *et al.* (1990). The scanning laser ophthalmoscope: basic principles and applications. *Journal of Ophthalmic Photography*, **12**, 17–23.

Yannuzzi L. A. *et al.* (1986). Fluorescein angiography complications survey. *Ophthalmology*, **93**, 611–17.

Yannuzzi, L. A. *et al.* (1994). Indocyanine green videoangiography: current status. *European Journal of Ophthalmology*, **4**, 69–81.

1.6.8 Anterior segment vascular imaging

Paul Meyer

Introduction

The conjunctival microcirculation, lying under a clear epithelium, is the most accessible in the body. Its vascular architecture, calibre, blood flow, and competence can be observed with higher resolution than in any other site. In contrast, the episcleral circulation may be somewhat obscured by the opalescent Tenon's capsule of younger patients and iris vessels lie beneath a pigmented epithelium which impedes both clinical and contrast examinations in most subjects.

Clinical slit lamp (SL) examination is a powerful method for demonstrating these circulations but the techniques of anterior segment fluorescein angiography (ASFA) and haemoglobin video imaging (HVI) enhance it considerably. Each has its particular merits: ASFA times arterial flow and tests the competence of vessels; HVI best characterizes flow in capillaries, venules, and veins. Whenever possible, all three should be used in combination (Fig. 1(a–c)).

Techniques

Clinical slit lamp examination (SL) (Fig. 1(a))

Slit lamp examination illustrates more than the architecture and calibre of a microcirculation. Transparent, but refractile, vascular walls can be demonstrated by an oblique, offset beam of white light, reflected off the sclera or iris to give bright or dark field retroillumination. This can reveal blood vessels through

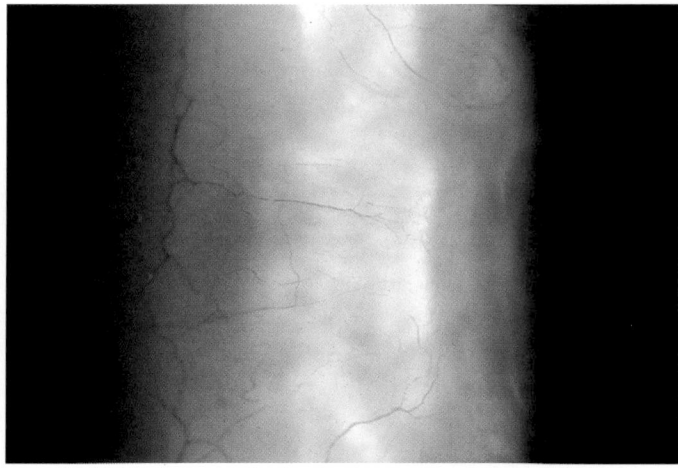

(a)

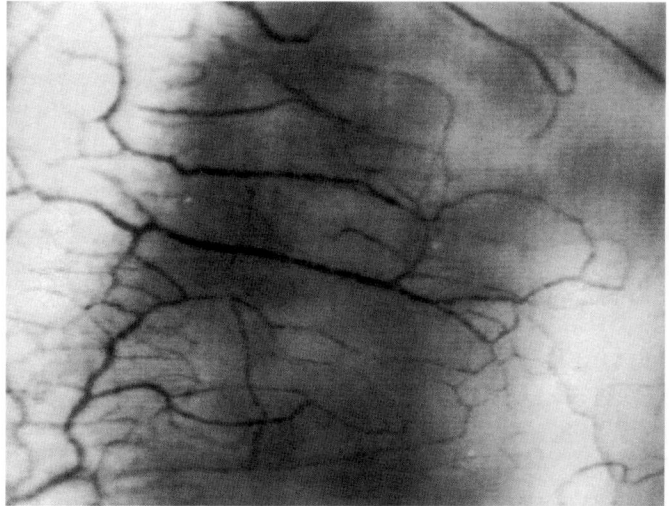

(b)

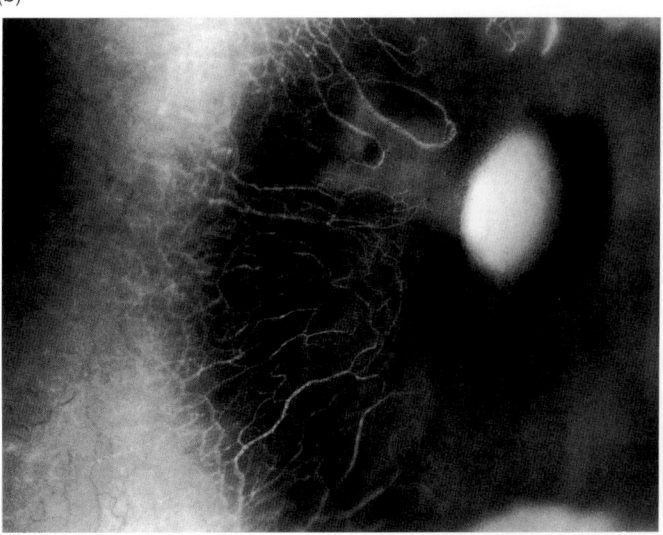

(c)

Fig. 1 Corneal new vessels: sclerokeratitis in a 57-year-old man with rheumatoid arthritis. (a) Slit lamp photograph of corneal new vessels, illustrating dark-field retroillumination of peripheral cornea and bright-field retroillumination more centrally. (b) The same field, demonstrated by haemoglobin video imaging. (c) The same vessels during photographic low-dose fluorescein angiography (1 min).

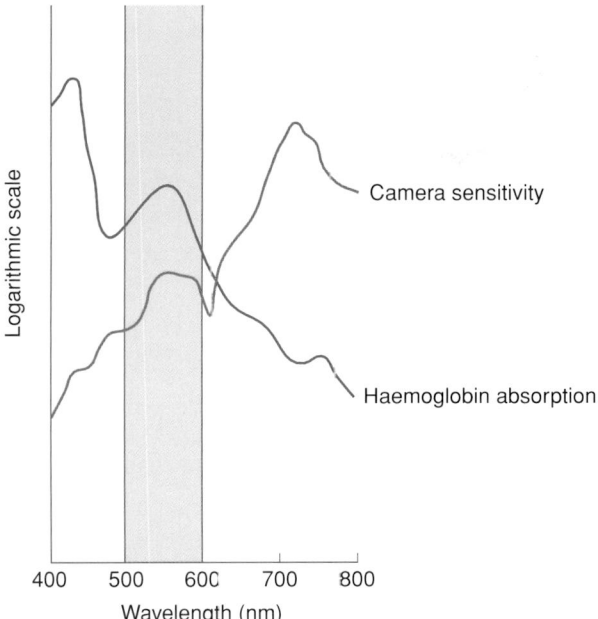

Fig. 2 Haemoglobin video imaging: Overlapping semilogarithmic plots to demonstrate correspondence between the haemoglobin long wavelength absorption peak, camera sensitivity, and illumination waveband.

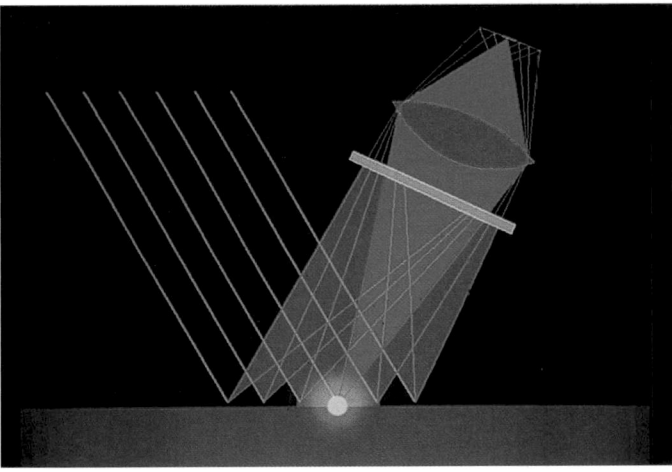

Fig. 3 Fluorescein angiography: The entire field is illuminated by light from which wavelengths greater than the fluorescein excitation peak have been excluded. A 'barrier' filter obscures all this illumination, but transmits the longer wavelength fluorescence.

which erythrocytes may not be flowing, both at the normal limbus and in inactive interstitial keratitis.

Furthermore, red blood cells act as quanta of contrast in vessel lumina. Haemoglobin has an absorption peak at about 520 nm and appears black when illuminated by green light. Most clinical slit lamps have a suitable green filter and the clinician can expect to resolve single erythrocytes flowing through the capillaries and venules of the conjunctival and limbal microcirculations.

Haemoglobin video imaging (HVI) (Fig. 1(b))

Conjunctival and episcleral vessels are illuminated by a waveband which spans the long-wavelength absorption peak of haemoglobin, and a video camera with a corresponding peak in its sensitivity spectrum images light which has been reflected by sclera (Fig. 2). The optics are arranged so that a single erythrocyte covers at least two pixels in the video image.

Perfusion is a cyclical phenomenon and this technique extends slit lamp examination to record changes in erythrocyte flow over time. It is particularly valuable for demonstrating laminar flow or erythrocyte aggregation in the capillary and venous phases of the circulation, and the diversion of blood though venous shunts.

Fluorescein angiography (ASFA) (Fig. 1(c))

Method

A fluorophore absorbs light in a particular waveband and re-emits it at longer wavelength. For fluorescein, the absorption and emission peaks are 495 nm and 520 nm, respectively.

During fluorescein angiography, the field is illuminated by a source from which all wavelengths greater than the absorption peak have been excluded by an 'excitation' filter. It is observed through a 'barrier' filter which obscures all the illuminating radiation, but transmits any longer-wavelength fluorescence, thereby demonstrating the injected fluorescein with high contrast against a dark background (Fig. 3).

Images are recorded by rapid sequence flash photography (1–2 s intervals), giving exquisite capillary detail, or by a sensitive CCD video camera, which achieves high temporal resolution (0.04 s intervals) at the expense of some spatial resolution: an advantage in most clinical situations (compare Figs 7 and 8).

Fluorescence intensity and leakage

Fluorescein is a small molecule (375 Da), which crosses endothelial fenestrations in the conjunctival and episcleral circulations, but is retained by limbal, iris, and retinal capillaries. However, it binds ionically to circulating albumin and, when this binding is not saturated, its distribution mirrors that of albumin in the early frames of a study. Therefore, when the dose of fluorescein is restricted, angiograms demonstrate better the integrity of conjunctival and episcleral vessels (low dose ASFA).

Fluorescence from intraluminal fluorescein is normally attenuated due to quenching by albumin and the absorption of exciting and emitted light by haemoglobin (Fig. 4). Once fluorescein has extravasated, these constraints no longer apply: fluorescence is much brighter and little dye need leak to overwhelm the image of surrounding vessels.

The brightness of extravascular fluorescence makes ASFA a particularly sensitive technique for distinguishing foci of inflammation or neovascularization, in which vessels retain albumin poorly and fluorescein leaks profusely. There is disproportionate leakage from affected vessels in the early frames of such a study, while the late frames show excessive staining of the surrounding sclera.

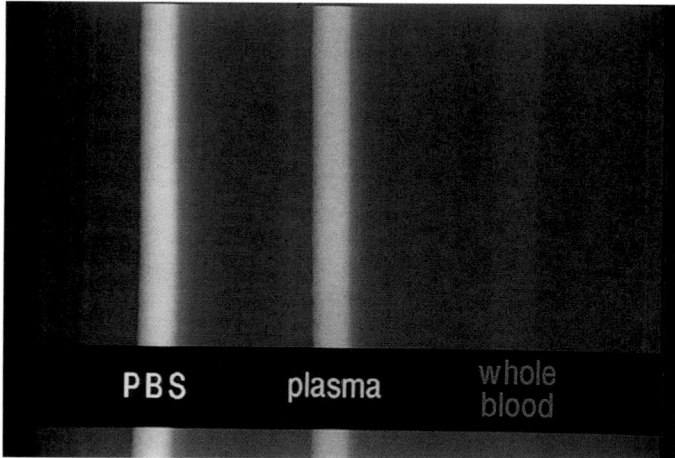

Fig. 4 Fluorescein angiography: the influence of blood and plasma upon vascular fluorescence. Fluorescein video-angiogram of three capillary tubes. Each contains the same concentration of fluorescein, dissolved in buffered saline, plasma, or whole blood.

Artefacts

Specular reflection of exciting light can overwhelm a barrier filter, giving highlights in angiographic images. Extravascular fluorescence may also arise when tissues, such as sclera (see Fig. 8(a,b)) and lens (see Fig. 1(c)), themselves fluoresce (autofluorescence). Both specular reflexes and autofluorescence can be seen in control frames and remain equally bright throughout a study.

Certain structures, such as corneal infiltrates, reflect fluorescence generated elsewhere in the eye (pseudofluorescence). Such fluorescence increases throughout a study, as the source fluorescence brightens, and its interpretation is often problematic.

Blood or pigment mask fluorescence. The masking of scleral autofluorescence by overlying vessels can be valuable for demonstrating vascular anatomy in the control frames of an angiogram (see Fig. 8). By contrast, masking by pigment frequently interferes with iris fluorescein angiograms and these must always be interpreted in conjunction with corresponding colour photographs.

Timing

A bolus of fluorescein is introduced intravenously, creating an advancing dye front, which demonstrates a single cycle of the circulation. Since the entire globe and the anterior conjunctiva are supplied by the ophthalmic artery, differences in circulation time within the orbit are represented by variations in the timing of first fluorescence in different perfusion fields. However, the timing of arteriovenous transit and leakage are unique to each lobule of the microcirculation and are calculated from the first appearance of dye.

Normal blood flow

The interpretation of anterior segment angiograms demands an understanding of normal anterior ocular blood flow, particularly interarterial and intervenous communications.

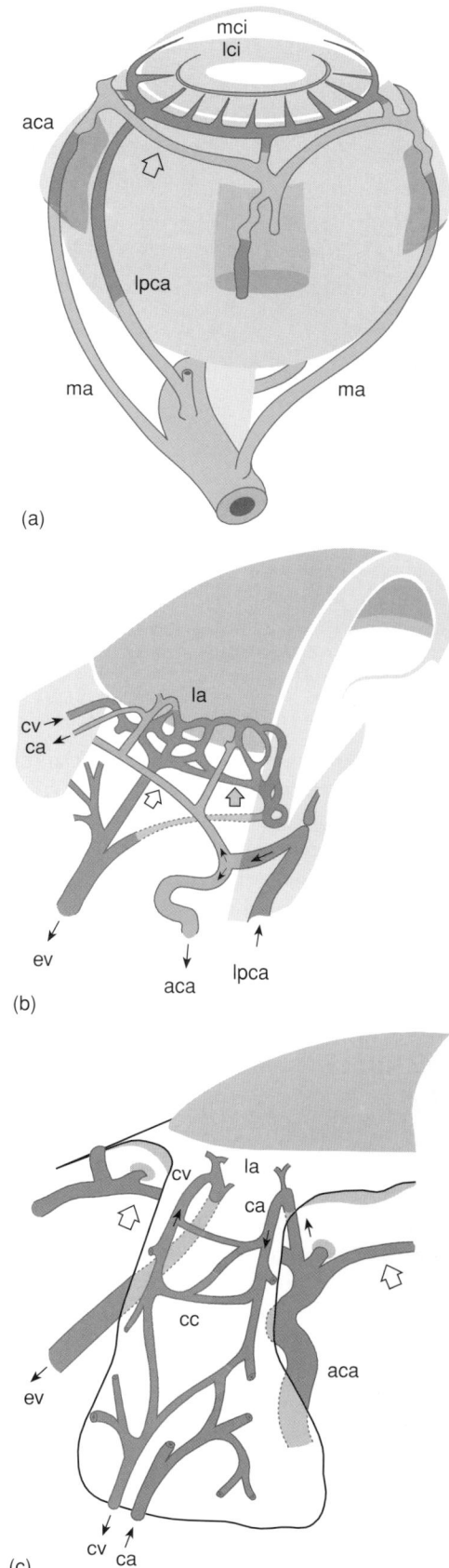

Fig. 5 Blood supply of the ocular anterior segment (see text and Tables 1, 2, and 3): (a) delivery. (b) distribution to episclera and limbus.(c) Distribution to conjunctiva.

Table 1 Haemoglobin video imaging (Figs 5(a–c), 6(a–d))

Small arteries (eg. aca, eac)	Tortuous. Homogeneous blood column (Fig. 6(a,b))
Terminal arterioles	Straight. High velocity, flow often pulsatile
Capillaries (cc)	Erythrocytes transmitted singly or in convoys (Fig. 6(b)). Intermittent flow
Small collecting venules (cv)	Erythrocytes aggregate. Halting or periodic flow (Fig. 6(b))
Limbal arcades (la)	Blood delivered to apices by fine arterioles from anterior roots of eac. Erythrocytes aggregate in venules which drain into the lvc (Fig. 6(c))
Limbal venous circle ((lvc; ♦)	Erythrocyte aggregation inconstant. Flow direction may reverse as pressure gradients between collecting veins change
Episcleral collecting veins (ev)	Laminar flow. If aqueous is carried, this flows in a discrete lamina, within or at the edge of the blood column (Fig. 6(d))

Table 2 Fluorescein angiography of conjunctiva and episclera (Figs 5(a–c), 7, 8, 9)

Anterior ciliary arteries (aca)	Radial. Tortuous. 50–100um diameter. Fill from scleral perforators or over muscle insertions. May flow away from, or towards, the limbus. Rapid flow (<100mm/s). Well-defined front of uniform fluorescence. Empty to leave a dark centre and marginal fluorescence. No leakage
Episcleral arterial circle (eac; ♀)	Circumferential arterioles, close to the limbus (Figs. 7, 8). Interarterial communications between adjacent ACAs are seen as pulsating non-fluoresceinated blood columns, which fill late (Fig. 9). Fine anterior roots supply the conjunctival arterioles and limbal arcades (Fig. 8). No leakage
Anterior conjunctival arterioles (ca)	Fine, recurrent, radial vessels. Arise from anterior roots of eac and loop back at the limbal reflection of conjunctiva. Homogeneous fluorescence with sharp dye front: flow away from limbus (Fig. 7). Gradually become submerged in extravascular fluorescence. No leakage
Conjunctival capillaries (cc)	Branching, lace-like network, arrayed between radial arterioles and venules. Become submerged in extravascular fluorescence. Multifocal leakage
Anterior conjunctival venules (cv)	Radial. Usually flow towards the limbus. Granular masking of fluorescence by aggregated erythrocytes, particularly when flow is slow. Multifocal leakage
Limbal arcades (la)	Delicate, circumferential microcirculation in peripheral cornea, but often incomplete in horizontal meridian. Visible throughout study. No leakage
Limbal venous circle (lvc)	Single or duplicate, circumferential channels. Receive blood from conjunctival venules and limbal arcades. Fluorescence usually homogeneous, but may show granular masking. No leakage
Episcleral collecting veins (ev)	Rapid venous flow. No granular masking. No leakage
Posterior conjunctival circulation	Arteriovenous loops, derived from the posterior tarsal circulation. They serve the posterior bulbar conjunctiva, out of phase with the anterior circulation. Rapid arterial flow. No leakage from arteries or veins

Table 3 Fluorescein angiography of iris (Figs 5(a), 10)

Major circle (mci)	Circumferential vessels close to iris root. Normally hidden behind limbus, but short arcs sometimes visible. Brisk, uniform fluorescence. Gives rise to long and short radial arteries (Fig. 10(a))
Long radial arteries (l)	Radial vessels, supplying the circulation of the sphincter (Fig. 10(a)). Pass directly, branching little, to a site close to the pupil, where they join, forming the lesser circle (Fig. 10(c)). The timing of their fluorescence may vary by up to 10 s in different sectors of iris
Short radial arteries (s)	Vascular loops arising from the major circle of iris (Fig. 10(a)). Supply peripheral iris
Lesser circle (lci)	Arterial circle (sometimes incomplete), formed from circumferential branches of long radial iris arteries. Supplies iris sphincter and some recurrent vessels to the dilator muscle (Fig. 10(b, c))
Iris veins	Long, straight centrifugal vessels, passing radially or obliquely from central iris. Discrete from the long radial arteries. May drain the lesser circle directly (Fig. 10(c))

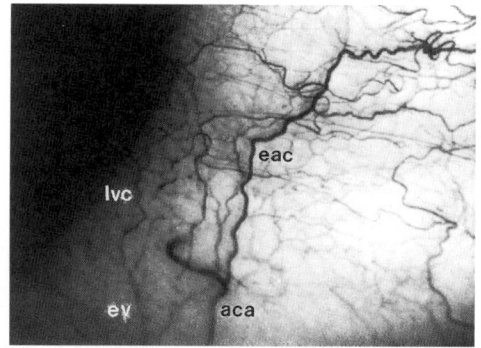

(a)

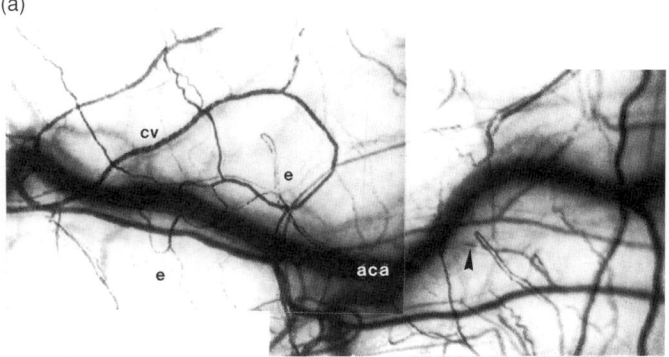

(b)

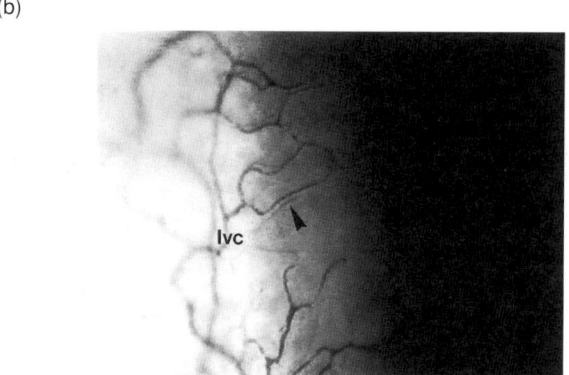

(c)

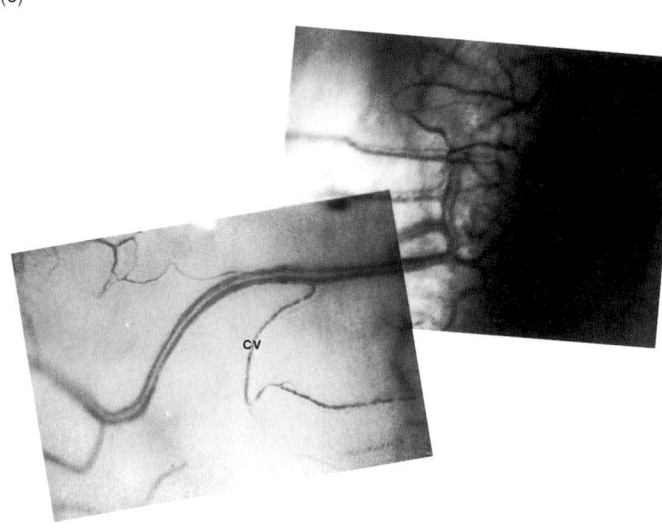

(d)

Interarterial communications (Fig. 5(a-c))

Blood is delivered to the anterior segment of the eye from the ophthalmic artery by two routes. On the surface of the globe, the muscular arteries (ma) continue as anterior ciliary arteries (aca), which join to form the episcleral arterial circle (eac; ↻). Within the globe, the medial and lateral long posterior ciliary arteries (lpca) pass forward in the suprachoroidal space to supply the major circle of the iris (mci). The episcleral arterial circle and major circle of the iris are joined by arteries which perforate the sclera, completing trans-scleral arcades: the sagittal arterial ring.

Blood is distributed to the conjunctival, limbal, and episcleral circulations on the anterior surface of the globe by the episcleral arterial circle (eac: ↻), and to the iris, ciliary body, ciliary processes, and anterior choroid by the major and lesser circles of the iris (mci, lci).

These circulations form a network of axial and circumferential interarterial communications, throughout which blood flow can freely reverse. There is also arterial continuity between the anterior and posterior conjunctival circulations (Fig. 5(c)) making this a site of internal–external carotid communication.

Intervenous communications (Fig. 5(b, c))

The venous equivalent of the episcleral arterial circle is the circumferential limbal venous circle (lvc; ◆), which receives venules draining the anterior conjunctiva and limbal arcades and freely redistributes venous blood from one sector of the globe to another. It drains into radial episcleral collecting veins (ev), the superior and inferior ophthalmic veins and the cavernous sinus.

Posterior conjunctival veins join the posterior tarsal circulation, which drains into the facial and external jugular systems. Venous continuity across the conjunctival watershed (Fig. 5(c)) makes this a site of internal–external jugular communication.

Angiographic characteristics (Tables 1, 2, 3)

Pathological blood flow

(The preferred method for demonstrating each sign is shown in parentheses.)

General

Inflammation

In inflamed microcirculations, capillary and venular dilation, and the disruption of endothelial tight junctions, are followed

Fig. 6 Haemoglobin video imaging. (a) Inferonasal limbus (low magnification): eac: episcleral arterial circle; aca: anterior ciliary artery; lvc: limbal venous circle; ev: episcleral collecting vein. (b) Conjunctival circulation, 5 mm behind left temporal limbus: aca: anterior ciliary artery; (◆): fusiform bolus of erythrocytes within arteriole. e: fragmentation of capillary blood column into individual erythrocytes; cv: erythrocyte aggregation in collecting venule. (c) Normal limbus: arrow: boluses of erythrocytes pulsed to apices of limbal arcades. lvc: limbal venous circle. (d) Laminar flow in an aqueous vein: erythrocytes entering an episcleral vein from a conjunctival vein (cv) join the peripheral lamina of blood.

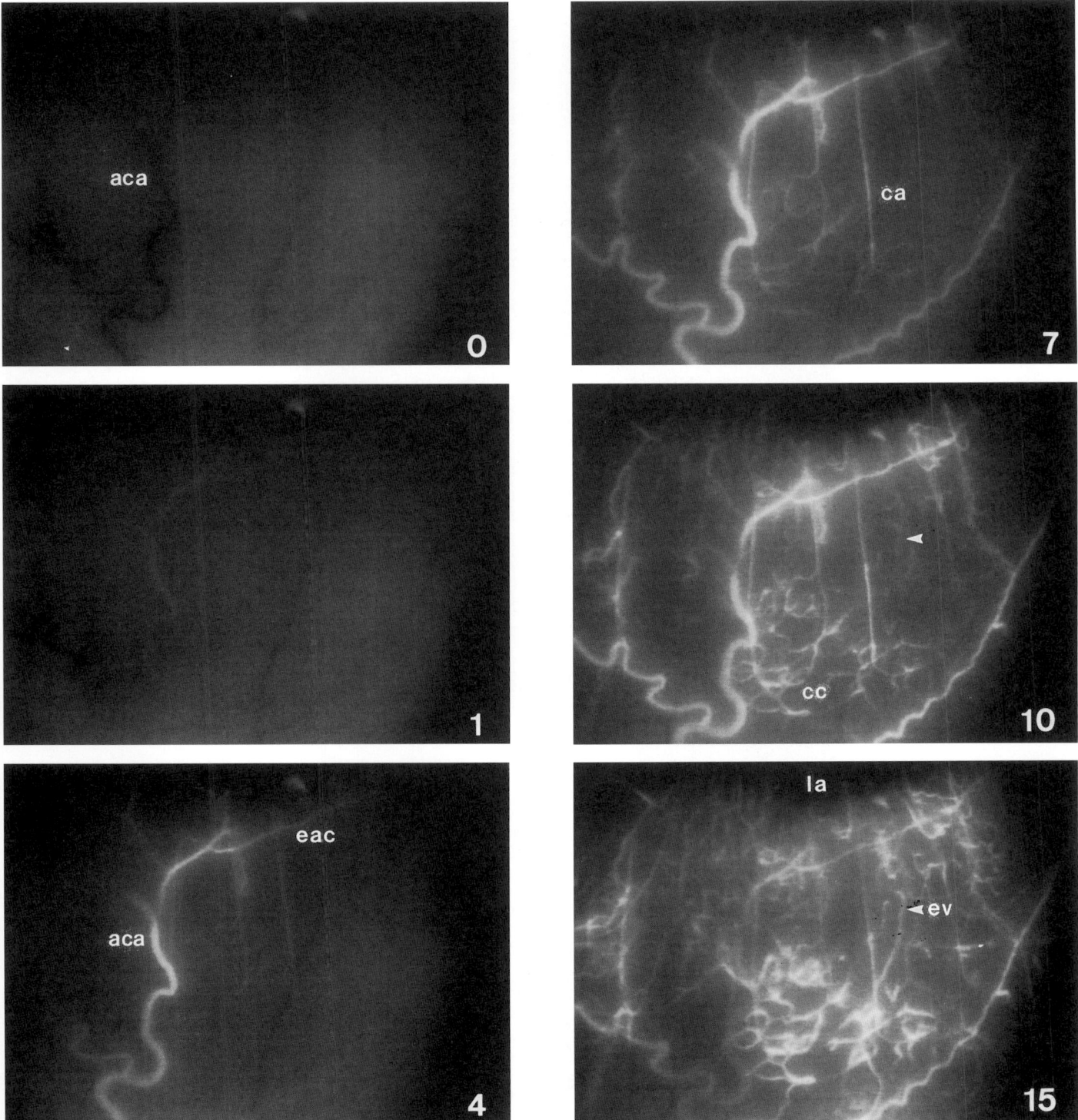

Fig. 7 Normal low-dose fluorescein videoangiogram (timings in seconds). An anterior ciliary artery (aca) fills from a trans-scleral perforating artery close to the limbus and feeds the episcleral arterial circle (eac). This gives anterior roots, which pass forward to the reflection of conjunctiva, supplying conjunctival arterioles (ca) and the limbal arcades (la). Conjunctival capillaries (cc) leak fluorescein about 4 s after they perfuse. An episcleral vein (ev ◆) flows away from the limbus late in the angiogram.

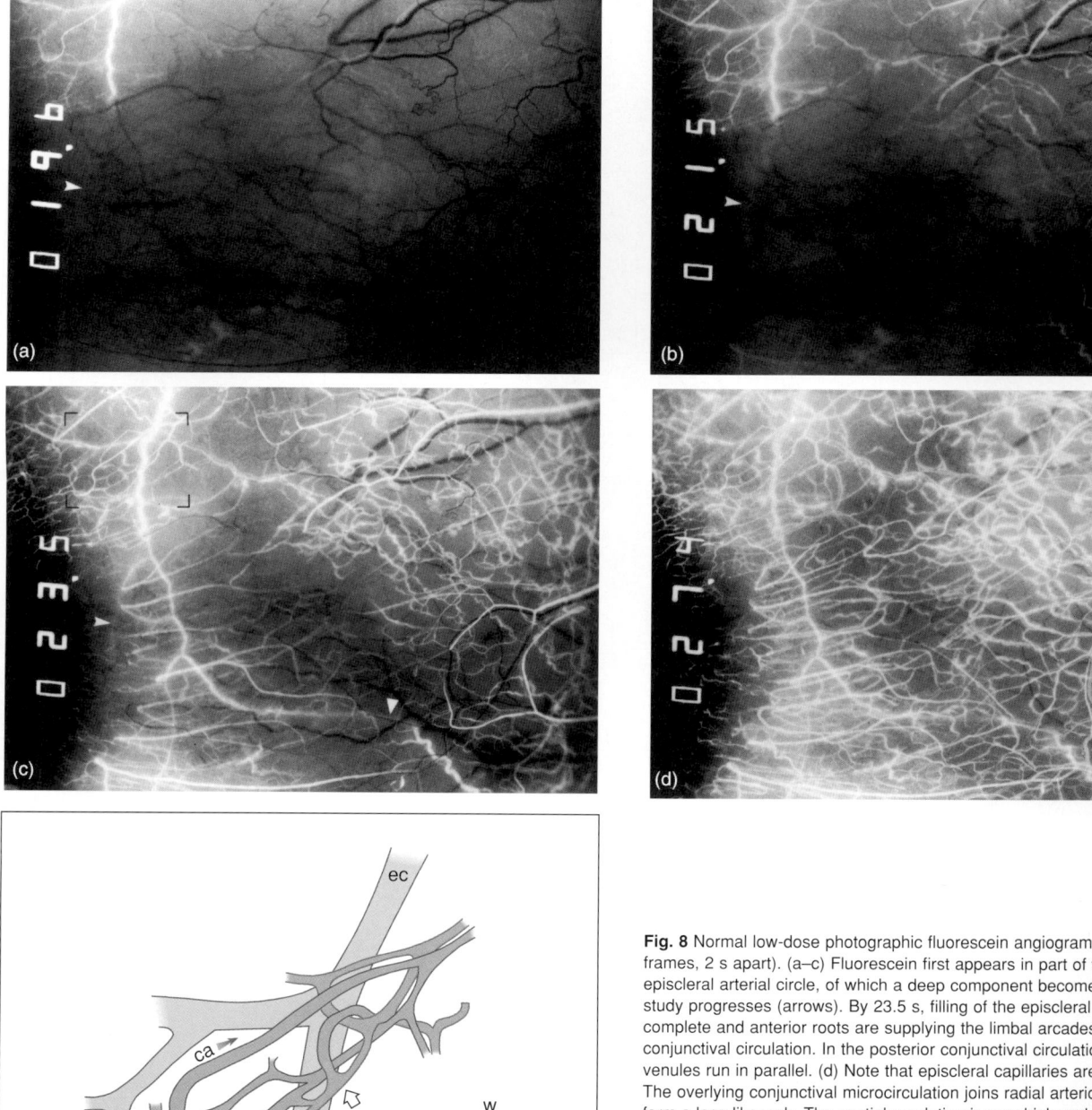

Fig. 8 Normal low-dose photographic fluorescein angiogram (consecutive frames, 2 s apart). (a–c) Fluorescein first appears in part of the anterior episcleral arterial circle, of which a deep component becomes visible as the study progresses (arrows). By 23.5 s, filling of the episcleral arterial circle is complete and anterior roots are supplying the limbal arcades and anterior conjunctival circulation. In the posterior conjunctival circulation, arterioles and venules run in parallel. (d) Note that episcleral capillaries are arrayed in a net. The overlying conjunctival microcirculation joins radial arterioles and venules to form a lace-like web. The spatial resolution is very high and fluorescein leakage from capillaries never obscures vascular detail. (e) Diagrammatic representation of area bracketed in Fig. 8(c). Close to the limbal reflection of conjunctiva, lie small arteriovenous communications (◊) which divert blood from the anterior conjunctival circulation. This explains why anterior conjunctival venules may fill before capillaries. ec = episcleral arterial circle; ca = conjunctival arteriole; cv = conjunctival venule; w = watershed between anterior and posterior conjunctival circulations.

by hypoperfusion due to endothelial oedema. This sequence of events can be staged by anterior segment vascular imaging: the early events are described here; the late stages under 'ischaemia'.

Slit lamp examination and *HVI* demonstrate increased capillary, venular and venous calibre, and tortuosity. On account of the greater volume and velocity of blood, the erythrocyte aggregation which normally characterizes venules is reduced or absent. At the apices of affected limbal arcades, characteristic opalescent subepithelial halos form, which rapidly evolve into dense, yellow deposits (Fig. 11(a)). These become crystalline in appearance as they resolve (Fig. 11(b)).

Fluorescein angiography shows rapid arteriovenous transit, with intense, early leakage of the dye from capillaries and venules (Fig. 12). The normally competent limbal arcades leak fluorescein into the peripheral cornea. When iris vessels are damaged, the surrounding stroma develops a bright, fluorescent glow.

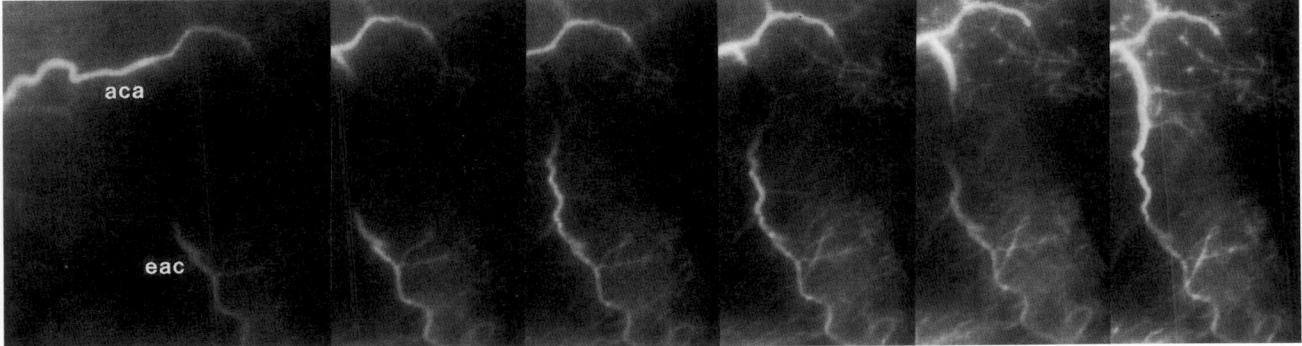

Fig. 9 The episcleral arterial circle (eac) receives blood from two adjacent anterior ciliary arteries, of which one is shown (aca). The intervening blood column pulsates and drifts to and fro, before fluorescing late in the angiogram. (Images captured at 2-s intervals.)

Ischaemia

Conjunctiva and sclera

The vascular communications in the anterior segment of the globe are so extensive that arterial or venous closure is usually followed, not by ischaemia, but by the redirection of blood flow. After anterior ciliary artery occlusion, the episcleral arterial circle fills from an adjacent artery, or by reversed flow through the sagittal arterial ring (ASFA). Similarly, episcleral venous closure diverts blood through the limbal venous circle to an adjacent episcleral collecting vein, or into the conjunctival circulation (SL, HVI). Therefore, most cases of capillary closure result from direct inflammatory or chemical insults.

Slit lamp examination and *haemoglobin video imaging* show oedema of vessel walls and surrounding tissue; and haemorrhages, particularly where venous flow has been interrupted. Erythrocytes aggregate within venules and small veins and may remain static for days or weeks (see Figs 17, 20). New haemorrhages can accompany re-perfusion.

At *fluorescein angiography* the episcleral arterial circle, being an arcade, fills normally from any undamaged contributing vessels. Perfusion of the affected microcirculation is absent or delayed (see Fig. 16). When capillaries and venules do perfuse, there is brisk fluorescein leakage with staining of sclera, and plasma between the aggregated erythrocytes in venules fluoresces intensely. Both ASFA and HVI may also show impaired venous return, with erythrocyte aggregates persisting into episcleral collecting veins (see Fig. 20).

Iris

Closure of anterior or long posterior ciliary arteries is followed by the immediate redistribution of iris blood flow through the major or lesser circles (iris FA). The affected sector fills with delay and remote sectors may also perfuse slowly due to arterial steal (Fig. 13). After a recovery phase, the major circle adapts to accommodate the shunted blood, and flow through the lesser circle returns to normal.

When iris vessels become inflamed, iris FA shows paravascular hyperfluorescence, with fluorescein staining of iris stroma. There may also be accelerated leakage of fluorescein from the ciliary apparatus into the anterior chamber, with obscuration of vascular detail.

Neovascularization

Whether as a complication of inflammatory disease or during the resolution of ischaemia, the earliest stage of neovascular budding is represented by a delicate, refractile tube, contiguous with a pre-existing venule (SL: bright field retroillumination). Solitary erythrocytes are frequently trapped at the apices of such vessels (SL, HVI) and these become mobile as circulation is established. All immature new vessels leak fluorescein and fluorescein angiography shows bright, focal hyperfluorescence, with spreading, dense staining of surrounding tissues (Fig. 14).

As neovascular circulations mature, they gradually acquire the leakage characteristics of the tissues in which they lie (Fig. 14).

Pathological blood flow

Specific

Conjunctiva and sclera

Scleral inflammatory disease

Scleritis is associated with a spectrum of vascular damage, from mild inflammation of superficial scleral circulations to closure of large sectors of the scleral blood supply. By defining the nature and distribution of this damage, anterior segment vascular imaging may be used to stage the disease.

Episcleritis/diffuse scleritis (inflammation) (Fig. 12(a, b)) There is dilation of the circulations of Tenon's capsule/superficial sclera. Capillaries, venules, and veins are engorged, dilated and convoluted, and there is loss of erythrocyte aggregation in venules (SL, HVI). Arteriovenous transit is very rapid compared with control circulations in the same eye and leakage of fluorescein from capillaries and venules is intense and almost instantaneous (<4 s: ASFA). Treatment completely reverses these changes (Fig. 12).

Nodular/necrotizing scleritis (arteriovenous shunts and capillary closure) (Fig. 15) Surrounding an area of diffuse scleritis, dilated arteriovenous communications form (pulsatile reversal of blood flow: SL, HVI; perfusion of veins before surrounding capillaries: ASFA), and the affected sclera

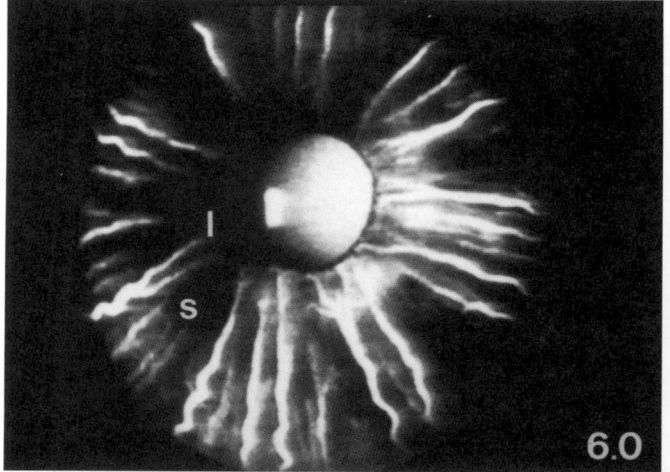

(a)

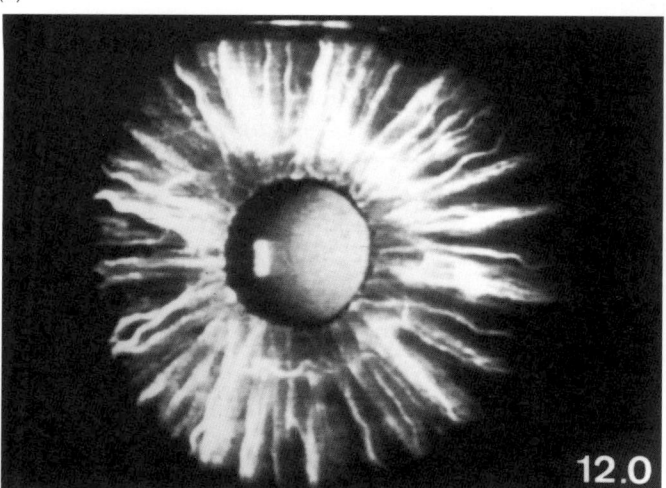

(b)

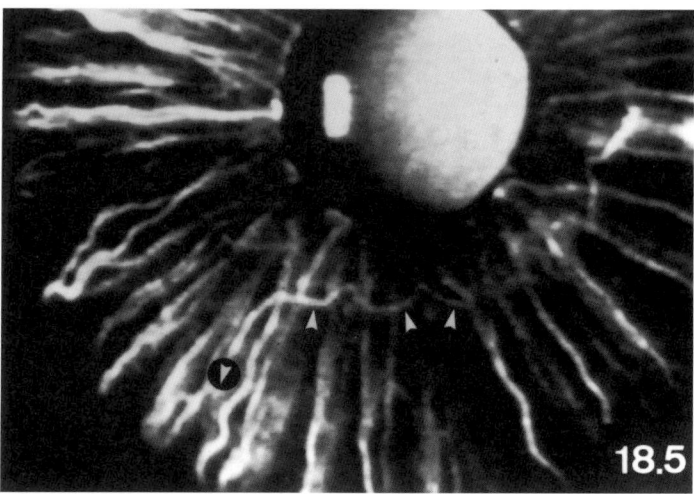

(c)

Fig. 10 Normal iris fluorescein videoangiogram (timed in seconds after first flush of fluorescence). (a) Arterial flow: long (l) and short (s) radial arteries, both arising from the major arterial circle, flow simultaneously in each sector. However, up to 10 s may separate perfusion of different sectors. (b) Capillary phase. (c) Arrows show the lesser arterial circle, and its drainage into a radial iris vein.

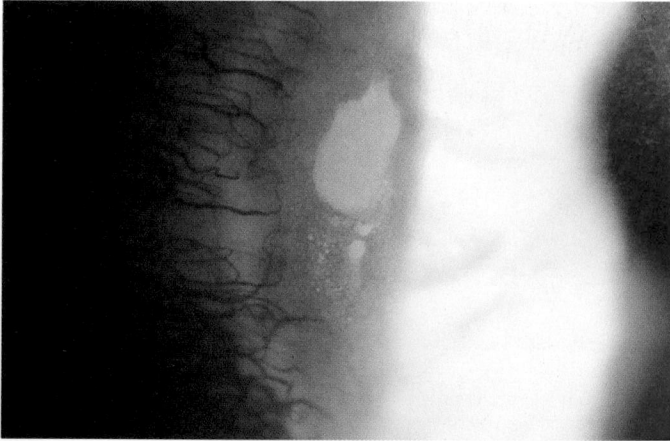

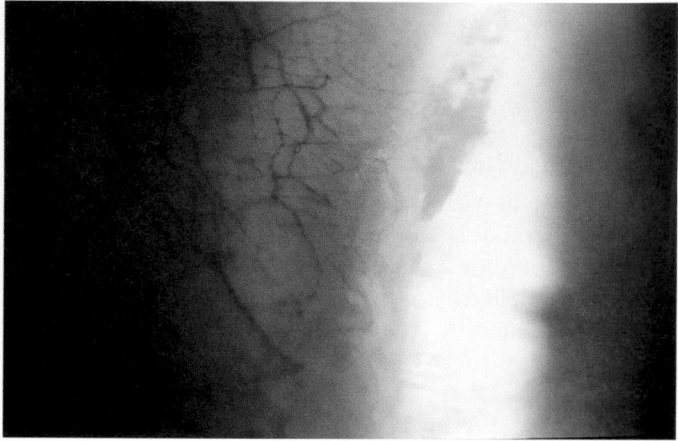

Fig. 11 Subepithelial corneal infiltrates at the apices of the limbal arcades in different subjects with systemic vasculitis: (a) acute (< 24 h), (b) resolving (16 months).

becomes oedematous (SL) and hypoperfused (ASFA). The vascular reorganization is permanent.

Necrotizing scleritis/scleral sequestra (non-perfusion) (Fig. 16) Within an area of scleritis, an island of sclera exhibits no blood flow (ASFA). It may accumulate mucus and discharge necrotic scleral debris (through breaches in ischaemic conjunctiva). Veins often remain engorged for long periods after they have ceased to flow and fluorescein angiography (ASFA) is necessary to establish non-perfusion.

Resolution As episcleritis and diffuse scleritis resolve, vascular tortuousity declines and there is normalization of capillary and venular flow (SL, HVI) and fluorescein leakage (ASFA). However, once arteriovenous communications have developed, circulations do not recover. The shunt vessels of nodular and necrotizing scleritis remain (SL, HVI, ASFA) and scleral necrosis resolves with neovascularization (ASFA).

Acid and alkali burns (Fig. 17)

Chemical injuries damage exposed microcirculations, but must be severe to harm the arcades of the episcleral arterial circle, which lie deep to the conjunctiva. At slit lamp microscopy, the affected conjunctival circulation may appear perfused, but

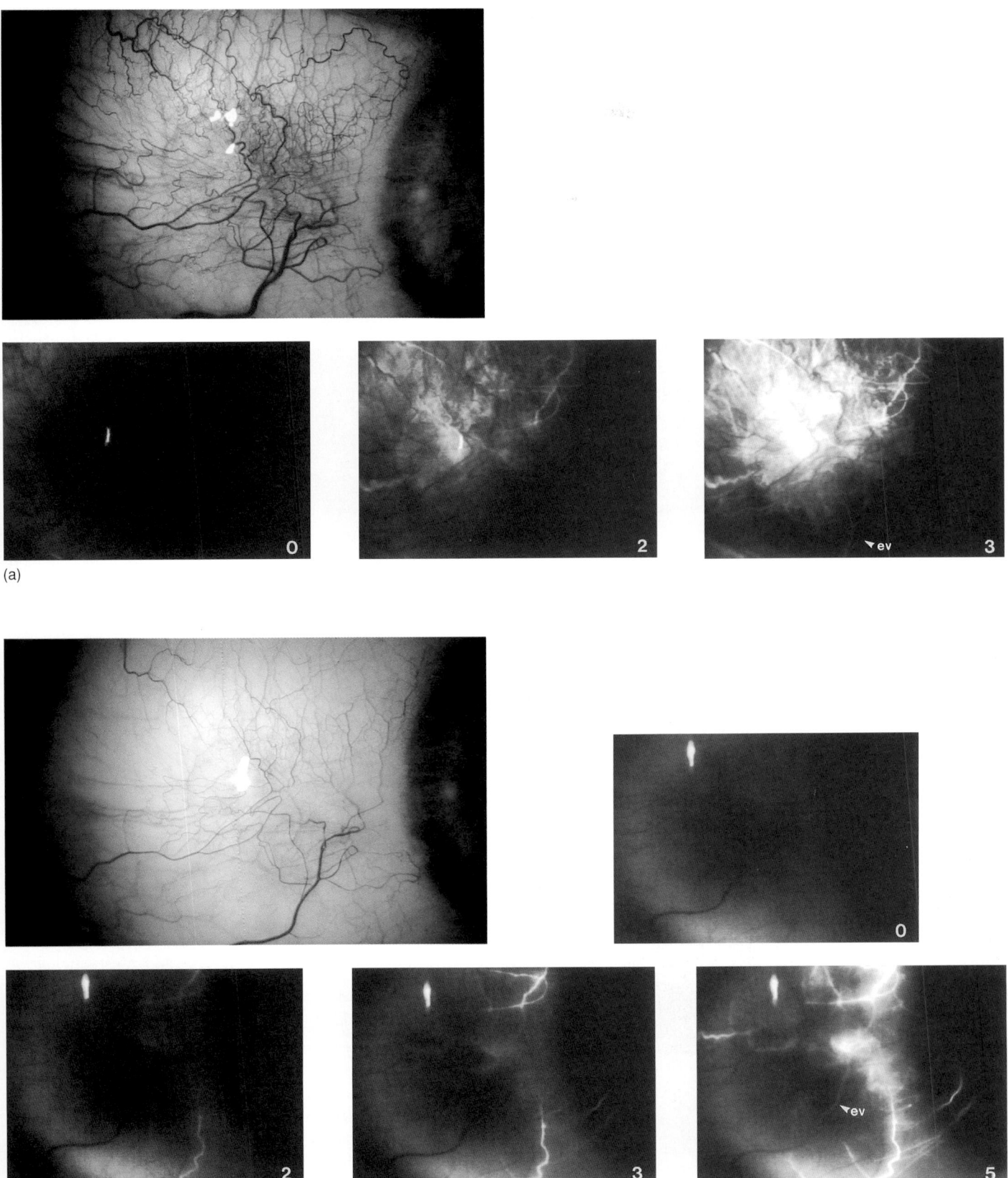

(a)

(b)

Fig. 12 Diffuse anterior scleritis in a 67-year-old woman: (a) Active: the scleritis is centred on a field of venous drainage (ev = episcleral vein). Angiography shows rapid arteriovenous transit and instantaneous fluorescein leakage from episcleral and conjunctival circulations. (b) The same field, 3 weeks after two intravenous injections of methylprednisolone, followed by oral prednisolone and cyclophosphamide: the location of her scleritis is marked by increased scleral translucency. Arteriovenous transit has slowed and capillary integrity is recovering. Normal vascular architecture is preserved. (Captured images timed in seconds after first flush of fluorescence.)

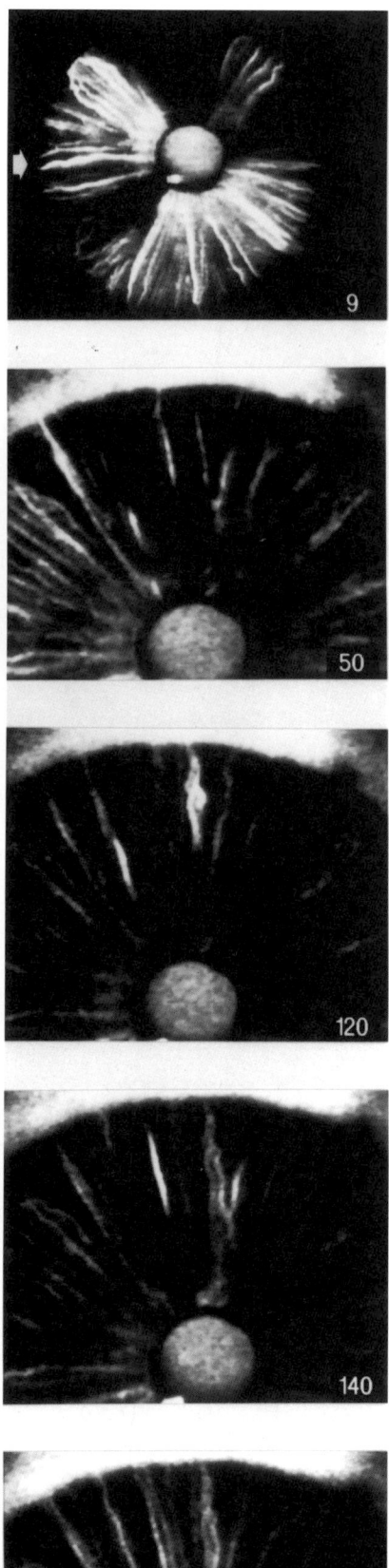

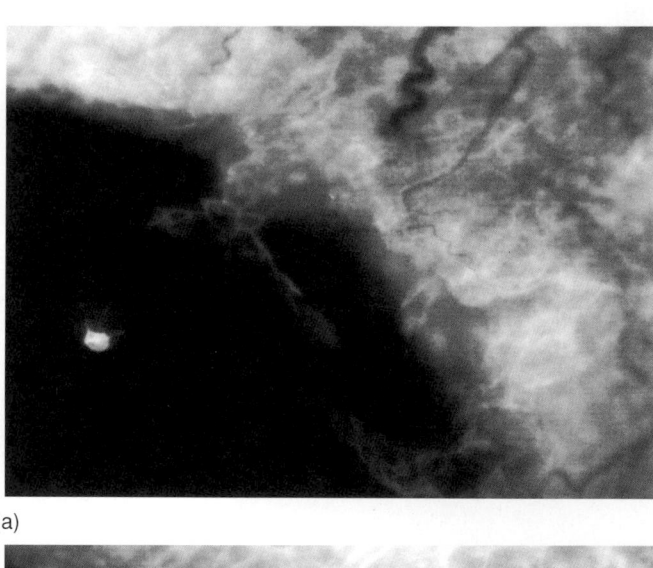

(a)

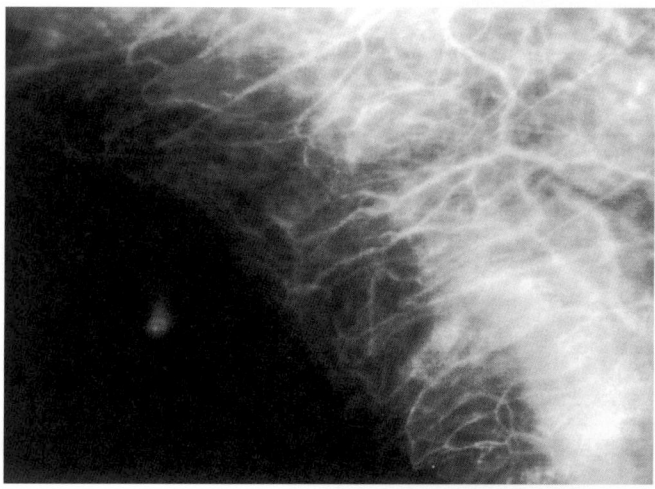

(b)

Fig. 13 Right intraoperative iris videoangiogram after clamping of lateral rectus (◆): Preoperatively, the inferolateral and superomedial sectors had filled last; however, surgical closure of the *lateral* anterior ciliary arterial supply delayed perfusion of *superior* iris. Iris blood flow returned to its preoperative state at 24 h. The most likely explanation is arterial steal, with diversion of blood from superior to lateral iris, through the major arterial circle. (Captured images timed in seconds after first flush of fluorescence.)

Fig. 14 Fluorescein videoangiography of right superonasal limbus in a 65-year-old woman with Wegener's granulomatosis: (a) Active disease: corneal and episcleral new vessels, showing local extravasation of dye. (b) Six months after control of her systemic disease with the humanized monoclonal antibody, CAMPATH 1H. A mature neovascular circulation forms a false limbus, from which fluorescein leakage into cornea is minimal. (Both images captured at 15 s after first flush of fluorescence.)

careful SL examination with a green filter, or HVI fail to demonstrate erythrocyte flow. Fluorescein angiography may confirm rapid perfusion of the episcleral arterial circle, but absent anterior conjunctival flow. The periphery of the lesion shows the characteristic features of inflammation.

Venous shunting
The venous communications between the anterior and posterior conjunctival circulations form a potential site for internal/

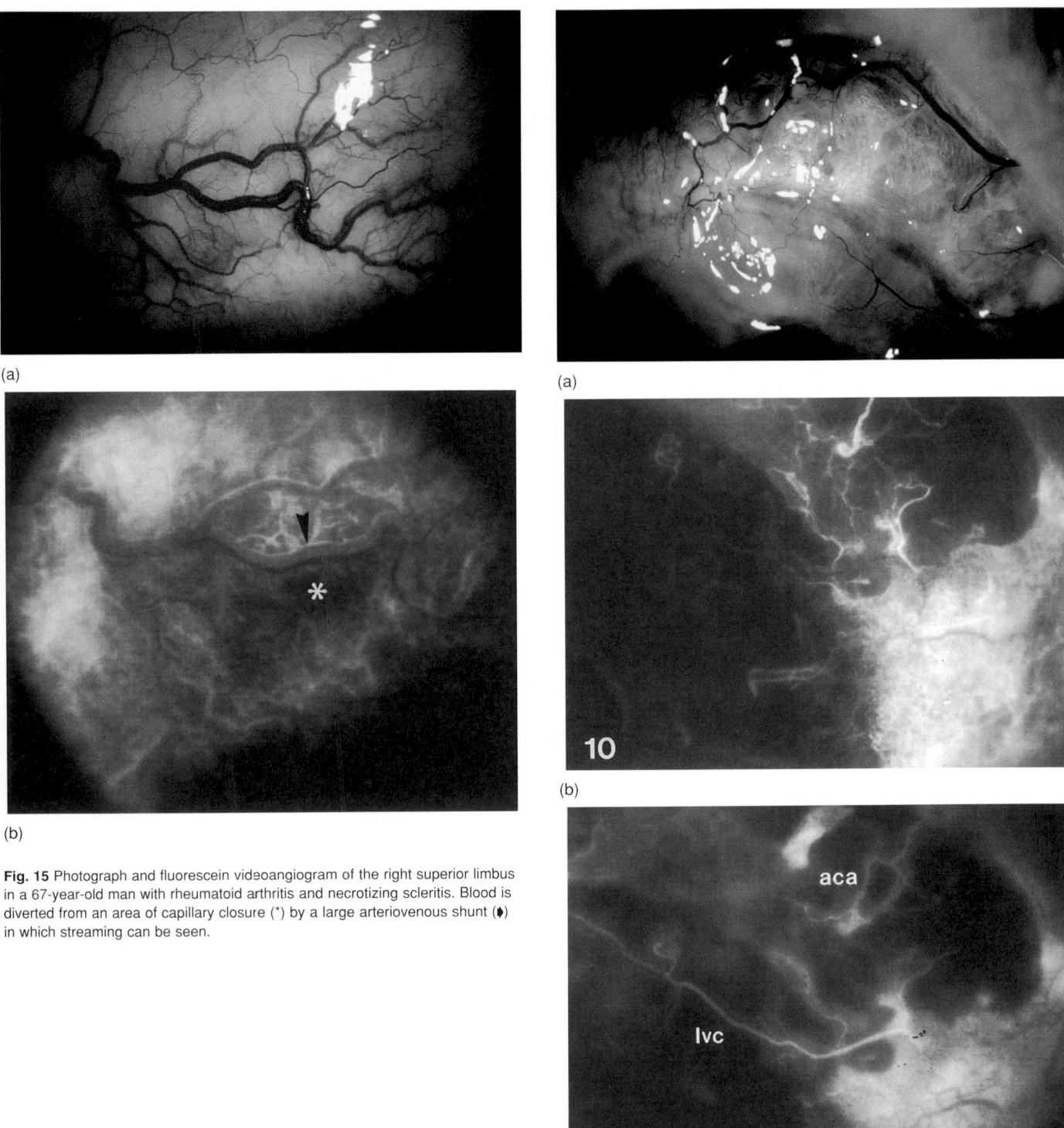

Fig. 15 Photograph and fluorescein videoangiogram of the right superior limbus in a 67-year-old man with rheumatoid arthritis and necrotizing scleritis. Blood is diverted from an area of capillary closure (*) by a large arteriovenous shunt (♦) in which streaming can be seen.

Fig. 16 Fluorescein videoangiogram from an 84-year-old woman with surgically-induced necrotizing sclerokeratitis, arising 5 months after a cataract extraction by phakoemulsification. The affected sclera fails to perfuse throughout the angiogram. There is, however, brisk perfusion of surrounding inflamed sclera and conjunctiva; and of scleral and corneal neovascular circulations, which leak progressively. Note that the anterior ciliary artery (aca) and limbal venous circle (lvc) serving this area are unscathed. (Captured images timed in seconds after first flush of fluorescence.)

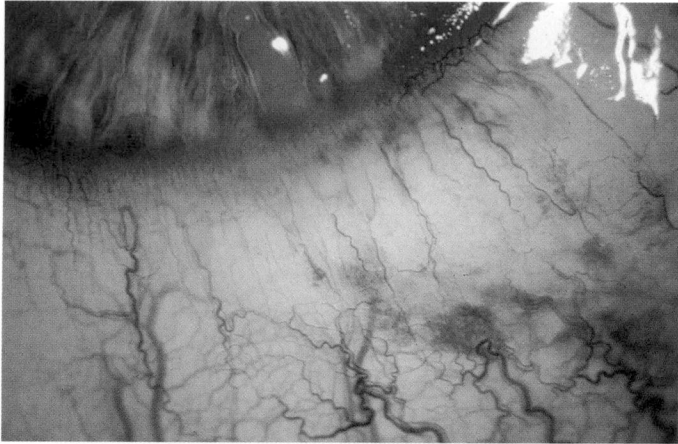

(a)

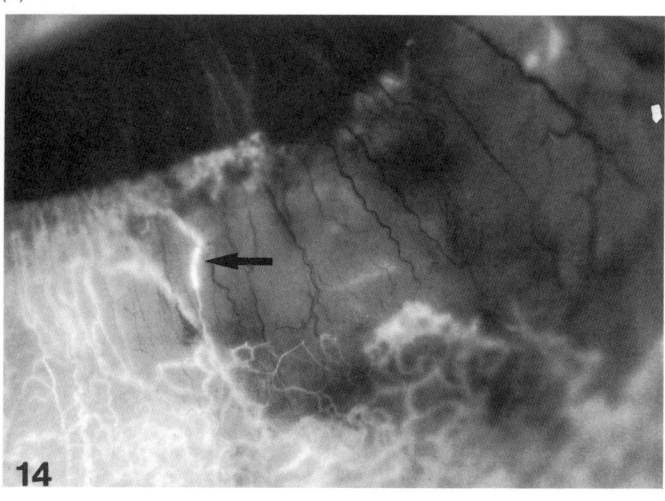

(b)

(c)

Fig. 17 Alkaline burn: photographic fluorescein angiogram. The colour photograph shows a pale area of conjunctiva and episclera, fringed with haemorrhage. Vessels within this zone appear intact. There is oedema of contiguous corneal epithelium. Fluorescein angiography shows conjunctival blood flow to be absent and the limbal arcades to be sparsely perfused. Nevertheless, blood flow in the episcleral arterial circle is just discernible (◊) and the clinical prognosis is, therefore, good. Note the brisk perfusion of surrounding inflamed circulations and leakage from a conjunctival vein at the edge of the burn (♦). (Images timed in seconds after first flush of fluorescence.)

external jugular shunting. This becomes manifest clinically when general or focal rises in orbital venous pressure occur (thyroid eye disease, orbital myositis, posterior scleritis, Wegener's granulomatosis, pseudotumours, lymphomas, and metastatic carcinoma). It also occurs in cases of raised cavernous sinus pressure (caroticocavernous fistulae and cavernous sinus thrombosis).

Blood from the anterior conjunctiva normally drains towards the limbal venous circle and into radial episcleral veins, the superior and inferior ophthalmic veins and the cavernous sinus. When orbital venous pressure rises, flow in episcleral veins is impeded (and may even reverse). The anterior conjunctival venules then drain away from the elevated pressure of the limbal venous circle and into the posterior conjunctival circulation (SL, HVI). It is reversal of blood flow in anterior conjunctival venules which is easiest to discern clinically (SL), since all radial anterior conjunctival vessels – arterioles and venules – now flow away from the limbus.

Iris

Rectus muscle surgery (iris FA)

The dual supply of the iris from the anterior and long posterior ciliary circulations, and the availability of circumferential shunting by the major and lesser arterial circles, explains its resilience to strabismus and retinal surgery. Fluorescein angio-

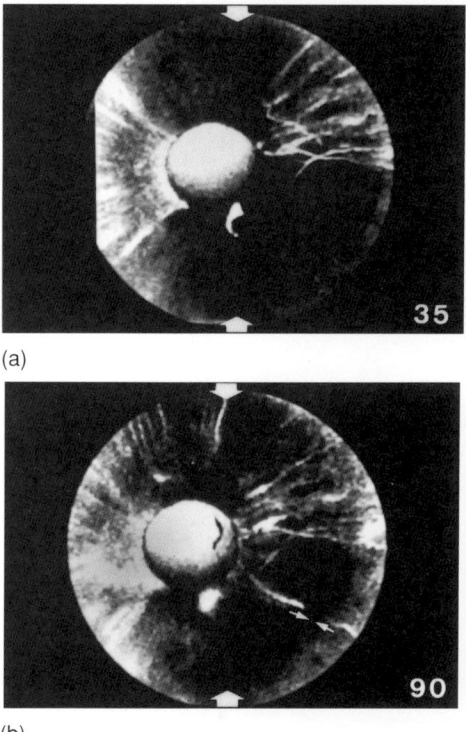

(a)

(b)

Fig. 18 Intraoperative fluorescein videoangiogram of the left iris during the clamping of both vertical rectus muscles (◊). Perfusion of superior and inferior iris is delayed and blood from adjacent iris reaches the affected inferior sector through the lesser arterial circle. The long radial artery, which delivers this blood retrogradely, shows convergence of opposing blood columns, with delayed fluorescence (arrows).

grams often show the filling of long radial arteries to be delayed in the sector(s) of iris corresponding with the transected muscle(s) (Fig. 18). Flow through adjacent or remote sectors may also be attenuated due to arterial steal (Fig. 13). Acutely, it is common for affected vessels to fill retrogradely, from the lesser arterial circle (Fig. 18); however, perfusion patterns usually normalize within 2 weeks.

Shunting through the MCI and LCI is usually effective through 90°, but may be inadequate for larger arcs. Therefore, damage to a horizontal rectus muscle and subjacent long posterior ciliary artery may be followed by iris ischaemia if the vertical anterior ciliary arteries are also cut. This risk cannot be predicted by patterns of iris blood flow in preoperative fluorescein angiograms.

Iritis or iris ischaemia? (iris FA)

In anterior uveitis, foci of perivenular iris hyperfluorescence are common and leakage of fluorescein from the ciliary apparatus into the anterior chamber rapidly obscures vascular detail. The technique becomes of clinical value when an alternative diagnosis of anterior segment ischaemia is suspected: the affected segment of iris then fails to perfuse or fills with a delay exceeding 10 s.

Abnormal circulations

Neovascularization

New vessels have uncharacteristic anatomy (SL) and leak fluorescein when immature (ASFA). In the iris, they grow over the pigmented epithelium; therefore, their fluorescence is less attenuated than the normal circulation.

Tumours

Tumour circulations have all the characteristics of immature new vessels and there is clear demarcation from adjacent, competent vessels. Pigmented melanomas intensely absorb exciting and fluorescent radiation; however, leakage still occurs, and late frames of an angiogram can be used to demonstrate the true extent of infiltration of surrounding tissue.

Vascular anomalies

These are usually convoluted, with arteriovenous transit times similar to parallel, normal circulations. They have the leakage characteristics of the surrounding mature blood vessels.

Iris arteriovenous malformations arising at the pupil margin (Cobb's tufts), are not covered by pigmented epithelium, and fluoresce with particular intensity.

Planning of corneoscleral surgery

The success of complex corneoscleral surgery may depend upon careful, preoperative appraisal of disease activity. After necrotizing sclerokeratitis, reconstructive surgery should be delayed until inflammatory activity has been controlled, in order to minimize the risk of recurrent collagen melting. This activity is best demonstrated by ASFA.

Pre- or intraoperative ASFA and HVI can also be used to select vessels which are to be preserved at surgery,

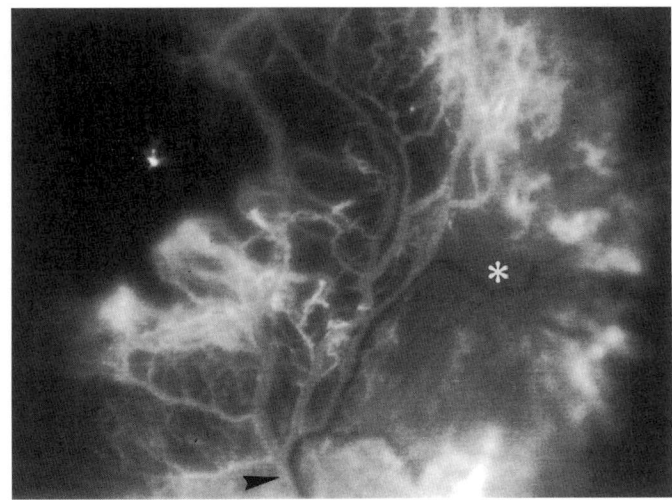

Fig. 19 Corneoscleral fluorescein videoangiogram of a 57-year-old man, 15 years after an alkali burn and immediately prior to corneal grafting. The study was performed to identify venous drainage from a conjunctival stem cell allograft (*); particularly, to learn whether a large vein (◊) merited preservation at surgery. ASFVA showed that this vessel carried the graft's entire venous outflow. A potential collateral circulation was identified superior to the graft; however, the vein in question was preserved, since perfusion of the graft was critically slow and may not have survived a further fall in the pressure gradient across it.

particularly when the perfusion of a tissue is known to be critical (Fig. 19).

The conjunctiva in systemic disease

The conjunctival microcirculation shows little specialization and may be considered to be a visible sample of many hidden microcirculations elsewhere in the body. Anterior ciliary arteries become attenuated in atheroma and systemic sclerosis (SL, HVI, ASFA). Wegener's granulomatosis, microvascular polyarteritis, and rheumatoid vasculitis may all be associated with the aggregation of erythrocytes into particularly large particles, which interfere with arteriovenous transit (SL, HVI, ASFA) (Fig. 20). In these, and other vasculitic diseases, fluorescein angiograms may show foci of intense leakage from small arterioles or venules. Individual limbal arcades can become involved, and subepithelial corneal infiltrates form at their apices (SL, ASFA) (Fig. 11(a, b)).

Summary

The anterior segment circulations are best studied by slit lamp examination, haemoglobin video imaging and fluorescein angiography in combination. Slit lamp examination and haemoglobin video imaging characterize the flow of erythrocytes and their interactions with each other and with vessel walls throughout the circulatory cycle. As fluorescein angiography demonstrates a circulation, the advancing dye front also times blood flow and tests vascular integrity.

Interpretation of angiograms requires a clear understanding of anterior segment vascular patterns and of actual and potential vascular communications.

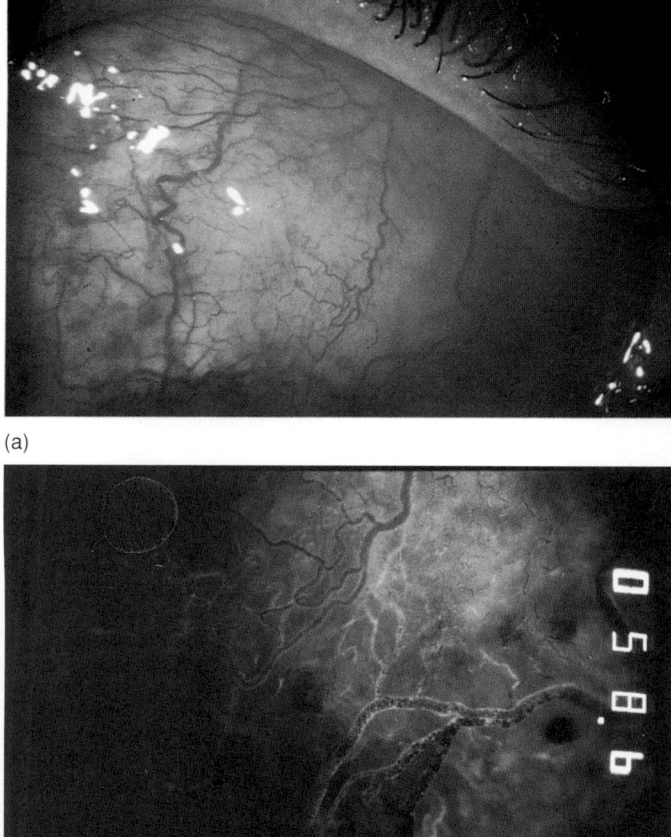

(a)

(b)

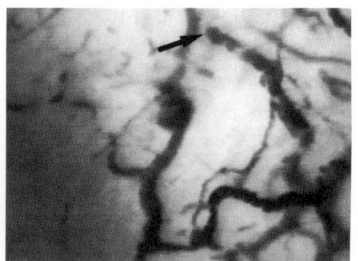

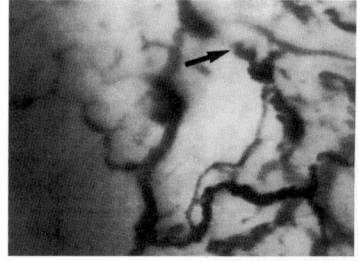

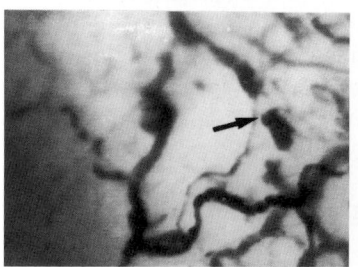

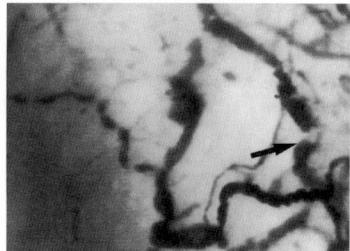

(c)

Fig. 20 Active systemic Wegener's granulomatosis in a 54-year-old man: (a) Anterior scleritis. There is multifocal scleral thickening and disorganization of the limbus. The conjunctiva and episclera are studded with small haemorrhages from damaged venules. (b) Photographic fluorescein angiogram. An episcleral collecting vein shows marginal hyperfluorescence and masking of the blood column by erythrocyte aggregates. Conjunctival haemorrhages mask episcleral fluorescence. (c) Haemoglobin video imaging of the conjunctival circulation in the same subject. Erythrocytes in venules collect into large aggregates, which impede blood flow. (Arrows indicate the trailing edge of such an aggregate.) (Images captured at 3-s intervals.)

These techniques have particular value when investigating inflammatory eye disease, anterior segment ischaemia, abnormal circulations, and raised orbital venous pressure. They can also assist with the diagnosis of systemic microcirculatory disorders.

Further reading

Hayreh, S.S. and Scott, W.E. (1978). Fluorescein iris angiography I: normal pattern. *Archives of Ophthalmology*, **96**, 1383–9.

Hayreh, S.S. and Scott, W.E.(1978). Fluorescein iris angiography II: disturbances in iris circulation following operation on the various recti. *Archives of Ophthalmology*, **96**, 1390–400.

Henkind, P., Hansen, R.I., and Szalay, J. (1979). Ocular circulation. In *Physiology of the human eye and visual system. Biomedical Foundations of Ophthalmology* (ed. T.D. Duane and E.A. Haeger), vol. 2 ,ch. 5, pp.1– 54. Harper and Row, Hagerstown.

Meyer, P.A.R. and Watson, P.G. (1987). Low dose fluorescein angiography of the conjunctiva and episelera. *British Journal of Ophthalmology*, **71**, 2–10.

Meyer, P.A.R. (1988). Patterns of blood flow in episcleral vessels studied by low-dose fluorescein videoangiography. *Eye*: **2**, 533–46.

Meyer, P.A.R. (1989). The circulation of the human limbus. *Eye*, **3**, 121–7.

Morrison, J.C. and van Buskirk, E.M. (1983). Anterior collateral circulation in the primate eye. *Ophthalmology*, **90**, 707–15.

1.6.9 Visual electrodiagnosis (diagnostic psychophysiology)

Demetrios Papakostopoulos

Visual electrodiagnosis is a medical discipline enabling the application of the structural, functional, and psychophysical knowledge of the neurosciences to the clinical management of individual patients and clinical research, by providing objective and non-invasive quantification of function. The technical foundations of visual electrodiagnosis are based on the integration of electronic engineering, computer programming, statistics, and more recently telecommunications.

The primary variables investigated by visual electrodiagnosis are electrical fields or waves picked up at a distance from the area of their origin. The origin of these bioelectrical fields, related to the neurochemical and neurophysiological transactions underlying visual function, can be located in the depth of the eye or brain. The waves associated with these bioelectrical currents generated in the depth of the eye or brain are picked up by electrodes acting as small aerials attached to the face or scalp. The radio waves, for example, are generated by currents moving across the transmitter of a remote broadcasting station and picked up by the aerial of a radio.

In this chapter, the shape or waveform of each potential will be illustrated and described together with the methodology of recording and normative values. The origins of each potential and its relationship to anatomy, neurochemistry, and cellular biocurrents are discussed. This is followed by a review of the clinical and research applications of each potential, and its modifications, according to stimulus or environmental change.

The purpose of this chapter is to introduce the reader to the use of these waveforms as a tool to infer the state of the anatomical, histological, neurochemical, and neurophysiological background of the functioning visual system. Examples from clinical and research applications are used to explain the elements of visual electrodiagnosis.

Methodological issues

The instrumentation used in visual electrodiagnosis, the methodology of its application, and the results obtained are subject to many extensive publications (see reading list; for an in-depth analysis of principles and analytical techniques see Regan 1989).

The main elements needed for visual electrodiagnosis are amplifiers, stimulators, electrodes, and computers arranged in an environment which allow control of illumination and audiovisual contact with the individual under examination. Figure 1 shows the recording area of a laboratory. Figure 2 shows raw and processed data obtained during a typical recording. The top trace in Fig. 2 shows the output of the amplifier recorded on paper as a prolonged trace with deflections going

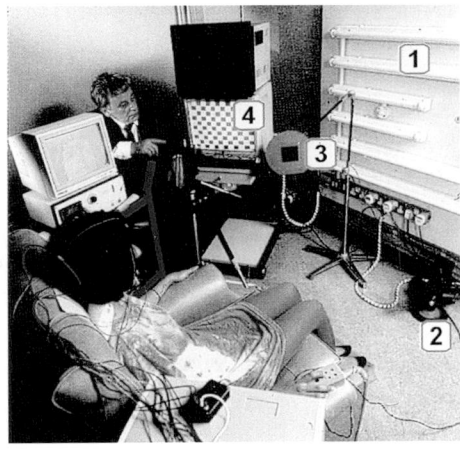

Fig. 1 The recording section of an electrodiagnostic centre. (1) The fluorescence lights used for electro-oculogram illumination are in front of the subject who is sitting in a comfortable chair listening to some instructions, with the scalp and face electrodes attached. (2) The infrared video camera monitors the subject in both light and dark from an adjacent room where the data are displayed and processed. (3) The flash stimulator. (4)The computer screen providing the pattern reversal visually evoked potential stimuli.

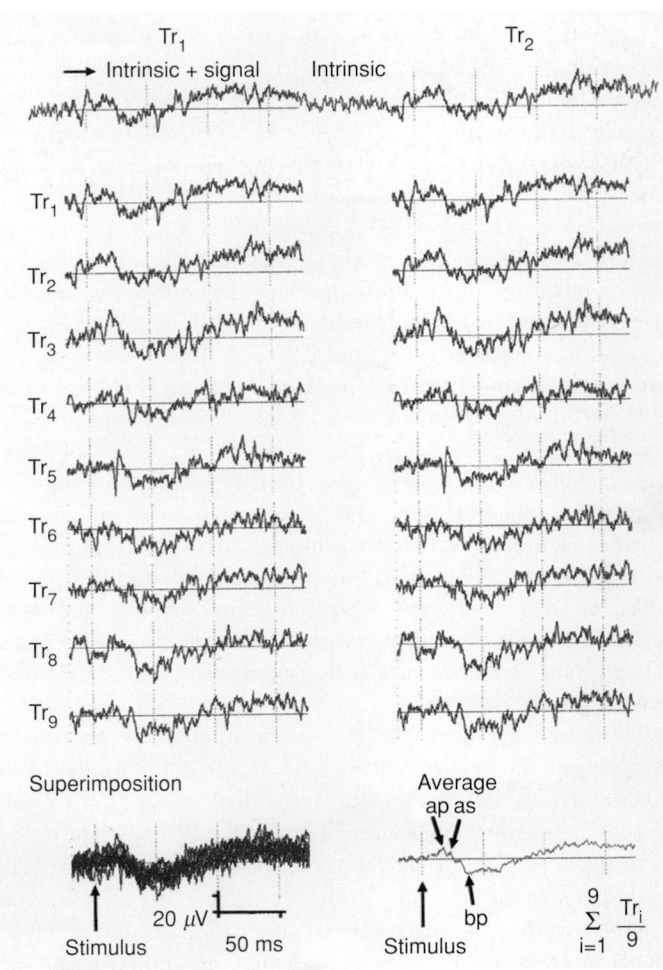

Fig. 2 Top trace: data of intrinsic bioelectrical signals containing activity (signal) due to stimulation. Traces Tr1 to Tr8: 200-ms sections of activity commencing 20 ms before stimulus presentation (arrow). The Tr1 to Tr8 sections are superimposed (last trace left) and averaged (last trace right).

up or down due to changes in the field potentials picked up (waves). The amplitude of these waves is usually very small, measured in microvolts (μV). The number of times that these deflections change direction determines their frequency. The trace can be seen to contain fast changing deflections and more slowly changing ones (fast and slow frequencies). Correct representation of the amplitude and the frequencies of an electrobiological field potential is determined by the gain and frequency characteristics of the amplifier. Incorrect setting of the amplifier with respect to the amplitude and frequency characteristics of the studied field potential will lead to distorted and thus misleading recordings. The amplitude of certain field potentials is large enough to permit their recognition and measurement the moment that they are recorded as traces on paper or on the oscilloscope screen. The electrocardiogram (ECG), with an amplitude of a few hundred μV, is such a potential; the electroencephalogram, with an amplitude of approximately 100 μV, is another. Both the ECG and the electroencephalogram are continuous bioelectrical phenomena referred to as intrinsic activities or intrinsic potentials. The intrinsic activities can be modified by external events but are not evoked by environmental (exogenous) or organic (endogenous) changes (stimulation). However, other electrobiological activities are the direct result of stimulation and they are referred to as evoked potentials. In general the amplitude of the evoked potential is much smaller than the intrinsic activities that are continuously present. This amplitude difference between the two types of electrobiological activity makes the evoked potential virtually undetectable and certainly unmeasurable amongst the intrinsic ones. Dawson (Dawson 1951) established a new era in human neurophysiology and electrodiagnosis when he proposed the technique of superimposition for the detection of evoked potentials which led to the development of methods of summation and averaging of electrodiagnostic results. The effect of superimposition is shown in Fig. 2 where instances Tr1 to Tr8 of 200 ms duration of intrinsic and evoked potentials, following the delivery of a stimulus, were collected and then superimposed. This superimposition was initially made photographically. It is apparent from the superimposed traces that the intrinsic activities, which have no reason to be synchronized with the stimulus, are losing their identity whereas an upward followed by a downward deflection seems to be a consistent feature (the signal) of this otherwise amorphous (noise) trace. The upward and downward deflections or peaks are the desired evoked potentials.

However, photographic superimposition soon became a cumbersome procedure and in 1962 Manfred Clynes designed a computer to handle the data. Individual traces (Tr1 to Tr8 in Fig. 2) are continuous electrobiological potentials referred to as analogue signals. Analogue signals cannot be recognized by a computer as they can only deal with discrete, digital, electrical events. It is therefore necessary to take samples of the analogue signal at frequent intervals to measure the amplitude of the sample, for instance once every millisecond, and to store this number in an electronic register as a digit. This process of transforming the analogue waveform into a string of digits (digitalization) is performed by analogue to digital converters

(A/D converters). The rules upon which the rate of sampling depends are dealt with by the Nyquist equation. As a rule of thumb the sampling rate should be at least twice the highest frequency expected to be present in the data. Failure to obey these rules may result in missing features or creating non-existent ones (aliasing).

The string of numbers of the waveforms Tr1 to Tr8 are plotted as graphs in Fig. 2. Any one of these numbers in each string has its equivalent in time in all strings. These numbers sampled at the same time in each string can be summed and the product divided by the number of strings or 'trials'. This procedure is repeated with all of the numbers in the trial and the new averaged string of numbers displayed as a graph showing the average evoked potential (bottom right in Fig. 2). The mathematical or graphical manipulations that can be applied to the average evoked potential and indeed the single trials that underlie its calculation are restricted only by the limits imposed by mathematics, imagination, and the degree of co-operation of the people of the different disciplines involved—that is, electronic engineers, computer specialists, mathematicians, neurobiologists, and clinicians.

Potentials evoked by retinal stimulation are known as electroretinograms. Potentials recorded from brain structures after visual stimulation are referred to as visually evoked potentials. Such potentials are further subdivided according to various attributes of the stimulus. For example presentation of brief flashes of diffuse light elicit the flash electroretinograms, and visually evoked potentials while reversing checkerboard-like stimuli elicit the pattern reversal electroretinograms or visually evoked potentials. Briefly appearing or disappearing similar stimuli elicit the stimulus onset or offset electroretinograms or visually evoked potentials. The start of a shift of a stimulus on the computer screen leads to the development of the motion potentials. High frequency of stimulation drives the retinal or brain electrical activity at the same frequencies and their higher harmonics, a phenomenon referred to as the steady state or flicker following electroretinograms or visually evoked potentials. The subdivisions mentioned are further expanded according to the colour of the stimuli and their intensity. In the case of patterned stimulation with vertical stripes, for example, the contrast between the stripes is important as well as the number of stripes per unit of space, referred to as spatial frequency. Furthermore, the same subject's electroretinograms or visually evoked potentials to a specified stimulus recorded simultaneously from many locations may be different in waveform or latency and amplitude of components. The study of this topographic development of evoked potentials is extensive; however, it is fundamental to ensure accurate calibration of all amplifiers over time.

It becomes apparent from the above discussion that for clinical or research purposes the use of the term electroretinogram or visually evoked potential may be meaningless unless there is explicit specification of the stimulus parameters and the recording location and convention.

Stimulus parameters are mainly dependent on the type of stimulator used and the type of stimulus it generates. The recording procedures are dominated by the type of electrodes

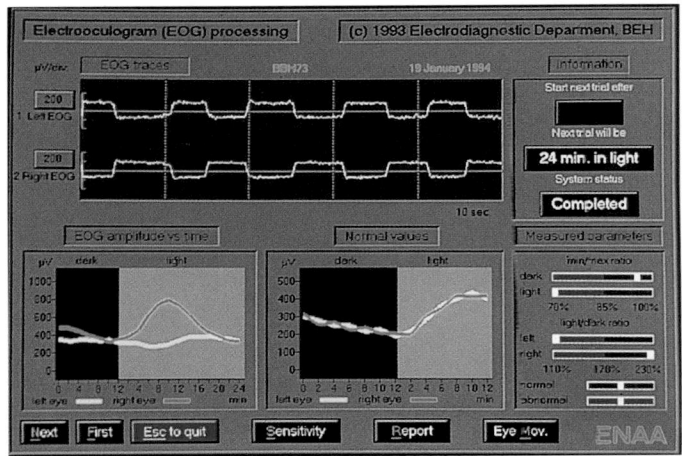

used, their placement, and their mode of connection. For stimulation by brief diffuse flashes, photic stimulators such as those produced by Grass or SLE are used, or specially made reflecting domes referred to as Ganzfeld stimulators. Use of neutral or colour filters with such stimulators can control the relevant parameters. For patterned stimulation, computers are programmed to generate shape with different forms, contrast, luminance, and colour on screen, thus presented to the subject at the desired frequency. There are many types of electrodes ranging from those which are attached directly to the retina like the Burian Allen electrode, to those made from gold or carbon which are hooked to the lower lid and again directly touch the retina. Another electrode is based on a silver chloride coated string placed across the eye, known as the DTL-type electrode. In a number of laboratories electrodes which do not touch the cornea are used, and these are referred to as skin electrodes. The skin electrodes are universally used for visually evoked potential recordings. This variability between electrodes generates great variability among normative values therefore efforts have been made to counteract this situation by publishing standards for recordings.

Generally, reference to electroretinograms and visually evoked potentials implies that the stimulus is a visual event and the visually evoked potential an electrical field; however, this is not necessarily the case. The stimulus may be an electrical or magnetic pulse and the electroretinograms or visually evoked potentials may be recordings of the magnetic fields accompanying the same currents which are registered as electrical fields. The study of the retinal and brain biocurrents by registering and processing the related magnetic fields on the surface is referred to as electromagnetography.

Electro-oculography

The electrical fields of the left and right eye recorded from a patient with uniocular central retinal vein occlusion, performing horizontal eye movements, are shown in the upper panel of Fig. 3. Such potentials are known as the electro-oculogram. The electro-oculogram has been extensively used to register spontaneous or induced eye movements with the subject either asleep or awake and engaged in some kind of visual search or reading. An alternative use of the electro-oculogram has been developed for application in ophthalmology. In this, the span of eye movements is fixed and the subject performs them first in a dark and then in a bright environment. For eye movements of fixed span the amplitude of the potential is different in the dark than in the light conditions (Fig. 3). The degree of amplitude difference during dark and light conditions provides valuable information on retinal function. The technique generally employed for recording the electro-oculogram and its change during darkness and subsequent light exposure is based on that of Arden and Kelsey (Arden and Kelsey 1962). Recording standards have recently been proposed (Marmor and Zrenner 1993).

In our laboratory (Electrodiagnostic Department, Bristol Eye Hospital, UK), in order to ensure consistent horizontal eye movements spanning an angle of 30°, two red light-emitting

Fig. 3 Raw electro-oculogram traces from one subject at the 12th min in light (top panel) electro-oculogram amplitudes throughout the test (left bottom panel), normal values from a group of 14 subjects (right bottom panel), 'information' on the status of the recording, the 'measured parameters' (extreme right panels), and the menu choices during electro-oculogram recordings (extreme bottom series of panels).

diodes are positioned in front of the subject, at eye level, separated by a distance of 0.82 m. The distance from the eyes to the mid-point between the light-emitting diodes is 1.5 m. The light-emitting diodes are controlled by a computer which is toggling them at a rate of 1 per second in counter phase, hence only one light-emitting diode is on at any one time. The subject is instructed to shift the direction of the gaze quickly towards the activated light-emitting diode and then maintain it steadily as long as the light-emitting diode stays on.

The electro-oculogram recording session consists of 13 trials of 10 s duration each, separated by 2-min intervals. In each trial a 10-s fragment of electro-oculogram potential is recorded. The first trial starts immediately after all the lights in the subject's room are switched off and the following six trials are also recorded in the dark. After the seventh trial the bright lights (3000 cd/m²) are switched on in the subject's room, and the remaining six trials are recorded in bright light. All timing of the trials is performed automatically by a stimulus and environment control computer.

Chlorided silver electrodes are attached to the bridge of the nose and each outer canthus. The electrode resistance should be less than 5 kΩ measured with a 40 Hz resistance meter. The signals are amplified with a time constant of 10 s, an upper frequency response of 100 Hz (3 dB down), and a gain of 20 µV/mm. However, because the diagnostically valuable information is contained in the slow component of the recorded potential, the data sampling rate is set at 50 samples/s.

The amplitude of electro-oculogram traces recorded every 2 min in the dark and light conditions are automatically calculated and displayed as a graph as on the lower left panel of Fig. 3. Similar graphs obtained from 14 normal subjects have been produced, averaged, and displayed in the lower right panel of Fig. 3. It should be noted that in Fig. 3 additional trials have been collected for a further 12 min in the light. In spite of the presence of light the electro-oculogram amplitude

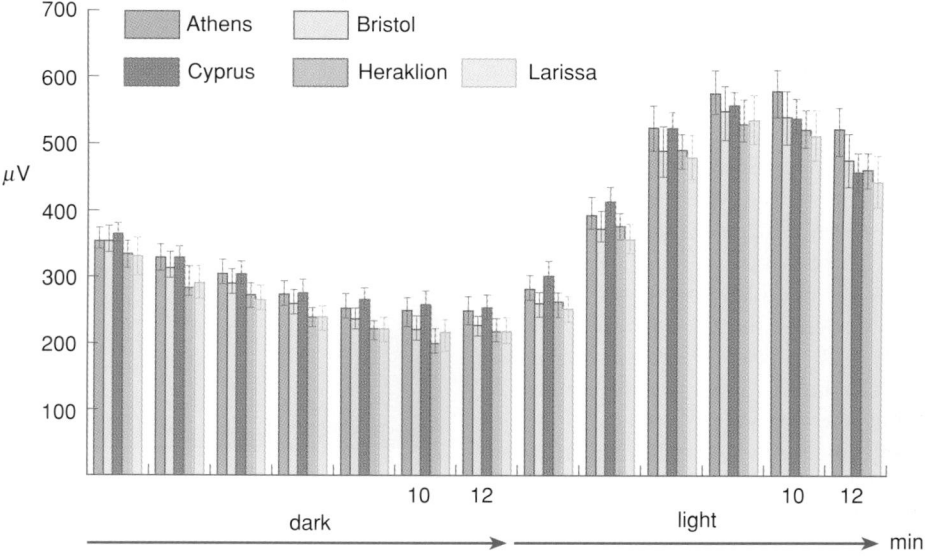

Fig. 4 Mean and standard error values of the electro-oculogram amplitude (in µV) from each of the five laboratories during 12 min of exposure to darkness followed by 12 min exposure to light. Notice the similarity of mean and standard error for each satellite station for each measurement.

diminishes to the level of the dark trough after about 10 min of the additional time. If the recording continues even further in time a second rise of the electro-oculogram amplitude takes place followed by a new drop. These spontaneous oscillations are repeated and referred to as electro-oculogram oscillations.

Comparisons of electro-oculogram records between laboratories reveals significant variability noticed by many authors. However, if care is taken to replicate precisely the electrode position, head position of the subject, and environmental illumination, electro-oculogram variability between laboratories is very small. To demonstrate the degree of consistency of electro-oculogram amplitude between laboratories, the data of 14 subjects examined with undilated pupils, in five different laboratories are presented in Fig. 4. The standard error for each location and time throughout the test are also shown. Statistical analysis of the results did not reveal significant differences between laboratories and between eyes. However, there were significant sex differences ($P > 0.001$) with female subjects developing higher potentials than males.

The ratio of the maximum electro-oculogram value, called the light peak (Lp), after exposure to intense illumination (3000 cd/m^2) and the lowest electro-oculogram value, called the dark trough (Dt), multiplied by 100 ($Lp/Dt \times 100$), calculated for each eye separately is called the light to dark (L/D) or Arden ratio.

The electro-oculogram originates in the pigment epithelium. The pigment epithelium is the layer of cells interposed between the choroidal circulation and the photoreceptors. The choroidal or outer part of the pigment epithelium cells is referred to as the basal part. The inner part of the cells support the photoreceptors within the invagination of their membrane and is referred to as the apical part. Between the basal and apical parts there is a continuous difference in the magnitude of the membrane potential, known as transepithelium potential, with a value of about 15 mV in the dark. The transepithelium potential is the main contributor to the standing potential, which in the apical part is more positive (hyperpolarized) than the basal part. The value of this difference is influenced by the level of illumination, the time of exposure to a particular illumination, and certain metabolic factors leading to hyperosmolarity.

The relatively large value of the standing potential permits other electrical fields generated by structures in front of the pigment epithelium to be ignored and the eye can be considered as a single generator, like a dipole, positive at the front.

A considerable period of time, about 8 min, is necessary before the maximum values of the dark trough and light peak are developed. This prolonged period indicates that the processes underlying are chemical and not neuronal in nature. Substances released by the cones and rods as well as from deeper retinal structures have been suggested as influencing the changes of the standing potential during dark and light conditions, and dopamine is considered as one of these (Williams and Papakostopoulos 1995).

In the above discussion, the light used for the electro-oculogram recordings is white. Coloured light may also be used for certain special research purposes. Alternatively, non-photic techniques may be used to induce electro-oculogram changes. These techniques of non-photic stimulation employ injection of substances which induce metabolic changes leading to a decrease of the standing potential. These are manifested as an additional drop of the dark trough value a few minutes after application (Mori *et al.* 1991).

The electro-oculogram has considerable value in the diagnosis, prognosis, follow-up, and further understanding of many retinal disorders from vascular to degenerative and from traumatic to metabolic disorders. Low values of electro-oculogram light rise is the most sensitive index to detecting the onset of certain retinal diseases before any other sign during clinical or laboratory examination is noted. These diseases include retinitis pigmentosa and some homozygotic carriers of this disease, traumatic effects of blunt instruments, metalosis, and toxic effects of drugs like chloroquine.

Prognosis is poor for developing rubeosis if the electro-oculogram ratio between the affected and non-affected eye is less than 50 per cent. The results of treatment of detachment are poor if the between-eyes ratio is less than 35 per cent. A normal electro-oculogram is associated with stationary retinal dystrophies except Best's disease where it has an abnormally low light rise.

The diagnosis of certain unusual disorders like retinitis sine-pigmentation or unilateral retinitis pigmentosa may be confirmed. Its normality in retinoschisis contributes to the diagnosis. An abnormal light rise is found in Stargardt's disease and dominant drusen.

The treatment of opacities of the ocular media may be guided by the electro-oculogram results as they provide objective means of retinal function when ophthalmoscopy may not be possible.

Its sensitivity to toxic drug effects provides means to monitor their side-effects.

Electroretinography

Stimulation of the eye with a diffused bright flash of white light leads to a sequence of fluctuation of electrobiological activity of the retina, known as the electroretinogram (Fig. 5).

There are two outstanding features in trace 1 in Fig. 5, an upward going deflection (the a-wave) and a downward one (the b-wave). The convention of displaying the a- and b-waves varies between laboratories. In many publications the a- and b-waves are displayed as downwards and upwards deflections, respectively. The results can in no way be affected whichever display convention is adopted.

The electroretinogram in Fig. 5 was recorded simultaneously with corneal contact electrodes and skin electrodes, with the subject tested in a dark room. The data from both recordings are superimposed. From this superimposition it can be seen that the obtained waveforms are virtually identical. In Fig. 6 similar recordings are shown using a gold foil electrode and a skin electrode with the subject tested in a well-illuminated room. Again the waveforms are virtually identical. The only difference between the corneal and skin recordings is the amplitude of the potentials. The corneal recordings are considerably larger than the skin ones, as can be seen from the value of the calibration bar for the two types of recording.

In Fig. 5 the traces marked (1) were recorded within the first 3 min in the dark and those marked (2) between the eighth and 11th min in the dark. Both skin and corneal electrode recordings show that the peak of the b-wave recorded during the first three minutes—the 'b' photopic (b_p)—is followed by an additional peak after the eighth minute which is larger in amplitude and has longer latency—the 'b' scotopic (b_s). A similar distinction between photopic and scotopic elements is

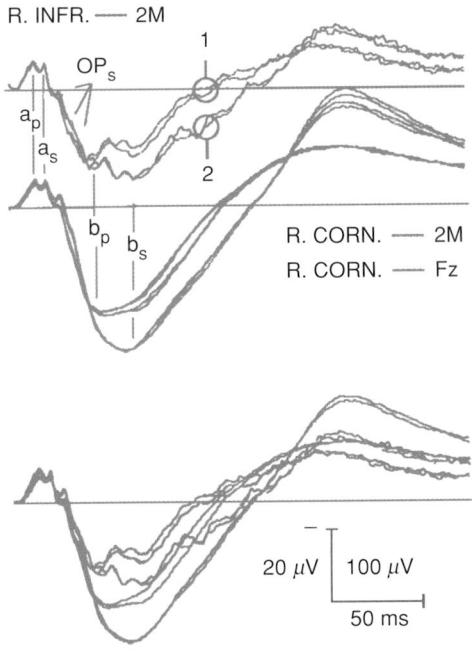

Fig. 5 Superimposed electroretinogram averages (*n* = 100) recorded from the right eye simultaneously with skin (*upper traces*) and corneal (*middle traces*) electrodes. Both groups of data are shown superimposed (*lower traces*). The skin data obtained with an infraorbital electrode referred to two linked mastoid electrodes (R. INFR–2M). The corneal electrode was referred either to the mastoid (R. CORN–2M) or to Fz (R. CORN–Fz) electrodes. The separate averages obtained are superimposed and are nearly identical. For both skin and corneal averages the traces encircled were obtained 1–3 min (1) and 8–11 min (2) after preadaptation. Peaks and troughs are as follows: a_p (a photopic), a_s (a scotopic), OP (oscillatory potentials), b_p (b photopic), and b_s (b scotopic). In this and all following figures negativity of the active electrode appears as an upward deflection for both electroretinograms and visually evoked potentials.

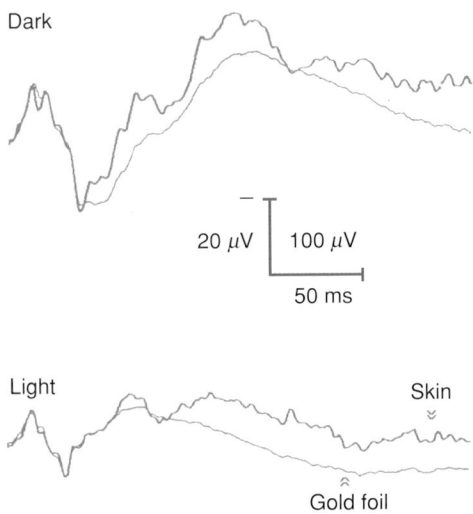

Fig. 6 Superimposed electroretinogram averages (*n* = 100) recorded from the right eye simultaneously with skin (*thick traces*) and gold foil (*thin traces*) electrodes during dark (*upper traces*) and light (*lower traces*) conditions.

responsible for the two peaks of the photopic (a_p) and scotopic (a_s) peaks of the a- wave in Fig. 1. Stimulation with flashes of blue light makes the b scotopic wave more prominent while red flashes favour the development of the b photopic wave. The receptors responsible for the development of the a_p and the b_p waves are the cones while the a_s and the b_s waves are the rods. However, while the a-waves represent potentials originating in the biocurrents of the photoreceptors the b-potentials are generated by currents developing in the Müller cells under the influences of activity of the bipolar cells. On the descending part of the b-wave small fluctuations can be observed which are known as the oscillatory potentials. Current experimental evidence suggests that all the oscillatory potentials originate in the vicinity of the inner plexiform layer with the depolarizing amacrine cells considered as the main candidates. Recording standards for the electroretinogram have been published (Marmor and Zrenner 1995).

When the rate of stimulation increases, the electroretinogram features described fade out gradually and a sinusoidal-like waveform develops known as flicker following electroretinogram or steady state electroretinogram. The frequency of the flicker following electroretinogram is similar to the stimulation rate or multiples of it. Beyond the rate of 20 Hz the flicker following electroretinogram reflects only cone activity as the rods do not follow high rates of flickering. To activate the rods preferentially, the colour of the stimulus is altered to blue by appropriate filter and recordings take place while the subject has been dark adapted. Under conditions of dark adaptation the intensity of the stimulus can be varied and the minimum amount of light eliciting an electroretinogram permits the determination of the threshold of dark adaptation. Very strong stimuli and special recording conditions reveal potentials with shorter latency than the a-wave, known as 'early receptor potentials'.

So far, the stimuli used are diffused or unpatterned. Stimuli can be created in the form of stripes or checkerboards and presented to the subject on a computer screen. These patterned stimuli may be switched on, switched off, or reversed. In the last instance, the potentials elicited are referred to as pattern reversal electroretinograms. The rate of reversal may also be varied, and the pattern reversal steady state electroretinograms are recorded. The pattern reversal electroretinogram originates partly in the inner retinal layers and significantly in the ganglion cell layer.

A low value of the b scotopic wave is the most sensitive index in detecting the onset of certain retinal diseases before any other clinical or laboratory examination. Amongst these diseases retinitis pigmentosa, retinal detachment, central vein occlusion, ocular trauma, or diabetic retinopathy are included. Because of the minimum co-operation needed by the subject to record the various types of electroretinogram a mean is provided to assess retinal function of newborns, infants, and subjects unable to co-operate.

Prognosis is poor for developing diabetic retinopathy if the oscillatory potentials or the b scotopic wave to blue flashes are low or absent. The electroretinogram is reported as a good prognostic indicator for the result of operations in cases of opaque media due to vitreous haemorrhage. Low electroretinogram in central retinal vein occlusion is a prognostic index for neovascularization of the iris.

The diagnosis of certain unusual disorders such as retinitis sine-pigmentation or unilateral retinitis pigmenosa may be confirmed. In retinoschisis, a preserved a-wave with a low or absent b-wave contributes to the diagnosis. This particular anomaly in the waveform is referred to as negative electroretinogram. An abnormal scotopic negative electroretinogram is associated with night-blindness and rod dystrophies in general and an abnormal photopic positive electroretinogram is associated with cone dystrophy. A preserved electroretinogram in macular disorders confirms the local nature of the disease, while its abnormality, in spite the presence of only local abnormality clinically, suggests generalized disease of the retina.

The treatment of opacities of the ocular media may be guided by the electroretinogram results as they provide objective means of retinal function when ophthalmoscopy may not be possible.

The electroretinograms sensitivity to toxic drug effects provides means to monitor the side-effects. A low or absent b scotopic wave is associated with vitamin A deficiency, administration of which improves the electroretinogram abnormality.

Visually evoked potentials

Any stimulus applied to the visual system evokes a change in electrobiological brain activity. This change is referred to as visually evoked potential. This term has been used by authors in different ways. In many publications the term refers to any type of electrical activity recorded by a variety of electrodes in the anaesthetized or awake animal or human and evoked by any stimulus which can influence the state of any part of the visual system. Other authors restrict the term to the field potential following a particular stimulus, like a flash of light, recorded with scalp electrodes and made distinguishable from the much larger electroencephalogram by averaging procedures using a computer. Within this second approach, a further development is in progress which defines the stimulus explicitly, for example flash or pattern reversal visually evoked potential, or defines the origin of the visually evoked potential, for example cortical, and refers to the procedural means of revealing it, for example averaging. The need for such explicit terminology has emerged from the realization that each particular stimulus condition generates visually evoked potentials with different waveforms, different anatomical and neurophysiological substratum, and different clinical significance. This will become apparent from the visually evoked potential in Fig. 7 obtained from the same electrode from the same subject by stimulation with a diffuse flash, a reversing checkerboard pattern, and a flickering light at 20 Hz. This diversity of waveforms is much broader if it is taken into consideration that simultaneous recordings from other brain locations generate visually evoked potentials with different waveform characteristics, or that a small change in a stimulus parameter generates apparently similar potentials, generated by different parts of the visual pathway. This last point is demonstrated in Fig. 8 where a reversing checkerboard

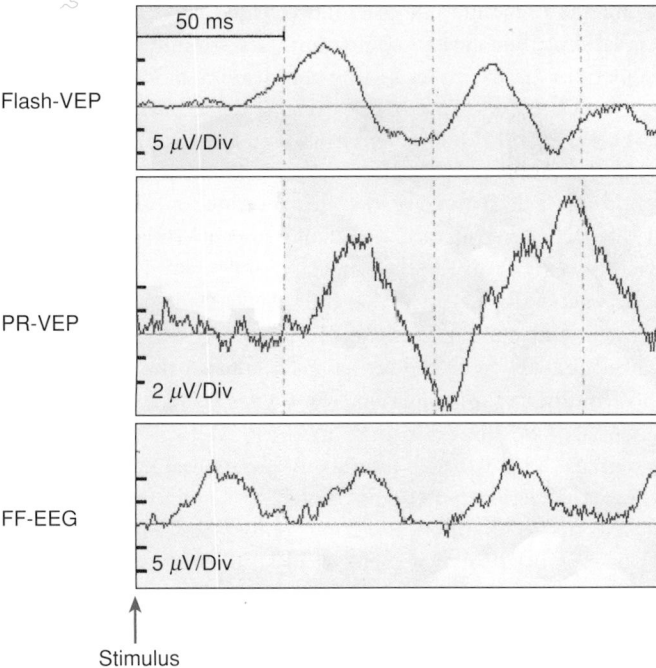

Fig. 7 Visually evoked potentials to a diffuse flash stimulus (flash visually evoked potential, F-VEP), a reversing checkerboard (pattern reversal visually evoked potential, PR-VEP), and flickering at 20 Hz (flicker following electroencephalogram, FF-EEG).

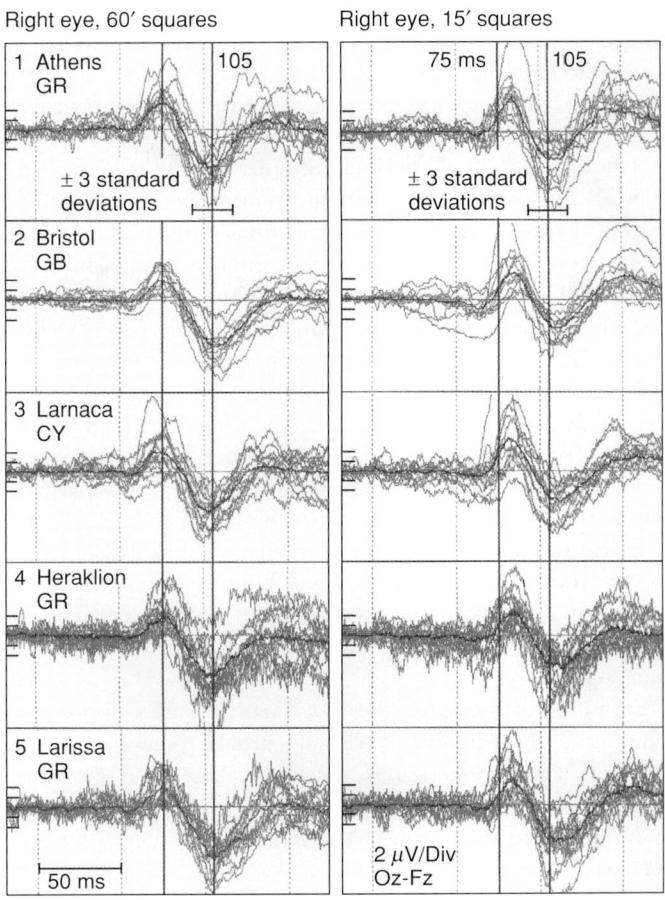

Fig. 8 Superimposed pattern reversal visually evoked potential averages after right eye stimulation. Each trace is the average ($n = 100$) of one subject. Its set of averages (top to bottom) shows the results of the five (labelled 1–5) different laboratories in three European countries (Greece, United Kingdom, and Cyprus). Left column: stimulation with 60-min squares. Right column: stimulation with 15-min squares. Note the similarity of the traces across subjects, laboratories, and countries in term of latency (vertical lines) and amplitude. Also note the consistent differences in latency and amplitude to the two stimulus conditions.

pattern with the same luminance and contrast has been used but the size of the squares was different. The overall waveforms to 60-min and 15-min squares (Fig. 8) appear deceptively similar; however, close inspection reveals latency differences and different amplitude changes for each component to each stimulus. Two main components dominate the pattern reversal visually evoked potentials in Fig. 8. The first appears as an upward deflection (negative) with latency of about 75 ms, known in the literature as the N70 component and a second downward deflection (positive) with a latency of 105 ms known as the P_{100} component. Both the N70 and the P_{100} components are consistently more delayed when 15-min squares are used, and the smaller squares also generate higher N70 amplitudes in comparison with the 60-min squares. These differences are the result of different pathways activated by the two stimuli. Small squares activate macular fibres which are thinner and conduct at lower speeds compared with the thick fibres of the peripheral retina which have faster conduction and different cortical destination, activated by the larger squares. It is this sensitivity to apparently small experimental variations combined with the rigidity of the response under similar stimulation conditions which gives the current clinical values of the pattern reversal visually evoked potentials and predicts an important expansion for visual electrodiagnosis in the future.

The data in Fig. 8 have been obtained by using a black and white checkerboard pattern, subtending the visual angle of 60° or 15° at 95 per cent contrast and reversing every 500 ms, presented to a subject, at each eye separately, on the screen of a computer monitor which was subtending 15° of the visual arc. The luminance of the white squares was 50 cd/m².

The pattern reversal visually evoked potentials were recorded simultaneously from three occipital deviations (O_z, O_1, O_2) referred to a frontal electrode (Fz) within the frequency range of 0.1 to 500 Hz. The data sampling rate was 2000 samples/s. The analysis time was 200 ms including a 20-ms prestimulus epoch. Two runs of $n = 100$ reversals were recorded for each eye. Fourteen normal subjects, seven males and seven females aged between 18 and 34 years, were tested in five different laboratories.

The visually evoked potentials are valid indexes of conductivity across the visual pathway if the retinal function is normal. Cone dystrophies, for example, and retinoschisis are consistently associated with delayed pattern reversal visually evoked potentials.

Visually evoked potentials provide a sensitive and objective index in assessing visual acuity in infants.

Prognosis is good for developing normal vision in infants with delayed maturation who have normal visually evoked potentials. Flash visually evoked potential is reported as the best prognostic indicator for the result of operation in cases of opaque media due to cataract. In cases of ocular trauma a preserved electroretinogram accompanied by an absent flash visually evoked potential suggest optic nerve damage and poor prognosis.

The diagnosis of demyelinating optic neuritis and multiple sclerosis has improved substantially since it was shown that the pattern reversal visually evoked potentials remain abnormal in latency even when the visual acuity, after an attack, has been restored. A normal electro-oculogram, abnormal b-wave of the electroretinogram, and delayed pattern reversal visually evoked potentials are characteristic in retinoschisis. The abnormal decussation in the chiasma in albinism can be established by visually evoked potentials and the diagnosis confirmed. Chiasmal and retrochiasmal lesions can be detected using pattern reversal visually evoked potentials. The pattern reversal visually evoked potential is one of the means by which malingering and excessive functional overlays can be investigated. It is also one of the tools used to assess cortical blindness. Differences in pattern reversal visually evoked potential amplitude (exceeding 10 per cent), to uniocular stimulation, are encountered in amblyopia.

Surgical treatments on the visual pathway may improve by monitoring the stability of visually evoked potentials during orbital or cardiac operations, thus provoking early corrective action which could avoid, for example, obstruction of blood flow and brain anoxaemia. Vitamin B_{12} deficiency leads to delayed pattern reversal visually evoked potentials.

The origin of field potentials

The bioelectrical fields recorded with surface electrodes as electro-oculogram, electroretinogram, or visually evoked potentials are generated by currents related to the maintenance and changes of the membrane potential of the cell body and its dendrites. Changes of the membrane potential may be induced by external physical energy, when they are referred to as receptor potentials, or may be the result of the activity of other cells, when they are referred to as synaptic potentials. The receptor potentials in the visual system emerge from the neurochemical phototransactions in the cone and rod outer segments. The early and late a-waves are such examples. The synaptic potentials in the retina, the geniculi, the visual cortex, and the other brain structures related to vision, are mainly the results of chemicals released by the axon terminals of the pathways involved in the receptor areas of the receiving cell. The visually evoked potentials are examples of this. The membrane potential does not necessarily have identical values across various parts of a cell leading to the development of bioelectrical fields. The photoreceptors and the cells of the pigment epithelium are an example of cells displaying continuous differences in the value of the membrane potential between the peripheral and the proximal parts of their cell body. As a result of this difference, referred to as polarization, bioelectrical fields are generated around the cell body which are additional to the receptor or synaptic potentials, or indeed the continuous intrinsic fluctu-

ations of the membrane potential referred to as diamembranic oscillations. The electro-oculogram dark trough, light rise, and oscillations are examples of this polarization and its modulation by various factors. Another reason for these bioelectrical fields is the change of the ionic environment due to synaptic activity leading to diamembraning change of cells sensitive to this new condition. The b-wave of the electroretinogram is an example of this, reflecting membrane change of the Müller cells due to synaptic activity of the bipolar cells.

It is generally accepted that only electrobiological changes in the cell body and dendrites contribute to the generation of evoked potentials. In the retina and the brain the electrical signals conducting information via the cells axons—the action potentials—do not contribute to the waveform of the evoked potentials. This is in contrast to the peripheral nervous system where the action potentials travelling along the nerves are picked up as compound action potentials. The compound action potential following electrical stimulation of the median nerve in the wrist, for example, may be picked up by electrodes positioned in the clavicle and referred to as brachial plexus potential. The brachial potential as well as all the compound potentials are envelopes of action potentials.

The use of evoked potentials as a non-invasive method of studying the human visual system has emerged from the existing neurohistochemical knowledge, the development of specialized stimulators, the use of multichannel recording systems permitting appropriate electrode arrangements, and the development of enhanced means of analysis. The guidelines for this work derive from the understanding of the multiplicity of sensory channels, multiple cortical representation, and parallel processing. To demonstrate this approach, colour visually evoked potentials could be used. The retinal ganglion cells which synapse onto the four parvocellular layers in the lateral geniculate nucleus are called P-type cells, while retinal ganglion cells that synapse onto neurones in the two magnocellular layers in the lateral geniculate nucleus are called M-type cells. The distinction between these two 'streams' seems to be maintained at entry into the striate cortex and beyond. Most of the parvocellular cells in lateral geniculate nucleus have small receptive fields which may be colour opponent, and receive input and conduct to the striate cortex in medium velocities. The M-type cells, however, have large receptive fields, no colour sensitivity, conduct at high velocity, and have greater contrast sensitivity. Each one of these pathways may be studied by visually evoked potentials elicited by the appropriate stimulus.

The depth of information that is needed depends upon the purposes of the particular case. However, it is important to note that evidence from neurophysiological experiments as well as Golgi staining and electron microscopy indicates that in cat, monkey, and human retina the synaptology is the same, at least for the rod pathways. The neurotransmitters are very similar. Consequently, the application of laboratory results in the animal may be diagnostically applicable to individual patients in helping to locate the damage and in applying the precise treatment.

Maturation

Changes in the newborn's numerous biological systems and their functions as it matures and ages is reflected by changes in the biopotentials which provide the basis of electrodiagnosis. The waveforms of the visually evoked potential or the electroretinogram potential at birth scarcely resemble the waveforms of the adult and change significantly as the subject ages. As far as the retinal potentials are concerned their major changes take place in the first postnatal year. The same holds for the visually evoked potentials. The implications of these changes are both in clinical practice and research. In the case of recordable potentials, serial testing will reveal maturation proceeding, or its arrest due to damage. In old age the electroretinogram and visually evoked potential amplitude is gradually decreasing while the latency is prolonged. Both these effects are not a result of the small pupil size associated with ageing.

Clinical electrodiagnosis

Clinical electrodiagnosis is the link between information technology, patients, clinicians, basic laboratory research, and health care within a particular socioeconomic environment.

There is a basic difference between electrodiagnostic and other laboratory tests. Electrodiagnosis deals with the quantification of the many neurobiological processes which underlie everyday terms such as dark adaptation, visual acuity, colour vision, depth perception, and many others.

The clinician may suspect, for example, demyelination and ask for pattern reversal visually evoked potentials, a test which reveals deterioration of conduction across the visual pathway. In other cases, such a precise request cannot be formulated. The clinician simply requires support to evaluate 'an unexplained loss of vision'. In this latter case a battery of tests is necessary in order to establish the existence of dysfunction and to isolate the precise mechanism affected (Papakostopoulos 1982). In the author's experience 85 per cent of referrals by 50 consultants for a period of 15 years fell within this category.

It cannot be overemphasized that the issue is not to list the electrophysiological findings, for example in retinoschisis, but to answer the question 'Can you help to explain the drop of visual acuity, in this patient, by performing electrodiagnostic tests?' For example, a particular clinical problem may be summarized as follows: 'restriction of visual fields, some pigmentation, perhaps difficulty in night vision and normal visual acuity. Otherwise, nothing remarkable except that a distant relative suffers from retinitis pigmentosa which is a cause of enormous anxiety to this 23-year-old design engineer'. An abnormal electroretinogram to white flashes under photopic and scotopic conditions will make retinitis pigmentosa very probable but the results might be within the normal range (better than two standard deviations of the means of amplitude and latency for each component). Such a result does not exclude Best's diseases. An abnormal electro-oculogram ratio (less than 170 per cent or 1.7) would solve the problem, but it may be normal. The possibility of rod dystrophy has not been excluded. It is necessary to proceed with dark adaptation electroretinogram

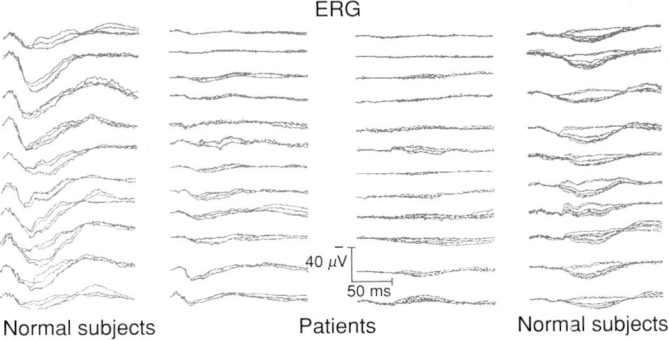

Fig. 9 Superimposed electroretinogram averages of 10 normal subjects (first column) during stimulation with white flashes of light, and similar data from 10 patients with retinitis pigmentosa (second column). Data from the same patients stimulated with blue flashes of light (third column) and corresponding data of 10 normal subjects (fourth column).

using blue flashes of light which is much more sensitive than white light electroretinogram (Fig. 9). If the results are positive, cone dysfunction has to be excluded. This can be done by recording the steady state electroretinogram response to various frequencies of flickering light up to at least 48 Hz. But the results may still be within the normal range. In this case the possibility of optic nerve atrophy has to be investigated. Flash visually evoked potentials, steady state electroencephalogram, and especially pattern reversal visually evoked potentials to high and low special frequencies may show abnormality.

Research electrodiagnosis

The theoretical issues and the clinical problems related to human behaviour urge the development of appropriate methods. Electrodiagnostic techniques have certain unique features to address some of these issues. It is the only methodology which provides non-invasive, continuous, on-line, quantifiable information about nervous system function in a given individual when asleep, awake, or under anaesthesia from the time of birth to any age.

Conditions with wide socioeconomic implications can be studied using electrodiagnostic techniques including drug abuse, the effects of pharmacological agents in the treatment of cardiovascular or infectious diseases, and the effects of some tranquillizers and antiepileptic drugs. Insecticides or smoking may damage visual function and this can be studied by applying electrodiagnostic techniques.

Many of these waveforms have already been recognized as having undisputed diagnostic value. Some of them also have prognostic value. Others are suitable for research in understanding and improving the action of various drugs, or revealing the adverse effects of pharmaceutical treatment. Evoked potentials are useful in monitoring the integrity of nervous structures during surgery. Other types of evoked potentials reveal the processes underlying cognitive brain function such as the execution of skilled visuomotor tasks.

Telematic electrodiagnosis

So far the contribution of electrodiagnosis in bringing the knowledge of psychophysics, neurophysiology, neurohistology, and neurochemistry to clinical practice and the individual patient has been discussed. It has been shown that electrodiagnosis is possible, beneficial, and continuously advancing. To make these benefits available to a wider population is an additional problem with new and particular demands attached.

Only during the last few decades have individuals, governments, and international institutions recognized that the avoidance of rationing medical care depends upon the formulation of a new approach in the management of the available technical, economic, and human resources. The key factor in this approach is information technology. Current levels of telecommunications and computing provide the means to bring electrodiagnostic and other psychophysiological research and clinical services to populations with restricted scientific, technical, and economic resources. User-friendly equipment capable of automated test configuration and administration, self-calibration, equalization, environmental control, single trial storage, and teletransfer of results to a specialized centre for evaluation is necessary. The Electrodiagnostic Neurophysiological Automated Analysis system, developed within the Eureka 1026 project does this (Papakostopoulos *et al.* 1996, 1997).

To validate its performance Electrodiagnostic Neurophysiological Automated Analysis was installed in Bristol, three Greek cities, and Cyprus and set up to transmit data to the central station in Bristol. Pattern reversal visually evoked potentials were chosen as a test potential, requiring accurate control of stimulus luminance and contrast, accurate timing, multichannel recordings, and various modes of signal processing. Recordings were made in 70 subjects of between 18 and 34 years of age (seven male and seven female in each laboratory) with silver chloride electrodes attached to occipital locations and referred to a frontal electrode. Two-tailed *t*-statistics did not reveal significant differences in latency or amplitude of the main features of the waveform between laboratories, referred to as N70 and P_{100} components, thus validating the ability of the system for standardized recordings between and within countries (see Fig. 8). Similar procedures have been adopted for the electrooculogram (see Fig. 4) and electroretinogram (Fig. 10) potentials and again no significant differences were found between laboratories.

Further reading

Arden, G.B. and Kelsey, J.H. (1962). Changes produced by light in the standing potential of the human eye. *Journal of Physiology*, **161**, 189–204.

Armington, J.C. (1974). *The electroretinogram*, pp. 86–8. Academic Press, New York.

Babel, J., Stangos, N., Kordol, S., and Spiritus, M. (1977). *Ocular electrophysiology*. Thieme, Stuttgart.

Carr, R.E. and Siegel, I.M. (1982). *Intramuscular visual electrodiagnostic testing: a practical guide for the clinician*. Williams & Wilkins, Baltimore.

Chiappa, K.H. (ed.) (1989). *Evoked potentials in clinical medicine*. Raven Press, New York.

Chiarenza, G.A. and Papakostopoulos, D. (ed.) (1982). *Clinical application of cerebral evoked potentials in paediatric medicine*. Excerpta, Amsterdam.

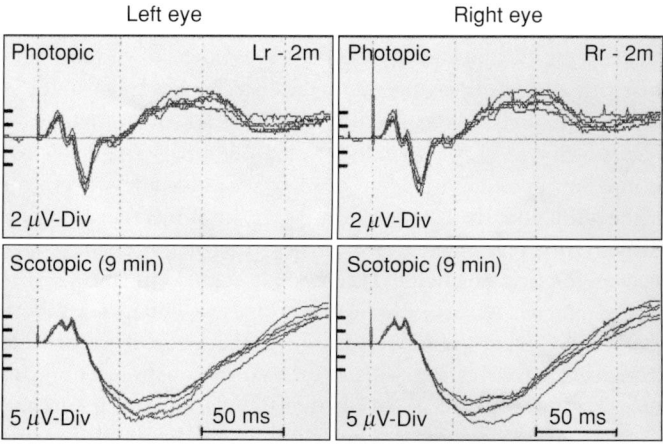

Fig. 10 Superimposed electroretinogram grand averages after left eye and right eye stimulation. Each trace is the average of all subjects (*n* = 14) in each laboratory (*n* = 5) in three European countries (Greece, United Kingdom, and Cyprus). Upper traces: photopic condition. Lower traces: scotopic condition. Notice the similarity of the traces across laboratories and countries in terms of waveform latency and amplitude. Also note the consistent differences in waveform latency and amplitude in the two stimulus conditions.

Clynes, M. (1962). CAT: computer of average transients. *Instruments and Control Systems*, **35**, 87–91.

Dawson, G.D. (1951). A summation technique for detecting small signals in a large irregular background. *Journal of Physiology*, **115**, 2–3.

Galloway, N.R. (1981). *Ophthalmic electrodiagnosis*. Lloyd-Luke Medical, London.

Halliday, A.M. (ed.) (1982). *Evoked potentials in clinical testing*. Churchill Livingstone, Edinburgh.

Harding, G., Janday, B., and Armstrong, R. (1992). The topographic distribution of the magnetic P_{100} M to full- and half-field stimulation. *Documenta Ophthalmologica*, **80**, 63–73.

Heckenlively, J.R. and Arden, G.B. (ed.) (1991). *Principles and practice of clinical electrophysiology of vision*. Mosby Year Book, St Louis.

Hennessy, M.P. and Vaegan. (1995). Amplitude scaling relationships of Burian Allen, gold foil, and Dawson, Trick and Litzkow electrodes. *Documenta Ophthalmologica*, **89**, 235–48.

Marmor, M.F. and Zrenner, E. (1993). Standard for clinical electrooculography. *Documenta Ophthalmologica*, **85**, 115–24.

Marmor, M.F. and Zrenner, E. (1995). Standard for clinical electroretinography (1994 update). *Documenta Ophthalmologica*, **89**, 199–210.

Mori, T., Marmor, M.F., Miyoshi, K., and Tazawa, Y. (1991). Combined photic and non-photic electro-oculographic responses in the clinical evaluation of the retinal pigment epithelium. *Documenta Ophthalmologica*, **76**, 315–22.

Papakostopoulos, D. (1996). Telematic electrodiagnosis. *Journal of Telemedicine and Telecare*, **2** (suppl 1), 30–3.

Papakostopoulos, D., Barber, C., and Dean Hart, J.C. (1993). The sampling properties of different types of ERG electrode. *Clinical Vision Science*, **8**, 481–8.

Papakostopoulos, D., Everingham, M., Gogolitsyn, Y., Dodson, K., Papakostopoulos, S., and Dean-Hart, J.C. (1997). Comprehensive standardized ophthalmic telemedicine. *Journal of Telemedicine and Telecare*, **3** (suppl. 1), 49–52.

Regan, D. (1989). *Human electrophysiology*. Elsevier, New York.

Williams, C. and Papakostopoulos, D. (1995). Electro-oculographic abnormalities in amblyopia. *British Journal of Ophthalmology*, **79**, 218–24.

1.6.10 Visual field analysis

Anath C. Viswanathan and F. W. Fitzke

It has long been realized that human visual function is not uniform across the visual field. As early as 150 BC Ptolemy attempted to measure the visual field. Damian, writing in the fifth century, describes 'sharp central vision' as opposed to 'blurred peripheral vision'. From these beginnings techniques for measuring visual fields have greatly increased in complexity: the need for precise, quantifiable, reproducible estimates of the visual field has resulted in a variety of perimeters which are used to examine the visual field under standardized conditions. Manual perimeters require the operator to determine many of the components of the examination such as where and when stimuli are presented to the subject, and evaluation of the reliability of the subject's responses. In automated perimeters, however, these factors are controlled by computer, and the role of the examiner is to encourage and motivate the subject to produce a reliable test result.

Manual perimetry

Before the advent of computerized perimeters the most reproducible estimates of the visual field were made with manual hemispherical bowl perimeters such as the Goldmann perimeter (Fig. 1(a) and (b)). This instrument has the great advantage over the earlier arc perimeters and tangent screens that the visual field may be examined in conditions of constant background illumination, and thus fixed light adaptation state of the eye. This has a critical bearing on the properties of the visual field: for example, in photopic conditions the fovea has a higher light sensitivity than the parafoveal area whereas in scotopic conditions it is relatively depressed.

Kinetic testing

Although the Goldmann perimeter may be used either for static or kinetic testing, its main use is in the latter. Kinetic testing involves moving a target of fixed size and luminance from the periphery of the visual field towards the centre until it is seen. This strategy relies on the fact that the central visual field is usually more sensitive to a given target than the peripheral field. The process can be repeated for targets of different sizes and luminances: each target yields an isopter on the visual field chart which corresponds to a contour of the 'hill of vision' (Fig. 2(a–c)).

The benefit of the Goldmann perimeter is that an experienced operator can perform fast, flexible testing for a variety of visual field abnormalities in subjects who might not be able to produce reliable tests under the more rigorous, not to say tedious conditions imposed by an automated perimeter. Thus it is invaluable in the determination of the presence, absence, or

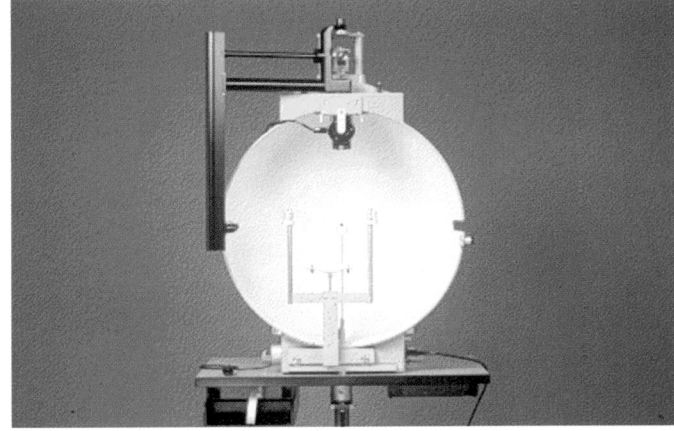

(a)

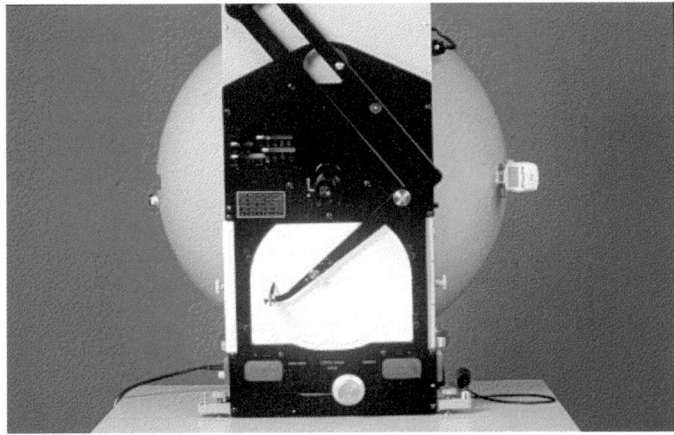

(b)

Fig. 1 The Goldmann perimeter.

progression of visual field defects in patients with neurological disease.

However, the versatility of manual perimetry may also limit its effectiveness, since it is a source of variation and bias. The examiner may neglect areas of the field which are not thought to be important. The pattern of visual field abnormalities may be 'forced' to comply with preconceived ideas. The result of the test is highly dependent upon the level of training of the examiner. Furthermore, kinetic testing gives poorly reproducible results in the central field and at the edges of gradually deepening scotomas such as those found in glaucoma. For these reasons, when quantifiable, reproducible results are required, automated perimetry is used.

Automated perimetry

Although some automated perimeters, such as the Humphrey field analyser II (Fig. 3), may be used to perform kinetic testing, they are usually used to test a grid of retinal locations in a static manner.

Static testing

The term 'static testing' encompasses a variety of disparate testing strategies, all of which share the feature that the stimuli

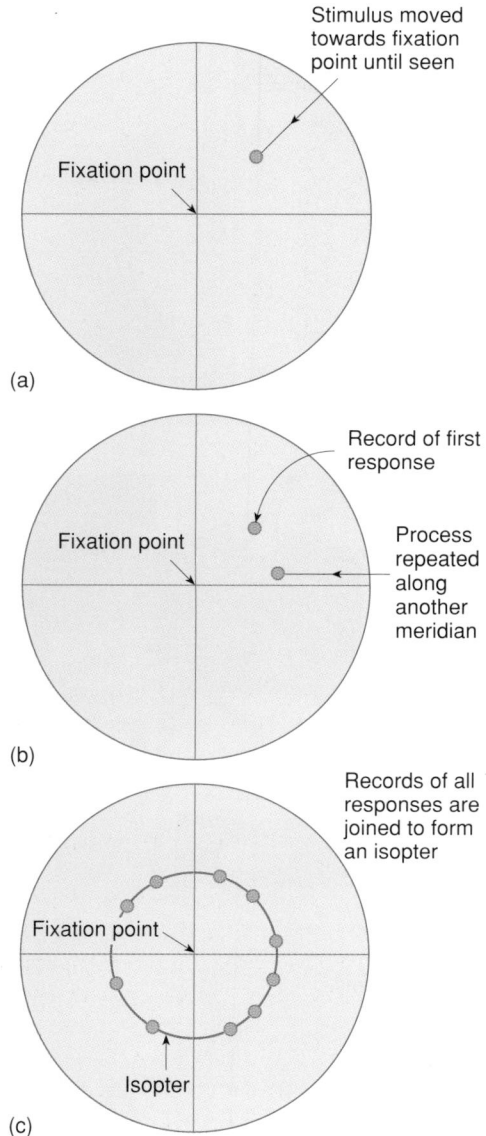

Fig. 2 Diagram of kinetic strategy and the construction of an isopter.

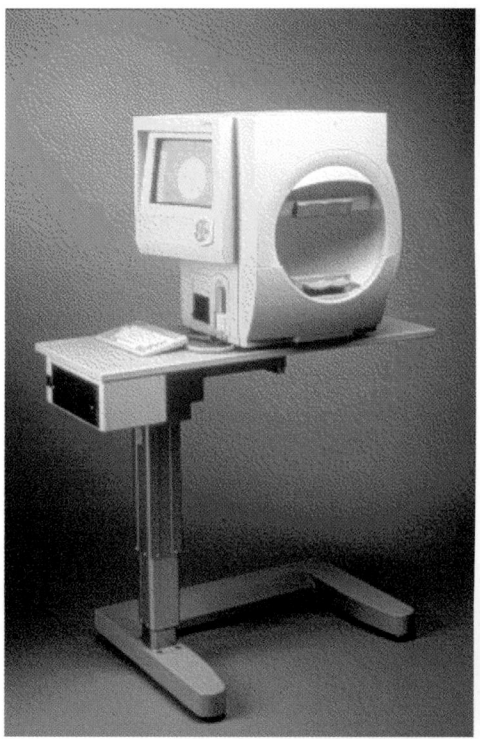

Fig. 3 The Humphrey field analyser II.

presented to the subject do not move. Static testing attempts to estimate the luminance sensitivity at fixed test locations, rather than moving a stimulus until it is seen. The combination of automated perimetry with static testing has the advantages that it is operator independent and yields numerical data relating to the spatial co-ordinates of the test locations and sensitivities at those locations: these data are amenable to sophisticated statistical analysis, unlike the results of kinetic perimetry. Static testing strategies may be divided into full threshold strategies and suprathreshold strategies.

Full threshold strategies

If kinetic testing may be imagined to give rise to a contour map of the hill of vision, full threshold static testing produces a grid of numbers representing estimates of the height of the hill at various fixed points. The most widely used strategy for estimat-

ing the sensitivity at a given test location is the 4–2 dB 'two reversal staircase' bracketing strategy (Fig. 4). An initial stimulus is presented whose brightness depends on the results of tests on nearby points, or on age-matched normal values. If this is seen, the next presentation at that location is 4 dB less intense. If this is also seen, the following stimulus at that location is reduced by a further 4 dB in intensity, and so on until the subject fails to see a stimulus presentation. This is the 'first reversal'. The stimuli following this are increased in intensity by 2 dB each time until the subject again reports a stimulus as seen. This is the 'second reversal'. The sensitivity is estimated as the mean of the final and the penultimate presentation intensities. If the initial presentation is not seen, intensities of subsequent presentations are increased by 4 dB until one is

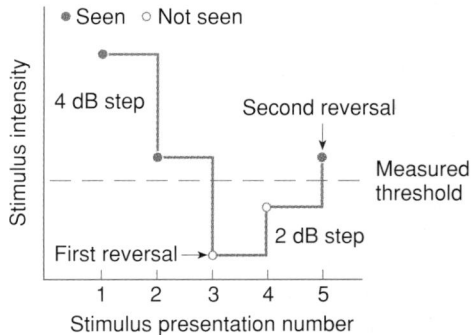

Fig. 4 Diagram of 4-2 dB 'two reversal staircase' bracketing strategy.

seen ('first reversal') then decreased by 2 dB until one is missed ('second reversal').

Suprathreshold strategies

Pure suprathreshold strategies are simpler and faster than full threshold strategies. Instead of ascribing a numerical estimate of sensitivity to a test location, they merely record whether it is normal or abnormal. This is done by presenting a stimulus calculated to be slightly more intense than the patient's sensitivity threshold. This calculation requires an estimate of the patient's threshold: the various methods by which this is obtained provide the names for the various suprathreshold strategies. The fixed intensity suprathreshold test assumes that all patients have a similar threshold. Thus the same test intensity is used for all patients. The age-related suprathreshold test takes account of the fact that sensitivity declines with age by approximately 1 dB per decade, and uses a table of normal data along with the patient's age to calculate the test intensity. The threshold-related suprathreshold test precedes the suprathreshold test with a determination of the patient's threshold, usually by means of a brief full threshold examination using a greatly reduced set of test points. The test intensity is then calculated relative to this threshold.

The amount by which the stimulus of a suprathreshold test is more intense than the patient's threshold, the suprathreshold increment, must be such that a 'missed' point truly represents abnormality (i.e. the stimulus must not be too dim) and a 'seen' point truly represents normality (i.e. the stimulus must not be too bright). Most perimeters use a suprathreshold increment of between 4 and 6 dB. In addition, most suprathreshold strategies in use compensate for the relatively reduced sensitivity of the peripheral visual field compared to the central field under the conditions in which perimetry is performed (lower photopic). These eccentrically compensated strategies derive an approximation of the hill of vision from their estimates of the patient's threshold, and thus vary the stimulus intensity to maintain a constant suprathreshold increment for all test locations.

Full threshold versus suprathreshold strategies

Full threshold strategies provide more detailed information than suprathreshold strategies since they indicate the depth of scotomas rather than merely their presence or absence. However, full thresholding is more time-consuming, which has important implications for resource allocation. It is also more wearisome for the patient, which can affect the reliability of test results. Many patients exhibit pronounced learning effects: their performance in full threshold testing improves with repeated attempts.

For these reasons, suprathreshold testing is best used when a rapid distinction between normality and abnormality is required, whereas full thresholding is better for the long-term follow-up of patients whose visual fields are known to be abnormal and may be slowly deteriorating. For example, suprathreshold testing is commonly used to 'screen' for glaucoma, but patients with established glaucoma are followed with full threshold tests.

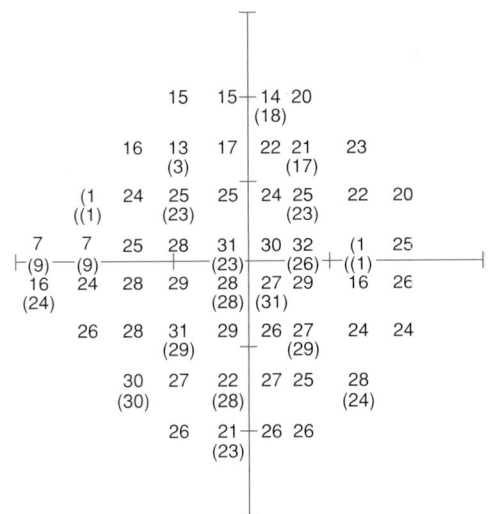

Fig. 5 Humphrey field analyser raw sensitivity plot (24-2 strategy).

Graphical display of results

The precise format of the display varies according to which brand of perimeter is used. However, the print-outs of almost all automated perimeters have some features in common.

Numerical threshold data

Numbers representing the thresholds measured at all the test locations are displayed diagrammatically as in Fig. 5. The intersection of the two axes represents fixation, and each number represents the threshold at that test location. For this particular figure (the Humphrey 24-2 strategy), the separation of the locations, both vertically and horizontally, is 6°.

Numerical displays such as that in Fig. 5 may show either the 'raw' thresholds at each location, or they may show the difference in sensitivity between the measured threshold and a threshold obtained from a normal, age-matched database. For the Humphrey field analyser this latter display is called the total deviation plot. The Humphrey field analyser also displays a numerical pattern deviation plot: this is a plot in which any generalized shift away from the age-matched norm is removed, and only more localized defects are shown.

Grayscales

Although the numerical displays mentioned above provide much useful information, they are rather dry and difficult to interpret at a glance. The grayscale provides an image which is more readily understood: thresholds are first interpolated to give a denser grid of values than the numerical display, then these are coded according to a key (Fig. 6(b)) and displayed as in Fig. 6(a), which is the grayscale corresponding to the numerical display in Fig. 5. The Humphrey field analyser also provides grayscale displays for the total deviation and pattern deviation plots.

Suprathreshold tests

Since only one of two categories ('seen' or 'not seen') is attached to each test location, numerical displays are not appro-

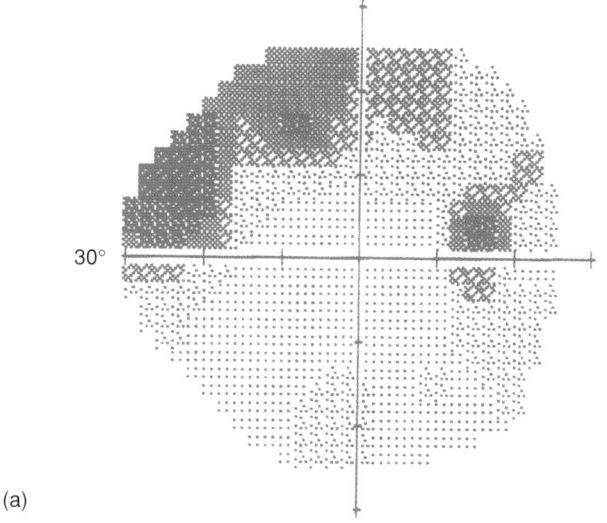

(a)

Graytone symbols

SYM										
ASB	0.8 to 0.1	2.5 to 1	8 to 32	25 to 10	79 to 32	251 to 100	794 to 316	2512 to 1000	7943 to 3162	≥ 10000
DB	41 to 50	36 to 40	31 to 35	26 to 30	21 to 25	16 to 20	11 to 15	6 to 10	1 to 5	≤ 0

(b)

Fig. 6 (a, b) Humphrey field analyser grayscale and legend.

priate: each location is instead represented by a symbol indicating whether the stimulus at that location was seen or not.

Factors affecting automated visual fields

When interpreting the results of automated visual testing, it is important to be aware of several factors which may greatly influence the test before ascribing any deviation from the normal or from previous tests to pathological change.

Pupil size

A reduction in pupil size results in a decrease in threshold values, especially in the peripheral visual field, and in an increase in the variability of threshold measures. These effects are particularly relevant with regard to miotic therapy for glaucoma: for example, an apparent worsening of a patient's visual field may be found to coincide with the start of a course of pilocarpine drops. If this patient's pupil is dilated with a short-acting topical mydriatic administered before the visual field test (if this is clinically appropriate) the result will be free from the adverse effects of the miotic and a fairer comparison with previous tests may be made.

Refractive error

Uncorrected refractive error causes defocusing of the retinal image of the test stimulus. The effect of 5.00 dioptres of simulated hyperopic blur on a Goldmann size III stimulus (commonly used in the follow-up of glaucoma patients) is to reduce the central sensitivity by approximately 6 dB. The effect

of defocus on sensitivity varies with the degree of refractive error and the eccentricity of the stimulus, and depends on the individual patient. Refractive errors greater than 1.00 dioptre should be corrected. Many perimeters use a testing distance for which a presbyopic correction will also be necessary.

Unfortunately, the correction of refractive errors itself poses problems. Many perimeters incorporate a holder for a standard trial lens in order to correct the eye under test, but the small diameter of these lenses may mean that the edge of the lens may encroach upon the visual field and cause a lens rim artefact. This appears as a defect at the edge of the central visual field. It does not usually respect either the horizontal or vertical meridians but may mimic a nerve fibre bundle defect. Lens rim artefacts are more common in elderly people and in hypermetropes. They may be avoided by ensuring that the patient's eye is as close to the correcting lens as possible and well centred behind the lens. The patients' own spectacles should be used if possible (unless they are bi-, multi-, or varifocal or inappropriate to the testing distance) since they give a larger field of view than a trial lens. If the correcting lens is powerful (either plus or minus) the visual field will show evidence of the prismatic effect of the lens. Light entering the lens paraxially will be subject to this effect: a strong plus lens (such as that worn by an aphakic patient) will cause an apparent constriction of the field with the blind spot diminished in size and shifted centrally, whereas a strong minus lens will cause an apparent increase in size and peripheral shifting of the blind spot.

Lid artefacts

Apparent losses in the superior visual field may result from slight ptosis, prominent eyelashes, dermatochalasis, or prominent brows. Incorrect positioning of the patient at the perimeter may be a contributory factor. These artefacts may be extremely difficult to distinguish from incipient arcuate scotomas. If the cause is ptosis, however, the problem is easily solved: if the lid is gently lifted with adhesive tape for the duration of the test, so as to abolish the ptosis but still allow the patient to blink fully, the artefact disappears.

Media opacities

Opacities in the cornea, the aqueous, the lens (or posterior capsule following extracapsular cataract surgery), or the vitreous may adversely affect the results of visual field testing since they lead to degradation of the retinal image through a combination of filtering and scattering. Media opacities usually cause a generalized reduction of sensitivity across the whole field: this may be difficult to distinguish from diffuse glaucomatous loss. Occasionally localized lens opacities may cause focal visual field defects but these are rarely as well defined as nerve fibre bundle defects. Examination of the ocular media will reveal any opacities dense enough to affect the visual field.

A special case of scattering occurs through iatrogenic disruption of the tear film: this is particularly marked when viscous coupling medium is used as part of an examination with a goniolens. Such examinations are better left until after the field test.

The learning effect

Some subjects show a marked increase in sensitivity from the initial test to subsequent tests. This tends to be more marked in the superior and peripheral parts of the field. Other subjects, however, do not show any learning effect and produce reliable tests from the outset. Most learning effects have disappeared after the first two visual field tests. If learning effects are suspected, the results of visual field tests should be ignored until a stable baseline is achieved.

Retinal adaptation

Perimetric examinations are usually performed in low photopic conditions: it is essential that the patient's eyes are allowed sufficient time to adapt to these lighting levels before the test is begun. In most cases, if the room lights are dimmed before the patient is seated at the perimeter and while a brief instruction and demonstration are given, adaptation will have occurred by the time the test starts. If, however, the patient has been examined with an ophthalmoscope the retina will be 'bleached' and adaptation will take much longer. Thus it is not advisable to perform ophthalmoscopic examination before visual field analysis.

Statistical analysis

Since automated perimetry generates numerical results, a huge number of methods of statistical analysis have been applied to visual fields in order to characterize individual fields, and to attempt to identify trends in visual field series. Most of these efforts have been directed at the visual fields of glaucoma patients and glaucoma suspects. The following discussion is restricted to the more widely used analyses, and applies particularly to the Octopus and Humphrey perimeters.

Reliability indices

Before statistical analysis of an automated field test may be considered, some account must be taken of its reliability. This involves attention to the factors mentioned in the previous section. In addition, perimeters calculate reliability indices which are shown on the output display. Fixation losses are measured by the Heijl–Krakau technique: once the position of the physiological blind spot has been ascertained, stimuli are presented within this area. Any reported as seen represent inaccurate fixation. False positives are recorded when the machine behaves exactly as if a stimulus were about to be presented, but none is, and the subject reports the (non-existent) stimulus as seen. False negatives are detected when a stimulus known to be above the threshold at a particular location is presented at that location and the subject does not record the stimulus as seen.

Visual fields which have a large proportion of fixation losses, false negatives, or especially false positives are likely to be unreliable. Automated perimeters may alert the examiner to this: for example, the Humphrey field analyser displays a 'low patient reliability' message. These messages should be interpreted with caution, however, as there is no proven association between machine-generated reliability indices and actual patient reliability. If the machine fails to determine the location of the physio-

$$ SF = \left[\frac{1}{n} \sum_{i=1}^{n} \frac{\sum_{j=1}^{r} (x_{ij} - \overline{x_i})^2}{r - 1} \right]^{\frac{1}{2}} $$

SF = short-term fluctuation
r = number of repeat determinations (usually 2)
$\overline{x_i}$ = mean sensitivity at location i
x_{ij} = sensitivity at location i for repeat determination j
n = number of locations with repeat determinations

Fig. 7 Formula for the calculation of short-term fluctuation (Octopus).

logical blind spot correctly, the Heijl–Krakau technique will record a large number of fixation losses even though the subject's fixation is steady. Furthermore, early glaucoma may be associated with an increased proportion of false negatives in some patients: in these cases false negatives are an index of disease rather than reliability.

Single visual fields

Information relating to the amount of visual field loss, and whether the loss is generalized or focal, is encapsulated in a set of summary measures known as global indices. For the Octopus perimeter these are mean defect, short-term fluctuation, loss variance, and corrected loss variance. The corresponding measures for the Humphrey perimeter are mean deviation and short-term fluctuation. The Octopus indices will be described first as they are more readily understood and the Humphrey indices are more complex versions of them.

Mean defect is calculated by taking the difference between the threshold measured at each test location and a value obtained from a normal age-matched database. The mean defect is the mean of these differences. It is more sensitive to generalized or diffuse loss than to small, focal scotomas. It is of more value in the follow-up of patients with established visual defects than in the detection of early disease. The validity of the mean defect is critically dependent upon the validity of the comparison between the test data and the normal data set. In other words, the sample used to compile the normal database must be truly representative of the population from which the subject under test is drawn. This comment applies to all measures which involve a comparison with a 'normal' database.

Short-term fluctuation is a measure of the intratest variation. It is calculated by testing a set of locations more than once during each visual field examination and analysing the variance of these repeat measures. The formula for short-term fluctuation for the Octopus is shown in Fig. 7. Short-term fluctuation is increased in glaucoma.

Loss variance is an index of the amount of focal loss in the field. It depends on the fact that, if there are areas of the field with large defects (i.e. differences from normal values) and

$$\mathrm{SF} = \left[\left[\frac{1}{n}\sum_{i=1}^{n} s^2{}_i\right] \times \left[\frac{1}{n}\sum_{i=1}^{n} \frac{\sum_{j=1}^{r}(x_{ij} - \overline{x_i})^2}{r-1}\right]\right]^{\frac{1}{2}}$$

SF = short-term fluctuation

$s^2{}_i$ = number intratest variance at location i

r = number of repeat determinations (usually 2)

$\overline{x_i}$ = mean sensitivity at location i

x_{ij} = sensitivity at location i for repeat determinations j

n = number of locations with repeat determinations

Fig. 8 Formula for the calculation of short-term fluctuation (Humphrey field analyser).

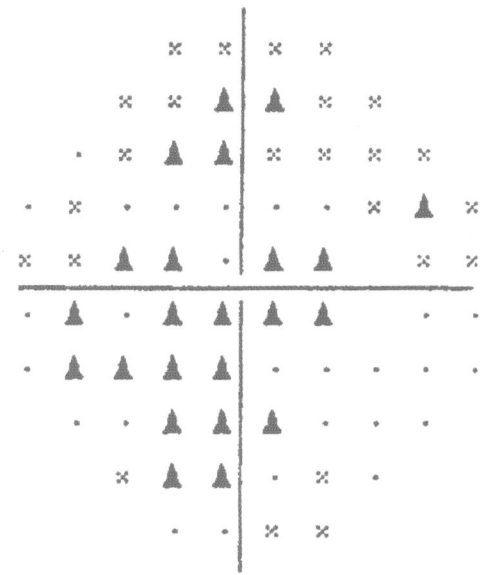

Fig. 9 Statpac 2 display (detail).

other areas with small defects, the variance of the defects will be larger than if the field were uniformly normal or uniformly depressed.

Since variability is inherent in visual field testing, there will always be some loss variance. The concept of corrected loss variance was introduced to obtain a zero-based measure of focal loss. Corrected loss variance is calculated by subtracting from the value of loss variance a measure of the subject's intratest variability. This measure is the square of the short-term fluctuation.

The global indices provided by the Humphrey field analyser have a similar theoretical basis to the Octopus indices, but there are some important differences. In the Humphrey field analyser, the formula for the calculation of a global index includes a term which accounts for the normal variance at each location. This can be seen by comparing Fig. 8, which is the formula for short-term fluctuation for the Humphrey field analyser, with Fig. 7. The Humphrey indices of focal loss, and pattern standard deviation are related to the Octopus loss variance and corrected loss variance, respectively. However, the Humphrey indices are measures of standard deviation (square root of variance) as their names suggest, and they incorporate measures of normal variance at each location as mentioned previously. In addition, corrected pattern standard deviation includes a constant factor to adjust for the non-uniform fluctuation pattern across the field. The greater complexity of the Humphrey indices does not greatly affect their usefulness as summary measures of visual field behaviour.

Visual field series

If a subject has undergone a series of visual field examinations a further dimension may be added to the statistical analysis: the diagnosis of the presence or absence of progressive visual field loss may be attempted. Comparison of serial global indices by means of linear regression, or statistical methods such as t-testing or analysis of variance, does not provide a good indica-

tion of progression. There are statistical objections to many of these methods, and the spatial information gathered in perimetry is lost during the formulation of global indices: new scotomas in previously undamaged areas of the field are missed as evidence of progression.

There are two commercially available software packages for the Humphrey field analyser which evaluate progression on a point-by-point rather than a field-by-field basis: Statpac 2 and Progressor.

Statpac 2 (and, more recently, Statpac for Windows) is the 'native' statistical glaucoma change probability software available as an add-on for the Humphrey field analyser. The program uses the thresholds from the first two fields in the series as a baseline (if they are reliable): each subsequent field is compared on a point-by-point basis to this baseline and points are labelled with a black triangle (Fig. 9), if $P < 0.05$ for the null hypothesis of no glaucomatous change. A problem with this analysis is that the particular field under study is compared only with the baseline, so artefact or fluctuation in the baseline fields will have a large effect, and information in any intervening fields after the baseline does not contribute to the analysis. Furthermore, points are frequently labelled as deteriorating purely by chance: several consecutive fields showing consistent abnormality are necessary for a reliable diagnosis.

Progressor performs linear regression of sensitivity on time for each test location over the whole field series. Results are presented as a cumulative graphical display (Fig. 10(a)). Each test location is represented as a small bar graph, with one bar for each test. The length of each bar corresponds to the sensitivity of the location at that test: the longer the bar, the lower the sensitivity. The colour of the bar relates to the significance of the slope of the regression line at that test (Fig. 10(b)). Thus undamaged locations are seen as series of short grey bars, damaged but stable locations are seen as long series of long grey

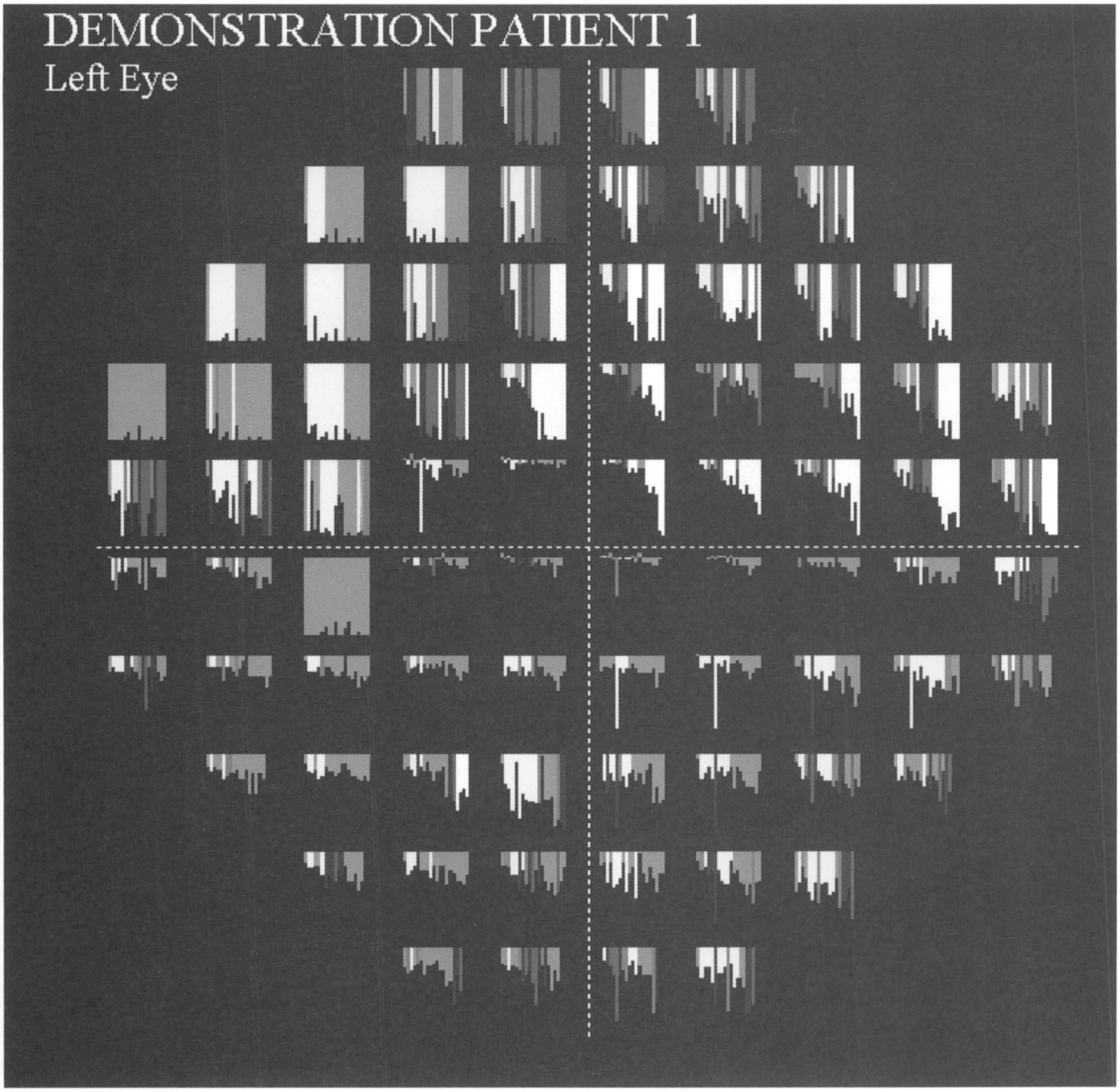

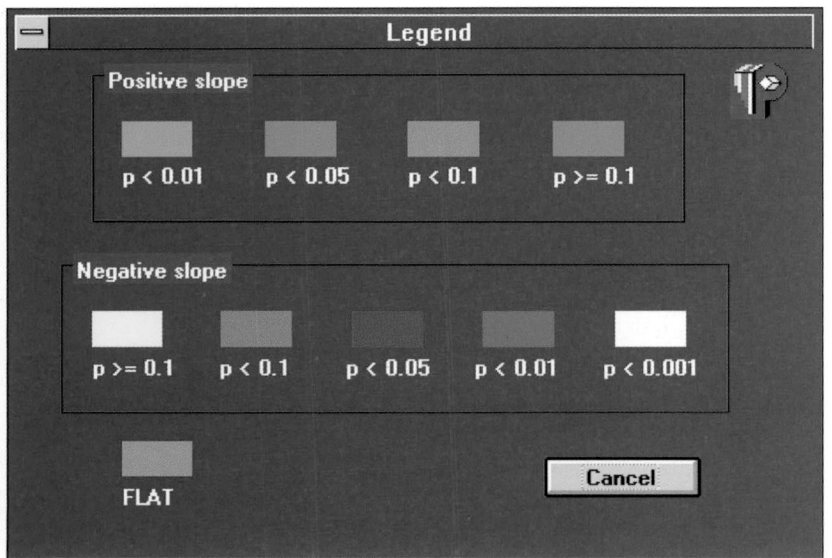

(a)

(b)

Fig. 10 (a, b) Progressor display and legend.

bars, and progressing locations are seen as series of progressively lengthening bars which change colour as the regression slope becomes more significant.

Progressor has been shown to detect progression earlier than Statpac 2 in ocular hypertensives and normal-tension glaucoma patients, but both algorithms produce 'false positives' compared to clinical judgment. However, clinical judgment is an inadequate gold standard against which to compare these algorithms: there is a great deal of disagreement over the diagnosis of visual field progression even amongst expert observers. Furthermore, clinical judgment does not provide a consistent theoretical basis upon which to compare the effects of different treatments, so it is not of use in clinical trials. Although the current methods of automated analysis of serial visual fields leave room for improvement, they are a useful adjunct to the clinical decision-making process. Refinements to the software are likely to improve the algorithms and widen their use.

Further reading

Henson, D.B. (1993). *Visual fields*. Oxford University Press, Oxford. [A detailed overview of the principles and practice of perimetry, including reviews of commercially available perimeters and the application of perimetry to various clinical situations.]

Humphrey, A. (1987). *The field analyzer primer*. San Leandro. [A user-friendly guide to the interpretation of results from the Humphrey field analyser.]

Lachenmayr, B.J. and Vivell, P.M.O. (1993). *Perimetry and its clinical correlations*, (trans. F.C. Blodi). Thieme Medical, New York. [A detailed overview of the principles and practice of perimetry, including reviews of commercially available perimeters and the application of perimetry to various clinical situations.]

2

Clinical ophthalmology

2.1 Orbital disease

2.1.1 Anatomy of the orbit and lacrimal apparatus

C.D. Illingworth

The orbit consists of bony walls and their contents. It is pear-shaped, narrowed toward the apex with the optic canal as the stalk, and has a volume of approximately 30 ml. For ease of description the main orbital cavity may be considered as a pyramid which is tilted when viewed from the front, so that the medial wall lies in the anteroposterior plane, while the lateral wall lies at a 45° angle to the sagittal plane. The bony walls are comprised of the frontal bone, zygomatic bone, maxilla, lacrimal bone, sphenoid, ethmoid, and palatine bone. The contents consist of the globe, striated muscle (the extraocular muscles), smooth muscle (Müller's muscles), the main and accessory lacrimal glands and the lacrimal drainage apparatus, the optic nerve, peripheral sensory and motor nerves, autonomic nerves, the ciliary ganglion, arteries and veins, cartilage (the trochlea), and lastly a complex arrangement of fascia. This chapter discusses the anatomy of all except the globe and the muscles which are included in other chapters.

Bony anatomy

The margins of the orbit are as follows. The superior margin is formed by the frontal bone, which posseses a supraorbital notch or foramen and a supratrochlear notch (rarely foramen) to allow the passage of the supraorbital and supratrochlear neurovascular bundles. The supraorbital notch is found at the junction of the medial one-third and the lateral two-thirds of the superior orbital rim, while the supratrochlear notch is situated a variable distance medially. The lateral margin is formed by processes of the frontal and zygomatic bones. The inferior margin is formed by the zygomatic bone and maxilla. A suture which closes in adulthood leads from the inferior margin to the infraorbital foramen. The foramen is situated approximately 9 mm below the mid-point of the inferior margin, and the infraorbital artery and nerve pass through it. The medial margin is formed by processes of the maxilla and the frontal bone. The anterior and posteror lacrimal crests, running

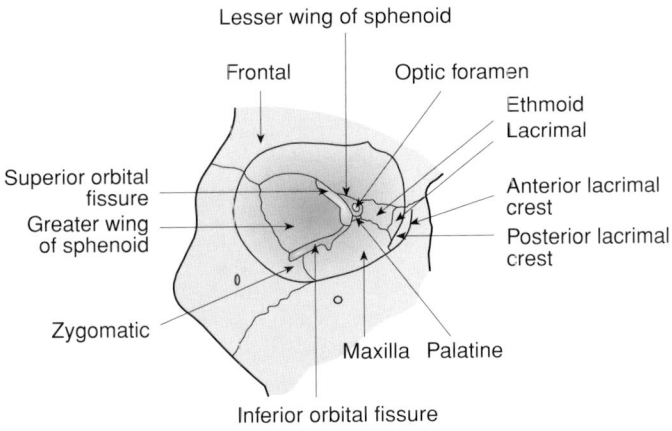

Fig. 1 Bones of the orbit.

upward and downward respectively, overlap at the medial margin.

The roof of the orbit is formed by the thin orbital plate of the frontal bone, which separates the orbit from the anterior cranial fossa. Posteriorly the roof is composed of the lesser wing of the sphenoid. Anteriorly the frontal bone is split to form orbital and cranial plates, between which lies the frontal sinus. A shallow depression in the anterolateral aspect of the roof marks the site of the orbital part of the lacrimal gland. The trochlear spine (when present) is situated at the junction of the roof and the medial wall, just behind the orbital margin. At the apex of the roof is the optic foramen, which is the opening of the optic canal. The canal is formed by the two roots of the lesser wing of the sphenoid arising from the body of the sphenoid, and is 4 to 9 mm long. It transmits the optic nerve, ophthalmic artery, and sympathetic nerve fibres (Fig. 1).

The medial wall is formed anteriorly by the frontal process of the maxilla, with the anterior lacrimal crest protruding from it. Posterior to this is the lacrimal bone, marked by the posterior lacrimal crest. Between anterior and posterior lacrimal crests lies the lacrimal fossa, from which leads the nasolacrimal canal. The remainder of the medial wall is formed by the thin orbital plate of the ethmoid (lamina papyracea), which articulates with the body of the sphenoid close to the optic foramen. At the junction of the ethmoid and the frontal bone are the anterior and posterior ethmoid foramina, through which pass the anterior and posterior ethmoidal nerves and arteries. The medial relations of the orbit are the ethmoid sinuses anteriorly, the sphenoid sinus posteriorly, and the cavity of the nose inferiorly.

The floor of the orbit is formed mainly by the orbital plate of the maxilla, which separates the orbit from the maxillary antrum. The floor is first grooved and then canalized by the course of the infraorbital nerve and artery. The nerve is vulnerable to damage by fracture of the floor of the orbit, which will often result in infraorbital anaesthesia. Anterolaterally the zygomatic bone forms a small part of the floor, and at the apex the orbital process of the palatine bone makes up a small component. The orbit is related to the maxillary sinus inferiorly.

The lateral wall is formed by the zygomatic bone anteriorly and the greater wing of the sphenoid posteriorly. Whitnall's tubercle lies just within the lateral margin at about its midpoint. The superior orbital fissure, which is a gap between the greater and lesser wing of the sphenoid, separates the lateral wall from the roof and is itself separated from the optic foramen by a thin strip of bone, while the inferior orbital fissure separates the lateral wall from the floor. The two fissures are interconnected at their medial ends. The superior orbital fissure leads to the middle cranial fossa and transmits the superior ophthalmic vein, lacrimal nerve, frontal nerve, trochlear nerve, superior division of the oculomotor nerve, nasociliary nerve, inferior division of the oculomotor nerve, and abducent nerve. It also transmits sympathetic fibres, sensory root of the ciliary ganglion, anterior meningeal branch of the ophthalmic artery, inferior ophthalmic vein, and often the anastomotic branch from the middle meningeal artery to the lacrimal artery. The inferior orbital fissure leads to the pterygopalatine and infratemporal fossa, and transmits the infraorbital nerve, zygomatic nerve, and ascending branches from the pterygopalatine ganglion, as well as the infraorbital artery and sometimes an inferior ophthalmic vein. It is covered with Müller's muscle, which is of unknown function, although since it is more developed in other species it may be vestigial. The zygomatic foramina, which transmit the zygomaticotemporal and zygomaticofacial neurovascular bundles, are found on the lateral wall a short distance behind the orbital margin. The lateral relations of the orbit are the skin anteriorly, then the temporal fossa, and the middle cranial fossa posteriorly.

The thinnest parts of the orbital walls are the inferior wall and the lamina papyracea of the ethmoid. These are vulnerable in the case of a direct blow to the eye when the orbital contents are suddenly compressed, leading to a blow-out fracture with extrusion of fascia and sometimes muscle at the fracture site. Another important clinical correlation is that infection can spread from the sinuses through the lamina papyracea, resulting in orbital cellulitis.

Fascia of the orbit

The arrangement of the orbital fascia is complex and it is not only important in providing support for the globe, but is intrinsic to the correct function of the extraocular muscles. The three main forms of fascia in the orbit are Tenon's capsule, the periorbital fascia, and the fat-enclosing septae that are present between Tenon's and periorbital fascia.

Tenon's capsule (the fascia bulbi or episcleral fascia) is attached to the globe from the corneoscleral limbus to the optic nerve. Its thin inner layer is closely associated with the sclera, while the outer layer sheaths the tendons of the muscles that attach to the globe. Laterally the outer layer is attached to Whitnall's tubercle on the zygomatic bone just behind the orbital margin, to form the lateral check ligament, while medially it is attached to the posterior lacrimal crest, forming the medial check ligament. Inferiorly the fascia between the two ligaments is thickened to form the suspensory ligament of Lockwood which supports the globe, probably in conjunction with other elements of the orbital fascia.

The periorbital fascia is in fact the loosely attached periosteum that covers the walls of the orbit. Posteriorly it blends with the dura mater covering the optic nerve sheath, and anteriorly it is continuous with the periosteum covering the bones of the face. The fascia divides to surround the lacrimal sac.

Numerous connective tissue septae appear to connect Tenon's capsule to the periorbital fascia, and also attach to the extraocular muscles. The work of Koornneef has shed new light on this area. He found that the septae are arranged in a circumferential pattern in the anterior orbit, while more posteriorly in the region of the muscle 'cone' they are arranged radially. They enclose adipose tissue, and a complex vascular arrangement may be found within them. The inferior rectus and inferior oblique muscles are connected by a connective tissue mass containing smooth muscle, that is also attached to the periosteum of the floor of the orbit. This may explain the observation that the motility disorder found after orbital floor fractures often resembles a combined inferior rectus and inferior oblique palsy, and also the frequent finding during surgery for blow-out fractures that only fascia is entrapped in the fracture site. The superior and inferior oblique muscles are connected to Tenon's capsule by similar septae, and all of the muscles are connected to the periorbit. Koornneef also found a strong attachment between medial and lateral rectus muscles and the annulus of Zinn and optic nerve sheath, while in the case of the other muscles the attachment was much less strong. It was concluded from these studies that the septae form an important element of the support of the globe.

Lacrimal gland

The lacrimal gland is located in a shallow fossa in the lateral part of the roof of the orbit. It weighs approximately 80 g and its average dimensions are $20 \times 12 \times 5$ mm. The gland is supported by fascial septae which attach to the periorbital fascia of the orbital roof. It is separated into a larger orbital part and a smaller palpebral part by the lateral horn of the aponeurosis of the levator palpebrae superioris, around which it extends posteriorly so that the two parts are usually joined by a narrow isthmus. The orbital part is deeper and is separated from the globe by orbital fascia and Tenon's capsule, while the palpebral part can by seen through the lateral part of the superior conjunctival fornix on everting the upper lid. Approximately 12 ducts open into the fornix 5 mm above the lateral tarsal

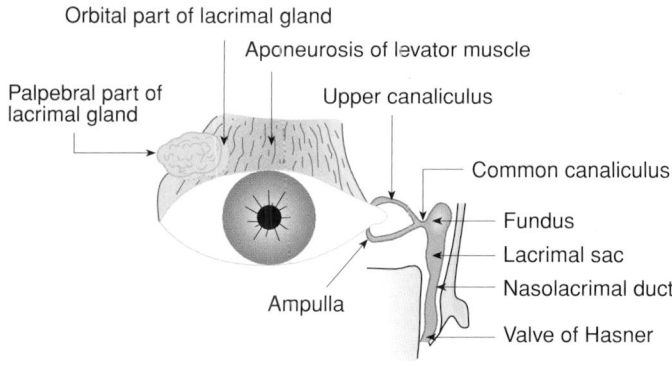

Orbital part of lacrimal gland
Aponeurosis of levator muscle
Palpebral part of lacrimal gland
Upper canaliculus
Common canaliculus
Fundus
Lacrimal sac
Nasolacrimal duct
Ampulla
Valve of Hasner

Fig. 2 Lacrimal gland and drainage apparatus.

margin. The ducts originate from the orbital part and pass through the aponeurosis and then through the palpebral part.

The gland is classically said to be of serous type, although it has recently been found that the gland contains mucopolysaccharide granules. It is of lobulated tubuloalveolar form, and has acini lined by columnar cells containing basophilic granules. The columnar cells are surrounded by a myoepithelial layer.

The parasympathetic secretomotor nerve fibres derive from the superior salivatory nucleus of the pons and pass via the greater petrosal nerve to synapse in the pterygopalatine ganglion. The postganglionic fibres travel to the gland either via the zygomatic and then lacrimal nerves, or by small nerves that pass directly from the ganglion. The gland has a sensory supply from the lacrimal nerve and derives its blood supply from the lacrimal artery.

There are also a number of accessory lacrimal glands. The glands of Krause number 20 in the upper fornix and six to eight in the lower fornix, while three glands of Wolfring are located in the superior tarsus. The accessory glands are thought to be the main providers of basal tear secretion in contrast to reflex secretion which is produced by the lacrimal gland, although the lacrimal gland may also have a role in basal secretion (Fig. 2).

Lacrimal drainage system

Tears drain through the upper and lower lacrimal punctae, which are located at the apex of the lacrimal papillae. They are situated 6 mm from the medial canthus, are approximately 0.3 mm in diameter, and are directed slightly backward. The punctae drain into the upper and lower canaliculi, of which the vertical first part, the ampulla, is 2 to 3 mm wide and 2 mm long. The canaliculi are collapsed if empty and can expand to a diameter of 2 mm. They are approximately 8 mm long and sweep medially, usually to join for the last 2 mm to form the common canaliculus before entering the lacrimal sac. The sac is surrounded by fascia derived from periosteum, which splits into two, the superficial layer bridging the anterior and posterior lacrimal crests to cover the sac. The upper part of the superficial layer is covered by the medial palpebral ligament (medial canthal tendon), which has a free edge inferiorly and attaches to the anterior lacrimal crest. The height of the sac is 10 to

15 mm, of which the part that extends above the entry of the common canaliculus is termed the fundus and is usually 3 to 5 mm in height. It may often appear to be absent due to compression by the medial palpebral ligament.

The nasolacrimal duct extends from the inferior part of the sac through the bony nasolacrimal canal, passing downward and slightly posteriorly. The canal is approximately 12 mm in length, and the duct usually extends for 5 mm beyond the termination of the canal, lying within the mucous membrane of the lateral wall of the nose, to open at the ostium lacrimale between the anterior third and the middle third of the meatus beneath the inferior turbinate.

The ostium is about 30 mm behind the lateral margin of the anterior nares. The lacrimal drainage system is lined by pseudostratified columnar epithelium and the walls of the canaliculi and lacrimal sac are rich in elastic tissue. The mucous membrane is folded at certain points to form valves. The valve of Rosenmueller is found at the entry of the common canaliculus into the lacrimal sac, and the valve of Hasner (plica lacrimalis) is situated at the opening of the nasolacrimal duct under the inferior turbinate. At birth the duct is often closed at the level of the valve of Hasner, but usually canalizes during the first few months of life. There are also valves at the opening of the sac into the nasolacrimal duct and along the course of the duct.

The lacrimal fossa is related to the ethmoid sinus posteriorly while the duct is related to the ethmoid sinus medially in its upper part and then to the maxillary antrum laterally. This area is subject to much anatomical variation. The lacrimal punctae may be absent, stenosed, or duplicated, and fistulae are not uncommon. Other surgically important variations are enlargement of the ethmoid sinus to interpose between the lacrimal fossa and the lateral wall of the nose, anterior extension of the middle turbinate, and a lower opening of the nasolacrimal duct. Rarely the duct may open in the middle meatus of the nose.

Tears drain from the ocular tear film through the canaliculi to the lacrimal sac and then to the nose via the nasolacrimal duct. Drainage is split approximately equally between the upper and lower canaliculi. It appears that the process is facilitated by means of an active pump mechanism activated by blinking. During eyelid closure the punctae are occluded by the lid margin, preventing reflux of tears. Further action of the superficial and deep heads of the pretarsal orbicularis oculi muscle compresses the ampullae and canaliculi, and also shortens the canaliculi, forcing fluid into the lacrimal sac. When the eyelids open, negative pressure in the canaliculi and ampullae refills them. This theory, first suggested by Jones, also proposes that the pull of the deep head of the preseptal orbicularis muscle (which has part of its origin from the lacrimal fascia) opens the lacrimal sac when the lids close during blinking and creates a negative pressure, further aiding emptying of the canaliculi into the sac. The latter component of the pump mechanism cannot be essential for tear drainage, since negative pressure cannot occur in the sac after the surgical procedure of dacryocystorhinostomy, yet tear drainage is usually effective.

Other factors that may aid tear drainage are the effect of gravity on fluid in the sac, capillary action, and microscillation in the nasolacrimal duct. In addition, evaporation of tears from the surface of the eye is probably of importance.

Blood vessels of the orbit

The ophthalmic artery is the main blood supply of the orbit. It usually arises from carotid artery above the diaphragma sellae and under the optic nerve. Occasionally it is derived mainly or solely from the middle meningeal artery. The ophthalmic artery enters the optic canal under the optic nerve, and on emerging at the orbital apex is inferolateral to the nerve and medial to the lateral rectus muscle within the muscle cone. It then turns sharply (the 'angle') to pass medially above the optic nerve (below in 15–20 per cent) and then passes forward above the medial rectus muscle and under the superior oblique to meet the medial orbital wall close to the anterior ethmoidal foramen.

The orbital and ocular branches of the ophthalmic artery mainly arise in the retrobulbar area. The following is their usual order (Fig. 3):

1. The central artery of the retina most commonly arises close to the angle of the ophthalmic artery and passes forward under the optic nerve, before turning upward at a point approximately 10 mm from the globe to pierce the dural and arachnoid sheaths. It usually lies inferomedial to the nerve at this point and then runs forward as the intravaginal part of the artery. After a variable distance it invaginates the pia mater and enters the central part of the optic nerve, where it passes forward as the intraneural part to divide into the retinal arteries, its terminal branches, at the nerve head. It is closely related to the central retinal vein during its course through the nerve. It gives off branches to the pia from the intravaginal part, and branches to the nerve from the intraneural part. It is generally held that the pial branches of the central retinal artery anastomose with pial branches of the ciliary circulation and with pial branches of the ophthalmic artery.

2. The posterior ciliary arteries arise in a variable number of trunks that divide into 15 to 20 branches, which pierce the sclera around the optic nerve.

3. The lacrimal artery has a variable origin and passes forward along the lateral wall of the orbit at the upper margin of the lateral rectus muscle. After reaching the lacrimal gland it divides to form two lateral palpebral arteries, having given off branches to the lateral and often to the superior rectus muscles, in addition to zygomatic branches which pierce the zygomatic bone. The lacrimal artery often sends a recurrent meningeal branch to join the anastomotic branch of the middle meningeal artery, passing through the superior orbital fissure or occasionally through a separate foramen in the greater wing of the sphenoid. There may be anastomotic connections via both routes. In some cases the lacrimal artery is entirely derived from the anastomosis, and occasionally the ophthalmic artery is derived mainly or solely from it.

4. Branches to the pial plexus of the optic nerve and chiasm.

5. The muscular branches generally take the form of a superior trunk which supplies the superior rectus, superior oblique and levator palpebrae superioris, and an inferior trunk which supplies the medial rectus, inferior rectus, and inferior oblique. The branches to the muscles give off long ciliary branches which run along the muscles to the globe.

6. The posterior ethmoidal artery leaves the orbit through the posterior ethmoidal foramen approximately 5 mm anterior to the optic canal, to supply the posterior ethmoidal sinus, the sphenoidal sinus, and part of the lateral wall of the nose. It frequently gives a branch to the superior oblique. The artery is occasionally absent.

7. The supraorbital artery passes forward along the medial border of the levator and then between the levator and the roof of the orbit to leave the orbit via the supraorbital notch or foramen. It gives branches to the superior rectus and levator muscles.

8. The anterior ethmoidal artery passes through the anterior ethmoidal foramen and supplies the anterior and middle ethmoidal sinuses, frontal sinus, and the side of the nose.

9. The anterior meningeal artery runs back through the superior orbital fissure.

10. The medial palpebral arteries usually take the form of a superior and inferior branch and supply the medial lids and lacrimal sac.

11. The supratrochlear (frontal) artery is one of the ter-

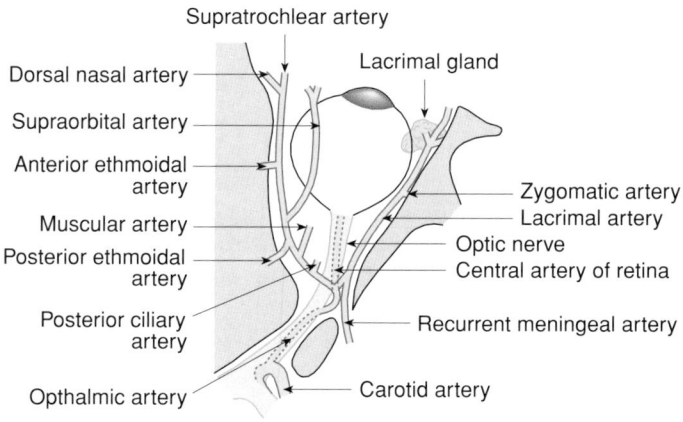

Supratrochlear artery

Dorsal nasal artery

Lacrimal gland

Supraorbital artery

Anterior ethmoidal artery

Muscular artery

Posterior ethmoidal artery

Posterior ciliary artery

Opthalmic artery

Zygomatic artery

Lacrimal artery

Optic nerve

Central artery of retina

Recurrent meningeal artery

Carotid artery

Fig. 3 Arteries of the orbit.

minal branches. It pierces the orbital septum and leaves the orbit through the supratrochlear notch.

12. The dorsal nasal artery, the other terminal branch, leaves the orbit between the trochlea and medial palpebral ligament, and anastomoses with the angular artery (which is derived from the facial artery).

However, the branches of the ophthalmic artery are variable, especially in the case of the posterior ciliary and muscular arteries, which may be derived from the lacrimal artery. The arrangement of the arteries is invariably different if the optic nerve is undercrossed. If this occurs, the first branch is usually a posterior ciliary artery, followed by the central retinal, medial muscular, and lacrimal arteries.

The infraorbital artery supplies a small part of the orbit. It is one of the terminal branches of the maxillary artery and enters the orbit from the pterygopalatine fossa via the inferior orbital fissure. It passes through the infraorbital canal to emerge on the face through the infraorbital foramen. It gives off one or more orbital branches, which divide to supply the inferior rectus and inferior oblique muscles, lacrimal gland, and lower lid.

Veins of the orbit

The superior ophthalmic vein is formed from the union of branches of the supraorbital and angular veins posterior to the reflected tendon of the superior oblique muscle. It passes posterolaterally inferior to the superior rectus muscle and above the optic nerve within the muscle cone, until it reaches the lateral border of the superior rectus. It then proceeds posteriorly above the lateral rectus muscle, and enters the cavernous sinus via the superior orbital fissure, usually passing outside the annulus of Zinn. Its tributaries accompany the branches of the ophthalmic artery.

The inferior ophthalmic vein arises from a venous rete in the anteromedial part of the orbit. Through the rete the veins of the orbit communicate with the facial vein and the rete also connects to the superior ophthalmic vein. The inferior ophthalmic vein passes posterolaterally to leave the orbit via the inferior part of the superior orbital fissure to empty into the cavernous sinus or join the superior ophthalmic vein. There is also a second inferior vein in some cases, which empties through the inferior orbital fissure into the pterygoid venous plexus, and there may also (in approximately 40 per cent of individuals) be a medial ophthalmic vein. This arises from the superior ophthalmic vein and passes posteriorly close to the medial orbital wall, entering the cavernous sinus inferior to the superior ophthalmic vein. A number of collateral veins connecting the superior ophthalmic vein with the inferior vein and rete are described, passing either inside or outside the muscle cone.

The central retinal vein may either join the superior or inferior ophthalmic veins, or occasionally enter the cavernous sinus separately.

The connections between ophthalmic and facial veins are

important clinically, since infection may spread from the face to the cavernous sinus, resulting in cavernous sinus thrombosis.

Lymphatic vessels

The orbit contains no lymph nodes, and lymph vessels have not been convincingly demonstrated in the human orbit, although they have been found in primate orbits.

Nerves of the orbit

The optic nerve emerges from the optic foramen sheathed in pia, arachnoid, and dura mater, which continue until the nerve meets the eye. In this sense the nerve may be considered as an extension of the brain. The nerve courses laterally and inferiorly as it passes forward to meet the globe 3 mm medial to the posterior pole. The length of the nerve in the orbit is approximately 25 mm, and it has a sinuous course, with the result that it is approximately 6 mm longer than the distance from the optic foramen to the globe. It is crossed superiorly by the ophthalmic artery, superior ophthalmic vein, and nasociliary nerve.

One-third of the way along the course of the optic nerve from the foramen to the eye the ciliary ganglion lies laterally. The ganglion receives roots from the nasociliary nerve and from the nerve to the inferior oblique as detailed below, and also receives sympathetic fibres from the cavernous plexus that enter the orbit in the lower part of the superior orbital fissure. It gives off 12 or more short ciliary nerves which pierce the sclera around the optic nerve.

The infraorbital nerve and zygomatic nerve are branches of the maxillary nerve that pass through the inferior orbital fissure. The infraorbital nerve, together with the infraorbital artery, runs forward on the orbital floor before entering the infraorbital canal to subsequently emerge through the infraorbital foramen. The zygomatic nerve runs forward on the lateral wall and divides to form the zygomaticotemporal and zygomaticofacial nerves which enter foramina in the lateral wall from where they traverse the zygomatic bone accompanied by small branches of the lacrimal artery. Before entering the foramen the zygomaticotemporal nerve sends a communicating branch to the lacrimal nerve carrying secretomotor fibres to the lacrimal gland, although doubt has been cast upon the importance of this branch (Fig. 4).

The other main nerves of the orbit pass through the superior orbital fissure. In order from above to below the lacrimal, frontal, and trochlear nerves pass outside the annulus of Zinn, while the upper division of the oculomotor, the nasociliary, the lower division of the oculomotor and the abducent, lie within the annulus. The lacrimal, frontal, and nasociliary nerves are branches of the ophthalmic division of the trigeminal nerve.

The lacrimal nerve runs along the upper border of the lateral rectus muscle and gives branches that enter the lacrimal gland. The nerve pierces the orbital septum to supply a small area of the lateral part of the upper lid. It also gives branches to the upper fornix of the conjunctiva.

The frontal nerve runs between the levator muscle and the

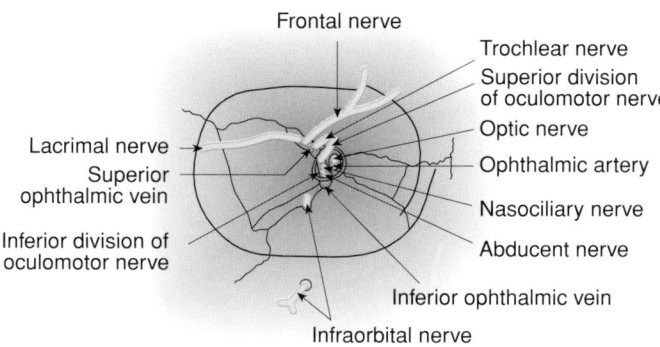

Fig. 4 Relationship of nerves and blood vessels to the orbital fissures.

roof of the orbit to divide into two terminal branches, the supraorbital and supratrochlear nerves, which accompany the corresponding arteries. It gives a branch to the mucous membrane of the frontal sinus.

The trochlear nerve (IV) passes forward and medially over the levator muscle to enter the upper surface of the superior oblique muscle.

The superior division of the oculomotor nerve (IIIs) runs forward between the optic nerve and the superior rectus muscle before piercing the superior rectus and then entering the levator, supplying both muscles.

The inferior division of the oculomotor nerve (IIIi) gives three branches. The nerve to the medial rectus passes inferior to the optic nerve before entering the muscle. The branch to the inferior rectus runs on the upper surface of the muscle before entering it. The branch to the inferior oblique runs along the lateral edge of the inferior rectus, giving a motor (parasympathetic) branch to the ciliary ganglion before entering the inferior oblique.

The nasociliary nerve passes forward lateral to the ophthalmic artery, crossing the optic nerve (which runs laterally underneath), before dividing into its terminal branches. The branches of the nasociliary nerve are:

1. The sensory root of the ciliary ganglion leaves the nasociliary nerve either in the superior orbital fissure or immediately within the orbit. It passes forward lateral to the optic nerve to enter the ciliary ganglion.

2. The long ciliary nerves, usually two in number, leave the nasociliary nerve as it crosses the optic nerve and pass on the medial side of the optic nerve to pierce the sclera medial to the short ciliary nerves. They carry sympathetic fibres to the dilator pupillae muscle and sensory fibres to the cornea.

3. The posterior ethmoidal nerve accompanies the posterior ethmoidal artery to pass beneath the superior oblique muscle and then enters the posterior ethmoidal foramen, to supply the posterior ethmoidal and sphenoidal sinuses.

4. The infratrochlear nerve is one of the terminal branches. It arises near the medial wall of the orbit to

pass forward and beneath the lower border of the superior oblique and the trochlea. It passes above the medial palpebral ligament, supplying conjunctiva, the lacrimal sac, and an area of skin of the upper lid.

5. The anterior ethmoidal nerve (VI) is the other terminal branch, entering the anterior ethmoidal foramen. It supplies the anterior and middle ethmoidal sinuses, frontal sinus, and cavity of the nose before emerging to supply the skin of the lower part of the nose.

The abducent nerve (VI) passes forward and laterally away from the optic nerve to enter the medial surface of the lateral rectus muscle.

Summary of the autonomic nerves of the orbit

Parasympathetic

1. Secretomotor fibres to the lacrimal gland, derived from the superior salivatory nucleus of the pons, passing via the greater petrosal nerve to synapse in the pterygopalatine ganglion, and postganglionic fibres entering the gland either directly, or via the zygomatic and lacrimal nerves.

2. Motor fibres to the sphincter pupillae and ciliary muscles, derived from the Edinger–Westphal nucleus and passing via the oculomotor nerve to synapse in the ciliary ganglion, with postganglionic fibres passing via the short ciliary nerves.

Sympathetic: (derived from the cavernous plexus)

1. Motor fibres to the dilator pupillae muscle that pass via the nasociliary nerve and long ciliary nerves

2. Motor fibres to Müller's component of the levator palpebrae superioris that pass via the superior division of the oculomotor nerve.

3. Vasomotor fibres that accompany arteries, and also pass through the ciliary ganglion and enter the globe via the short ciliary nerves. Vasomotor nerves reach the lacrimal gland via the lacrimal nerve.

Further reading

Duke-Elder, S. and Wybar, K.C. (1961). *System of ophthalmology*, Vol. II. *The anatomy of the visual system*. Henry Kimpton, London.

Hayrey, S.S. (1962). The ophthalmic artery. III. Branches. *British Journal of Ophthalmology*, **46**, 212–47.

Hayrey, S.S. and Dass, R. (1962). The ophthalmic artery. I. Origin and intracranial and intracanalicular course. *British Journal of Ophthalmology*, **46**, 65–98.

Iwamoto, T. and Jakobiec, F. (1982). Lacrimal glands. In *Ocular anatomy, embryology and teratology*, (ed. Jakobiec F), pp. 762–4. Harper & Row, Philadelphia.

Jones, L.T. (1973). Anatomy of the tear system. In *The preocular tear film and dry eye syndromes*, Vol. 13, (ed. F.J. Holly and M.A. Lemp), pp. 3–22, *International ophthalmology clinics*.

Koornneef, L. (1982). Orbital connective tissue. In *Ocular anatomy, embryology and teratology* (ed. F. Jakobiec), pp. 835–57. Harper & Row, Philadelphia.

Whitnall, S.E. (1932). *The anatomy of the human orbit and accessory organs of vision*. Oxford University Press, Oxford.

Williams, P.L., Warwick, R., Dyson, M., and Wing, J.K. (1989). *Gray's anatomy*, (37th edn). Churchill Livingston, London.

2.1.2 The investigation of orbital disease

Garry Davis

The patient with orbital disease presents infrequently to the general ophthalmologist and, for this reason, many clinicians feel uncomfortable when dealing with such a patient. This chapter introduces an approach to the clinical evaluation of orbital disease and provides a rationale for investigation.

Frequency of disease

In order to evaluate the orbital patient one should understand the relative frequency with which conditions are likely to be encountered (Table 1). Many large series report the frequency of orbital conditions, but bias in the pattern of referral, or the nature of the series being reported (clinical versus pathological) ensures that the figures often do not represent the true incidence of the different orbital diseases.

Clinical evaluation

The detailed clinical assessment of the patient presenting with orbital disease is of prime importance. Currently available radiological and laboratory techniques provide valuable, sometimes diagnostic, information, but this should be viewed as supplementary to the information derived from a systematic history and careful examination.

Characterizing the disease process

In order to characterize the abnormality, two essential elements must be addressed: location and pattern of disease.

Location

Disease location is a clue to the site of origin and, hence, possible aetiology (Table 2). Although the majority of orbital processes exert a mass effect on surrounding structures by displacing them away from the site of pathology, others may exert a 'negative' effect by drawing the orbital contents towards them:

Table 1 Frequency of orbital diseases

Paediatric
Cystic: dermoid, epidermoid
Inflammatory: orbital cellulitis, idiopathic
Vascular: capillary haemangioma, venous anomaly
Optic nerve glioma
Primary neoplasia: rhabdomyosarcoma, histiocytosis X
Secondary/metastatic: neuroblastoma,* myeloid leukaemia
Neurofibroma
Fibrous dysplasia

Adult
Thyroid eye disease*
Secondary/metastatic
Inflammatory: idiopathic, infective, specific (Wegener's, sarcoidosis*)
Vascular: venous anomaly, cavernous haemangioma
Lymphoproliferative: benign reactive lymphoid hyperplasia, lymphoma
Cystic: mucocele, dermoid
Lacrimal gland neoplasia: pleomorphic adenoma, adenoid cystic carcinoma
Other primary neoplasia: optic nerve sheath meningioma, peripheral nerve
Bone lesions: cholesterol granuloma, fibrous dysplasia, osteoma

*Diseases often presenting bilaterally.
Note: diseases are presented in approximate descending order of frequency and only the more common conditions within each category are listed.

Table 2 Diseases by location

Superotemporal
Lacrimal gland—infection, inflammation (idiopathic, specific), lymphoproliferative (benign reactive hyperplasia, lymphoma), epithelial neoplasia; *dermoid cyst; neurofibroma, cholesterol granuloma

Superior/superonasal
Sinus mucocele; *dermoid cyst; venous anomaly; *meningoencephalocele; subperiosteal abscess; *rhabdomyosarcoma

Inferior/inferonasal
Lacrimal sac—mucocele, tumour; paranasal sinus carcinoma; *microphthalmos with cyst

Intraconal
Cavernous haemangioma; schwannoma (neurilemmoma); optic nerve—*glioma, meningioma; *rhabdomyosarcoma

Diffuse
Thyroid eye disease; inflammation (idiopathic, specific); orbital cellulitis

*Diseases usually presenting in childhood or adolescence.

examples include aplasias (absent greater wing of sphenoid in neurofibromatosis), cicatrization (sclerosing inflammation, metastatic breast carcinoma), or destruction (trauma). Infiltrative processes may exert little effect on structure, but their location can be deduced by the nature of the functional impairment produced.

Table 3 Patterns of disease

Structural
Asymmetry, proptosis, enophthalmos, painless, associated
   developmental anomalies, variable effect on function
Examples: previous trauma, craniofacial dysostoses, fibrous dysplasia

Inflammatory
Pain, swelling, erythema, warmth, impaired function
Examples: cellulitis, thyroid eye disease, acute idiopathic inflammation

Mass
Proptosis, displacement, compression, congestion, variable effect on
   function
Examples: neoplasia, mucocele, dermoid cyst

Infiltrative
Impaired function
Examples: cicatrizing neoplasia, sclerosing inflammation

Vascular
Dynamic change (pulsation, positive Valsalva manoeuvre),
   haemorrhage, vascular engorgement, compressible mass, variable
   effect on function
Examples: venous anomaly, arteriovenous malformation, arteriovenous
   shunt

Pattern of disease

Five characteristic patterns of orbital disease are evident (Table 3). These are not mutually exclusive, although one pattern usually predominates in a particular clinical setting.

History

Presenting complaint

Careful elucidation of the duration, rate of onset, and nature and rate of progression of the abnormal process is essential in order to arrive at a logical differential diagnosis.

The duration may, in some cases, be longer than the symptoms suggest; examination of old photographs is valuable, as is the opinion of a reliable witness. The temporal nature of the onset is often typical for a particular category of disease (Table 4). The rate and nature of progression is a useful guide to the underlying condition: steady progression suggests neo-

Table 4 Temporal onset

Catastrophic (minutes to hours)
Vascular—haemorrhage, fulminant infection

Acute (days)
Infection, inflammation, vascular—haemorrhage

Subacute (weeks)
Thyroid eye disease, inflammation, vascular, fulminant malignancy

Chronic
Months: vascular, benign and malignant neoplasia
Years: congenital, structural, vascular, benign neoplasia

Table 5 Pain in orbital disease

Frequently painful	*Infrequently painful*
Cellulitis	Thyroid eye disease
Subperiosteal abscess	Vascular malformations, neoplasia
Acute idiopathic inflammation	Lymphoma
Fulminant neoplasia	Benign neoplasia
Adenoidcystic carcinoma	Sclerosing inflammation
(lacrimal gland)	Cystic lesions
Acute haemorrhage	Rhabdomyosarcoma
	Structural lesions
	Bone lesions

plasia, with fulminant malignancy evolving more rapidly than benign tumours or low-grade malignancy. Orbital haemorrhage progresses rapidly over a period of hours to days, usually followed by a gradual resolution. Diurnal fluctuation, with swelling and diplopia worse in the morning, is suggestive of thyroid eye disease, whilst dynamic changes, either with the Valsalva manoeuvre or a change in posture, are suggestive of a venous anomaly.

The presence and nature of pain can be a guide to the possible diagnosis (Table 5). The possibility of referred pain from an intracranial, nasopharyngeal, or dental source should be considered.

Symptoms related to functional impairment—visual loss, diplopia, or sensory changes—may suggest disease location. Where a patient is vague as to the duration or degree of visual loss, information may be gained from other sources, such as the patient's optometrist, general practitioner, or employer.

Whilst the patient may have noted a loss of symmetry between the two orbits, one should be aware that perceived proptosis or enophthalmos may be due to alterations in lid position. If swelling of the lids has been noted, it is important to determine whether or not this is progressive and if there is any fluctuation.

Alterations in sensation or tear secretion, subjective cranial bruits, orbital pulsation, or gaze-evoked amaurosis may be symptoms not volunteered by the patient and should be specifically sought.

Additional history

A full ocular history must include reference to known refractive errors (unilateral myopia presenting as pseudoproptosis), changes in refraction (hypermetropic shift due to retrobulbar compression), or previous intraocular or eyelid tumours. The general medical, surgical, family, drug, and social history should identify symptoms or past history of thyroid or metabolic disease, systemic vasculitis, autoimmune disease, upper or lower respiratory tract disease, renal disease, skin lesions, previous trauma, or neoplasia (Table 6).

Examination

Before focusing on the detail of the examination, it is important to gain an overall impression of the patient in general, and the

Table 6 Systemic associations

System	Disease	Manifestation
Endocrine	Thyroid disease	Thyroid eye disease
ENT/respiratory	Sinusitis	Cellulitis; mucocele
	Sarcoidosis	Lacrimal gland enlargement
	Wegener's granulomatosis	Orbital inflammation
Autoimmune	Sjögren's disease	Lacrimal gland enlargement; lymphoma
Malignancy	Lymphoma, lung, prostate, breast, gastrointestinal, melanoma	Orbital metastasis
Immune system	AIDS	Lymphoma; Kaposi's sarcoma
Phacomatoses	Neurofibromatosis	Optic nerve—glioma, meningioma; peripheral nerve sheath tumour; sphenoid wing aplasia
Metabolic	Diabetes mellitus	Mucormycosis
Dietary	Parasitic infection	Myositis; muscle cyst

face and orbit in particular. In this way it is less likely that facial asymmetry (congenital anomalies, trauma), subtle lid retraction or lag (thyroid eye disease), temporal fullness (sphenoid wing meningioma), or generalized debility (malignancy, acquired immune deficiency syndrome—AIDS) will be overlooked.

The examination should begin with the assessment of visual acuity, both uncorrected and best corrected, or pin-hole. Signs of optic neuropathy—colour desaturation (using pseudoisochromatic charts) and relative afferent pupillary defect—must be sought. Pupillary abnormalities, such as light–near dissociation or Horner's syndrome, should be documented.

Visual field examination to confrontation is sufficient for screening purposes, but formal perimetry (Goldmann or computerized) must be performed where there is any question of involvement of the visual pathways.

The range of ocular motility should be assessed in all cardinal positions of gaze; the traction and the force-generation test are performed to differentiate restrictive from paretic ophthalmoplegia.

The eyelids should be inspected for colour, swelling, contour, ptosis, retraction, lag on downgaze, and levator function. Eyelid retraction and lag on downgaze are characteristic of thyroid eye disease, an S-shaped deformity of the upper lid, with ptosis laterally, is usually due to lacrimal gland disease, whilst a medial deformity is typical of a venous anomaly. The conjunctival fornices should be inspected routinely, as the 'fish-flesh' lesions of lymphoma commonly occur in this location.

The orbit should be palpated, noting the size, location, firmness, and mobility or fixity of any masses. Congenital or traumatic structural abnormalities may be evident. An increase in proptosis, or in the size of an eyelid mass, with the Valsalva manoeuvre or postural change suggests a venous anomaly. Pulsation, due to an arteriovenous malformation, absent greater wing of sphenoid, or highly vascular tumour such as capillary haemangioma, may be apparent by palpation, by careful inspection of the globe from the lateral aspect, or by applanation tonometry. Auscultation may reveal orbital or cranial bruits in high-flow vascular lesions such as caroticocavernous fistula or arteriovenous malformation.

Sensation in each branch of the ophthalmic (supratrochlear, infratrochlear, supraorbital, lacrimal, nasociliary), and maxillary (infraorbital, zygomaticofacial, zygomaticotemporal) divisions of the trigeminal nerve should be examined systematically.

In order to assess proptosis and globe displacement accurately, an exophthalmometer which corrects for parallax (Hertel-type) and a clear millimetre rule must be used. The exophthalmometer is placed firmly on the lateral orbital rims, and the eye to be examined regards the opposite eye of the examiner (patient's left eye fixes examiner's right eye and vice versa), with the fellow eye occluded by the examiner's thumb. The intercanthal distance is recorded for future reference. Vertical globe displacement is determined with the ruler, using the medial or lateral canthi as reference points and comparing the relative positions of each eye as they fix in turn (as described above for the measurement of proptosis), to ensure that any manifest deviation is accounted for. The centre of the nasal bridge and the medial limbus of each eye are used as reference points in the assessment of horizontal displacement.

In addition to the routine slit lamp examination, the conjunctival vessels should be inspected, noting injection over the muscle insertions in myositis, venous prominence over the lateral rectus in thyroid eye disease, or episcleral venous engorgement in arteriovenous malformation or caroticocavernous fistula. Chemosis (thyroid eye disease, infection, non-specific inflammation) or infiltration (lymphoma, amyloid) should be documented. A change in intraocular pressure, between the primary and upgaze positions, of greater than 10 mmHg, suggests a markedly enlarged inferior rectus due to thyroid eye disease; whilst a raised intraocular pressure, with a large pulse variation, is found in caroticocavernous fistula and some arteriovenous malformations. A misdiagnosis of glaucoma can be made in the thyroid patient when using the Goldmann tonometer; the Perkins-type portable tonometer obviates this by not requiring the patient to maintain the forced primary position, as is necessary with the Goldmann tonometer.

A complete examination of the fundus is essential: the optic disc should be examined for oedema or atrophy; optociliary shunt vessels and optic atrophy are typical features of long-standing optic nerve compression due to optic nerve sheath meningioma; posterior uveitis or retinal vasculitis suggests a diagnosis of sarcoidosis; retinal vascular malformations may occur in association with an orbital arteriovenous malformation. Retinal or choridal masses (retinoblastoma, melanoma, metastatic deposits), choroidal folds, or posterior uveitis should be documented photographically, and with fluorescein angiography as indicated.

The parotid and cervical lymph nodes must be examined where orbital malignancy is suspected. A directed systemic examination should identify generalized lymphadenopathy in lymphoma, skin lesions in cutaneous melanoma, systemic vasculitis, or neurofibromatosis (café-au-lait spots, cutaneous neurofibromas), black palatal eschar in mucormycosis, palatal vascular anomalies associated with orbital venous malformations, or generalized debility in malignant disease or AIDS. Blood pressure measurement and urinalysis should be performed when indicated. A more complete evaluation may require consultation with a physician, neurologist, oncologist, otolaryngologist, or neurosurgeon.

It is important for both future reference and medicolegal purposes to obtain clinical photographs of all patients.

Radiological investigation

The radiological investigation is integral to the assessment of orbital disease; this discussion will serve to introduce the important aspects of the commonly used modalities.

Computed tomography (CT) remains the investigation of choice in the majority of cases. Magnetic resonance imaging (MRI) has not superceded CT, but is indicated in specific circumstances. Ultrasonography is of limited value in the assessment of orbital disease when compared to CT and MRI.

Plain radiology, air and contrast orbitography, conventional tomography, and orbital venography are outmoded techniques.

Computed tomography

Air and orbital fat are of low attenuation on CT, and provide excellent natural contrast to water-containing tissues (extraocular muscles, neoplasms, inflammatory tissue), sclera, and bone. Current-generation CT scanners offer excellent resolution and very fine cuts with rapid acquisition times. The orbital bones and surrounding structures are imaged directly, and, with bone-window settings, subtle bony erosion can be appreciated. Calcification within lesions such as optic nerve sheath meningiomas, malignant lacrimal gland tumours, and venous anomalies (pleboliths) is best demonstrated with CT.

Direct axial and coronal sections should be obtained in all patients. Reconstructions can be performed in the coronal and sagittal planes, but lack the resolution of direct images.

The major disadvantages of CT are that the optic nerve is not well imaged at the orbital apex due to bone artefacts, dental metals can produce severe artefacts, and wooden foreign bodies may be invisible. Although there is some concern regarding the radiation hazard, this is not of significance unless frequent follow-up examinations are required.

Magnetic resonance imaging

In most cases, MRI of the orbit provides no more information than current-generation CT. The cost is high, it is generally less widely available, and there is less experience in its interpretation when compared to CT. Only in certain circumstances, therefore, is it the radiological investigation of choice.

Optic nerve lesions are best demonstrated with MRI, particularly where there is a need to examine the intracanalicular or intracranial segments of the optic nerve, as there is no artefact from surrounding bone. Special T_2 and fat-suppression techniques are able to demonstrate oedema within the muscles of patients with active thyroid eye disease, thereby enabling a prediction as to those patients most likely to benefit from radiotherapy. Orbital wood foreign bodies are more likely to be detected with MRI than CT. Due to the lack of ionizing radiation, those patients requiring frequent examinations are best imaged using MRI.

Angiography

Contrast angiography is indicated in the assessment of selected arteriovenous malformations or shunts (for example high-flow caroticocavernous fistula), in order to determine the origin of feeder vessels, and whether or not the lesion is amenable to selective embolization. Non-contrast magnetic resonance angiography (MRA) has now largely superceded invasive contrast studies in centres where it is available.

Ultrasonography

Orbital ultrasound is unable to provide the anatomical detail of CT or MRI. It is, however, able to provide valuable information in real-time about the internal properties of lesions located in the anterior half of the orbit. Doppler studies can demonstrate the blood flow characteristics of orbital vascular lesions. Recent studies suggest that, with A-scan ultrasonography, the internal reflective properties of extraocular muscles in patients with thyroid eye disease can be used to differentiate 'active' from 'burnt-out' disease.

The information obtained from the ultrasound examination is very much dependent upon the experience and ability of the ultrasonographer.

Laboratory investigation

The appropriate laboratory investigations should be selected on the basis of information derived from the clinical assessment. Some investigations may be indicated only once a tissue diagnosis has been made, in order to evaluate the extent of sys-

Table 7 Laboratory investigations

Serum biochemistry
Calcium: sarcoidosis, multiple myeloma
Acid/alkaline phosphatase: metastatic bone deposits (prostate, breast)
Liver function tests: liver metastasis
Angiotensin-converting enzyme: sarcoidosis

Complete blood picture
Lymphoproliferative disease, leukaemia

Thyroid function
Thyroxine, thyroid-stimulating hormone, antithyroid antibodies

Immunological profile
Antineutrophil cytoplasmic antibody: Wegener's granulomatosis
Serum protein electrophoresis: multiple myeloma, blood dyscrasia
Autoimmune profile (rheumatoid factor, antinuclear antibody, anti-DNA
    antibody): rheumatoid arthritis, polyarteritis nodosa, systemic lupus
    erythematosus

Tumour markers
Prostate specific antigen: prostatic carcinoma
Carcinoembryonic antigen: gastrointestinal malignancy

Chest radiograph
Sarcoidosis, bronchogenic, and oat cell carcinoma

Urinalysis
Bence-Jones protein: multiple myeloma, amyloidosis
Glycosaminoglycan excretion: active thyroid eye disease

Further reading

De Potter, P., Flanders, A.E., Shields, C.L., *et al.* (1993). Magnetic resonance imaging of orbital tumours. *International Ophthalmology Clinics*, **33**, 163–73.

Glasgow, B.J., Goldberg, R.A., Gordon, L.K., *et al.* (1995). Fine needle aspiration of orbital masses. *Ophthalmology Clinics of North America*, **8**, 73–82.

Hiromatsu, Y., Kojima, K., Ishisaka, N., *et al.* (1992). Role of magnetic resonance imaging in thyroid-associated ophthalmopathy: its predictive value for therapeutic outcome of immunosuppressive therapy. *Thyroid*, **2**, 299–305.

Ho, H.B., Laitt, R.D., Wakeley, C., *et al.* (1994). The STIR sequence MRI in the assessment of extraocular muscles in thyroid eye disease. *Eye*, **8**, 506–10.

Just, M., Kahaly, G., Higer, H.P., *et al.* (1991). Grave's ophthalmopathy: role of MR imaging in radiation therapy. *Radiology*, **179**, 187–90.

Klimer, L., Wenzel, M., and Mosges, R. (1993). Computer-assisted orbital surgery. *Ophthalmic Surgery*, **24**, 411–17.

Krohel, G.B., Stewart, W.B., and Chavis, R.M. (1981). *Orbital disease: a practical approach.* Grune & Stratton, New York. [A concise book providing a logical approach to the evaluation of the orbital patient.]

Leib, M.L. (1994). The continuing utility of computed tomography in ophthalmolgy. *Ophthalmolgy Clinics of North America*, **7**, 271–6.

Prummel, M.F., Suttorp-Schulten, M.S., Wiersinga, W.M., *et al.* (1993). A new ultrasonographic method to detect disease activity and predict response to immunosuppressive treatment in Grave's ophthalmopathy. *Ophthalmology*, **100**, 556–61.

Rootman, J. (1988). *Diseases of the orbit: a multidisciplinary approach.* Lippincott, Philadelphia. [A comprehensive textbook of orbital disease with excellent chapters describing the assessment of the orbital patient.]

Rose, G.E. (1993). Orbital imaging. *Current Opinion in Ophthalmology*, **4**, 70–5.

Spencer, W.H. (1986). *Ophthalmic pathology*, (3rd edn). Saunders, Philadelphia.

Wright, J.E. (1988). Doyne Lecture: current concepts in orbital disease. *Eye*, **2**, 1–11.

temic involvement. Relevent investigations and their clinical implications are summarized in Table 7.

When faced with a condition that requires a tissue diagnosis, one must decide whether to proceed with an open or fine-needle biopsy. It is the author's practice to perform an open biopsy whenever possible, in order to provide the pathologist with sufficient material so that the structural morphology of the lesion can be properly assessed, and a variety of special stains (cytochemical, immunohistochemical) performed.

Tissue should be placed immediately into 10 per cent buffered formalin for routine paraffin sections, a fresh pot (for freezing) for immunohistochemical and other special stains, and glutaraldehyde for electron microscopy. Biopsy using frozen section can be misleading in some cases and is not recommended.

Lesions likely to be malignant should be biopsied through the orbital septum; under no circumstances should the periosteum be breached, as this acts as a barrier to tumour spread. Clinically and radiologically benign lesions are, where possible, excised intact; this is essential when a pleomorphic adenoma of the lacrimal gland is suspected.

Fine-needle biopsy is of particular value in diagnosing possible metastatic spread to the orbit in patients with a history of malignancy. A non-diagnostic biopsy necessitates open biopsy. CT and ultrasound are of value in localizing the needle and the area to be biopsied if the lesion is not palpable. New technologies which permit CT- or MRI-guided frameless stereotaxic biopsy have been reported and may prove to be of value in selected cases.

2.1.3 Inflammatory conditions of the orbit

*Kenn A. Freedman and
Gregory B. Krohel*

Orbital inflammation often represents a clinical urgency which can pose a serious threat to both the vision and life of the affected patient. Inflammation of the tissues of the orbit can arise from a large spectrum of disease processes. These include infections, neoplasms, trauma, systemic inflammatory and immunological disorders, and idiopathic processes. This chapter discusses the differential diagnosis of orbital inflammatory disorders and their management. Topics such as orbital trauma, thyroid orbitopathy, and orbital neoplasms are detailed elsewhere.

Differential diagnosis

A list of the causes of orbital inflammation is given in Table 1. This table, while not exhaustive, demonstrates the major categories of disease processes that can present with the character-

Table 1 Differential diagnosis of orbital inflammation

Infections (e.g. bacterial, viral, fungal, parasitic)

Thyroid-related immune orbitopathy

Idiopathic inflammatory pseudotumour
    local (e.g. myositis, dacryoadenitis, perineuritis)
    diffuse

Vascular
    systemic vasculitis (e.g. Wegener's granulomatosis)
    orbital thrombophlebitis/cavernous sinus thrombosis
    lymphangioma with haemorrhage

Systemic granulomatous disease (e.g. sarcoidosis)

Reactive orbital inflammation (e.g. retained foreign body, sinusitis, ruptured dermoid, etc.)

Aggressive neoplasms (e.g. rhabdomyosarcoma, metastatic tumours, malignant lacrimal gland tumours, lymphangioma (with haemorrhage)

Trauma

istic signs and symptoms of orbital inflammation. Infectious processes and thyroid-related immune orbitopathy account for the majority of cases (90–95 per cent). Other aetiologies include orbital neoplasms that can present aggressively, systemic vasculitides, granulomatous processes, foreign body reactions, and also idiopathic inflammation (also known as orbital pseudotumour). Inflammation within the orbit can be diffuse in nature or confined to a specific structure (e.g. lacrimal gland inflammation or dacryoadenitis).

In the evaluation of a patient with suspected orbital inflammation a thorough history is imperative, including past medical history, medications, and a review of systems. A careful eye examination must include exophthalmometry and orbital palpation. The characteristic symptoms and signs of orbital inflammation can include pain, diplopia, proptosis, periorbital oedema and erythema, conjunctival injection and chemosis, and impairment of ocular motility.

Acute onset of symptoms suggests orbital cellulitis or orbital pseudotumour, although in children aggressive orbital tumours must also be considered. Symptoms can appear in hours to days. In subacute inflammation, the signs and symptoms can appear over the course of weeks to months. This pattern of presentation is more characteristic of thyroid orbitopathy. The presence of pain can be useful in differential diagnosis. Orbital cellulitis and pseudotumour frequently present with pain, whereas thyroid orbitopathy rarely does. Bilateral involvement is more suggestive of a systemic disorder such as thyroid orbitopathy (although thyroid disease can present unilaterally), vasculitis, and granulomatous diseases.

Signs of localized inflammation can be useful in the diagnostic process. Occasionally, orbital abscesses will present with localized tissue swelling and point tenderness externally. Swelling in the superior temporal quadrant of the orbit is suggestive of lacrimal gland inflammation such as dacryoadenitis. Injection and chemosis over the extraocular muscles and their insertions indicate myositis or thyroid disease.

Initial laboratory evaluation is dependent on clinical suspicion. In most instances, proptosis or other signs of an orbital disease process warrants imaging studies. Computed tomography (CT) scanning is usually preferred over ultrasound or magnetic resonance imaging (MRI) as the initial radiological study. CT scanning is better at defining sinusitis, bony abnormalities, and calcifications. If any infectious aetiology is suspected, a temperature chart, a complete blood count, and blood cultures are necessary. A blood sugar may be useful to detect diabetes mellitus. This is important as diabetics are more susceptible to orbital infections including mucormycosis. Other useful laboratory tests include thyroid function studies, and the antineutrophilic cytoplasmic antibody if Wegener's granulomatosis is suspected. If sarcoidosis is suspected, an angiotensin-converting enzyme level and a chest radiograph may be useful. Incisional biopsy for pathological investigation or culture may be necessary.

Orbital cellulitis and orbital abscess

Infection of the orbital tissues can be classified by the location of the infectious process. Preseptal cellulitis involves the tissues lying only anterior to the orbital septum. This disease process is more commonly seen in children less than 2 years of age. Orbital cellulitis is defined as an infectious inflammation which involves the soft tissue posterior to the orbital septum. This occurs more commonly in older children and adults. Orbital abscesses can be found anterior to the orbital septum, but more frequently are located posterior to the orbital septum. In addition, they can also be located underneath the periosteum of the orbital walls. The most common location for subperiosteal abscesses is along the medial wall of the orbit adjacent to the ethmoid sinus.

Aetiology

The microbiology of orbital infectious diseases is detailed in Chapter 2.1.3. The most frequently encountered organisms include *Staphylococcus*, *Streptococcus*, *Haemophilus influenza*, and anaerobes. Viral infection of the orbit is possible with organisms such as herpes zoster. Fungal orbital cellulitis occurs with systemic mucormycosis and *Aspergillus* infection.

Orbital cellulitis is most commonly related to sinus disease. More than 50 per cent of all cases of orbital cellulitis are secondary to ethmoidal sinusitis. Spread from the adjacent sinus is thought to occur through congenital or traumatic dehiscences in the thin orbital walls or through pre-existing foramina. Retrograde spread through the valveless orbital vein is also possible. Polymicrobial (mixed) infections are generally found. Spread from other adjacent structures is possible. Orbital infections may follow dental infections or extractions, metastatic endophthalmitis, local osteomyelitis, mid-facial infections, and dacryocystitis. Haematogenous spread from more distant structures has been reported.

Post-traumatic and postsurgical orbital cellulitis is seen after violation of the orbital septum. The most common causative organism is *Staphylococcus aureus*, although anaerobic and mixed infections are possible. Gram-negative rods can be seen with orbital foreign bodies.

Medically compromised patients are at a greater risk for certain orbital infections. Patients in metabolic acidosis (e.g. diabetic ketoacidosis) have a higher incidence of mucormycosis. Patients who are immunocompromised, such as human immunodeficiency virus (HIV) positive individuals and those on steroids have been shown to have a high incidence of orbital *Aspergillus* infection.

Clinical evaluation

Orbital infection commonly presents with symptoms of eye pain, headache, and fever. Children may also have nausea and vomiting. It is very important to differentiate preseptal cellulitis from orbital cellulitis. Both conditions can exhibit periocular tissue oedema and erythema. Orbital involvement is indicated by the additional presence of chemosis, limitation in ocular motility, proptosis, and visual loss (Fig. 1). The onset of the signs and symptoms of bacterial orbital cellulitis is often acute, while fungal infections are usually more chronic and insidious. Partially treated bacterial orbital infections can also be present subacutely. In orbital mucormycosis, the clinical presentation is frequently that of an orbital apex syndrome with multiple cranial nerve involvement (e.g. decreased vision, ophthalmoplegia, and hypaesthesia). Dark necrotic lesions can be seen on the skin, nasal mucosa, or the palate.

Laboratory evaluation should include a CT scan of the orbit and brain to rule out or confirm any orbital and central nervous system involvement. A complete blood count and blood cultures should be obtained. Cultures of the conjunctiva and nasopharynx usually have little value as there is often no correlation between these cultures and organisms cultured at the time of surgical drainage. With development of meningeal or cerebral signs, a lumbar puncture for culture and cell counts may be indicated.

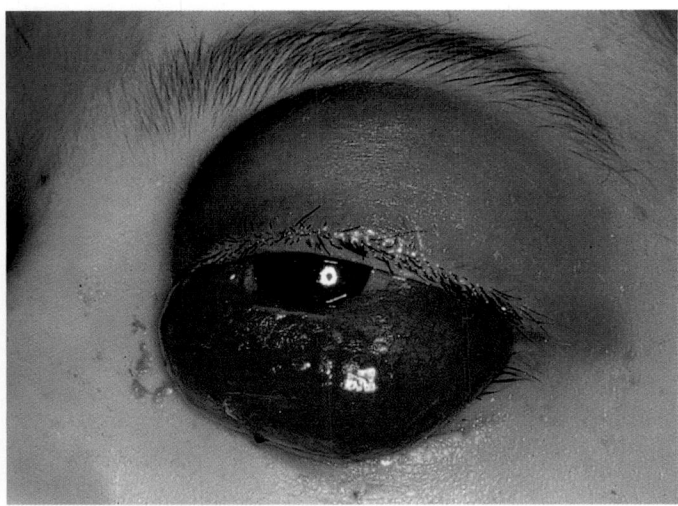

Fig. 1 Proptosis, chemosis secondary to orbital cellulitis. In addition, visual loss and decreased ocular motility can be present.

Management

Preseptal cellulitis in an infant or child requires hospital admission with intravenous antibiotics. CT scanning of the orbits should be performed to look for postseptal involvement. Most adult cases of preseptal cellulitis can be treated with oral antibiotics on an outpatient basis. Antibiotic coverage (usually a cephalosporin) should cover common causative agents including *Haemophilus influenza* in children and *Streptococcus pneumonia* and *Staphylococcus aureus*.

If orbital cellulitis is suspected in any age group, it should be considered an emergency situation with prompt hospital admission. Intravenous antibiotics must be started as soon as possible. An initial antibiotic choice might be cefuroxime for broad Gram-positive and Gram-negative coverage. Gentamicin or tobramycin might be added for Gram-negative rod coverage if a foreign body were present. Changes in therapy would be contingent on clinical response, blood cultures, or direct culture if an abscess is drained. Frequent patient follow-up is absolutely necessary to monitor clinical improvement. It is important to monitor for complications including visual loss, cavernous sinus thrombosis, and/or intracranial extension. If there has not been any improvement in 24 to 48 h, repeat scanning or surgical drainage to rule out an abscess may be warranted.

Other treatment considerations in a patient with orbital cellulitis include treatment for any corneal exposure due to proptosis. Topical ocular antibiotics may be necessary. In addition, intraocular pressures should be measured periodically to monitor for any increase in the ocular pressure secondary to the orbital process. Appropriate therapy for the increased orbital pressure (e.g. cantholysis or decompression) should be undertaken when appropriate.

Surgical intervention may become necessary in various instances. In sinus-related orbital cellulitis, surgical drainage of the involved sinus must be considered if the clinical response to medical treatment is poor. Cultures can be taken from the sinus and may modify antibiotic therapy.

Subperiosteal abscesses can pose a threat to the patient's vision. Frequently, they are located along the medial wall (Fig. 2) and can compress the optic nerve near the orbital apex. Another mechanism of visual loss would be the development of increased orbital pressure leading to ischaemic optic neuropathy. In any event, acute visual loss in the presence of an orbital infection is a surgical emergency and drainage of the abscess with medial wall decompression is usually necessary. Cultures from the drained abscess may also prove useful in modifying antibiotic therapy.

The treatment of subperiosteal orbital abscesses in children is more controversial. Many orbital abscesses in children have been observed to resolve with only medical treatment, and have not required surgical drainage.

If orbital mucormycosis is suspected, biopsy of the orbital tissue or periorbital area is necessary. A fungal stain is used to demonstrate the characteristic large, non-septate, branching hyphae. Treatment includes administration of intravenous amphotericin B and appropriate surgical debridement as necessary. It is important to correct the patient's underlying predis-

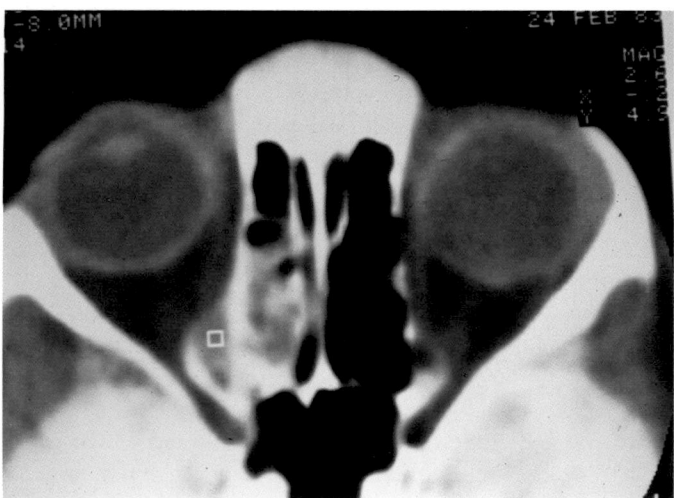

Fig. 2 CT scan with ethmoid sinusitis and contiguous subperiosteal orbital abscess.

posing risk factor, such as diabetic ketoacidosis. Despite aggressive therapy, many of these cases are fatal.

Non-infectious orbital inflammation

Apart from orbital infections, there are a wide variety of disease processes that can cause orbital inflammation (see Table 1). Thyroid-related immune orbitopathy represents the largest majority of cases of non-infectious orbital inflammation. Idiopathic orbital inflammation (orbital pseudotumour) accounts for the majority of remaining cases once infection and thyroid disease have been ruled out.

Orbital pseudotumour is the term used to describe non-specific idiopathic orbital inflammation. It is often associated with pain, proptosis, chemosis, lid oedema, decreased ocular motility, and problems with vision. This orbital inflammation can be diffuse in nature or involve specific orbital structures, such as the extraocular muscles (myositis).

Orbital pseudotumour affects a wide age range from children under the age of 5 years to elderly adults. There does not appear to be a predilection for either males or females, nor is there a racial preference. The condition in adults often involves only one eye, whereas bilateral pseudotumour is more frequently seen in children (up to one-third of the cases). Bilateral inflammation in adults is more suggestive of a systemic inflammatory condition or a neoplastic lymphoproliferative process.

The aetiology of orbital pseudotumour remains unknown. Non-specific markers of inflammation, such as fever and increased erythrocyte sedimentation rate are not found in this condition, suggesting that this disease is not usually a systemic autoimmune process. When localized to the extraocular muscles, the disease does have some clinical features of thyroid-related immune orbitopathy. Experimentally, serum antibodies to various eye muscle membrane proteins have been demonstrated in patients with pseudotumour.

Histopathologically, these lesions can show a variety of patterns. There is frequently a mixed inflammatory infiltrate including lymphocytes, plasma cells, eosinophils, and macrophages. A combined B-cell and/or T-cell lymphocytic infiltrate can be seen, and differentiation from lymphoma at times can be difficult. Other histopathological variations include perivascular infiltration with vasculitis, extensive fibrosis, or a combination of the above. When granulomatous inflammation is seen, another disease process must be suspected (such as foreign body reactions, sarcoidosis, or Wegener's granulomatosis).

Clinical and laboratory evaluation

The clinical presentation of orbital pseudotumour depends on the orbital structures involved. Patients commonly present with a rapid onset of pain and proptosis (usually over hours to days, although sometimes over weeks). There is also often chemosis and swelling over the extraocular muscle insertion, lid oedema, and possibly ptosis. In children, the presenting symptoms may be accompanied by nausea, vomiting, abdominal pain, and headache. Orbital pseudotumour can mimic orbital cellulitis. An elevated eosinophil count can be noted in children in 20 per cent of cases.

The orbital location of the inflammatory process will further determine any of the presenting signs and symptoms. Acute anterior orbital inflammation can involve the globe, particularly the sclera and Tenon's capsule. There can be an associated uveitis, exudative retinal detachments, and papillitis. When the inflammation is more evenly distributed throughout the entire orbit the condition is termed diffuse idiopathic orbital inflammation. The symptoms include diplopia, visual loss from optic nerve involvement, and choroidal folds. When the optic nerve and its coatings are involved, the term perineuritis is used. Orbital thrombophlebitis has been described with idiopathic inflammation of the orbital veins. Orbital myositis is characterized by pain on eye movement, diplopia, and injection over the muscle insertions. This disease typically involves one muscle, but multiple extraocular muscles can be involved to varying degrees. Forced ductions are positive.

Dacryoadenitis usually presents with swelling over the superior lateral aspect of the orbit and upper eyelid (Fig. 3). There is usually a palpable tender mass in the lacrimal gland fossa. There is no proptosis with strict lacrimal gland involvement, but the globe can be displaced downward and/or medially. In addition to idiopathic orbital pseudotumour, the lacrimal gland can also be frequently involved in cases of sarcoidosis with granulomatous inflammation. In contrast to pseudotumour, these patients usually do not have significant pain and bilateral involvement is more common.

Orbital inflammation can be confined to the orbital apex. This is often associated with deep orbital pain but minimal proptosis. There can be a restriction in ocular motility, an afferent pupillary defect, and loss of vision due to involvement of cranial nerves II, III, IV, and VI. The Tolosa–Hunt syndrome is an inflammatory condition which involves the superior orbital fissure and cavernous sinus. Along with multiple cranial nerve palsies, there can be eyelid swelling and chemosis due to

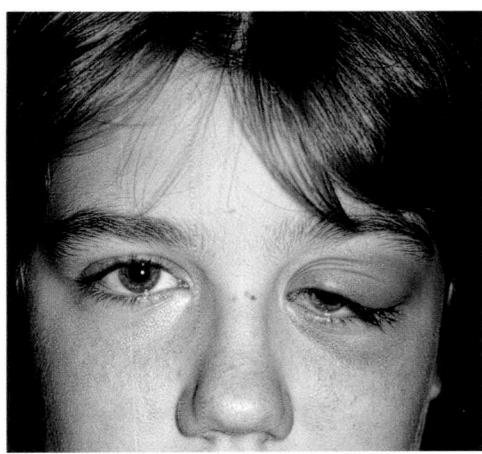

Fig. 3 Superior lateral eyelid erythema and oedema secondary to dacryoadenitis.

obstruction of venous outflow. In the diagnosis of this syndrome, other conditions must be ruled out including cavernous sinus neoplasm, aneurysm, meningioma, and metastatic disease.

Orbital imaging is necessary in all cases of suspected orbital pseudotumour. CT or MRI scanning can provide additional information to support the diagnosis of pseudotumour. For example, in Fig. 4 a CT scan reveals orbital myositis with involvement of the medial rectus muscle, contiguous involvement of the tendinous insertion, as well as the intraconal adipose tissue. This contrasts with thyroid immune orbitopathy where only the extraocular muscle belly is involved.

Orbital imaging can also be useful in the diagnosis of dacryoadenitis where the enlarged lacrimal gland moulds to the globe and orbital wall without any evidence of bony erosion. Orbital imaging can show scleral thickening due to posterior scleritis and can also be useful in localizing inflammation located in the orbital apex. Intracranial extension of orbital pseudotumour is occasionally seen.

The diagnosis of idiopathic orbital pseudotumour is usually established by biopsy. Patients with myositis or deep apical lesions may be given a diagnostic trial of corticosteroids. Patients who do not have a prompt and complete remission of their disease are then considered biopsy candidates. In most patients who are surgical candidates, an open biopsy of the abnormal tissue under direct visualization is recommended. This technique allows for an adequate amount of specimen for pathological study. Fine-needle aspiration biopsy is recommended only in patients who are poor surgical candidates or where the lesion is difficult to approach surgically (orbital apex).

In many instances light microscopy is not adequate in the analysis of the specimen. Lesions with significant numbers of lymphocytes require further testing in an attempt to separate benign from malignant lymphoid lesions. This distinction is often difficult since there is no single definitive test for the presence of malignant lymphoma.

There are two types of lymphocytes, B and T cells. Immuno-histochemical staining techniques can be useful in identifying cell types such as in the identification of immunoglobulins present on the surface of B lymphocytes. In addition, tests determining the clonality or similarity of the lymphocyte cell types are necessary. Flow cytometry and gene rearrangement studies determine whether the cells are monoclonal or polyclonal. Benign lesions are often polyclonal whereas malignant lesions are usually monoclonal and predominantly B cells. Fresh tissue specimens not preserved in formalin are necessary for these last two techniques.

A flow scheme for further evaluation and treatment of patients with suspected orbital pseudotumour is shown in Fig. 5. Those with biopsy specimens diagnosed as lymphoma need referral for systemic evaluation. It should also be noted that even those who are diagnosed with benign lymphocytic lesions need to be carefully followed as a significant number have been noted to develop lymphoma over time.

Management

In confirmed or suspected cases of orbital pseudotumour a trial of systemic corticosteroids is appropriate in the initial management. Patients with myositis have been noted to respond particularly well to systemic steroids. A high starting dosage of daily oral prednisone is appropriate. There is usually a dramatic improvement in symptoms noted over days to weeks. The dosage is tapered carefully over weeks, and it often takes months to get the patient completely off the steroids without recurrence of symptoms. Local injection of corticosteroids should be considered in patients who are poor candidates for systemic steroids. Palpable lesions located in the anterior orbit (e.g. dacryoadenitis) are most appropriate. A suspension of triamcinalone is frequently used. In some milder cases of inflammation or in patients who cannot tolerate corticosteroids, a course of non-steroidal anti-inflammatory agents (such as ibuprofen) can be considered. Those patients who are relatively asymptomatic without pain or disturbances of vision can be carefully followed without further treatment. Patients with

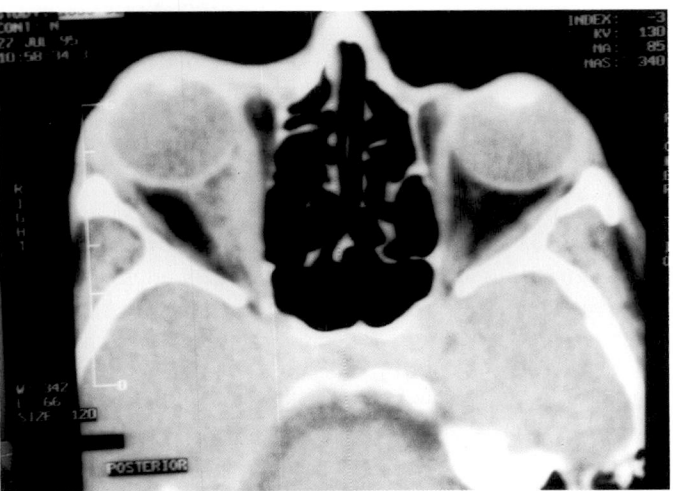

Fig. 4 CT scanning shows enlarged medial rectus muscle and orbital fat involvement consistent with pseudotumour of the extraocular muscle (myositis).

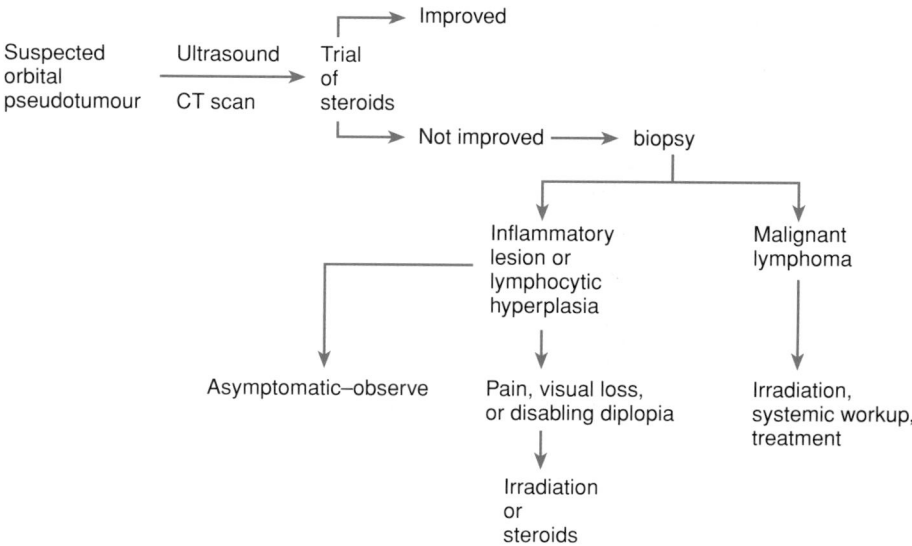

Fig. 5 Flow diagram for the management of suspected orbital pseudotumour. (Krohel *et al.* 1981.).

lymphoid hyperplasia and those who respond incompletely or cannot tolerate steroids are candidates for radiation treatment. Patients with primary lymphocytic hyperplasias have been noted to respond particularly well to localized extended beam radiation.

Idiopathic sclerosing inflammation of the orbit is predominantly composed of fibrotic tissue elements. This particular type of orbital pseudotumour presents a difficult challenge as it has been shown to have an incomplete response to both corticosteroid and radiation treatment. This disease can be visually disabling and early aggressive immunosuppressive therapy may be warranted.

Finally, another possible treatment option would be surgical resection or debulking of an accessible lesion. This technique has been shown to be successful in selected patients. Good surgical candidates might include those who have anterior localized lesions and are not able to take systemic steroids.

Further reading

Char, D.H., and Miller, T. (1993). Orbital pseudotumor. Fine needle aspiration biopsy and response to therapy. *Ophthalmology*, **100**, 1702–10.

Harris, G.J. (1994). Subperiosteal abscess of the orbit, age as a factor in the bacteriology and response to treatment. *Ophthalmology*, **101**, 585–95.

Krohel, G.B., Krauss, H.R., and Winnick, J. (1982). Orbital abscess, presentation, diagnosis, therapy and sequelae. *Ophthalmology*, **89**, 492–8.

Krohel G.B., Stewart W.B., and Chavis R.M. (1981). *Orbital disease: a practical approach*, p. 128. Grune & Stratton, New York.

Lanciano, R., Fowble, B., Sergott, R.C. *et al.* (1990). The results of radiotherapy for orbital pseudotumor. *International Journal of Radiation Oncology and Biological Physics*, **18**, 407–11.

Rootman, J., McCarthy, M., White, V., Harris, G., and Kennerdell, J. (1994). Idiopathic sclerosing inflammation of the orbit, a distinct clinicopathologic entity. *Ophthalmology*, **101**, 570–84.

Steinkuller, P.G. (1991). Focal points, orbital cellulitis in *Clinical Modules for Ophthalmologists*, Vol. IX, Module II. American Academy of Ophthalmology, San Francisco, CA.

2.1.4 The orbit in neuro-ophthalmology

P. Blake and Neil R. Miller

Diseases that affect the orbit often produce ocular manifestations, such as proptosis, chemosis of the conjunctiva, and generalized limitation of eye movement from mechanical restriction of the extraocular muscles. Orbital disease can also produce neurological manifestations from damage to nerves within the orbit. The optic nerve, oculomotor nerves, branches of the trigeminal nerve, and nerves to the pupillary sphincter and dilator muscles can all be damaged by orbital disease. In this chapter, we discuss the clinical symptoms and signs that result from disease within the orbit that damages these nerves.

Damage to the optic nerve (optic neuropathy)

Visual loss that results from damage to the optic nerve can take many forms: intermittent, acute and stable, stuttering, rapidly progressive, or slowly progressive. The pattern of visual loss depends primarily on the type of damage suffered by the nerve.

Transient visual loss may occur when the optic nerve is intermittently compressed by an orbital mass. In such cases, the patient may experience profound loss of vision in one eye only when the eye is moved in a particular direction. This gaze-evoked amaurosis is usually caused by compression of the blood vessels supplying the optic nerve, resulting in transient ischaemia. The most common lesions that produce gaze-evoked

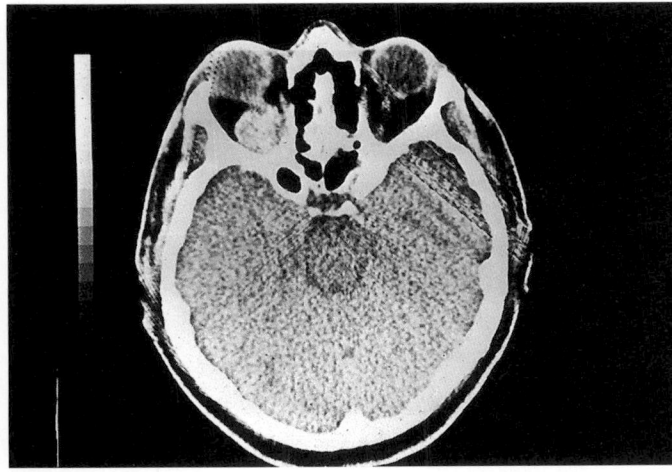

Fig. 1 Axial CT scan in a patient with gaze-evoked amaurosis in the right eye showing a well-circumscribed mass displacing the right optic nerve medially in the orbit.

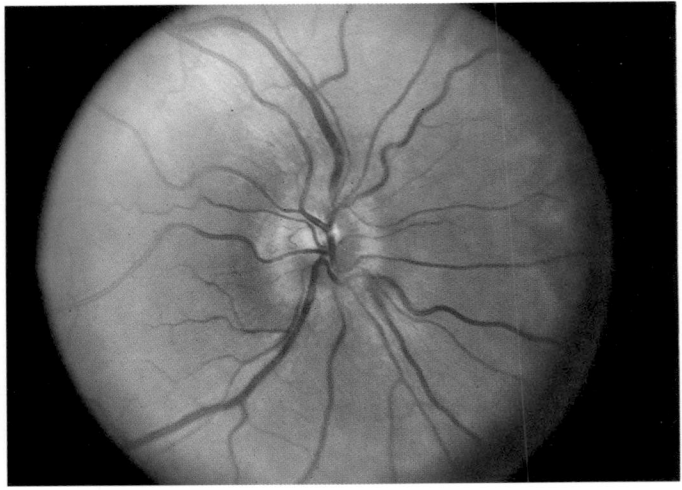

(a)

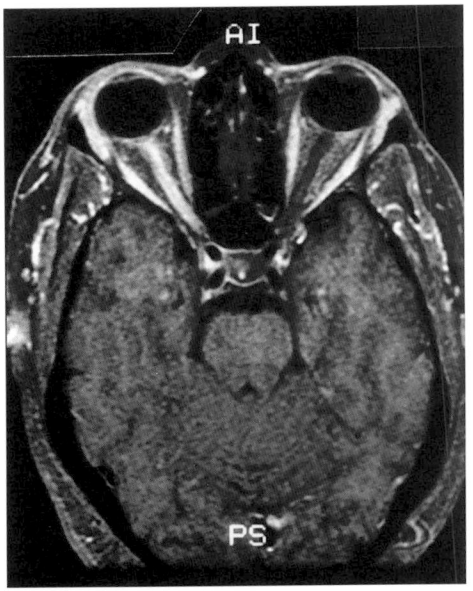

(b)

Fig. 2 Anterior optic neuritis. (a) The right optic disc is hyperaemic and mildly swollen. Note absence of haemorrhages. (b) MRI in axial view after intravenous injection of paramagnetic contrast material reveals marked hyperintensity of the entire orbital portion of the right optic nerve.

amaurosis are optic nerve sheath meningiomas, cavernous haemangiomas, and schwannomas (Fig. 1).

Acute visual loss from optic neuropathy that occurs in the setting of orbital disease is usually caused by ischaemia or inflammation. Pain is more common in patients with inflammation of the optic nerve (optic neuritis), but it may also be present in patients with ischaemic optic neuropathy. When the intraocular or proximal orbital portion of the optic nerve is affected, optic disc swelling is present. In cases of optic neuritis, the disc swelling usually is hyperaemic and unassociated with haemorrhages or exudates, unless there is an underlying systemic infectious process (Fig. 2). In cases of anterior ischaemic optic neuropathy, the disc swelling may be hyperaemic or pallid, and there are often small flame-shaped haemorrhages on or just adjacent to the swollen disc (Fig. 3). When the distal orbital portion of the optic nerve near the apex of the orbit is affected by ischaemia or inflammation, the disc appears normal and either remains normal in appearance or eventually becomes pale (Fig. 4).

Progressive visual loss from optic neuropathy that occurs in the setting of orbital disease usually is caused by compression or infiltration. As is the case with ischaemia and inflammation, compression and infiltration of the optic nerve generally produce swelling of the optic disc when they affect the intraocular or proximal orbital portion of the optic nerve (Fig. 5); however, in rare cases, compression of the distal orbital portion of the optic nerve can also produce optic disc swelling. The severity and rate of progression of visual loss from compression or infiltration are extremely variable. Visual acuity may be normal or nearly normal for weeks, months, or even years. As a rule, infiltrative processes, such as lymphoma, sarcoidosis, and so on, produce more rapidly progressive visual loss than do most compressive lesions. Colour vision is usually affected early, however, and there may be an overt reduction in colour sensation in the affected eye, or there may simply be evidence of desaturation of colours, particularly when tested using a red

object. Any type of visual field defect may be present in eyes with an infiltrative or compressive optic neuropathy, and a relative afferent pupillary defect is invariably present regardless of the severity of visual loss, unless there has been previous damage to the contralateral optic nerve or there is a concomitant process affecting the nerve at that time.

Optic atrophy eventually develops in most eyes that experience any type of damage. The appearance of the atrophy tends to be non-specific, and it is almost impossible to determine exactly what process has caused the atrophy. In some cases, associated narrowing of retinal arteries suggests a previous ischaemic process, whereas in others, the observation of a prominent or resolving macular star figure composed of hard exudate suggests an inflammatory process (Fig. 6). In still other cases, the presence of corkscrew-shaped 'optociliary shunt vessels'

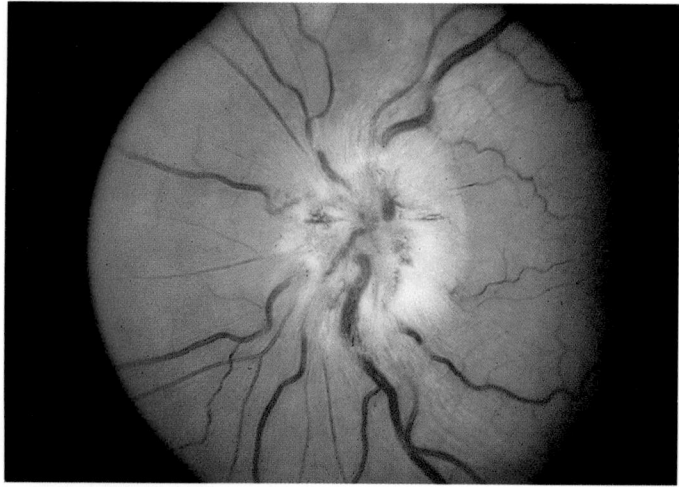

Fig. 3 Anterior ischaemic optic neuropathy. The left optic disc is swollen. There are numerous small haemorrhages and cotton-wool spots on and adjacent to the disc.

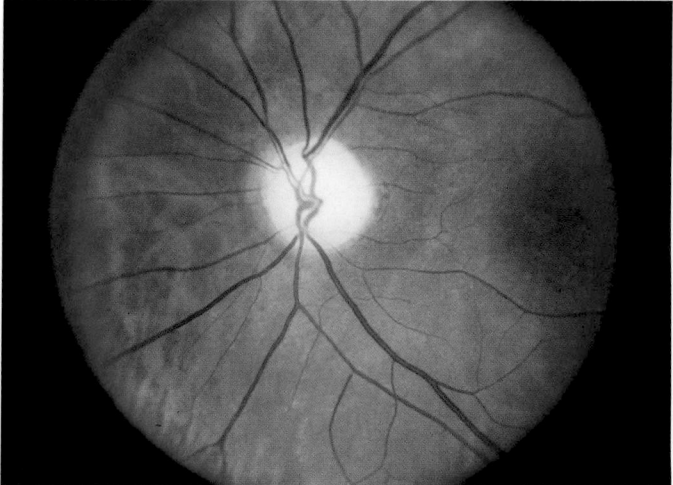

(a)

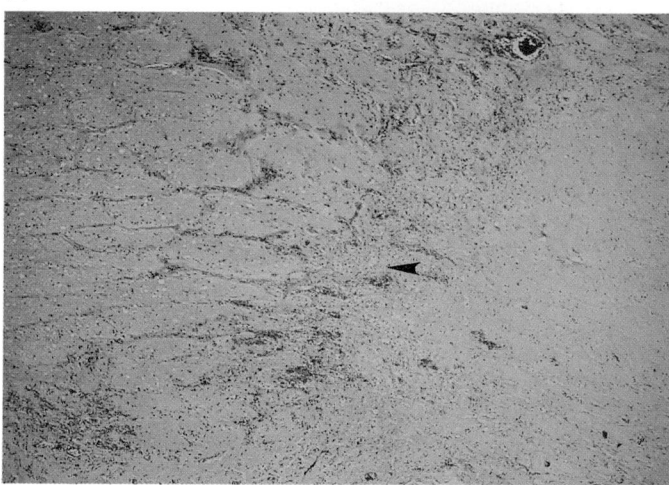

(b)

Fig. 4 Optic atrophy from retro-orbital ischaemia. The patient was a 65-year-old man with diabetes mellitus who lost vision abruptly in the left eye. The optic disc initially appeared normal despite visual acuity of no light perception. A CT scan revealed enlargement of the left optic nerve in the posterior orbit. (a) Six weeks after onset of visual loss, the left optic disc is diffusely pale. The retinal arteries are moderately attenuated. (b) Because of concern that the patient had a tumour of the optic nerve, the posterior orbit was explored. The optic nerve was noted to be swollen and hyperaemic. A biopsy of the abnormal portion was obtained. Longitudinal section through the posterior left optic nerve reveals marked ischaemia. Note interface between normal and abnormal appearing portions of the nerve (*arrowhead*). Haematoxylin and eosin, ×150.

(also called 'retinochoroidal shunt vessels') on the surface of the optic disc in an eye with progressive visual loss and optic atrophy is virtually pathognomonic of a compressive lesion that has an orbital component (Fig. 7). These vessels are congenital veins that connect the choroidal and retinal venous circulations, that dilate under certain circumstances, such as when there is chronic compression of the optic nerve, preventing normal retinal venous outflow through the central retinal vein. Under such circumstances, the vessels shunt venous blood from the retinal to the choroidal circulation, permitting it to leave the eye via the vortex veins that coalesce to form the superior and inferior ophthalmic veins.

Damage to the oculomotor nerves (oculomotor nerve pareses)

Diseases that arise in or spread to the orbit may produce limitation of eye movement and diplopia by damage to one or more of the extraocular muscles; however, such diseases may also produce ophthalmoparesis and strabismus by damaging one or more of the oculomotor nerves. Oculomotor, trochlear, and abducens nerve palsies may all be caused by orbital disease. When the oculomotor nerve is damaged, the resultant paresis may be complete or incomplete. When incomplete, it often takes the form of a divisional palsy. Damage to the superior division of the oculomotor nerve produces only an ipsilateral ptosis and limitation of elevation of the eye from involvement of the nerves to the levator palpebrae superioris and superior rectus muscles. Damage to the inferior division of the nerve produces limitation of adduction and depression of the eye, a dilated pupil, and only minimal limitation of elevation of the eye (from involvement of the nerve to the inferior oblique muscle). In other cases, the disease may cause damage to nerves supplying individual muscles, including the levator palpebrae superioris and the iris sphincter. Involvement of these latter two muscles (producing ptosis and a dilated, poorly reactive

pupil, respectively) is particularly helpful in determining that the ophthalmoparesis is neuropathic rather than myopathic. Damage to the trochlear and abducens nerves may be complete or incomplete. In our experience, it is more common for an orbital process to damage more than one oculomotor nerve than to produce an isolated oculomotor, trochlear, or abducens nerve paresis (Fig. 8). It should also be emphasized that patients in whom orbital disease has produced ophthalmoparesis from damage to one or more oculomotor nerves often have ipsilateral facial numbness, reduced corneal sensation, facial pain, or a combination of these manifestations from concomitant damage to the ophthalmic and maxillary branches of the trigeminal

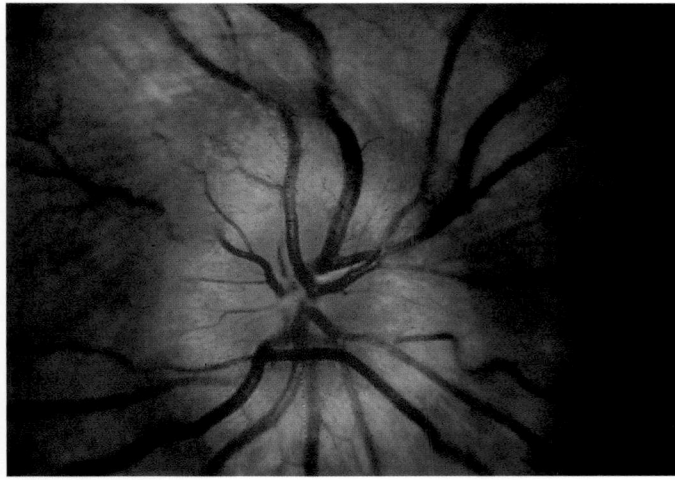

(a)

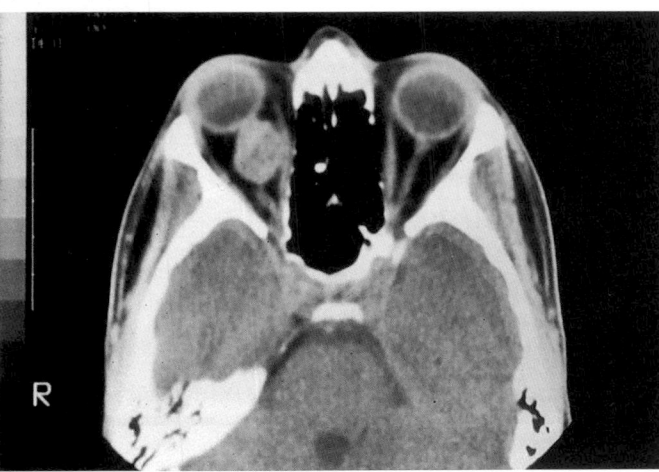

(b)

Fig. 5 Anterior compressive optic neuropathy. (a) Appearance of right optic disc in a 35-year-old man with progressive visual loss in the right eye. The disc is swollen and hyperaemic. (b) CT scan in axial view, after intravenous injection of contrast material reveals a well-circumscribed mass in the anterior portion of the right orbit. Note that the mass is adjacent to the globe and superior to the right optic nerve, which is displaced downwards and laterally.

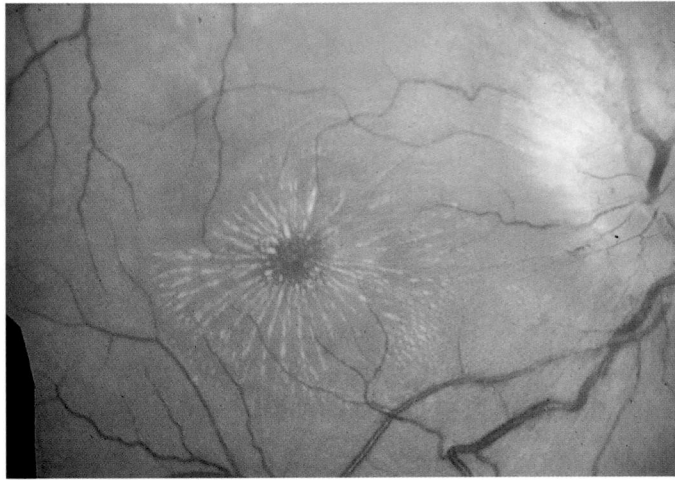

(a)

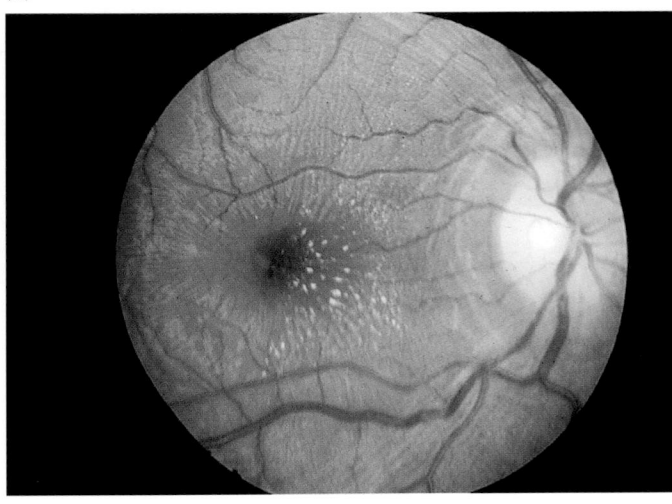

(b)

Fig. 6 Anterior inflammatory optic neuritis with macular star (neuroretinitis). (a) In the acute phase of the condition, the right optic disc is swollen and hyperaemic. There is a star figure in the macula, composed of hard exudate (lipid). (b) At a later stage of the condition in a different case, the right optic disc is pale, and the star figure is beginning to resolve. In this setting, the presence of the macular star figure in an eye with optic atrophy indicates that the cause of the atrophy was probably inflammation of the anterior (proximal) portion of the optic nerve within the orbit.

nerve (see below). Such patients may also have ipsilateral loss of vision from damage to the optic nerve in the apex of the orbit.

Damage to the trigeminal nerve (trigeminal neuropathy)

Both the ophthalmic and maxillary divisions of the trigeminal nerve have branches within the orbit. Thus, orbital disease may produce a trigeminal sensory neuropathy. The neuropathy may be characterised by diminished or absent corneal sensation; pain, numbness, or both in the cutaneous distributions of the ophthalmic and maxillary nerves; or both corneal and cutaneous manifestations. Since the mandibular division of the trigeminal nerve does not provide any branches to the orbit, neither pain or numbness in the cutaneous distribution of this branch of the trigeminal nerve nor evidence of a trigeminal

motor neuropathy are part of the trigeminal manifestations of orbital disease. Their presence in a patient with other evidence of orbital disease indicates that the condition either originated or has spread beyond the confines of the orbit.

Damage to the fibres for pupillary constriction (tonic pupil)

Orbital disease that damages the ciliary ganglion or the short ciliary nerves that originate within the ganglion and transmit parasympathetic impulses to the pupillary sphincter muscle produces a tonic pupil (Fig. 9(a)). The affected pupil is generally moderately or markedly dilated. In the acute period, it may be completely non-reactive to both light and near stimulation; or a portion of the pupillary sphincter may remain intact and

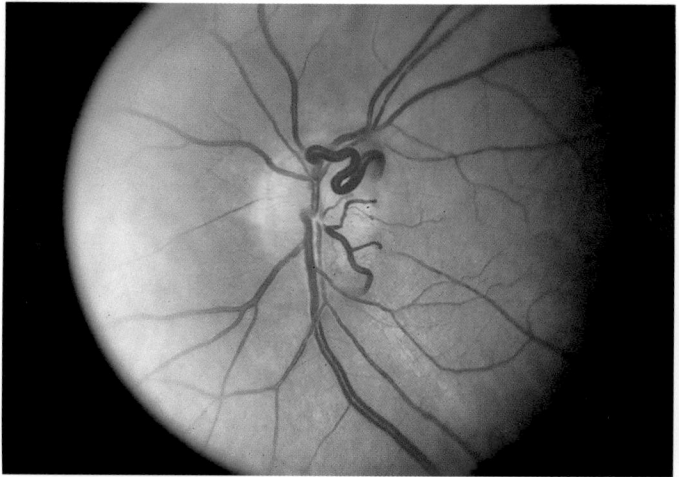

(a)

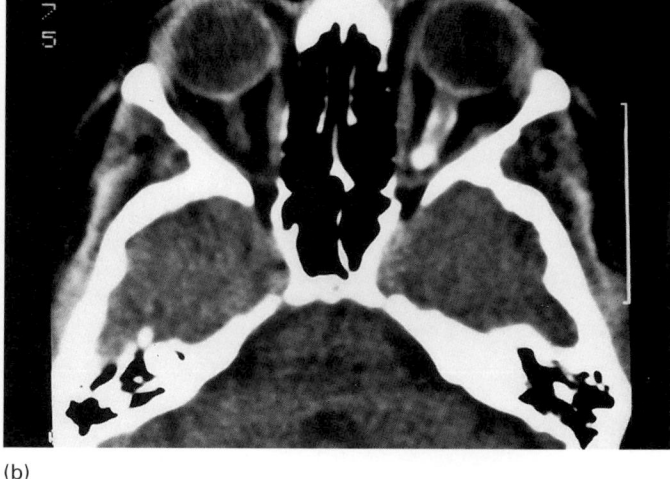

(b)

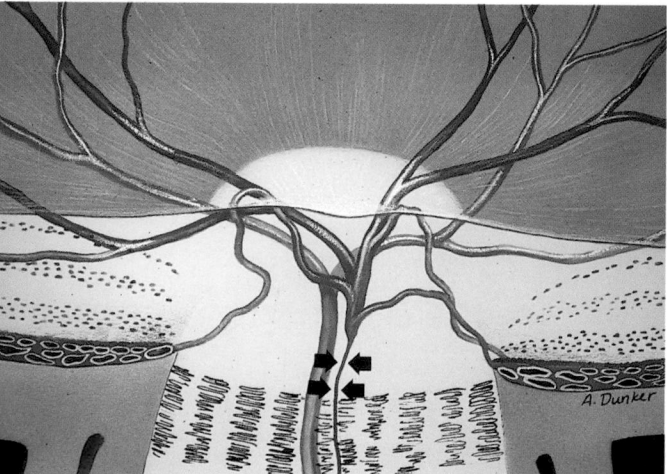

(c)

Fig. 7 Optociliary (retinochoroidal) shunt vessels from chronic compression of the orbital portion of the optic nerve. (a) Appearance of left optic disc in a 45-year-old woman with a 1-year history of progressive visual loss in the left eye. The left optic disc is diffusely pale. Note two irregular vessels that extend from the optic disc to the peripapillary region. (b) Unenhanced CT scan in axial view reveals thickening of the orbital portion of the left optic nerve, with areas of increased density consistent with calcification along its surface. The patient had an optic nerve sheath meningioma. (c) Optociliary shunt vessels connect the retinal and choroidal venous circulations. When there is chronic compression of the anterior orbital portion of the optic nerve that prevents outflow of retinal venous blood through the central retinal vein (arrowheads), these pre-existing vessels dilate, thus allowing retinal venous blood to be shunted to the choroidal circulation and to exit the eye via the vortex veins.

relatively reactive, whereas the remaining portions of the pupil are non-reactive. With time, the pupil may develop light–near dissociation, characterised by a poor (or no) reaction to light stimulation and an intact but sluggish constriction to near stimulation, following which there is a slow (tonic) redilation of the constricted pupil. Tonic pupils show evidence of denervation supersensitivity of the pupillary sphincter muscle to acetylcholine and other similar parasympathomimetic substances, such as pilocarpine (Fig. 9(b)). This phenomenon can develop as early as 24 h after damage to the ciliary ganglion or short ciliary nerves. The diagnosis of a tonic pupil thus can be made by placing 2 drops of a solution of 0.1 per cent pilocarpine in the lower cul-de-sac of each eye. A tonic pupil with denervation supersensitivity should show marked constriction within 45 min after instillation of the solution of pilocarpine, whereas the normal pupil generally will not constrict in this setting (although exceptions occasionally occur).

Damage to the fibres for pupillary dilation (Horner's syndrome)

Damage to the long ciliary nerves in the orbit, which transmit sympathetic impulses to the pupillary dilator muscle, produces

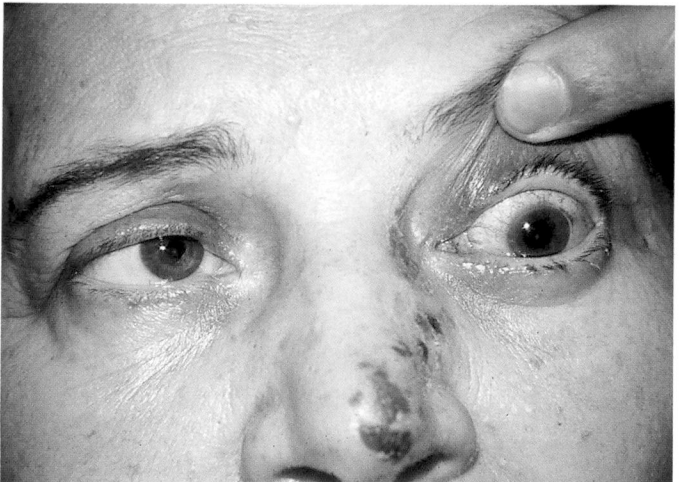

Fig. 8 Ophthalmoplegia from herpes zoster ophthalmicus. The patient has a left oculomotor nerve paresis that occurred about 2 weeks after the onset of left-sided herpes zoster ophthalmicus. Note left exotropia and dilated left pupil. The left eyelid is being elevated manually because the patient has a left ptosis. The patient had limited adduction, elevation, and depression of the left eye. She also had mild abduction weakness of the left eye caused by a concomitant left abducens nerve paresis.

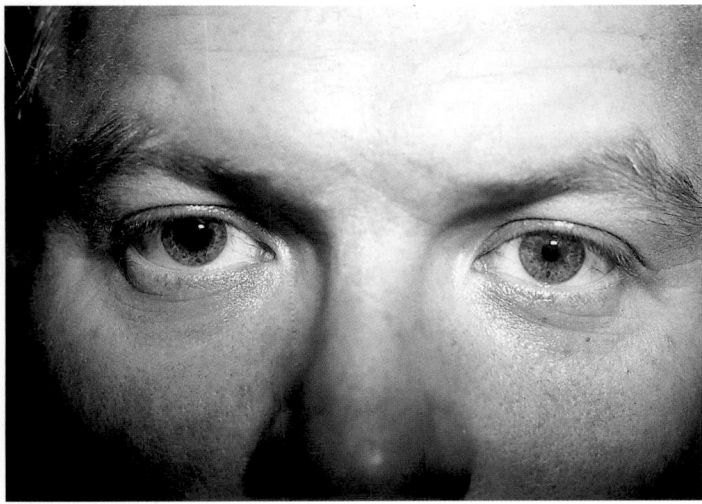

(a)

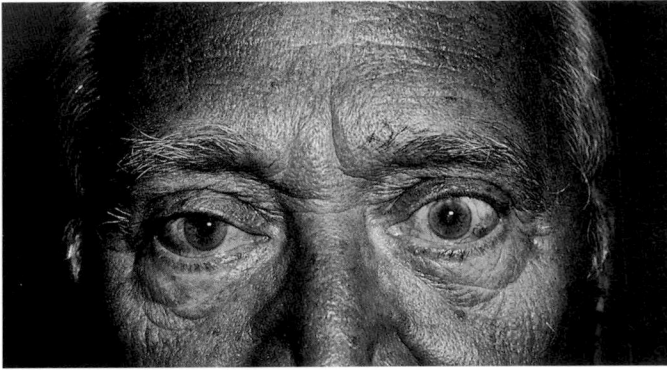

Fig. 10 Horner's syndrome. Note mild right ptosis and anisocoria, with right pupil smaller than left. Both pupils reacted normally to both light and near stimulation.

Further reading

Anderson, D.R. (1970). Vascular supply to the optic nerve of primates. *American Journal of Ophthalmology*, **70**, 341–51.

Burde, R.M., Savino, P.J., and Trobe, J.D. (1992). *Clinical decisions in neuro-ophthalmology*, (2nd edn), pp. 379–416. Mosby, St Louis. [Chapter 15 in this excellent textbook of neuro-ophthalmology describes the approach to the diagnosis and treatment of orbital lesions that produce neuro-ophthalmological manifestations.]

Glaser, J.S. (1990). Orbital diseases and neuro-ophthalmology: an overview. In *Neuro-ophthalmology*, (ed. J.S. Glaser), 2nd edn, pp. 437–57. Lippincott, Philadelphia. [An outstanding primer on neuro-ophthalmology, the 14th chapter of which describes neuro-ophthalmological manifestations of orbital disease.]

Miller, N.R. (1982). *Walsh and Hoyt's clinical neuro-ophthalmology*, (4th edn), Vol. 1. Williams & Wilkins, Baltimore. [This volume of a definitive textbook of neuro-ophthalmology describes the various orbital and non-orbital causes of optic neuropathy, with and without optic disc swelling.]

Miller, N.R. (1985). *Walsh and Hoyt's clinical neuro-ophthalmology*, (4th edn), Vol. 2, pp. 652–707. Williams & Wilkins, Baltimore. [Chapter 35 of this volume of a definitive textbook of neuro-ophthalmology describes the various orbital and non-orbital causes of oculomotor nerve pareses.]

Miller, N.R. (1988). *Walsh and Hoyt's clinical neuro-ophthalmology*, (4th edn), Vol. 3, pp. 1143–9. Williams & Wilkins, Baltimore. [The first chapter of this definitive textbook of neuro-ophthalmology describes the neuro-ophthalmological manifestations of orbital disease in more detail.]

Orcutt, J.C., Tucker, W.M., Mills, R.P., and Smith, C.H. (1987). Gaze-evoked amaurosis. *Ophthalmology*, **94**, 213–18.

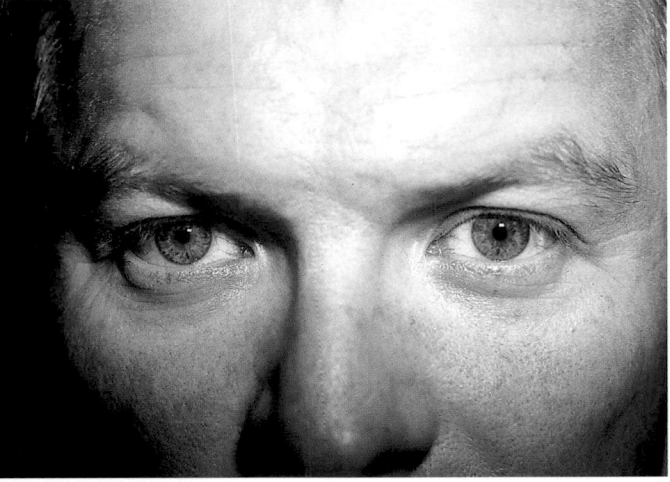

(b)

Fig. 9 Tonic pupil with parasympathetic denervation supersensitivity. The patient was a 45-year-old man who developed a dilated right pupil associated with mild headache and blurred near vision. He denied diplopia. (a) There is anisocoria, with the right pupil being larger than the left. The right pupil was non-reactive to both direct and consensual light stimulation. The left pupil reacted normally to both direct and consensual light. Both eyes moved fully in all directions, and there was no evidence of strabismus. Note absence of ptosis. (b) Forty-five minutes after instillation of 2 drops of 0.1 per cent pilocarpine in each inferior cul-de-sac, the right pupil is constricted, whereas the left pupil is unchanged in size.

a pupil that is small and normally reactive. If the sympathetic fibres to the eyelid are also affected, the patient will develop a true Horner's syndrome (Fig. 10). In fact, orbital disease that damages the sympathetic fibres in the orbit usually also damages parasympathetic fibres to the pupil (see above). The resultant pupil may be larger or smaller than the opposite pupil, depending in part on the amount of surrounding light and in part on the severity of damage to the sympathetic versus the parasympathetic fibres. It typically does not react normally, as would be expected with a typical Horner's pupil. We have never observed a pure Horner's syndrome in a patient with orbital disease.

2.1.5 Orbital disease; overview

Devron H. Char

A myriad of benign and malignant orbital tumefactions can cause a mass effect, displacement of globe, or inflammation and infiltration of orbital structures. This chapter provides an overview of the differential diagnosis of orbital proptosis, discusses a rationale evaluation schema, and reviews the treatment options for most orbital tumours. Discussion of subspeciality details that impinge on orbital tumour management such as neuro-ophthalmology, radiological techniques, radiation therapy, and chemotherapy are discussed elsewhere and in separate textbooks.

Various approaches can be used to characterize lesions that affect the orbit. A division into paediatric versus adult orbital tumefactions is effective for several reasons. Different diseases involve infants and children as compared to adults. In the former group, orbital proptosis from both benign and malignant aetiologies can progress with sufficient rapidity to require emergency intervention to prevent severe ocular morbidity. In adults the most common cause of either unilateral or bilateral proptosis is thyroid ophthalmopathy; usually adult proptosis can be routinely evaluated without an increased risk of ocular damage.

A diagnostic accuracy that approaches 97 per cent should be possible with modern, non-invasive techniques prior to obtaining histological confirmation. The evaluation of orbital disease includes a complete patient history and review of systems, clinical ophthalmological examination, visual field testing, imaging studies which may include computed tomography (CT), magnetic resonance imaging (MRI), occasionally ultrasonography, and in select cases CT-controlled fine-needle aspiration biopsy.

Symptoms and signs

A thorough history and review of systems is imperative in patients with orbital disease. As in any other body site, the rapidity of onset and the progression of both signs and symptoms are very useful to establish the nature of the lesion. Of almost equal import is the relationship between the orbital findings and other systemic symptomatology. As an example, over two-thirds of patients with thyroid-related orbitopathy have a history consistent with hyperthyroidism. Such patients usually have, in addition to the eye findings, nervousness, tremulousness, heat intolerance, and other findings of Graves' disease. Similarly, while some patients with Wegener's granulomatosis, and other collagen vascular diseases, present with orbital involvement, usually such patients have a history of generalized malaise, joint symptoms, cutaneous rashes, and other stigmata typical of these syndromes. A thorough review of systems in all patients with orbital processes should be obtained with emphasis on symptomatology that could be associated with endocrine abnormality, collagen vascular disease, infection, or systemic malignancy.

Several clinical features are helpful to establish the correct diagnosis of a patient with orbital disease. Orbital tumefactions can produce (a) alterations in the eyelid position (ptosis, eyelid retraction, or changes in the lid shape); (b) alterations of the conjunctival vascular pattern (increased vessels over the insertion of the extraocular muscles, diffuse injection, or arterialization of the vessels); (c) corneal oedema due to exposure; (d) intraocular findings (uveitis, choroidal folds, or optic nerve changes); (e) alteration in extraocular motility; and (f) various malpositions of the eye. Three patterns of eyelid malposition

are diagnostically useful. (a) Bilateral eyelid retraction and proptosis is almost always associated with thyroid-related orbitopathy. (b) Eyelid inflammation, ptosis, induration, and erythema is most commonly found in benign inflammatory diseases such as either idiopathic orbital pseudotumour or systemic inflammatory, infectious, or collagen vascular diseases with secondary orbital involvement. Occasionally patients with metastatic orbital tumours have secondary eyelid inflammation. (c) An 'S-shaped' upper eyelid with lateral droopiness is typical for an inflammatory or neoplastic process involving the lacrimal gland. Similarly, three conjunctival changes are useful to establish a differential diagnosis, with the caveat that the cornea does not have sufficient exposure and damage to produce secondary conjunctival findings. (a) With thyroid eye disease there is often increased prominence of vessels over the insertions of the recti muscles. (b) With orbital inflammation there is often an associated scleritis manifested by diffuse episcleral vascular prominence. (c) With a dural-cavernous or a carotid-cavernous fistula there is arterialization of the conjunctival vessels.

Intraocular findings associated with orbital processes include uveitis if there is sufficient contiguous orbital inflammation, optic nerve swelling or atrophy due to pressure on the nerve by extrinsic tumour, or involvement of that structure by an intrinsic neoplasm, and choroidal folds due to pressure on the eye by a large mass.

The nature and pattern of ocular displacement by an orbital process is useful to establish both a differential diagnosis and determine the location of the orbital tumefaction (Table 1). A vascular process such as an arteriovenous fistula or a venous varix will often produce marked increase in proptosis with manoeuvres that increase venous pressure to the orbit such as the patient bending over, being placed in a prone position, or performing a Valsalva manoeuvre. Tumours that are in the intraconal portion of the orbit (optic nerve masses or neoplasms that are inside the extraocular muscle cone) will generally produce axial, or direct forward, displacement of the globe. In contrast, tumours involving the lacrimal gland and its fossa will produce a downward and medial displacement of the globe. Tumours of either the ethmoid sinus or medial orbit will displace the globe laterally. Tumours that involve the maxillary sinus will displace the eye superiorly. Neoplasms that arise from the superior orbit and contiguous brain displace the globe inferiorly. Finally, scirrhous carcinoma, sinusitis, some mucoceles, and blow-out fractures can produce enophthalmos. A number of orbital neoplasms have a propensity for particular areas of the orbit and therefore the patterns of globe displacement help to focus the differential diagnosis. Table 1 lists some of the more common types of adult orbital tumefactions as a function of the area of the orbit they most typically involve.

The measurement of globe displacement can be performed with several different exophthalmometers. In the United States, the Hertel exophthalmometer is the most commonly used instrument. Some other devices, such as the Naugle exophthalmometer, have the advantage of not requiring positioning on the orbital rim (especially useful if the rim has been surgically removed). In most studies of normal subjects there have been distinct differences in ocular prominence between

Table 1 Location of common orbital tumours

Optic nerve and nerve sheath
Optic nerve glioma
Optic nerve sheath meningioma
Extraocular extension of retinoblastoma
Leukaemic infiltrate
Metastic carcinoma
Inflammatory lesions (pseudotumour)

Extraocular muscles
Metastatic tumours
Rhabdomyoma
Rhabdomyosarcoma
Lymphoma
Alveolar soft part sarcoma
Thyroid-related myositis
Idiopathic myositis
Amyloidosis
Cavernous sinus-carotid or dura-sinus fistula
Lymphoma

Lacrimal fossa
Epithelial tumours
  benign mixed tumour (pleomorphic adenoma)
  adenoid cystic carcinoma
  mixed carcinoma
Lymphoid tumours
  pseudotumour
  lymphoma
Metastases
Dermoid cysts

Intraconal lesions
Benign tumours
  cavernous haemangioma
  haemangiopericytoma
  neurofibroma
  neurilemmoma
Malignant tumours
  malignant haemangiopericytoma
  metastases
  optic nerve and sheath tumours (see above)

Extraconal lesions
Leukaemia
Epidermoids
Capillary haemangioma
Varices
Lymangiomas
Inflammation from contiguous sinusitis
Lymphoma
Metastases
Infectious inflammation (syphilis, tuberculosis, mumps, viral, etc.)
Pseudotumour

Orbital bones
Developmental bone abnormalities/alterations
  axial myopia
  fibrous dysplasia
  osteopetrosis
  craniofacial malformations
  neurofibromatosis
Mass lesions
  epidermoid and dermoid cysts
  haematic bone cyst
  aneurysmal bone cyst
  ossifying fibroma
  mucocoele
  osteosarcoma
  fibrosarcoma
  metastases
  contiguous sinus malignancies
  benign and malignant histiocytosis syndrome

Source: Char, D.H. (1989) *Clinical ocular oncology* (1st edn). Churchill Livingstone.

various races and at different ages. Usually for a novice examiner, a serial difference of less than 2 mm in ocular prominence is not reproducible. Devices that avoid parallax, and measurements done with the same base setting, diminish the variability of measurements; with increased observer experience the accuracy of proptosis measurement is also improved.

The appropriate medical evaluation of patients with orbital disease represents a distinct challenge to the ophthalmologist. Some studies should be obtained by the eye specialist to establish a diagnosis, while other investigations are in the realm of the paediatrician or medical consultant. Several laboratory investigations may be important to rule out systemic inflammatory processes that can involve the orbit, systemic malignancies that can metastasize to ophthalmic structures, or infectious processes that may simulate an orbital tumour. In most centres, the metastatic evaluation of a patient once a primary orbital malignancy has been diagnosed is the responsibility of either the paediatric or medical oncologist.

Causes of orbital disease

In children under 2 years of age, capillary haemangiomas, cystic lesions, optic nerve gliomas, and metastatic tumours, especially neuroblastoma, or acute myelomonocytic leukaemia can involve the orbit (see Table 1). Appropriate studies in consultation with the paediatrician should be obtained to rule out these systemic processes. Usually, the sinuses are not completely formed and air-filled until approximately 24 to 36 months of age so an orbital abscess secondary to acute ethmoid sinusitis is unlikely. In slightly older children the possibility of an infectious process, usually originating in the ethmoid sinus with a break through the medial orbital wall is not uncommon.

In adults, thyroid-related eye disease is the most common cause of proptosis. As an ophthalmologist managing such patients, two issues should be resolved with laboratory studies. The first is whether the patient is currently hyperthyroid. The most sensitive screening test is the thyroid-stimulating hormone assay. In hyperthyroid patients, the thyroid-stimulating hormone level should be quite low. A three- to four-fold change in the serum T3 or T4 level produces an approximately 50-fold change in the thyroid-stimulating hormone, explaining why it is a more sensitive assay. Unfortunately a significant number of patients the author has evaluated with thyroid eye disease have had spontaneous involution of the systemic hyperthyroidism. In such patients the second issue is the identification of a thyroid-related autoimmunity and this includes studies of thyroid-stimulating immunoglobulins, antithyroid peroxidase, and antithyroglobulin antibodies.

The possibility of a systemic process as an aetiology for the orbital findings should especially be sought in patients with bilateral orbital disease. A myriad of different inflammatory and infectious processes can produce bilateral orbital involvement including the collagen vascular diseases (systemic lupus erythematosus, Wegener's granulomatosis, Sjögren's disease, and so on), and infectious diseases ranging between tuberculosis, upper respiratory viral infections, and idiopathic systemic conditions such as sarcoidosis and necrobiotic xanthogranuloma.

Sarcoid in African–American patients will often present with orbital involvement and tests such as the serum angiotensin-converting enzyme and gallium scans are diagnostic in most patients, if patients are not currently taking systemic corticosteroids.

In patients who have symptoms consistent with the above processes, a complete blood count with white cell differential and appropriate immunological tests should be obtained. Some of these include anti-DNA antibodies, antineutrophil cytoplasmic antibodies, and appropriate studies for microbes.

The orbit can be secondarily involved either from a systemic lymphoma or a metastatic tumour. In breast carcinoma, 90 per cent of patients have a known primary, while in some other systemic malignancies, orbital metastases are the initial presentation of the primary neoplasm. Studies to assess the likelihood of a metastatic malignancy should be especially undertaken in very young children or older patients with a known history of a primary neoplasm. These may include imaging studies such as breast mammography, chest–abdominal CT and a gastrointestinal series. Several serological tests are useful including prostate-specific antigen studies and carcinoembryonic antigen; newer molecular biological approaches will probably be both more specific and sensitive. In patients with possible systemic lymphoma that secondarily involves the orbit, bone marrow biopsies and chest–abdominal imaging are indicated.

In the author's experience, better imaging data for the evaluation of most orbital lesions is obtained with either CT or MRI as compared with ultrasonography. The problem with ultrasonography is three-fold. (a) While it is a reasonably good technique with a very experienced ultrasonographer for lesions isolated to the anterior and mid orbit, the accuracy of ultrasonography is much lower in less experienced centres. In contrast, a superb quality CT or MRI scan can be obtained in any centre using standardized programs, with the proviso that good equipment is available. (b) Many processes that involve the orbit also involve adjacent sinuses or the central nervous system; these areas are not adequately imaged with ultrasonography. (c) In many settings in addition to establishing a diagnosis, imaging studies are used to determine the optimal surgical approach for each patient. Thus multiplanar MRI or CT images with computer reformation yield far better data for treatment planning than is possible with ultrasonography.

As a general rule, high quality CT with high resolution, thin section (1.0–1.5 mm) scans are adequate for most studies. While the anatomical detail available with thin section high resolution, high field strength MRI using head or surface coils is superior to CT, the added cost of that imaging modality versus the improvement in diagnosis or management decisions is minimal. There are at least four settings where either CT or MRI have definite advantages over the other imaging modality. (a) In children, the rapidity of helical (spiral) CT has allowed imaging to be performed without anaesthesia. In contrast to conventional CT or MRI which usually requires sedation or anaesthesia in children under 3 years of age, helical CT is rapid enough to obtain an entire orbit and brain scan in under 90 s. (b) In orbital processes that involve either the optic nerve and its sheath, or the contiguous central nervous system, MRI is more sensitive at detecting such lesions than CT. Several reports have described patients with small optic nerve sheath meningiomas, or meningiomas that arose from the sphenoid wing and secondarily involved the orbit, not detectable with CT but easily demonstrable on MRI scans. (c) In the diagnosis of patients with compressive thyroid optic neuropathy, MRI is much more sensitive than CT. (d) In patients with orbital bone lesions CT is the preferable technique. For most orbital processes, data available with thin section, high resolution CT is adequate, sufficient, and more cost-effective for patient management.

Fine-needle aspiration biopsy has had major impact on the evaluation of many orbital processes. Over 100 000 fine-needle aspiration biopsies have been reported from various body sites; there have been extremely few cases of tumour spread documented when a 25-gauge or smaller needle is used. The major indications for orbital fine-needle aspiration biopsy are disease processes that requires cytological confirmation prior to treatment, but are not going to be managed by surgical removal. Fine-needle aspiration biopsy requires several ancillary skills. It is a superb technique if a well-trained cytopathologist is available; otherwise it is quite dangerous. The author routinely performs fine-needle aspiration biopsies under CT control for non-palpable lesions. The reasons for this are two-fold. (a) CT facilitates optimal placement of the needle in the middle to outer third of the lesion thus avoiding necrotic debris that can occur in the centre of a tumour. (b) By placing a needle and verifying its position in the lesion, a negative as well as a positive result can have some import.

This technique has been especially useful not only in patients referred with metastatic tumours to the orbit but also, when combined with flow cytometry, in patients with orbital lymphoid processes. Obviously, as with any invasive technique, fine-needle aspiration biopsy should not be used if the results will not influence patient management.

Management of orbital processes

The management of orbital processes varies from serial observation without intervention in some benign incidental lesions detected by neuroimaging studies for other problems, to aggressive wide field surgery, chemotherapy, or radiation.

A discussion of surgical techniques, with appropriate illustrations, is well summarized elsewhere (see Char 1997). Tumour locations and optimal surgical approaches for these lesions are shown in Figs 1 to 5. Neoplasms that involve the lateral or intraconal orbit are approached through a lateral orbitotomy (Fig. 1). This incision is also used as an ancillary approach to create space for removal of a large medial tumour. Performing a lateral orbitotomy in the latter instance allows the eye to be moved away from the tumour and provides sufficient space for removal of the neoplasm. Tumefactions that involve the medial or medial superior orbit are approached through a vertical eyelid splitting incision lateral to the upper canaliculus (Fig. 2). Lesions involving the floor of the orbit can be approached through either a swinging lower lid or a conjunc-

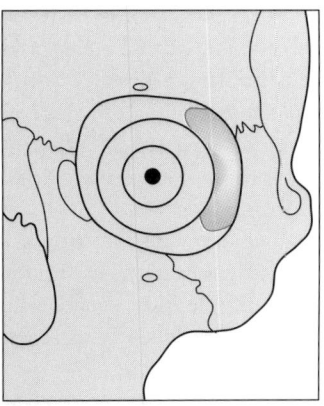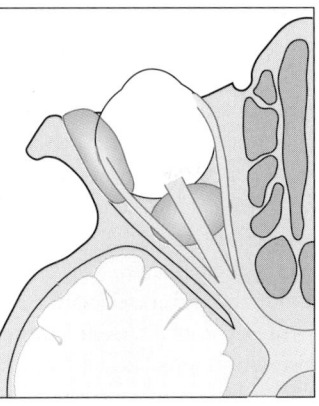

Fig. 1 Location of lesion optionally approached with a lateral orbitotomy.

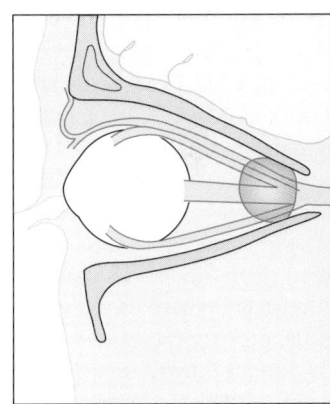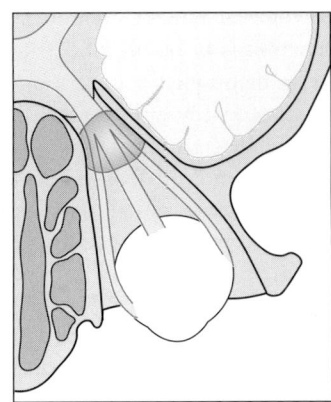

Fig. 4 Combined neurosurgical–ophthalmic approach for posterior apical tumours.

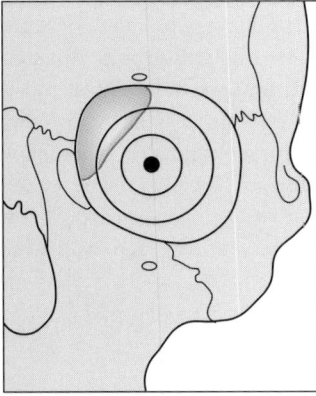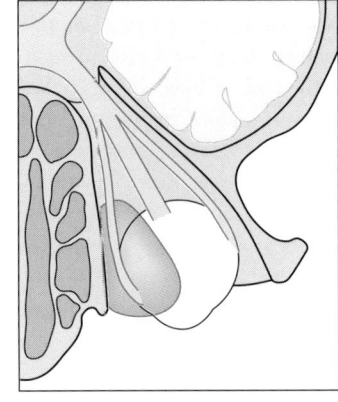

Fig. 2 Schematic approach; lesions removed with a medial vertical lid splitting procedure.

tival incision. Processes that involve both the orbit and contiguous sinuses are reached through a modified Lynch incision (Fig. 3). Tumours at the orbital apex and optic nerve canal are usually approached through a combined ophthalmic–neuro-

surgical procedure using craniotomy (Fig. 4). Small lesions at the superior middle or anterior superior orbit are approached through a brow (Benedict's) incision (Fig. 5).

A detailed discussion of surgical techniques for the orbit are beyond the scope of this chapter. Three general points should, however, be stressed. (a) CT or MRI scans are quite useful to determine the optimal approach to an orbital tumour. There have been several cases in which the physical findings would have led the author to enter an orbit with one approach that would not have been the most appropriate to biopsy or remove a neoplasm. (b) It is often useful to obtain a frozen biopsy of a diffuse orbital process to ensure that a representative sample has been obtained. At the time of biopsy, it is also imperative that the surgeon discusses the differential diagnosis with the pathologist so that appropriate handling and fixation of biopsy material is done. This is especially germane for tumours such as small round cell neoplasms or lymphomas that may be studied with molecular biological techniques. As an example for some primitive neuroectodermal tumours, chromosomal studies can be quite helpful and the performance of those studies requires some forethought. (c) As a general rule, while benign discrete space-occupying processes that impinge on visual function can be removed *in toto* from the orbit, for malignant

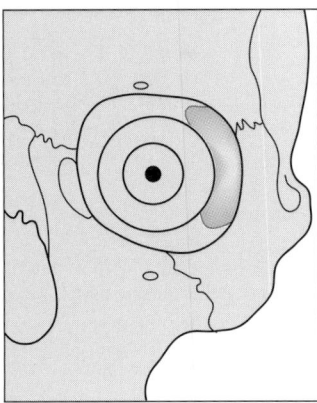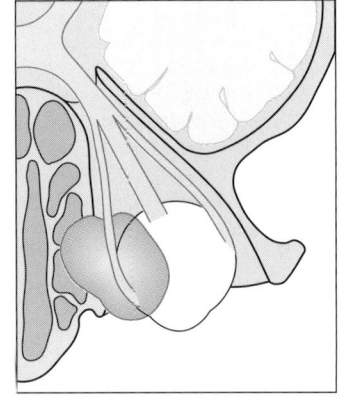

Fig. 3 Lynch incision for medial tumours that involve the sinuses.

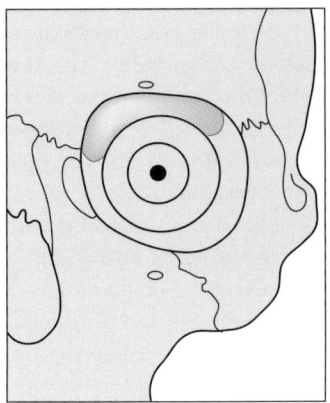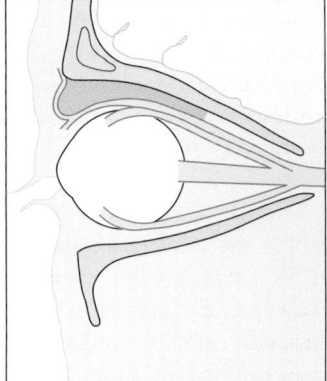

Fig. 5 Benedict's incision for superior orbital tumours.

tumours debulking and ancillary treatment is necessary if visual function is to be retained.

As mentioned above, some orbital processes can be serially evaluated without intervention. In most cases, these are patients with a discrete small non-symptomatic lesion detected when either a brain MRI or CT has been performed for other reasons. For example the author has several cases of presumptive cavernous haemangiomas of the orbit that are non-symptomatic and have not changed with up to 15 years of follow-up. Similarly, in capillary haemangiomas diagnosed in infancy that do not produce proptosis, ptosis, or anisometropia, these lesions will spontaneously involute in 6 to 12 months and can be followed without intervention. Likewise, while up to 90 per cent of patients with Graves' disease have ocular findings, less than 5 per cent will require treatment with corticosteroids, radiation, or surgical intervention.

As a general rule, most orbital processes that require therapeutic intervention should have histological confirmation of their aetiology. Exceptions to this rule occur and these include patients with thyroid orbitopathy, acute idiopathic orbital myositis, and some patients with the inflammatory orbital apex syndrome (Tolosa–Hunt).

Corticosteroid therapy is used in several disease processes and can be delivered either systemically or as a periocular injection. In infants with symptomatic capillary haemangiomas, usually the initial treatment is an intralesional injection of steroids. Often these children will respond to either the first or second injection with marked reduction in the size of the vascular lesion. Similarly in children with focal histiocytosis syndromes, intralesional injection has been demonstrated to be efficacious. In adults with orbital inflammatory processes, a short course of high dose oral corticosteroids is often indicated. The relative morbidity of long-term systemic corticosteroids as compared with low dose radiation has led the author to use the latter therapy in patients who have thyroid orbitopathy or orbital pseudotumours that do not respond to 100 mg of oral prednisone daily for 1 week.

Radiation therapy is used in the management of several orbital processes. The spectrum of these processes include thyroid orbitopathy, inflammatory and benign lymphoid lesions, and malignancies that are either primary or metastatic to the orbit. It is imperative that patients have radiation care in an optimal setting. Studies have shown that radiation treatment prior to the routine use of CT planning resulted in up to a 30 per cent error rate in dose delivery. The ability to computer plan and use multiple beams plus the availability of newer treatment techniques that include charged particles and γ-knife delivery systems have improved our ability to treat orbital lesions with less morbidity than previously possible.

Radiation therapy is most commonly used in children with orbital rhabdomyosarcoma. In contrast to the historic survival of 50 per cent when exenteration was used, a combination of chemotherapy and radiation has had over 93 per cent long-term survival in several co-operative intragroup rhabdomyosarcoma studies. In adults the most common use of orbital radiation is for benign diseases, including severe thyroid orbitopathy or orbital pseudotumours that have not been responsive, or recur after short-term oral corticosteroids. Radiation therapy is also used extensively for orbital metastases which are either a solitary focus of secondary malignancy or in patients whose other metastatic deposits have failed to respond to chemotherapy. Radiation therapy is also used as adjuvant treatment in a number of primary orbital malignancies that have been removed without adequate margins.

Chemotherapy is mainly indicated for specific primary malignancies such as orbital rhabdomyosarcoma, metastatic tumours, and rare benign systemic disease that secondarily involve the orbit such as the diffuse histiocytosis syndromes, and contiguous spread of intraocular retinoblastoma.

A number of experimental approaches may impact on the diagnosis, monitoring, and therapy for orbital diseases. Currently both MRI spectroscopy as well as proton emission tomography are experimental. Both these techniques may improve our ability to delineate the treatment response with various agents as well as allow early identification of therapeutic complications. Several new chemotherapeutic agents may affect the management of both benign and malignant orbital diseases. Molecular biology may bring about improvements both to the diagnosis and management of orbital processes. At present while molecular biological techniques, especially polymerase chain reaction, have started to improve the diagnostic evaluation of some ophthalmological diseases, gene therapy for malignant processes remains a hope rather than a proven modality.

Further reading

Alfred, P. and Char, D.H. (1996) Orbital cavernous hemangioma. *Orbit*, **15**, 59–66.

Arora, R., Rewari, R., and Betharia, S.M. (1992). Fine-needle aspiration cytology of orbital and adnexal masses. *Acta Cytologica*, 36, 483–91.

Char, D.H. (1997). *Thyroid eye disease*, 3rd edn. Butterworth–Heinemann.

Char, D.H. (1997). *Clinical ocular oncology*, 2nd edn. Lippincott–Raven Press, 1996.

Char, D.H. and Miller, T. (1993). Orbital pseudotumor: fine-needle aspiration biopsy and response to therapy. *Ophthalmology*, **100**, 1702–10.

Cousins, J.P. (1995). Clinical MR spectroscopy: fundamentals, current applications, and future potential. *American Journal of Roentgenology*, **164**, 1337–47.

Croce, C.M. (1993). Molecular biology of lymphomas. *Seminars in Oncology*, **20**, 31–46.

Das, D.K., Das, J., Bhatt, N.C., *et al.* (1994). Orbital lesions: diagnosis by fine-needle aspiration cytology. *Acta Cytologica*, **38**, 158–64.

DeRemee, R.A. (1995). Sarcoidosis. *Mayo Clinic Proceedings*, **70**, 177–81.

Doz, F., Neuenschwander, S., Plantaz, D., *et al.* (1995). Etoposide and carboplatin in extraocular retinoblastoma: a study by the Societé Française d'Oncologie Pediatrique. *Journal of Clinical Oncology*, **13**, 902–9.

Dunsky, I.L. (1992). Normative data for Hertel exophthalmometry in a normal adult black population. *Optometry and Vision Science*, **69**, 562–4.

Egeler, R.M. and D'Angio, G.J. (1995). Langerhans' cell histiocytosis. *Journal of Pediatrics*, **127**, 1–11.

Font, R.L. and Ferry, A.P. (1976). Carcinoma metastatic to the eye and orbit. III. A clinicopathologic study of 28 cases metastatic to the orbit. *Cancer*, **38**, 1326–35.

Frueh, B.R. and Musch, D.C. (1985). Positional effects on exophthalmometer readings in Graves' eye disease. *Arch Ophthalmol*, **103**, 1355–6.

Heiken, J.P., Brink, J.A., and Vannier, M.W. (1993). Spiral (helical) CT. *Radiology*, **189**, 647–56.

Henderson, J.W. (1994). *Orbital tumors*, 3rd edn. Raven Press.

Kallenberg, C.M., Brouwer, E., Mulder, A.L., *et al.* (1995) ANCA-pathophysiology revisited. *Clinical Experimental Immunology*, **100**, 1–3.

Kennerdell, J.S., Dubois, D.J., Dekker, A., *et al.* (1980). CT-guided fine-needle aspiration biopsy orbital optic nerve tumor. *Ophthalmology*, **87**, 491–6.

Kijlstra, A. (1990) The value of laboratory testing in uveitis. *Eye*, **4**, 732–6.

Lindblom, B., Truwit, C.L., and Hoyt, W.F. (1992). Optic nerve sheath meningioma. Definition of intraorbital, intracanalicular, and intracranial components with magnetic resonance imaging. *Ophthalmology*, **99**, 560–6.

Musch, D.C., Frueh, B.R., and Landis, J.R. (1985). The reliability of Hertel exophthalmometry. *Ophthalmology*, **92**, 1177–80.

Neumaier, M., Gerhard, M., and Wagener, C. (1995). Diagnosis of micrometastases by the amplification of tissue-specific genes. *Gene*, **159**, 43–7.

Pappo, A.S., Shapiro, D.N., Crist, W.M., *et al.* (1995). Biology and therapy of pediatric rhabdomyosarcoma. *Journal of Clinical Oncology*, **13**, 2123–39.

Rootman, J. (1988). *Diseases of the orbit*. Lippincott.

Rosenman, J. and Cullip, T. (1992). High-performance computing in radiation cancer treatment. *Critical Reviews in Biomedical Engineering*, **20**, 391–402.

Spencer, C.A. (1988). Utility and cost-effectiveness of sensitive thyrotropin assays and ambulatory and hospitalized patient. *Mayo Clinic Proceedings*, **63**, 1214–22.

Taylor, C., Patel, K., Jones, T., *et al.* (1993). Diagnosis of Ewing's sarcoma and peripheral neuroectodermal tumour based on the detection of t(11;22) using fluorescence *in situ* hybridization. *British Journal of Cancer*, **67**, 128–33.

Walker, R.S., Custer, P.L., and Nerad, J.A. (1994). Surgical excision of periorbital capillary hemangiomas. *Ophthalmology*, **101**, 1333–40.

Weber, A.L. (1992). Comparative assessment of diseases of the orbit using computed tomography and magnetic resonance imaging. *Israel Journal of Medical Science*, **28**, 153–60.

2.1.6 Orbital lacrimal disease

2.1.6.1 Lacrimal gland neoplasms

G. T. Fahy

Inflammatory, neoplastic, and structural lesions are the principal causes of tumour formation in the lacrimal fossa. This chapter is primarily concerned with neoplastic tumours of the lacrimal gland. Inflammatory lesions are covered elsewhere.

Lymphoproliferative lesions

Lymphoproliferative lesions in the orbit represent a spectrum of disorders from benign through dysplastic to malignant. Malignant lymphomas form the largest group. They have a predilection for the anterior orbit, particularly the lacrimal gland, and occur mainly in the sixth and seventh decades of life. Twenty-five per cent are bilateral.

Presentation is one of a painless, slow-growing mass in the lacrimal fossa associated with proptosis, downward and medial displacement of the globe, and occasionally lateral ptosis. The lacrimal gland is frequently palpable, firm, and smooth or slightly nodular. There may be lymphomatous subconjunctival infiltration present, manifested by salmon-pink subconjunctival infiltration (Fig. 1). Orbital lymphomas in children and young adults are rare and more rapidly growing high-grade tumours but tend not to occur in the lacrimal gland.

Orbital CT scans (axial and coronal views) reveal a homogeneous, well-defined mass moulding to the lacrimal fossa and the eye (Fig. 2). Low-grade tumours typically do not involve bone.

Diagnosis is established by biopsy of the lacrimal gland. Primary lymphomas of the lacrimal gland are invariably of B-cell type and follow an indolent clinical course with a good long-term survival. Systemic evaluation is essential to determine the extent of disease. Approximately 35 per cent of patients have, or will develop, systemic lymphoma.

Treatment is tailored by the oncology team to take into consideration the histopathological type, the age of the patient, the extent of orbital involvement, and the extraorbital extent of the

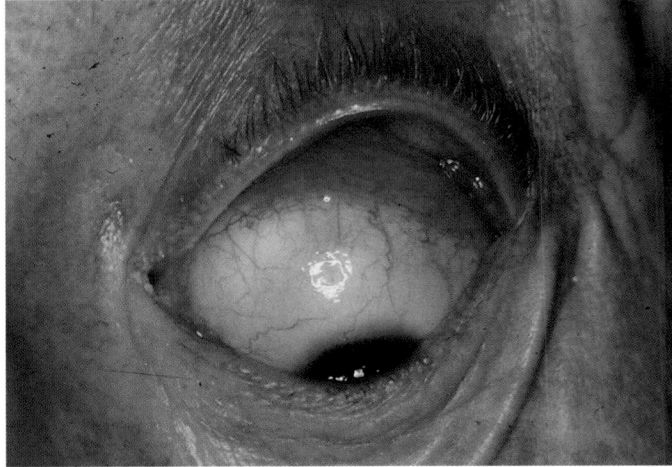

(a)

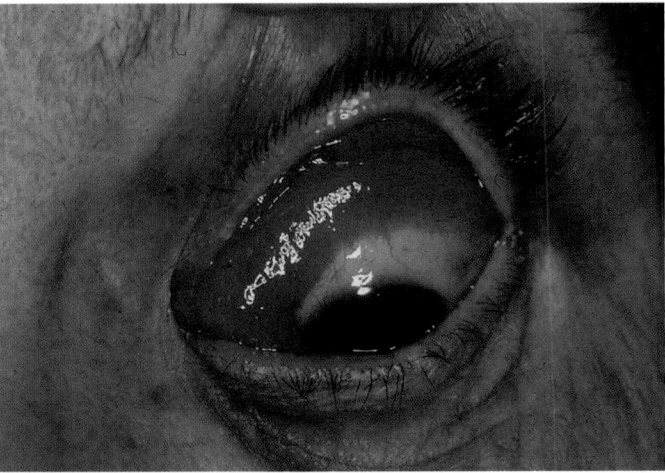

(b)

Fig. 1 Conjunctival lymphoma: (a) lymphomatous subconjunctival infiltration in the superior fornix in a patient with a lacrimal gland B-cell lymphoma; (b) florid B-cell lymphoma of the conjunctiva.

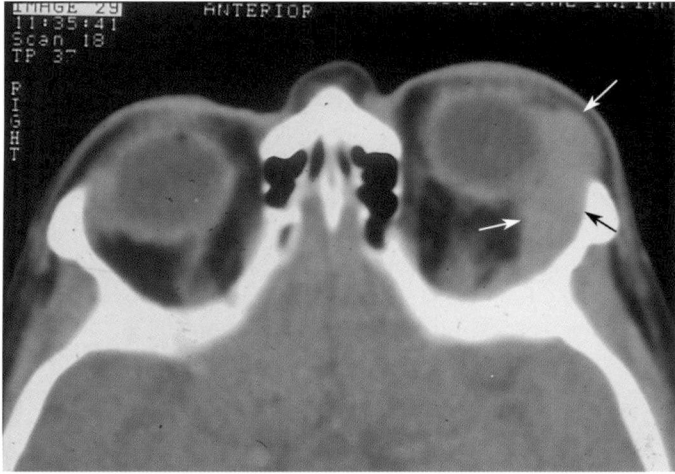

(a)

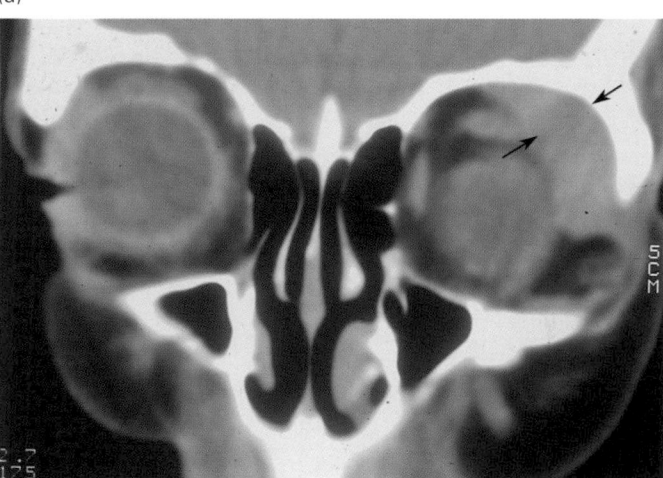

(b)

Fig. 2 Lymphoma of lacrimal gland: axial (a) and coronal (b) CT scan of orbit shows an enlarged left lacrimal gland that moulds to the shape of the orbit and eye.

lymphoma. Isolated B-cell lymphomas respond extremely well to orbital radiotherapy. Poorly differentiated orbital lymphomas and systemic lymphoma are treated with systemic chemotherapy and occasionally adjunctive radiotherapy.

Epithelial tumours

It is essential to distinguish pleomorphic adenoma from other neoplasms of the lacrimal gland because it requires total excision as the primary surgical procedure whereas the others should be biopsied first.

Pleomorphic adenoma

Pleomorphic adenomas (benign mixed tumour) are rare. They represent 50 per cent of epithelial tumours of the lacrimal gland and 10 to 25 per cent of all tumours of that gland. They present in the third to the fifth decades as a painless, slow-growing mass, typically over more than 1 year, in the orbital lobe of the lacrimal gland. Old facial photographs may be very helpful in demonstrating gradual downward and medial dis-

placement of the globe. The patient is asymptomatic in the early stages. Proptosis and downward and medial displacement of the eye typically occurs, and a firm smooth mass may be palpable in the superolateral orbit. Globe displacement can be substantial but, because of the slow growth, visual impairment or diplopia are unusual. There are no signs of inflammation. Rarely, these tumours occur in the palpebral lobe of the lacrimal gland, in which case they present earlier as a lump in the lateral upper lid.

The essential investigation is an axial and coronal orbital CT scan with bone views. CT provides better bony detail than MRI. The tumour is well-circumscribed, frequently bosselated, and the orbit is excavated (Figs 3 and 4). There should be no bony destruction. Calcification is unusual and more typical of malignancy.

The goal is to establish the diagnosis from clinical and radiological investigations and completely excise the tumour without biopsy. Open biopsy before definitive, extirpative surgery is associated with multiple orbital seeding and recurrent disease

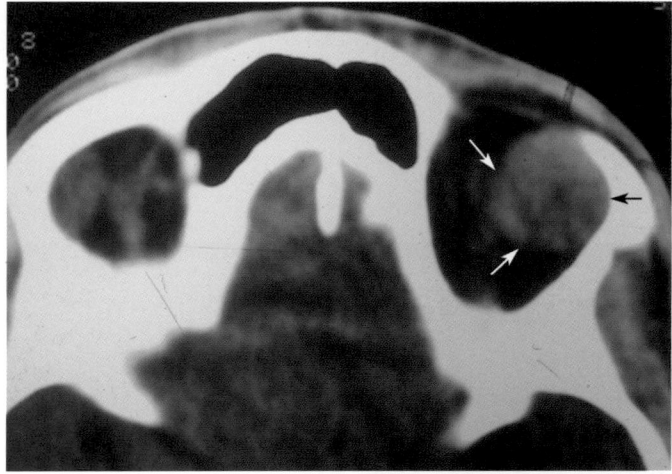

(a)

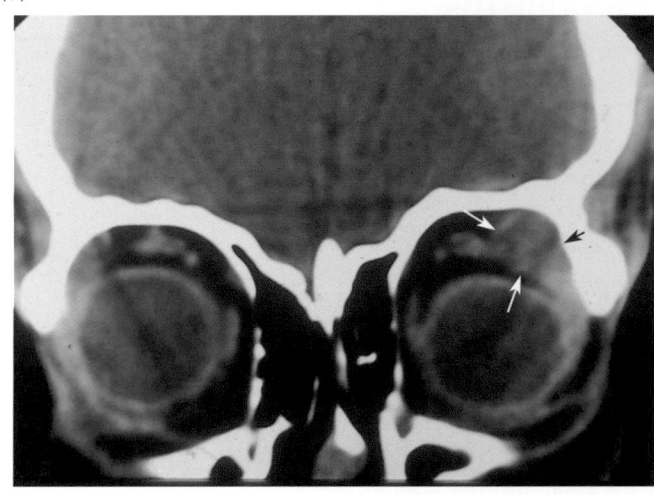

(b)

Fig. 3 Pleomorphic adenoma of lacrimal gland: axial (a) and coronal (b) CT scan shows a well-circumscribed mass in the lacrimal fossa with associated bony excavation; no bony destruction is present.

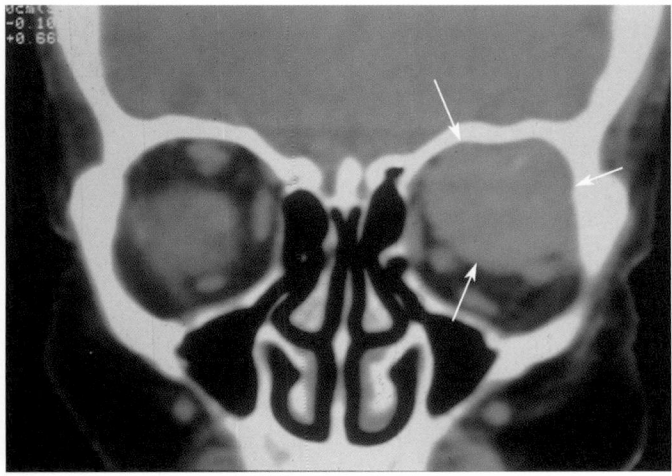

Fig. 4 Large pleomorphic adenoma of lacrimal gland: coronal CT scan of a very large, long-standing tumour shows marked orbital excavation with no destruction; there is calcium in the tumour, which is unusual.

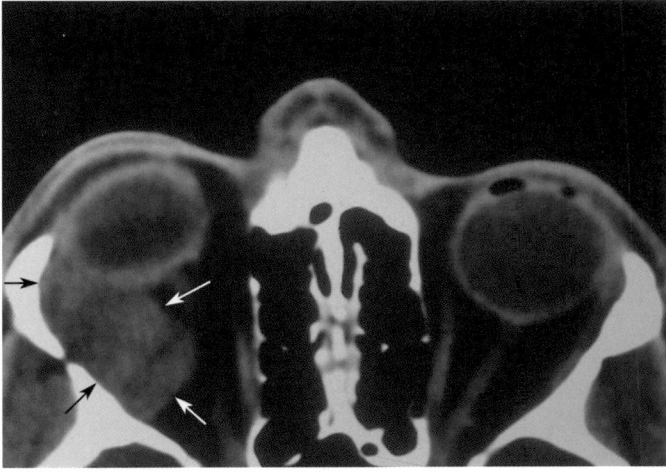

(a)

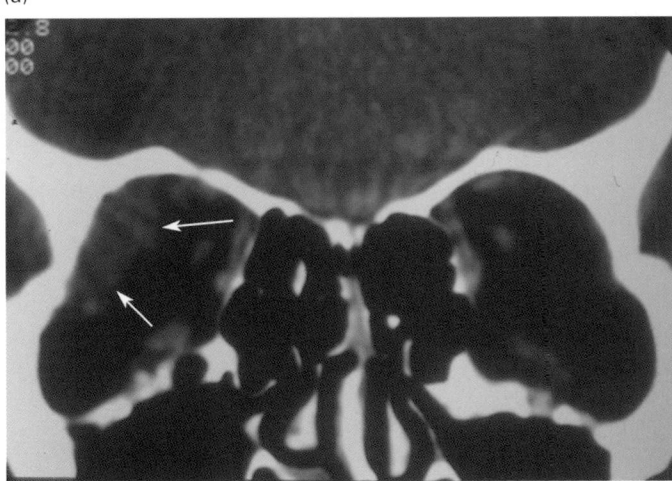

(b)

Fig. 5 Adenoid cystic carcinoma of lacrimal gland: axial (a) and coronal (b) CT scan of orbit reveals a large mass in the right lacrimal fossa with adjacent bony irregularity; the patient was 35 years old with a 5-month history of orbital pain and globe displacement; tumour was infiltrating bone at the time of surgery.

that is difficult to manage. Fine-needle biopsy may present problems with representative tumour sampling and pathological interpretation. Total excision is associated with 99 per cent cure. The tumour is approached via a modified lateral orbitotomy to provide wide exposure. Total excision is the aim, accomplished by including lateral periosteum and an adequate excision margin of surrounding tissues.

Histopathologically there are two main components to this tumour, an epithelial component with ductal structures in irregular islands and a stromal component composed of myxomatous, amorphous tissue with spindle cells. There may be calcification present and pseudocartilage. A pseudocapsule surrounding the tumour usually has microscopic extensions of tumour into and through it at various sites, indicating the importance of excising an adjacent cuff of normal tissue at surgery.

Carcinoma

Carcinomatous tumours of the lacrimal gland are rare, and account for 50 per cent of epithelial tumours of the gland, of which over half are adenoid cystic carcinoma. Other, less common tumours are carcinoma within pleomorphic adenoma (malignant mixed tumour), mucoepidermoid carcinoma, *de novo*-arising adenocarcinoma, and squamous-cell carcinoma.

There is a peak incidence during the fourth to fifth decades. Symptoms include a mass or swelling, pain (particularly with adenoid cystic carcinoma), globe displacement, diplopia, and ptosis of typically less than 10 months' duration. Clinically all have some evidence of a mass in the lacrimal fossa that is usually palpable and frequently associated with globe displacement. Less frequently, limitation of ocular movement (30 per cent) and altered facial sensation (20 per cent) occurs.

Carcinoma arising in a pleomorphic adenoma (malignant mixed tumour) may present either as a rapid enlargement of a pre-existing mass in the lacrimal gland, or as an enlarging mass in association with pain and bony infiltration, or as rapid recurrence of a mass in the lacrimal fossa at the site of a previously excised pleomorphic adenoma.

High-resolution axial and coronal orbital CT scans demonstrate a moulding mass in the lacrimal fossa, frequently with irregular margins extending towards the orbital apex, and with adjacent bony erosion (80 per cent), irregular bony destruction (33 per cent), and calcification within the tumour (20 per cent) (Fig. 5). Occasionally these tumours are well-circumscribed without evidence of bony destruction. Bony excavation may occur more easily in young patients and therefore distinction from pleomorphic adenoma may be difficult. Biopsy of the lacrimal gland is performed to establish the diagnosis.

The microscopic features of adenoid cystic carcinoma deserve special mention. It is composed of densely packed, small cells with a scanty cytoplasm. Five histopathological patterns (basaloid, cribriform, sclerosing, tubular, comedo-carcinomatous) have been described, all of which may occur within one tumour. Predominantly basaloid pattern has been associated with a poorer prognosis. The tumour has a propensity to invade nerves and surrounding structures. Bone adjacent to tumour is frequently involved (even in the presence of a normal CT scan) and perineural invasion may be present several centimetres beyond the apparent tumour margins. This biological behaviour helps, in part, to explain the very poor prognosis associated with these tumours.

Treatment is controversial. Extensive surgery involving cranio-orbital resection has not been shown to improve survival or reduce recurrence compared with exenteration of the orbital contents and removal of the lateral wall of orbit, followed by orbital radiotherapy. Exenteration and removal of the lateral wall followed by radiotherapy are most frequently performed. Prognosis is poor for all these carcinomas, which are plagued by local recurrences and distant metastasis.

Other soft-tissue tumours

Cavernous haemangioma and peripheral nerve tumours rarely occur in the lacrimal gland; they are slow-growing.

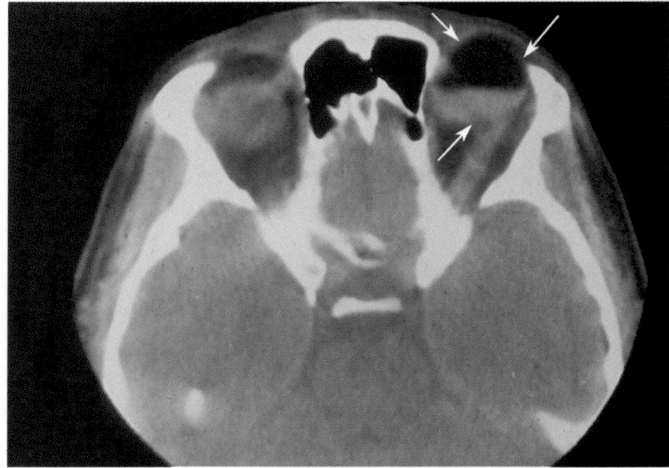

(a)

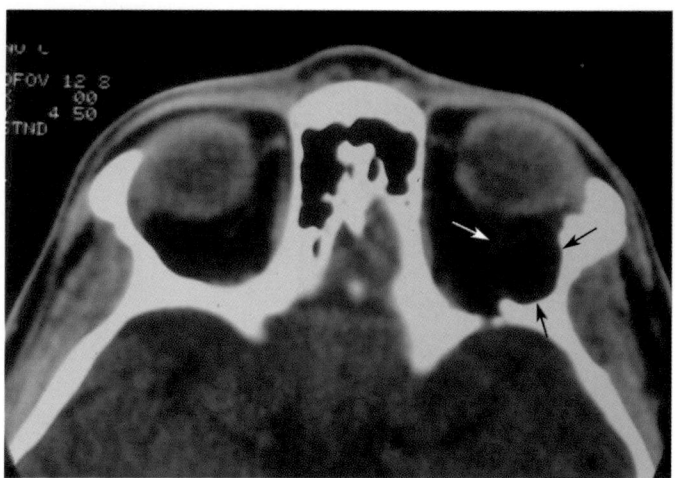

(a)

(b)

Fig. 6 Deep lateral orbital dermoid: axial (a) and coronal (b) CT scan of orbit reveals a low-density (fat-containing) mass in the lacrimal fossa with associated bony excavation and adjacent irregular notched bony edges.

(b)

Fig. 7 Deep lateral orbital dermoid: axial (a) and coronal (b) CT scan of orbit; low- (fat) and high-density areas are present within a superior orbital mass; the axial scan with the patient lying down demonstrated a fat-fluid level.

Other tumours of the lacrimal fossa

Deep dermoid cysts in the lacrimal fossa are the 'tumours' most likely to be confused with a neoplasm of the lacrimal gland. They present in adulthood as a slow-growing mass in the lacrimal fossa. There may be episodes of more rapid growth due to intermittent release of contents into the surrounding area. An orbital CT scan may be diagnostic if there are multiple, low-density areas of fat within the tumour, rim calcification, and a full-thickness bony defect with irregular, notched borders that extend only to the frontozygomatic suture (Figs 6 and 7).

Further reading

Font, R. L. and Gamel, J. W. (1978). Epithelial tumours of the lacrimal gland: an analysis of 265 cases. In *Ocular and adnexal tumours* (ed. F. A. Jakobiek), pp. 787–805. Aesculapius, Birmingham, Alabama.

Rootman, J. (1988). *Diseases of the orbit. A multidisciplinary approach.* Lippincott, Philadelphia.

Rose, G. E. and Wright, J. E. (1992). Pleomorphic adenoma of the lacrimal gland. *British Journal of Ophthalmology*, **76**, 395–400.

Shields, C. L., Shields, J. A., Eagle, R. C., and Rathmell, J. P. (1989). Clinico-pathologic review of 142 cases of lacrimal gland lesions. *Ophthalmology*, **96**, 431–5.

Wright, J. *et al.* (1992). Primary malignant neoplasms of the lacrimal gland. *British Journal of Ophthalmology*, **76**, 401–7.

2.1.6.2 Investigation of lacrimal disease

Frank V. Buffam

Diagnosis and successful treatment of lacrimal disease requires an appropriately directed history and examination of involved areas. It presupposes knowledge of basic anatomy of both lacrimal secretory and excretory systems and their relationship to the eye and the lateral wall of the nose. This chapter concentrates on diseases of the excretory system. Treatment of lacrimal gland disease is covered in Chapter 3.7.

Embryology

The nasolacrimal groove forms in the 6-week-old embryo as ectoderm becomes progressively buried between the meso-dermal maxillary and lateral nasal swellings. At about the same time grooves start to appear in the lateral nasal wall which develop into the turbinates. The solid core of epithelium trapped in the nasolacrimal groove fairly quickly grows laterally into the developing lids. At about the fourth month of gestation, canalization begins to occur, initially in the area of the lacrimal sac and progressively towards the puncta and down towards the nose. Patency is usually complete at the puncta by 7 months when the lids have separated, while 60 to 70 per cent of newborns have a residual membrane at the lower end of the nasolacrimal duct beneath the anterior end of the inferior turbinates. In most infants this opens spontaneously within the first month after birth. Zeis and meibomian glands become identifiable late in the third and early in the fourth months. They appear as epithelial buds in the eyelids and develop over the next months. The lacrimal gland is evident by week 8 as epithelial cords grow from the surface conjunctiva in the upper fornix into the orbit. Mesoderm condenses and proliferates about these cords and by week 12 a lumen begins to appear in each cord. By the fifth month the levator aponeurosis indents the gland producing orbital and palpebral lobes. The gland is fully developed by 3 to 4 years postpartum.

Anatomy

The lacrimal secretory system includes basic and reflex secretors. Basic tear secretors lie in the tarsal plate and conjunctiva. Each tarsus has roughly 25 meibomian glands (more in the upper tarsus than the lower) which produce lipid. This lipid forms the anterior layer of the tear film and reduces tear film evaporation. Glands of Krause (in the upper and lower conjunctival fornices) and Wolfring (in the upper tarsus and adjacent conjunctiva) produce the middle aqueous layer. This comprises 98 per cent of the tear film and contains water, electrolytes, proteins including albumin, antibodies (immunoglobulin A and E), and various amino acids. The aqueous layer protects the eye by washing away foreign bodies and through direct immunological and antibacterial activity. Goblet cells throughout the conjunctiva produce the posterior mucin layer containing glycoprotein which stabilizes the tear film and prolongs tear film break-up time.

Reflex secretors lie in the lacrimal gland. Lacrimal gland secretion has a similar composition to that of the glands of Krause and Wolfring. The lacrimal gland is almond shaped and lies in the upper outer orbit, held in place by fibrous septae extending from the capsule of the gland to the periosteum of the orbital roof. The gland is indented by the lateral expansion of the levator aponeurosis and Whitnall's ligament, dividing it into larger orbital and smaller, more superficial, palpebral lobes. Ten to 12 ductules originate in the orbital lobe and perforate the palpebral lobe and aponeurosis to open in the upper lateral fornix 4 to 5 mm above the upper tarsal border. With age it is common for the gland to prolapse increasingly into the lid and fornix producing a pinkish mass which should not be confused with yellowish orbital fat.

The palpebral fissure slants slightly downward with the lateral canthal angle lying 1 to 2 mm above the medial canthal angle. The lacrimal excretory system lies in the medial canthus and lateral wall of the nose. It comprises puncta, canaliculi, lacrimal sac, and nasolacrimal duct. The lower punctum lies slightly lateral to the upper. Both are 0.5 to 1.5 mm in diameter and normally turn inward to receive tears and are therefore not visible to direct inspection. The canaliculi pass medially along the lid margin and lie immediately anterior to the caruncle. At the medial canthal angle they form a common canaliculus which passes deeply to enter the lacrimal sac roughly 5 mm behind the anterior limb of the medial canthal tendon. The fundus and upper body of the sac are contained by the tendon so that swelling or tumefaction of the sac presents below the medial canthal angle. The sac measures roughly 12 to 15 mm in length and lies within a fossa bounded anteriorly by the medial canthal tendon in its upper part. The relationship of the sac to the cribriform plate and ethmoid air cells varies considerably. The plate may lie as close as 3 mm or as much as 30 mm above the medial canthal tendon. Vigorous bony manipulation during surgery may result in fracturing the cribriform plate and result in cerebrospinal fluid leak. Whitnall by dissection, and Blaylock *et al.* by computed tomography (CT), have shown ethmoid air cells lying medial to the lacrimal sac in roughly 50 per cent of individuals. The nasolacrimal ducts parallel the nasojugal fold passing downwards and backwards at a 15° angle to enter the nose under the anterior end of the inferior turbinate.

The orbicularis muscle is important in normal lacrimal excretion. It has been described by Jones as having three portions—pretarsal, preseptal, and orbital. The puncta are surrounded by slips of pretarsal orbicularis (muscle of Riolan). The pretarsal muscle divides into superficial and deep heads, the former enveloping the canaliculi to insert on the anterior end of the medial canthal tendon and along the frontal process of the maxilla and frontal bone in the region of the anterior lacrimal crest. The deep tarsal head inserts on the posterior lacrimal crest and adjacent lacrimal fascia. The preseptal orbicularis similarly divides into two—the superficial head inserting along the medial canthal tendon and adjacent bone, the deep head inserting on the lacrimal fascia. The attachment of these heads and their relation to both canaliculi and lacrimal sac is felt to be important in 'pumping' tears along to the nose and in properly positioning the nasal eyelids and medial canthal angle against the globe. Laterally, the orbicularis originates in a less complex fashion from Whitnall's tubercle posterior to the lateral orbital rim, drawing the eyelids against the globe in that area.

The canaliculi are lined with stratified non-keratinized squamous epithelium. The lacrimal sac is similarly lined with squamous epithelium but in addition contains many goblet cells and foci of columnar ciliated (respiratory) epithelium. This respiratory type epithelium becomes more prevalent lower in the nasolacrimal duct. The duct occupies 75 per cent of the 3 to 4 mm wide bony lacrimal canal. The remainder of the canal is filled with a vascular plexus resembling that covering the inferior turbinate. Many 'valves' have been described in the nasolacrimal duct which are in fact mucosa and which may retard tear flow if swollen or inflamed. Inspection of the nasal cavity reveals the nasal septum centrally, dividing the nose in half with inferior, middle and superior turbinates occupying the lateral wall of each side of the nose. The turbinates have a bony core covered with respiratory epithelium. In addition, the inferior turbinates are covered with a vascular plexus which can become engorged, altering air flow in the nose. The inferior and middle turbinates are visible on direct rhinoscopy, although it is not possible to see beneath either with a simple headlight and nasal speculum. Nasal endoscopy using both 0 and 30° mirrors permits such visualization and is a valuable adjunct in assessing suspected disease beneath either turbinate. The nasofrontal duct, the maxillary sinus, and anterior ethmoidal sinus all enter the nose beneath the middle turbinate. Patients with chronic inflammation or allergic sinusitis often develop polyps presenting as shiny smooth masses as they grow into the nose from the maxillary or ethmoidal sinuses. Disease of the lacrimal excretory system produces symptoms and signs due to mass effect, obstruction to tear flow, inflammation, or infection.

History

Certain questions should be asked of patients complaining of epiphora or presenting with medial canthal pain or swelling.

Congenital causes of tearing include canalicular agenesis and accessory canaliculi which open on the skin below the medial canthal tendon (lacrimal anlage duct syndrome). Previous sinus disease raises the possibility of nasal polyps with secondary nasal obstruction. Nasoethmoid trauma may damage canaliculi or transect the nasolacrimal duct. Tearing following nasal surgery may be due to an inappropriately placed nasoantral

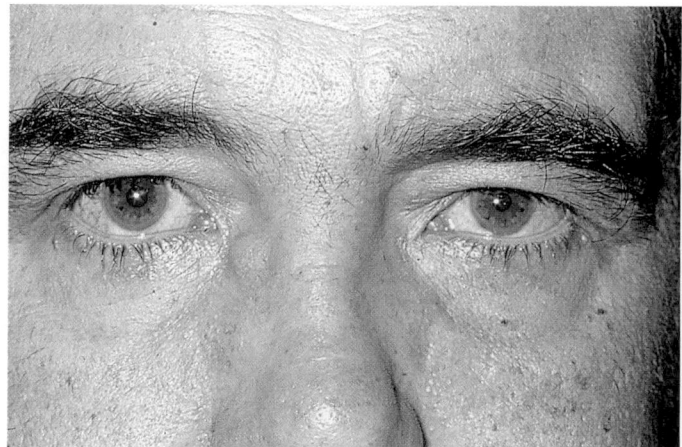

(a)

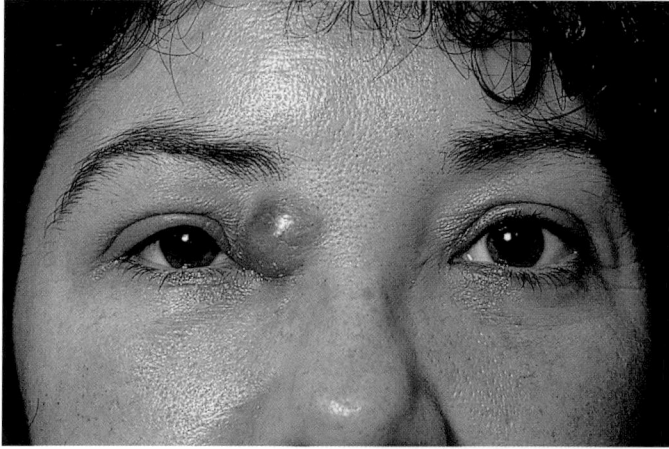

(b)

(c)

Fig. 1 (a) Patient with chronic right dacryocystitis with lacrimal sac mucocele (swelling below right medial canthal tendon). (b) Acute right dacryocystitis with acutely inflamed mucocele. (c) Acutely inflamed ethmoidal mucocele showing swelling above medial canthal tendon. Contrast this with position of lacrimal swelling in (a) and (b).

window destroying the lower end of the nasolacrimal duct. Seasonal or environmental allergies frequently produce tearing.

Certain topical medications (e.g. strong miotics such as phospholine iodide, antiviral drugs), and systemic chemotherapeutic agents (such as 5-FU), viruses (*Herpes simplex*), and medial canthal radiation may produce canalicular stenosis or obstruction. Bacterial infection more commonly produces nasolacrimal duct obstruction, *Staphylococcus aureus* being the most common pathogen. *Actinomyces*, a filiform bacterium, produces unilateral epiphora and conjunctivitis due to retained concretions in the affected canaliculus. These 'sulphur granules' partially obstruct either the involved canaliculus or lacrimal sac. Concretions may also contain fungi such as *Candida*. Fungal dacryoliths are typically softer and 'cheesier' than those produced by *Actinomyces*. Recurrent dacryocystitis in young adults suggests a retained dacryolith in the sac or duct. Systemic diseases such as thyroid and Sjögren's syndrome may cause reflex tearing.

Examination

Inspection and examination of the lacrimal excretory system and nasal cavity should be part of a complete eye examination in symptomatic patients. Swelling below the medial canthal tendon is usually caused by a dilated lacrimal sac whereas isolated swelling above the tendon suggests a non-lacrimal cause, most often ethmoidal sinus mucocele (Fig. 1). Rarer causes of superior swelling are frontal sinus mucocele and meningocele. Punctal malposition (ectropion, entropion) or occlusion produce epiphora. An accessory canaliculus (anlage duct) presents as a fistula below the medial canthal tendon through which tears drain to the skin surface. Assess lid tone and canthal laxity by pulling the lid both off the globe and laterally. A normal lid will spring smartly back when pulled off the globe and released, and will not permit punctal displacement lateral to the nasal limbus when the lid is pulled laterally. Slit lamp examination will reveal local irritants (trichiasis, foreign body) or the pout-ing, inflamed punctum with a tell-tale wisp of pus suggesting a contained canalicular concretion. Intranasal inspection will reveal polyps or other tumours if present, a laterally impacted turbinate, or traumatic displacement of the nasal septum. Objective tests of secretory and excretory components of the lacrimal system permit precise identification of the cause of tearing in most patients. Secretory tests include Schirmer's test, basal tear secretion, tear film break-up time, and primary dye test.

Secretory tests

Secretory tests determine adequacy of basal and reflex tear production as well as functional patency of the lacrimal excretory system. The Schirmer test is performed by placing a 5-mm wide strip of filter paper over the lid margin of the unanaesthetized eye. Although imprecise, less than 5 mm of wetting after 1 min suggests hyposecretion from basal and reflex secretors. The basal tear secretion test differentiates reflex from basal hyposecretion and is of greater clinical value. The conjunctiva is anaesthetized with topical anaesthetic and a filter paper strip applied as described for the Schirmer test. Wetting of less than 5 mm for 1 min indicates hyposecretion caused by failure of basal secretors alone. The difference between the basal secretion and the Schirmer's test give some indication of the effort of the reflex secretors to compensate for the failure of basal secretion. The tear film break-up time test is performed by observing the fluorescein-stained cornea with the slit lamp while holding the lids apart. Dry spots appearing in the precorneal tear film in less than 10 s suggest abnormal corneal wetting or dispersion. The primary dye test (Jones test) is the only test which proves hypersecretion (Table 1). If a wisp of cotton placed beneath the inferior turbinate is stained with fluorescein placed in the eye the test is positive. This indicates a normally patent and functioning lacrimal excretory system. In many normal individuals, dye passage may occur within 2 to 3 min

Table 1 Investigation of tearing

Primary dye test	Dye disappearance test	Secondary dye test	Other tests	Diagnosis
+ (Dye reaches nose)	+	Unnecessary	Unnecessary	Normal
− (No dye in nose)	−	+	DCG, normal; Tc99, hold-up at level of duct	Functional
−	−	(−) Fluid reaches nose unstained	DCG, normal; Tc99, hold-up at punctum	Punctal stenosis
−	−	(−) No fluid reaches the nose but refluxes through the opposing punctum	DCG shows site of obstruction; Tc99 unnecessary	Obstruction
−	−	(−) No fluid refluxes through opposing punctum		Canalicular obstruction

DCG, dacryocystogram; Tc99, technetium-99.

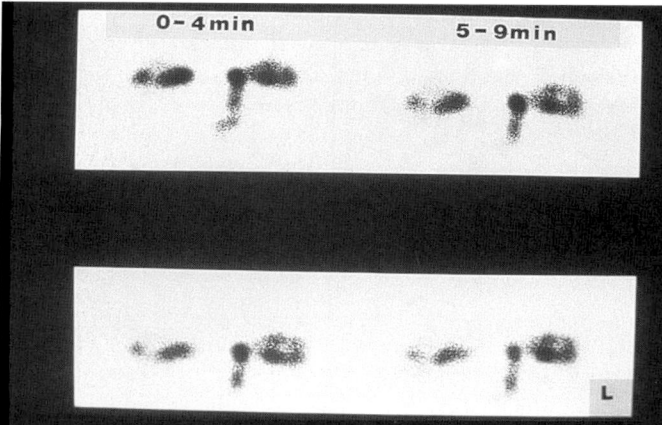

Fig. 2 Representative technetium scan showing complete obstruction on the right in the region of common canaliculus; normal left drainage.

Fig. 3 (a) Normal bilateral dacryocystogram showing normal canaliculi with prompt and regular uniform filling of sac and duct. (b). Dacryocystogram showing obstruction at the sac–duct junction and secondary lacrimal sac mucocele formation. (c) Filling defect in lacrimal sac which proved surgically to be a dacryolith. (d) Dacryocystogram showing nasal lacrimal duct narrowing (arrow) in a patient who presented with tearing, negative primary dye test, and positive secondary dye test.

so that cotton placed after instilling fluorescein in the eye can be checked then to save time. As dye passage can be affected by variables such as volume of dye instilled in the fornix, however, one should wait 10 to 12 min before declaring the test negative. If the cotton is unstained, dye either has not flowed down the duct or the probe has been incorrectly placed. Wipe along the floor of the nose and beneath the under surface of the inferior turbinate to rule out the latter possibility.

Excretory tests

These tests investigate the anatomical patency of the lacrimal excretory system and include the primary dye test (see above), secondary dye test, the dye disappearance test, canalicular and nasolacrimal duct probing, technetium scan, and dacryocystogram. When dye instilled in the fornix disappears from the eye without running down the cheek, one has indirect evidence of

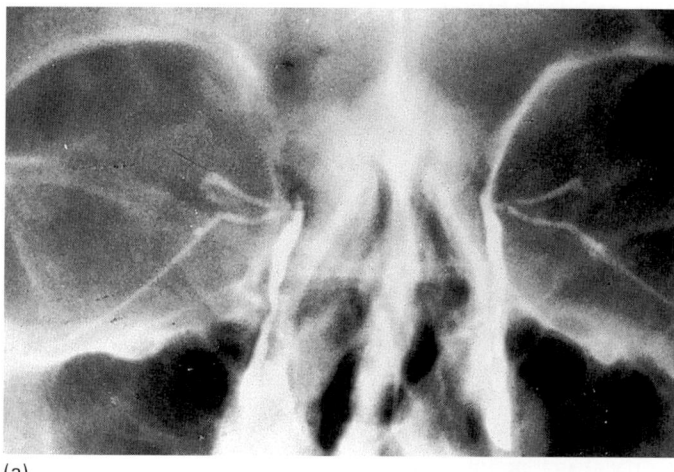

(a)

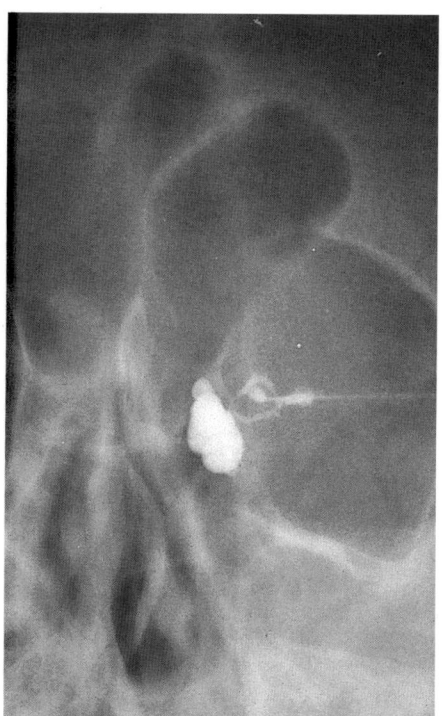

(b)

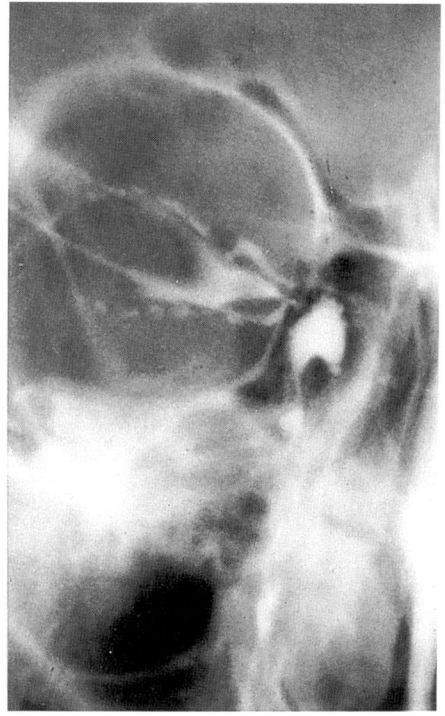

(c)

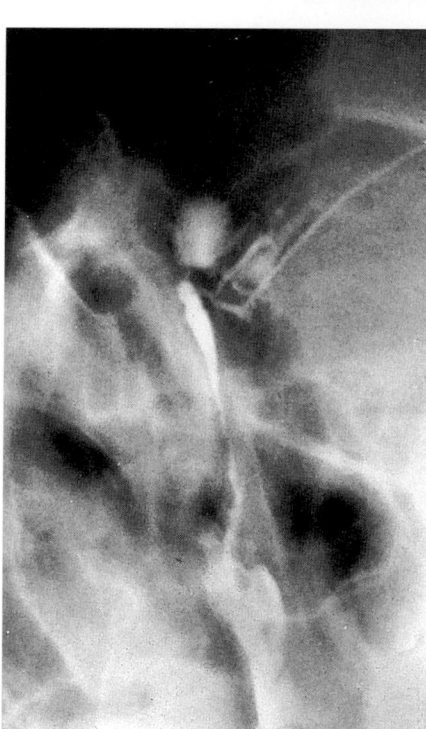

(d)

lacrimal excretory function. This dye disappearance test is useful in conjunction with the primary and secondary dye tests. A similar test based on the taste of saccharin has been popularized by Hornblass. If a patient can taste saccharin solution placed in the conjunctival fornix, this is supportive evidence of the system's patency. The test must be done on separate occasions for each eye, however, as the taste of saccharin is so intense that a positive test on one side precludes effective evaluation on the other. If the primary dye test is negative, a secondary dye test should follow. Clear saline is irrigated through a cannula inserted to the level of the lacrimal sac while the patient bends forward holding a bowl beneath the nostril. If nothing emerges through the nostril on syringing, a complete obstruction exists distal to the needle tip. If fluid regurgitates through the opposing punctum (positive canaliculus test), patency exists at least to the internal common canaliculus. Fluid coming from the nose unstained (negative secondary dye test) suggests a blockage to flow between the punctum and the needle point, that is to say somewhere between the punctum and sac. Finally, if fluid emerges from the nostril stained by fluorescein the secondary dye test is positive indicating passage of dye to the sac but not beyond. This is the condition seen in 'functional tearing'. If fluid does not come from the nose, it is useful to pass a Bowman probe along each canaliculus to measure the distance from the punctum to the obstruction. This is important preoperatively as a dense obstruction encountered less than 8 mm from either punctum makes an internal punctoplasty with insertion of tubing less likely to work, and the need for a conjunctivorhinostomy likely. Lacrimal scintillography (technetium scan) provides information useful in diagnosing 'functional' tearing and canalicular dysfunction (Fig. 2). Delayed passage down the canaliculi or duct is reflected by prolonged pooling of the radioisotope at the site of obstruction. This has been suggested to be a sensitive and reproducible test of canalicular function but unreliable as a test of nasolacrimal duct function.

In patients with unexplained tearing in whom surgery is contemplated, or in whom a lacrimal sac tumour is suspected, intubation dacryocystography is valuable (Fig. 3). Obstruction in the common canaliculus, evidence of a shrunken sac, or canalicular irregularity from previous inflammation indicates the need for silicone intubation at surgery, and implies slightly higher failure from drainage surgery. Obstruction due to tumour or dacryolith will be evident. Ancillary tests, useful in specific individuals, include cultures (if infection is suspected) and CT scanning in cases of nasoethmoid or facial trauma.

Further reading

Blaylock, W.K., Moore, C.A., and Linberg, J.V. (1990). Anterior ethmoid anatomy facilitates dacryocystorhinostomy. *Archives of Ophthalmology*, **108**, 1774–7.

Carter, K.C., Nelson, C.C., and Martony, C.L. (1988). Size variation of the lacrimal punctum in adults. *Ophthalmic Plastic and Reconstructive Surgery*, **4**, 231–3.

Chavis, R.M., Welham, R.A.N., and Maisey, M.N. (1978). Quantitative lacrimal scintillography. *Archives of Ophthalmology*, **96**, 2066–8.

Hornblass, A. (1973). A simple test for lacrimal obstruction. *Archives of Ophthalmology*, **90**, 435–6.

Hurwitz, J.J., Welham, R.A.N., and Lloyd, G.A.S. (1975). The role of intubation macrodacryocystography in the management of problems of the lacrimal system. *Canadian Journal of Ophthalmology*, **10**, 361–6.

Hurwitz, J.J., Welham, R.A.N., and Maisey, M.N. (1976). Intubation macrodacryocystography and quantitative scintillography—the complete lacrimal assessment. *Transactions of the American Academy of Ophthalmology and Otolaryngology*, **81**, 575–82.

Jones, L.T. (1961). An anatomical approach to problems of the eyelids and lacrimal apparatus. *Archives of Ophthalmology*, **66**, 111–24.

Jones, L.T. and Wobig, J.L. (1976). *Surgery of the eyelid and lacrimal system*, pp.160–73. Aesculapius Publishing Co., Birmingham, Alabama..

Kaplan, L.J. (1984). Embryology of the bifunctional lacrimal system. *Advances in Ophthalmic Plastic and Reconstructive Surgery*, **3**, 1.

Kurihashi, K. and Yamashita, A. (1991). Anatomical consideration for dacryocystorhinostomy. *Ophthalmologica*, **203**, 1.

Langman, J. (1963). *Medical embryology*, pp. 303–5. Baltimore, Williams & Williams.

Linberg, J.V. and McCormick, S.A. (1986). Primary acquired nasolacrimal duct obstruction—a clinicopathologic report and biopsy technique. *Ophthalmology*, **93**, 1055–63.

Ozanics, V. and Jakobiec, F. (1982). Prenatal development of the eye and its adnexa. In *Ocular anatomy, embryology and teratology*, (ed. F. Jakobiec). Harper & Row, Philadelphia.

Records, R.E. (1995). The tear film. In *Duane's biomedical foundation of ophthalmology*, Vol. 2, Chapter 3. Lippincott, Philadelphia.

Sevel, D. (1981). Development and congenital abnormalities of the nasolacrimal apparatus. *Journal of Pediatric Ophthalmology and Strabismus*, **18**, 5, 13–19.

Tucker, N.A. and Codere, F. (1994). The effect of fluorescein volume on lacrimal outflow transit time. *Ophthalmic Plastic and Reconstructive Surgery*, **10**, 256–9.

Whitnall, S.E. (1911). The relations of the lacrimal fossa to the ethmoidal cells. *Ophthalmology Review*, **30**, 321–5.

2.2 Oculomotility and strabismus

2.2.1 Anatomy of the extraocular muscles and associated cranial nerves

Michael Cole

There are three pairs of extraocular muscles responsible for rotating each eye: two horizontal rectus, two vertical rectus, and two oblique muscles. The movement of one eye from one position to another is sometimes called duction and these movements may be considered to occur around three imaginary primary axes (of Fick) which pass through the centre of rotation all at right angles to one another (Fig. 1).

Internal (intorsion or incycloduction) and external (extorsion or excycloduction) rotation of the eye describes the movement of the superior limbus as the eye rotates around the anteroposterior (visual) axis. The eye rotates laterally (abduction) and medially (adduction) around the vertical axis, and is elevated (supraduction) or depressed (infraduction) around the horizontal axis. Each eye movement results from a combination of contracting and relaxing muscles acting concurrently, best understood by studying the individual muscle's primary action

which is the greatest movement that occurs when the muscle contracts in the straight ahead position (the primary position), and then their secondary actions in specific positions.

The four rectus muscles

Origins and insertions

The rectus muscles all originate from a common tendinous ring (the annulus of Zinn), a thickening of the periosteum at the orbital apex which surrounds the optic foramen and middle third of the superior orbital fissure (Fig. 2). They are inserted into the sclera 5.6 to 7.8 mm from the limbus the distance increasing from the medial rectus round to the superior rectus to form the spiral of Tilau, and the muscle bellies are 40 to 41 mm long in the primary position (Table 1). All measurements and angles referred to in this chapter are averages for adults with no refractive error.

Fascial system

The rectus muscles penetrate Tenon's capsule, an elastic connective tissue coating which surrounds the globe from optic nerve to limbus, at 12 to 15 mm from the insertions splitting the muscle into its intracapsular and extracapsular components. The extracapsular portions are surrounded by sheaths which spread laterally, fusing to form the intermuscular septa and these, with the rectus muscles, form the muscle cone separating

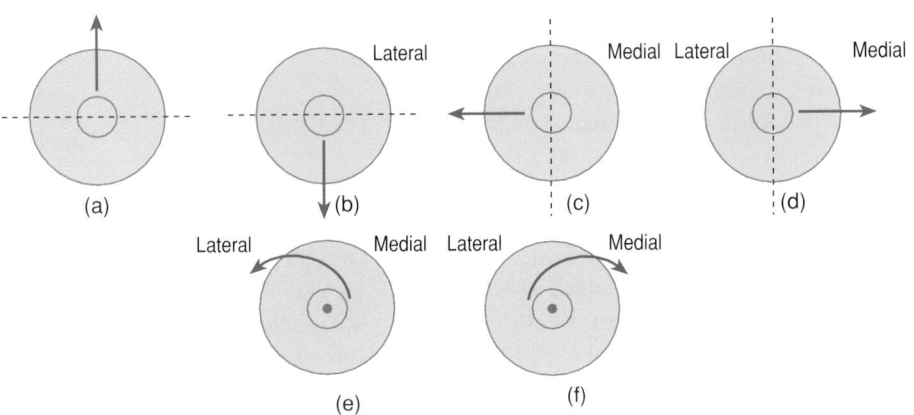

Fig. 1 Different eye movements around the three axes of Fick. Transverse axis (a) elevation; (b) depression. Vertical axis (c) abduction; (d) adduction. Sagittal (visual) axis (e) extorsion; (f) intorsion. (From Snell and Lemp 1989, with permission.)

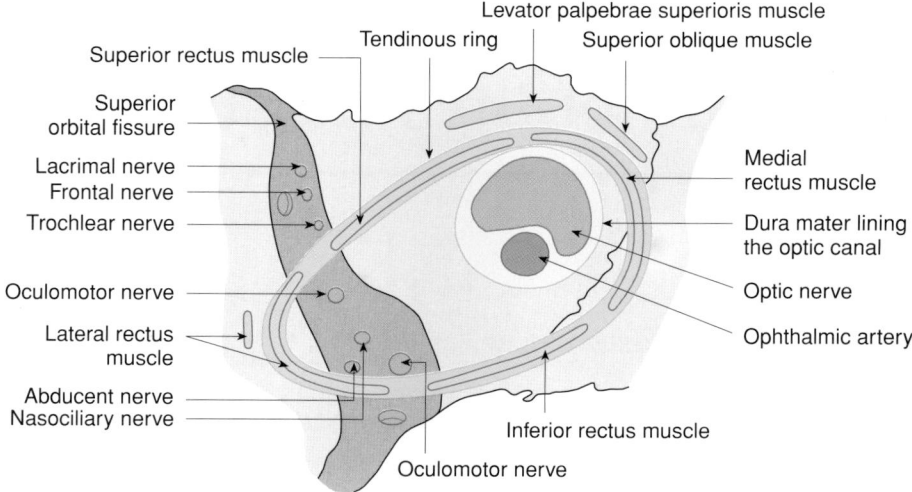

Fig. 2 The orbital apex: this shows the common tendinous ring which gives origin to the four rectus muscles, the origins of levator palpebrae superioris and superior oblique, and positions of the nerves and blood vessels entering the orbital cavity. (From Snell and Lemp 1989, with permission.)

Table 1 Anatomical features of extraocular muscles

Muscle	Length of muscle belly (mm)	Tendon length (mm)	Insertion distance from limbus (mm)	Nerve supply	Angle of vertical plane (°)
Medial rectus	40	3.6	5.6	III (inf)	
Inferior rectus	40	5.0	6.6	III (inf)	23
Lateral rectus	40	8.4	7.0	VI	
Superior rectus	41	5.4	7.8	III (sup)	23
Superior oblique	32	Tendon from 10 mm before trochlea	Lateral aspect. Post-superior quadrant	IV	54
Inferior oblique	34	Very short	Posterolateral quadrant	III (inf)	51

the contents of the orbit into the retro-orbital and peribulbar compartments.

Fascial spaces

The spaces separating Tenon's capsule from the conjunctiva (subconjunctival space) and sclera (subtenon's space) are sites which can be used for anaesthetic, antibiotic, and steroid injections.

Check and suspensory ligaments

The fascial sheaths of the medial and lateral recti send an expansion to the adjacent orbital wall (medial and lateral check ligaments) which need to be freed during surgery on these muscles. The Tenon's capsule inferiorly including that surrounding the inferior rectus and oblique muscles is thickened and with the check ligaments creates the suspensory ligament of Lockwood. Additional fine connective tissue radial septae which attach the muscle sheaths to the orbital wall periorbita also help to support the globe (sometimes they can become

entrapped within orbital fractures to restrict the movements of the involved muscle) (Fig. 3). The Tenon's capsule, ligaments, and bands described prevent retraction of the globe during eye movements, maintain the centre of rotation fairly constant, and enable the movements to be smooth and graduated.

Surgical points

1. The intermuscular septae fuse anteriorly with Tenon's capsule 3 mm from the limbus and then with the conjunctiva 1 mm from the limbus. A limbal incision brings the surgeon immediately down to sclera allowing all three tissues to retract away undisturbed exposing the muscle insertions.

2. The motor nerve supply enters the internal muscle surface at the junction of the posterior one-third and anterior two-thirds. Botulinum toxin injections aimed to weaken these muscles have their greatest action in

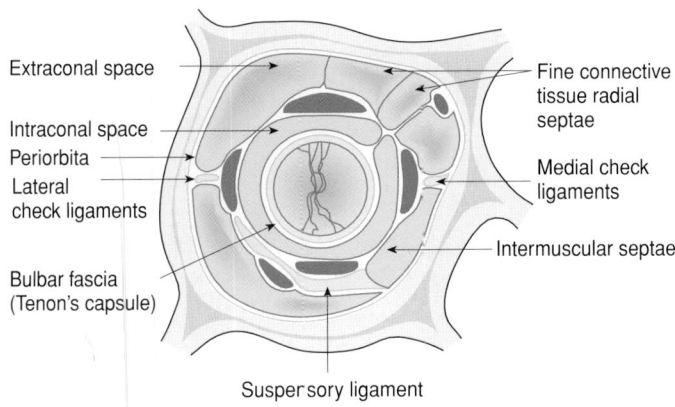

Extraconal space

Intraconal space

Periorbita

Lateral
check ligaments

Bulbar fascia
(Tenon's capsule)

Fine connective
tissue radial
septae

Medial check
ligaments

Intermuscular septae

Suspensory ligament

Fig. 3 Connective tissue septae, fascial sheaths, and ligaments at the equator. (From Forrester *et al.* 1996, with permission.)

the muscle belly at this point where there is the greatest concentration of nerve endings.

3. The muscular branches of the ophthalmic artery supply blood to the rectus muscles and continue to form the anterior ciliary arteries which supply the anterior sclera, and contribute to the great arterial circle of the iris. Surgery to more than two rectus muscles at one operation can therefore cause anterior segment ischaemia and should be avoided.

4. The muscle insertions can be up to 1.5 mm wide and its site appears to creep forward after disinsertion. Occasionally tendinous slips leave the muscles to be reattached to the sclera and may be missed at squint surgery.

Medial rectus

The two medial orbital walls lie parallel to each other and the medial rectus lies adjacent to this wall. Its origin is attached to the dural sheath of the optic nerve as is the superior rectus origin which is the reason why eye movements are often painful during an attack of optic neuritis. Just above the muscle lies the ophthalmic artery, the superior ophthalmic vein, and the nasociliary nerve.

Actions

As the muscle follows the horizontal meridian of the globe, its primary action is to adduct the eye so the limbus meets the medial canthus, but also has a secondary vertical action in upgaze or downgaze.

Surgical points

1. The vertical action can be brought into play during surgery on this muscle by transposing the muscle insertion up or down to produce a heightening or lowering effect respectively.

2. Under normal circumstances, the medial rectus is a tight muscle and has limited contact with the globe;

hence the terminal tendinous portion is only 4 mm long. Resections of the muscle cause more bleeding and, if greater than 6 mm, can limit abduction, narrowing of the palpebral fissure, and retraction of the globe. Recessions can limit adduction if greater than 6 mm.

3. The insertion varies in its position in relation to the limbus and equator in early life thus influencing the effect of a recession especially during the first 6 months of life when the growth of the eye is greatest.

Lateral rectus

This muscle lies adjacent to the lateral orbital wall, runs at an angle of 56° from the medial rectus and visual axis, and is not so tight. Its primary action is to abduct the eye, until the limbus meets the lateral canthus. Its secondary vertical actions are identical to the medial rectus. Just above the muscle lies the lacrimal artery and nerve.

Surgical points

1. The two horizontal rectus muscles together can be transposed so the upper limit of their insertions meet the temporal border of the superior rectus muscle to create upward movement where no superior rectus function exists (the Knapp procedure).

2. A recession of the lateral rectus of greater than 7 mm can limit abduction. Resections can limit adduction if greater than 8 mm.

3. The prolonged contact of the muscle with the globe also influences the position a faden suture must be placed in relation to the insertion for it to hamper abduction in lateral gaze or prevent upshoots in Duane's syndrome. (This suture is more commonly used on the medial rectus for convergence excess esotropia and the superior rectus for dissociated vertical deviations (DVDs) where the position required to limit their action without inhibiting their effect in the primary position likewise varies.)

4. There are attachments between the lower border of the lateral rectus and the inferior oblique which must be dissected free during resections to prevent damage of the oblique muscle or anterior dragging of the muscle.

Superior rectus

This muscle subtends an angle of 23° with the visual axis in the primary position and its insertion is slightly curved and oblique straddling the vertical meridian.

Actions

If the eye is abducted by 23°, the superior rectus acts solely by elevating the eye—its primary action. In adduction, whilst the principal action remains as elevation, the secondary actions of adduction and intorsion become more significant.

Surgical points

1. Recessions of 5 mm or more can limit upgaze (usually 30 to 40° though this gradually recedes in the elderly), but may be necessary in treating patients with dissociated vertical deviation. In recessing the muscle, there are fascial attachments between the muscle and the superior oblique which must be divided for the procedure to be effective. Resections of 5 mm or more can limit downgaze.

2. Embryonically the superior rectus stems from the same mesoderm as the levator muscle which lies above and runs parallel to the superior rectus. The origin of the levator lies just above the annulus and its muscle capsule is partially fused with the superior rectus. They act concurrently. A further slip of fascia also connects the sheath to the superior fornix conjunctiva allowing the fornix to rise during elevation. Children with congenital ptosis may also have united elevation of the globe from malfunction or absence of the superior rectus. Resections of the superior rectus greater than 5 mm can produce a ptosis.

Inferior rectus

Actions

This muscle subtends an angle of 23° with the visual axis. With the eye abducted 23° the muscle purely causes downward movement—its primary action. In adduction, the secondary actions of adduction and extorsion become more significant.

Surgical points

1. The capsule is connected to lid structures through check ligaments as far back as the vortex veins and through attachments to Lockwood's ligament, all of which must be freed during recession to limit lower lid retraction.

2. Recessions of greater than 5 mm can limit downgaze. Resections of greater than 5 mm can draw up the lid and narrow the palpebral fissure.

3. Transposition of the two vertical rectus muscles to the insertion of the lateral rectus muscle is used to create an abducting force in patients with sixth nerve palsy.

Oblique muscles

The oblique muscles run posteriorly to insert behind the equator countering some of the retracting forces of the rectus muscles.

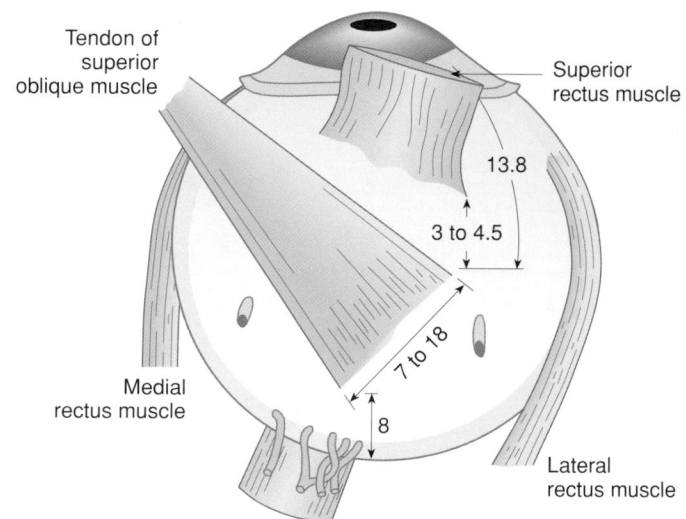

Fig. 4 Insertion of the superior oblique (measurements in millimetres). (From Von Noorden 1990, with permission.)

Superior oblique muscle

This muscle originates from the body of the sphenoid bone above and medial to the optic canal just outside the annulus of Zinn (see Fig. 2) and runs along the nasal wall above the medial rectus for 40 mm becoming tendinous for 9 mm before passing through a fibrocartilaginous pulley (the trochlea) which is attached to the trochlear fossa of the frontal bone just inferior to superonasal anterior orbital margin. The tendon is surrounded by a vascular sheath as it passes through the trochlea and, after emerging from this structure, passes back, subtending an angle of 54° with the visual axis for 20 mm. The tendon passes through Tenon's capsule half way to track underneath the medial border of the superior rectus muscle 3 to 4.5 mm behind its insertion. In downgaze the muscle slips back to 8 mm away from the insertion and the tendon is best identified at this point before it splays out to a paper thin transparent layer before its wide convex insertion 7 to 18 mm wide posterolateral to the superior rectus with its posterior limit only 5 mm from the optic nerve (Fig. 4). The supratrochlear nerve lies above and lateral to the muscle and lateral to the trochlea.

Actions

The primary action of the superior oblique is intorsion. With the eye in 51° of adduction, it acts purely to depress the globe, though still secondary to the inferior rectus muscle. With 39° of abduction, the muscle acts mainly as an intorter but also with some degree of abduction as the insertion lies posterior to the equator.

Surgical points

1. The anterior fibres of the tendon are mechanically responsible for much more of the intorting effect of the muscle. This can be enhanced by the Harada Ito procedure which advances these fibres anteriorly and temporally.

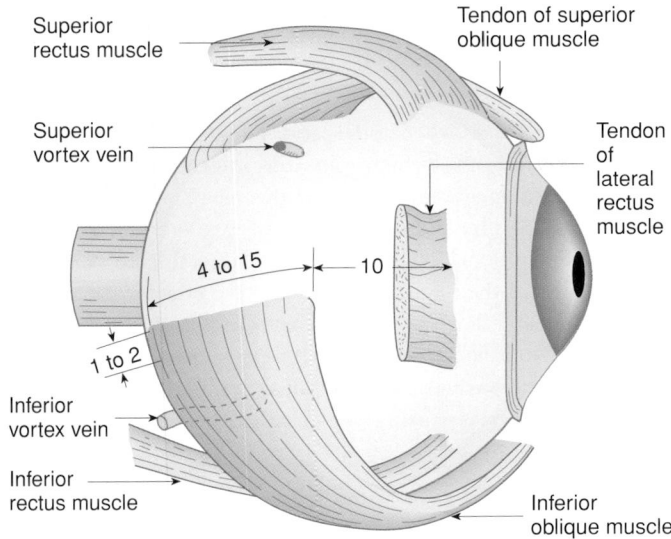

Fig. 5 Insertion of inferior oblique muscle (measurements in millimetres). (From Von Noorden 1990, with permission.)

poral border, loops just posterior to the inferior oblique, and must be avoided.

2. Anterior transposition of the inferior oblique insertion to a point along the spiral of tilau just lateral to the inferior rectus insertion causes the muscle to become a functional depressor and is useful when inferior oblique overactivity and dissociated vertical deviation occurs concurrently.

Third, fourth, and sixth cranial nerves

The motor nerves to the extraocular muscles are the third, fourth, and sixth cranial nerves. The oculomotor nerve supplies all these muscles except the lateral rectus and superior oblique muscles. It also transmits the parasympathetic nerve fibres for the choroid, sphincter pupillae, and ciliary muscles. Afferent nerves, mainly from the muscle spindles and tendon organs, are also transmitted through these nerves leaving them to join

2. Weakness of the muscle is best detected clinically by assessing the extent of downgaze when the eye is adducted. As an abductor, weakness also causes an A pattern because of the greater effect of the muscle in the downward positions.

3. The superior temporal vortex vein leaves the sclera at the posterior tip of the superior oblique insertion under the superior rectus muscle hidden from view. To avoid this during retinal detachment surgery, it is best identified by approaching the tendon from the nasal side (see Fig. 4).

Inferior oblique muscle

This muscle is 37 mm in length and originates from the floor of the orbit just posterior to the orbital margin and just nasal to the nasolacrimal canal from the nasal corner of the orbital floor. It passes posteriorly and temporally, external to the inferior rectus, to pass through Tenon's capsule and then under the lateral rectus, inserting just anterior to the macula (Fig. 5).

Actions

The primary action of the inferior oblique is extorsion. With the eye adducted by 57°, the muscle acts purely to elevate the globe and overaction is clinically apparent if the inferior limbus of the adducting eye is higher than the inferior limbus of the abducting eye, especially when the eyes are elevated. With the eye abducted by 39°, the muscle extorts mainly, with some degree of abduction. As an abductor, overaction produces a V pattern as its greatest effect is seen in elevation.

Surgical points

1. The inferior vortex vein leaves the sclera 8 mm posterior to the inferior rectus insertion along its tem-

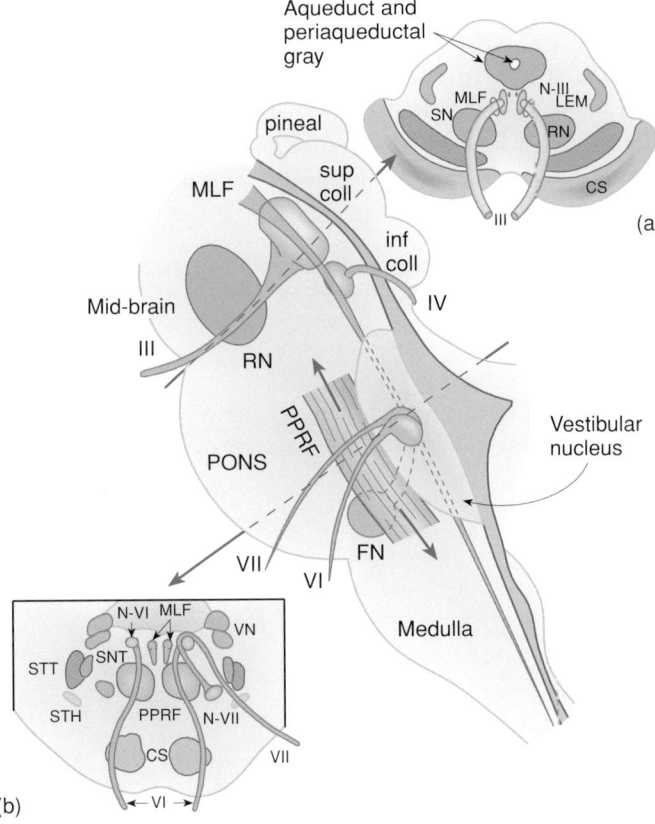

Fig. 6 Brainstem: position of third, fourth, and sixth nerve nuclei and fasciculi. (a) Cross-section at level of superior colliculus. N-III, oculomotor nucleus; MLF, medial longitudinal fasciculus; LEM, medial lemniscus; RN, red nucleus; SN, substantia nigra; CS, corticospinal tract. (b) Cross-section at level of abducens nucleus (N-VI). PPRF, pontine paramedian reticular formation [note that reticular formation continues rostrally and caudally (*arrows*)]; N-VII (FN), facial nucleus; VN, vestibular nuclear complex; SNT, spinal nucleus of trigeminal; STT, spinal tract of trigeminal; STH, spinothalamic tract. (From Glaser 1990, with permission.)

the fifth nerve either in the wall of the cavernous sinus or in the brainstem. The cell bodies are situated in the mesencephalic nuclei although some have been traced to the Purkinje cells in the cerebellum. Sympathetic fibres to the globe also pass with these nerves from the cavernous sinus (Fig. 6).

Oculomotor nerve

Nuclei

The oculomotor nerve nuclei lie in the midbrain at the level of the superior colliculus in the ventral region of the periaqueductal grey matter extending cranially into the floor of the third ventricle. There are separate nuclei for each muscle supplied, and in addition the Edinger–Westphal nucleus which supplies parasympathetic fibres to the eye. The nucleus for the superior rectus is on the contralateral side and its nerve fibres decussate at the caudal end of the complex. Hence nuclear lesions may affect both superior recti, and can be mistaken for a vertical gaze palsy. There is a single midline nucleus which supplies both levator palpebrae muscles; therefore nuclear lesions cause bilateral ptosis or irritation manifested as lid nystagmus or retraction. Nerves fibres from the remaining nuclei for the medial rectus, inferior rectus, and inferior oblique muscles do not decussate.

Dorsal midbrain fasciculi

The efferent fibres from the third nerve nuclei pass through the red nucleus, where an infarct affecting the nerve may produce contralateral involuntary movements (Benedikt's syndrome).

Ventral midbrain

The fasciculi then pass through the medial aspect of the cerebral peduncle where an infarct affecting the nerve may produce a contralateral hemiplegia (Weber's syndrome).

Roots

The fasciculi leave the midbrain as a series of rootlets to pass into the subarachnoid space in the interpeduncular fossa where they fuse. The nerve then passes between the origins of the posterior cerebral and superior cerebellar arteries.

Basilar part

The nerve then runs parallel and lateral to the posterior communicating artery which joins the internal carotid artery, the site where aneurysms affecting the nerve most frequently occur (Fig. 7). The pupillomotor fibres are superficial in the oculomotor trunk which makes them vulnerable to compression. The nerve then runs between the free edge of the tentorium and the lateral aspect of the posterior clinoid process. The temporal lobe can herniate between this free edge and the midbrain when pushed down by an extradural haematoma to compress the nerve causing the pupil to become dilated and unreactive.

Cavernous sinus

The nerve pierces the dura to enter the superior aspect of the cavernous sinus and runs in the upper part of the lateral wall (Fig. 8).

Superior orbital fissure

The nerve splits into superior and inferior divisions which both enter the intraconal space through the superior orbital fissure (i.e. inside the annulus of Zinn).

Orbit

Superior division

The superior division passes upwards, lateral to the optic nerve to supply the superior rectus which it pierces to reach the levator superioris.

Inferior division

The inferior division splits into three branches which supply the medial rectus, inferior rectus, and inferior oblique. The branch to the inferior oblique passes forward close to the orbital floor and lateral to the inferior rectus to enter the posterior

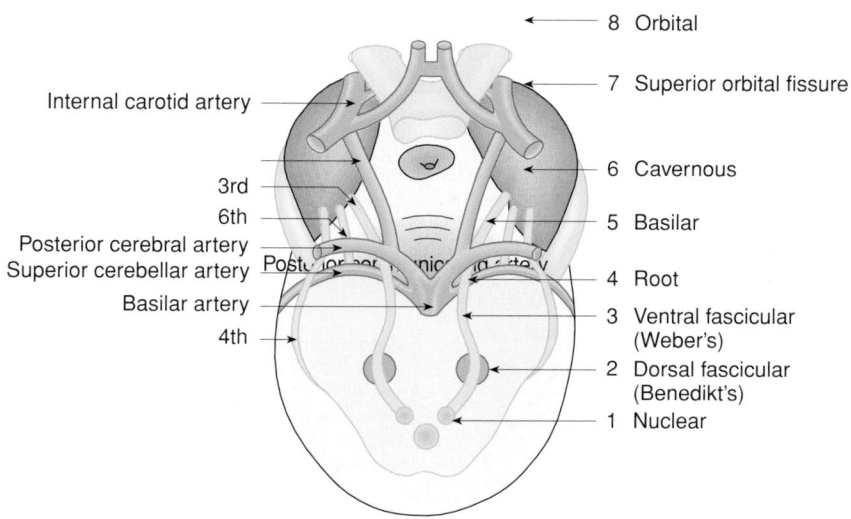

Fig. 7 Anatomy of the third nerve. (From Kanski 1994, with permission.)

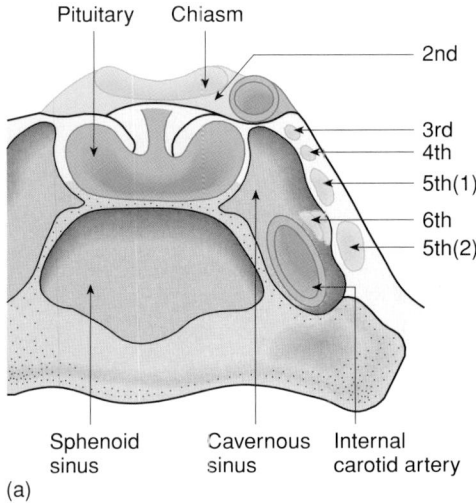

Fig. 8 Location of cranial nerves in the cavernous sinus. (From Kanski 1994, with permission.)

border of the oblique muscle. It sends parasympathetic nerve fibres to the ciliary ganglion. The postganglionic neurones travel to the eye in the short ciliary nerves.

Trochlear nerve

Nucleus

The fourth nerve nucleus lies in the anterior part of the periaqueductal grey matter at the level of the inferior colliculus in line with the other oculomotor nuclei (Fig. 9).

Decussation

The fibres first pass posteriorly and medially before decussating through the superior medullary velum (part of the roof of the fourth ventricle).

Posterior cranial fossa

It then emerges uniquely as the only cranial nerve through the posterior surface of the brainstem in the subarachnoid space of the posterior cranial fossa. The nerve then continues around the cerebral peduncles of the midbrain, crosses the superior cerebellar artery, and reaches the free edge of the tentorium.

Cavernous sinus

It then enters the dura and runs forward in the wall of the cavernous sinus initially inferior, but eventually superior and lateral to the third nerve (see Fig. 8)

Superior orbital fissure and orbit

The nerve enters the orbit through the superior orbital fissure above the annulus (see Fig. 2) and medial to the frontal nerve which runs with the fourth nerve passing medially above the origin of the levator. It then enters the upper surface of the superior oblique.

Abducent nerve

Nucleus

The sixth nerve nucleus lies in the mid pons. The seventh nerve fibres pass over the nucleus to create an elevation on the floor of the fourth ventricle (the facial colliculus). The nucleus contains two groups of neurones, one to the lateral rectus and a group of interneurones which cross the midline to pass up the medial longitudinal fasciculus to connect with the third nerve nucleus. Damage to the nucleus therefore causes an asymmetric gaze palsy, and damage to the medial longitudinal fasciculus crossing from the other side produces the one and a half syndrome with abduction of the contralateral eye as the only remaining horizontal movement. Nuclear lesions frequently involve the seventh nerve as it encircles the sixth nerve nucleus (see Fig. 6).

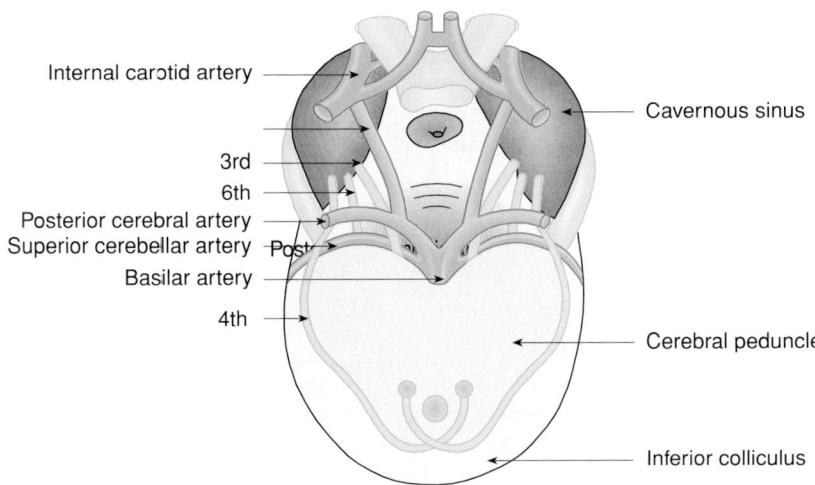

Fig. 9 Anatomy of fourth nerve from brain stem to cavernous sinus. (From Kanski 1994, with permission.)

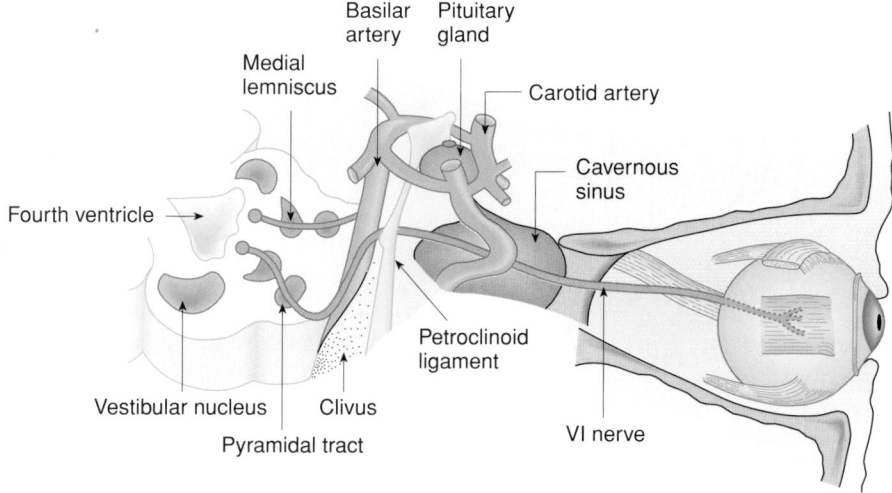

Fig. 10 Anatomy of the sixth nerve. (From Kanski 1994, with permission.)

Fasciculus in the pons

The emerging fasciculus passes ventrally through the pontine paramedian reticular formation and then through the pyramidal tract where an infarct affecting the nerve can produce a contralateral hemiplegia (Millard–Gubler syndrome).

Clivus

The nerve then leaves the brainstem at the lower border of the pons in the subarachnoid space (susceptible here to compression from acoustic neuroma) and ascends on the clivus ridge where the nerve can be compressed by the pons when the intracranial pressure is elevated (Fig. 10).

Apex of the petrous tip

The nerve then pierces the dura lateral to the dorsum sella of the sphenoid bone. It then passes through Dorello's canal at the apex of the petrous tip anchored by the petroclinoid ligament making the nerve prone to traction here during closed head injuries. It is also susceptible to spread of infection from the middle ear and spread from malignancies in the body of the sphenoid bone.

Cavernous sinus

The sixth nerve then passes into the cavernous sinus lying freely covered by endothelium lateral to the internal carotid artery.

Superior orbital fissure and orbit

The nerve then passes into the orbit through the superior oblique fissure within the annulus of Zinn (see Fig. 2) to enter the lateral rectus.

Oculomotor system

The purpose of the oculomotor system is to place and maintain the image of regard on the fovea. This is accomplished by input from both visual and non-visual systems.

Visual

Input from the retina initiates various types of ocular movements which originate in the supranuclear cerebral centres and superior colliculus. Smooth pursuit movements maintain the image of a moving target on to the fovea. Saccadic movements place the image of an object of interest in the peripheral visual field quickly on to the fovea. Fine fixation movements place retinal images on to adjacent photoreceptors at regular intervals to prevent the image from fading from persistent bleaching of their pigments (Troxller's phenomenon).

Non-visual

Eyes are kept stable through subcortical vestibulo–ocular and cervico–ocular reflexes. These influences are channelled into the oculomotor nucleic both directly and through the so-called gaze centres as follows.

1. The paramedian pontine reticular formation controls horizontal gaze

2. The rostral interstitial nucleus of the median longitudinal fasciculus controls vertical gaze.

The nuclei are connected by interneurones in the median longitudinal fasciculus (lesions here cause internuclear ophthalmoplegia). The resulting co-ordinated action of muscle groups produce:

1. Conjugate movements in the same direction

2. Disjugate movements in the opposite direction, the eyes turning in (convergence) and turning out (divergence).

The muscle fibres are highly specialized functionally containing three main types:

● type A producing rapid movements (e.g. required for saccadic movements)

- type B producing slow movements required for smooth pursuit movements

- type C producing tonic contractions required to align both visual axes.

All muscles are constantly involved through two fundamental principles of innervation:

1. Hering's law of equal innervation states that when a nervous impulse is sent to a muscle causing it to contract, an equal impulse goes to its contralateral synergist in order to maintain parallelism of the visual axes. Yoked muscles therefore contract together to rotate both eyes in the same direction. For example, the right lateral rectus and left medial rectus both rotate the eyes to the right. The right superior oblique and the left inferior rectus have their greatest effects rotating the eyes down and to the left. The right inferior oblique and left superior rectus have their greatest effects rotating the eyes up and to the left. (The cardinal positions of gaze.) Paretic muscles require extra innervation to bring about contraction and excessive action of the contralateral synergist results.

2. Sherington's law of reciprocal innervation states that when an extraocular muscle receives an impulse to contract, an equivalent inhibitory impulse is sent to its antagonist which relaxes. If a muscle becomes paretic, the unopposed action of the antagonist can, with time, lead to contracture.

Afferent fibres from the extraocular muscles come mainly from:

1. Muscle spindles (responses increase as the muscle relaxes)

2. Golgi tendon organs (responses increases as the tension in the tendon rises).

This information plays an important role in the positional sense and control of ocular movements.

Further reading

Bron, A.J., Tripathi, R.C., and Tripathi, B.J. (1997). *Wolff's anatomy of the eye and orbit* (8th edn). Chapman and Hall Medical, London.
Forrester, J. *et al.* (1996). *The eye, basic sciences in practice.* Saunders, London.
Glaser, J.S. (1990). *Neuroophthalmology.* Lippincott, Philadelphia.
Kanski, J.J. (1994). *Clinical ophthalmology*, pp. 471, 472, 475, 477. Butterworth–Heinemann, Oxford.
Morris, R. (1997). Strabismus surgery. In *Paediatric ophthalmology* (ed. D. Taylor), chapter 67. Blackwell Science, Oxford.
Porter, J.D., Baker, RS, Ragusa, R.J. and Bruecker, J.K. (1995). Extraocular muscles: basic and clinical aspects of structure and function. *Survey of Ophthalmology*, **39**, 451–84.
Snell, SS. and Lemp, M.A. (1989). *Clinical anatomy of the eye.* Blackwell Scientific Publications, Boston.
Swan, K.C. and Wilkins, J.H. (1984). Extraocular muscle surgery in early infancy—anatomical factors. *Journal of Paediatric Ophthalmology and Strabismus*, **21**, 44–9.
Von Noorden, G.K. (1990). *Binocular vision and ocular motility.* Mosby, St Louis.

2.2.2 Binocularity

Suzanne P. McKee and Julie M. Harris

Binocularity is the study of how the human brain combines the information provided by the signals coming from the two retinas. Each eye sees almost, but not quite, the same view of the world. The substantial overlap between the visual fields creates a problem in visual processing, namely how to assign a unique visual direction to the edges and markings that define visible objects and surfaces. A simple demonstration reveals the nature of the problem. Hold a pencil about 20 cm in front of your nose, and fixate on the point. As you cover each of your eyes in succession, the objects behind the pencil appear to jump from one location to another. This apparent shift occurs because each monocular image specifies a slightly different visual direction for any feature lying beyond (or in front of) the fixation point. Ambiguous information about visual location would undoubtedly impair our ability to act quickly, so the binocular system 'fuses' the monocular visual directions of each feature into a single direction as though we were looking at the world through one cyclopean eye. The differences, or disparities, between the monocular visual directions are also a valuable source of information about depth—about the relative distances to objects in front of the head, and their three-dimensional shapes. Binocularity can be roughly divided into two related topics: fusion, the study of how the binocular system combines the monocular visual directions, and stereopsis, the study of how the binocular system uses the difference between the visual directions to generate information about depth.

Visual direction and fusion

The study of visual direction begins with the simple geometry of binocular viewing. Figure 1 shows the monocular visual directions (or lines of sight) for two points, when viewed from above (plan view). The eyes are fixating on point *F*. The visual axis is the line of sight that passes from the fovea through the optical nodal point (*np*) to the fixation point. The angle at the point *F* where the visual axes cross is the vergence angle. Lines of sight, drawn through the nodal points of each eye to point (*P*), define the binocular parallax angle of this point lying beyond the fixation point. The difference in these angles gives the relative disparity of points *F* and *P*. By convention, points lying beyond fixation are said to have 'uncrossed' horizontal disparity, while points lying in front of fixation have 'crossed' disparity. The reason for this nomenclature is that, when one eye is covered, features beyond fixation appear to move toward the open eye, while features in front of fixation move toward the closed eye.

How are these parallax angles related to differences in visual direction? The two monocular images, drawn in the boxes at the bottom of Fig. 1, show the locations of the points in each

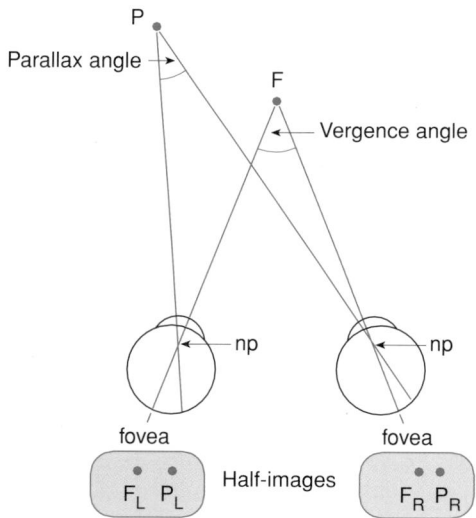

Fig. 1 A geometric diagram of the parallax angles and monocular visual directions (lines of sight) associated with two points presented at different distances. The boxes at the bottom show the monocular images (called 'half-images') of the points on the retina.

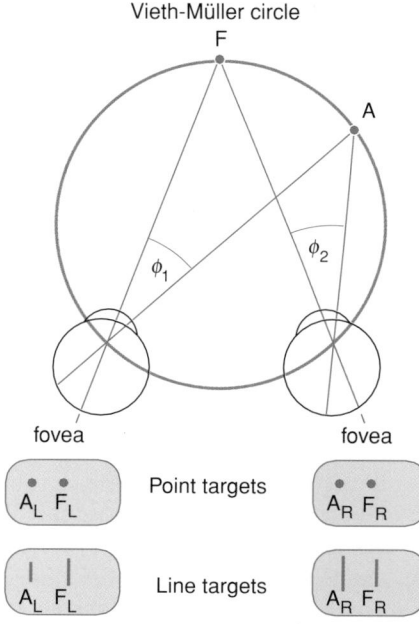

Fig. 2 The Vieth–Müller circle is a theoretical longitudinal horopter derived from simple geometry. The angle between the lines of sight for points F and A is the same in both eyes ($\varnothing_1 = \varnothing_2$), so theoretically, the monocular visual directions associated with each point are the same in the two eyes. All points in space that fall on this circle have the same visual direction in each eye, and therefore have zero disparity.

eye. These paired monocular images are often called 'half-images' in studies of stereopsis. The fixation point is imaged in the fovea, so the visual direction (or location) of point F is necessarily the same in the two eyes. Clearly, the visual direction of point P is not the same in the two eyes, because the lines of sight intersect the retinae at different places. This difference between the visual directions is readily apparent in the half-images where the distance separating the points in the left image is larger than the distance in the right image.

The horopter

Spatial positions that have the same visual direction in both eyes are said to fall on 'corresponding points' of the two retinas. The locus of points in space that fall at retinal correspondence is known as the horopter. Theoretically, corresponding points occupy the same anatomical position in each eye, as though the two retinas were superimposed. If this idea were strictly correct, then the horopter could be determined geometrically for any vergence angle. Figure 2 shows the predicted horopter for the case where the eyes are symmetrically converged on point F. The angle between the lines of sight for points F and A is the same in both eyes ($\varnothing_1 = \varnothing_2$), so the horizontal distances between these points are equal in the monocular half-images for the point targets. The monocular lines of sight for point A intersect at a circle drawn through the nodal points of the two eyes and the fixation point (F). The angle between the fixation point and any point on this circle will be the same in both eyes, so the visual directions for all points on the circle are the same in both eyes; all points on this circle have zero disparity. By similar reasoning, it is possible to show that all points on a vertical line passing through the circle at the midline also have zero disparity. In the special case drawn in Fig. 2, the eyes are converged symmetrically at the midline, so the vertical horopter passes through point F. The geometric construction

shown in Fig. 2 is known as the Vieth–Müller circle after the physiologists who described it in the nineteenth century.

A complexity in this simple circular scheme becomes apparent if we consider targets other than points, for example vertical lines. A line at point A is closer to the right eye than to the left, so its vertical extent in the right half-image is necessarily magnified when compared to the left half-image (see boxes at the bottom of Fig. 2); the ends of the lines cannot have the same visual direction in the two eyes. The predicted horizontal disparity of these lines is zero, but there is a vertical disparity associated with the ends of the lines.

Numerous empirical studies have determined which spatial positions have the same perceived horizontal direction in the two eyes (the longitudinal horopter). In one commonly used paradigm, the observer is asked to align nonius lines presented at various lateral positions in the visual field, while fixating a point at the midline. Nonius lines consist of a pair of vertical lines, presented one above the other, in which only one line is visible to each eye. When the nonius pair appear aligned, the horizontal visual directions of the lines must be the same in two eyes. Experimental data, based on this paradigm as well as others, have shown that the empirical horopter deviates systematically from the Vieth–Müller circle. The measured points on the empirical horopter lie outside the Vieth–Müller circle, falling on an arc of shallower curvature which passes through the fixation point. This observed deviation can be explained by assuming that, neurally, the angular distances on the nasal retina have a different scaling factor from the distances on the temporal retina. If, for every pair of corresponding points, the angular distance on the nasal retina was magnified compared to the distance on the temporal retina, then the horopter would have the measured shape.

Panum's area

Binocular fusion refers to the percept of singleness that is generated when similar monocular images fall at retinal correspondence. In other words, a single objective feature that stimulates the same visual direction in the two eyes looks like a single feature. Disparate images also appear fused if the difference between their monocular visual directions is not too large. The largest horizontal and vertical disparities that permit fusion define the limits of Panum's fusional area (named after another nineteenth-century physiologist). When these disparity limits are exceeded, two images of the same feature are visible—a condition called diplopia (double vision). Panum's fusional range is greater for horizontal than for vertical disparities. In the fovea, thin bright bars will appear fused if the horizontal disparity is 10 minutes of arc or less, while a vertical disparity of only 5 minutes of arc produces diplopia. Panum's area varies with retinal eccentricity; the horizontal disparity limit for thin bars increases to over 30 minutes of arc at an eccentricity of 12°. The fusional range also depends on the characteristics of the stimulus; fuzzy or blurred images have a much larger fusional range than images with sharp edges. For example, very fuzzy targets (composed of very low spatial frequencies) may appear fused even with disparities as large as 2°.

In natural surroundings, many visual features lying far from the fixation point will exceed the disparity limits of Panum's area, and thus should appear double. Most individuals are unaware of these double images, unless their attention is directed to features beyond the point of fixation. Thus, diplopia is only a serious problem in those pathological cases where features near the fixation point are not fused, thereby hampering reading or visually directed actions. It is interesting that diplopic images have an apparent depth. Normal observers can correctly identify whether a briefly flashed feature is in front or behind the fixation point for disparities ranging upwards of 5°. Fusion is not a prerequisite for depth perception.

Binocular visual direction

What is the visual direction of a binocularly fused, but disparate, feature? If the monocular half-images have the same contrast, the perceived binocular direction lies roughly half-way between the monocular directions. However, if one of the half-images has a higher contrast that the other, the apparent location of the fused image will be shifted in the direction of the higher contrast half-image. This result shows that binocular visual direction is not based on a fixed geometry of retinal local signs, but instead depends on the relative signal strength of the monocular signals that are combined in the fusion process.

Binocular summation and rivalry

In fusing the two monocular images, the binocular system sums together the signals from the two eyes, thereby improving signal quality. The result is that generally two eyes are better

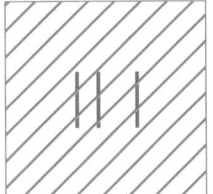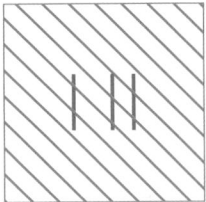

Fig. 3 A perceptual demonstration of binocular rivalry, showing that stereopsis is possible in the presence of a rivalrous background. Converge on a point in front of this figure to fuse the outer frames. When the two images are fused, the central black line should appear at a different depth from the pair of black lines flanking it.

than one. How much better depends on the relative strength of the eyes. For example, binocular visual acuity is better than monocular visual acuity, provided the monocular visual acuities are similar. If not, the binocular visual acuity is roughly the same as the better of the two eyes. In normal subjects, almost all binocular measurements of visual performance are superior to comparable monocular measurements, provided that the targets are presented at or near retinal correspondence so that the signals can be summed. A concomitant effect of binocular summation is that a strong signal in one eye will usually mask (or suppress) a much weaker signal at retinal correspondence in the other eye.

If two very different monocular images are presented to the eyes at retinal correspondence, the resulting percept is a fairly rapid alternation between the two conflicting images. This percept is called rivalry. Large differences in colour, brightness, orientation, or contour shape can all induce rivalry. The binocular system is not alternating between eyes, shutting down all signals first from one eye and then the other. Instead rivalry occurs between local patches of the two images, as though the alternation represented a competition between neurons serving corresponding regions of the visual field. Indeed, stereopsis, which depends on combining the signals from the two eyes, is possible even in the presence of a rivalrous background. Readers capable of free fusion can confirm this observation for themselves by converging in front of the two square pictures shown in Fig. 3.

Disparity and stereopsis

Stereopsis is the perception of depth generated by differences in horizontal disparity. In special circumstances, vertical disparity can influence perceived depth, but this topic is outside the scope of this section. In normal human infants, the ability to respond to stereopsis first appears at about the age of 4 months. The important scientific issue is how the binocular system encodes disparity, since there are several ways to represent the disparities of binocularly visible points. In Fig. 1, the difference in the parallax angles of points F and P is one valid measure of relative disparity. The only problem with this representation is that it suggests that parallax measurements are important in judging relative depth. In principle, the binocular system could use a kind of range-finding system based on triangulation: converge on point F and measure the angle between the visual axes, then converge on point *P*, measure the new vergence angle, and take the difference between the angles. However, measuring parallax angles is certainly not necessary because relative depth can be judged accurately for stimulus durations too brief to permit changes in convergence. Moreover, judgements of binocular parallax are very imprecise when compared to the best estimates of human stereoacuity. Stereoacuity is the smallest detectable difference in disparity where the sign of the depth can be correctly identified, for example point *P* is behind point *F*.

In the conceptual framework based on visual direction, the absolute horizontal (or vertical) disparity of any point in the image, for example point *P* in Fig. 1, is given by the difference between the monocular visual locations ($PL - PR$ in the half-images). Recall that points at retinal correspondence have zero absolute disparity ($FL - FR = 0$). If the binocular system could encode absolute disparity with high precision, then observers could readily judge the depth of features presented sequentially. For example, point *F* could be presented for one-fifth of a second and followed immediately by point *P* presented for an equally brief time. Stereoacuity for sequentially presented targets is much poorer than for simultaneously presented targets, for example *F* and *P* both presented together for one-fifth of a second. This result means that the binocular system uses relative disparity to make the most precise judgements of relative depth. Relative disparity is defined as the difference between the absolute disparities of any pair of points; the relative disparity of points *F* and *P* is ($FL - FR$) − ($PL - PR$). Absolute disparity drives oculomotor convergence, but relative disparity is the basis of fine depth judgements.

Stereoacuity

The best thresholds for detecting a difference in disparity are less than 5 seconds of arc. At arm's length, this difference amounts to roughly 1/10 of a millimetre, showing the remarkable human ability to discern the surface relief of hand-held objects. Stereoacuity falls off more steeply with retinal eccentricity than visual acuity. It is also best near the fixation plane, falling off steeply with the distance from the horopter.

Random dot stereograms

It is now common practice to use images formed of randomly positioned points to test for stereopsis because the monocular cues to relative depth are almost completely obscured by the random positioning. Figure 4 shows a sparse random dot stereogram. Readers who can free-fuse these images by verging away from the picture plane will see a central cloud of dots hovering at a different depth from the surrounding dots which appear in the same plane as the square frame. Compare the monocular half-images of the random dot stereogram to the three bars of the stereogram shown in the centre of Fig. 3. Individuals lacking stereopsis could use the relative position of the black bars in either half-image of Fig. 3 to detect a change in depth. Of course, the points in the centre of the random dot stereogram are also in different relative locations in the two

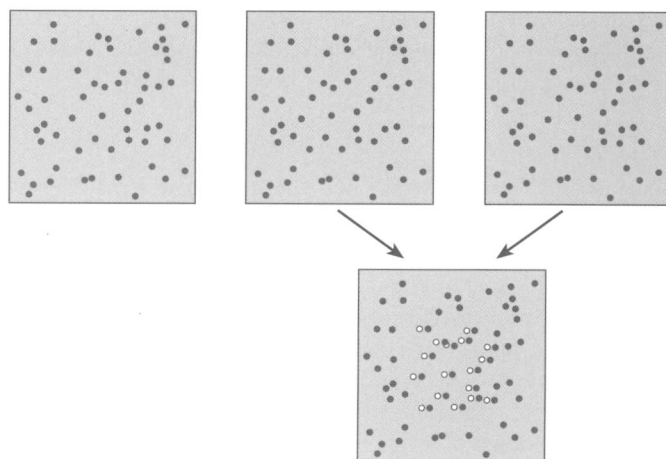

Fig. 4 A perceptual demonstration of a random dot stereogram. The upper row of squares can be fused by either converging or diverging the eyes. When fused, the central region of dots should appear at a different depth from the surrounding dots. The lower square in the right corner shows how a random dot stereogram is generated. One set of dots (shown for illustrative purposes as unfilled circles) is displaced with respect to the others, creating a relative disparity between different sets of dots when the squares are fused.

monocular half-images, but it is very hard to detect this shift by examining either half-image. A diagram showing the shift in the relative monocular location is presented in the box in the lower right corner of Fig. 4, where the position of the centre points in one half-image is shown by unfilled circles so that their relative disparity is obvious.

Further reading

Howard, I. and Rogers, B.J. (1995). *Binocular vision and stereopsis*. Oxford University Press, Oxford. [An outstanding text containing all available information on human binocular vision.]

Mansfield, J.S. and Legge, G.E. (1996). The binocular computation of visual direction. *Vision Research*, **36**, 27–41. [An excellent paper on the neural basis of binocular visual direction, containing a brief summary of previous theory, some recent experimental work, and a novel theoretical framework for this important issue.]

Ogle, K.N. (1950). *Researches in binocular vision*. Saunders, Philadelphia. [A classic text containing studies of the empirical horopter, fusion, stereoacuity, and vertical disparity.]

Schor, C.M. (1991). Binocular sensory disorders. In *Binocular vision*, (ed. D. Regan), pp. 179–223., Vol. 9 of *Vision and visual dysfunction* (general ed. J.R. Cronly-Dillon). CRC Press, Boston. [A very thoughtful compendium of abnormalities in binocular vision and their relation to normal binocularity.]

Shimojo, S. (1993). Development of interocular vision in infants. In *Early visual development, normal and abnormal*, (ed. K. Simons), pp. 201–23. Oxford University Press, New York. [A good summary of the development of binocular vision.]

Tyler, C.W. (1991). The horopter and binocular fusion. In *Binocular vision*, (ed. D. Regan), pp. 19–38, Vol. 9 of *Vision and visual dysfunction*, (general ed. J.R. Cronly-Dillon). CRC Press, Boston. [A clear, succinct description of the geometry of binocular vision and its relation to fusion.]

2.2.3 Introduction to childhood strabismus

Arvind Chandna and Rowena McNamara

Introduction

The importance of childhood strabismus and amblyopia is reflected in its prevalence. Approximately 5 per cent of the population has strabismus and/or amblyopia. Monocular visual loss due to amblyopia is the leading cause of visual impairment in childhood and has a higher prevalence than conditions such as glaucoma and diabetic retinopathy in the adult population (20–70 year age group).

The study of childhood strabismus provides an opportunity to obtain a fascinating insight into the developing visual system. Rapid developmental changes are taking place in sensory functions such as acuity, contrast sensitivity, stereopsis; motor aspects such as ocular alignment, smooth pursuit eye movements; anatomical changes in ocular growth and organization of the visual cortex. The time course of these changes has been defined as the critical or sensitive period and extends from birth to approximately 5 years with rapid development in the early months. It now appears that there is a great deal of interdependence for all these factors in order to come together as a mature visual system.

A disturbance in any one of the mechanisms during the critical period will have an effect on other aspects of visual development. It is not known whether there is an innate defect in the visual system where the system is not programmed for normal development or whether abnormal development of one or more visual functions leads to a disturbance in the entire visual system. It is possibly a combination of both. The visual system responds in different ways to these disturbances. The commonest clinical manifestation is strabismus. Another important feature is poor visual acuity or amblyopia in one or uncommonly in both eyes. Unequal visual input to the visual cortex results in a 'switching off' of the deviating eye and is called suppression. A refractive error may coexist leading to further difficulties for the developing visual system. Although the system is sensitive to such disturbances it also responds to treatment of the visual defect when detected within the critical period. Amblyopia responds to occlusion therapy, ocular alignment can be achieved by optical or surgical means, and occasionally suppression may be eliminated with restoration of binocularity.

The purpose of this chapter is to provide a structured introductory overview of the assessment of childhood strabismus. The approach outlined here refers mainly to practice in the United Kingdom which differs in certain points of detail from that used in the United States.

History

Listen carefully to the parents' version of events. A parent convinced that he or she has noticed a turn in the eye in the absence of an obvious squint at the time of examination suggests an intermittent squint. Family photographs are helpful in resolving the doubt in the examiner's mind. However, describing a squint in lateral gaze is more often associated with pseudostrabismus due to epicanthus.

Table 1 Key points in the history of a child with strabismus

Age of onset	*At birth* Esotropia – suggests central neurological insult Exotropia – suggests ocular pathology Vertical deviation – suggests neurology e.g. skew deviation *By 6 months – 1 year* Esotropia – early onset esotropia syndrome Exotropia – uncommon *By 18 months – 6 years* Intermittent esotropia – often accommodative Intermittent exotropia – distance type most common Vertical deviation – suggests neurology e.g. IV Nerve palsy
Mode of onset	Sudden – suggests neurological cause Intermittent – decompensation of a heterophoria at a particular time or fixation distance Constant – may be unilateral and indicate amblyopia Alternating – suggests equal in both eyes
Duration	Long-standing and unilateral – suggests dense amblyopia Recent and alternating – suggests equal vision
Associated symptoms and signs	Diplopia – child may shut one eye usually to compensate for diplopia or nystagmus Compensatory head posture Blurring and asthenopia – suggests refractive error or decompensating heterophoria Nystagmus – may be associated with manifest or latent strabismus; compensatory head posture Improved visual behaviour within the first 12 weeks – suggests delayed visual maturation
Previous treatment	Spectacles, occlusion, strabismus therapy, surgery, orthoptic exercises
Birth history	Problems during pregnancy, labour, prematurity, neonatal problems e.g. asphyxia
General health	Milestones, medications previous surgery, diagnosed syndromes
Family history	Strabismus in children varies between 30 and 70% in families with history of childhood squint

Table 1 summarizes the key points to be covered when taking the history for a child with strabismus.

Examination

The child should be watched throughout the consultation. The examination can be considered in terms of a number of components. These can be described as general observation, assessment of vision (Table 2), examination and measurement of the strabismus itself (Table 3), and assessment of sensory status in terms of binocular functions such as stereoacuity and fusion (Table 4). Where indicated, certain additional more specific tests may be appropriate (Table 5).

The examination findings should be recorded in an orderly and structured format. Figure 1 provides a suitable proforma for this information. Figure 2 illustrates the principles of cover tests, Fig. 3 the Bagolini striated glasses test, and Fig. 4 Worth's four dot test for sensory status.

Table 2 Examination: general observation and assessment of vision

Observation	Dysmorphic features
	Interocular size difference between the eyes
	Ptosis
	Epicanthic folds (pseudostrabismus)
	Compensatory head posture
Assessment of vision	*Visual acuity* assessed by method appropriate for age
	Observation of visual behaviour may be only method possible in very young and multiply handicapped children
	Qualitative assessment of vision
	Fixation and following of interest targets, location of small objects
	Optokinetic nystagmus
	Comparative behaviour when using monocular occlusion
	Quantitative assessment of vision
	Behavioural tests
	(infants and toddlers)
	Preferential looking e.g. Teller or Keeler
	Acuity cards
	Cardiff Acuity cards
	Recognition tests
	(older children and toddlers)
	Picture/Shape tests
	Kay picture test (uncrowded)
	Lea-Hyvärinen acuity test – (geometric progression)
	Optotype tests
	Sheridan Gardiner single letters (uncrowded)
	Sonksen-Silver acuity system – (crowded)
	Cambridge crowding cards
	LogMAR letters and chart – (geometric progression)
	B-VAT acuity tester – (screen display)

Table 3 Examination of the strabismus

Assessment of deviation	Cover–uncover test
	Alternate cover test at 33 cm; 6 m, noting fixation pattern in heterotropia, rate of recovery in heterophoria
Assessment of ocular movement	Versions
	Ductions
	Cardinal positions of gaze noting any A or V patterns
	Monocular occlusions/rotation to assess abduction
Measurement of deviation	*Methods*
	Hirschberg test
	Krimsky test/prism reflection test
	Prism and alternate cover test
	Simultaneous prism and cover test in microtropia
	Measure deviation for
	Distance: 6 m
	Near: 33 cm
	Up and downgaze: 6 m
	Right and left gaze: 6 m
	Tilting head to
	right and left: 6 m
	Analyse the strabismus by comparing measurements for
	Distance and near to determine abnormal accommodation and/or convergence
	Up and downgaze to assess A or V patterns
	Right and left gaze to look for incomitance
	Right and left head tilt for additional vertical deviations

Table 4 Examination of sensory status

Responses for the following tests should be obtained for distance (6 m) and near (33 cm) fixation with an appropriate target. Sensory tests are valuable in children presenting with latent strabismus, asthenopia symptoms, and microtropia. They have very little if any value in manifest strabismus.

Fusion	*Sensory*: presence or absence fusion
	Bagolini striated lenses: least dissociative therefore, ideal but obtaining reliable responses difficult in young children.
	Worth 4 dot test: most dissociative therefore, not ideal but obtaining responses easier in young children
	Motor: fusional amplitudes –
	(strength of fusion)
	measured by prisms in the presence of sensory fusion for
	Convergence: baseout:
	Divergence: base in:
	Upvergence: basedown:
	downvergence: baseup:
	Cyclovergence:
	Intorsion:
	Extortion:
Suppression	*Area*: measured by sequentially increasing strengths of prism in manifest strabismus including microtropia until diplopia appreciated
	Density: measured by sequentially increasing density of neutral filter (Sbiza bar) in front of deviating (suppressed eye) until fixation changes to fellow eye
	Area helpful in determine outcome of surgery with regards to possible postoperative diplopia
	Density helpful in planning occlusion therapy and determining outcome
Stereoacuity	*Near stereopsis test* (range in seconds of arc)
	Non-dissociative
	Frisby
	Lan
	Dissociative
	TNO
	RANDOT
	Wirt (Titmus Fly)
	Distance Stereopsis Test
	A/O Vectograph slides
	B-VAT Acuity tester

Note: children may have stereopsis for near and not for distance i.e. distance exotropia. These tests are not interchangeable and serial examination should be carried out using the same test.

Table 5 Additional tests

Major amblyoscope	Limited use in children because of responses required
	Limited use in strabismus because of possibility of simulating proximal convergence and getting false results
	Useful for measuring torsion and assessment of fusion and stereopsis
Near point of convergent/ accommodation	Useful in children with asthenopic symptoms
Accommodation convergence AC/A ratio	To assess whether the change in deviation between distance and near is due to abnormal accommodative effort
Diagnostic monocular occlusion	To assess maximum deviation under conditions of complete dissociation, i.e. to differentiate between distance, exotropia, and simulated distance exotropia
Binocular visual acuity (Bar reading)	To assess the strength of binocular single vision while reading a near target with moderate dissociation

(a) Visual acuity

	Right eye	Left eye	Method
With glasses			
Distance			
Near			
Without glasses			
Distance			
Near			

Spectacle prescription

Cover test

Cover/uncover

Alternate cover

Comments

Fixation pattern

	Grade	Percentage
Distance		
Near		

(Fixation pattern (FP) is assessed repeatedly for a detailed target in the distance and for near. FP may vary according to target size and motivation. Therefore, it is essential to standardize the target size and assessment of grade is repeated until at least 75% of responses are of a particular grade. For example; a grade 3 response must be obtained 3 out of 4 or 4 out of 5 times before a decision is made. The target size should be within acuity levels of the amblyopic eye.)

Grade 1: holds fixation from either eye even after a blink (true alternation)
Grade 2: switches fixation to preferred eye with a blink
Grade 3: switches fixation before a blink
Grade 4: switches fixation immediately

(b) Measurement of deviation

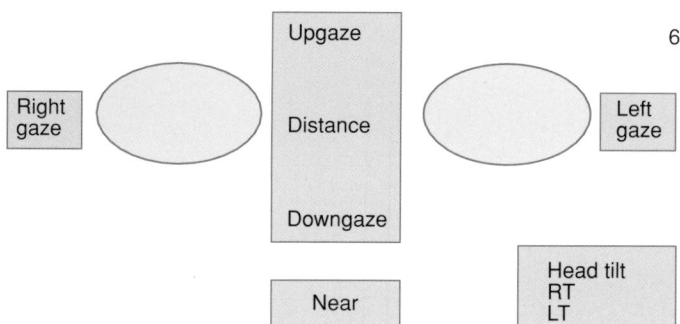

(c) Assessment of ocular movements

Underactions

The area of limited version is represented by a grid and comparison with duction indicated by a solid line. In this example the right eye shows an equally limited version and duction indicating a mechanical limitation due to a tight medial rectus as in entrapment with a medial wall blow out fracture. The left eye shows as a separate example the duction to be better than the version indicating a partial left lateral rectus palsy.

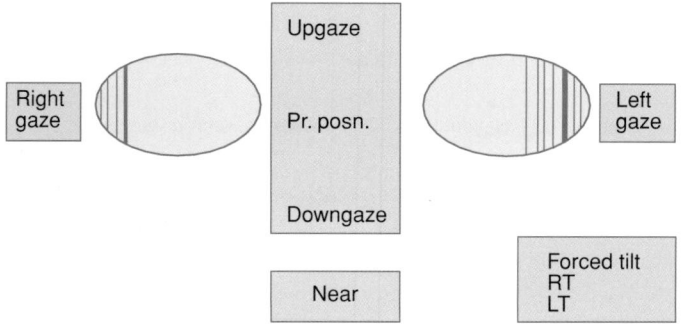

Overactions

Overactions are shown by arrows. The arrow begins at the point at which the overaction is evident and ends with the arrowhead indicating the extent of the overaction. In this example of a bilateral superior oblique palsy, overaction of the inferior oblique muscle in the right eye begins in the primary position with a manifest hypertropia with an increasing deviation as the right eye is brought into adduction where the right hypertropia is maximal.

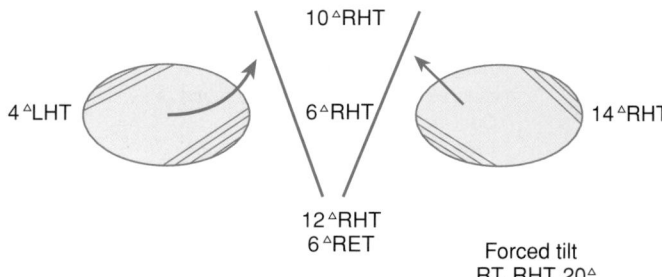

A similar representation is shown for the left eye but of a lesser degree indicating an asymmetrical bilateral superior oblique palsy. The resulting V-pattern esotropia is indicated in the centre with a continuous line.

(d) Other graphics

The examiner is free to add other graphics such as

for nystagmus

The arrows indicate direction and the amplitude. The circles indicate null point

6 RHT

Narrowing of the palpebral fissure

and for DVD

and torsion

(e) Assessment of sensory status

Bagolini striated lenses

Worth lights

Fusional amplitudes

	Break point	Recovery point	Method
Distance			
Base out (convergence)			
Base in (divergence)			
Base up (upvergence)			
Base down (downvergence)			
Near			
Base out (convergence)			
Base in (convergence)			
Base up (upvergence)			
Base down (downvergence)			

Stereopsis	Seconds of arc	Method

Comments:

Diagnosis

Management plan

Fig. 1 Examination of strabismus—a proforma for recording examination findings

(a) Cover–uncover test (for a manifest deviation)

On inspection an inward turn of the left eye is noted.
Using a pen-torch left corneal reflection is displaced temporally.

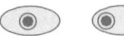

Cover the right eye. The left eye takes up fixation by moving outwards and the right eye is driven inwards under the cover.

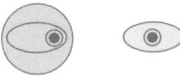

Uncover the right eye. The right eye may resume fixation indicating amblyopia and poor acuity in the left eye (A) or the left eye may continue fixation (even after a blink) indicating equal acuity in both eyes. Between A and B there may be other grades of fixation.

A   B

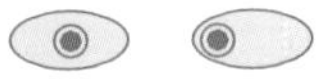

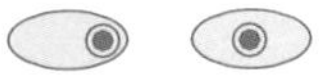

(b) Alternate cover test (for a latent deviation)

On inspection no manifest deviation is seen, corneal reflections are symmetrical.

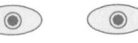

Cover one of the eyes. The other eye does not move but the eye under the cover moves e.g. inwards.

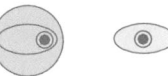

Place the cover over the other eye without an interval. Now the previously covered eye moves outwards to take up fixation and the eye now under cover turns inwards.

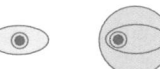

Repeat the alternate cover test and observe for the movements described above. On removing the cover both eyes resume fixation and no manifest deviation is observed. This diagnoses a latent deviation (esophoria in the example shown), the speed at which the eyes resume fixation on removal of the cover is the rate of recovery.

Fig. 2 Cover tests

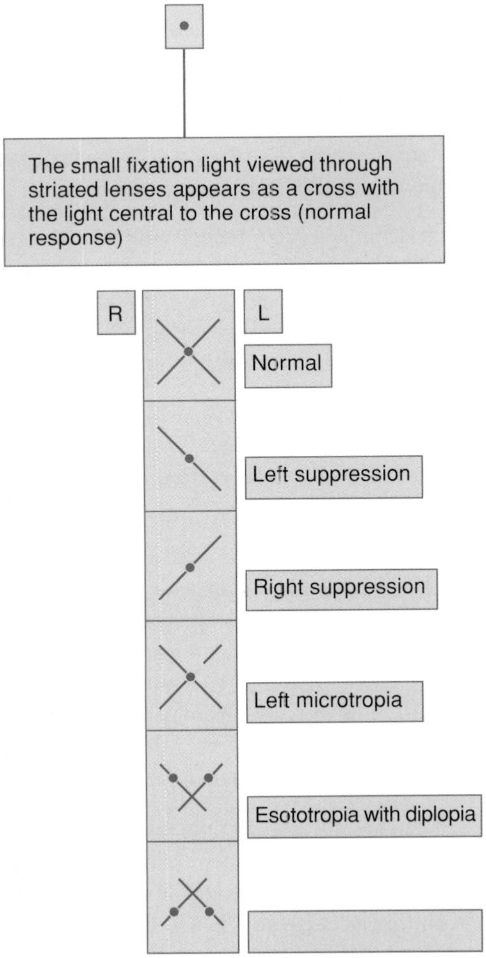

Fig. 3 Bagolini striated glasses test. The normal response is cross with the fixation light at the centre of the cross. In the presence of a manifest deviation the presence of cross indicates abnormal retinal correspondence. In suppression the child will describe a single line and the orientation will indicate the fixing eye. In microtropia a small gap will be described indicating foveal suppression. In a manifest deviation, if suppression is absent the child will report two lights and in the above example the lines will intersect below the lights in exotropia (crossed diplopia) and above the light in esotropia (uncrossed diplopia). (Modified from Pratt-Johnson and Tillson 1994.)

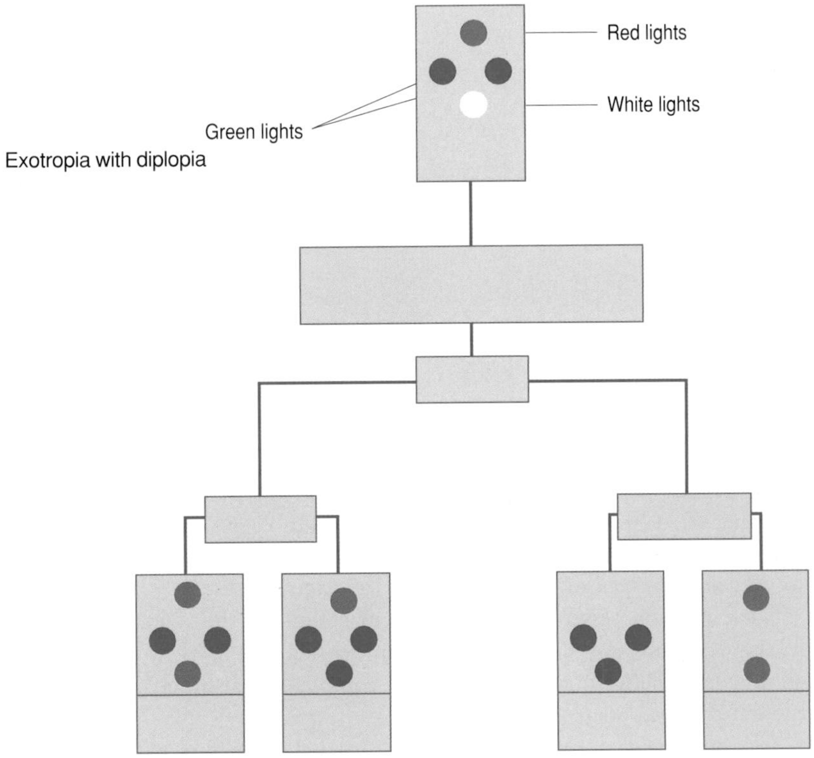

Fig. 4 Worth four dot test. The right eye (red glass) views the top red light and the left eye (green glass) views the two green lights. The dominant eye will see the white light in the corresponding colour (see normal response). In children with suppression of the right eye, the red light will not be seen; alternatively they will be unable to see the green light with left suppression. Five lights may be seen in children with heterophoria which has decompensated by wearing the complementary colours or in rare cases of pathological diplopia due to a sudden onset of strabismus. This is a dissociative test and the results may not represent normal viewing circumstances. However, the presence of fusion under such dissociative conditions indicates fusion under normal conditions but the converse is not true.

Further reading

Helveston, E.M. (1993). *Surgical management of strabismus. An atlas of strabismus surgery* (4th edn). Mosby, St Louis. A good account of considerations in strabismus before proceeding to surgery. Case reports discussed in detail are helpful for the surgeon.

Jampolsky, A.J. (1971). A simplified approach to strabismus diagnosis. In *Symposium on strabismus. Transactions of the New Orleans Academy of Ophthalmology*, pp. 34-92. Mosby, Saint Louis. A seminal thought-provoking paper, essential reading for every clinician dealing with strabismus.

Leigh, R.J. and Zee, D.S.(1991). *The neurology of eye movements* (2nd edn). F.A. Davis, Philadelphia. A timeless book on the control of eye movements and eye movement disorders.

Mein, J. and Trimble, R. (1991). *Diagnosis and management of ocular motility disorders* (2nd edn). Blackwell Scientific Publications, Oxford. A standard textbook in orthoptic practice in the United Kingdom. A useful textbook for general reading and understanding orthoptic examination of children with amblyopia and strabismus.

Pratt-Johnson, J.A .and Tillson, G. (1994). *Management of strabismus and amblyopia. A practical guide* (1st edn). Thieme Medical Publishers Inc., New York. A practical guide with details of methods and interpretation of tests in strabismus for the uninitiated. A good book for starting in strabismus.

Veronneau-Troutman, S. (1994). *Prisms in the medical and surgical management of strabismus* (1st edn). Mosby, St Louis. A detailed account of the principles of prisms and their use in the diagnosis and treatment of strabismus. A well written textbook with excellent illustrations.

van Noorden, G.K. (1995). *Binocular vision and ocular motility theory and management of strabismus* (4th edn). Mosby, St Louis. A comprehensive survey of strabismus with numerous references for further reading.

2.2.4 Sensory adaptations to strabismus

Richard Harrad

For primates, eyesight is the most important of the five senses for survival. Constant diplopia is a serious handicap and the developing visual system has a series of adaptations designed to prevent diplopia, often at some cost to vision.

Soon after the onset of a strabismus in childhood the vision in the deviating eye is suppressed. Suppression affects a part of the visual field but it may be nearly complete, sparing only the temporal monocular crescent.

In some patients remapping of the visual field of one eye takes place, such that under binocular viewing conditions noncorresponding points on the two retinas register an object in the same position in visual space. This is known as abnormal retinal correspondence.

Binocular fusion may be completely absent or substantially reduced in strabismus. (It is traditional to test for fusion using Worth's four dots and if present the fusion range is measured using base in and base out prisms of increasing strength.)

The extent to which binocular vision is degraded is related to the age of onset and the direction and extent of the strabismus. Very small angle esotropia (also known is microtropia or monofixation syndrome) is compatible with stereoacuity of 200 to 400 arc. With larger angles of esotropia, gross stereopsis may be present. In intermittent exotropia, stereoacuity is usually normal when the eyes are straight and in constant exotropia good stereoacuity may be achieved following surgical realignment.

Suppression

Clinical measurement of suppression

Measurement of suppression is most commonly carried out in patients who are suffering from diplopia or who are at risk of developing diplopia after surgery. Prisms are used to realign the visual axes prior to testing (postoperative diplopia test).

The following techniques are available for measuring suppression.

1. Bagolini glasses are plano glasses which have been scratched to produce diagonal striations. When the glasses are worn a bright line that passes through fixation is seen by each eye. If either line is interrupted suppression is present. This test has the advantage of not dissociating the two eyes.

2. Prims may be used to realign the visual axes and measure the range of ocular alignment within which suppression occurs in free space. Fresnel prisms may be applied to glasses to assess the effect of changing ocular alignment over a long period of time.

3. Suppression slides may be used in the synoptophore. This test is dissociative which is likely to mean that it is less accurate than a test carried out in free space.

4. The depth of suppression when present may be measured using a Spizer bar or neutral density filter bar. When placed over the fixing eye, the illumination is progressively reduced until diplopia occurs. Alternatively, the filters may be placed over the deviating eye in patients with diplopia and the density of filters required to abolish diplopia may be assessed. Banggarter developed a range of filters which may be applied to spectacles in order to facilitate suppression.

5. Where it is thought that diplopia may develop following surgery, ocular realignment may be achieved using botulinum toxin. The transient effect of toxin means that if diplopia does result it will be short lived.

Fortunately patients who have intractable diplopia are rare, but the most common group are those patients who initially had an esotropia and have developed diplopia either following surgery or over the course of time. In some cases the patient may have to decide between an unsightly squint and single vision or straight eyes and diplopia. Neuroplasticity in the visual system is thought to cease after 7 years. However, temporary loss of vision in one eye may lead to loss of binocular function in older children and younger adults and prolonged monocular cataract may lead to intractable diplopia in some cases. Conversely, some patients seem to be capable of suppressing diplopia even when it begins in adult life.

Area of suppression

Where there is a large misalignment between the two eyes that is beyond the scope of any facilitatory interaction such as in alternately fixating strabismic patients the entire visual input of one eye may be suppressed. With smaller angles of strabismus the area is smaller. It has been suggested that the fovea of the deviating eye is suppressed 'in order to prevent diplopia' but a more physiological explanation of central suppression is that selective suppression of fine detail represented by small ganglion cell receptive fields occurs. This allows fusion of the rest of the scene (peripheral fusion) represented predominantly by large ganglion cell receptive fields.

In exotropia some authors maintain that there is suppression of the area of overlap of the visual fields of the two eyes, others have suggested that there is remapping of the retinotopic organization of the deviated eye.

Depth of suppression

Holopigian et al. found that the strength of suppression was inversely proportional to the depth of amblyopia suggesting that profound amblyopia obviates the need for interocular suppression. Another interpretation of their data is that the depth of suppression varies with the type of amblyopia: anisometropic amblyopes suppressing weakly, strabismics suppressing more strongly, and alternate fixators suppressing the most powerfully of all.

Anisometropic amblyopes are able to make use of residual binocular interactions to bring about suppression which then need not be more powerful than that seen in binocular rivalry in normal subjects, of the order of 0.15 to 0.2 log units. Similarly in small angle strabismus some binocular interactions persist. However, in strabismus with alternate fixation the normal binocular interactions can no longer be used and a functionally different type of powerful suppression comes into play.

When the angle of strabismus changes either spontaneously or as a result of surgery, suppression may be broken down leading to diplopia. For many years it has been recognized that a change in the angle of the strabismus from an esotropic to an exotropic position or vice versa is likely to lead to loss of suppression. Schor measured suppression in a group of small angled esotropes and exotropes and found that suppression occurred only for uncrossed disparity in esotropes and crossed disparity in exotropes. He proposed that suppression depended upon whether an object subtended crossed or uncrossed disparities at the retina rather than an area of retina being suppressed. Jampolsky and Schor have found that it is stimuli of similar orientation that lead to suppression in strabismus whilst stimuli of different orientation provoke rivalry and in normal subjects and lead to diplopia.

Physiology of suppression

The psychophysical literature on the subject of suppression is apparently confusing but if it is accepted that several mechanisms are operating, that confusion may be resolved.

In anisometropic amblyopia and small angle strabismus, dichoptic masking, fusional suppression, or disparity-dependent suppression are operating.

In large angled strabismus suppression is probably a form of binocular rivalry suppression. Suppression of cellular activity has been found in primary visual cortex when dissimilar stimuli are independently presented to the two eyes in strabismic cats; it seems likely that this suppression is based upon inhibitory interaction between neighbouring ocular dominance columns.

Abnormal retinal correspondence

When the lower vertebrates move their eyes independently, the presumed visual direction of each eye is computed in order to assign an object a position in space. It is suggested that this primitive system comes into play when the onset of strabismus causes the failure of the fusion mechanism. This use of the two eyes as two independent detectors is known as utrocular vision. Abnormal retinal correspondence does not impair accurate spatial localization, since despite the strabismus, the eyes are yoked (Hering's law) and eye position may be deduced from the motor discharge. If positional disparities are introduced between the eyes in cats by means of prism and lenses, these changes can be completely compensated for by changes in binocular neurones. It is thought that changes such as these underlie the process of abnormal retinal correspondence in humans. Enlargement of Panum's fusional area to accommodate disparities equal to the angle of strabismus allows fusion to maintain single vision. The presence of squint does not upset the judgement of relative disparities (otherwise the fluctuating state of convergence would lead to fluctuating depth in the visual world).

Stereoanomalies

Since stereopsis is possible off the horopter, a small angle strabismus is compatible with stereopsis at low spatial frequencies while binocular cells tuned to high spatial frequencies have been lost. Such a person would show abnormal retinal correspondence at high spatial frequency and normal fusion at low spatial frequency. Static depth discrimination sensitivity is limited by crowding effects at high spatial frequency in strabismus. Dynamic stereopsis is similarly limited by crowding effects in strabismus; Sireteanu has found that although stereomotion may be lost in the centre of the visual field in strabismus, it may still be retained in the periphery.

Stereovision with reduced stereoacuity is the norm in anisometropic amblyopia and small angle strabismus.

Further reading

Harrad, R.A. (1996). Psychophysics of suppression. *Eye*, **10**, 270–3.

Harrad, R.A., Sengpiel, F., and Blakemore, C. (1996). Physiology of suppression in strabismic amblyopia. *British Journal of Ophthalmology*, **80**, 373–7.

Holopigian, K., Blake, R., and Greenwald, M.J. (1988). Clinical suppression and amblyopia. *Investigative Ophthalmology and Visual Science*, **29**, 444–51.

Schor, C. (1991). Binocular sensory disorders. In *Vision and visual dysfunction* (ed. J.R. Cronly-Dillon), Volume 9, pp. 179–223. Macmillan, London.

Sengpiel, F., Blakemore, C., Kind, P.C., and Harrad, R.A. (1994). Interocular suppression in the visual cortex of strabismic cats. *Journal of Neuroscience*, **14**, 688–71.

Sireteanu, R. and Fronius, M. (1981). Naso-temporal asymmetries in human amblyopia: consequence of long-term interocular suppression. *Vision Research*, **21**, 1055–63.

von Graefe, A. (1896). *Das Sehen der Schielendedn. Eine ophthalmologisch-physiologische Studie*. Wiesbaden.

2.2.5 Strabismus

Eugene M. Helveston

Definition and description

Strabismus is a misalignment of the visual axes where the object of regard falls on the fovea of one eye called the fixing eye and on an extra foveal area of the other eye called the deviating eye. When the object of regard falls on the fovea of each eye simultaneously manifest strabismus is not present. This absence of strabismus results in parallel visual axes when the eyes are fixating at infinity (6 m and beyond) and convergent visual axes when the eyes are fixating nearer objects. Strabismus is usually described by one or more of its characteristics as follows:

1. According to direction

Eso – deviating inward – convergence
Exo – deviating outward – divergence
Hyper (hypo) – deviating vertically either upward (or downward)
Cyclo – deviated in a torsional or wheel-like way around the pupil axis (Y axis) (There is no typical external appearance for cyclotropia. The diagnosis is made either from reports by the patient of a cyclodiplopia (subjective) or after testing with a projection screen or a double Maddox rod (objective). Torsion of the fundus can be determined with the indirect ophthalmoscope. Patients with torsional diplopia often assume a head tilt to achieve fusion (Fig. 1).)

2. According to when the strabismus is present

Tropia – a constant deviation
Intermittent – a deviation which is sometimes present and sometimes not

Phoria – a latent deviation. This deviation occurs only when the eyes are dissociated. The eyes return to normal alignment when the dissociation ends.

3. According to time of onset

Congenital – born with the strabismus or with the tendency to develop the strabismus later at a certain time during maturation.
Acquired – developing after birth from an event occurring after birth.

4. According to sameness of the deviation

Comitant – size of deviation is the same in all directions of gaze
Incomitant – size of deviation different in different directions of gaze

5. According to mechanics

Restricted ductions (confirmed by positive passive duction testing)
'Overaction' of a muscle (overaction of a muscle in the field of action of the muscle may be an inaccurate description of either 'under checking' or a muscle acting slightly out of its usual field, especially the oblique muscles)
Free ductions (either spontaneous or confirmed by finding unrestricted passive ductions in a case of paresis)

Restricted passive ductions are always caused by a physical restriction. They can also coexist with a long-standing paresis.

6. According to preference for fixation

Alternation – the patient uses either eye for fixation without preference (amblyopia is not present with free alternation)
Preferred fixation with one eye – amblyopia or some other reason for reduced vision is inferred in the non-preferred eye. The depth of amblypopia is related to the degree of preference. Fusion – the patient uses the two eyes together producing a solitary image out of the separate input from the two eyes. This is called 'motor fusion'. The fused images may be enhanced by unique perception of the combined images seen by the two eyes which are actually seeing a slightly different view of the same object because they are separated by a distance of approximately 6 cm (the normal interpupillary distance). Combining these slightly different views which are disparate images is the basis for stereopsis, which is the fusion of objects falling on disparate retinal areas but within Panum's fusional space and producing stereoscopic depth perception. Stereopsis is the key factor in 'sensory fusion'.

The characteristics listed above provide the basis for what could be called the 'signature' of the strabismus. For example; a 4-year-old boy has a congenital (tendency for the strabismus present at birth) esotropia (a constant in-turning) with a 'V' pattern (incomitance) overaction of the inferior obliques (muscle overaction in their field of action), and

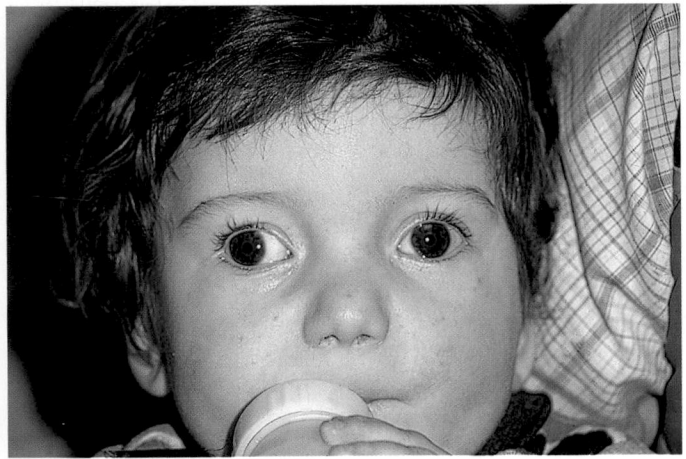

(a)

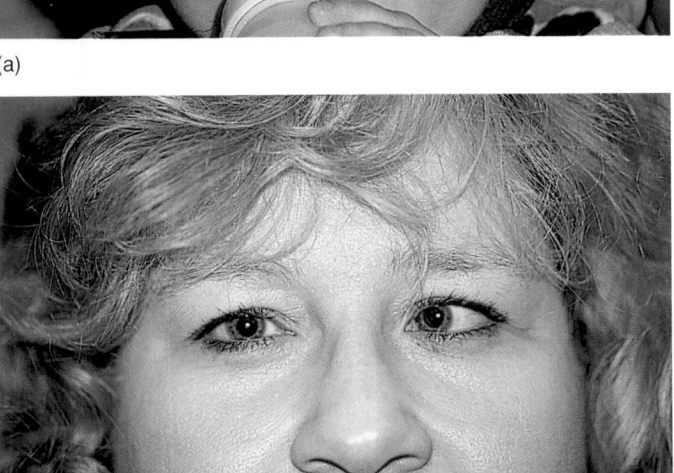

(b)

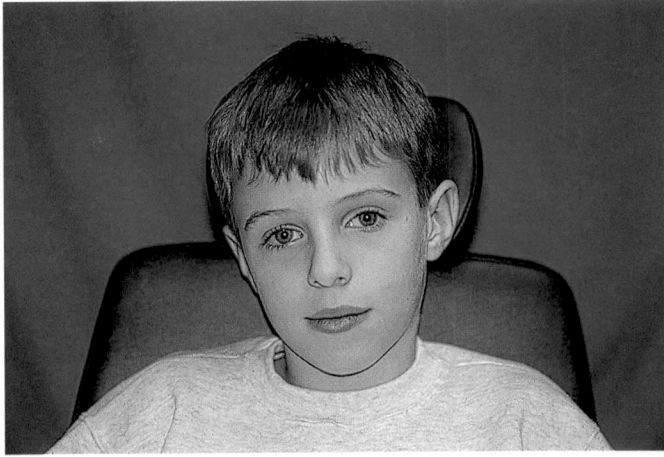

(d)

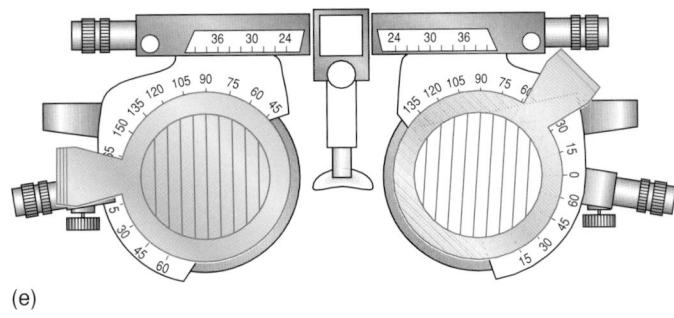

(e)

Fig. 1 (a) Three-year-old boy with right exotropia. (b) Thirty-five-year old woman with left exotropia. (c) Twelve-year-old boy with left hypertropia. (d) Torsional strabismus usually presents with a head tilt. (e) Tortional diplopia is measured with a test such as the double Maddox rod.

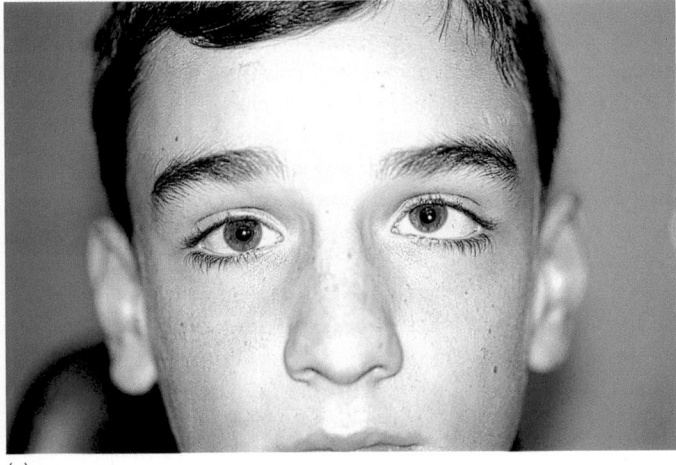

(c)

preference for fixation with the right eye (amblyopia of the left eye).

Any type of strabismus can be described by listing the several characteristics found in the patient. Some strabismus signatures are more complicated than others.

Initial approach to the strabismus problem

The deductive process

The diagnosis of strabismus can be accomplished using one or more of several techniques depending on the examiner's experience and personal preference. Two techniques will be described here. The first is called the 'gestalt' approach. With this technique, the strabismus patient is observed in a casual setting – often while obtaining the history from the patient or parent. The patient is evaluated by simply observing the patient and his/her strabismus as a whole picture. The preliminary diagnosis arises from the total picture or 'gestalt'. This method is used consciously or unconsciously in most cases by the experienced strabismologist. For the experienced strabismologist this method is a fast and accurate way to make a qualitative diagnosis. In a few instances of complex or rare vertical strabismus, an inferior oblique palsy, for example, the experienced strabismologist will arrive at a tentative diagnosis after observation knowing only that a vertically acting muscle is paretic. In such a case, a more didactic or inductive approach is required to identify the paretic muscle.

After labelling the strabismus, or establishing the 'gestalt', the 'traditional' strabismus work-up is used to quantify it. This both confirms the observation 'gestalt' diagnosis and establishes the size of the deviation or the 'quantitative' factor. This quantitative part of the testing starts with a series of questions dealing with the patient's symptoms, and past medical and family history, part of which may have been covered during observation, and continues with a series of measurements.

Work-up of the strabismus patient

History

(1) Onset of the strabismus

(2) Family history for strabismus – or other significant diseases including malignant hyperthermia associated with general anaesthesia

(3) Birthweight – growth and development (for infants and children)

(4) Symptoms experienced by the patient (diplopia, asthenopia, etc.)

(5) Prior surgery and/or orthoptic treatment

(6) Present glasses (bifocal – prism – contact lenses)

Examination

(1) Visual acuity distance and near with and without correction

(2) Prism and cover testing: (a) cover/uncover test for latent deviation – (phoria), (b) alternate prism and cover for maximum deviation – (tropia), and intermittent strabismus – (c) simultaneous prism and cover for deviation in casual seeing. Alternate prism/cover testing is done with and without spectacle correction in the primary position and in the diagnostic positions of gaze. Testing is also done with head tilted to either side (Bielschowsky) in patients with vertical strabismus.

(3) Ductions or monocular movements of each eye

(4) Versions (screen comitance) – this is the binocular movement of the eyes comparing the action of yoked muscles, looking for over- or under-action

(5) Stereoacuity

(6) Worth four lights test if the stereoacuity test is failed and in younger patients with aligned or nearly aligned eyes.

(7) Torsion as measured with the projection screen, double Maddox rod, or the Awaya torsion test – in appropriate cases

(8) Head posture and facial symmetry is noted as part of the external examination including comment on epicanthal folds, ptosis, intercanthal distance, etc.

(9) Fusional amplitudes measured with a haploscope or with prism in free space in cases where the eyes are or have been aligned and in the presence of asthenopia.

(10) Refraction – manifest initially especially in myopic and cycloplegic patients, especially important with refractive esodeviations. Cycloplegia is achieved with cyclopentolate, 0.5 per cent under 1 year and 1 per cent over 1 year. One or two drops in each eye 3 to 5 min apart are sufficient in most cases. Repeat doses of cyclopentolate or use of atropine 0.5 per cent or 1 per cent drops usually given at home for 2 days before the examination may be required in heavily pigmented eyes.

(11) Ocular examination – anterior segment (biomicroscope), media, and fundus (indirect ophthalmoscope)

A preprinted sheet can be very useful for compiling data, but it should be understood that in most instances this type of 'shorthand' is useful only for the individual who designed the form and uses it on a regular basis, being confusing and bordering on incomprehensible to those unfamiliar with the form. Having another strabismologist's data sheet thrust in front of you with all sorts of information that is useful only to the person who gathered it can be frustrating even for the experienced examiner. A generic data collection form is shown below (Fig. 2).

The less experienced examiner encountering a strabismus patient may take a slightly different approach to that of the experienced examiner. The less experienced examiner first gathers a set of historical facts and then obtains a set of strabismus measurements. After this the history and measurements are analysed, enabling the examiner to arrive at a diagnosis by means of a 'best fit' approach. Some examples of the gestalt and the inductive methods will be shown.

The infant illustrated in Fig. 3 sitting on the parent's lap appears to be 6 months old and has obviously crossed eyes. The child appears otherwise normal, a fact that is quickly confirmed by the parent. To the experienced examiner this patient has congenital esotropia. The experienced examiner anticipates that this infant will have physical characteristics and sensory findings appropriate for the diagnosis, and that the patient will require a specific course of action. To confirm the 'gestalt' diagnosis, the examiner gently turns the infant's head from side to side in a 'doll's head' or oculocephalic manoeuvre confirming full abduction and ruling out the first of two possible but rarer causes of infantile esotropia, sixth nerve palsy, and Duane syndrome, a type of sixth nerve palsy. A cycloplegic refraction of +3.00 dioptres or less rules out the second cause of esotropia in the infant and young child, refractive esotropia (+3.00 dioptres is an arbitrary figure which deals with probability. If an esotropic infant has hyperopia of +3.00 dioptres or more this correction is prescribed. Some children treated originally as non-refractive esotropia may require hyperopic correction

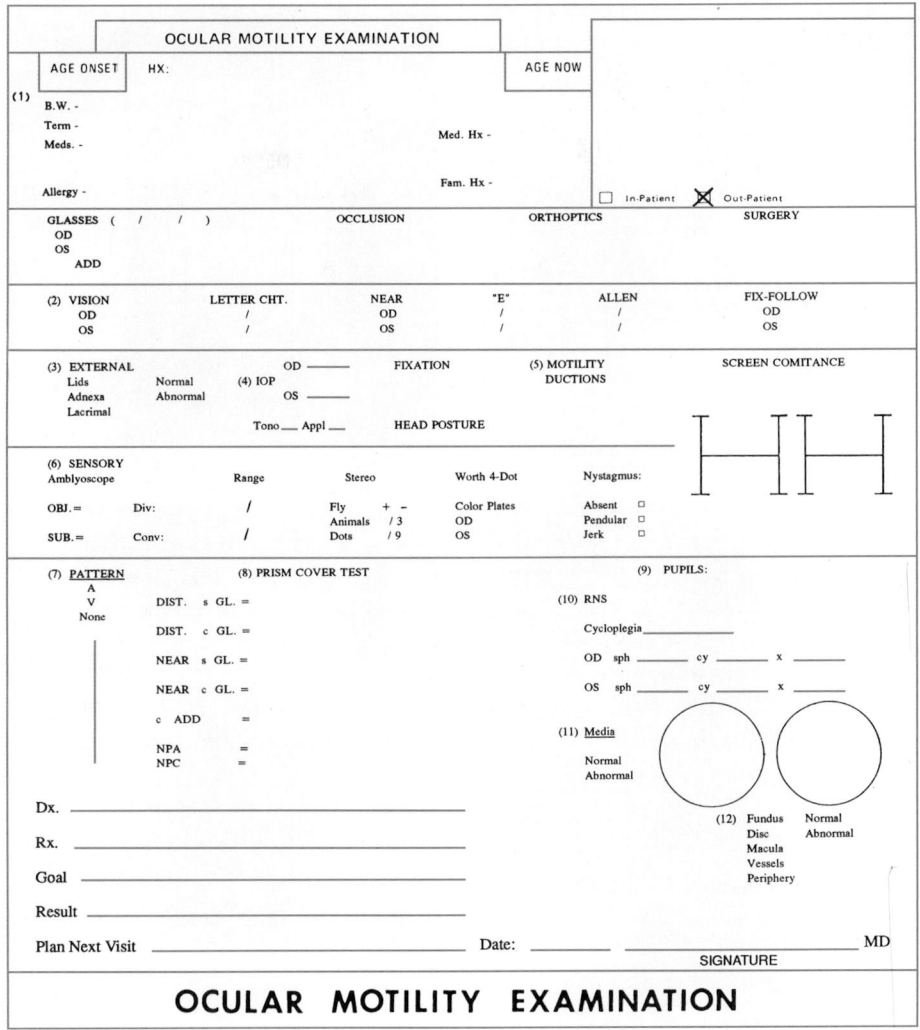

Fig. 2 A form such as this can be used to record data from an examination of ocular motility.

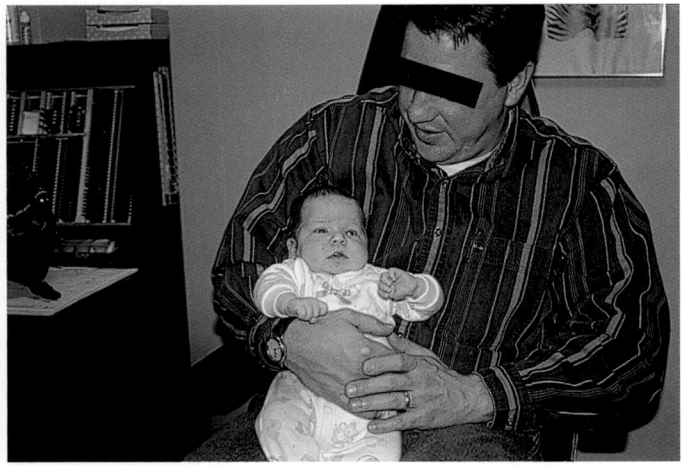

Fig. 3 This 1-month-old presents with the 'gestalt' of congenital exotropia. Further evaluation suggested a diagnosis of class I Duane syndrome, left eye.

for a refractive component with hyperopia less than, or which later increases to, +3.00 dioptres or more.) Moebius syndrome, a rare combination of congenital sixth and seventh nerve palsy is characterized by flat facial expression with absence of nasolabial folds and atrophy of the distal one-third of the tongue, causing feeding difficulty. The diagnosis is made in most cases by simply observing this dull facial expression in an esotropic infant, certainly not present in our example.

In another example, a 40-year-old male patient presents with a left head tilt and chin depression as illustrated in Fig. 4. The examiner observes the left head tilt and chin depression in a relaxed state as the patient begins telling his story to the doctor. It is important at this time to observe the patient while he/she is at ease and not 'on guard'. A tendency to assume an anomalous head posture, in nearly every case, will be accentuated in the relaxed state making the abnormal posture and its diagnostic clues more obvious. The patient shown (Fig. 4(a)) has a right superior oblique palsy based on the head posture and this is the diagnosis or in computer language the 'default' until ruled out. Furthermore, the palsy in this case is, in all likeli-

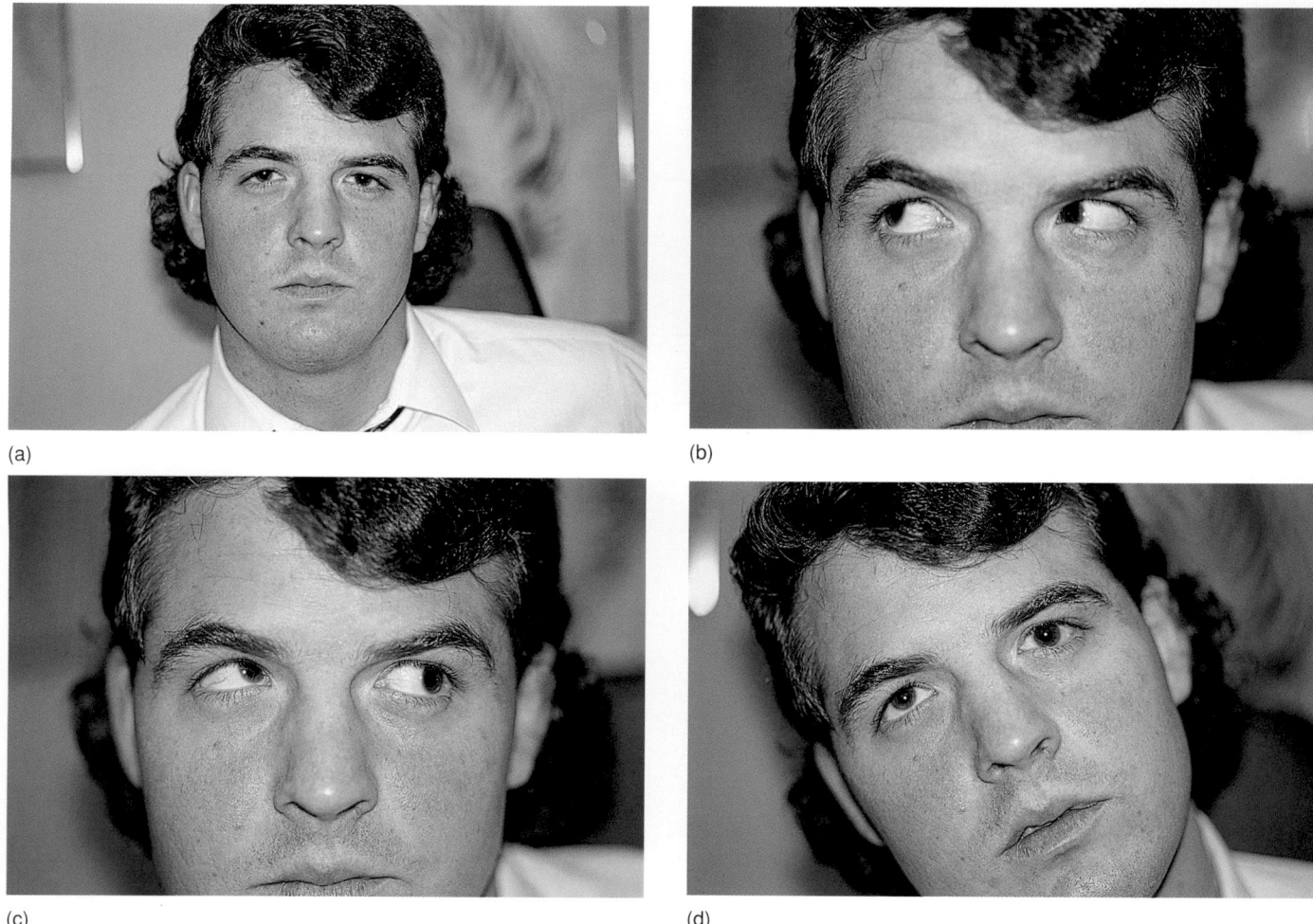

(a)

(b)

(c)

(d)

Fig. 4 (a) Left head tilt and chin depression typical in a patient with right superior oblique palsy. (b) Small right hypertropia in right gaze. (c) Large right hypertropia, overaction of the right inferior oblique in left gaze. (d) Increased right hypertropia, positive Bielschowsky test in right head tilt. These findings combine to confirm the diagnosis of right superior oblique palsy.

hood, congenital, because when the head is straightened the patient has a fuller face on the right while the left face is smaller with an almost pinched expression. The diagnosis is confirmed as the motility examination is begun by noting a larger right hypertropia on left gaze and an increasing right hypertropia on right head tilt (the Bielschowsky head tilt test). Prism and cover testing in the diagnostic positions combined with testing with the double Maddox rod provides quantitative information useful in design of the surgical procedure. The diagnosis was therefore suspected with a high degree of probability, based on the patient's appearance and well before measurements were taken.

If instead of using the observation or 'gestalt' method, the inductive technique is used, the process of work-up proceeds exactly in the reverse. A patient presents with a strabismus problem, the measurements are done carefully, and a 'best fit' is established. The patient in Fig. 4(b) has a definite head tilt which was subsequently determined to be caused by a right superior oblique weakness. The practitioner who must resort to this technique in anything but a learning situation or in the

rare case such as that presented by, for example, an inferior oblique palsy would find the practice of strabismus very trying indeed.

The techniques of measurement for the strabismus patient

Visual acuity

Visual acuity should be measured at distance and at near with and without correction, using the highest grade, most demanding, and therefore most accurate test (visual demand) suitable for the patient, progressing more or less as described below.

Fixation and following of interesting objects

This is used for infants and the preliterate child and includes testing with the optokinetic drum or tape in horizontal and vertical directions. In the normal infant an OKN drum should elicit a slow following movement followed by rapid refixation. Forced choice preferential looking (FPL) tests an infant's preference to fixate a square wave grating rather than a homogenous target of equal luminance. The FPL test has some value as a research tool and for quantifying the depth of amblyopia in an infant, especially in following up treatment.

If during the examination a very young infant keeps the lids shut, turn off the lights. In nearly every case the eyes will open and in most cases even with dim illumination in the room a satisfactory evaluation of vision can be accomplished. Rotating an infant from side to side should produce a few beats of post-rotary nystagmus. Prolonged nystagmus is a poor prognostic sign for vision.

Pictures simulating Snellen optotypes

This test is suitable for children who do not know their letters. A variety of picture charts are suitable for testing preliterate children but they are more useful for comparing visual acuity between the eyes than determining absolute values for visual acuity. No pictures are universally culturally ideal and none is as sensitive as Snellen optotypes.

Snellen optotypes

Snellen letters are the 'gold standard' for vision testing. For research purposes spacing of the optotypes has been shown to be critical but for the usual clinical setting, separation of optotypes is not critical. In the clinical setting a computer generated array with random presentation of optotypes speeds and adds confidence to vision testing.

When amblyopia is suspected, threshold vision should be determined with a full line of optotypes and then repeated using single optotypes to determine the effect of the crowding phenomenon. Patients with amblyopia have visual acuity one or more lines better using single optotypes compared with a full line. Amblyopes also accurately identify the first and last optotypes in a full line when testing at threshold while missing optotypes in the middle, also because of crowding. In the United Kingdom Sheridan Gardiner 'singles' are routinely used to assess Snellen equivalent acuity in an uncrowded situation. In cases with latent nystagmus, the non-tested eye can be fogged with a high plus lens to allow testing of the non-fogged eye which may have no or reduced nystagmus. It is important to check vision in patients who have latent nystagmus with both of their eyes open in order to obtain accurate measurement of binocular vision, a test which tells how the patient will function in ordinary situations. Test of near vision is done with text or optotypes reduced for 36 cm. Nearpoint of accommodation may also be tested at this time.

Versions

Versions are a test of binocular pursuit in the principal field of action of the yoked muscles. This is also called the screen comitance test. The patient is asked to follow a slow moving target in what are called the diagnostic positions of gaze. Movement of the eyes in these positions demonstrates the relative action of yoked muscles. The action of the muscles can be recorded in a diagram as shown in Fig. 5.

The screen comitance test recorded on the form illustrated in Fig. 5 provides a graphic representation of over- and under-

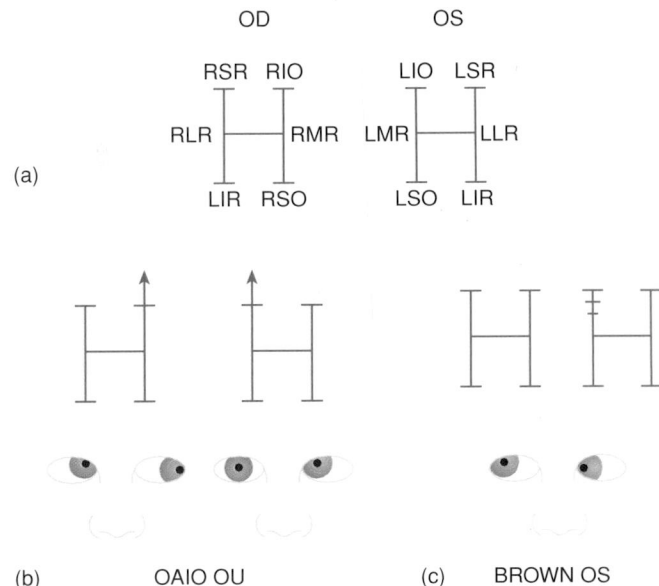

Fig. 5 (a) The actions of the extraocular muscles individually and yoked. (b) Diagram of bilateral overaction of the inferior oblique muscles. (c) Diagram of left Brown syndrome.

action of the paired extraocular muscles. Comparison of the yoked muscles is a more sensitive test for identifying over- or under-action of a muscle even if subtle.

Ductions

Ductions are monocular movements normally tested in four directions, abductions, adduction, elevation, and depression. A deficiency of a duction suggests a more profound defect of ocular movement. Measurement of the deviation is done with prism and cover testing or with the light reflex test with or without prism.

Observation of the corneal light reflex produced by a point source of light held approximately 1 m in front of the patient at the patient's eye level allows estimation of the direction and angle of strabismus. For each millimetre of decentration of the corneal light reflex of the non-fixating (deviated) eye, approximately 15 prism dioptres of strabismus is recorded. Since the average corneal diameter is approximately 12 mm, a light reflex appearing halfway between the centre of the pupil and the limbus is 3 mm displaced representing 45 prism dioptres of strabismus. A light reflex at the limbus is 6 mm displaced and represents approximately 90 prism dioptres of strabismus. This estimation of the deviation is called the Hirschberg test.

The prism light reflex test of Krimsky is a variation of the above test. With the Krimsky test a correcting prism is placed before the fixing eye; that is, the eye with the reflex centred in the pupil. The amount and orientation of prism that must be placed before the fixing eye to centre the light reflex passively in the formerly deviated eye is the Krimsky measure of the deviation.

The Hirschberg test is useful in very young infants, in patients with paretic or paralysed muscles, or in otherwise unco-operative patients. The Krimsky test is useful in patients who have difficulty in taking up fixation with the deviated eye because of poor vision in that eye from any other cause. If movement is restricted in the deviated eye, the prism is held before the deviated eye in the Krimsky test.

The alternating prism and cover test

The prism and cover test employs two basic examination tools: the hand-held prism and the occluding cover or paddle. The prism and the cover are used together to neutralize movement in the misaligned eyes while the eye(s) fixate a specific target in the distance or at near in the primary position and also in various directions of gaze. The simplest prism and cover measurement is done by first placing a prism before each eye with the prism power estimated to be that needed to neutralize the deviation and then alternately covering the two eyes while increasing or decreasing prism power until movement of the eyes either stops, is slightly reversed in direction, or results in an equal movement away from and then toward the apex of the prism. This test may require the examiner to select several prisms of different power until the correct one, the prism that neutralizes the movement of the eyes, is found. The alternate prism and cover test measures the maximum deviation and does not separate a tropia or manifest deviation from a phoria or latent deviation.

The cover – uncover test

A phoria is measured by covering and then uncovering one eye, noting both the direction and amplitude of the re-fixation movement. The eye is then re-covered and a prism estimated to be the power needed to neutralize the movement previously observed is placed behind the cover. The eye is then uncovered. When prism power has been selected sufficient to eliminate movement when the cover is removed, the size and direction of the phoria has been established.

The simultaneous prism and cover test

Some deviations increase in size during dissociation with the alternate cover test. In order to measure the manifest deviation present during casual seeing (the minimum deviation) as opposed to that deviation which can be built up by prolonged alternate cover testing (the maximum deviation), the simultaneous prism and cover test is used. With this test, the examiner determines which eye the patient is using for fixation. The examiner then simultaneously covers the fixing eye with an occluder and places a prism of the estimated size and direction before the deviated eye to anticipate and eliminate the need for refixation. With the simultaneous prism and cover test it may be necessary to select several prisms on a trial-and-error basis until the deviation is neutralized.

Of all these tests, the alternate prism and cover test is the most important for deciding how much surgery is required. The findings from this test are the objective data most commonly used to determine how many millimetres the extraocular muscles must be recessed, resected, or shifted to restore alignment. On the other hand, the simultaneous prism and cover test may be the one most important in deciding whether or not to carry out surgery. A non-symptomatic patient with only a 5 prism dioptre deviation on the prism and cover test but a 25 prism dioptre deviation on the alternate prism and cover test may not need surgery because his/her appearance will be acceptable and the patient is comfortable. However, if the patient is symptomatic, complaining of asthenopia, and surgery is carried out, it would be more likely that the surgery will be carried out with more consideration for the 25 prism dioptre deviation found with alternate prism and cover test than the five prism dioptre deviation found with the simultaneous prism and cover test.

Other tests

A cycloplegic refraction is carried out in all patients with strabismus or suspected of having strabismus using 0.5 per cent cyclopentolate, one drop in each eye for children under 1 year and 1 per cent cyclopentolate, one drop in each eye for children over 1 year. When atropine is selected for cycloplegia, drops are given, starting 2 days before the examination. One drop is given in one eye in the morning and in the other eye in the evening for 2 days before the examination; one drop is then given in each eye on the morning of the examination for a total of three drops in each eye. Parents are cautioned to use only one drop at each instillation and to use pressure over the punctum for a few seconds after giving the drop to avoid systemic absorption of the atropine. They must be warned that the drops should be stopped and the physician consulted immediately if the child becomes flushed, agitated, and febrile.

The Worth four light test

This test determined the presence or absence of peripheral fusion, gives an estimation of the size of the scotoma, and, when strabismus is present, confirms fixation preference for one eye or the other or demonstrates anomalous retinal correspondence. To perform this test, the patient wears glasses with one green and one red lens while viewing a flashlight with four small spots of light: two green, one red, and one white. Seeing two green and two red lights with aligned eyes means that fusion is present. The size of the target lights on the face of the flashlight and the distance that the flashlight is held from the patient determine the size of the retinal image. This variation also enables estimation of the size of the scotoma if present. The farther away the flashlight is from the eyes, i.e. the smaller the retinal area stimulated, the more central the fusion or smaller the scotoma, and vice versa. When the patient sees three green lights it means that the eye behind the green lens is preferred. If the patient sees two red lights it means that the eye behind the red lens is preferred. If the patient sees five lights there is diplopia. If the patient sees four lights with manifest strabismus, anomalous retinal correspondence is present.

The Bagolini test

The Bagolini test is done by placing two lenses with microstriations producing a Maddox rod effect at 90° before the patient's eyes while he or she views a point source of light. This test provides information about sensory behaviours in the non- or minimally-dissociated state. With normal binocular vision patients will see two complete streaks of light crossing at the point light source. Strabismic patients also see a cross but often with a segment missing at the centre of the line seen by the deviating eye. In strabismic patients this visual response is interpreted as harmonious anomalous retinal correspondence with a relative scotoma of the deviating eye. Diplopia is rarely seen with this test.

Translucent occluders

Spielmann described translucent occluders which dissociate eyes while allowing a full view of motility for the examiner. These occluders may be used over one or both eyes. They are an important tool for the study of dissociated phenomena, including dissociated vertical deviation (DVD) and dissociated horizontal deviation (DHD) and for planning of surgery for these patients.

Stereo testing

The stereoacuity test utilizing polarized lenses and polarized targets may be done quickly and accurately in the clinical setting. The ability to see the stereo offset targets as a single object in three dimensions means that fusion of disparate objects is occurring within Panum's fusional space. This polarized viewing of two real displaced polarized images has been called local stereopsis. If the target is seen flat, it means that suppression is present in one eye and that the patient lacks stereopsis, at least on that test. A more sensitive test for stereopsis is done with the random dot test of Julesz. This test has no 'real picture' which could be seen without analysing glasses, meaning it is devoid of monocular cues making it more demanding and possibly a more reliable test for stereopsis than the Titmus test of local stereopsis. The Julesz test measures global stereopsis. The Lang test and the Frisbee test measure stereopsis without the need for polarized glasses. The two–pencil test popularized by Lang is a simple test for stereopsis where the examiner holds a pencil pointing upward and the patient tries to touch the examiner's pencil by thrusting his pencil downward. Patients with normal stereopsis and with both eyes open can accurately place their pencil on top of the examiner's pencil at the first attempt. With one eye closed these normal patients and also patients who lack stereopsis cannot easily place their pencil on the examiner's pencil, requiring several 'localized' thrusts before accomplishing the task.

Other factors in the strabismus examination

Angle kappa

When the pupil axis is displaced from the visual axis the angle between the visual axis and the pupillary axis creates an angle and direction of pseudostrabismus. If the visual axis is displaced nasally from the pupillary axis an exodeviation is simulated. If the visual axis is displaced temporally from the pupillary axis an esodeviation is simulated. The former is called a positive angle kappa and the latter a negative angle kappa. A

small positive angle kappa is physiological. A large 'pathological' angle kappa is seen in patients with retinopathy of prematurity who have temporal dragging of the macula. Obviously, strabismus surgery is not indicated for the apparent or pseudostrabismus resulting from an abnormal angle kappa. Painted portraits invariably depict an exaggerated positive angle kappa in the normal subject. A painting without a positive angle kappa makes the subject appear esotropic. Comparison of mediaeval with modern paintings emphasizes this point.

External examination

External examination of a patient with strabismus provides important information .

Epicanthus

An epicanthal fold can obliterate or reduce the amount of 'white' seen medial to the limbus. This can give the appearance of an esotropia, especially in an infant and during lateroversion. When a patient with a pseudostrabismus from epicanthus is presented for examination, the parent(s) should be shown the centred pupillary light reflex, the lack of movement on cover testing, and the 'straightening' effect produced by pulling forward the skin over the bridge of the nose. This latter manoeuvre must be done last and looked for quickly, because it often elicits a howl from the infant followed by a turn of the head, ending an otherwise happy examination session.

Facial symmetry

Facial symmetry is common in congenital superior oblique palsy and in other conditions which lead to a head tilt. With superior oblique palsy the face is fuller on the side of the paretic muscle because the head is tilted away from it. In other strabismus conditions that occur in early childhood and which cause a head tilt, the face is smaller on the lower side and fuller on the higher side. Facial symmetry may occur in any patient with head tilt and does not imply strabismus. This occurs in some patients with a tight sternocleidomastoid muscle producing an 'orthopaedic' head tilt. Any infant with head tilt should have strabismus ruled out before orthopaedic treatment is undertaken.

Ptosis

Ptosis may be true ptosis or pseudoptosis. True ptosis occurs with reduced levator function. If severe ptosis is present, the upper lid may obstruct the pupil (visual axis) causing amblyopia or inducing chin elevation, a posture to enable the patient to look under the ptotic lid. Pseudoptosis has normal levator function and the lid margin does not obstruct the pupil. Pseudoptosis occurs in the normal eye when fixation is taken up by the eye with a paretic depressing muscle; for example, if a patient has right superior oblique palsy and habitually fixates with the right eye, a hypotropia with ptosis will be seen in the left fellow-normal eye. Infants with ptosis who have a backward head thrust in order to see under the lids may have delayed motor development, sitting up and walking later than normal.

Fixation (a monocular phenomenon)

In cases of amblyopia or in some cases of macular disease, suppression or poor vision at the macula forces use of a retinal area other than the fovea of fixation (eccentric fixation). This 'fixation' is usually imprecise compared with normal foveal fixation and has an area rather than a discrete point for fixation. Eccentric fixation is always associated with reduced vision in that eye.

Tests for torsion

Torsion is measured after dissociation of the eyes by placing a red Maddox rod which is vertically oriented before one eye and a white Maddox rod also oriented vertically before the fellow eye. The patient views a point source of light through these Maddox rods, seeing a red horizontal line and a white horizontal line. If torsion is present, one or both line(s) will be seen at an angle to the horizon. To measure the angle, the rod producing the tilted line is rotated until the patient reports that the lines are parallel and vertically separated indicating a residual vertical deviation or fused into a reddish or pink line indicating that there is no vertical deviation only torsion. The amount of torsion can be determined by noting the degrees of rotation of the vertical Maddox rod. The most common torsional strabismus is the extorsion found with superior oblique palsy.

Torsion can also be measured with a Hess or Lees projection screen using a linear pointer. An ingenious test for torsion devised by Awaya employs red and green halved discs presented in gradual degrees of tilt. These discs are viewed haploscopically with red and green glasses. The two half discs which are seen vertically parallel indicate the amount of torsion and the direction. If no torsion is present, the two discs which are printed parallel and vertically oriented will be seen as such through the dissociating glasses.

Measurement for generated force by comparison of saccades

The contractile power of the muscles can be inferred simply and non-invasively by estimation of saccadic velocity. This is done by asking the patient to switch fixation from one extreme of lateral version to the opposite. The speed of movement of the two eyes is compared. In the presence of a paresis, there will be a difference in the speed of movement. The slower eye will have what is called a 'floating saccade'. A 'floating saccade' indicates the presence of a paresis in the eye with the slower floating movement. Normal saccades are approximately 400° per second. A paretic eye with a floating saccade may have a movement of half that speed or less and is easily observed.

Passive or forced ductions

Passive or forced ductions are measured to determine whether an ocular movement is limited because of mechanical restraints or because of paresis or paralysis. This test, done in the outpatient clinical setting, requires topical anaesthesia to the conjunctiva using proparacaine hydrochloride, xylocaine 5 per cent, or equivalent drops. After this, the limbus is grasped with fine toothed forceps while the patient attempts to look in the direction of the gaze to be tested, i.e. if passive abduction is to be tested in the right eye, the patient is asked to look to the right. The eye is then gently rotated around the centre of rotation of the globe ('Z' axis). It is important in this manoeuvre to avoid retropulsing the globe and creating the impression that passive ductions are free or less restricted than they actually are. In a pure paresis with no mechanical restriction, passive ductions will be free. When a mechanical restriction is present passive ductions will be stiff and restricted, meaning that the full duction cannot be completed even with assistance. In some cases, there is coexistence of a paresis and a mechanical restriction. In this case the patient will have a floating saccade within the range of the limited movement. If forced duction testing is done, the examiner can also do a generated force test.

Generated force test

Generated force is tested after the conjunctiva has been anaesthetized as with passive duction testing. The patient looks first in the direction opposite from the muscle action to be tested. The globe is then grasped at the limbus and the patient is asked to look slowly in the direction of the muscle to be tested. The force in the muscle to be tested is estimated by feeling the tug or traction on the forceps stabilizing the globe. This test takes some practice to be able to quantify accurately the force generated. The examiner should monitor eye movement during this test by noting that the fellow eye completes the intended version. In patients with normal force generation, conjunctiva can break free from the stabilizing forceps causing bleeding. If the examiner feels an impending tear of conjunctiva, the forceps should be released immediately.

In most cases, estimation of generated force with inference about the muscle's ability to contract determined after observation of saccadic velocity provides sufficient information for diagnosis and planning of surgery. Passive duction testing need only be done in the operating theatre in most cases because this information is used more for the design of surgery than for diagnosis and requires no patient co-operation. The decision to free a restriction or the lack of need to free a restriction need only be made at the time of surgery. Generated force may be ?quantified with a strain gauge or equivalent device, but this is usually reserved for research purposes.

Classification of strabismus

There are several possible schemes for classifying strabismus, but none is sufficient to encompass its complexity satisfactorily. An arbitrary, but logical classification starts by considering aetiology as the prime factor. This scheme initially groups patients into those who are born with a capacity for motor fusion and those who are not. Those born lacking the capacity for normal motor fusion have the congenital esotropia syndrome and are considered separately. In the other branch of the classification, those patients born with the capacity for motor fusion are subdivided according to (1) mechanical versus neural strabismus, (2) sensory versus motor strabismus, and (3) supranuclear versus nuclear and intranuclear strabismus (Fig. 6).

Congenital esotropia

A working theory for the aetiology of essential infantile esotropia is that it occurs because of an inborn absence of, or defi-

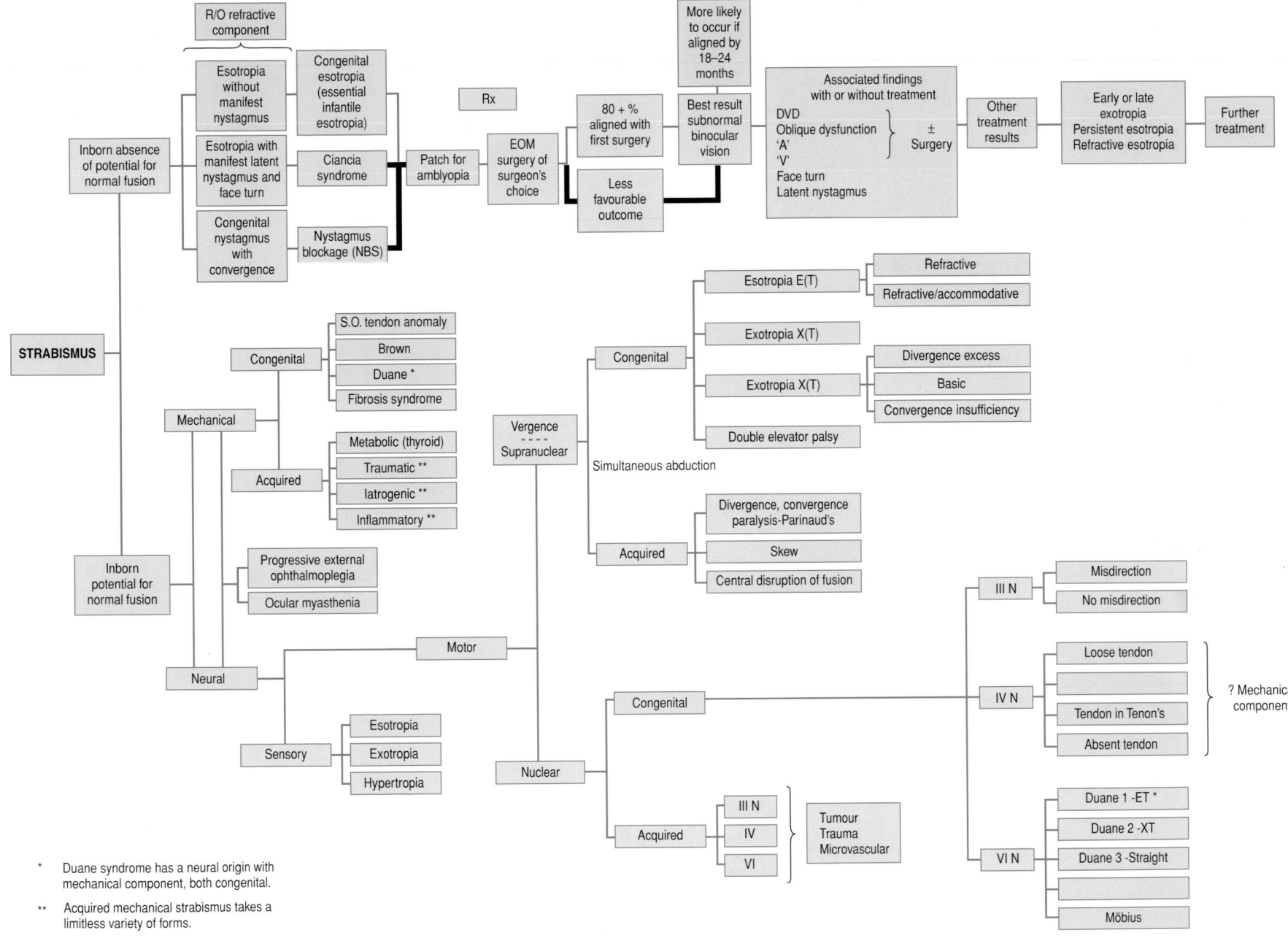

Fig. 6 A comprehensive classification of strabismus.

*   Duane syndrome has a neural origin with mechanical component, both congenital.

** Acquired mechanical strabismus takes a limitless variety of forms.

ciency in, normal motor fusion. Alternative theories for the cause on congenital esotropia have been proposed and may play some role in the clinical picture (congenital abnormality in motion processing manifested as OKN asymmetry and nasal retinal predominance manifest as nasal eccentric fixation with micronystagmus are thought by some to be the cause of congenital esotropia) but the theory of motor fusion deficiency, originally described by Worth as the 'fusion faculty' makes sense. At birth, motor control of the neonate's eyes is unstable. Study of infants between 3 hours and 3 days of age showed two-thirds of infants had intermittent exodeviations while less than 5 per cent had intermittent esodeviation. Unsteady alignment resolves in the normal neonate during the first few months of life. Then between the age of 2 and 4 months alignment of the eyes becomes stable and stereoacuity can be confirmed, at least in the laboratory setting. To achieve this, an optokinetic stimulus of moving stripes is viewed haploscopically producing OKN only if stereopsis is recognized.

In the first few months of life, normal infants and those with congenital esotropia have asymmetric OKN. This means that OKN is robust when following targets moving from a temporal to nasal direction and is diminished when following targets from a nasal to temporal direction. This motion processing defect is thought by some to be an aetiological factor in congenital esotropia, but others believe that OKN asymmetry is a sign of immaturity and/or strabismus and not the cause of congenital esotropia. Among current theories, the motor fusion defect theory as the initial event in the occurrence of congenital esotropia is sound and supportable.

The defining diagnostic characteristics of congenital esotropia are:

(1) Esodeviation confirmed by 4 months of age and ranging in size from 10 to 90 prism dioptres.

(2) Lack of a refractive component as cause of the esodeviation. (In practice, a hyperopia of +3.00 dioptres or more calls for a trial of spectacles to rule out a refractive component.)

(3) The above occurring in a neurologically normal infant.

At the time of initial diagnosis of congenital esotropia in an infant, full abduction in each eye should be confirmed. This usually requires carrying out the doll's head test where the head is gently rotated form side to side, noting the extent of abduction of each eye. Full abduction rules out sixth nerve palsy, including that associated with Duane syndrome and Moebius syndrome. Fixation preference should be evaluated in all infants with congenital esotropia. Is the right eye or the left eye preferred, or is free alternation between the eyes present? Free alternation virtually assures that no amblyopia is present. Preference for fixation with either eye indicates, or at least strongly suggests, presence of amblyopia or an organic cause of poor vision in the non-preferred eye. Infants with amblyopia will strenuously object to occlusion of the preferred eye while demonstrating little or no objection to occlusion of the non-preferred eye. The fundus of both eyes then must be carefully evaluated for any abnormality. A common cause for an organic vision deficit in an infant is optic nerve hypoplasia, but other organic defects such as coloboma, inflammatory lesions, and even retinablastoma can occur.

If amblyopia is diagnosed by observing fixation preference and ruling out an organic lesion, a patching programme is begun. A safe programme for an infant, as suggested by von Noorden, is to occlude the preferred eye fulltime for 2 or 3 days and then occlude the amblyopic eye fulltime for 1 day, repeating this pattern until alternation is established. This procedure makes it safe to pursue a slightly less rigorous follow-up programme compared with that necessary when fulltime patching of the preferred eye is carried out. Fulltime patching of the preferred eye can result in occlusion amblyopia in a very young child. This can be avoided by employing the safer but just as effective procedure of unequal alternating patching. Patching the amblyopic eye on alternate days eliminates any need for suppression which would enforce amblyopia.

When the diagnosis of congenital esotropia has been established and amblyopia has been ruled out or successfully treated, surgical treatment of the esodeviation can be undertaken. This means that surgery can and probably should be done at the earliest reasonable time after confirmation of diagnosis (Fig. 7). Since normal alignment is established between 2 and 4 months, the earliest surgery for a confirmed diagnosis of congenital esotropia is during the fourth month. Surgery at this time requires competent paediatric anaesthesia and good surgical shape. At 4 months of age, the medial recti are sufficient large to undergo surgery. The axial length of the eye of a 4-month-old infant is about 19.5 mm—large enough to allow recession of the medial recti to 10.5 mm from the limbus. This axial length of 19.5 mm compares with 17 mm at birth and approximately 23.5 mm at age 3 to 5 years.

Surgical 'formulas' should be given with appropriate disclaimers such as 'in my hands', and 'in most cases', etc. Most texts contain surgical tables and most readers demand them.

Table 1 shows a guide for surgical treatment of congenital esotropia. The figures are examples only of surgical values that have been effective for the author. They should always be subject to modification based on each surgeon's experience. Some surgeons prefer an approximate size recession of one medial rectus and a resection of the antagonist lateral rectus. For deviations greater than 50 prism dioptres some surgeons prefer to do three muscles using a formula such as that used by the prism adaptation study.

The surgical formula uses the limbus as a reference for the measurement of medial rectus recession, the rationale being that the medial rectus insertion has been found to vary between 3 and 6 mm from the limbus in infants and young children with congenital esotropia and this insertion distance has no relationship to the angle of strabismus. On the other hand, the corneal diameter (used for defining the location of the limbus) and the axial length (defining the location of the equator) are reliable, age-related landmarks independent of the angle of strabismus. The scheme shown in Table 1 calls for sufficient recession to treat a given angle of esotropia while at the same time avoiding excessive recession of the medial recti.

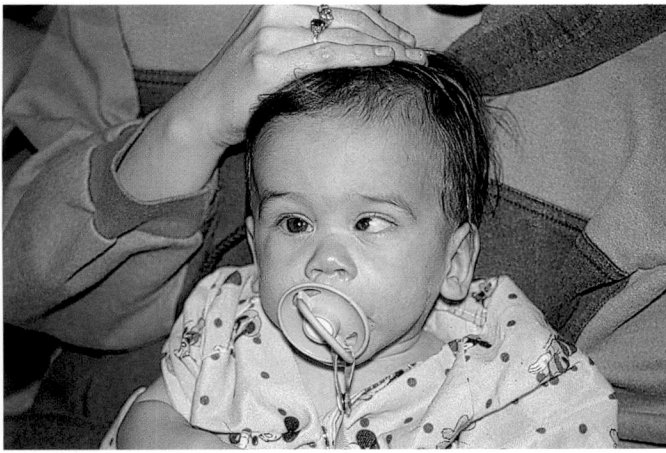

(a)

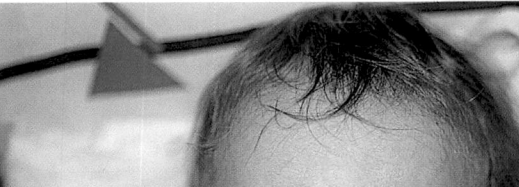

(b)

Fig. 7 (a) Esotropia in a 6-month-old preoperative. (b) The same patient with eyes aligned 2 months postoperatively.

Table 1 Bimedial rectus recessions measured from the limbus

Deviation	mm	<1 year	>1 year	>5 years
Small	20–30	8.5	9.0	9.0
Medium	30–45	9.5	10.0	10.5
Large	45+	10.5	11.0	11.5

Using the above formula, 80 to 85 per cent of patients treated with bimedial recession for congenital esotropia would be expected to have less than 10 prism dioptres of residual esotropia after their initial procedure. When a bimedial rectus recession is carried out the best early postoperative result is orthotropia. An exodeviation of 10 prism dioptres or more, especially with limited adduction in the first few days postoperatively, is a sign that the patient may develop a larger exodeviation, producing an overcorrection requiring later medial rectus advancement. In other cases a small exodeviation with normal adduction present in the first few weeks after surgery can result

in good alignment. If a recession–resection procedure is done as the initial procedure for congenital esotropia, an early exotropia is common and is a good prognostic sign. An esodeviation persisting 8 weeks after bimedial recession usually persists or increases in size.

For about half of patients treated surgically for congenital esotropia, the initial bimedial rectus recession is only the beginning of the story. These patients can develop some or all of the following conditions.

Dissociated vertical deviation (DVD)

This is an upward deviation of either eye when occluded; it sometimes occurs spontaneously when the eye is suppressed. DVD may be asymmetrical or even unilateral in some cases. If this upward deviation is unacceptable cosmetically it can be treated surgically with recession of the superior rectus muscle up to 7 mm or more from the original insertion. Surgery should be bilateral and unequal if the DVD is unequal, thus avoiding increased DVD in the unoperated eye. Residual DVD persisting after superior rectus recession is treated with inferior rectus resection. If a patient with DVD also has inferior oblique overaction and a 'V' pattern, inferior oblique anterior transposition, always bilateral, can be performed.

DVD may also occur as a primary condition without esotropia and may be an expression of the congenital motor fusion defect syndrome which is the basis of congenital esotropia itself. DVD occurring primarily can also appear with 'A' pattern and overaction of the superior obliques. This primary condition is treated with bilateral superior oblique weakening and lateral rectus weakening if required. A secondary form of the 'A' exotropia triad occurs after larger bimedial rectus recession. In this case the 'A' pattern and the exodeviation are treated with advancement of the medial recti and the DVD is treated with recession of the superior recti.

'V' pattern with overaction of the inferior obliques

This condition is treated by bilateral weakening of the overacting inferior oblique muscles.

Refractive esotropia

A recurrent esotropia can occur as the result of an uncorrected hyperoptic refractive error in a patient who had early surgery for a congenital esotropia but who later develops a refractive component. Careful cycloplegic refraction should be repeated and appropriate hyperoptic correction prescribed.

Overcorrection

An exotropia can occur after bimedial rectus recession of any surgery for congenital esotropia, either early, after a few months to a year, or after several years. This secondary exotropia is treated with either bimedial rectus advancement or bilateral lateral rectus recession. The former is employed in cases where the previous recession has resulted in reduced adduction. If a recession–resection procedure is done, the reoperation should be tailored to the deviation and eye movements.

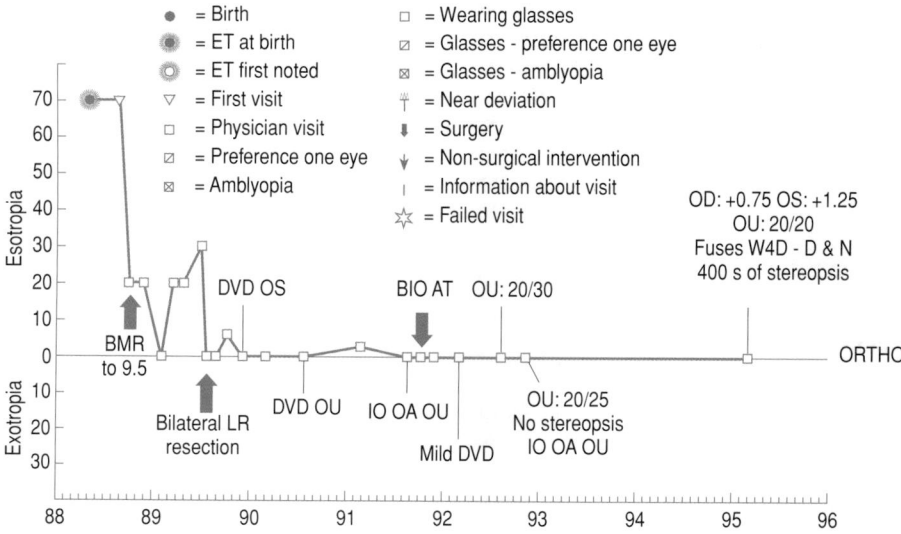

Fig. 8 The time line is a graphic description of a congenital esotropia examined and treated with 21 outpatient visits in 6.5 years. Two additional surgical procedures were required, one for recurrent exotropia, bilateral lateral rectus resection at age 1 year and bilateral inferior oblique anterior transposition at age 3.5 years for dissociated vertical deviation. At age 6.5 years the patient's eyes were aligned, vision was good, and peripheral fusion was recorded. X-axis—date (year); Y-axis deviation in prism dioptres.

Persistent esotropia

Persistent esotropia often occurs in patients who have manifest patent nystagmus, abduction nystagmus, rotary nystagmus, and face turn preoperatively and in patients with a very large angle preoperatively. Some of these make up the Ciancia syndrome which is a congenital esotropia with marked manifest latent nystagmus causing face turn and cross fixation, that is, fixing to the left with the esodeviated right eye and vice versa.

Amblyopia

After surgical treatment of congenital esotropia it can be more difficult to detect obvious fixation preference for one eye in a preliterate child because of the much smaller or even absent angle of strabismus. Such children should be observed closely for evidence of fixation preference and, as soon as possible, with visual acuity testing. When amblyopia is found, a careful occlusion programme should be undertaken.

Results of surgical treatment for congenital esotropia are satisfactory in most instances. However, careful attention to detail during follow-up is essential. A 'time line' showing sequential treatment of a patient with congenital esotropia demonstrates graphically the typical dynamic postoperative course. Figure 8 shows a patient who had successful realignment of the eyes after several 'mid-course corrections' and who now demonstrates sensory fusion.

There is no single 'correct' or universally agreed-upon formula for either the timing or the technique in treatment of congenital esotropia. However, weight of evidence suggests that early alignment results in more patients attaining sensory fusion. In a prospectively-studied series of 12 patients aligned before 6 months of age and followed carefully for 6 years, 50 per cent had measurable stereopsis denoting sensory fusion.

Early surgery for congenital esotropia with alignment before

18 months reported in several series shows a higher number of patients achieving fairly good levels of binocularity as evidenced by measurable stereoacuity. Better sensory fusion results from early alignment which allows expression of an innate response that has not been degraded by long-standing strabismus. Stereoacuity, when present, is the result of alignment in the normal binocular state; it is not the enabler or cause of alignment. There is no reason to delay surgery for congenital exotropia until the child is older and attains what has been called the 'orthoptic age' at approximately 5 years. Arguments about inaccurate measurements and surgical complications caused by immature muscles are invalid.

Congenital esotropia and its sequelae account for about 50 per cent of cases of strabismus requiring treatment. In the United States, as a rule, a patient with congenital esotropia needs to be followed through adolescence to deal adequately with the potentially varied course of this complex strabismus.

Refractive esotropia

Uncorrected hyperopia leads to an esodeviation if appropriate accommodation is exerted by a patient who lacks sufficient fusional divergence. Refractive esotropia can occur as early as 4 to 6 months of age in a few cases, but is usually seen at about 2 to 2.5 years. The treatment of refractive esotropia is prescription of the full cycloplegic refraction, resulting in alignment of the eyes if the esodeviation is due entirely to accommodative effort and if the accommodation convergence/accommodation ratio (AC/A) is normal or near normal. Refractive esotropia can be as low as 5 to 15 dioptres or as high as 70+ prism dioptres. Some patients with refractive esotropia will have a high AC/A ration causing a larger esodeviation at near. Not all patients with high AC/A and a near esodeviation have

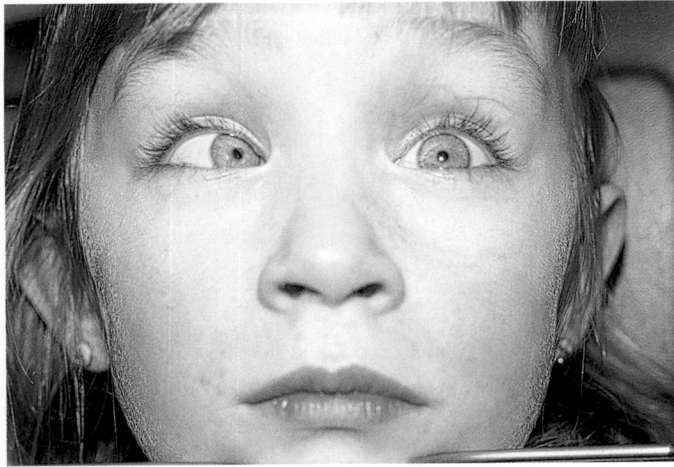

(a)

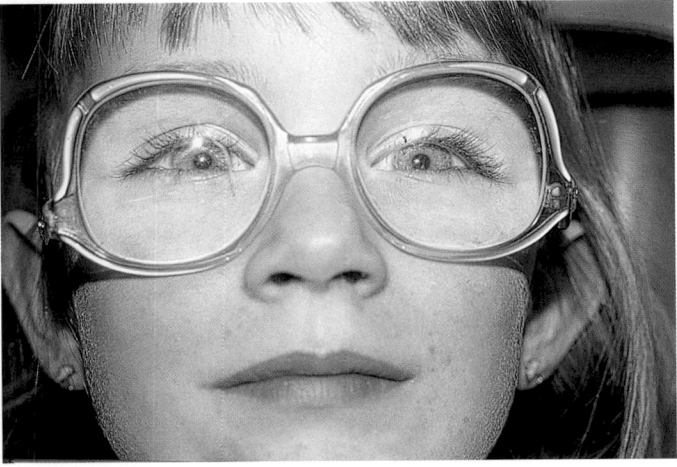

(b)

Fig. 9 (a) Esotropia without spectacles. (b) Eyes are aligned wearing +3.00 spectacles in a patient with refractive esotropia.

Table 2 Scheme for surgical treatment of exodeviation

Bilateral lateral rectus recession
5.0 mm OU/20–25 prism dioptres
6.0 mm OU/25–30 prism dioptres
7.0 mm OU/30–40 prism dioptres
8.0 mm OU/40–50 prism dioptres

Recession lateral rectus – resection medial rectus
5.0 mm – *5.0 mm/20–25 prism dioptres
6.0 mm – *6.0 mm/25–30 prism dioptres
7.0 mm – *8.0 mm/30–40 prism dioptres
8.0 mm – *10.0 mm/40–50 prism dioptres

Three-muscle surgery
8.0 mm – *8.00 mm – 8.0 mm/50–60 prism dioptres
8.0 mm – *10.0 mm – 8.0 mm/60–75 prism dioptres

Four-muscle surgery
8.0 mm – *8.0 mm – *8.00 mm – 8.00 mm/75–80 prism dioptres
8.0 mm – *10.0 mm – *10.0 mm – 8.0 mm/85–100 prism dioptres

* Medial rectus resection

A controversial treatment for refractive esotropia advocates discarding glasses in favour of surgical treatment. Surgery is said to produce a change in the convergence–accommodation/convergence ratio. This can result in asthenopia and blurred vision requiring reinstitution of glasses and causing a secondary exotropia. Surgical treatment of refractive esotropia as a replacement for spectacle correction has no sound theoretical basis, little convincing clinical support, and should be avoided.

Intermittent exotropia

Patients with intermittent exotropia appear to be perfectly normal when they are aligned. However, to achieve an enlarged peripheral field when the eyes are exodeviated they have reduced quality of binocularity with central suppression. When the eyes are dissociated after occlusion during testing or spontaneously, bifoveal fusion is 'turned off'. The deviation in intermittent exotropia can be small, as little as 10 to 14 prism dioptres, or as large as 50 prism dioptres or more. The eyes may be deviated infrequently, less than 10 per cent of the time, or, often, more than 80 per cent of the time. The deviation may be greater at distance (divergence excess), at near (convergence insufficiency) or be the same at distance and near (basic).

The decision whether to operate for intermittent exotropia is based on consideration of how often the eyes are deviated, the size of the deviation, or on the degree of asthenopia. For example, a patient with 50 prism dioptres of intermittent exotropia manifest about 5 per cent of time may not require surgery while a patient with 20 prism dioptres of intermittent exotropia manifest 80 per cent of the time would require surgical treatment. If the duration of the tropia is reversed in the above example, the larger deviation would require a larger amount of surgery. A reasonable surgery schedule for intermittent exotropia is listed in Table 2. In general, bilateral lateral rectus recessions is done for a deviation greater at distance, or

refractive esotropia. Patients with high AC/A and a near esodeviation have refractive esotropia. High AC/A with greater near esodeviation can be present in a myopic patient (Fig. 9).

A few patients with moderate to high hyperopia of +4.00 to +8.00 dioptres or more will retain aligned eyes at the expense of a chronically blurred image. In this situation, bilateral ametropic amblyopia can occur. With normal AC/A and moderate to high hyperopia, a patient who accommodates sufficiently to produce a clear retinal image and who has less than exuberant fusional divergence will have an esotropia from normal accommodative convergence. Traditionally, patients with greater esotropia at near with a high AC/A, have been treated with bifocals with a power of up to +3.00 dioptres or slightly more. The bifocal add is usually flat-topped and is placed high in the lens to bisect the pupil. Older patients, more adept at bifocal wear, can use a blended, 'no line' bifocal, often with a reduced power. Long-term use of bifocals in the young can lead to premature presbyopia. For this reason, bifocals are not used by some ophthalmologists if fusion is present at distance fixation. The issue of bifocal use for high AC/A is unresolved as yet.

when the distance near deviation is equal and vision is equal. A recess–resect procedure is also done when the deviation is equal distance and near, when the deviation is greater at near and when vision is poorer in one eye and surgery is to be limited to that eye.

The term binocularity is used loosely and not always accurately in strabismology. Binocular vision means that both eyes are used simultaneously , at least within the confines of retinal rivalry. For example, the 'competitive' part of the non-fusible binocular visual field which is modified by harmonious anomalous retinal correspondence is suppressed in the non-preferred eye but does receive some stimulation. The peripheral monocular field is useful and in the exotrope creates an enlarged binocular peripheral field. Patients whose eyes are aligned following large angle exodeviation frequently say that they have 'tunnel vision' which may be disturbing immediately after alignment of their eyes. This sensation always disappears in a matter of days or weeks without sequelae.

Convergence insufficiency intermittent exotropia presents a difficult therapeutic challenge. In most cases it should be treated initially with orthoptics. Nearpoint of convergence 'push up' exercises are done by holding a small accommodative target at arm's length, fusing the target, and then bringing it towards the nose, keeping the accommodative component in focus and fused until the image is seen doubled, signifying that the eyes are exodeviated. This event signals that motor fusion is lost. The target is then moved further away until the image is re-fused and seen singly and the 'push up' exercise is repeated. The ten-repetition exercise is done two or three times a day. This treatment, if initially successful, can be carried out in a maintenance programme for weeks or months. If orthoptics fails to achieve comfort, base-in prism may be used either over the entire lens or the lower half for near use. Failing success with exercises and prism, surgery (bimedial rectus resection or recession of one lateral rectus and resection of one medial rectus) may be carried out. In either case, the patient should be warned of the certainty of postoperative diplopia at least in the short term and often permanently in lateroversion on the side of the operated eye when a recess–resect has been done. Long-term attention to follow-up is needed for patients who have surgical treatment for convergence insufficiency.

Exotropia

Constant exotropia occurs on a sensory basis as a result of poor vision in one eye, from a decompensated intermittent exotropia, or from a congenital exotropia (which is probably congenital exotropia in the 'other' direction). It also occurs with third nerve palsy, Duane syndrome II, medial rectus paresis, and as a secondary manifestation after other strabismus or orbital surgery. Exotropia is usually treated with a recession of the lateral rectus and resection of the medial rectus, including addition of a third and sometimes a fourth muscle according to the angle of the deviation and the status of passive ductions. When only two muscles are treated, the chronically deviated eye is usually treated. As a rule, any deviation with free and full ductions can be aligned with appropriate recession and resection

Table 3 The characteristics of congenital and acquired superior oblique palsy

Characteristic	Congenital	Acquired
Facial asymmetry	+	−
History acute onset	−	+
Loose superior oblique tendon	+	−
Large angle	+	+
Large fusion amplitudes	+	+
Torsion response – double Maddox	+	+

of two horizontal recti. Those patients requiring three or four muscle surgery will usually demonstrate limited ductions of one or more horizontal recti.

Superior oblique palsy

Superior oblique palsy is the most commonly occurring isolated cranial nerve palsy affecting the extraocular muscles seen in a strabismus practice. The three salient features of superior oblique palsy are (1) head tilt to the opposite shoulder with chin depression, (2) hypertropia greater to the side opposite the palsied muscle in lateral versions, (3) hypertropia greater when the head is tilted to the same side as the paretic muscle (the Bielschowsky head tilt test). The diagnosis of superior oblique palsy for the experienced strabismologist is made literally from 'across the room', is confirmed by the Bielschowsky test, and is quantified by careful prism and cover testing in the diagnostic positions together with testing for torsion with the double Maddox rods or equivalent.

The unique anatomy of the superior oblique tendon is a prime factor in the surgical management of superior oblique palsy. The size of the deviation is also important because small deviations can be treated successfully with prism in some cases especially if they are comitant or nearly so. Larger incomitant deviations are best treated with surgery.

Acquired superior oblique palsy in an adult causing vertical diplopia with a small, nearly comitant hypertropia is best treated initially with temporary Fresnel prism. In older patients superior oblique palsy may be the result of a microvascular event. Such a patient should be evaluated by a general physician and treated for hypertension, diabetes, or other systemic disease as required. Imaging with computed tomography (CT) or magnetic resonance imaging (MRI) is not required in these patients. The vertical tropia usually resolves. If it does not, permanent prism can be prescribed.

Other patients with superior oblique palsy (the majority) are grouped according to whether they are congenital or acquired (usually from trauma), then according to the size of deviation, and finally according to the pattern of the deviation which in long-standing cases may become nearly comitant. Table 3 compares the characteristics of congenital and acquired superior oblique palsy .

A scheme for surgical treatment of superior oblique palsy

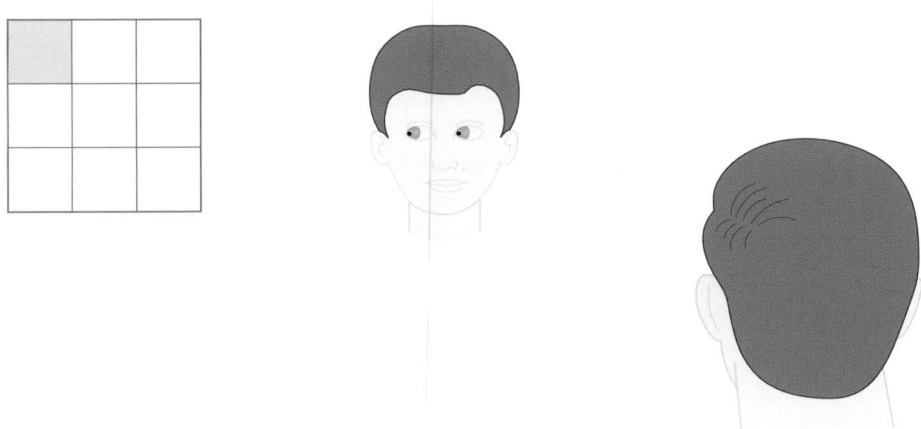

Fig. 10 This patient has greatest left hypertropia in upright gaze representing class I superior oblique palsy.

follows, modified from one originally proposed by Knapp. The examples are for left superior oblique palsy.

Surgical treatment for class I: weaken ipsilateral inferior oblique (Fig. 10).

Surgical treatment for class II: if small, +8 prism dioptres, avoid surgery—use appropriate prism; if larger than 8–10 prism dioptres—superior oblique tuck if the superior oblique is loose or contralateral inferior rectus recession if the tendon is tight. This class is rarely seen (Fig. 11).

Surgical treatment for class III: for a hypertropia less than 25 prism dioptres—inferior oblique myectomy, if the deviation is 25 prism dioptres or more add superior oblique tuck if the tendon is loose or a contralateral inferior rectus recession if the superior oblique tendon is tight (Fig. 12).

Surgical treatment for class IV: this class is usually larger

than 25 prism dioptres—surgical treatment consists of inferior oblique myectomy on the involved side with ipsilateral superior rectus recession. Also if the deviation is greater than 35 prism dioptres a loose superior oblique tendon is tucked or resected or if the superior oblique tendon is tight small recession of the contralateral inferior rectus is carried out (Fig. 13).

Surgical treatment for class V: recess ipsilateral superior rectus and recess contralateral inferior rectus (Fig. 14).
Bilateral superior oblique palsy is characterized by the following:

Chin down—gaze up
'V' pattern
Bilateral superior oblique underaction
Bilateral inferior oblique overaction
Spontaneous cyclodiplopia
Torsion often measured greater than 15°

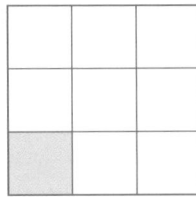

Fig. 11 Class II superior oblique palsy. Greater deviation in opposite downgaze field.

Fig. 13 Class IV superior oblique palsy. Deviation also present in same side downgaze field.

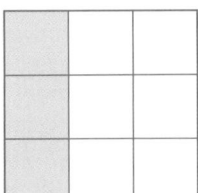

Fig. 12 Class III superior oblique palsy. Larger deviation in entire opposite gaze field.

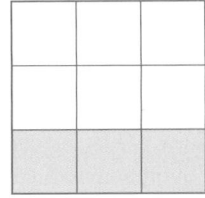

Fig. 14 Class V superior oblique palsy. Greater deviation in downgaze.

Table 4 Duane syndrome*

Class	Primary position	Head turn	Ductions	Fissure narrowing	Upshoot/downshoot
I	Esotropia	Toward involved	↓ ABD	+	±
II	Exotropia	Toward normal	↓ ADD	++++	++++
III	Orthotropia	None	↓ ABD and ADD	++	++
Simultaneous abduction	Exotropia	Toward involved	↓ ADD	0	0

* May be bilateral

Surgical treatment for class VI: bilateral superior oblique palsy requires some or all of the following:

(1) Bilateral inferior oblique weakening—for inferior oblique overaction—for superior oblique underaction – for 'V' pattern

(2) Bilateral inferior rectus recession with small nasal shift – for 'V' pattern (eso in downgaze)

(3) Medial rectus downshift for the 'V' pattern – eso in downgaze

(4) Bilateral superior oblique Harada-Ito – for torsion (avoid Brown with small shift)

(5) Small bilateral superior oblique tuck (or resection) – for torsion—superior oblique underaction (avoid Brown with small tuck (or resection))

Surgical treatment of bilateral superior oblique palsy is demanding in that a variety of options is available. In general, it is best to achieve alignment or undercorrect at the first surgery.

Class VII superior oblique palsy is the so-called 'canine tooth' syndrome of Knapp. It is a combination Brown syndrome and superior oblique palsy on the same side. It may occur after trauma producing mechanical restriction of up and downgaze or the eye may be mechanically restricted on upgaze with paresis on downgaze or it may be iatrogenic after a superior oblique tuck for superior oblique palsy where there is mechanical limitation of upgaze from the superior oblique tuck and residual superior oblique underaction. The best treatment for canine tooth syndrome, class VII superior oblique palsy, is to ignore the Brown and treat the superior oblique palsy with recession of the contralateral yoke inferior rectus or to create a total superior oblique palsy, by superior oblique tenectomy near the trochlea, and then treat this superior oblique palsy according to the pattern of deviation.

Superior oblique palsy after sinus surgery occurs in some cases when the Lynch incision is used with subperiosteal displacement of the trochlea. This displacement of the trochlea can produce superior oblique underaction which is indistinguishable from superior oblique palsy. These patients are best treated with recession of the yoke inferior rectus, recession of the ipsilateral superior rectus, weakening of the ipsilaterial inferior oblique, and for torsion, a Harada-Ito procedure on the affected superior oblique.

Duane syndrome

Duane syndrome is caused by aberrant innervation in the orbit, occurring when fibres innervating the medial rectus also innervate the lateral rectus. This occurs with nuclear hypoplasia of the sixth nerve. Duane syndrome can be unilateral or bilateral, is found slightly more often in females and left eyes and is fairly common. The consistent feature of Duane's syndrome is sixth nerve paralysis. This may be masked or completely over-ridden by variations in the degree of aberrant regeneration to the lateral rectus with fibres from the third nerve. Duane syndrome is divided into classes I, II, III, and simultaneous abduction.

Table 4 compares the various classes of Duane syndrome illustrated in Fig. 15.

If treatment of Duane syndrome is elected the choice is surgical. The aim is to align the head by aligning the eyes, reduce the upshoot, downshoot, and enophthalmos associated with cocontraction and/or align the eyes in the primary position. In class I the medical rectus on the side involved is recessed. In other cases combined medial rectus and lateral rectus recessions are employed in varying degrees to balance and align the eyes and to reduce the up and downshoot in adduction. A faden or posterior fixation suture of the contralateral medial rectus may be done to enhance abduction of the eye involved as a type of 'laudable' secondary deviation. Resection of any muscle in Duane syndrome should not be done, and muscle transfer should be carried out only in cases with little or no enophthalmos. In the final analysis, surgical treatment of Duane syndrome is a compromise at best and is, in nearly every case, a recession or other weakening procedure.

Brown syndrome

Brown syndrome is a mechanical limitation of elevation in adduction which may be congenital or acquired. The acquired form may be from trauma, inflammation, or be iatrogenic. Several weakening techniques for the superior oblique tendon have been employed to treat Brown syndrome, none with complete success. Superior oblique tenotomy medial to the superior rectus is the most effective technique, but unfortu-

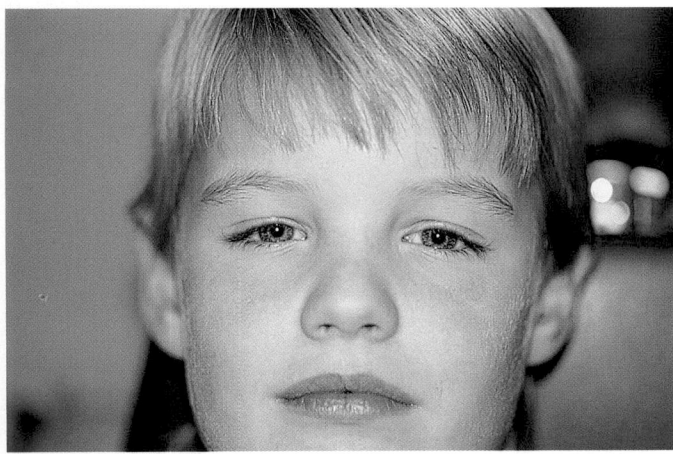

(a)

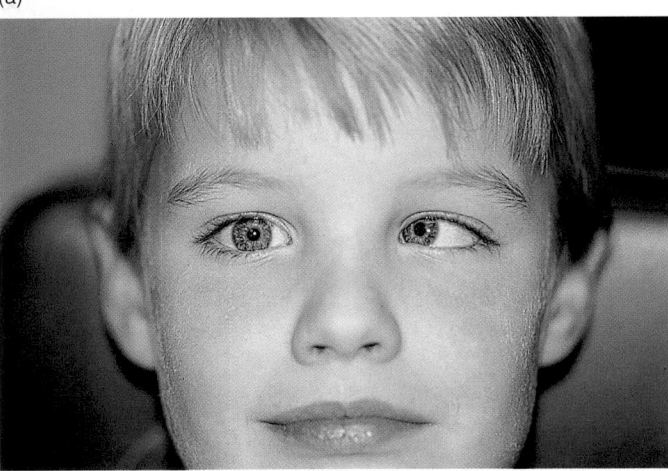

(b)

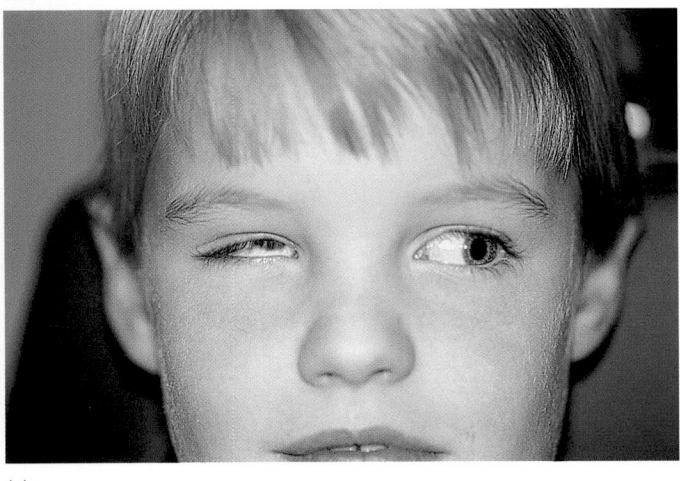

(c)

Fig. 15 (a) Duane I with small angle left exotropia. (b) Cocontracture in right gaze with narrowing of the fissure and enophthalmus. (c) Larger exotropia in left gaze with limited abduction.

nately this tenotomy is the treatment most likely to produce a superior oblique palsy. In one-third of cases where this is done, superior oblique underaction equalling superior oblique palsy occurs and this requires a second operation, usually weakening of the ipsilateral inferior oblique. This secondary

procedure should not be carried out primarily. If Brown syndrome is mild with only minimal chin elevation in a young child, surgery should not be carried out. As a child with Brown syndrome grows taller, the implications of limited elevation in adduction become significantly less as more of the environment is straight ahead and downward, not above. A cyst of the superior oblique tendon nasal to the superior rectus can cause Brown syndrome. Surgical removal can free ductions, but the Brown syndrome frequently recurs. A silicone band may be used as a spacer to lengthen the superior oblique tendon nasal to the superior rectus and prevent the ends of the superior oblique from reuniting. Wright and others have reported good results but complications have also been reported including extrusion of the silicone band and return of the Brown syndrome.

Sixth nerve palsy

Sixth nerve palsy is characterized by limited abduction of the involved eye which may be unilateral or bilateral and is usually acquired. A head turn toward the involved side is common in unilateral cases. The acquired form may be from tumour (compression), vascular insufficiency, inflammation, increased intracranial pressure, or trauma. The long course of the sixth nerve makes it particularly vulnerable to diffuse intracranial pressure. The treatment of sixth nerve palsy if elected must be guided by history and other physical findings suggesting the most obvious cause. There is no preferred, single treatment to follow. The treatment of sixth nerve palsy depends on the amount of lateral rectus function remaining, and whether the palsy is unilateral or bilateral. Residual function can be estimated by evaluation of forced ductions and generated force usually determined by observed saccadic velocity or, occasionally, by determination of isometric contraction with the generated force test. Table 5 shows a suggested surgical scheme.

Recession of the medial rectus on the uninvolved side in a case of unilateral sixth nerve palsy should be avoided because this can reduce the total binocular visual field by creating an exodeviation in gaze to the side opposite the paresis.

In cases where there is a need to weaken the medial rectus muscle antagonist to the paretic muscle, when doing an extraocular muscle transfer shifting the superior and inferior recti to the lateral rectus, botulinum α-toxin can be used to produce a temporary weakening of the medial rectus muscle. This technique may spare the anterior ciliary vessels in the medial rectus.

Third nerve palsy

This nerve palsy presents a challenge because four of the six extraocular muscles are paretic and in addition aberrant regeneration occurs in two-thirds of cases with innervation shared between the medial rectus and levator, superior rectus and inferior rectus, and inferior rectus and levator. With peripheral compressive nerve lesions the pupil remains dilated and accommodation is weak or absent. This occurs most often with tumour and aneurysm and with inflammatory lesions at the orbital apex.

Table 5 Sixth nerve palsy*

	ABD	Generated force	Forced ductions	Surgery
I Paresis	↓	+	Free DD	Recess medial rectus Resect lateral rectus
II Paralysis	↓↓	−	Free	Extraocular muscle transfer Inferior rectus and superior rectus to lateral rectus ± Oculinum medial rectus
III Paralysis	↓↓	−	Restricted	Recess medial rectus Extraocular muscle Inferior rectus and superior rectus to lateral rectus

* May be bilateral

Determination of aetiology is important in third nerve palsy because this condition is frequently associated with serious vascular disease. An important guide is pupil sparing in third nerve palsy, because this suggests an intrinsic microvascular lesion and does not require imaging (CT, MRI). In contrast, acute lesions involving the pupil do require imaging because of the threat of serious intracranial disease. Traumatic third nerve palsy work-up is dictated by the overall physical condition. Both congenital and acquired third nerve palsy from trauma or compression result in aberrant regeneration about two-thirds of the time. Occasionally a patient with congenital third nerve palsy chooses to fix with the paretic eye because vision in this eye is better. This fixation with the paretic eye produces a huge secondary deviation with exotropia and hypertropia in the

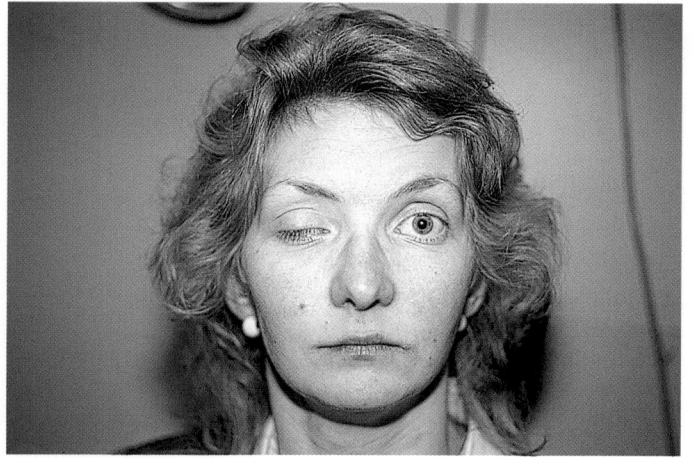

(a)

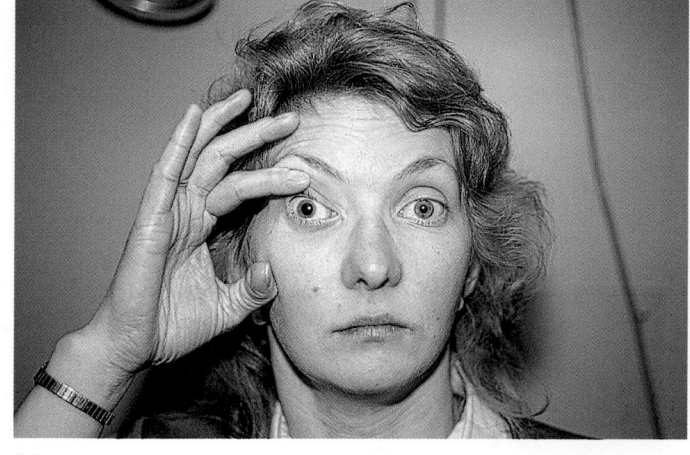

(b)

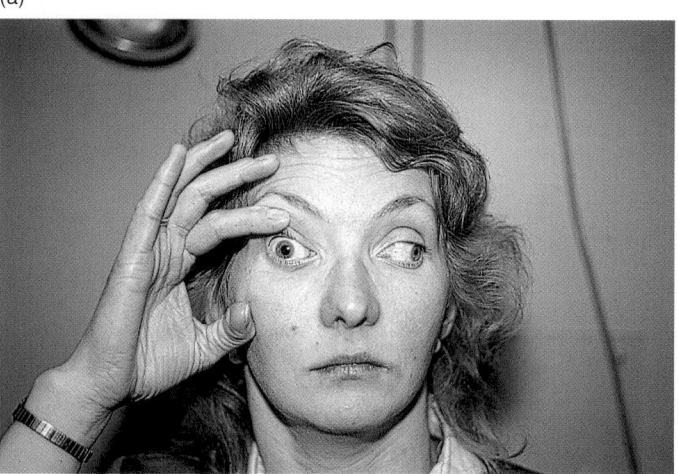

(c)

Fig. 16 This patient has third nerve palsy of the right eye. (a) Ptosis of the right eye. (b) Small exotropia and hypophoria of the right eye in primary position. (c) No adduction of the right eye.

fellow eye. Acquired third nerve palsy from trauma produces an eye which is down and out with complete ptosis. The pupil is usually dilated and fixed (Fig. 16).

The surgical treatment of third nerve palsy consists of lateral rectus recession, medial rectus resection, and in some cases superior oblique tenectomy or transfer to the medial rectus. If there is no aberrant regeneration, the superior rectus can be resected and the inferior rectus recessed. However, in cases of aberrant regeneration the eye is usually fairly well aligned vertically. When surgery is done for third nerve palsy at least one anterior ciliary artery should be spared. The ptosis in third nerve palsy should be undercorrected to maintain corneal protection. This usually requires a frontalis suspension procedure.

The decision whether or not to treat third nerve palsy resulting from trauma must be guided by the patient's expectations about postoperative diplopia. Suppression of the paretic eye is by far the best sensory status for such a patient. If suppression is present, simply aligning the eye in the primary position is the best possible treatment together with undercorrection of the ptosis. If diplopia persists, it may be necessary to occlude one eye. This can be done with a patch, frosted glasses, or best of all with an opaque contact lens.

In congenital third nerve palsy diplopia is not a factor. If the eye involved has vision potential, careful occlusion is needed to avoid amblyopia. Spectacles should be use to correct any refractive error and bifocals should be given if accommodation is affected. Patching should be stopped short of creating a situation where diplopia will occur or fixation switched to the paretic eye.

Other strabismus with acquired mechanical restriction

Thyroid myopathy

Thyroid myopathy is characterized by acquired strabismus in a patient with Graves' disease or sometimes in a patient who is euthyroid and who has never shown signs of hyperthyroidism. The muscle most frequently affected is the inferior rectus. followed by the medial rectus, superior rectus, and least commonly, the lateral rectus. Several muscles can be involved. If this is the case, the usual finding is a restrictive hypotropia and esotropia in the eye involved. While one eye is usually more severely involved, thyroid myopathy is usually bilateral.

Treatment of thyroid myopathy is surgical and includes recession of the involved muscle(s). Adjustable recession is the logical surgical plan, but care must be exercised when carrying out an adjustable recession of the inferior rectus because slippage after recession for thyroid myopathy is common. When needed (for example, if esotropia and hypotropia are present) both the medial and inferior rectus muscles can be recessed with an adjustable suture on each. In addition, bilateral surgery can be carried out. This is especially important if some restriction to elevation is present in the second, less affected eye. Doing an adjustable recession on the more affected eye and no surgery on the less affected eye can produce an overcorrection on the basis of secondary deviation. Surgery for the strabismus

of thyroid myopathy should always be deferred until the patient is past the 'wet' stage of active disease.

Diplopia after cataract

Acquired strabismus, usually with restriction, can result after any surgery around the eye and orbit. With the advent of intraocular lenses for treatment of cataracts carried out primarily with local anaesthesia often early in both eyes, a large number of patients are being seen with acquired vertical strabismus. This usually results in very bothersome diplopia, the symptom that brings the patient to seek treatment. After bilateral cataract surgery resulting in good vision, patients are intolerant of diplopia and resistant to treatment with prism, possible because these cases often do very well without glasses.

The cause of diplopia after cataract is thought to be myopathy related to local anaesthesia or possibly in some cases to injection of antibiotic or steroids into the extraocular muscle. In a few cases, pre-existing strabismus may be uncovered after surgery and this may be the cause.

Treatment is surgical. In most cases this can be accomplished with an adjustable recession of the inferior rectus or appropriate rectus muscle(s). In a few cases, recession of the superior rectus is required. In these cases, surgery is effective and patients are usually satisfied after one operation under minimal local anaesthesia.

Strabismus after retinal detachment repair

The removal of one or more muscles, dissection around muscles that are not detached, and the placement of various support elements around the globe in the process of retinal detachment repair can produce strabismus. When this occurs, initial treatment should be with prisms. If strabismus persists for 6 to 8 months after retinal surgery, the patient may be a candidate for strabismus surgery. If surgery is carried out, the first requirement is to free any restrictions. If this requires removal of support elements, they can be removed safely after approximately 8 months, but to be certain of the safety of this option the retinal surgeon should be consulted. With or without this consultation, redetachment after strabismus surgery with or without removal of support elements is extremely rare. Because of the wide variety of strabismus types that could follow retinal surgery, no specific recommendations can be given.

Strabismus in myasthenia gravis

Strabismus is common in myasthenia gravis. There is no specific pattern for this strabismus and treatment can be very difficult. For example, while resolution of the ptosis during the Tensilon test is a reliable diagnostic sign, there is often little or no change in the strabismus during this test even in patients who clearly have myasthenia and strabismus. The most effective treatment of strabismus associated with myasthenia is systemic steroids usually in fairly low doses such as 5 to 20 mg of prednisone every other day given for a period of several weeks, tapering off when the acute phase is over. Because of incomitance, prisms are often ineffective, but they may be tried in some cases. Occasionally, surgery is carried out. If elected, either recession, resection or both may be done, but only in long-standing strabismus which is refractory to non-surgical treatment.

Double elevator palsy

Double elevator palsy is a condition where the eye elevates poorly, often with ptosis. Because the eye is elevated by muscles which are innervated by different branches of the third nerve, it is not easy to determine if a discrete neurological deficit causes this condition. It may be due to a brainstem defect which affects gaze rather than specific muscle weakness. Supporting this is the common finding of an intact Bell phenomenon indicating soundness of muscle function and innervation. When this occurs with free ductions, a muscle transfer is a logical surgical option, but this should be undertaken bearing in mind that a large and essentially unexplained exodeviation can occur after what is thought to be a well performed shift of the horizontal recti to the superior rectus. A vertical recession/resection procedure can be effective, especially in cases with mechanical restriction to elevation. If ptosis persists, a small levator resection may be required.

Fibrosis syndrome

Fibrosis syndrome is characterized by bilateral, but sometimes unequal, hypotropia, ptosis, chin-up position, and convergence on attempted upgaze. Of all of the strabismus entities, this condition has the most obvious hereditary pattern, usually being transmitted as an autosomal dominant with nearly complete penetrance. The treatment of fibrosis syndrome is surgical and consists of recession of the inferior and medial recti with a ptosis procedure most appropriate for the degree of levator function. In most cases this turns out to be frontalis suspension.

Sensory esotropia

Strabismus frequently develops when vision is very poor in one eye. The eye may be esotropic or exotropic regardless of the age at which vision is lost. However, when strabismus occurs in the case of unilateral cataract either without treatment or after removal with persistence of deep amblyopia, strabismus is usually a large angle esotropia. This may be associated with vertical downbeating nystagmus only in the affected eye, Heimann-Bielschowsky phenomenon. Sensory esotropia is treated very effectively with an appropriate recession of the medial rectus muscle and resection of the lateral rectus muscle.

Esotropia with high myopia

Patients with very high axial myopia frequently develop large angle esotropia early, occasionally in their twenties but usually later in the fifth decade and beyond. These patients often have very large eyes with refraction of -20 dioptres and more and with globe axial lengths of up to 30 mm. CT scan of the orbits in these patients shows them to be filled with the globe with a thin lateral rectus compressed between the large globe and the lateral wall of orbit. Lateral rectus paresis is easy to infer with this clinical picture. In addition, these patients are likely to have restricted passive abduction. Surgery is the only effective treatment. In such a case the amount of surgery should be increased, being nearly doubled with appropriate bimedial rectus recession and bilateral lateral rectus resection because of the coexistence of mechanical restriction to abduction and lateral rectus weakness.

Guidelines for the management of over- and under-corrections after strabismus surgery

In spite of efforts to produce the best attainable alignment after strabismus surgery, it does occasionally result in an over-orrection, an under-correction, or the appearance of a new problem unrelated to the original strabismus. In each case the patient must be dealt with in a forthright manner which includes prompt and accurate diagnosis and effective timely treatment. The wide variety of problems which could occur after surgery preclude offering a systemic approach to the management of this complex situation. As a rule, a very large and unexpected change in the deviation including a large over-correction or a large under-correction suggests the possibility of a 'lost' muscle, i.e., a muscle which has become detached from the sclera. In addition to the over- or under-correction, this condition is characterized by severely reduced saccadic velocity and reduced generated force in the opposite direction to the over-correction. Muscles that have become detached from the globe require early surgical retreatment. Likewise, severe mechanical restrictions occurring from a resection or a muscle transfer which is too tight also benefit from early reoperation. In cases of mild over- or under-correction, the patient should be observed for approximately 8 weeks. This has been a benchmark for 'final' results of strabismus surgery. If at this time the patient's results are not satisfactory, the strabismus should be assessed as through it were a new case, the findings carefully evaluated, and a surgical plan decided upon. However, when the time comes for surgery, the patient should not be looked upon as an entirely new case because it is obvious that certain muscles have been detached and reattached. As a general rule, at least one anterior ciliary artery should remain intact to avoid the occurrence of anterior segment ischaemia.

This is a very conservative approach. Some surgeons will detach all four muscles in a child, provided the surgery is done in two stages with a reasonable timetable of, for example, 1 year between operations. The likelihood of anterior segment ischaemia increases with the age of the patient, but fortunately is rarely encountered.

When dealing with a new problem after strabismus surgery, that is, a problem unrelated to the strabismus surgery itself, it is simply dealt with in the normal way. In most cases, this new problem is either a conjunctival cyst, scarring, or ptosis. The recognition of an unfavourable surgical result from the first procedure by the surgeon and conveying appropriate concern together with a positive plan for remedying it is very effective in allaying fears and instilling confidence in the patient for the next procedure, whether carried out by the same surgeon or by a consultant.

Further reading

Calhoun, J.H., Nelson, L.B., and Harley, R.D. (1987). *Atlas of paediatric ophthalmic surgery*. Saunders, Philadelphia.
Campos, E.C. (1994). *Manuale di strabismo*, Milan.
Gonzalez, C. (1983). *Strabismus and ocular motility*. Williams and Wilkins, Baltimore.
Helveston, E.M. (1994). *Surgical management of strabismus: an atlas of strabismus surgery*, (4th edn). Mosby, St Louis.
Lang, J.D. (1984). *Strabismus*. Charles B. Slack, Thorofare, NJ.
Lennerstrand, G,. ed. (1994). *Update on strabismus and paediatric ophthalmology*. CRC Press, Boca Raton.
Mein, J. and Harcourt, B. (1986). *Diagnosis and management of ocular motility disorders*. Blackwell, Oxford.
Parks, M.M. (1983). *Atlas of strabismus surgery*. Harper and Row, New York.
Pratt-Johnson, J.A. and Tillson ,G. (1994). *Management of strabismus and amblyopia*. Thieme, New York.
Spielmann, A. (1989) *Les strabismus: de l'analyse clinique a la synthesis chirurgicale*. Masson, Paris.
von Noorden, G.K. (1983). *Atlas of strabismus*, (4th edn). Mosby, St Louis.
von Noorden, G.K. (1995). *Binocular vision and ocular motility*, (5th edn). Mosby, St. Louis.
von Noorden, G.K. and Helveston, E.M. (1994). *Strabismus: a decision making approach*. Mosby, St Louis.
Wright, K.W. (1991). *Color atlas of ophthalmic surgery*. Lippincott, Philadelphia.

2.2.6 Mechanically restricted ocular movements and myopathies

Peter Fells

Brown's syndrome

Harold Brown in 1950 wrote about failure of elevation in adduction of one eye in children which did not show the usual sequelae that would have been expected from paresis of the inferior oblique muscle. He found that this elevation in adduction movement was restricted when attempted under general anaesthesia with forceps—a positive traction test. Because stripping what Brown called the anterior tendon sheath of the superior oblique from the tendon cured his patient he named the condition 'the superior oblique tendon sheath syndrome'. Other surgeons were not able to confirm that this surgical method worked. The condition is now known as Brown's syndrome, but until a positive traction test has been found (and Brown insisted that this was essential) the diagnosis can only be presumed Brown's syndrome. It is not justifiable to carry out the traction test under a general anaesthetic unless there is consent to proceed to surgical treatment if that test is positive. As yet there is no agreed surgical approach so the criteria for intervention must be considered.

1. A marked compensatory head posture of chin elevation and/or face turn towards the opposite side

2. Abandonment of a previously well-documented compensatory head posture

3. A cosmetically noticeable strabismus in primary position.

If there is only a slight or minimal compensatory head posture, or the appearance is acceptable, the child should be assessed every 6 to 12 months. From around 7 years up to 12 years of age there is usually spontaneous improvement in these cases of presumed Brown's syndrome with pain on attempting to elevate the eye in adduction together with a palpable 'click' over the trochlea. This so-called click syndrome is a stage in the spontaneous resolution of Brown's syndrome.

When operation is indicated the diagnosis is first confirmed by a positive traction test; the superior oblique tendon is exposed at the medial border of the superior rectus and the whole tendon and its sheath is transected (Fig. 1). The traction test is repeated and any remaining posterior fibres of superior oblique are cut. This manoeuvre is carried out as many times as necessary until the traction test is normal. Mere improvement is not enough as postoperatively the voluntary excursion of the eye would be as limited as ever. In some 25 per cent of patients a permanent superior oblique palsy results and after 4 to 6 months these patients will benefit from ipsilateral inferior oblique recession.

The aetiology of Brown's syndrome is not fully understood. In some cases the superior oblique muscle and tendon is too short, and in a few patients it is so short that its insertion is medial to the superior rectus. In others the fault probably lies within the trochlea. Not all cases are present at birth and it is best described as a developmental rather than congenital anomaly. Sevel's concept of delayed lysis of the radially running trabeculae between the tendon and the trochlea supports the most common outcome of spontaneous improvement by 12 years of age.

Trauma to the trochlea leads to acquired Brown's syndrome which is very resistant to treatment including surgery.

Orbital blow-out fractures

Blunt trauma to the orbit in addition to producing the classical 'black eye' can cause fractures of the orbital walls. If the orbital rim is intact they are called pure blow-out fractures and the inferior, medial, and, rarely, superior walls may be affected. Symptoms of sensory infraorbital nerve involvement, diplopia due to trapped connective tissue septa and signs of enophthalmos (after initial bruising and swelling have subsided), limited ocular rotations with retraction of the globe on attempted elevation or abduction, and orbital emphysema make the diagnosis. Formal orthoptic assessment of ocular

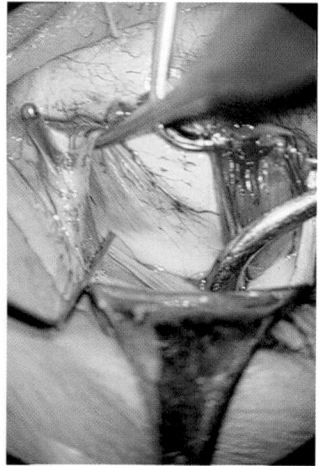

(a)

Surgeon's view from head of table, behind patient's head, of right eye.

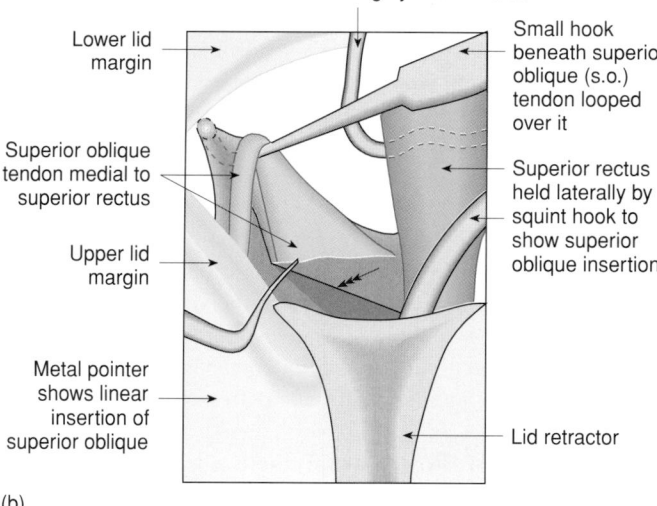

(b)

Fig. 1 (a) View through operating microscope of a shorter than normal superior oblique tendon inserted anteriorly and medially to superior rectus. (b) A shorter than normal superior oblique muscle inserted anteriorly and medial to the superior rectus muscle. The triple arrow indicates where the small hook would be inserted several times to pick up any missed posterior tendon fibres, all of which must be severed before the traction test returns to normal.

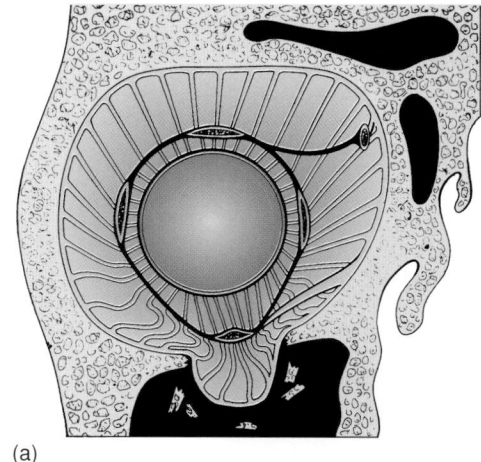

(a)

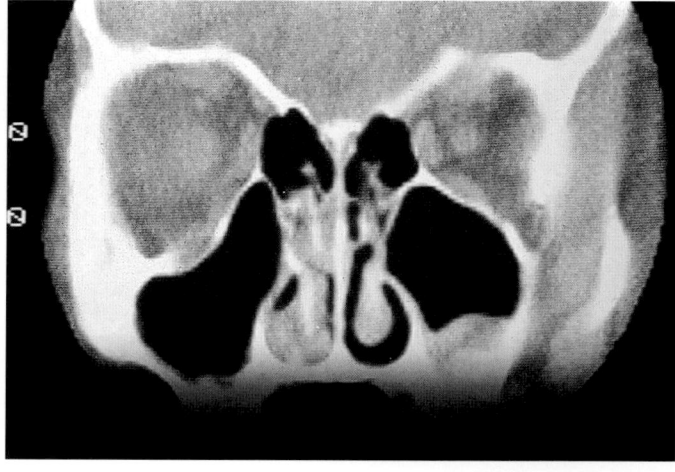

(b)

Fig. 2 (a) Diagram of right orbit with blow-out fracture of the floor showing orbital fat and connective tissue septa herniating into the antrum. The inferior rectus is pulled towards, but not into, the antrum and the medial rectus is dragged downwards by the connective tissue septa. (Reproduced with permission from Koorneef 1982.) (b) CT scan showing fractured floor of right orbital and medial rectus being dragged towards the fracture.

movements, including Hess charts and field of binocular fixation can document any improvement in the early days after injury.

Indications for surgery are 3 mm or more of enophthalmos, marked retraction of the globe on attempting elevation or abduction, and limited ocular movements with diplopia showing no improvement over 10 to 14 days. This group of patients, where surgery is planned, should have CT scans (Fig. 2). There is no place for routine plain radiographs of the orbit for patients suffering blunt injury to the orbit.

For orbital floor fracture surgery should be performed by the ophthalmologist via a skin incision beneath the lower lid. The periosteum is elevated from 4 mm below the inferior orbital rim and the fracture identified beneath the periosteum. Prolapsed orbital fat and trapped connective tissue are returned to the orbit to restore movement and volume and reduce enophthalmos. Connective tissue septa should be freed until the traction test shows full upward movement. The rectus muscles themselves are almost never incarcerated. A thin silicone sheet, shaped to fit and cover the whole orbital floor and not just the fracture, is inserted. The periosteum is sutured over the inferior orbital rim to retain the implant and the skin closed.

If the orbital floor is displaced downwards over a wide area, or is comminuted, it is preferable to do a combined operation with an ear, nose, and throat surgeon. Direct access to the antrum through its anterolateral wall allows freeing of trapped connective tissue septa until the ocular traction test is normal. Bone fragments are repositioned and then supported by an antral pack of ribbon gauze soaked in Whitehead's varnish (pigmentum iodoform compound). Oral antibiotic cover is given for 1 week and the pack removed (after a second general anaesthetic) 2 weeks later.

When the medial wall is fractured with trapped orbital contents combined surgery with an ear, nose, and throat colleague is advised.

Some patients have limited infraduction as well as poor elevation. This may be due to direct damage to the inferior rectus and/or its nerve against the posterior convexity of the orbital floor at the time of the original injury. If there is no improvement in downward movement over 3 months an inverse Knapp procedure, transferring both horizontal recti towards the inferior rectus insertion, should be performed, following which the range of vertical movement increases gradually over a period of several weeks without loss of horizontal movement.

Thyroid eye disease

The enormously enlarged extraocular muscles in thyroid eye disease may cause optic nerve compression as well as restricting ocular rotations with diplopia. If active orbital inflammation cannot be suppressed by retrobulbar radiotherapy and high-dose corticosteroids, surgical decompression via the medial and inferior orbital walls may be needed. Diplopia may change after decompression because of the different tensions within the ocular muscles and the tight medial recti often pull the eyes further into esotropia. Disinsertion of the inferior obliques from their attachment to the anteromedial floor of the orbit during decompression often adds A-pattern to this esotropia. Later, recessions of both medial recti using adjustable sutures correct the esotropia and partial posterior disinsertion of the superior obliques reduces the A-pattern.

If proptosis is greater than 26 mm and ocular movements have remained stable but limited then decompression should be considered first, even in the absence of optic nerve compression, because recessing tight recti will increase the proptosis. Restricted elevation, abduction, and depression are the most common limitations caused by tight inferior recti, medial recti, and superior recti, respectively. Once ocular movements have been shown to be stable, by Hess chart and field of binocular fixation, for at least 6 months surgery can be undertaken (Fig. 3). Tight muscles are confirmed by the traction test and recessed using adjustable sutures. The aim is to undercorrect the hypotropia slightly as further improvement occurs over the next few weeks. The surgeon should not operate on three recti of one eye at the same time in order to avoid anterior segment ischaemia.

If the vertical deviation is more than 20 dioptres this will usually be due to a tight inferior rectus and a tight superior rectus of the fellow eye and both need recessing. Even if the fellow superior rectus is not tight it is better to recess it to correct a large vertical strabismus instead of resecting the ipsilateral superior rectus.

All necessary ocular muscle surgery must have been completed before adjusting lid positions.

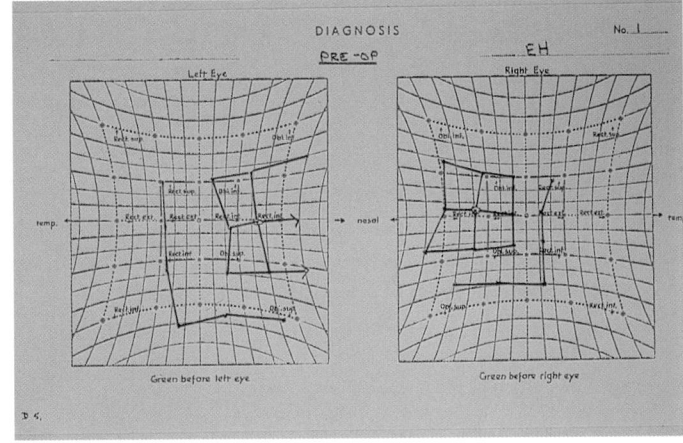

(a)

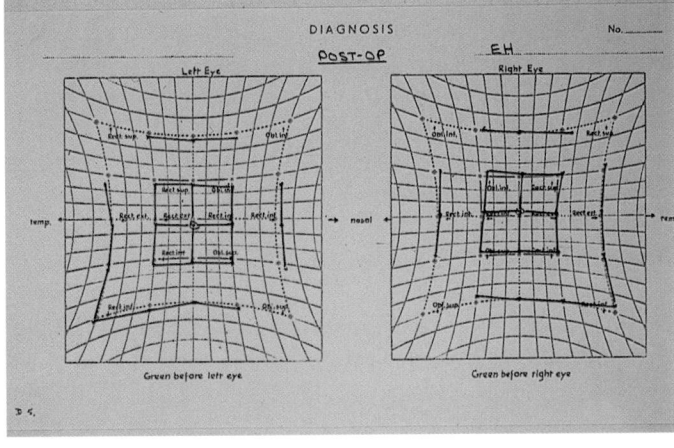

(b)

Fig. 3 (a) Hess chart of patient with thyroid eye disease and a large esotropia of 35 prism dioptres, right hypertropia of 8 prism dioptres, and bilateral inability to elevate the eyes. (b) After surgery to the two tight medial recti and tight inferior recti when all four muscles were recessed, the two muscles on the right side having adjustable sutures. Before the operation there was no area of fusion, but surgery restored a field of binocular single vision to 71 per cent of normal.

Other diseases of ocular muscles

There are a number of primary diseases of muscle which involve systemic and sometimes ocular muscles.

Congenital myopathies

A group of congenital myopathies has been defined structurally with central core myopathy, rod myopathy, myotubular myopathy, multicore disease, and congenital fibre type disproportion. Ptosis and external ophthalmoplegia may occur occasionally in all these conditions to a variable extent.

General fibrosis syndrome

This rare congenital, sometimes familial, condition with autosomal dominant inheritance may also be sporadic. There is a marked compensatory chin elevation with ptoses, often asymmetrical, and the eyes are held in downgaze. Ocular movements are very limited vertically with a wide, shallow A-pattern. Attempting upgaze shows esotropia, while downgaze produces wide exotropia with obvious incyclotorsion (Fig. 4). The eye with the worse ptosis is usually amblyopic. Surgery is difficult with strongly positive traction tests into elevation due to both inferior rectus and superior oblique tightness. Despite maximal inferior rectus recession, more than one operation may be needed to move the fixing eye towards the primary position. Ptosis surgery should be a cautious sling procedure because of absent Bell's phenomenon and high risk of corneal exposure.

Strabismus fixus

Fortunately this is a very rare congenital condition in which both eyes are firmly locked in adduction. Even when the medial recti have been detached from the globe there is no improvement until the deeper and more posteriorly attached fibrous cords have been severed.

Acquired forms of strabismus fixus, either esotropic or exotropic, have been described.

Muscular dystrophies

The muscular dystrophies are a group of genetically determined disorders that cause increasing weakness and wasting of skeletal muscles. Myotonic dystrophy with autosomal dominant inheritance is the commonest. Myotonia (delayed muscle relaxation) is shown typically by slow release of the grasp when shaking hands. Muscle wasting of the face gives a characteristic appearance of ptoses with an open mouth suggesting mental retardation which is often present too. The commonest ocular feature is a multicoloured cataract with minute dot opacities. Testicular atrophy is a late sign.

There is an oculopharyngeal dystrophy occurring in French-Canadian families presenting usually in the fifth decade with dysphagia, and the ptoses and reduced eye movements following years later.

Mitochondrial cytopathies

Chronic progressive external ophthalmoplegia or 'ophthalmoplegia plus' is the commonest type, starting with ptosis and proceeding slowly to complete ophthalmoplegia. There is no diplopia because of the gradual and symmetrical loss of movement. Pigmentary retinopathy of the posterior fundus and cardiac conduction involvement, sometimes with systemic muscle weakness, comprise the Kearns–Sayre syndrome.

Ocular myasthenia gravis

Ocular myasthenia gravis is a form of myasthenia that is limited to the extraocular muscles, the levator palpebrae superioris, and the orbicularis oculi muscles. If there is no evidence of systemic muscle involvement within 2 years it is called ocular myasthenia and will probably stay localized to the eyes. Fifty per cent of patients present with ocular involvement but in only 12 to 15 per cent does the condition remain localized to the eyes.

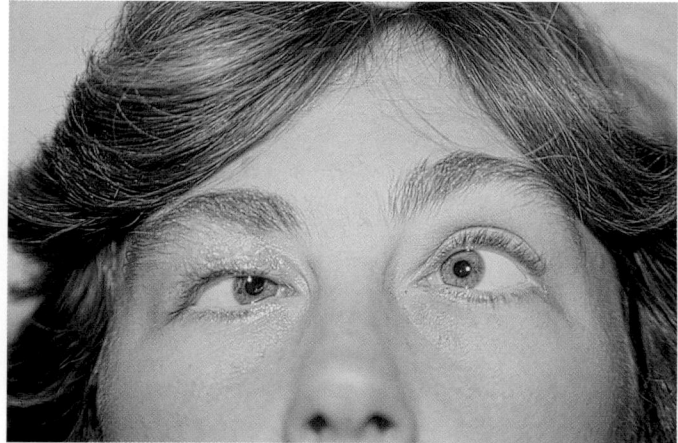

(a)

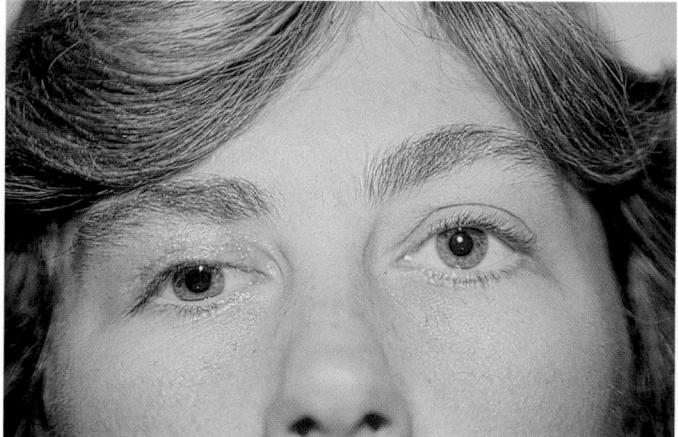

(b)

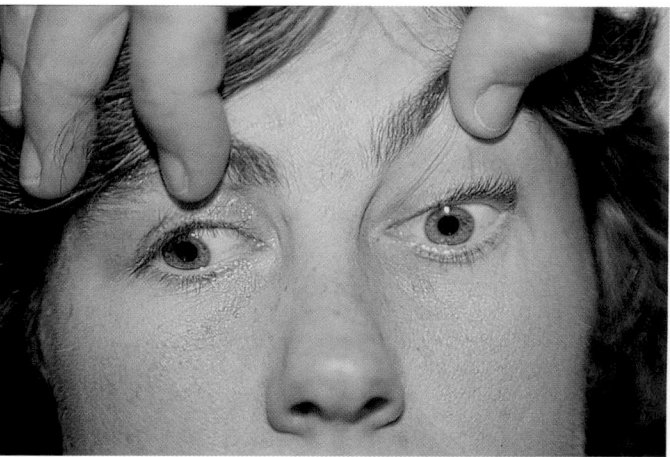

(c)

Fig. 4 A patient with general fibrosis syndrome: wide, shallow A-pattern where the eyes go from large esotropia to wide exotropia with only a very limited total vertical range. The ptotic right eye is amblyopic. (Reproduced with permission from the Medical Illustration Department, Moorfields Eye Hospital, London.)

Between 10 and 20 per cent of patients with ocular myasthenia may show complete or temporary remission over a period of years. These remission rates are improved by corticosteroid therapy.

Ocular muscle paresis (ophthalmoparesis) eventually occurs in 90 per cent of patients with myasthenia gravis. Any muscle may be involved and any type of ocular paresis mimicked, including internuclear ophthalmoplegia. Ptosis may be unilateral or asymmetrically bilateral and shows a lid twitch (Cogan's sign) when the eye moves from downgaze to the primary position. The orbicularis oculi is weak bilaterally. The symptoms may show variation during the day, and sustained fixation in full upgaze becomes fatigued and ptosis increases. The Tensilon test, where edrophonium chloride is injected intravenously, produces an immediate improvement in ptosis and ocular movement.

Some patients can be symptomatically relieved with Fresnel prisms. If the ocular movements are reasonably stable for 6 months or longer built-in prisms or ocular muscle surgery may be used with benefit in selected cases.

Further reading

Bhattacharya, J., Moseley, I.F., and Fells, P. (1997). The role of plain radiography in the management of suspected orbital blow-out fractures. *British Journal of Radiology*, **70**, 29–33.

Fells, P. (1993). Management of thyroid eye disease. In *Surgical Endocrinology* (ed. J. Lynn and S.R. Bloom), pp. 312–23. Butterworth-Heinemann, London.

Fells, P., Waddell, E., and Alvares, M. (1984). Progressive, exaggerated A-pattern strabismus with presumed fibrosis of extraocular muscles. In *Strabismus*, Vol. II, (ed. R.D. Reinecke), pp. 335–43. Grune & Stratton, New York.

Helveston, E.M., Merrian, W.W., Ellis, F.D., Shellhamer, R.H., and Gosling, C.G. (1982). The trochlea. A study of the anatomy and physiology. *Ophthalmology*, **89**, 124–33.

Koornneef, L. (1982). Current concepts on the management of orbital blow-out fractures. *Annals of Plastic Surgery*, **9**, 185–200.

Miller, N.R. (1985). Myopathies and disorders of neuromuscular transmission. In *Walsh and Hoyt's clinical neuro-ophthalmology*, Vol. 2, (4th edn) pp. 785–891. Williams & Wilkins, Baltimore, MD.

Rave, N.L. and Williams, J.Ll. (1994). Fractures of the zygomatic complex and orbit. *Rowe and Williams maxillofacial injuries*, (2nd edn) (ed. J.L.I. Williams), Vol. 1, pp. 475–590. Churchill Livingstone, Edinburgh.

Sevel, D. (1981). Brown's syndrome—a possible etiology explained embryologically. *Journal of Pediatric Ophthalmology and Strabismus*, **18**, 26–31.

Waddell, E. (1982). Brown's syndrome revisited. *British Orthoptic Journal*, **39**, 17–21.

Waddell, E., Fells, P., and Koornneef, L. (1982). The natural and unnatural history of a blow-out fracture. *British Orthoptic Journal*, **39**, 29–32.

Weinberg, D.A., Lesser, R.L., and Vollmer, T.L. (1994). Ocular myasthenia: a protean disorder. *Survey of Ophthalmology*, **39**, 169–210.

2.2.7 Botulinum toxin

Sarah Vickers

Clostridium botulinum is a ubiquitous Gram-negative organism, which under anaerobic conditions produces seven toxins. Ingestion of food containing these toxins produces the disease of botulism, an acute symmetrical descending paralysis.

At the neuromuscular junction the toxin binds to a specific receptor site on the terminal non-myelinated axon, and prevents the release of acetylcholine from the nerve terminals. Paralysis of the muscle then follows by the exhaustion of the vesicular acetylcholine. The affected neuromuscular junctions are permanently inactivated, and muscle function returns only once new junctions are established by a process of sprouting from presynaptic axons; clinically this takes approximately 8 weeks.

Clinical use of botulinum toxin A

In the 1970s Alan Scott pioneered the clinical use of botulinum toxin A by injection into extraocular muscles with the aim of providing an alternative to strabismus surgery. As a spin-off from this work he also suggested it might be of use for conditions such as blepharospasm. The efficacy of this treatment has led to the use of botulinum toxin A in many focal dystonias, such as spasmodic torticollis, hemifacial spasm, spasmodic dysphonia, and writer's cramp.

The small quantities of botulinum toxin used for treating eye movement disorders preclude systemic intoxication and no incidences have been reported in over 40 000 treatments.

Toxin for squint

Technique

The commercial preparation of botulinum toxin A is stable until reconstituted into solution. It must be used within hours as its effectiveness rapidly deteriorates. The standard unit of measuring potency is derived from mouse assays. The potency of botulinum toxin A varies with the manufacturer and accompanying directions should be consulted for appropriate dosages. The dose used in strabismus is less than 1/100 of the estimated human median lethal dose (LD_{50}), and at these low dosages the formation of antibodies is not of clinical significance.

To obtain the best results, the botulinum toxin A is injected into the rectus muscle near the motor end plate, which is approximately 2.5 cm behind the muscle insertion. To localize the needle point position an electromyograph response from the tip of the needle is monitored. Once the needle has been advanced into the muscle to be injected, the site of maximal muscular activity is located by asking the patient to look in the direction of the muscle being injected and observe the resulting increase in the electromyograph signal. As the toxin is then injected slowly, the electromyograph signal will diminish as the muscle tissue is pushed away from the needle tip by the entering fluid. The needle is then left *in situ* for 30 seconds to minimize the efflux of toxin back along the needle track which otherwise may cause ptosis (Fig. 1).

Anaesthesia

In co-operative adults and children over the age of 10 years topical anaesthesia provides sufficient anaesthesia prior to injection. When sedation is required in children, ketamine anaesthesia is recommended as it preserves the electromyograph signal required to monitor the injections for strabismus.

Indications for treatment

In common with the basic principles of strabismus treatment, results are most effective if the potential for fusion is present; and for strabismus measuring less than 50 dioptres, larger angles may require several injections.

Botulinum toxin is particularly useful in the treatment of paralytic strabismus, in postoperative small residual angles, in the prediction of the presence or absence of postoperative diplopia, and for the investigation of fusional areas and suppression. Botulinum toxin A is also of value where further strabismus surgery is inappropriate due to multiple previous operations, were they for squint, retinal detachment, or orbital trauma.

Botulinum toxin as a first line of treatment in children remains controversial; many patients require more than one injection with its attendant general anaesthesia, and a significant number require further surgery.

Horizontal strabismus

Horizontal strabismus responds well to toxin injections reducing the deviation by approximately 70 per cent in the majority of cases although the effect is short-lived. In the cases of small surgical over- and undercorrections, botulinum toxin can be very useful producing adequate alignment in 87 per cent of patients.

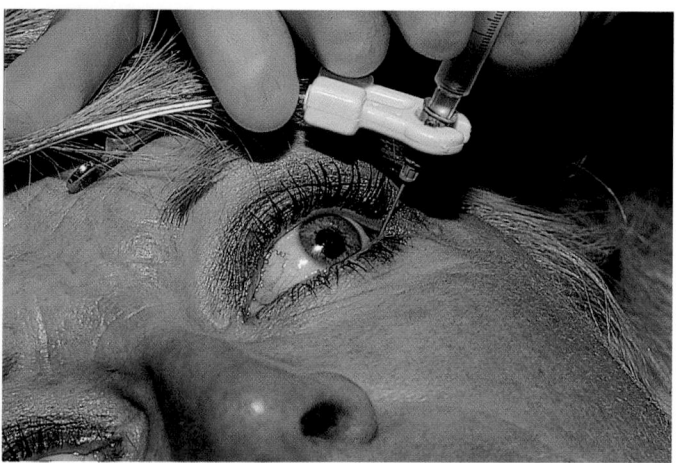

Fig. 1 Botulinum toxin A injection into lateral rectus muscle.

Paralytic squint

In an unrecovered sixth nerve palsy, where medial rectus contracture may be masking lateral rectus recovery, botulinum toxin A is a useful diagnostic tool. An injection of botulinum toxin A into the ipsilateral medial rectus may reveal one of three things: (a) following one injection full recovery of the lateral rectus and binocularity may result; (b) following a medial rectus injection a partial recovery of lateral rectus function may be evident, in which case a simple medial rectus resection and lateral rectus recession operation may be curative. (c) After paralysis of the medial rectus with toxin, if there is no abduction of the eye beyond the midline, the indication is that there is no lateral rectus recovery (Fig. 2).

In this case temporal transposition of superior and inferior rectus (Hummelsheim) can be performed in conjunction with a preoperative medial rectus botulinum toxin A injection. This procedure reduces the incidence of anterior segment ischaemia by limiting incisional surgery to two rectus muscles. Immediately postoperatively a marked exotropia may occur, but with the recovery of medial rectus function, binocularity hopefully will be re-established (Fig. 3).

Occasionally a subsequent ipsilateral medial rectus recession may be required if a degree of esotropia returns and this surgery can be safely performed 6 months later, once anterior segment perfusion is re-established.

In third nerve palsies toxin is useful in exploring fusion potential, contracture development, and in assessing the potential for useful surgery.

Fourth nerve palsies present a problem. It is difficult to paralyse the ipsilateral inferior oblique without affecting the inferior rectus and therefore the assessment of the toxin injection result becomes complex.

Vertical strabismus

The inferior rectus muscle is the only muscle that is routinely injected for vertical deviation. In uncomplicated cases an average of 30 dioptres of height may be corrected, technically this is easier to achieve using a transdermal as opposed to a transconjuntival approach (Fig. 4).

The results of the injection of superior muscles have proved disappointing because of the complication of ptosis.

Childhood strabismus

There is now evidence that botulinum toxin A can offer an alternative to incisional surgery in children; the change in alignment being more stable than that achieved in adults, presumably due to the establishment of binocular fusion. Some authors believe best results are achieved in under 6 months of age where contracture has not had a chance to develop in the ipsilateral antagonist. Others dispute the increased efficacy of botulinum toxin A over incisional surgery in this age group.

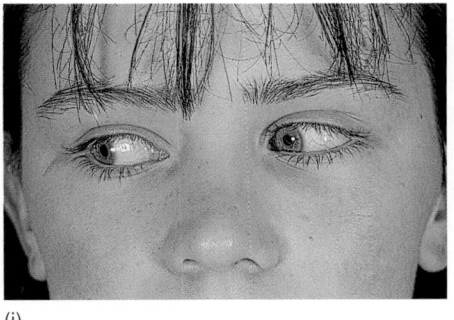 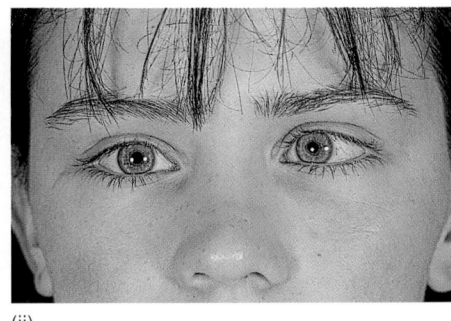 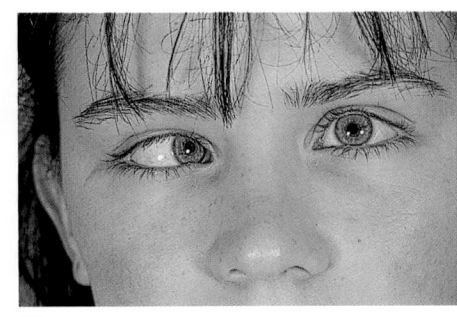

(i) (ii) (iii)

Fig. 2 (a) Left sixth nerve palsy before toxin.

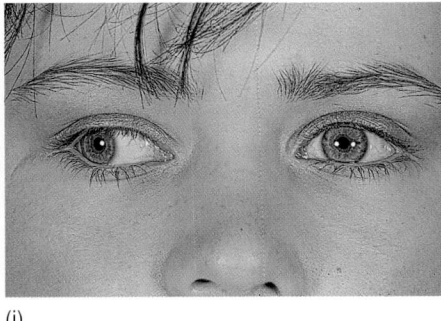 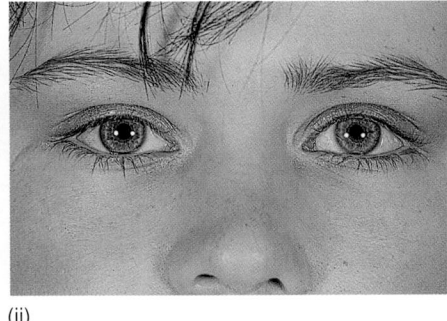 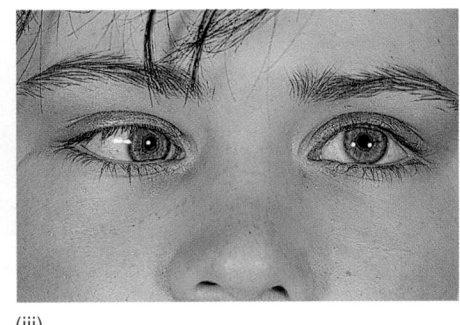

(i) (ii) (iii)

Fig. 2 (b) Left sixth nerve palsy after toxin with paralysed left medial rectus and still no abduction.

Complications of botulinum toxin A injection

Short-lived complications include:

- spread of botulinum toxin A to adjacent muscles causing ptosis or unwanted induced vertical or horizontal deviations

- subconjunctival haemorrhage

- retrobulbar haemorrhage.

Accidental scleral puncture

In this instance the electromyograph signal will go silent. In the suspected cases of scleral puncture the pupil will be dilated for careful retinal examination and any retinal holes appropriately treated. In a reported 8600 injections, nine scleral punctures resulted, in which there have been no adverse visual sequelae.

Limitations of treatment

The effect of botulinum toxin A on ocular deviation is temporary, lasting 2 to 6 months and maintenance of the altered ocular position requires repeated injections, although in most cases a small permanent reduction in angle of 10 dioptre or less can occur following injection.

Treatment of the medial and lateral rectus and inferior rectus and oblique are routine but attempts to treat the superior rectus and oblique usually result in ptosis.

Established muscle contracture, for example in cases of dys-thyroid ophthalmopathy, will limit the extent of flaccid paralysis produced.

Nystagmus

In a case of intractable oscillopsia caused by nystagmus or ocular flutter, botulinum toxin A has proved to be moderately effective; either by retrobulbar injection into the muscle cone, or by direct rectus muscle injection, to reduce the amplitude and frequency of the ocular oscillation. Bilateral injection produces an incomitant strabismus; therefore only one eye is treated and the other occluded.

Eyelid disorders and abnormal facial movements

Essential blepharospasm is an involuntary bilateral closure of the eyelids, commonly presenting to ophthalmologists. Blepharospasm may be isolated, or part of a more extensive dystonia. Some patients may have coexisting blepharitis or dry eyes which may act as a trigger for the dystonia and these should be treated appropriately. Blepharospasm may also occur in association with Parkinson's and Wilson's disease, and evidence of these should be sought. Prior to the introduction of botulinum toxin for the treatment of essential blepharospasm, the procedure of choice was the stripping of the facial nerve, but botulinum toxin has proved to be so effective that this approach has been largely abandoned. Adjunctive therapy with centrally acting anticholinergic therapy may be necessary (Fig. 5).

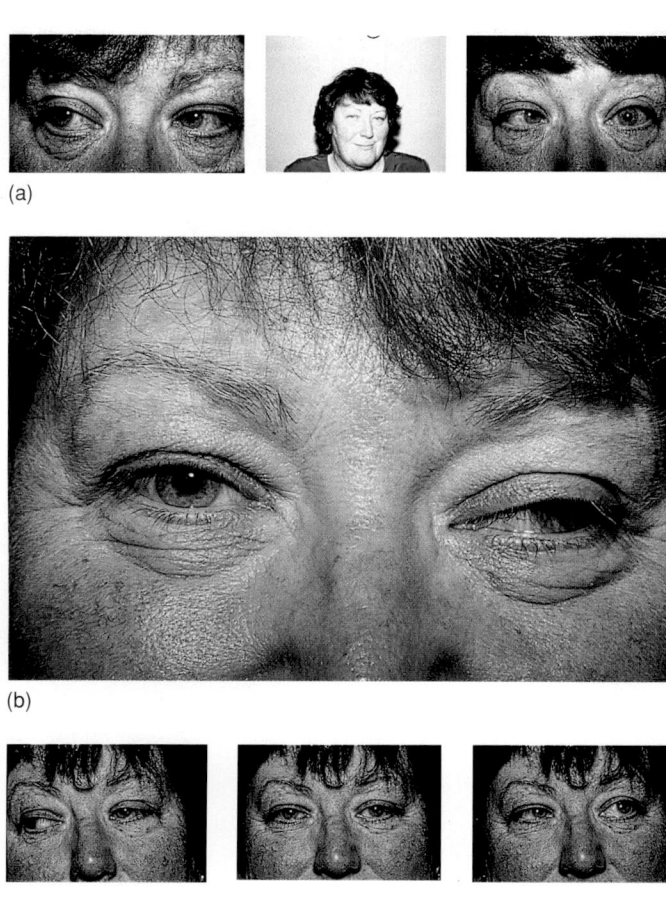

(a)

(b)

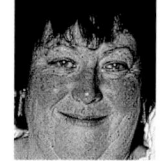

(c)

Fig. 3 (a) Left sixth nerve palsy. (b) Left sixth nerve palsy after transposition and left medial rectus botulinum toxin A with exotropia. (c) Once medial rectus botulinum toxin A worn off.

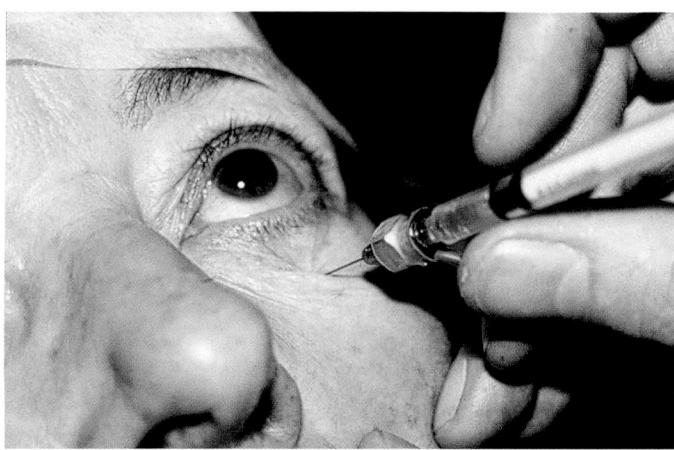

Fig. 4 Translid approach to the inferior rectus or inferior oblique.

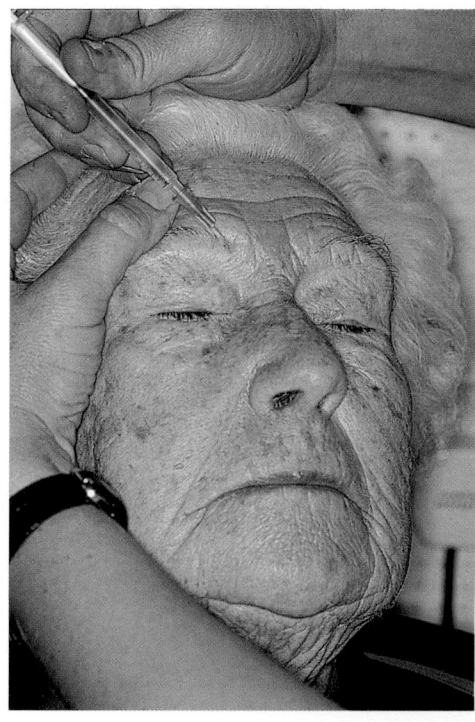

Fig. 5 Technique of injection for blepharospasm or hemifacial spasm.

The technique is by local injection of toxin solution in divided doses into the affected orbicularis oculi muscles, which being superficial do not require electromyograph monitoring. The injections are given at the junction of the orbital and pre-septal orbicularis. The injections into the upper lid are directed away from the levator, to minimize the chances of ptosis as an unwanted side-effect. Clinical improvement is usually noticed by the patient in 12 to 24 h.

Complications

Complications include:

- periorbital oedema
- Ptosis
- spread to extraocular muscles producing unwanted, usually vertical muscle imbalance, which is short lived and can be treated temporally with prisms
- lower facial weakness.

Limitations

Injections for a blepharospasm have to be repeated about every 3 to 4 months.

Hemifacial spasm

This is an involuntary unilateral synchronous contraction of those muscles innervated by the facial nerve, often caused by compression of the facial nerve in the posterior fossa by an aberrant arteriole. However, other cranial nerves should be examined carefully to exclude other aetiological factors. The definitive treatment, if appropriate, is that of a posterior fossa microvascular decompression of the facial nerve. However, in those patients who would be at significant risk of a neuro-surgical procedure, botulinum toxin treatment is used with good effect.

Chemical ptosis

In corneal disease where corneal cover is required, or during the recovery phase of a facial nerve palsy, for example, following an acoustic neuroma resection, botulinum toxin can be used to produce a 'protective' chemical ptosis. The advantages are that such a procedure is reversible and does not damage the lid margin, which may in turn compromise the tear film at a later date. The disadvantages are that the superior rectus is usually also paralysed, causing disruption of the protective Bell's phenomenon and on occasions a hypotropia.

Further reading

American Academy of Ophthalmologists (1989). Ophthalmic procedures assessment: botulinum toxin therapy of eye muscle disorders. *Ophthalmology*, 2, 37–41.

Buckley, E.G. (1993). Chemodeviation of extraocular muscles. *Duane's clinical ophthalmology*, Vol. 6, pp.1–14. Lippincott Raven, New York.

Campos, E.C. (1993). New indications for BTXA in strabismus and medical treatment of amblyopia. *Current Opinions in Ophthalmology*, 4, 34–6.

Elston, J.S. (1988). The clinical use of botulinum toxin. *Seminars in Ophthalmology*, 3, 249–60.

Ing, M.R. (1993). Botulinum alignment for congenital esotropia. *Ophthalmology*, 3, 318–22.

Kao, I., Drachman, D.B., and Price, D.L.(1976). Botulinum toxin: mechanism of presynaptic blockage. *Science*, 193, 1256–8.

Lee, J., Elston, J., *et al.* (1988). Botulinum therapy for squint. *Eye*, 2 (part 1), 24–8.

Scott, A.B. (1980). Botulinum toxin injection into extra-ocular muscles as an alternative to strabismus surgery. *Ophthalmology*, 87, 1044–9.

Scott, A.B., Rosenbaum, A., and Collins, C.C. (1973). Pharmacological weakening of extra ocular muscles. *Investigative Ophthalmology and Visual Science*, 12, 924–7.

Scott, A.B., Magoon, E.H., *et al.* (1990). Botulinum treatment of childhood strabismus. *Ophthalmology*, 97, 1434–8.

2.3 Clinical optics and refraction

2.3.1 Optical principles

Rachel V. North

The properties of light have been discussed elsewhere in this text. This chapter will outline some optical principles including reflection, refraction, and diffraction.

Reflection

Reflection occurs when light rebounds from a surface. Reflection at a surface may be classified as (a) regular (specular), from a good quality surface such as polished silver, when nearly all the light is reflected in definite directions; or (b) irregular (diffuse) when irregularity of the surface leads to reflection of light in different directions. Diffuse reflecting surfaces can be considered to be numerous randomly arranged regular reflectors.

Laws of reflection

There are two laws which relate to the reflection of light at any surface/interface. First, the incident ray, the reflected ray, and the normal to the reflecting surface all lie in the same plane. Second, the angle of incidence (i) equals the angle of reflection (r). Thus a ray of light AB (incident ray) will be reflected along the path BC (reflected ray) and the angle of incidence will be equal to the angle of reflection ($i = r$) (Fig. 1). These laws apply to both plane and curved reflectors.

Reflection at a plane surface

Point source

The light from a point source positioned at A will be reflected at the surface of a mirror. The image of object A is seen at point B and is known as a virtual image (not a real image). It is called a virtual image because the rays of light appear to intersect at point B but they actually do not (Fig. 2).

The virtual image will lie along a line which is perpendicular to the reflecting surface and at an equal distance behind as the real object is in front.

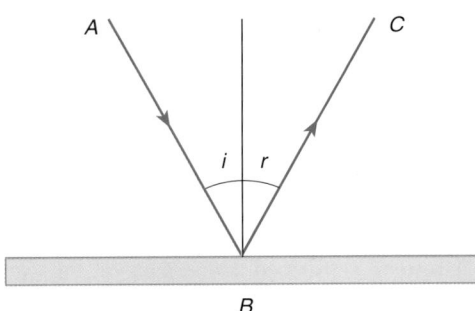

Fig. 1 Reflection of light at a plane surface (i = angle of incidence, r = angle of reflection).

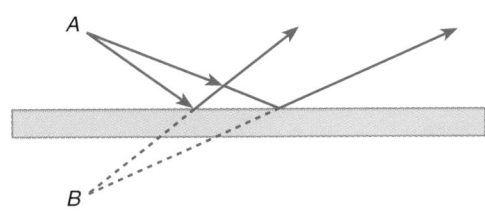

Fig. 2 Reflection of a point source at a plane surface.

Object

An object (larger than a point source) when viewed in a mirror will undergo what is known as lateral inversion. The image will appear horizontally reversed. This is the reason why Snellen chart letters are printed in reverse if they are to be viewed indirectly by a mirror.

Rotation of a mirror

If a plane mirror is rotated while the rays of light fall upon its centre of rotation then the reflected ray turns through twice the angle turned through by the mirror.

To summarize, the image formed by a vertical plane mirror can be described as follows:

- the distance of the apparent image behind the mirror is equal to the distance of the object in front of the mirror

- the object and image size are equal

- the image is virtual and upright

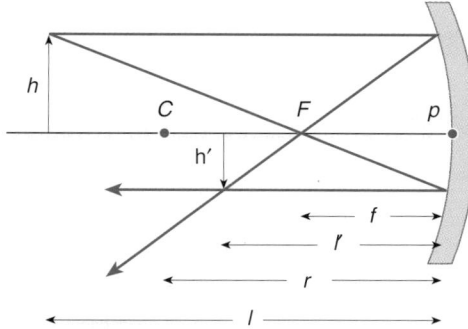

Fig. 3 Reflection from a concave spherical surface—object and image distance and heights.

• the image is laterally inverted.

Reflection of light at curved surfaces

A spherical mirror is formed from part of the surface of a sphere. Mirrors can be classified as (a) concave, if the inner surface of the sphere is coated with a reflecting surface; and (b) convex, if the outer surface of the sphere is coated with a reflecting layer. Curved mirrors can be used instead of lenses to form images of objects, for example they are used in slide projectors and reflecting telescopes.

Notation

Refer to Fig. 3. The following notation is used in this chapter:

C = centre of curvature of the spherical reflecting surface
P = pole (vertex) of the mirror (midpoint of the reflecting surface)
PC = principal axis of the mirror = radius of curvature of the mirror
F = principal focus of the mirror
FP = focal length of the mirror
$f = \dfrac{\text{radius of curvature}}{2}$

Any other axis (line passing through the centre of curvature) is known as a subsidiary axis.

The position, size, and orientation of the image formed by a spherical reflecting surface can be found by using the following two rules:

1. Rays of light parallel to the principal axis, *PC*, are reflected towards or away from the principal focus, *F*

2. Rays of light from the top of an object, passing through the centre of curvature, *C*, will be reflected back along the same path.

Light parallel to the principal axis, PC

1. A narrow pencil of light will be reflected from a concave surface and converged to pass through a real single point, known as the principal focus, *F*. If the mirror is convex, the rays diverge from an apparent point, *F*, which is a virtual point.

2. If a broad beam of light is reflected then the reflected rays do not all pass through a single point focus. This problem associated with a spherical surface is known as spherical aberration.

Calculation of the position of the image formed by a spherical mirror

This is given by the formula:

$$\frac{1}{l} + \frac{1}{l'} = \frac{1}{f} = \frac{2}{r}$$

where l = distance of the object from the mirror, l' = distance of the image from the mirror, f = focal length of the mirror, and r = radius of curvature of the mirror.

$$\text{Magnification} = \frac{\text{image size}}{\text{object size}}$$
$$= \frac{h'}{h}$$
$$= \frac{-l'}{l}$$

Table 1 summarizes the image position and characteristics created by concave and convex spherical reflecting surfaces.

The Cartesian sign convention which must be used is illustrated in Fig. 4.

A ray diagram should show light travelling from left to right and the focal length and radius of curvature will be positive values for convex mirrors and negative for concave mirrors (therefore the value of l, the distance from the object to the mirror, will be negative).

Table 1 Summary of the image location and nature formed by reflecting surfaces

Location of object	Position of image	Size of image	Nature of image
Concave mirror			
infinity (ω)	At *F*	Very small	
between ω and *C*	Between *F* and *C*	Smaller	
at *C*	At *C*	Equal size	Real and inverted
between *C* and *F*	Between *C* and ω	Larger	
between *F* and *P*	Behind surface	Larger	Virtual and upright
Convex mirror	Any position	Smaller	Virtual and upright

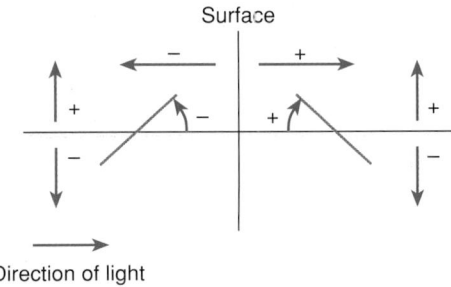

Fig. 4 The Cartesian sign convention (for reflection and refraction at curved surfaces).

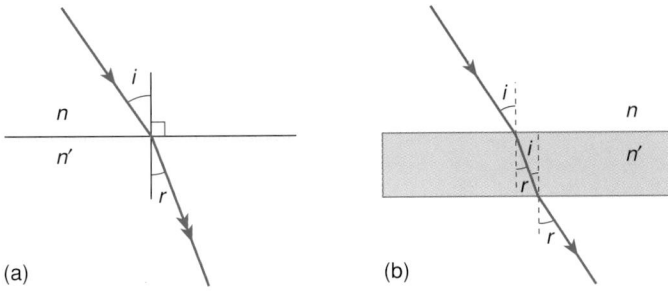

Fig. 6 Refraction of light (a) entering a medium of higher refractive index, and (b) through a plate of glass.

Refraction

Refraction is the change in direction of the path of light as it passes obliquely from one medium to another having a different index of refraction. Therefore when a ray of light in air falls on a glass surface, some light will be reflected, some will be absorbed, but most will be transmitted. The direction of the ray in glass will be different from that in the air. This change in direction is known as refraction. Plastics and glass are used to make ophthalmic lenses because of their refractive properties and transparency.

Refraction at a plane surface

Light travels more slowly in an optically denser medium. So, as can be seen in Fig. 5, when part of the beam of light falls on the glass surface, it slows down and as the beam in the air travels distance *AB* the same wave in the glass moves more slowly and will travel a shorter distance *CD*. The beam will deviate or be bent towards the normal.

The speed of light in a given medium depends upon the wavelength of light and consequently the index varies accordingly. The index of refraction is the ratio of the speed of light in a vacuum or in air to the speed of light in a given medium, referred to as the absolute and relative index respectively:

$$\text{Absolute index of refraction} = \frac{\text{speed of light in a vacuum}}{\text{speed off light in medium}}$$

$$\text{Relative index of refraction} = \frac{\text{speed of light in air}}{\text{speed of light in medium}}$$

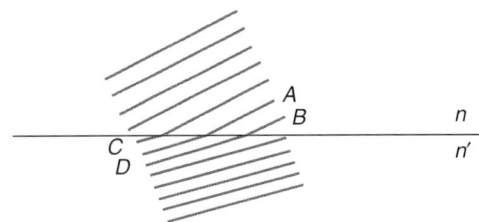

Fig. 5 Refraction of a beam of light entering a medium of higher refractive index.

Laws of refraction

The incident ray will make an angle of incidence, i, to the normal. The refracted ray will make an angle of refraction, r, to the normal (Fig. 6(a)). According to Snell's law the angles vary depending upon the refractive index of the media involved. The incident and the refracted ray lie in one plane which is normal to the refracting surface at the point of refraction. The angle of incidence and angle of refraction are related to the refractive index, n, of the media:

$$\text{Snell's law: } \frac{n'}{n} = \frac{\sin i}{\sin r}$$

where n and n' = the refractive index of the two media, that is

$$\frac{\sin i}{\sin i} = \text{constant}$$

This applies for monochromatic light.

Examples of refractive index

Vacuum = 1   lowest value
Air = 1.00027 (taken as 1)
Water = 1.33
Cornea = 1.37
Crystalline lens = 1.38–1.42
Crown glass = 1.523
Polycarbonate = 1.39
CR39 = 1.50
Diamond = 2.42   highest known value

Therefore, if the media are air and another:

$$n' = \frac{\sin i}{\sin r}$$

as $n = 1$.

The Reversibility Principle states that if a reflected or refracted ray be reversed in direction it will return along its original path.

If a ray of light passes through a sheet of glass, the light is bent/deviated laterally, as shown in Fig. 6(b). It then emerges

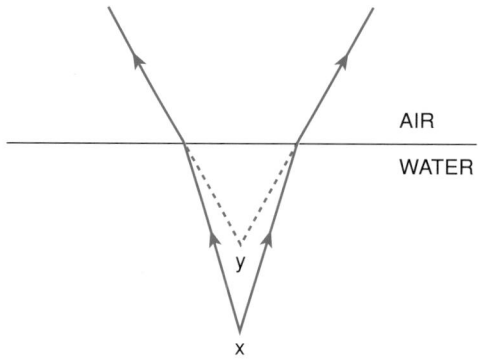

Fig. 7 Refraction: real and apparent depth.

in a direction parallel to the incident ray, so that the ray of light is laterally displaced but has not changed its direction.

Real and apparent depth

Objects positioned within a medium of greater refractive index appear to be closer than they actually are. Hence objects submerged in water appear to be closer to the surface than their true position. This is due to refraction of the emerging rays which diverge and appear to originate from a point closer to the surface. For example, in Fig. 7 an object located at x appears to be positioned at point y.

Refraction at a curved surface

When light travels from one medium to another of a higher refractive index then light rays will be bent towards the normal (Snell's law). When light travels from air through glass, if the surface of the glass is convex then the light will be converged and if it is concave the light will be diverged.

The power of the refracting surface, F, can be calculated:

$$F = \frac{n'-n}{r}$$

where F is measured in dioptres, n = refractive index of the first medium, n' = refractive index of second medium, and r = radius of curvature of surface (m).

Principal foci

For a converging spherical surface, as seen in Fig. 8, the following definitions apply:

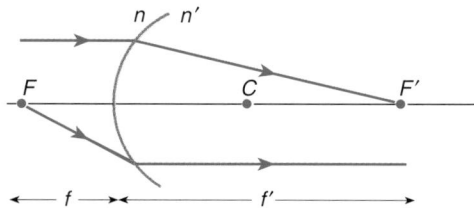

Fig. 8 Principal foci of a converging spherical refracting surface.

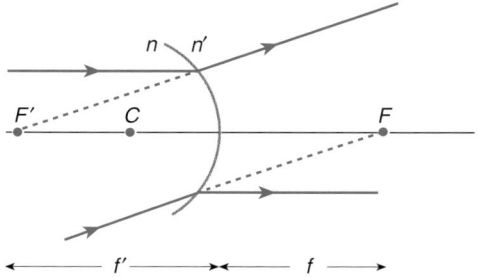

Fig. 9 Principal foci of a diverging spherical refractive surface.

- the first principal focus, F, is the point on the axis which creates an *image* at infinity

- the second principal focus, F', is the image corresponding to an *object* point at infinity.

Both, F and F', are *real* points with the refracted and incident rays being parallel to the axis, respectively.

For a diverging spherical surface as seen in Fig. 9 the same definitions apply except that F and F' are *virtual* object and image points, respectively.

The vergences of the incidence and refracted light can be referred to as L and L' respectively, where:

$$\text{Object vergence } L = \frac{n}{l} \text{ and image vergence } L' = \frac{n'}{l'}$$

The unit of vergence is the dioptre when the values of l and l' are given in metres. Therefore we can obtain what is known as the fundamental paraxial equation:

$$L' = L + F$$

This equation can be applied to mirrors, and single refracting surfaces.

The lateral magnification is the ratio of the size of the image to the size of the object:

$$\text{Magnification} = \frac{h'}{h}$$
$$= \frac{L'}{L}$$

where h' = image size and h = object size. If the value is positive then the image is upright and on the same side of the surface as the object. If the value is negative then the image is inverted and on the opposite side of the surface as the object. This applies to both refraction and reflection at a single surface.

Total internal reflection and the critical angle

When rays of light travel from a higher to a lower refractive index then rays will deviate away from the normal and hence

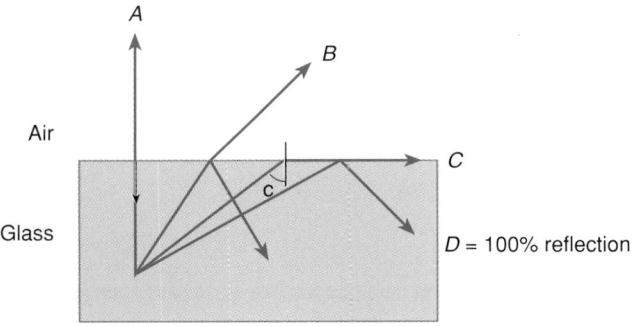

Fig. 10 Total internal reflection and the critical angle (c).

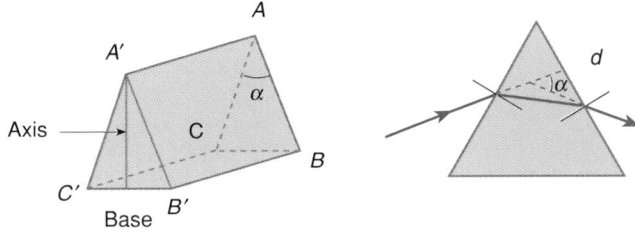

Fig. 11 Prism construction and the deviation of light (d = angle of deviation).

the angle of refraction is larger than the angle of incidence (Fig. 10). Rays of light will behave differently when they meet the interface depending upon the angle of incidence.

If the rays are incident normally at the interface, that is at 90°, then they will pass straight through without any deviation. Rays that meet the interface more obliquely will be refracted less and reflected more. Therefore the refracted ray becomes dimmer and the reflected ray brighter with increasing angle of incidence. At a certain angle, known as the critical angle (c), the refracted ray will run parallel to the interface.

If the angle of incidence is larger than the critical angle, then all the rays will be reflected back from the interface and this is known as total internal reflection. Therefore the minimum angle of incidence beyond which total internal reflection occurs is called the critical angle. Using Snell's law:

$$\sin i_c = \frac{n'}{n}$$

For a glass to air interface, the critical angle is:

$$\sin i_c = \frac{1}{1.523}$$
$$i_c = 41.2°$$

($n' = 1$ and $n = 1.523$). It is total internal reflection that prevents the angle of the anterior chamber from being viewed directly. Hence the use of a gonioscopy lens, a contact lens of a higher refractive index than the cornea, which permits a view of the angle as the cornea to air interface has been eliminated.

Refraction by prisms

A prism consists of two transparent surfaces inclined at an angle to one another. The two refracting surfaces of the prism are $AA'B'B$ and $AA'C'C$ which meet at the apex (refracting edge) of the prism. The face opposite the apex is the base (Fig. 11).

The angle between the refracting surfaces is called the apical angle, α. The axis of the prism is the line which bisects the angle. Once again, light traversing a prism will obey Snell's law at each surface. Therefore, a ray of light is bent/deviated towards the base of the prism and the image will appear to be

displaced towards the apex of the prism. The image will appear to be upright (erect) and virtual.

The angle of deviation of the light, angle d, produced by a prism will depend on the refractive index of the prism, the apical angle, and the angle of the incident light. For ophthalmic prisms where the apical angle is small (usually less than 15°), the angle of deviation $d = (n-1)\alpha$, where n is the refractive index of the prism. For a prism with a refractive index of 1.5, the angel of deviation is half the apical angle, as $d = (1.5-1)\ \alpha = \alpha/2$.

The power of a prism can be described in terms of its apical angle or the deviation of light produced. Ophthalmic prisms are usually marked with their deviation in prism dioptres or far less frequently in degrees. One prism dioptre (1 Δ), represents a deviation of 1 cm on a flat surface 100 cm (1 m) away from the prism (Fig. 12). A prism power of 5 Δ will produce a displacement of 5 cm on a surface 100 cm away.

The prism dioptre is a unit of angular measure being the angle whose tangent is 0.01 (1/100). Therefore the power (P) in prism dioptres and deviation (d) produced in degrees is:

$$P\Delta = 100 \tan d$$
$$1\Delta = 100 \tan d$$
$$\tan d = 0.01$$
$$d = 0.57°$$

that is 1 prism dioptre deviates the light by 0.57°.

A centrad (V) is a unit in which the image displacement is measured along an arc 1 m from the prism instead of on a flat screen. It therefore gives a very slightly larger angle of deviation compared to prism dioptres.

When prisms are prescribed for ocular muscle imbalances

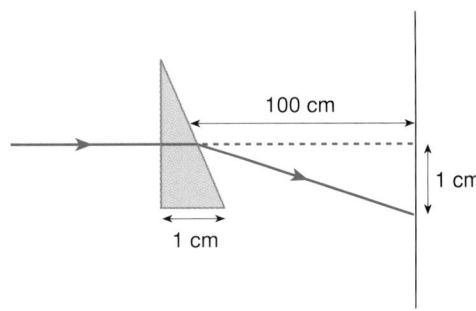

Fig. 12 Notation of prisms: the prism dioptre.

then the power of the prism is given and the direction of the prism, for example 6 Δ base out or 2 Δ base down.

Total reflection in a prism

There will be circumstances when the angle of incidence at the first surface of a prism will be such that the light will meet the second surface at an angle greater than the critical angle and therefore the light will be totally reflected.

Images viewed through a prism

The image viewed through a prism will appear upright, virtual, and shifted towards the apex. Light from a near object will diverge and meet the first surface at different angles. As the deviation of each ray of light depends upon the angle of incidence then the rays will be refracted by differing amounts. The light will not appear to be a point but a short line, an astigmatic image. However, the astigmatic image can be eliminated if the incident light is parallel, not diverging.

Another problem encountered when viewing through a prism is colour dispersion. The light, unless monochromatic, will be dispersed with each wavelength being deviated by different amounts. Hence a small white object will appear as a spectrum, with the shorter wavelengths being deviated the greatest amount. A larger object may appear to have coloured fringes with blue/violet at one side and red at the other. The colours from intermediate points of the object overlap and produce white.

Diffraction

When a wavefront of light meets the edge of an obstacle or a small opening the wave motion spreads out on the far side of the obstacle, that is the light is bent. The edge of the obstacle acts as the centre from which secondary wave fronts are produced. These secondary waves are out of phase with the initial (primary) waves. This is known as diffraction.

If light passes through a circular opening (aperture) then a circular diffraction pattern is produced. This is made up of a bright central area (known as the Airy disc) which is surrounded by alternate dark and light rings.

Diffraction effects are most apparent with small apertures and they occur with all optical systems including the eye and optical instruments. Diffraction phenomena are divided into two categories:

1. Fraunhofer diffraction—when the source of light and the screen on which the pattern is observed are effectively at infinity

2. Fresnel diffraction—when the source or the screen, or both, are at finite distances from the aperture. (For further details see Freeman 1990.)

Further reading

Elkington, A.R. and Frank, H.J. (1991). *Clinical optics*, (2nd edn), Chapters 2 and 3. Blackwell Scientific Publications, Oxford.

Freeman, M.H. (1990). *Optics*, (10th edn), Chapters 2,3, and 13. Butterworth-Heinemann, Oxford.
Jenkins, F.A. and White H.E. (1981). *Fundamentals of optics*, (4th edn), Chapters 1,2,3, and 6. McGraw-Hill, London.
Tunnacliffe, A.H. and Hirst, J.G. (1981). *Optics*, Chapters 2,5, and 14. Association of British Dispensing Opticians, 6, Hurlingham Park, London.

2.3.2 Retinoscopy

Gordon Sanderson

Retinoscopy is a clinical technique which enables a skilled observer to determine the refractive state of an eye objectively. It is normal practice to conduct the objective assessment of refractive error by either retinoscopy or an automated refraction technique prior to conducting a subjective refinement. Retinoscopy relies on the ability of the clinician to observe the movement of a small patch of illuminated retina, called the retinoscopy reflex. The illumination is provided by a source of light within the retinoscope. As this light is moved across the subject's pupil the image of the illuminated retina will be seen by the observer to be either moving in the same direction as the source (with) or in the opposite direction (against). Careful alteration of the power of lenses placed in front of the eye will enable the observer to 'neutralize' these with and against movements.

Retinoscopy

Types of retinoscopy

Retinoscopy can be performed with the subject fixing on a target at infinity (static retinoscopy), with the subject fixing on a target close to the sight hole of the retinoscope (dynamic retinoscopy), or with the subject's accommodation paralysed (cycloplegic retinoscopy).

Two types of illumination source are in common use: (a) the spot source which produces a beam from the retinoscope which is circular, not unlike the beam of an ophthalmoscope; and (b) the streak source where the beam is elongated (generally produced by a bulb with a straight horizontal filament) and capable of being rotated through 360°.

The original retinoscopes were circular mirrors, with a sight hole in the centre, held by means of a short handle. The illumination was provided by a Lister lamp placed behind the subject's head. The observer shone the reflected beam of light from the mirror into the subject's eye. There were two types of retinoscope in common use. One used a plane mirror and produced a divergent beam, and the other used a concave mirror and produced a beam which focuses between the observer and the subject. The terminology plane and concave mirror have been carried over into the modern self-illuminated retinoscope. The same effect is achieved by sliding the condenser lens inside the retinoscope up or down thus enabling the filament to be focused either behind the subject's head (equivalent to a plane mirror) or between the observer and the subject (equivalent to a concave mirror). The convention is that when the condenser is slid down it represents a plane mirror whilst when it is slid up it represents a concave mirror.

The patch of illuminated retina becomes the object in the observation system. The image is produced by the vergence of the subject's cornea and lens. When the object is at a point greater than the focal length of the subject's cornea and lens (such as in myopia) the image if virtual. Hence a movement of the object from right to left is seen by the observer to be moving from left to right (an against movement) whereas when the object is inside the focal length of the subject's cornea and retina combination (e.g. hypermetropia) the opposite applies and the image is seen to move with. By adding to or subtracting from the power of the cornea/lens combination with trial lenses, the observer can determine the point at which the image of the illuminated retina is formed at the observer's eye. This is known as the endpoint, or neutrality. In practice, since the observer is not at infinity but typically at two-thirds of a metre from the subject, neutrality represents a far point of two-thirds of a metre; this is called the working distance. In order to put the far point at infinity, 1.5 dioptres must be subtracted from the power of the trial lenses. This produces the distance correction and is known as taking off the working distance.

In the case of astigmatism it will be found that there are two endpoints, one in each principal meridian. The principal meridians are usually at 90° to one another. If the astigmatism is significant, that is more than 0.5 dioptre, the reflex will appear slightly oval. From the direction of the ovality it is possible to ascertain both principal meridians. If a spot retinoscope is being used then the neutralization is obtained by refracting along the axis of the ovality and at 90° to it. The cylindrical correction is the difference between the two spheres and the axis is determined by the orientation of the oval reflex. If a streak retinoscope is being used the streak should be aligned parallel to the oval reflex and the beam of the retinoscope moved at 90° to the direction of the streak. Again, neutralization is accomplished in both principal meridians, the streak being rotated through 90° in order to achieve this.

The advantage of the streak retinoscope is that it can enable a more accurate determination of the axis of astigmatism. The disadvantage is that it introduces an additional variable, since if the axis of a streak does not coincide with the axis of the oval reflex a misleading result may be obtained. It is usually considered easier for a novice to begin learning retinoscopy with a spot retinoscope as there is one less variable to contend with.

Accommodation in retinoscopy

Accommodation by the subject can produce misleading results in retinoscopy. In order to prevent this it is essential that the subject be asked to fixate a distant target even though at times the observer may cross the fixation axis. When refracting a myope accommodation is seldom a problem but in hypermetropia, particularly in the young, accommodation can lead to considerable inaccuracy. There are several ways of avoiding this: cycloplegia is the most common and is used routinely with very young children. For subjects older than 10 years of age cycloplegia should not be necessary, provided the fixing eye is 'fogged' with sufficient plus power to render the subject myopic. This fogging may need to be increased as the refraction proceeds. If cycloplegia has been used then a suitable allowance for ciliary muscle tone (latent hypermetropia) will need to be made before the results can be prescribed as spectacles. Alternatively, a further subjective test known as a postmydriatic test, can be performed in slightly older children, once the effects of the cycloplegia have worn off.

Accuracy of retinoscopy

Retinoscopy in competent hands can produce very accurate objective refraction. Most retinoscopists would claim to be accurate to within 0.25 dioptre. Such accuracy can only be obtained if the retinoscopy is performed precisely along the visual axis. One method of ensuring this is dynamic retinoscopy.

Dynamic retinoscopy

A small illuminated target, typically containing letters or similar patterns, is incorporated into the retinoscope very close to the optic axis. The subject is asked to fixate this target while the retinoscopy is performed, thus ensuring that the retinoscopy takes place along the visual axis. Although very great accuracy in determining the power and axis of the cylinder can be obtained with this method, a suitable allowance for accommodation must be made to the sphere once the refraction is complete. Dynamic retinoscopy can also be used as an objective method for determining the near point of accommodation. This is accomplished by gradually reducing the working distance until the reflex changes to a 'with' movement, while having the subject maintain fixation.

Optical principles of retinoscopy

The simplest way to consider the optics of retinoscopy is to consider the illumination system and the observation system as separate entities. The source of illumination is a bulb contained within the body of the self-illuminated retinoscope. In the case of a streak retinoscope this bulb is capable of being rotated through 360°. The image of the filament is reflected by a 45° mirror in the head of the ophthalmoscope and projected into the subject's pupil. In the 'plane' mirror position the image of the filament is between the subject's head and infinity. In the 'concave' mirror position the image is between the subject and the observer. It is the image of the filament, albeit out of focus, which produces the illuminated patch of retina.

Because the ray paths cross in the concave mirror position the movement of the patch of illuminated retina is reversed, hence what would have appeared as a with movement, for example in hypermetropia, is now seen as an against movement.

The illuminated patch of retina, or more properly, that reflected from the interface between the posterior limiting light membrane of the vitreous and the neural layer of the retina, becomes the object for the observation system. Neutrality is achieved when the image of the subject's retina is conjugate with the observer's entrance pupil. If this image is in front of the observer's pupil it is seen as real and inverted and will move in the opposite direction to the patch of illuminated retina. If the image is behind the observer's pupil it is a virtual image and will move in the same direction as the patch of illuminated retina.

A student can observe this effect by using their finger as the streak of illuminated retina and a 20-dioptre convex trial lens to represent the focal system of the eye. When the finger is less than 5 cm from the lens a with movement will be observed as the finger is moved from side to side. When the finger is greater than 5 cm from the lens an against movement will be observed. Neutrality is when the finger is approximately 5 cm from the lens, the exact distance being determined by the position of the observer from the lens. At the point of neutrality the lens will appear to fill with the image of the finger and no predictable movement will be observed. This is the endpoint which in the case of retinoscopy is seen as the pupil filling with light. Students of retinoscopy are advised not to begin by looking for an endpoint, but rather by bracketing with and against movements and reducing the difference in power between the two lenses required to achieve this, the endpoint being in the middle. Students should not be disheartened if their first attempts do not meet with success as skill in the art of retinoscopy is said by some to take a lifetime to acquire.

Other methods of objective refraction

Several more complex methods of obtaining an objective refraction exist: they range from refractometers, which provide the observer with an image on the subject's retina not unlike the image seen in a focimeter, through to computed automatic refractors. Some of these use Sheiner's double pinhole principle, others employ a form of retinoscopy using infrared light. These machines can provide accurate and repeatable results as well as an indication of the confidence factor which will enable the refractionist to assess the reliability. However, they should never be relied upon totally before prescribing lenses. Further refinement by subjective refraction is almost always necessary although not always possible.

A number of versions of photorefractors are becoming available, the quantitative type do not yet appear to have realized their full potential, but the qualitative photoscreeners are becoming more widely used, particularly for detecting refractive errors and other ocular anomalies in infants.

Subjective refraction

In order to refine the results of objective refraction it is helpful to think of the refractive error as the solution of an equation with three unknowns: (a) the sphere; (b) the cylinder; and (c) the axis. It is only by considering these as separate, though related, entities that an accurate and repeatable result can be achieved.

Refinement of the sphere

Spherical refinement consists of providing the subject with increased or decreased spherical power until they themselves choose which option produces the clearest image. The aim of spherical power refinement is to find the maximum amount of convex power or the minimum amount of concave power that still enables the subject to maintain optimal visual acuity. This is particularly important if the subject is young and has active accommodation. If a test chart is being used, constant reassessment of the acuity should be performed to confirm the subject's responses. While this is being performed the subject should be asked to look at the lowest visible line on the chart, changing as improvement takes place. Further confirmation of the subject's response can sometimes be achieved with the duochrome test (Fig. 1). This relies on the fact that short wavelength light is refracted more than long wavelength light thus letters on a green or blue background will focus in front of the subject's retina whereas letters on a red background will focus behind. A hypermetropic subject will therefore see green letters in preference to red and a myopic subject the opposite. However, the duochrome test should not be relied upon in every case since the subject's accommodation can enable them to switch their preference from green to red.

Good practice in subjective refraction is to alter the power of convex lenses by inserting the new lens before the old lens is removed with the opposite being the case with minus lenses. This will prevent the subject from accommodating while the spheres are being changed. Similarly the phenomenon of instrument myopia can be avoided if the other eye is fogged rather than being occluded.

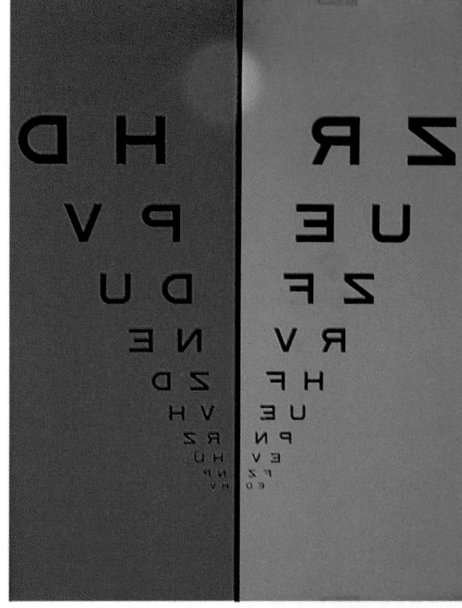

Fig. 1 The duochrome test.

Astigmatic refinement

There are three methods in common use for refining the cylindrical component of a patient's refraction. The first and most widely used is the Jackson crossed cylinder. This consists of a spherocylindrical lens, with the axes of the plus and minus component marked accordingly, held in a lens mount attached to a short handle. The crossed cylinder as originally described by Jackson was literally two cylinders of equal powers, one convex the other concave at 90° to each other. They are now typically manufactured as a spherocylindrical lens with the power of the sphere equal to half the power of the cylinder, the spherical equivalent thus being zero.

The other two methods for refining the cylindrical component of a patient's refraction are the stenopaeic slit and the astigmatic fan. Although less extensively used they still have a role to play in refraction, as they can both be used to detect a cylinder where none was thought to exist and they can both be used to illustrate the basic principles of correcting astigmatism.

Crossed cylinder

Although a Jackson crossed cylinder can be used to determine a cylinder which has not been found by objective refraction, the most common use of the crossed cylinder is to refine a previously determined cylinder. Before beginning a crossed cylinder test it is essential that the circle of least confusion lies on the subject's retina. To ensure this has occurred the subject should be rendered either equal or slightly green on the duochrome (in the latter case a small amount of accommodation by the subject will put the circle on to the retina). The accuracy of the crossed cylinder is considerably reduced if the circle of least confusion lies in front of the retina. Similarly the subject should be directed to look at a circular target. A linear target may induce a preference which will reduce the accuracy of the test.

Axis refinement

When both these prerequisites have been met the handle of the crossed cylinder is aligned along the axis of the cylinder in the trial frame. By rotating the handle of the crossed cylinder it will be seen that the orientation of the positive and negative components of the crossed cylinder can be transposed. These are described as position 1 and 2. The subject is then asked to determine whether, with the crossed cylinder in position 1 or 2, the circular target looks rounder and clearer. It is often important to alert the subject to the fact that neither may be as clear as without the crossed cylinder in place. When the subject makes a choice the cylinder in the trial frame is rotated towards the direction of the cylinder of like demonomination in the crossed cylinder, that is the axis of a plus cylinder is turned towards the plus sign on the crossed cylinder. The handle of the crossed cylinder is now realigned to coincide with the new position of the cylindrical axis and the procedure is repeated. The endpoint is reached when the subject is unable to distinguish between position 1 and 2.

Power refinement

To begin the power determination, the crossed cylinder is now repositioned with one of its axes aligned with the axis of the cylinder in the trial frame. Again by 'flipping' the crossed cylinder the patient is asked to choose between position 1 and 2. Once that choice has been made the power of the cylinder is adjusted in accordance with the power indicated on the crossed cylinder, that is if the patient prefers a position which provides more plus cylinder to an existing plus cylinder then the cylinder power must be increased. This is continued until the patient is unable to choose between position 1 and 2.

In order to maintain the circle of least confusion on the retina spherical adjustments of half the power of the cylinder must be made, that is if the cylinder is increased by +1.0 dioptres then −0.50 dioptres should be added to the sphere.

Generally speaking, if the retinoscopy has been reasonably accurate, the crossed cylinder can be used to refine the axis of the cylinder first, followed by the power. If there are any doubts as to the accuracy of the retinoscopy it is advisable to refine the power first followed by the axis and subsequently the power again.

Optical principles of the Jackson crossed cylinder

The Jackson crossed cylinder is designed to provide the subject with two choices. One choice expands the conoid of Sturm and the other contracts it. Neither has an effect on the position of the circle of least confusion. It can be shown from Stokes construction that this principle applies to both refinement of the power and refinement of the axis since in both cases the subject is being asked to look at two resultants. In the case of the axis determination these resultants are the product of obliquely crossed cylinders.

Stenopaeic slit

The stenopaeic slit consists of an opaque black disc into which has been cut a narrow slit approximately 1 cm long. This device can be used to determine a cylinder where none has previously been found by objective techniques. Clinically this can be very valuable for instance, when a distorted cornea has prevented accurate retinoscopy.

Method

The subject is asked to look at the test chart, a stenopaeic slit is placed in a trial frame and rotated until the subject indicates a preference for the optimal acuity. With the slit in this position the best sphere is determined subjectively. The power of the best sphere is noted, as is the axis of the stenopaeic slit. The slit is then rotated through 90° and the best sphere determined again.

Results

The original best sphere is the spherical component of the refraction, the difference between the first and second best sphere is the cylinder, and the axis is the first position of the stenopaeic slit.

Optical principles of the stenopaeic slit

The stenopaeic slit collapses one of the focal lines of the conoid of Sturm. Once this has occurred the other focal line is brought

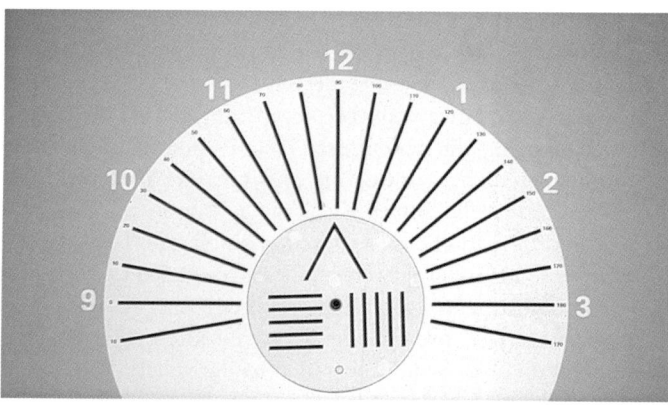

Fig. 2 The astigmatic fan.

to the retina by the use of spherical lenses. The difference between the first sphere and the second sphere represents the cylindrical difference between the two and since the stenopaeic slit has collapsed the focal line at 90° to its direction this then provides the axis of the cylinder.

Astigmatic fan (Fig. 2)

In common with the stenopaeic slit the astigmatic fan is generally used to ascertain the presence of a cylinder that has not been detected objectively. The astigmatic fan consists of a series of radial lines generally spaced 10° apart and marked with axes that are the complement of those on a trial frame. There is generally some sort of rotating device such as a Maddox V and/or a Maddox block which is used to help determine the axis.

Method

Before the astigmatic fan can be used it is important to ensure that the circle of least confusion lies in front of the subject's retina thus ensuring that the posterior focal line is closest to the retina. This is generally achieved by fogging the subject with convex lenses to approximately 6/18 on the test chart. The subject is then asked which of the radial lines appears the blackest. Assistance in determining this can be provided by the use of the Maddox V or block, the endpoint being where the V or block are seen by the subject as equally dark. Once the axis has been determined it is read off the astigmatic fan and negative cylinder is added to the prescription at that axis until all the lines on the astigmatic fan appear equally distinct. Thus both the power and the axis of the cylinder have been determined.

Optical principles of the astigmatic fan

Once the posterior focal line is adjacent to the retina, the optical state is that of myopic astigmatism. The addition of negative cylinder in the appropriate axis will move the anterior focal line back, towards the posterior focal line, the conoid of Sturm eventually collapsing to a single point as the two coincide.

Further reading

Brookman, K.E. (1993). The Jackson crossed cylinder: historical perspective. *Journal of the American Optometry Association*, **64**, 329–31.

Del Priore, L.V. and Guyton, D.L. (1986). The Jackson cross cylinder. A reappraisal. *Ophthalmology*, **93**, 1461–5.

Friedburg, D. (1990). Objective determination of refraction. *Fortschritte der Ophthalmologie*, **87**, S138–41.

Hanlon, S.D., Nakabayashi, J. and Shigezawa, G. (1987). A critical view of presbyopic add determination. *Journal of the American Optometry Association*, **58**, 468–72.

Kommerell, G. (1993). Streak retinoscopy. Optical principles and practical recommendations. *Klinische Monatsblätter für Augenheilkeidunde*, **203**, 10–8.

Locke, L.C. and Somers, W. (1989). A comparison study of dynamic retinoscopy techniques *Optometry and Visual Science*, **66**, 540–4.

Newell, F.W. (1988). Edward Jackson, MD—a historical perspective of his contributions to refraction and to ophthalmology. *Ophthalmology*, **95**, 555–8.

O'Leary, D.J., Yang, P.H., and Yeo, C.H. (1987). Effect of cross cylinder power on cylinder axis sensitivity. *American Journal of Optometry and Physiological Optometry*, **64**, 367–9.

Rutstein, R.P., Fuhr, P.D., and Swiatocha, J. (1993). Comparing the amplitude of accommodation determined objectively and subjectively. *Optometry and Visual Science*, **70**, 496–500.

Salvesen, S. and Kohler, M. (1991). Automated refraction. A comparative study of automated refraction with the Nidek AR-1000 autorefractor and retinoscopy. *Acta Ophthalmologica (Copenhagen)*, **69**, 342–6.

Saunders, K.J. and Westall, C.A. (1992). Comparison between near retinoscopy and cycloplegic retinoscopy in the refraction of infants and children. *Optometry and Visual Science*, **69**, 615–22.

Sims, C.N. (1987). The Jackson cross cylinder: a reappraisal. *Ophthalmology*, **94**, 891–4.

Velasco Cruz, A.A., Sampaio, N.M., and Vargas, J.A. (1990). Near retinoscopy in accommodative esotropia. *Journal of Pediatric Ophthalmology and Strabismus*, **27**, 245–9.

Whitefoot, H. and Charman, W.N. (1992). Dynamic retinoscopy and accommodation. *Ophthalmic Physiology and Optometry*, **12**, 8–17.

2.3.3 Spectacle and lens types

Gordon Sanderson

Spectacle frames

A spectacle frame is a device for holding optical prescription lenses at the correct location in close proximity to the eyes. They must fulfil the following criteria. The lenses must be held in a stable and precise location both relative to one another and relative to the visual axes and corneal vertices of the wearer. Frames must be made of a material which is non-irritating to the skin. They must conform as closely as possible to the wearer's anatomy. They must be of a pleasing cosmetic appearance.

To fulfil these various criteria a number of options are available both in terms of materials and design.

Materials

Spectacle frames can be made from a variety of both synthetic and naturally occurring materials, some of the earliest being made by jewellers of gold and other precious metals and also of horn and tortoiseshell. The appearance of the latter is imitated in contemporary frame design. Synthetic materials, generally plastics, include cellulose acetate, methyl methacrylate, polycarbonate, polyamide, and nylon. Frames from these materials are usually manufactured either by moulding or machine fabrication and reinforcement of plastic components with wire is frequently used to increase their strength.

Gold and other precious metals are still in use, although generally in the form of a plating or coating for base metal wire frames. Other metals such as nickel/silver alloys and titanium are also used. All these materials confer various advantages and disadvantages to the wearer. The ideal material combines strength, lightness, and pleasing aesthetic qualities.

Frame parameters

Frames are generally described by three parameters and are often marked accordingly: (a) the eye size; (b) the distance between the lenses; and (c) the temple length, the latter usually being written on the temple of the frame. A simple addition of the eye size and the distance between the lenses will provide the pupillary distance of the frame. This measurement becomes important in the centration of lenses and will be referred to later.

Optical considerations of the frame

The frame should hold the lens at a stable back vertex distance. Variations in the back vertex distance affect the ocular refraction. Although this may be used to advantage by the wearer, for instance sliding the frame down the wearer's nose will increase the effectivity of plus lenses or decrease the effectivity of negative lenses thus increasing the reading addition or producing one where one previously did not exist. For that reason, when prescribing lenses of power greater than 5 dioptres the back vertex distance must be measured and recorded on the prescription.

The frames must prevent any rotation occurring in the lenses which will alter the axis of a correcting cylinder. The frames may be used to introduce a tilt to lenses known as the pantoscopic tilt (typically around 10°) which will ensure that the optic axes of the correction coincides with the visual axes of the wearer for the majority of the wearing time.

Complications of spectacle frame wear

Apart from pressure sores which typically develop around the bridge of the nose or behind the ears, very few complications arise from the wearing of spectacles. Allergic dermatitis has been reported from frames containing nickel and from those made of cellulose acetate. Some anecdotal reports of basal cell carcinoma of the nose where pad pressure is exerted have also appeared in the literature.

Spectacle lenses

A spectacle lens is an optical component designed to correct spherical, astigmatic, or prismatic defects of one or both eyes, at a given distance from the eyes. The lenses must be of an optically homogeneous nature, able to provide, in combination with the wearer's eye(s), a sharp image at the retina. In order to achieve this, a number of optical conditions must be met. The surfaces of the lenses must be of high optical quality, the lenses must be maintained at the correct distance from the eye, they must be centred at the correct position relative to the subject's visual axis, and they must minimize aberrations.

Materials

The two materials in common use as spectacle lenses are glass and plastic.

Glass

A number of types of glass are used in spectacle lens manufacture, the most common being ophthalmic crown glass which has a refractive index of 1.523. It may be used in conjunction with flint glass ($n = 1.62$) to produce fused bifocals (see below). A number of higher index glasses are also used in spectacle corrections (up to $n = 1.8$) to reduce the thickness of the lenses and hence the weight. The weight of glass lenses is a considerable disadvantage particularly in the higher powers. However, although they are usually moulded, they can also be manufactured by surface grinding and produced individually to a minimum thickness. This technique is used extensively in the spectacle correction of aphakia. Glass lenses although relatively scratch resistant have the disadvantage of being easily broken. Injury can result from shards of glass penetrating the lids or globe. To minimize this risk various toughening procedures are available.

Thermal toughening

Glass can be annealed by rapid cooling and thus form very small crystals which on impact are likely to be less harmful to the eye and adnexae.

Chemical toughening

Immersion of the lenses into a bath containing molten potassium nitrate can provide a considerable degree of impact resistance to lenses. Having the advantage over thermal toughening of not requiring a minimum edge thickness of 2.5 mm before the toughening can be undertaken. However, molten potassium nitrate is not an easy substance to work with and not all laboratories are willing to provide this service, alternative methods of ion exchange toughening are available.

Lamination

Laminated or (Triplex) lenses consist of a thin parallel film of plastic material usually polyvinyl butyral sandwiched between two layers of annealed glass. The three layers are firmly bonded together. Although a laminated lens may be damaged on impact the splinters of glass remain adherent to the plastic film.

Plastic

Plastic, typically polymethyl methacrylate, is used extensively in spectacle lens manufacture. It has the advantage of being extremely light and virtually unbreakable. It has the disadvantage of being easily scratched. A number of surface-hardening processes exist for plastic lenses which can minimize the damage due to scratching. However, as a general rule, they are more easily scratched than glass lenses. Polycarbonate, which is occasionally used, is also extremely durable. Another disadvantage of plastic lenses is that they are usually moulded and hence manufactured in standard diameters; they also have lower refractive index than glass hence they are thicker at an equivalent power. The combination of these factors is that the lenses when cut to fit a frame significantly smaller than the diameter of the blank lens will either have thick edges or a large centre thickness or both, either of which are cosmetically undesirable. Like glass, plastic lenses can also be surface ground to reduce thickness. They are also available with a high refractive index (up to 1.66).

Quartz

Quartz has been used as a spectacle lens material and is still used in certain parts of the world.

Lens design

Lenses can be designed to minimize aberrations. This is typically achieved in two ways.

Bending

This ensures that, with the eye in an oblique direction of gaze, the visual axis is as near normal to the vertex of the lens as possible. This will reduce oblique astigmatism. A lens which simply corrects a spherical error and is bent in this way is referred to as a meniscus lens, the base curve being the flatter of the two. A lens which corrects both astigmatism and spherical error is referred to as a toroidal lens. The toroidal surface can be either on the front or the back.

Aspheric design

Reduction of the power of the lens periphery decreases spherical aberration and distortion and makes convex lenses thinner, hence lighter. The advantages, although obvious to some wearers, may be difficult to justify, due to the increased cost of these lenses. Flatter back surfaces can also give rise to increased reflections.

Optical considerations of spectacle lenses

A number of aberrations occur with the use of spectacle corrections for refractive error. Some are significant and can be minimized by careful lens design, others are insignificant, and still others cannot be corrected at all.

Spherical aberration

Spherical aberration can be minimized in spectacle lenses by the use of aspheric lenses. A number of aspheric designs are available for spectacle lenses. They rely on the principle of reducing the spherical power progressively towards the periphery of the lens. This has the effect of minimizing positive spherical aberration. The apparent disadvantage of a weaker periphery is offset by the fact that the eye when deviated from the primary position is at a greater vertex distance from the lens and the loss of vergence somewhat overcome by the increased effectivity that this produces.

Oblique astigmatism

Light incident on the lenses from an oblique axis will produce an astigmatic image. However, this can be minimized if the lens is curved in such a way that the incident light is normal to the surface of the lens. This curving of the lens is referred to as bending and it is a common device employed in the construction of ophthalmic spectacle lenses. A lens that is bent to minimize oblique astigmatism is referred to as a best form lens. The surface powers to produce this are computed by reference to Tscherning's elipse.

Distortion

This can also be reduced by the use of aspheric lenses but a certain amount of distortion will always persist. This may account for the phenomenon of 'getting used to new glasses' so frequently reported by spectacle lens wearers.

Coma and curvature of field

Neither can be corrected but they are not significant due to the fact that the retina is much less sensitive peripherally.

Chromatic aberration

This aberration cannot be corrected in spectacles either, but like the previous two effects it does not seem to greatly affect their optical efficiency.

The human eye is not corrected for chromatic aberration which may account for the popularity of tints which only permit the transmission of a relatively narrow band of light near the middle of the visible spectrum. The reduction in chromatic aberration combined with the loss of scattering normally caused by the shorter wavelengths could contribute to increased visual acuity.

Prismatic correction

The successful prescription of spectacle lenses occasionally calls for the incorporation of prism into the finished prescription. This can be accomplished in most cases by simple decentration of the lenses, the prismatic effect produced is calculated using Prentice's rule. When the power of the lenses is not great or the required prism is large, decentration may not be sufficient. In this case the prism will have to be worked into the lens at the time of manufacture at extra cost.

Prism should be specified by the location of the base in front of one eye. The spectacle laboratory will be able to decide which method of producing the prism is the most appropriate. They will also attempt to divide the prism equally between both eyes.

When checking for the presence of prism with a focimeter, vertical prism can be measured directly but horizontal prism can only be measured with reference to the patient's interpupillary distance. To maximize the amount of prism that can be achieved by decentration and minimize the centre thickness of the lenses a frame should be selected with a pupillary distance as close as possible to the patient's interpupillary distance.

Spectacle magnification

The positioning of a spectacle lens at the spectacle plane, that is some distance away from the eye, creates a telescopic system. This has the effect, in the case of a convex lens, of magnifying the image at the retina or minifying it in the case of a concave lens. Both are referred to as spectacle magnification. The exact amount of magnification is virtually impossible to calculate since it requires information about the individual optical constants of the eye under consideration, but there are two commonly accepted methods of estimating it.

Relative spectacle magnification

This method compares the size of the corrected ametropic image of a distant object with the image size of an emmetropic (schematic) eye.

(Absolute) spectacle magnification

This is a comparison of the sharp retinal image of the corrected image of a distant object with the blurred image of the same object in the uncorrected eye, although the measurements are taken from the centre of the blur circles, and at best it is only an estimate. This method is considered the most reliable.

Tints

There are many reports of actinic radiation leading to ocular damage, mostly attributed to the shorter wavelength light. Some degree of protection may be afforded by the prescription of tinted spectacle lenses. Various forms of tinted spectacle lenses are in use, the spectral transmission characteristics are usually made available for each tint.

Solid tints

By incorporating pigments at the time of manufacture lenses can be produced in a variety of tints. This is the oldest form of tinting. It has the advantage of providing consistency of colour and reproducibility of replacement lenses and solid tints are not damaged by scratching. The disadvantages are that the density of the tint may vary depending on the thickness of the lens and they are unpopular with manufacturers, as a large range of stock lenses has to be carried.

Surface-coated tints

These are produced by the vacuum chamber process. Various different colours can be added to the lenses by the use of different chemicals, usually metals. The advantages are that the depth of tint is uniform over the entire lens area. Further deposits can be added hence increasing the density of the tint (this can be useful in the management of cone dysfunction). The tints can be removed and they are inexpensive to produce. The disadvantages are that the tints are easily scratched and the consistency, hence the repeatability, can be difficult.

Dyed tints

Lenses can be dyed by immersion in a chemical bath. This process is particularly suitable for plastic lenses. By withdrawing the lens gradually from the dye the 'gradutint' effect can be produced. These lenses have the advantage of being inexpensive with the disadvantage of colour reproduction being inconsistent because the dye is taken up at different rates and the tint may vary as the lenses age.

Photochromic tints

Photochromic materials are made from glass or plastic containing microscopic crystals of silver halide. Changes in the orientation of these crystals cause the lenses to darken when exposed to ultraviolet light (300–400 nm). Transmittance ranges are quoted for example as 90/25, that is the transmission in the fully faded and the fully darkened phase, respectively. The advantage of these tints is that they enable tints to be worn indoors satisfactorily. The disadvantages are that they are affected by temperature, becoming unstable at high temperatures; they have a slow 'swing' time, particularly from dark to light; the tints age, hence matching replacement lenses becomes virtually impossible; and because they rely on ultraviolet to produce the conversion effect they do not work well when the ultraviolet is absorbed by glass, for example through a car windscreen. Like all solid tints they vary in density with the lens thickness; this can be overcome with surface coating which is available in photochromic form.

Antireflection coatings

A special type of tint known as an antireflection coating is used to minimize surface reflections from spectacle lenses. This is particularly important when the lens material has a high refractive index. Surface reflections can be reduced by coating lenses with a film of a material that has a lower refractive index than that of the lens. Reflections can almost be eliminated by meeting two conditions:

1. That the refractive index of the coating is the square root of the lens material

2. That the thickness of the coating multiplied by its refractive index is exactly one-quarter of the wavelength of light.

These two conditions can only be met for one wavelength of light. For high index glass, magnesium fluoride has almost the theoretically desired refractive index. Single layer coatings are designed to give the maximum effect in the middle of the spectrum. The characteristic purplish appearance of these coatings, due to a combination of the shorter and longer wavelengths of light being reflected, is usually called a bloom.

The limitations of the single layer antireflection coating can be overcome by multilayer coatings which are capable of almost totally eliminating surface reflections.

Antireflection coatings suffer from a number of disadvantages; they are easily scratched, they can craze, they are difficult to match, and they are difficult to keep clean, since grease from fingerprints and similar marks are very visible.

Presbyopia

The correction of presbyopia presents additional challenges particularly if the presbyopia is to be corrected in conjunction with ametropia. Confusion often exists in the minds of the public as to the distinction between correcting ametropia and supplementing the loss of accommodation which is known as presbyopia. The term magnifying glasses is often used to refer to lenses which correct for presbyopia. This term, although inappropriate, is understandable since a convex lens is required to supplement any lost accommodation. However, the true purpose of a correction for presbyopia is to bring the subject's near point up to a convenient reading distance. In the case of single vision lenses where presbyopia alone is to be corrected any coexisting ametropia must be fully corrected first.

A single vision correction for presbyopia can take the form of a full spectacle lens which in effect renders the subject myopic hence the correction cannot be worn satisfactorily for distance. Alternatively, a half eye or 'look-over' prescription can be provided which enables the subject to have an uninterrupted view of the distance while maintaining a near correction with the eyes in a position of downgaze.

Where a simultaneous correction for both distance and near is to be provided there are various options available. However, it would be wise to alert the patient that no spectacle correction will ever fully compensate for their own lost accommodation.

Types of presbyopic correction

Bifocals

Franklin

Benjamin Franklin invented a form of bifocal lens in 1870 which consists of two separate lenses held together by the rim of the frame. Generally the upper lens is the distance correction and the lower lens is the reading correction. The advantages of the Franklin bifocal is that they can easily have prism incorporated into the reading segment. The main disadvantage is that dirt tends to lodge in the junction.

Cemented bifocal

A wafer of glass or plastic containing the reading addition is cemented on to a distance lens. These lenses although largely superceded have the advantage of being able to be used as a temporary bifocal correction, when the subject is not sure that they wish to wear bifocals. A number of commercially available stick-on Fresnel segments are available for this purpose. The disadvantages of these are that the Fresnel optics are poor and do not provide the user with a realistic simulation of the near correction. The original glass wafers were cemented on to the distance lens by the use of Canada balsam which had a tendency to go brown with age.

Solid one-piece twin sights

These bifocals are manufactured by grinding the reading addition on to the front or back surface from one piece of glass or moulding the reading addition in plastic. The reading segment has a different radius of curvature to the distance portion. Plastic bifocals are always solid and the segment is incorporated

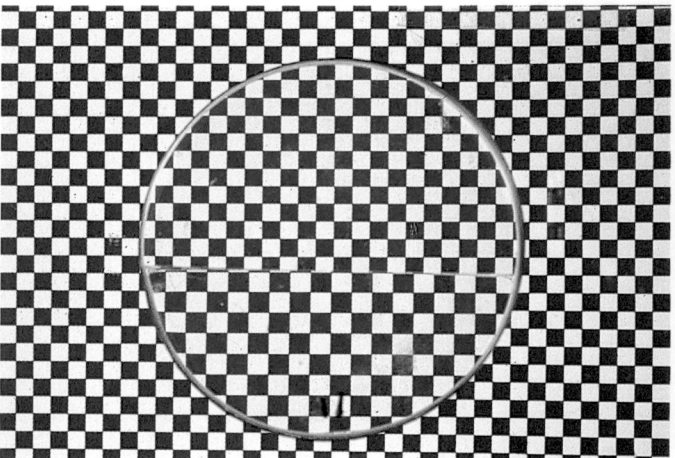

Fig. 1 Executive bifocals.

into the mould. The advantages are that they are the only bifocal available in photochromic glass and prisms can be incorporated into the reading segment. In the case of glass bifocals this is produced by tilting the axis of the machine used to grind the reading segment. This is known as prism control or centre control. The disadvantages of this type of bifocal is that they have a large and obvious reading segment and the round top segment is not easy to get used to.

Executive bifocals (Fig. 1)

This is a form of solid bifocal which provides the user with a flat top reading segment which generally occupies the entire lower half of the spectacle lens. It has the advantage of providing a wide field of vision for near and, because the optical centres are virtually coincident, there is no optical jump. The disadvantage of this type of bifocal is that the junction is very obvious and hence they can be cosmetically undesirable. Also, the front edge can chip and give rise to unwanted reflection. Executive bifocals are usually heavier than a fused segment bifocal and the reading segment cannot be decentred inward relative to the distance centre, therefore prismatic effects are more pronounced with the higher reading additions.

Fused bifocals

A plug of glass of high refractive index (e.g. flint glass) is placed into a depression in the front surface of a standard glass lens (ophthalmic crown) and fused at 770°C. The add in conjunction with the rest of the lens is polished smooth with an identical curvature all over. Because of the higher index of the plug of glass the bifocal segment has a greater surface power thus providing the reading addition. Fused bifocals are produced in two types, the rounded top (cryptok) and the flat top (D segment). The advantages of this type of bifocal is that they are the least visible, particularly the round top variety, and they are also the least expensive. The disadvantages are that they can produce chromatic aberration, especially if the distance prescription is a high minus; and the D segment type can cause reflections from the flat top though this can be reduced by the use of a C segment (a slightly curved top).

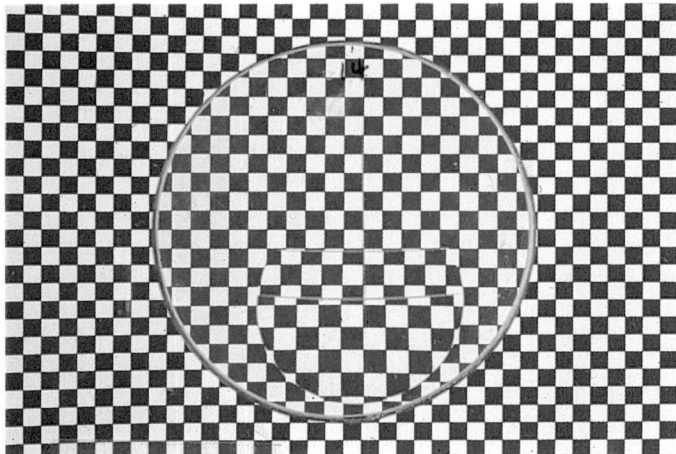

Fig. 2 Trifocals.

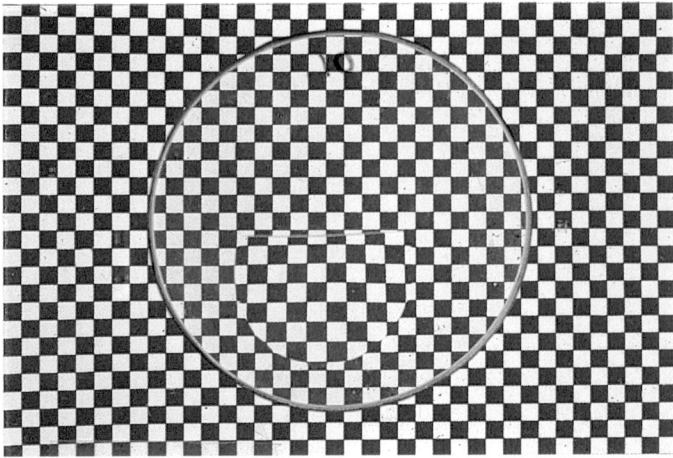

Fig. 4 The 'smart seg'.

Trifocals (Fig. 2)

When the subject requires an intermediate correction such as for a computer screen or a lathe this intermediate correction can be provided in addition to a distance and near correction in the form of a trifocal lens.

These can be either fused or solid and are available in either plastic or glass. Various intermediate additions can be produced. The advantage of this type of lens is that they provide an immediate correction for vocational or leisure reasons. The disadvantages are that they require the intermediate segment to be set comparatively high, they can be cosmetically unappealing, and tend to be expensive.

Progressive addition lenses (Fig. 3)

The focal length of this lens changes as the eye looks further down, thus the effect of a progressive addition is achieved. These lenses have the advantage of giving no sudden transition from one focal length to another. They also provide a good intermediate range and cosmetically are not detectable to the average observer. The disadvantages are that they have a restricted field of view for reading, this can be less than the width of a column of print. They have an 'hour-glass' reading field with marked peripheral astigmatism of up to 5 to 6 dioptres. This can be a great disadvantage for instance when the wearer is reversing a car and looking through the periphery of their lenses. They can be varied according to the patient's need as progressive addition lenses are available with, for instance, a large near zone and a small intermediate zone. An interesting variation of the progressive addition lens is available called the 'smart seg' (Fig. 4). It consists of a D segment bifocal in which the upper third or so of the segment is contructed as a progressive lens. This provides the wearer with a variable intermediate correction without compromising the field or quality of the near correction. They unfortunately tend to be more expensive than conventional bifocals

Progressive lenses are sometimes advocated for emmetropic presbyopes in the form of half eye look-overs, thus providing the wearer with an intermediate correction as well.

Optical considerations of bifocals

Prisms and bifocals Prisms are not easily incorporated into bifocal segments. However, with a fused segment type, a small amount of decentration relative to the distance optic centre can be produced by rotation. Prisms can be ground into solid bifocals. A certain amount of base down prism can be removed from concave lenses by using the slab-off technique at the time of manufacture (Fig. 5). If large prismatic corrections are required patients are often better advised to have a separate pair of reading glasses.

Image jump Image jump occurs when the object of regard is subject to the base down prismatic effect of the bifocal segment. The slightest movement of the head of the observer in a downward direction will allow the grazing ray from the object to pass through the distance portion unobstructed. This has the effect of making the object appear to 'jump' from one position to another. In Fig. 6 the patient looking at object P_1 will observe the object in its true position; however, a slight movement of the observer's head which then makes the light from

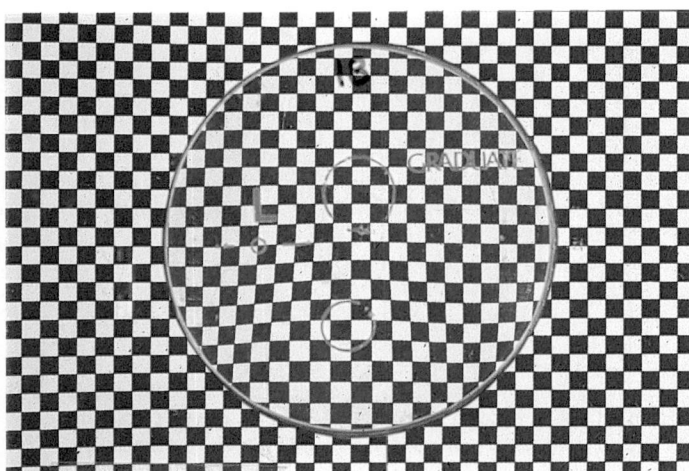

Fig. 3 The progressive addition lens.

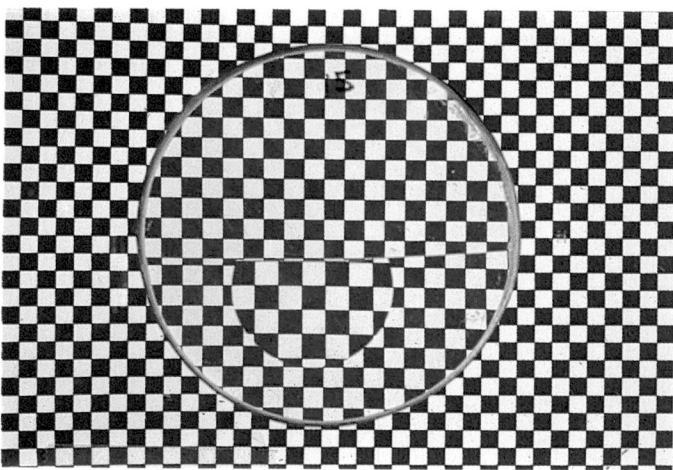

Fig. 5 A slab-off lens.

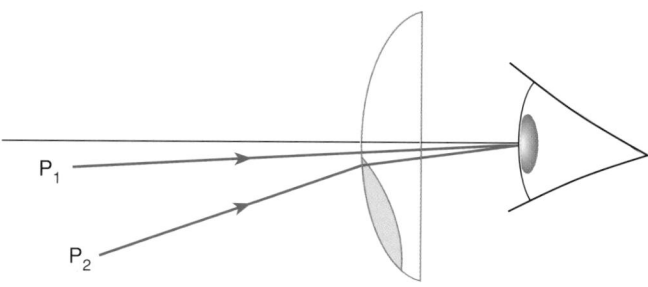

Fig. 6 The patient is looking at object P_1. When the visual axis passes through the bifocal segment a base down effect is produced - hence a shift of the object up (image jump). P_2 will appear at P_1; therefore the space between P_1 and P_2 is optically collapsed (cf. ring scotoma).

the object pass through the edge of the bifocal segment will produce an image which is optically displaced downwards at P_2. To eliminate or reduce the jump effect the optical centre of the reading lens must be at or near the top of the bifocal segment. This can really only be achieved with a D segment type of bifocal.

Object displacement When an object is not viewed through the optical centre of a lens, the prismatic effect produces an apparent displacement of that object. This increases with lenses of higher power. Bifocals can either increase or reduce the apparent object displacement caused by the distance lens in that area where the bifocal is superimposed. For instance a convex lens produces a base up prism in the lower field and this may be counteracted by the base down effect of an appropriate bifocal segment with its optical centre positioned down. This arrangement equalizes the prismatic displacement but only for one specific area.

Object displacement can become a problem and lead to symptoms if the distance corrections are unequal. A vertical prismatic difference between the two lenses, combined with constant downward gaze through the bifocal segments produced by prolonged reading, can produce symptoms of asthenopia very quickly in some subjects.

Choice of bifocal segments

A person who needs to change constantly from distance to near vision requires the image jump to be minimized, whereas a person who looks mostly through the lower segment, and is doing sustained reading, needs the object displacement to be minimized.

In practical terms this means that a hypermetropic presbyope must have the optimal system chosen for them, whereas myopes can have both image jump and object displacement reduced simultaneously by placing the near optical centre at the top of the bifocal segment.

Induced prism difference

There is an induced prism difference at comparable reading points on two spectacle lenses of unequal power for example, when correcting anisometropia or oblique astigmatism. This can often be reduced by using two different types of bifocal segments in each eye, or by grinding compensating prisms into solid bifocals, or in the case of concave lenses by the use of the slab-off (bicentric grind) to correct vertical prismatic differences (see Fig. 5).

Further reading

Atchison, D.A. and Tame, S.A. (1993). Sensitivity of off-axis performance of aspheric spectacle lenses to tilt and decentration. *Ophthalmic Physiology and Optometry*, **13**, 415–21.

Barth, R. (1985). New special eyeglass lens for emmetropic presbyopes. *Klinische Monatsblätter für Augenheilkeidunde*, **187**, 73–5.

Bennett, A.G. (1966). *Optics of contact lenses*. Association of Dispensing Opticians.

Chan, O.Y. and Edwards, M. (1994). Comparison of cycloplegic and non-cycloplegic retinoscopy in Chinese pre-school children. *Optometry and Visual Science*, **71**, 312–18.

Duke-Elder, S. (1970). *System of ophthalmology*, Vol. V. Henry Kimpton.

Freeman, M.H. (1990). *Optics*. Butterworths.

Guilino, G. (1986). Aspherical single-strength eye glasses with improved wearing comfort. *Klinische Monatsblätter für Augenheilkeidunde*, **189**, 73–7.

Huismans, H. (1991). Artificial compression of the superficial temporal artery by faulty eyeglasses (frame) position. A hemodynamically significant phenomenon. *Klinische Monatsblätter für Augenheilkeidunde*, **199**, 118–19.

Jain, N.K. and Rawal, U.M. (1986). Morphophysiological changes in ultraviolet irradiated crystalline lens—*in vitro* study. *Indian Journal of Ophthalmology*, **34**, 145–7.

Jain, N.K. and Rawal, U.M. (1992). The long-term effects of visible light on the eye. *Archives of Ophthalmology*, **110**, 99–104.

Jain, N.K., Rawal, U.M., Taylor, H.R., *et al.* (1990). Visible light and risk of age-related macular degeneration. *Transactions of the American Ophthalmology Society*, **88**, 163–73; discussion 173–8.

Jenkins, A.J. and White, H.E. (1957). *Fundamentals of optics*. McGraw-Hill.

Kratzer, B.J. (1987). Use of aspherical and atoric surfaces in the optics of eyeglasses. *Klinische Monatsblätter für Augenheilkeidunde*, **190**, 72–6.

Le Texier, F., Lenne, W., and Mercier, J.L. (1987). Generalization of the Tscherning theory: optimization of aspheric ophthalmic lenses. *Ophthalmic Physiology and Optometry*, **7**, 63–72.

Maclachlan, A., Yale, S., and Wilkins, A. (1993). Open trial of subjective precision tinting: a follow-up of 55 patients. *Ophthalmic Physiology and Optometry*, **13**, 175–8.

Prevost, G. (1988).Eyeglasses and prismatic effects. *Agressologie*, **29**, 697–8.

Schutten, G. and Reim, M. (1987). Eye injuries caused by eyeglass lenses. *Klinische Monatsblätter für Augenheilkeidunde*, **191**, 237–9.

Sonnex, T.S. and Rycroft, R.J. (1986). Dermatitis from phenyl salicylate in safety spectacle frames. *Contact Dermatitis*, **14**, 268–70.

Wehmeyer, K. (1987). Centering of eyeglasses with special reference to aspheric single-power lenses. *Klinische Monatsblätter für Augenheilkeidunde*, **191**, 69–73.

Wehmeyer, K. (1990). Aberrations of spherocylindrical ophthalmic lenses. *Optometry and Visual Science*, **67**, 268–76.

2.3.4 Contact lenses in adults

John K.G. Dart

Contact lenses are currently worn by 7 to 9 per cent of the adult population in many developed countries with an estimated 3.5 million users in the United Kingdom. Contact lenses are used most widely for the correction of low refractive errors and, increasingly, for early presbyopia. However, there are also important medical applications in diagnosis, for the improvement of vision, cosmesis in unsightly eyes, and the therapy of anterior segment disorders. The aims of this chapter are to familiarize the ophthalmologist with the lenses that are available, the indications for their use, and the principles of lens fitting, care, and maintenance, to enable constructive interac-

tion with the contact lens practitioner in a multidisciplinary service. In addition to well-known conditions for which the epidemiology and disease course have been modified by lens wear, the ophthalmologist is also faced with a number of new anterior segment disorders caused by contact lens wear. The diagnosis and management of this new area of corneal and external disease is also summarized. The essential information in this chapter is contained in the figures which are referred to throughout.

Contact lens types

Classification

Contact lenses may be classified by their materials, design, wear schedule, and disposal frequency and these are summarized in Table 1.

Contact lens wear was developed in the late nineteenth century with glass scleral lenses by Fick and Müller in Germany. The introduction of polymethylmethacrylate as a lens material in the 1940s resulted in the rapid development of both scleral and corneal rigid lenses because of the ease and flexibility of manufacture and the light weight compared to glass. The development of soft hydrogel materials led to the widespread introduction of soft contact lenses in the 1970s because of the suitability of the material for mass manufacture, the ease with which the lenses could be fitted, and their comfort. Silicone

Table 1 Classification of contact lenses (from Dart 1996)

	Hard	Soft	Hybrid
Materials	Gas permeable Polymethylmethacrylate	Hydrogel Silicone rubber	Gas-permeable/hydrogel sandwich[1]
Design	Corneal[2] Semiscleral[3] (sometimes called extralimbal) Scleral[4]	Semiscleral[3]	Semiscleral[3]
Wear schedule	Daily wear Extended wear[5] Flexible wear[6]	Daily wear Extended wear[5] Flexible wear[6]	Daily wear
Disposal frequency	Reusable[7]	Reusable[7] Planned replacement[8] Disposable extended wear[9] 'Disposable' daily wear[10] Disposable daily wear[11]	Reusable[7]

[1]The Softperm lens (Pilkington Barnes-Hind Ltd, Southampton, UK).
[2]Fitted within the cornea. This is the usual fit for hard lenses.
[3]Fitted over the cornea and limbus. This is the usual fit for soft lenses. Hard lenses fit in this way are used when a corneal lens is unstable.
[4]Hard lenses fitted over the cornea and limbus and stabilized by extensive contact with sclera. These are used when a corneal or semiscleral lens is unstable or as therapeutic lenses to provide maximal ocular surface cover.
[5]A minimum period of 24 h continuous wear with 7 days of continuous wear commonly recommended and up to 3 months or more for some users.
[6]Continuous wear and daily wear as required.
[7]Reused for more than 6 months.
[8]Planned replacement of the lens every 1 to 6 months.
[9]Replaced after each use. Lenses usually worn for 7 days of continuous wear.
[10]Lenses removed at the end of each day, stored overnight and replaced after 1–4 weeks. This usage regimen is not truly disposable but rather a frequently replaced reusable lens.
[11]Replaced after 1 day of use.

rubber lenses were developed in the early 1970s but the problems of maintaining a hydrophilic surface and consistent fit have precluded their widespread use despite an excellent physiological performance.

Oxygen availability

The importance of oxygen availability to the cornea as a major factor, determining both tolerance to contact lens wear and some of the complications of lens wear, has been widely accepted since the 1970s and has led to the development of materials and lens fits that optimize oxygen supply. Polymethylmethacrylate is impermeable to oxygen and the lens fit is critical to maintain the interchange of oxygen-laden tears over the surface of the cornea underneath the lens. This has led to the fitting of scleral lenses that maintain clearance at the limbus and which may be fenestrated, or channeled, to improve the exchange of tears from the front surface to the corneal surface of the lens; however, this type of lens cannot transmit enough oxygen for most corneas so that the wearing time is limited by the resulting corneal oedema and reduced tolerance (comfort). Corneal polymethylmethacrylate lenses are fitted with edge clearance away from the corneal surface, to encourage tear exchange, and are also reduced in diameter to minimize their effect on corneal oxygen availability. A reduced diameter results in instability and polymethylmethacrylate corneal lenses have to be fitted larger (extralimbal) than the cornea, on very astigmatic or irregular corneas, to improve stability at the expense of corneal oedema and reduced tolerance. This problem has been overcome since the 1970s by the introduction of rigid gas permeable materials which have made use of polymers, principally of methacrylate and silicone (siloxymethacrylates) and/or fluorine (fluoroalkylmethacrylates), to increase the oxygen permeability at the expense of reduced wettability, increased tendency to deposit, and less dimensional stability. The development of these materials has allowed the use of lenses with a larger overall diameter, to improve stability, without compromising corneal oxygen availability. This has been particularly useful in the fitting of lenses to irregular and scarred corneas. It has also permitted the use of rigid lenses for continuous and flexible wear although lens awareness has limited these applications. Oxygen permeability for the soft hydrogel materials is broadly proportional to their water content. This has been increased by polymerizing hydroxyethylmethacrylate, the first described soft hydrogel material, with more hydrophilic materials such as vinyl pyrrolidone. These high water content hydrogels are more fragile, in the absence of surface modification, and deposit more quickly than the lower water content hydrogels but reduce the frequency of occurrence of corneal oedema and related complications; their oxygen transmission permits their use for reasonably successful continuous wear although this is still only approximately half of the minimum requirement. Optimal levels of oxygen transmission can only be provided by silicone rubber.

Disposal frequency

The problem of hydrogel lens spoilage, because of the build-up of deposits, has been addressed by replacing hydrogel lenses more frequently. This has been made possible by automating manufacturing techniques to allow the economic production of low cost lenses with stable parameters, permitting a reproducible fit, so that replacement lenses can be issued without the need for an assessment of fit. Disposable extended wear lenses were introduced in 1990 in a limited range of materials and parameters. These were intended for replacement after each period of wear of up to a week. Because of the increased risks of extended wear for some complications these lenses are also used as frequent replacement daily wear lenses; inaccurately referred to as daily wear disposable lenses. Truly disposable daily wear lenses only became widely available in 1995.

Advantages and disadvantages of different lens types

These many different lens types have been developed principally for the benefit of the large population of healthy individuals, with low refractive errors, seeking good sight without the inconvenience of spectacles. Although the older materials and lens fitting techniques have become irrelevant for this group of users, the patient with a medical indication for contact lens use may still benefit from them. This has given the medical contact lens practitioner a large armamentarium to treat these often challenging problems; the ophthalmologist must be aware of these potential solutions to provide the optimum management for this group of corneal and external disease problems. Table 2 summarizes the advantages and disadvantages of the different types of lens that are currently available and Table 3 the more common medical indications for their use.

Requirements for lenses used to treat medical conditions

Contact lens users with low refractive errors are now almost exclusively fitted with rigid gas permeable lenses (approximately 20 per cent in the United Kingdom) or daily wear soft, disposable, reusable, or frequent replacement lenses, (70 per cent in the United Kingdom) with the remainder using extended wear, disposable, or reusable soft lenses. Patients with medical conditions requiring contact lenses for visual indications place different optical and physiological demands on contact lens correction, because of their high refractive errors and high or irregular astigmatism. The optical demands of high myopic corrections result in a thick lens edge with poor oxygen transmission, similarly the lens centre is thick in aphakic corrections. Figure 1 shows a rigid gas permeable lens fitted to a highly myopic eye which shows superior cornea neovascularization from previous soft lens use. In both situations rigid gas permeable lenses are preferable as the lens of first choice because the complication rate due to reduced oxygen transmission can be minimized.

The high or irregular astigmatism associated with the many medical indications for lens wear is usually more easily corrected with gas permeable rigid lenses than with soft toric lenses (Fig. 2). However, for those patients with reduced tolerance to rigid lenses a compromise with a soft lens for the spher-

Table 2 Advantages and disadvantages of different contact lens types

Lens type	Advantages and disadvantages	
	Visual indications	**Therapeutic indications**
Rigid corneal Polymethylmethacrylate	Rarely used except in high myopes (> 20 dioptres) when the stability of the material may provide better vision than with gas permeable materials	Occasionally useful for control of lens-related papillary conjunctivitis because it deposits less than gas permeable materials
Rigid gas permeable	Fewer complications than with reusable soft lenses. Optimal acuity for treating high or irregular astigmatism. Longer life than soft lenses. Wide range of materials and oxygen permeabilities useful in compromised eyes and suboptimal lens fits. High *Dk* lens materials may be unstable in high minus and toric powers. But more difficult to fit than soft lenses, less well tolerated. Spectacle blur[1] and need for adaption to wear limits use for occasional lens users	Daily wear therapeutic use in some patients with dryer eyes and ocular surface disease complicated by corneal scarring (i.e. pemphigoid and atopic keratoconjunctivitis). Large overall diameter lenses can give the optimal combination of stability, improved comfort and vision; these are often used postkeratoplasty
Soft hydrogel Daily wear soft lens	The lens of choice for occasional lens users, most low myopes and hypermetropes because well tolerated, easy to fit, readily supplied from stock, and cause little spectacle blur. However, hygiene more demanding for reusable lens users than with rigid lenses, costs higher, complications more frequent, and astigmatism difficult to correct using toric[2] designs	Useful for patients requiring relief from ocular surface pain during the day (i.e. Thygeson's keratitis, superior limbic keratoconjunctivitis, filamentary keratitis)
Low water content soft lens	More robust than high water content and deposit less easily but the lower *Dk* unsuitable for prolonged wearing times for many patients	Slower rate of spoilage and lower water content useful as daily wear therapeutics in patients with drier eyes or abnormal tear films. Thinner and tougher than high water content soft lenses providing moderate protection from lids and lashes and appose wound edges
High and medium water content soft lens	The lens of choice for most soft lens users with good comfort and adequate oxygen transmission for most users but deposit more easily and are more fragile than lower water content lenses	The most widely used type of therapeutic lens available in the widest fitting parameters. Used for extended wear and/or when the corneal epithelium is sick. Often dry out in aqueous tear deficiency
Extended wear soft lens	Complication rate higher both for minor problems and corneal infection. Risks particularly high in aphakic lens users. Only recommended for informed users with an indication for continuous wear	Use only when a continuous effect is required
Daily disposable soft lens	Expensive but may prove to be the safest option providing lenses are not reused	
Soft prosthetic (cosmetic) Tinted	Available	As cosmetic lenses well tolerated, with a wide range of tints, but cosmesis disappointing when matching pale irides. Reduced light transmission lenses available for occlusion
Laminated		Poor oxygen transmission, expensive and poorly reproducible but may give good cosmetic effect
Silicone rubber (soft)	Difficulty obtaining consistent fits, and maintaining the hydrophilic surface coating, has made these impracticable for most users. Occasionally useful for aphakic patients with compromised corneas requiring the very high oxygen transmission provided and in infantile aphakia	Can be very useful in dry eyes because no hydration is required. Also the relatively high rigidity provides good vision on irregular corneas and protection from damaged lids. Good for compromised corneas requiring high oxygen transmission. But difficult to fit and remove. Extended wear often impracticable because of deposits
Scleral Polymethylmethacrylate or gas permeable	Only indicated for very high corneal astigmatism when surgery is contraindicated (keratoconus with high risk of graft failure, Terrien's marginal degeneration, keratoglobus)	Protection from lids or hydration in exposure or for very dry eyes

Table 2 Continued

Lens type	Advantages and disadvantages	
	Visual indications	**Therapeutic indications**
Scleral ring	Not indicated	Maintenance of fornices after conjunctival reconstructive surgery or acutely ulcerated conjunctiva
Hybrid Gas permeable rigid lens sandwiched in a hydrogel lens	For astigmatism correction when toric soft lenses ineffective or in management of keratoconus when rigid lenses not tolerated	

Dk is the term describing oxygen permeability of a lens material and *Dk/l* the oxygen transmission is the lens where *l* is the lens thickness.
[1]Spectacle blur is the temporary blurring of spectacle vision because of moulding of the cornea, usually as a result of rigid lens wear. This may last 2 or more weeks after regular periods of daily wear.
[2]When the front surface of the lens is spherocylindrical.

Table 3 Summary of medical indications for contact lenses

Indication	Lens choice	
Improvement of acuity or field		
High myopia (more than −10 dioptres)	Rigid gas permeable; rigid PMMA	Lens of choice; PMMA more stable in prescriptions over 20 dioptre
	Daily wear soft	Neovascularization common due to thick lens edge but may be better tolerated by some
Aphakia	Rigid gas permeable	Safe but daily wear difficult in elderly. Comfort rarely a problem due to relative corneal anaesthesia
	Extended wear soft	Demanding after care and high complication rate but necessary for most elderly patients
Keratoconus	Rigid gas permeable	Lens of choice
Irregular astigmatism; corneal scarring	Scleral	For eyes where corneal lenses are too unstable and surgery is contraindicated. Large size useful when handling is poor
Corneal warping	High *Dk* rigid gas permeable	The condition will recover without discontinuation of lens wear providing the *Dk* is adequate
Diagnostic lenses	Large overall diameter PMMA	To permit a stable fit while visual acuity is assessed
Restoration of binocular vision		
Monocular aphakia; other anisometropias postgraft primary (above 4 dioptres)	Daily wear soft lenses; rigid gas permeable	Fit both eyes where indicated as lens wear less successful in one eye. Soft lens use to correct the spherical error with spectacles for the astigmatic element is often more helpful when unilateral rigid lens wear is not possible
Occlusion (reduction of incident light by opaque lens)		
Partial albinism	Daily wear soft	Stable fit but low light transmission lenses are almost black and therefore cosmetically poor
aniridia iris coloboma rod monochromatism	Rigid PMMA	A coloured iris can be painted on black PMMA for a cosmetic appearance but tolerance poor due to hypoxia
Complete intractable diplopia	Scleral	Scleral fit allows eccentric occlusion. Handling easy
Prosthetic (cosmetic lenses fitted primarily to improve appearance)		
Orbital volume deficit or squint	Scleral	Excellent cosmetic result obtainable but poor tolerance on normal corneas

Table 3 Continued

Indication	Lens choice	
No volume deficit or squint	Semiscleral PMMA	Good cosmetic result but also poor tolerance
	Tinted soft lens	Well tolerated, easy to fit and reproduce, but poor cosmetic result on pale eyes
	Laminated soft lens	Lens well tolerated than homogenous soft lens as *Dk* relatively poor but better cosmetic results on pale eyes although lenses difficult to reproduce
Central leucoma or cataract	Black pupil soft lens	Simple to fit and very effective
Therapeutic (to maintain integrity of ocular tissues; improving vision a secondary benefit)		

Mechanical protection
  lashes
  keratinized scarred tarsal conjunctiva
  or concretions
	All lens types may be indicated	For continuous wear slow water content soft lenses and silicone are more robust. Rigid lenses useful for daily wear. Lashes only treated by lenses as a temporizing measure

Promotion of epithelial healing
  persistent epithelial defects
  recurrent corneal erosion
	High water content soft lenses or silicone rubber	Soft lenses usually adequate but the better *Dk/l* of silicone may be more effective. Silicone is a better choice in dry eyes. Although some patients do well with recurrent erosions disease is exacerbated unpredictably in others

Apposition of corneal wound edges	Soft lenses	

Pain relief
  dry eye and/or filaments
  bullous keratopathy
	Soft or silicone rubber
	
	High water content soft lens
		Because soft lenses require hydration and increase tear film turnover these are not often successful in very dry eyes where silicone is useful Lens of choice. A period of continuous wear may result in prolonged symptomatic relief without the need for a lens in bullous keratopathy; a high risk of bacterial keratitis in long-term use for this

Thygeson's keratitis superior limbic keratoconjunctivitis		Daily wear safer and practicable for patients requiring relief of symptoms during the day only
Maintenance of epithelial hydration	Rigid or silicone rubber	Scleral lenses may be effective in very dry vascularized eyes (i.e. in pemphigoid and Stevens–Johnson). Hydrogels may help in moderately dry eyes but seldom in severe cases
Maintenance of fornices	Scleral ring	After conjunctival reconstructive surgery or to help maintain fornices during severe episodes of conjunctival ulceration (Stevens–Jonson syndrome or chemical burns)
Drug delivery	High water content soft	Occasionally useful as reservoir for water soluble drugs
Ptosis prop in myopathies	Scleral with shelf	When surgery is not possible

PMMA, polymethylmethacrylate; *Dk* is the term used to describe oxygen permeability of a lens material and *Dk/l* the oxygen transmission of the lens where *l* is the lens thickness.

ical error and an overcorrection with spectacles, for the astigmatic error, may be acceptable when there is less than 4 dioptres of regular corneal astigmatism. For these patients, with medical indications for contact lens wear, there is usually no short-term alternative to lens wear if they are to maintain useful vision, so that risk assessment plays an important role in balancing the disadvantages of a relatively poor physiological response to lens wear, with the improved stability or tolerance that may be provided by one of the older materials or lens fits. The rigidity of polymethylmethacrylate still has a small role in the management of highly myopic corrections where rigid gas permeable material flexing can reduce vision. Polymethylmethacrylate may also be useful in managing lens-related papillary conjunctivitis (Table 4), where the disadvantages of corneal warpage (Table 4) and hypoxia are outweighed by an increase in wearing time due to improved control of the conjunctivitis.

Other examples are the use of aphakic extended wear soft lenses, complicated by corneal neovascularization (shown in Fig. 3) and corneal microcystic epitheliopathy, in elderly aphakes intolerant of spectacles who are a high surgical risk; the corneal complications of lens wear in such patients would be unacceptable in a young myope but are outweighed, in this example, by the maintenance of a level of vision required for a normal existence. Scleral lenses are useful for correcting the astigmatism in patients with keratoglobus, or Terrien's or pellucid marginal degeneration; these conditions represent formidable and commonly insoluble surgical problems so that a compromise solution with scleral lenses, even with reduced lens wearing times, is often preferable. Scleral lenses may also be indicated for partially sighted patients because of their ease of handling and because they are more easily found if misplaced.

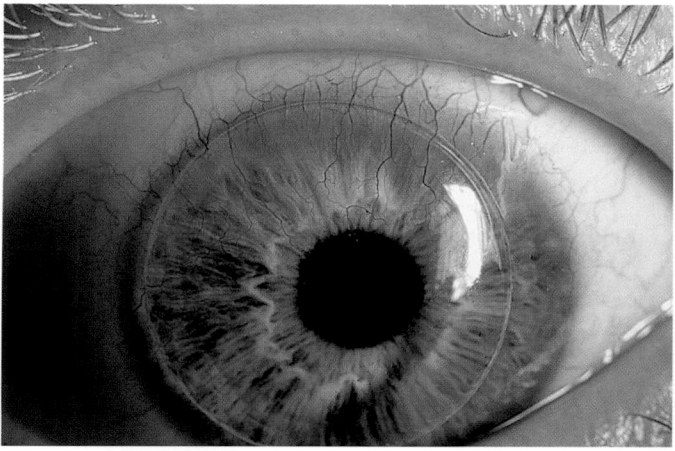

Fig. 1 A rigid gas permable lens fitted to a highly myopic eye. The superior cornea shows the new vessels resulting from the prolonged prior use of soft contact lenses.

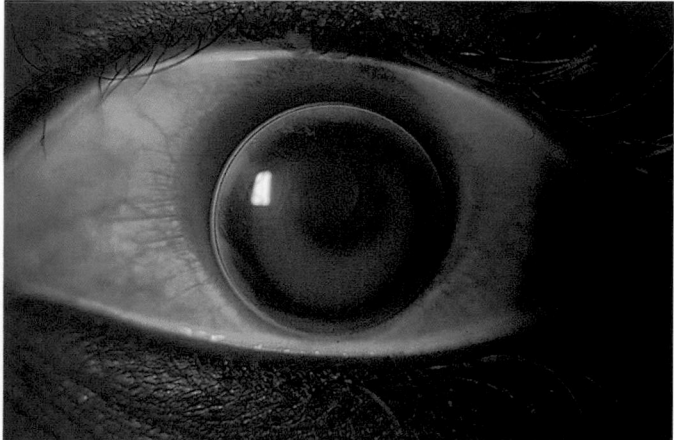

Fig. 2 Rigid gas permeable lens fitting for keratoconus showing the typical 'three-point touch' fluorescein pattern that is ideal on keratoconus corneas.

Requirements for lenses used for therapeutic reasons

The term therapeutic lens is often considered to be synonymous with the soft hydrogel extended wear lens but many of the other lens types may be used as therapeutic lenses to advantage. The daily wear of therapeutic lenses is practicable for those patients requiring relief of symptoms only during the day and avoids the increased risk of complications associated with continuous wear. Low water content soft lenses, rarely indicated for the treatment of low refractive errors because of reduced oxygen transmission, are useful as therapeutic lenses where their robustness, and reduced tendency to deposit and dehydrate, outweighs the disadvantage of their reduced oxygen transmission. The corneal oxygen requirement of diseased corneas is largely unstudied, except for aphakia in which it is lower, but those vascularized as a result of disease rather than contact lens wear, require less oxygen from the tear film to remain healthy. In these circumstances the continuous wear of poly-

methylmethacrylate scleral shells is possible. Alternatively, when the aim of therapeutic contact lens wear is to treat persistent corneal epithelial defects, a good oxygen supply is important and practitioners must be aware that failure to achieve healing with a hydrogel therapeutic may, in part, be due to this. In this situation silicone rubber is the only soft lens material that allows enough oxygen transmission (described by the term Dk/l, where Dk is the oxygen permeability of the material and l the lens thickness. Dk/l increases with increasing transmission) to meet normal corneal oxygen consumption.

Lens fitting care and maintenance

A detailed description of contact lens fitting is outside the scope of this chapter. Fitting rigid contact lenses, particularly for medical conditions with abnormal cornea may be very time-consuming and requires both a practical and scientific education. However, the goals of a stable and physiological lens fit should be understood by the general ophthalmologist together with the basic principles of lens maintenance.

Rigid lenses

The aims are to obtain a stable and physiological fit. To achieve both of these aims, compromises have to be made on some abnormal corneas. For rigid corneal lenses an overall diameter of about 9.0 mm is commonly chosen to optimize tear exchange whilst avoiding lens 'flare', resulting from the lens periphery overlapping the pupillary zone during lens movement. Stability may be difficult to achieve on astigmatic or irregular corneas and is usually achieved by increasing the overall diameter to as much as 10.0 or 11.0 mm and/or employing a toric periphery on the lens although in keratoconus reducing the overall diameter to as little as 8.0/8.5 mm can be successful. A physiological fit requires good tear exchange and alignment to the corneal surface to avoid microtrauma due to areas of heavy touch. The use of rigid gas permeable materials has allowed a greater latitude both in choosing the size of the lens and the tear exchange.

Fluorescein is used to assess the edge clearance of the lens periphery away from the cornea which assists tear exchange, as well as permitting a qualitative assessment of the rate of tear exchange by the speed of uptake and dilution of the dye under the lens. This requires movement of the lens with each blink. The intensity of fluorescein staining under the lens is used to assess the degree of lens touch and any areas of tear stagnation; an optimal pattern for keratoconus is shown in Fig. 2.

Scleral lens fitting is a specialized area but is assessed in a similar way; these lenses are all fitted with clearance to avoid compression of the limbal vasculature and to allow movement of the lens with blinking to encourage tears to be pumped under the lens. The ophthalmologist should ideally be able to assess these aspects with the contact lens practitioner.

Soft lenses

These are fitted over the limbus and little tear exchange occurs under the lens. However, some lens movement with blinking is necessary to avoid a red eye response as a result of limbal

Table 4 Classification of lens-related disorders (from Dart 1993)

Classification	Disease (synonyms)	Probable aetiology	Symptoms	Corneal signs	Conjunctival signs	Associated lens
Metabolic (hypoxia, hypercapnia and related effects)						
Epithelial	(1) Acute epithelial necrosis (overwear) syndrome	Epithelial cell necrosis; separation of cells and cell death due to hypoxia	Often blurred vision due to corneal oedema. Delayed pain and epiphora from necrosis. Resolves in hours, days if severe	Central punctate epithelial erosions may coalesce into an ulcer. Involved area larger in SCL wear. Stromal oedema in severe cases	Ciliary injection	PMMA-RCL and SCL
	(2) Microcystic epitheliopathy	Impaired epithelial metabolic activity	Asymptomatic or minor discomfort	Mini erosions during symptomatic episodes. Clear or opaque epithelial cysts and punctate keratitis	None	All types
	(3) Superior epithelial arcuate lesions	Multifactoral aetiology, including metabolic and mechanical effects	Often none	Superior arcuate epithelial staining	None	SCL
	(4) Corneal warpage	Metabolic and mechanical factors	Irregular astigmatism, vision good with lenses and poor with spectacles	Irregular keratometry and topography	None	PMMA-RCL commonest
	(5) Epithelial oedema (Sattler's veil)	Hypoxia and tear hypotonicity	Blurred vision after some hours of wear. May progress to acute epithelial necrosis	Dull corneal reflex due to epithelial oedema	None	All lens types but more common with PMMA and low Dk soft and rigid gas permeable lenses
Stromal	(6) Stromal oedema (striate keratopathy)	Stromal lactate accumulation, tear hypotonicity causing swelling	Blurring of vision in some cases only	Striae and stromal folds. Folds from corneal oedema, seen in severe acute epithelial necrosis	None except when associated with acute epithelial necrosis	Usually EW-SCL
	(7) Neovascularization (superficial and deep)	Hypoxia causes stromal oedema and release of vasogenic mediators	None unless lipid keratopathy or haemorrhage from deep vessels, causing loss of vision	Superficial/deep stromal vessels. Lipid keratopathy associate with deep vessels	None	Rare with RCL. Common with SCL
	(8) Deep stromal opacity	Probably due to prolonged hypoxia and hypercapnia	Asymptomatic or reduced acuity	Pre-Descemet's opacity in central cornea	None	Rare with RCL
Epithelial and stromal	(9) Tight lens syndrome	Lens tightening precipitated by hypoxia and reduced pH, also other factors	Starting during or after overnight wear. Vision usually affected	As above, but stromal oedema and an epithelial defect common	Ciliary injection and limbal indentation from the tight lens	EW-SCL
Endothelial	(10) Polymegethism and pleomorphism	Prolonged hypoxia and hypercapnia	None. Evidence of functional changes and slower deswell rates in polymegethism	Variations in endothelial cell size and shape	None	All
Mechanical/ traumatic						
	(11) Corneal abrasion	Trauma during lens handling or from trapped foreign bodies behind lens, deposits on lens or poor lens fitting	Sudden onset of pain and epiphora. Resolves in hours	Linear/sharply circumscribed epithelial defect	Hyperaemia	Commoner with RCL

Table 4 Continued

Classification	Disease (synonyms)	Probable aetiology	Symptoms	Corneal signs	Conjunctival signs	Associated lens
Toxic or allergic disorders						
	(12) Toxic keratopathy	Exposure to compounds adsorbed onto or absorbed by lens	Pain arising after inserting lens soaked in proteolytic enzyme/chemically preserved soaking solution	Widespread punctate stain	Ciliary injection	SCL
	(13) Thiomersal keratopathy (thiomersal keratoconjunctivitis or soft lens related superior limbic keratoconjunctivitis)	Preservatives act as haptens, causing a delayed hypersensitivity response	Irritation and redness soon after inserting lenses; symptoms increasing over 1–2 weeks. Rapid relief of symptoms after lens removal in early disease and recur within hours of restarting lens wear. Vision affected in severe cases	Keratopathy affecting superior quadrant and extending to visual axis in severe cases; changes include epithelial infiltrates, microcysts and anterior stromal opacity	Superior limbal hyperaenia, oedema and neovascularisation of limbus and superior cornea. Intense hyperaemia with lens *in situ*. Follicular changes remain when lens removed	SCL. Rare with RCL
	(14) Contact lens associated papillary conjunctivitis (giant papillary conjunctivitis or GPC)	Multifactoral aetiology; immune response to antigenic proteins on lenses, mechanical effects of lens edge. May be compounded by use of preserved solutions	Subacute onset. Increased discharge and greasing of lenses. Itching on lens removal in early stages, later severe irritation and tens intolerance. Acuity normal	None	Upper tarsal hyperaemia and fine papillary response. 'Giant' (compound) papillae > 1 mm in advanced disease with apical fibrosis. Clear mucous discharge	All lens types. Commoner with EW-SCLs and with prosthetic shells. Associated with spoiled lenses, poor lens hygiene and a history of allergy
	(15) Contact lens intolerance	Due to lens spoilation, chronic hypoxia, loss of adaption	Chronic redness, and/or discomfort and loss in tolerance. Vision may be blurred	Punctate stain common	Hyperaemia, papillae and follicles common	All types
Suppurative keratitis						
	(16) Sterile keratitis (aseptic keratitis, sterile corneal infiltrates)	Inflammatory response in the absence of infecting organism. Hypersensitivity to preservatives, bacteria or bacterial products, and tight lens fitting implicated	Discomfort, redness and discharge minimal and symptoms non progressive	Appearance similar to marginal keratitis. Usually peripheral infiltrates with/without ulceration. Peripheral lesions, occasionally central, may be multiple. Usually < 1 mm sometimes arcuate. Intact epithelium in early lesions, ulcerated in late	Hyperaemia	Common with reusable soft lenses, EWSCLs and some disposable soft lenses
	(17) Microbial keratitis	Multiple factors including increased ocular susceptibility and exposure to pathogens	Rapid onset, progressive pain hyperaemia and discharge in bacterial disease. Acanthamoeba slower onset but pain often a principle feature of early disease when signs are minimal	Epithelial ulcer with underlying stromal infiltrate. *Pseudomonas, Staphylococcus* and Acanthamoeba implicated. Lesions often central but may be in any location. Anterior chamber reaction in bacterial disease but not in early acanthamoeba for which radial keratoneuritis is pathognomonic	Cilliary injection in bacterial disease especially adjacent to affected corneal quadrant. In acanthamoeba keratitis anterior scleritis common	Bacterial keratitis most common in EW-SCL, rare in rigid lens use Acanthamoeba commoner in daily wear soft lens users either using chlorine disinfection, compared to other cold systems, or in those failing to use any disinfection system

Table 4 Continued

Classification	Disease (synonyms)	Probable aetiology	Symptoms	Corneal signs	Conjunctival signs	Associated lens
Tear resurfacing disorders						
	(18) 3 and 9 o'clock stain	Drying of corneal surface adjacent to lens edge and abnormal blink	Interpalpepral redness. Rarely discomfort	Punctate keratopathy at 3 and 9 o'clock. Severe cases; dellen formation and vascularized opacities	Interpalpebral hyperaemia	HCL
	(19) Inferior corneal strain	Incomplete blinking. Localized lens dehydration	Inferior limbal redness and discomfort	Inferior/interpalpebral punctate stain	Inferior limbal hyperaemia	SCL
	(20) Dimple veil	Static air bubbles under lens	Asymptomatic or blurred vision	Fluorescein pooling in epithelial depressions	None	HCL

PMMA-RCL, polymethylmethacrylate rigid contact lenses; SCL, soft contact lenses; EW-SCL, extended wear soft contact lenses; RCL, PMMA and rigid gas permeable contact lenses.

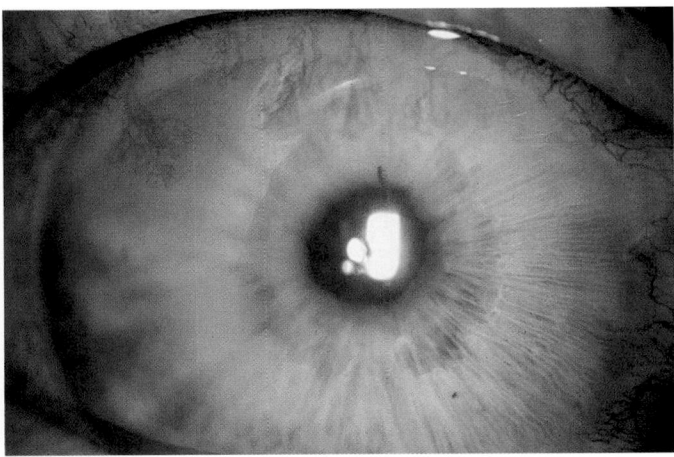

Fig. 3 Corneal neovascularization in an aphakic eye fitted with an extended wear soft contact lens. The vessels are engorged with blood and associated with corneal stromal oedema.

ischaemia and the build-up of debris under the lens. Because the parameters of hydrogel lenses alter in the eye, the fit should only be assessed after 30 min of lens wear and higher water content or high power lenses may require an hour to stabilize.

Lens maintenance

Good hygiene is critical to avoid many complications of lens wear. A discussion of the wide range of care systems available is outside the scope of this chapter. However, the same basic principles apply to the use of all systems. All lenses should be inserted and removed after hand washing. Truly disposable lenses should be disposed of whenever they are removed from the eye. All reused lenses require surfactant cleaning to remove debris and bacteria on the lens surface before disinfection. Tap water may be contaminated with both *Acanthamoeba* and bacteria and should never be brought directly into contact with the lens case or lens. The contact lens case must be kept clean and should be dried between each use to discourage the growth of Gram-negative bacteria and amoebae. Use of enzyme protein removing tablets once weekly is probably unnecessary for lenses replaced monthly but is otherwise advisable for most users.

Indications for different lens types

Some general principles of lens selection have been discussed. The medical indications for lens use are described in more detail here with guidelines for some of the more commonly encountered indications. Medical indications for lens fitting under the Hospital Eye Service in the United Kingdom and guidelines for lens types that may be useful are described in Table 3; additional notes are provided below.

Diagnostic lenses

The use of diagnostic lenses is often overlooked; the potential visual acuity is often underestimated by the use of a best spectacle correction with a pinhole overcorrection when there is substantial irregular corneal astigmatism. Although any rigid lens fitting set can be used as to assess visual acuity on scarred irregular corneas a bicurve lens set with an overall diameter of 10.5 to 12.0 mm will provide a lens fit that centres readily. The lens can be fitted with topical anaesthesia and the vision rapidly assessed with a spectacle over refraction.

Occlusion

Partial occlusion is the reduction of light entering the eye and can be achieved with tinted soft contact lenses although these may have to be very dark to achieve adequate reduction of light (Fig. 4). Scleral lenses can be made opaque with a layer of black polymethylmethacrylate which is painted to achieve a better cosmetic appearance and then covered with clear polymethylmethacrylate. Because scleral lenses depend for their stability on the scleral fit and not the corneal shape they can be used to occlude eccentric pupils. Complete occlusion with contact lenses, to treat intractable diplopia, is rarely tolerated but can be quickly assessed and treated with a soft lens having a black pupil.

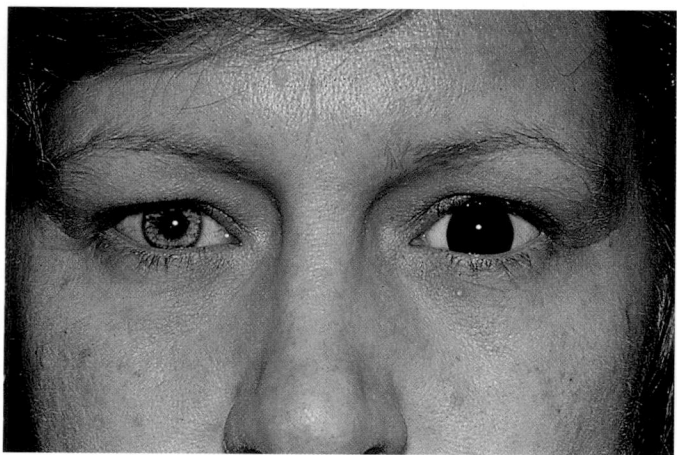

Fig. 4 A 2 per cent light transmission soft lens fitted to one eye of a patient with severe photophobia resulting from cone dystrophy. Lenses were worn in both eyes and successfully treated the symptoms as well as giving improved acuity.

Prosthetic

Lenses can be very valuable in helping to improve the appearance of unsightly eyes although the effect is limited by the need to place the pupil and iris on the surface of the eye and the difficulty of colour matching; therefore patients must be given realistic expectations. When the cornea is relatively normal soft lenses are usually the lens of choice although the colour matching is often disappointing for pale irides. Soft lenses with an artificial pupil may be very effective for patients with central corneal scars or mature cataracts in blind eyes (Fig. 5). Lamin-

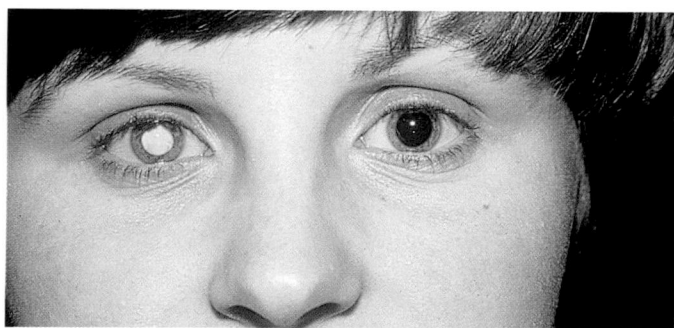

(a)

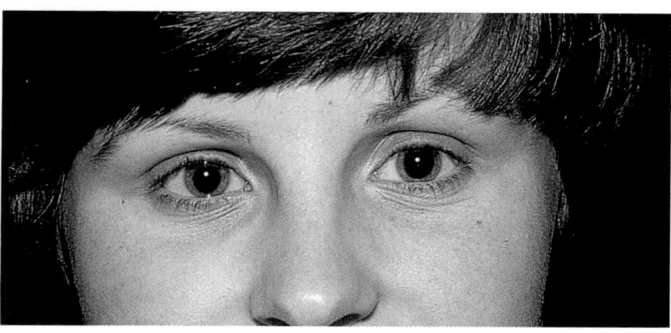

(b)

Fig. 5 (a, b) Soft daily wear cosmetic contact lens with a black pupil before and after fitting to a patient with a blind eye and mature cataract secondary to *Toxocara* chorioretinitis.

ated hand painted or printed soft lenses are available and can achieve a good cosmetic result but are expensive, difficult to fit and reproduce, and have poor oxygen transmission limiting wearing times on more normal corneas. Rigid corneal lenses in polymethylmethacrylate can be painted to give a realistic appearance but must be fitted large to achieve an acceptable effect and suffer from the same effects of hypoxia as laminated soft lenses. Scleral lenses can be similarly painted and are particularly indicated when the anterior segment disruption is severe and there is a volume deficit which can be corrected by increasing the lens thickness; squint can also be corrected with this type of lens as the artificial eye can be painted on the scleral lens in the primary position because the fit is independent of the position of the cornea.

Therapeutic

The use of therapeutic lenses should be regarded as invasive therapy with the potential for exacerbating the condition or precipitating bacterial keratitis. There is speculation as to how therapeutic lenses achieve their effect for many indications and this adds to the difficulty of predicting the results of treatment. Unpreserved topical medication is increasingly available and has simplified the use of therapeutic hydrogel lenses by eliminating preservative toxicity from the treatment equation.

Mechanical protection

Lenses should be used only for short-term protection and relief of pain in the management of conditions that can be treated surgically such as trichiasis because of the high risk of keratitis in these usually very compromised eyes.

Promotion of epithelial healing

Lenses are often inappropriately used for the management of indolent ulcers before correcting underlying predisposing factors such as keratoconjunctivitis sicca, drug toxicity, or corneal exposure. After these have been corrected a trial of therapeutic

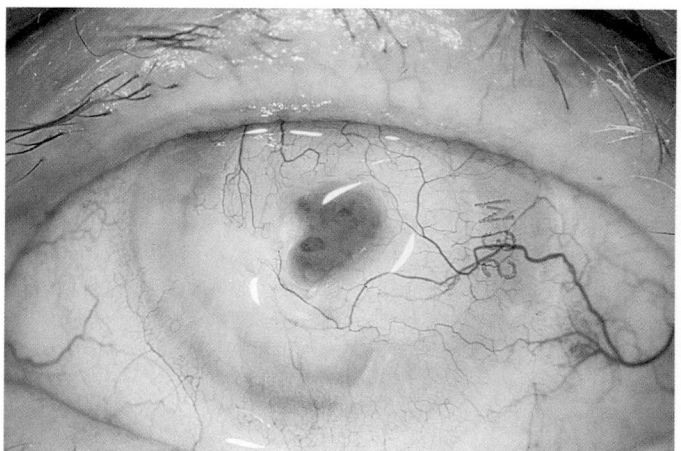

Fig. 6 A soft therapeutic lens fitted to seal a small central perforation in a conjunctival flap of an eye with chronic herpetic keratitis. Although this perforation did not heal the anterior chamber remained formed until graft surgery was performed several weeks later.

lens wear may be helpful but there is still a risk of microbial keratitis. For this reason prophylactic unpreserved antibiotics, other than the toxic aminoglycosides, should be used. The reduced corneal oxygen supply resulting from hydrogel lens wear may also account for some failures where a silicone rubber lens may succeed possibly because of better oxygen transmission.

Apposition of corneal wound edges

Many clean corneal lacerations or perforations may be treated with a contact lens with elimination of the astigmatism resulting from suturing. After the anterior chamber reforms the cornea usually needs to be refitted with a steeper lens. Figure 6 shows how a lens will mould to a very irregular cornea to seal a perforation succesfully.

Pain relief

In recurrent corneal erosion lenses may be a very effective form of treatment in some patients; unfortunately it is not possible to predict the outcome and 50 per cent of patients may develop an exacerbation soon after lens fitting. In successful cases, apart from improving comfort, a lens may provide resolution of symptoms and should be removed for a trial period after 2 months of continuous wear. In bullous keratopathy over 90 per cent of patients experience dramatic relief of symptoms but the risk of bacterial keratitis is high if lenses are used for prolonged periods. Pain relief may persist for some months after removing the lens. Daily or flexible wear of lenses is safe and practicable in many patients who only require relief of symptoms intermittently or during the day such as those with Thygeson's keratitis or superior limbic keratoconjunctivitis. Use of hydrogel lenses is helpful in some patients with moderate keratoconjunctivitis sicca and/or filamentary keratitis. However, hydrogels require hydration by the tear film, and also increase evaporation from the surface of the eye, so that they will dehydrate in many dry eyes leading to lens tightening and reduced oxygen

transmission. A silicone rubber lens is often effective in this situation.

Complications of contact lens wear

Contact lens wear has a wide range of effects on the eye the most important of which are on tear turnover, corneal and conjunctival epithelial metabolism, sensation, and corneal endothelial morphology (polymegethism). These are inevitable consequences of the use of current lens systems and affect all users to a variable extent. With the exception of endothelial polymegathism these effects are short term and recover soon after lens wear has ceased and are seldom of functional significance. Contact lens related disease develops in only some contact lens users and is distinguished from these inevitable consequences of lens wear by the development of symptoms, loss of function, or irreversible ocular changes. Contact lens related disease ranges from minor ocular adverse reactions such as corneal neovascularization, representing a suboptimal response to the stress

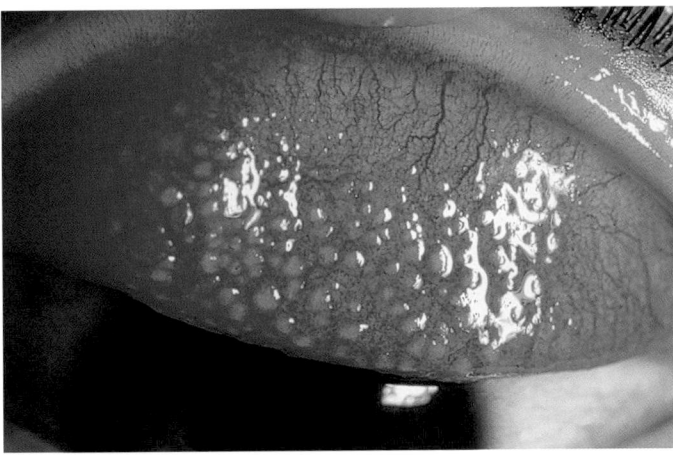

Fig. 8 Typical giant papillary conjunctivitis. This condition is better known as contact lens associated papillary conjunctivitis and may be symptomatic with minimal or absent papillae.

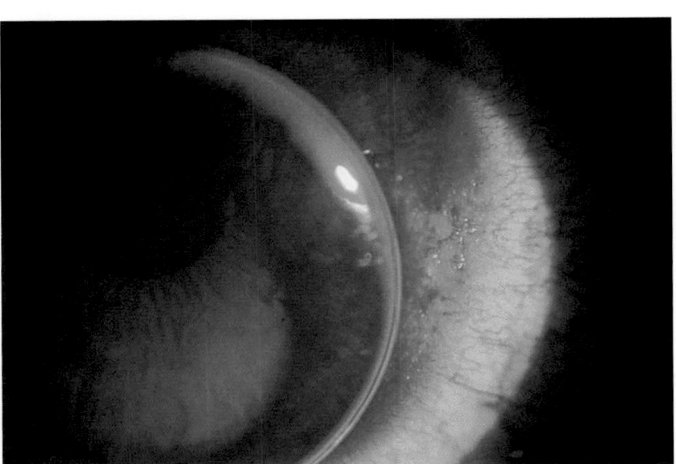

Fig. 7 Punctate keratopathy, demonstrated by fluorescein, in the 3 o'clock position in an eye with 3 and 9 o'clock keratopathy as a consequence of rigid gas permeable lens use. Note that the corneal epithelial disturbance does not extend beyond the lens edge.

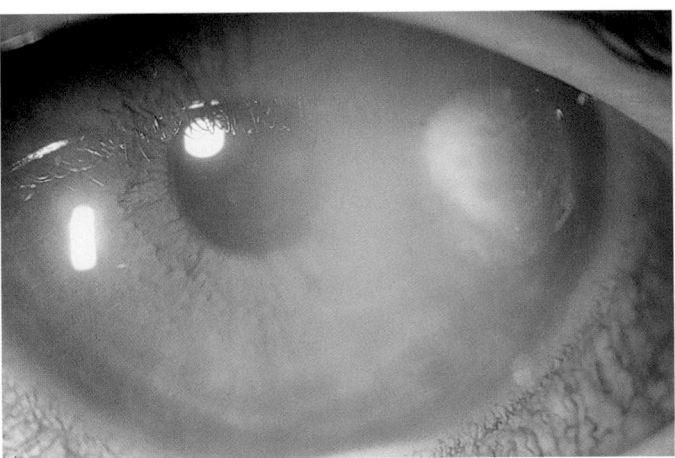

Fig. 9 *Pseudomonas* keratitis in a user of soft extended wear contact lenses for myopia.

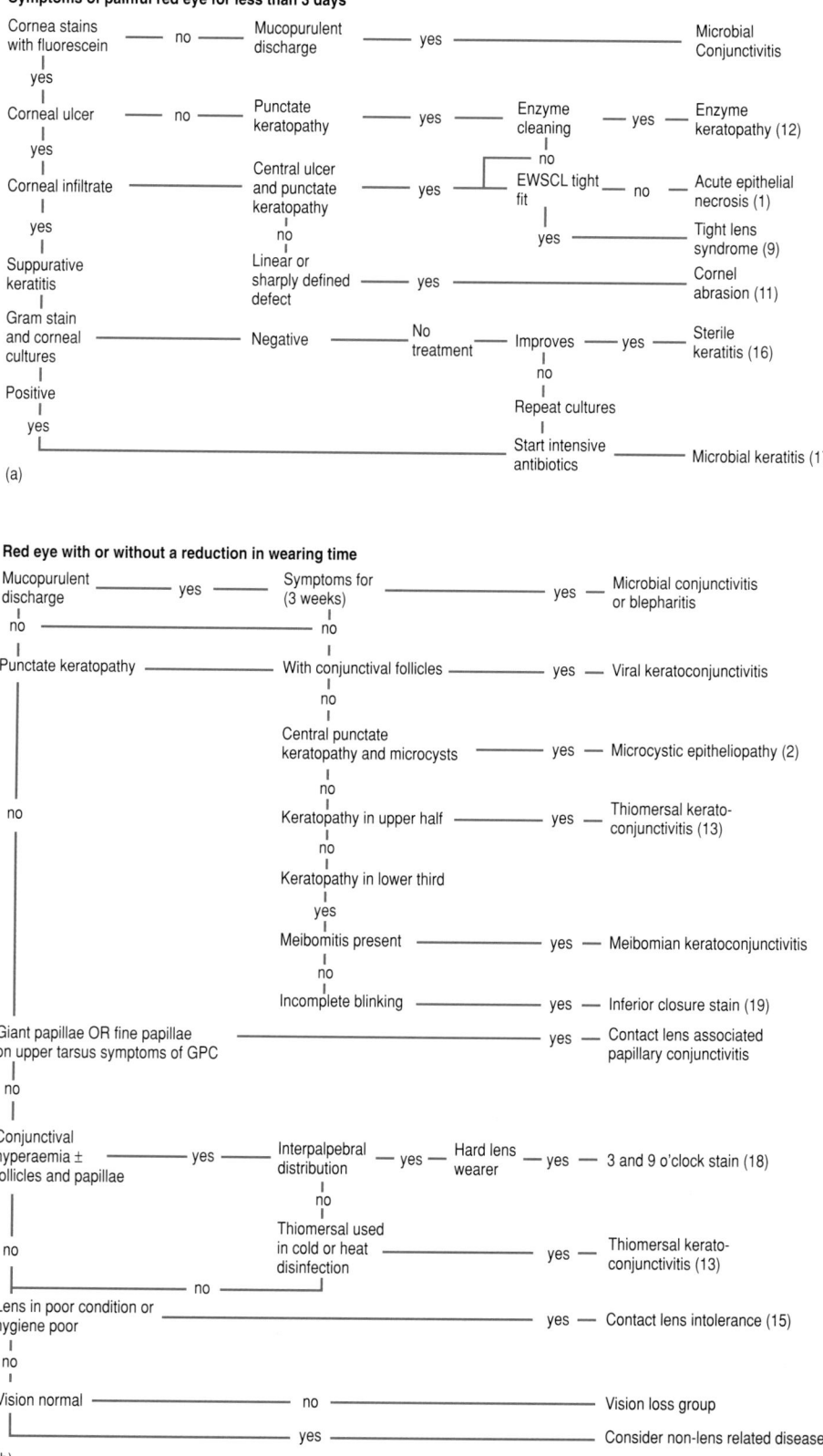

Symptoms of painful red eye for less than 3 days

Cornea stains with fluorescein — no — Mucopurulent discharge — yes — Microbial Conjunctivitis

yes

Corneal ulcer — no — Punctate keratopathy — yes — Enzyme cleaning — yes — Enzyme keratopathy (12)

yes — no — EWSCL tight fit — no — Acute epithelial necrosis (1)

Corneal infiltrate — Central ulcer and punctate keratopathy — yes — yes — Tight lens syndrome (9)

yes — no

Suppurative keratitis — Linear or sharply defined defect — yes — Cornel abrasion (11)

Gram stain and corneal cultures — Negative — No treatment — Improves — yes — Sterile keratitis (16)

no

Positive — Repeat cultures

yes — Start intensive antibiotics — Microbial keratitis (17)

(a)

Red eye with or without a reduction in wearing time

Mucopurulent discharge — yes — Symptoms for (3 weeks) — yes — Microbial conjunctivitis or blepharitis

no — no

Punctate keratopathy — With conjunctival follicles — yes — Viral keratoconjunctivitis

no

Central punctate keratopathy and microcysts — yes — Microcystic epitheliopathy (2)

no

Keratopathy in upper half — yes — Thiomersal kerato-conjunctivitis (13)

no

Keratopathy in lower third

yes

no — Meibomitis present — yes — Meibomian keratoconjunctivitis

no

Incomplete blinking — yes — Inferior closure stain (19)

Giant papillae OR fine papillae on upper tarsus symptoms of GPC — yes — Contact lens associated papillary conjunctivitis

no

Conjunctival hyperaemia ± follicles and papillae — yes — Interpalpebral distribution — yes — Hard lens wearer — yes — 3 and 9 o'clock stain (18)

no

Thiomersal used in cold or heat disinfection — yes — Thiomersal kerato-conjunctivitis (13)

no — no

Lens in poor condition or hygiene poor — yes — Contact lens intolerance (15)

no

Vision normal — no — Vision loss group

yes — Consider non-lens related disease

(b)

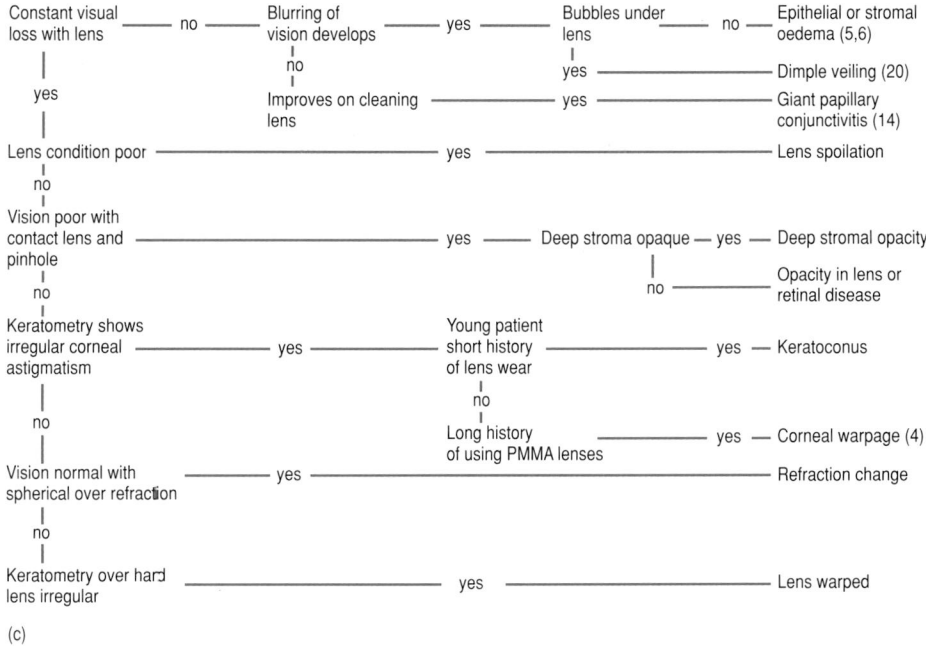

Fig. 10 Diagnosis of contact lens complications (numbers in brackets refer to diseases listed in Table 4). (a) Diagnosis of conditions causing a hyperacute presentation. (b) Diagnosis of conditions causing a chronic red eye and/or loss of lens tolerance. (c) Diagnosis of conditions causing loss of vision.

of lens wear, to severe complications such as microbial keratitis. The pathophysiology of contact lens related disease, like that of other biomaterials such as intraocular lenses and artificial joints, results from their physiological and anatomical effects in addition to the effect of their biologically active surface. Lens-related disease can be understood in these terms and some of the better characterized diseases illustrate this concept.

Corneal neovascularization (see Fig. 3) is principally a physiological effect resulting from reduced corneal oxygen availability, due to the relatively low oxygen transmission of some contact lenses. This is most often seen at the upper limbus, in soft contact lens wearers, where the cornea is already exposed to reduced oxygen tension levels, because of upper lid cover. These levels are further reduced by the presence of a lens.

A type of corneal dellen, 3 and 9 o'clock keratopathy (peripheral stain), is an anatomical effect resulting from interference by a rigid lens with tear resurfacing by the lid (Fig. 7). This is probably due to a combination, both of physical separation of the lid from the corneal limbus by the lens edge, and from the inhibitory effect of the lens on the blink reflex.

Contact lens associated papillary conjunctivitis (giant papillary conjunctivitis) is the result of the contact lens developing a biologically active surface in which there is an allergic response to ocular deposits that have accumulated on the lens surface (Fig. 8). In common with other biomaterials the lens surface rapidly becomes coated with materials derived from its environment including bacteria, cell debris, mucous, and proteins.

Many contact lens related disorders may be the result of complex interactions in which two or more of these effects are combined in the pathogenesis. An example is bacterial keratitis (Fig. 9). Important predisposing factors are the increased susceptibility of the contact lens wearing eye to bacterial infection resulting both from epithelial trauma and/or physiological stress; both are more common in extended wear lens use. Pathogenic organisms may be transferred to the cornea by adherence to the lens, colonization of the lens, or from a contaminated conjunctival sac. Reduced clearance of organisms from the ocular surface occurs, further increasing the risk of infection, due to interference with tear flow and tear resurfacing by the lids.

These concepts are useful in understanding how contact lens related disease differs from the established group of corneal and external eye disorders and has given rise to a new spectrum of diseases affecting these tissues.

Classification, clinical characteristics, and pathogenesis

Our current understanding of the pathogenesis of contact lens related disease is adequate for a clinical classification based on the adverse ocular effects of lens wear unlike more commonly used anatomical classifications. This approach assists in understanding both the development and management of this group of disorders. Twenty of the more common contact lens related diseases, their clinical characteristics, and probable pathogenesis are summarized in Table 4.

Diagnosis

Lens-related disease can be demanding to diagnose accurately. Interpretation of the symptoms and signs requires a detailed knowledge of the past history of lens wear. This should include the types of lens previously worn and for how long, problems related both to these and to previous lens hygiene systems, the current lens wearing cycle, age of the current lenses, and full details of the current hygiene regime. The inadequacies of the hygiene regime are often only clear if the clinician asks exactly what is done from the moment the lens is removed until next reinsertion. A direct inquiry about 'in eye' solutions that are being used will often reveal that preparations such as antihistamines or artificial tears are being used. This information, including the formulation of all these preparations and their preservatives may be vital to the diagnosis of conditions like thiomersal keratoconjunctivitis. The previous history is helpful in understanding the ocular changes that are present, which might be unexpected in relation to the current lens type, for example, peripheral corneal neovascularization in rigid lens users who have previously been wearing soft lenses or the opacities associated with 3 and 9 o'clock keratopathy in the converse situation. This information is also required when deciding on alternative lens wearing regimes.

Corneal and conjunctival disease in lens users is often related to lens wear and it is wise to assume that it is due to lens use until proved otherwise. Disorders usually present in three ways: as hyperacute conditions, with a red eye and/or lens intolerance, or visual loss. Guidelines to assist in the differential diagnosis of lens-related conditions and other common disorders in lens users are given in Fig. 10.

Suspension of lens wear is a useful diagnostic step when the diagnosis is unclear. The inflammatory symptoms of lens-related disease respond to this within a few days, although the physical signs may remain for many weeks (i.e. in contact lens associated papillary conjunctivitis and thiomersal keratoconjunctivitis). If the symptoms do not resolve, the disease is probably not lens related but an intercurrent disorder.

Viral and bacterial conjunctivitis are always associated with a discharge at onset and should not be diagnosed if this has not been present. Microbial keratitis is the principal lens-related condition that progresses after lens removal and must be investigated and managed urgently.

Table 5 Outline of principal management strategies for diseases in Figs 4 and 5

Disease number	Management strategy
(1–9) Epithelial and stromal metabolic disorders	Reduce wearing time. Supply more oxygen by looser fit, using a higher oxygen transmission hydrogel or GP material, refit soft lens users unresponsive to these measures with high Dk RGP lenses
(10) Polymegethism	Refit to provide better oxygen transmission only if changes are severe
(11) Corneal abrasion	Refit with soft contact lenses if this is a persistent problem
(12) Toxic keratopathy	Rinse lenses carefully before insertion
(13) Thiomersal keratopathy	Avoid thiomersal in all lens care materials including cleaner; purge soft lenses with multiple (10) overnight soaks in unpreserved saline and redisinfect using an unpreserved system prior to rewearing; resume lens wear when keratopathy has resolved — may take 9 months; no specific treatment
(14) Contact lens associated papillary conjunctivitis	Reduce the effect of the three major exacerbating factors: • mechanical trauma; improve lens edge, reduce lens size, improve lens surface • antigen on lens; try disposable or frequent replacement soft lens, improve lens cleaning, use enzyme cleaner, reduce wearing time, alter fit to reduce area of lens in contact with upper tarsal conjunctiva and alter material to reduce deposition • modify inflammatory response; mast cell stabilizers, steroids very rarely
(15) Contact lens intolerance	Refit with high water frequent replacement or disposable daily wear soft lens. Discontinue lens wear for 6–9 months and refit as new patient; frequently unresponsive to treatment
(16) Sterile keratitis	Improve lens hygiene, avoid overnight wear and some disposable lens types; change to RGP lenses if problem is recurrent
(17) Microbial keratitis	Intensive evaluation and treatment. Prevent by improving lens hygiene and reducing other risk factors by avoiding overnight wear and considering changing to RGP lens wear
(18) 3 and 9 o'clock stain	Alter lens size, improve lens edge, use thinner lens, increase edge clearance; may be difficult to eliminate. Fit with soft lens providing blink amplitude is satisfactory
(19) Inferior closure stain	Improve blinking characteristics, alter lens material, use thicker lens, use topical lubricants; if unsuccessful, change to RGP lens
(20) Dimple veil	Modify lens fitting. May be difficult to eliminate; treatment only indicated if associated corneal thinning is severe or if vision is affected

RGP, rigid gas permeable; Dk is the term describing oxygen permeability and Dk/l the oxygen transmission.

Management

When the diagnosis is clear and the symptoms are moderate, as in many of the metabolic disorders, early lens-associated papillary conjunctivitis, corneal warpage, and tear resurfacing disorders, it may be detrimental to lens tolerance to cease lens wear. In these cases, it is appropriate to institute treatment without suspending lens wear.

Discontinuation of lens wear is indicated as part of the management of infections, ulceration, or abrasion and when the symptoms are significantly exacerbated by lens wear. Management of disorders in patients using lenses for medical reasons, such as keratoconus and irregular astigmatism, who are incapacitated without lenses, requires specialized expertise to determine whether the risks of persisting with lens wear, are acceptable. The management of most lens-related disease is easily formulated, providing the diagnosis is correct and the pathogenesis is understood. Table 5 provides a brief outline of the principal management strategies for the diseases outlined in Table 4 and Fig. 10. The clinical and theoretical support for these is reviewed in the detailed description of each condition below.

Lens-related disease may provide challenging diagnostic dilemmas and it is not infrequent for the diagnosis to be obscure at the first attendance. In such cases, a step-by-step approach to the management, using remedies appropriate to each condition in a shortlist of differential diagnoses, is helpful. Ensuring that the lenses are in good condition and improving the lens hygiene regime are useful first steps when the symptoms are less than specific. Changing to a non-preserved system (such as hydrogen peroxide or heat) may also be worth a trial in these circumstances. Examination of the patient after a period of lens wear is essential to establish the diagnosis of a labile condition such as a tear resurfacing disorder.

Over the last 50 years the refinement of contact lenses has resulted in an alternative to spectacles for millions of users. For patients with medical indications contact lenses have provided an alternative to blindness as well as a revolutionary therapeutic modality. It is hoped that this chapter will provide doctors both with an introduction to this expanding field and to the diagnosis and management of the complications that are inevitable with the use of any biomedical device.

Further reading

Bacon, A.S., Astin, C., and Dart, J.K.G. (1994). Silicone rubber contact lenses for the compromised cornea. *Cornea*, 13, 422–8.

Dart, J.K.G (1993). Contact lens related disease: a review. *British Journal of Ophthalmology*, 77, 49–53.

Dart, J.K.G. (1996). Contact lens and prosthetic infections. In *Duane's foundations of clinical ophthalmology*, (ed. E. Jaeger and W. Tasman), Chapter 53.. Lippincott-Raven, Philadelphia.

Kastl, P.R. (ed.) (1995). *The CLAO guide to contact lenses*, (3rd edn), Vols I–III. Kendall/Hunt, Iowa.

Mackie, I.A. (1993). *Medical contact lens practice: a systematic approach*. Butterworth-Heinemann, Oxford.

2.3.5 Optics of aphakia and pseudophakia

Ben Parkin

Aphakia

The term aphakia is derived from the Greek meaning without a lens, and in an optical sense refers to any condition where the crystalline lens plays no part in the eye's refractive system. This is most commonly due to surgical removal of the cataractous lens. Other possibilities include traumatic dislocation, congenital absence, or ectopia of the lens.

In the aphakic eye there is recession of the iris and deepening of the anterior chamber. Clinically iridodonesis is noted, a tremulous movement of the iris on eye movement, and there is loss of the third and fourth Purkinje images normally formed by reflection from the lens surfaces.

Optics of emmetropia and aphakia

All parallel rays entering the eye by definition meet at the second principal focus F' of the eye. An unaccommodated eye which fails to bring parallel rays of light into sharp focus on the retina is said to be ametropic, and the second principal focus does not fall on the retina. Ametropia is divided into two main categories: spherical ametropia and astigmatism. In spherical ametropia the eye's refractive system is symmetrical about its optical axis, and therefore capable of forming a sharp image, but the retina is not in the corresponding position. Spherical ametropia is divided into myopia and hypermetropia, which may be subdivided into axial or refractive. In axial hypermetropia the eye is short relative to its focal power, whereas in refractive hypermetropia, the usual situation in aphakia, the refractive power of the eye is inadequate.

In the absence of the crystalline lens, rays of light entering the eye are refracted solely by the cornea, that is the equivalent power of the eye is that of the cornea alone. The principal points of the typical cornea very nearly coincide with one another and with the vertex of its front surface. Parallel rays of light are brought to a focus 31 mm behind the cornea, while the average length of the eye is only 23 to 24 mm (Fig. 1). The aphakic eye's optical system must therefore be supplemented by a positive lens (if the eye was previously emmetropic) to result in a clear retinal image.

Correction of aphakia

The ocular refraction (or principal point refraction) denoted by K is the reciprocal of the distance k (the distance to the eye's far point) in metres, that is it is the dioptric distance to the eye's far point. The axial length of the reduced eye is denoted by k', and if k' is regarded as an image distance then the corres-

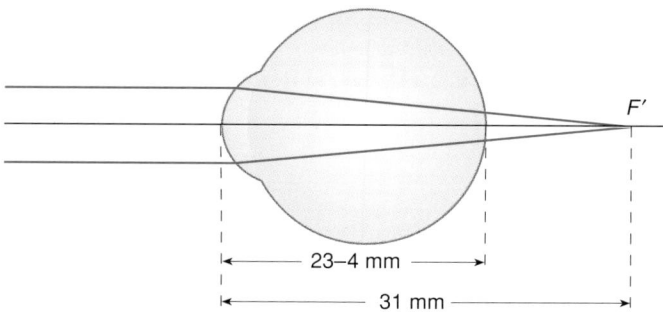

Fig. 1 Aphakia; an example of refractive hypermetropia. The average length of the globe is 23 to 24 mm, and the focal length in aphakia is 31 mm.

ponding image vergence K' is given by the formula $K = n'/k'$. K' may be called the 'dioptric length of the eye'.

Simple formulas can be used to calculate the aphakic correction required for any given eye. Here is an example using the figures for the schematic emmetropic eye of Gullstrand-Emsley to calculate the ocular retraction K (Fig. 2):

$$n = \text{refractive index of the air} = 1.0$$

$$n' = \text{approximation for the refractive index of aqueous/}$$
$$\text{vitreous} = 4/3 = 1.333$$

$$r = \text{radius of curvature of the cornea (m)} = 7.8/1000 \text{ m}$$

$$k' = \text{axial length (m)} = 23.89/1000 \text{ m}.$$

First the image vergence is calculated:

$$K' = n'/k' = 1.333 \times 1000/23.89 = +55.80 \text{ dioptres}.$$

Then the dioptric power of the whole eye (Fe), which in the aphakic eye is the power of the cornea, is calculated using the formula $Fe = n' - n/r$.

$$Fe = (1.333 - 1)/7.8/1000 = +42.69 \text{ dioptres}.$$

Then using the formula, $K = K' - Fe$, the ocular refraction K may be found:

$$K = 55.80 - 42.69 = +13.11 \text{ dioptres}.$$

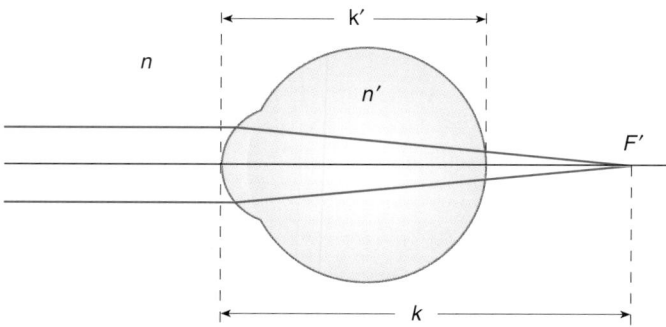

Fig. 2 Ocular refraction. n, n' = refractive indices of air and aqueous/vitreous, respectively; F', second principal focus; k, focal length; K', axial length.

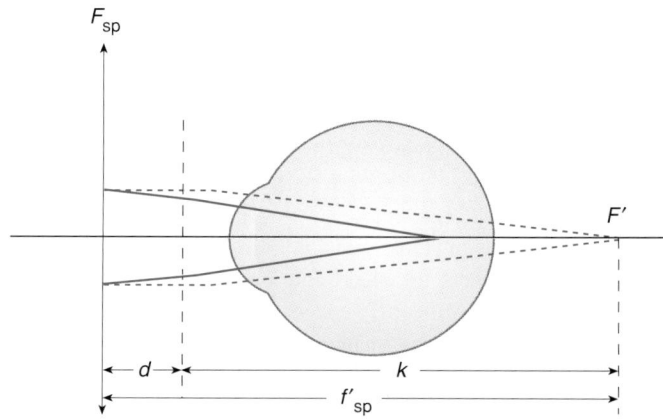

Fig. 3 Spectacle correction of aphakia. Spectacles at a distance d in front of the cornea.

This is the vergence required at the level of the cornea and therefore is the dioptric power of a correcting contact lens required for the aphakic reduced eye of Gullstrand-Emsley.

A spectacle lens is in a plane anterior to the cornea, and so the strength of correction required is less, as the effectivity of plus lenses increases with distance from the eye. The necessary correction may be calculated using the effectivity of lenses formula (see below), but it is simpler to make the calculation as follows (Fig. 3):

$$Fsp = \text{dioptric power of spectacle correcting lens}$$

$$d = \text{distance 12 mm in front of the eye}.$$

$$f's_p = \text{focal length of spectacle correcting lens}.$$

The distance to the aphakic eye's far point (k) in mm is the reciprocal of K calculated above:

$$k = 1/K = 1000/13.08 = 76.45 \text{ mm}.$$

If spectacles are worn 12 mm in front of the cornea, the focal length from the spectacles to the retina is

$$f'sp = k + d = 76.45 + 12 = 88.45 \text{ mm}.$$

So the focal power of spectacle correction required is less than the contact lens power,

$$Fsp = 1/f'sp = 1000/88.45 = +11.31 \text{ dioptres}$$

(from Bennett and Rabbetts 1989).

In contrast, the effectivity of an intraocular implant situated closer to the nodal point of the eye is less and so a greater power is required in order to obtain a clear retinal image.

Magnification

Spectacle magnification relates to the retinal image size in any given eye as a result of wearing either a spectacle or a contact lens. The relative spectacle magnification is the ratio of the retinal image size in the corrected ametropic eye to that in a specified emmetropic schematic eye. It thus compares the given corrected eye with a hypothetical standard.

The optical correction of refractive ametropia is always associated with a change in the retinal image size, whereas in axial ametropia, the relative spectacle magnification is unity if the correcting lens is placed at the anterior focal point of the eye. It is possible to calculate the different magnifications produced by the optical correction of aphakia (a refractive ametropia) by means of spectacles, contact lenses, or intraocular implants.

The percentage increase in retinal image size for spectacle aphakic correction is dependent on the previous spectacle correction, and there is a wide spread of possible values due to the number of different combinations of the eye's optical dimensions. If contact lens correction is used this effect may still be appreciable, but the possible spread of values is much narrower. The increase in retinal image size for pseudophakia also depends on the preaphakic spectacle correction. When aiming for emmetropia, neutralizing any previous spherical ametropia ranging from –8 to +8 dioptres, the corresponding magnification varies from 1.18 to 0.9, respectively. Whereas aiming to leave the patient requiring a –2 dioptre alteration to previous spectacle correction leaves the patient without any appreciable change in retinal image size.

Another factor in the level of magnification is the position of the correcting lens relative to the principal plane of the eye. As the distance of a convergent correcting optical device from the eye increases, so does the image magnification. An intraocular implant (intraocular lens) placed in the posterior chamber would theoretically induce minimal image magnification, but as the site of the intraocular lens moves forward to the pupillary plane or the anterior chamber, the induced image magnification increases to the range of 3 to 4 per cent.

Lens effectivity

The term effectivity denotes a change of vergence as light passes from one surface or reference point to another. The effectivity of a lens refers to the change in vergence power at the principal plane with distance from that plane (Fig. 4). For positive lenses, the effectivity increases with distance, which

explains why an aphakic spectacle lens worn at 12 mm in front of the eye requires less power than a correcting contact lens. Vergence of the lens in the new position is

$$L_2 = n/l_2.$$

Now,

$$l_2 = l_1 - d$$

therefore by substitution

$$L_2 = n/(l_1 - d).$$

As $L_1 = n/l_1$, again by substitution:

$$L_2 = n/[(n/L_1) - d] = n/[(n/L_1)(1 - L_1(d/n))]$$

$$So\ L_2 = L_1/1 - (d/n)L_1$$

In air $n = 1$, therefore

$$L_2 = L_1/(1 - dL_1)$$

(from Bennett and Rabbetts 1989).

Problems with correction of aphakia

Spectacles

There remain certain clinical situations in which it is not possible to correct aphakia with contact lenses or intraocular implants. However, there are many well-known optical, cosmetic, and physical disadvantages associated with aphakic spectacle correction.

Optical problems

The optical problems of spectacle corrected aphakia are well known and have been described eloquently by Woods, an aphakic ophthalmologist.

Magnification

Spectacle correction of aphakia produces a relative spectacle magnification of approximately 20 to 35 per cent. This causes considerable problems with altered depth perception, as optical perspective is changed and there is great difficulty in hand-eye co-ordination. In the case of unilateral aphakia, the aniseikonia, or unequal retinal image sizes between the two eyes, causes intolerable diplopia.

Image distortion

There is an increasing prismatic effect for rays of light passing through a spherical lens at a distance from the optical centre. The strength of the prism (in prism dioptres) can be calculated by Prentice's rule:

$$P = C \times F$$

where C is the distance from the optical centre in centimetres and F is the dioptric power of the lens. When an extended object is viewed through a high power plus spherical lens the edges of the object seen through the lens periphery are distorted in a 'pin cushion' fashion.

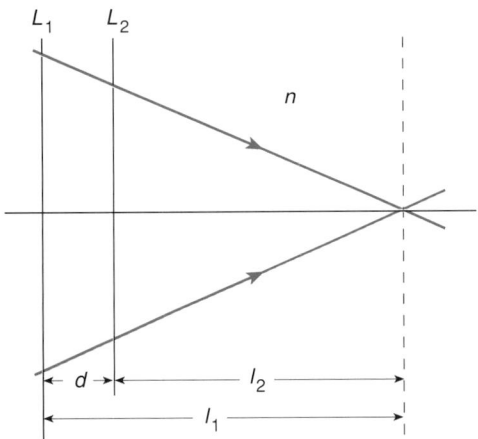

Fig. 4 Lens effectivity. L_1, vergence at original position; L_2, vergence at new position; d, distance moved; n, refractive index; l_1, object distance; l_2, new object distance; P, principal plane.

Ring scotoma

The prismatic effects at the periphery of the lens also produce a ring scotoma, which markedly reduces the visual field. The position of the scotoma changes with eye movement as it is dependent on the position of the nodal point of the eye relative to the spectacle lens. On attempting to take up fixation of an object in the peripheral field, the scotoma moves with the eye movement and the object disappears in a disconcerting manner. When the eye returns to the straight ahead position the object reappears, giving rise to the so-called 'jack-in-the-box' phenomenon.

Binocular single vision

In most cases it is impossible to maintain binocular single vision with spectacle correction of monocular aphakia, because of aniseikonia.

Other optical problems

Due to its high power the lens shows extreme sensitivity to minor changes in vertex distance and centration, which presents considerable difficulty in the fitting and wearing of aphakic spectacles.

Cosmetic problems

The eyes of the patient appear magnified, and may seem displaced when viewed obliquely because of prismatic effects. The lens itself is also thick and unattractive.

Physical problems

The lenses are heavy, and may slip down the patient's nose increasing the lens effectivity. This has partly been overcome with the use of modern, light, high refractive index materials, but these are plastic and therefore may easily be scratched.

Contact lenses

Contact lenses are situated closer to the nodal point of the eye and largely overcome the problems associated with the correction of aphakia described above. They do have many other associated potential difficulties and complications. Many elderly patients are unable to wear contact lenses because of arthritis, parkinsonism, or mental deterioration. The complications of contact lens wear include corneal vascularization, abrasions, superficial punctate keratitis, and corneal ulcers. The risk of complications is greatly increased with coincident dry eyes, blepharitis, or other lid disease.

Unilateral aphakia

In the typical case where emmetropia was present prior to surgery, unilateral aphakia presents an extreme example of hypermetropic anisometropia resulting from refractive ametropia. Spectacle correction produces an intolerable aniseikonia of about 25 per cent, while the equivalent figure for contact lenses is reduced to the order of 10 per cent (depending on the pre-aphakic refractive error). Attempts to attain binocular vision with spectacles usually result in diplopia, where the enlarged image of the aphakic eye has a smaller central inset representing the image of the phakic eye.

Aniseikonia may be reduced by adjusting the power of contact lenses and simultaneously worn spectacle lenses to provide the appropriate magnifying or minifying effect by the Galilean telescope principle. This principle may also be utilized in pseudophakia. The intraocular implant occupies a more anterior position than the crystalline lens, and if it is of incorrect power, an ametropic pseudophakic refraction results. Thus the intraocular lens and the required spectacle or contact lens correction form a Galilean telescope. Clinically for each dioptre of spectacle overcorrection at a back vertex distance of 12 mm, there is a 2 per cent magnification or minification for plus or minus lenses, respectively. A pseudophakic patient with a posterior chamber implant and a residual refractive error of 1 dioptre of myopia will therefore have a 2 per cent magnification from the intraocular lens and a 2 per cent minification from the spectacle lens resulting in no change in retinal image size.

Intraocular implants

The insertion of an intraocular implant within the aphakic eye overcomes the optical disadvantages of aphakic spectacles because it is situated very close to the position of the crystalline lens. The majority of aberrations and distortions from spectacles derive from their placement anterior to the nodal point of the eyes. In addition, the handling difficulties and potential complications of contact lenses described above are avoided.

Preoperatively, it is necessary to calculate an accurate prediction of the power of the intraocular lens required to produce emmetropia or the desired postoperative refractive error. Unlike the situation with contact lens or spectacle correction there is no opportunity to adjust the lens postoperatively, and the patient and surgeon must live with the result. Postoperative results are unreliable when the presurgical refraction alone is used for the determination of intraocular lens power. Calculation formulas for intraocular lens power are available for every lens style, and data suggest that the use of such calculations should produce a postoperative refractive result within 1 dioptre in 90 per cent.

Theoretical formulae

Formulae can be derived from first principles for calculating the required power of an implant. This is much simplified if the implanted lens thickness is ignored, and the postoperative aim is for emmetropia. The following is an example (Fig. 5).

The vergence power in the plane of the intraocular lens will be the combined effect of the refractive power of the intraocular lens and the cornea in this plane. With parallel incident light, the effective power of the cornea in this plane, that is the vergence at the implant, is calculated using the effectivity formula

$$L_2 = L'_1/[1 - (d/n)L'_1].$$

After refraction by the implant, the vergence L'_2 needed to place the focus on the retina is equal to the dioptric value of the distance between the intraocular lens and the retina:

$$L'_2 = n/(x - d).$$

Consequently, the required power of the implant is the

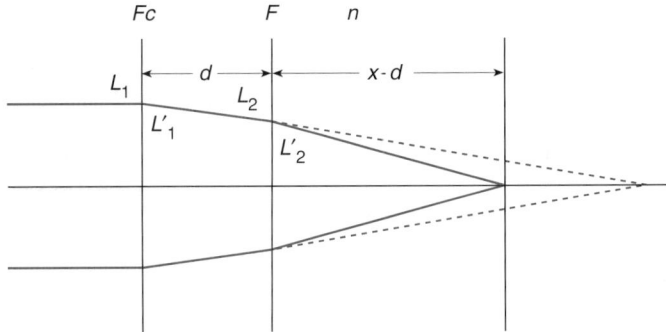

Fig. 5 Theoretical calculation of implant power. *Fc*, corneal power; *F*, implant power; L_1, vergence at cornea; L'_1, vergence after refraction by cornea; L_2, vergence at implant; L'_2, vergence after refraction by implant; *x*, axial length (mm); *d*, distance from vertex to implant (mm); *n*, refractive index of aqueous and vitreous.

required vergence at the plane of the intraocular lens less the effective power of the cornea at this plane:

$$F = L'_2 - L_2.$$

This equation can be adjusted in various ways to compensate for systematic inaccuracies arising in practices.

SRK formula

This formula, devised by Sanders, Retzlaff, and Kraff, was based on a statistical analysis of several thousand cases from various practitioners, covering many different implant designs. It is a regression formula, with the coefficients of corneal power and axial length calculated to give the best fit for the entire available sample. Its main advantage is that, being derived from case records, it takes account of systematic measuring errors and uncertainties such as postoperative corneal curvature changes and anterior chamber depth. The formula states that

$$P = A - B(AL) - C(K) - D(R)$$

where P = intraocular lens power, A to D are multiplication constants for the intraocular implant, the axial length (AL), the average keratometry reading (K), and the desired refraction, respectively.

Optical goals

The crucial requirement for comfortable and useful vision following cataract surgery is a clear retinal image with minimal aniseikonia. Most patients can tolerate aniseikonia of under 3 dioptres for a short period at least and this may be useful during the intervening period between first and second eye surgery.

The optimal result in the majority of patients is bilateral emmetropia. This is usually the goal when bilateral surgery is anticipated. Also in unilateral surgery, if the refractive error in the contralateral eye is +1.5 to +2.5 dioptres, then it is wise to aim for emmetropia as the image magnification of the intraocular lens is then matched by the magnification in the spectacle corrected contralateral eye. Equally, there will be minimal aniseikonia if a patient using a contact lens for the correction

of hypermetropia, myopia, or aphakia is left emmetropic in the operated eye. Finally, if there is no binocular vision present, for example due to amblyopia, bilateral cataracts, or age-related macular degeneration then emmetropia is the best result as there is no potential problem with aniseikonia.

However, there are some instances when ametropia may be the desired outcome. For example, some myopes prefer to retain their ability to read unaided and this option my be discussed with the appropriate patients. Also in unilateral pseudophakia, it may be preferable to calculate the power of the intraocular lens to duplicate the ametropia of the non-cataractous eye, so that the image magnification of the intraocular lens and supplementary spectacle lens is similar to that of the corrected fellow eye.

Control of postoperative astigmatism

Modern small incision surgery with phacoemulsification and foldable implants is becoming increasingly popular and patients normally have excellent visual acuity at an early stage due to the lack of postoperative astigmatism. In addition, it may be possible to lessen clinically relevant preoperative astigmatism by making an incision centred on the steeper meridian. This results in significant flattening in the steeper meridian as well as steepening in the flatter meridian.

Further reading

Bennett, A.G. (1968).The corrected aphakic eye: a study of retinal image sizes. *Optician*, **155**, 106–11, 132–5.

Bennett, A.G. and Rabbetts, R.B. (1988). Schematic eyes: time for a change? *Optician*, **196**, 14–15.

Bennett, A.G. and Rabbetts, R.B. (1989). *Clinical visual optics*, (2nd edn). Butterworths, London.

Binkhorst, R.D. (1975). The optical design of intraocular implants. *Ophthalmic Surgery*, **6**, 17–31.

Emsley, H.H. (1939). *Visual optics*, (2nd edn). Hatton Press, London.

Enoch, J.M. (1978). Restoration of binocularity in unilateral aphakia by non-surgical means. *International Ophthalmology Clinics*, **18**, 273–82.

Fyodorov, S.N., Galin, M.A., and Linksz, A. (1975). Calculation of the optical power of intraocular lenses. *Investigative Ophthalmology and Visual Science*, **14**, 625–8.

Hillman, J.S. (1983). Intraocular lens power calculation for planned ametropia. A clinical study. *British Journal of Ophthalmology*, **67**, 255–8.

Jaffe, N.S., Jaffe, M.S., and Jaffe, G.S. (1990). *Cataract surgery and its complications*, (5th edn). Mosby, St Louis.

Katsumi, O., Miyanaga, Y., Hirose, T., Okuno, H., and Asaoka, I. (1988). Binocular function in unilateral aphakia: correction with aniseikonia and stereoacuity. *Ophthalmology*, **95**, 1088–93.

Oguchi, Y. and V. Balen, A.TH. (1975). Determination of the expected power of the implant lens by ultrasound. *Ophthalmologica*, **171**, 281–3.

Retzlaff, J. (1980). Posterior chamber implant power calculation: regression formulae. *American Intraocular Implant Society Journal*, **6**, 268–70.

Sanders, D.R. and Kraff, M.C. (1980). Improvement of intraocular lens power calculation using empirical data. *American Intraocular Implant Society Journal*, **6**, 263–7.

Schechter, R.J. (1978). Image magnification, contact lenses, and visual acuity. *Annals of Ophthalmology*, **10**, 1665–8.

Volkmer, C., Pham, D.T., and Wollensak, J. (1996). On-axis cataract incisions for reducing postoperative astigmatism. A prospective study. *Klinische Monatsblätter für Augenheilkunde*, **209**, 100–4.

Welsh, R.C. (1961). *Postoperative cataract spectacle lenses*, (1st edn). Miami Educational Press, Miami.

Wirbelauer, C., Anders, N. Duy Thoai, Pham, and Wollensak, J. (1997). Effect of incision location on preoperative oblique astigmatism after scleral tunnel incision. *Journal of Cataract and Refractive Surgery*, **23**, 365–71.

Woods, A.C. (1952). The adjustment to aphakia. *American Journal of Ophthalmology*, **35**, 118–22.

2.3.6 The correction of aphakia in children

David Taylor

Technical success for surgery of congenital and acquired cataracts in childhood occurs in a very high proportion of cases. Surgical failure is usually serious and may result in such problems as glaucoma, retinal detachment, amblyopia, strabismus, irregular pupils, or endophthalmitis. There can be little doubt that the major difference in the results of treatment of congenital and acquired cataracts in childhood between now and 50 years ago is substantially due to the nature of the surgery employed. In developed countries it is now rare for children born with cataracts to become registered blind except as a result of complications of the disease which caused the cataract or the treatment.

Following the realisation of the importance of amblyopia during the development of the visual system and its effect on patients with congenital and acquired cataract, the management of the optical correction of aphakia in childhood has become paramount in achieving the best results. The optical treatment and the management of the amblyopia, not the surgery, is the most difficult for the child, the parents, and their doctor.

Factors determining the choice of optical correction

The choice between the different methods of treating the aphakia depend on a variety of factors:

1. The age of the child:

   (a) The developing visual system, after a period of relative insensitivity to a degraded image becomes exquisitely sensitive to defocus, which results in amblyopia. This sensitivity starts from the age of about 2 months or less rising in sensitivity to 6 to 12 months when it is at its zenith and then it gradually decreases in sensitivity over the next decade, more rapidly at first.

   (b) An enormous growth in the eye occurs in the first 2 years of life making any fixed optical correction used at birth incorrect by the age of 2 to 3 years. Contact lens power to achieve full optical correc-

tion can decrease from +34.0 to +18.0 in 2 years, due to an increasing axial length and a flattening of the corneal curvature.

2. The capability of the child and the parents.

3. The presence of any associated eye or systemic disease.

Methods of aphakic correction

Spectacles

For bilateral aphakia, spectacles are often very well tolerated even though the powers used are high. Sometimes, for a small infant, special frames are necessary and in these children the lens powers are usually highest, up to 20 dioptres being quite common. Bilaterally aphakic cases who have become intolerant to contact lenses, find that spectacles are a very useful alternative (Fig. 1). They have several advantages:

1. They improve the appearance of micropthalmic eyes because of the magnification factor.

2. Any strabismus may be manipulated by the prism effect.

3. Because of spectacle magnification they may acquire improved acuity.

4. The prescription can easily be changed as the child grows.

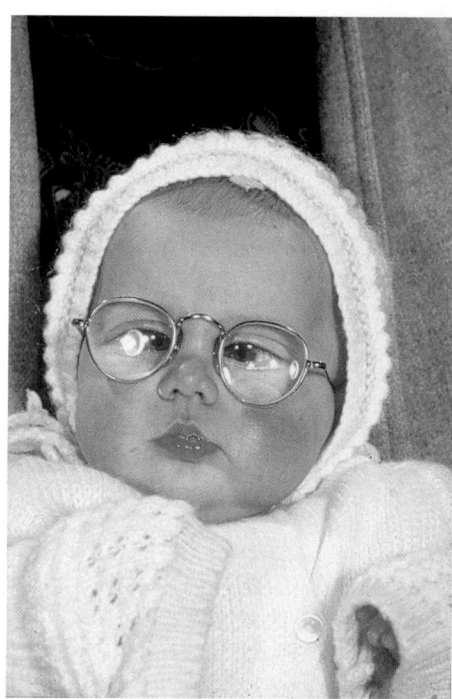

Fig. 1 Aphakic spectacles.

5. They can be inexpensive as long as they are not broken frequently.

The main disadvantages of spectacles are:

1. They are easily broken, and this may be expensive.

2. They are cosmetically unacceptable to some children and parents.

3. They are not good for unilateral aphakia because of aniseikonia.

4. The high powers used may cause difficulties with centration.

Whatever optical correction is used, bifocal or variable focus reading/distance glasses are used except in those who do not develop reading vision when a 'compromise' lens is chosen.

Contact lenses

For children under 2 years of age, whose eyes are going through a rapid period of growth, contact lenses are the most commonly used method of treatment of unilateral or bilateral aphakia from congenital cataract (Fig. 2). Various types of contact lenses are used; most frequently high water content soft contact lenses are used initially based on an empirical test consisting of refraction, estimation of corneal diameter, and the child's age, giving a lens of an appropriate power, diameter, and back optic radius for that age. If the lens fits well and the power is correct, it is left unchanged but if the fit is inappropriate the lens is removed and replaced with one that is likely to be more appropriate. If the lens fit is loose then a steeper back optic radius is used and a larger diameter. In this empirical way it is possible to avoid a further anaesthetic to fit the contact lenses. Continuous wear lenses are often used but the author feels that they increase the risks of complications and as soon as the parents handle the lenses well they use the lenses on a daily-wear basis (removing them at night) and then change to daily-wear lower water contact lenses.

Hard gas-permeable or silicone rubber lenses have also been

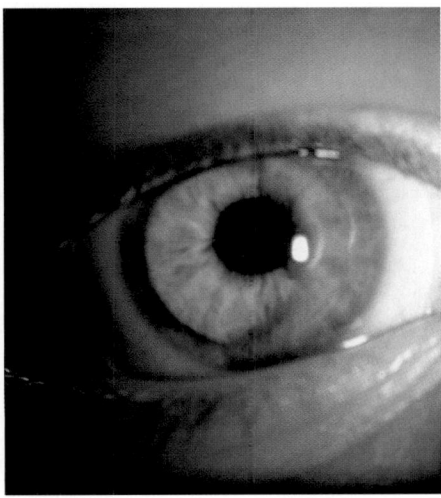

Fig. 2 A high water content aphakic soft lens *in situ* in an infant. Optic powers as high as +35, sometimes more, are required.

used in infants but may require a general anaesthetic for fitting; they are excellent for older children and may give better acuity than other types of optical correction. Lenses having nearly 100 per cent gas transmission are less likely to cause hypoxic ulceration but rarely, because they are silicone rubber lenses which are fitted flat, apical epithelial damage may occur.

Contact lenses have the following advantages:

1. They provide an easily changeable optical correction.

2. They can be used in eyes with corneal diameters of all sizes.

3. For unilateral aphakia the amount of aniseikonia is substantially less, which is better for the achievement of binocular vision which may be obtained in acquired cataract, rarely in congenital cases.

4. If there is a corneal scar, a rigid lens may help correct astigmatism.

5. The lenses can easily be tinted with a dark tint or ultraviolet and infrared barrier without becoming a cosmetic problem.

6. The squint angle may be reduced in unilateral aphakia.

Contact lenses do have substantial disadvantages however:

1. The frequent loss of lenses and/or changes in lens power require lens replacement, which may be a major financial burden.

2. Eyes fitted with soft contact lenses are at significantly greater risk of infection, hypoxic ulceration, and subsequent corneal scarring. To reduce this a daily-wear regime is often advised. This is burdensome for the parents and may be impossible if the parents are blind.

3. Soft contact lenses give rather inferior optical images compared with either hard contact lenses, spectacles, or intraocular lenses.

4. They may be difficult to wear if the corneas are irregular or astigmatic—especially in traumatic aphakia.

5. The contact lenses, and the eyes themselves need to be monitored frequently. This requires relatively frequent hospital visits which can be costly and time-consuming for the parents.

Contact lenses can be successfully worn in more than 90 per cent of infants (Moore 1993), but this usually takes a dedicated staff, a special clinic which is well equipped and with a large stock of lenses, and good communication with the parents who need to be quite dedicated to the treatment.

Epikeratophakia

Epikeratophakia is the use of a lens-shaped donor corneal button which is sutured or glued into a preformed circular

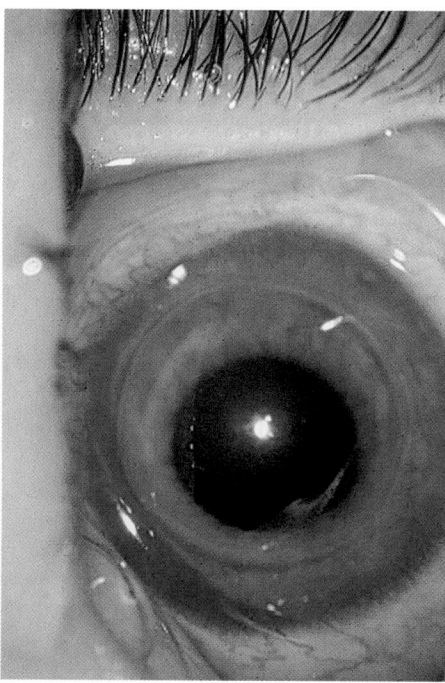

Fig. 3 Epikeratophakia grafts may be useful in some patients who fail to wear contact lenses or in traumatic cases.

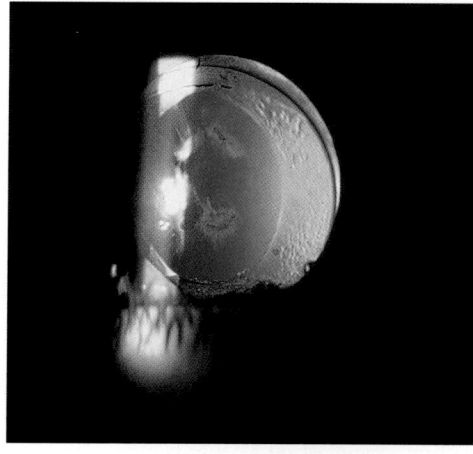

Fig. 4 Intraocular lenses are probably safe for children over 2 years of age. In this 3 year old, the lens is 'in-the-bag', and the crescentic edge of the anterior capsulorhexis can easily be seen; there are opacities in the posterior capsule.

groove in the recipient cornea of children who are intolerant of contact lenses or spectacles, usually in unilateral aphakia (Fig. 3). Since the graft takes some time to clear, this in turn gives rise to amblyopia. The visual results have generally been disappointing so that it has largely been abandoned, but it may be a useful procedure in some children with late contact lens intolerance in unilateral aphakia, that is those patients who have been tolerant until the age of about 2 and then become intolerant.

Intraocular lenses

Intraocular lenses cannot safely be used in patients who have had the whole of the lens removed by a lensectomy technique, and since it is an immutable form of optic correction, it is used with care for a child of less than 2 years. Since postoperative examination is difficult in some 2- to 4-year-old children it is also of limited application in this age group. However, in older children an 'in-the-bag' placement of the lens where it is safe and not directly irritating uveal or other tissue is an appropriate procedure with good visual results (Fig. 4). In unco-operative children, the power can be predicted either preoperatively by A- and B-scan ultrasonography and an estimation of corneal curvature, or intraoperatively by keratometry and A-scan ultrasonography. Most people aim for a small degree of postoperative hypermetropia in a child under 6 years, some for emmetropia, and all aim for emmetropia after the age of 10. Newer types of lenses such as foldable lenses are not yet appropriate except as an experimental procedure. One must remember that the recipient eyes are likely to last for 80 years and it is therefore inappropriate to use new lenses, however excellent they seem at the time, until a considerable period of evaluation has been

possible. Many previous generations of lenses that were thought to be excellent at inception have not withstood the test of time. The author recommends the use of only one-piece polymethylmethacrylate lenses implanted in-the-bag.

In older children and young adults, intraocular lenses may be implanted as a secondary procedure using the residual lens capsule for support; this is a treatment option that can be offered to older children who have had an aspiration procedure. The problem here is that aspiration procedures in very young infants are probably not appropriate because the posterior capsule frequently opacifies with subsequent amblyopia. The infant eye produces a strong inflammatory response and this may further complicate the procedure.

The use of watertight incisions reduces the need for sutures and reduces the likelihood of postoperative flat anterior chambers in children who have intraocular lens implants.

References

Amaya, L.G., Speedwell, L., and Taylor, D. (1990). Contact lenses for infant aphakia. *British Journal of Ophthalmology*, **74**, 150–4.

Amos, C.F., Lambert, S.R., and Ward, M.A. (1992). Rigid gas-permeable contact lens correction of aphakia following congenital cataract removal during infancy. *Journal of Pediatric Ophthalmology and Strabismus*, **29**, 243–5.

Baker, J.D., Hiles, D.A., and Morgan, K.S. (1990). Viewpoint: visual rehabilitation of aphakic children. *Surveys in Ophthalmology*, **34**, 366–84.

Cutler, S.I., Nelson, L.B., and Calhoun, J.H. (1985). Extended wear contact lenses in pediatric aphakia. *Journal of Pediatric Ophthalmology and Strabismus*, **22**, 85–91.

Gordon, R.A. and Donzis, P.B. (1985). Refractive development of the human eye. *Archives of Ophthalmology* **103**, 785–9.

Moore, B.D. (1993). Pediatric aphakic contact lens wear: rates of successful wear. *Journal of Pediatric Ophthalmology and Strabismus*, **30**, 253–8.

Morris, J. (1979). Contact lenses in infancy and childhood. *Contact Lens Journal*, **8**, 15–18.

Nelson, L.B., Cutler, S.J., Calhoun, J.H., *et al.* (1985). Silsoft extended wear contact lenses. *Ophthalmology*, **92**, 1529–31.

Neumann, D., Weismann, B.A., Isenberg, S.J., Rosenbaum, A.L., and Bateman, J.B. (1993). The effectiveness of daily wear contact lenses for the correction of infantile aphakia. *Archives of Ophthalmology*, **111**, 927–30.

Pollard, Z.F. (1991). Results of treatment of persistent hyperplastic primary vitreous. *Ophthalmic Surgery*, **22**, 48–52.

2.3.7 Low vision aids

Julian F. Giltrow-Tyler

It is estimated that about 1.5 million people (about 2.5 per cent of the population) in the United Kingdom have some form of vision impairment that is not adequately corrected by spectacles or contact lenses alone. In the United Kingdom the number of people who are registered blind or partially sighted (a BD8 form is completed by an ophthalmologist to signify registration) only totals some 188 000. The discrepancy between registrations and number of people estimated to be visually impaired is partly accounted for by some who could be registered but are not (estimated 959 000), with the remainder being made up of those people whose vision is impaired but is not bad enough to warrant registration.

From the data provided on completed BD8 forms the major reasons for vision loss are as follows:

Macular degenerations	49 per cent
Glaucoma	15 per cent
Diabetes	6 per cent
Cardiovascular disease	5 per cent
Muopia	4 per cent
Optic atrophy	4 per cent

These are primarily age-related problems; loss of vision in the United Kingdom is considered to affect people of retirement age (65 years) or older. They account for 83 per cent of all registrations. By way of contrast, loss of vision in developing countries is often associated with conditions that would be amenable to treatment in the developed world. In developing countries vision loss is more likely to occur at an age when the impaired person is being relied upon to provide an income, or a means of sustenance, to a family. Without an effective disability allowance the visually impaired person is reliant upon his or her family's support.

Fortunately most visually impaired people retain enough functional vision to benefit from low vision aids. The need for optical, illumination, and electronic devices to improve vision at distance or near vision should not be assessed in isolation. Other service providers, for example social, rehabilitation, counselling, and mobility services, may be of just as much, if not greater, importance than those who provide appropriate optical aids.

Examining the low vision patient

Ten to twenty per cent of patients referred to low vision clinics benefit from a change in prescription, some requiring only a change of glasses to achieve a good functional result. Improvements in vision allow patients a wider choice of magnifiers and have a positive effect upon their quality of life.

Optical solutions may be considered when the patient's symptoms indicate the following problems:

- image size of the object of regard is too small
- poor contrast
- glare.

Assessment routine

The refraction routine needs to be altered to accommodate visually impaired people. Part of the examination should include a full explanation of the disease causing the visual impairment. The final outcome is unlikely to be total blindness, and it is a great relief to many patients to be told this so that they can be more positive about their vision loss and rehabilitation.

History and symptoms

All too often the problems being experienced by visually impaired people are overlooked or, potentially worse, disregarded by clinicians. Many of their concerns will involve social, mobility, and domestic difficulties. Prompt referral to appropriate agencies should be made so that these problems can be addressed.

It is very easy to impose your ideas upon patients who may be looking for a simple solution. Closed questions like, 'Would you like to be able to read newsprint?' will often produce a positive response. However, reading newsprint might be inappropriate to a patient's needs and might also give the patient false expectations of what they are likely to achieve with optical aids. The question, 'What do you need to read?', is more likely to encourage a patient to address his or her principal problems.

Those who accompany patients, even though they mean well, might try and interpret what the patient really wants to do. Patients are unlikely to complain when this happens and inappropriate low vision aids might be prescribed as a result.

Areas of investigation are as follows.

Reading

Questions should investigate the size of print that a patient can already read, the size of print that the patient would like to be able to read, for how long the patient can read, and whether or not this is adequate. Questions also need to resolve which glasses, magnifiers, and lighting the patient uses to read.

Writing

It is useful to investigate what types of pen and paper patients are using (black fibre-tipped pens on white or pale yellow paper are recommended), whether they are able to read their own writing, and keep to a line (maybe consider a Millard writing frame or bold line paper). Special tasks, such as being able to complete a pension book, cheques, or bingo and lottery tickets should also be discussed.

Television

Many visually impaired people find it difficult to recognize people's faces on television, follow the action, and read captions. Many could sit closer to the television, which would make it appear larger; changing to a black and white set improves contrast.

Daily living

Optical devices may only have a limited use when aspects of daily living (e.g. cooking, washing, personal care, money) are being considered. It is important that any problems are identified so that patients can be referred to appropriate rehabilitation agencies. Better lighting and the removal of blocks to natural lighting such as net curtains at windows can dramatically improve visual efficiency.

Mobility

Patients who have difficulty moving around their own home or outside, specifically because of vision loss, may benefit from referral to specialist mobility rehabilitation services.

Social interaction

Some patients experiencing difficulties seeing other people's faces might benefit from advice about contrast. For instance, when talking to people in a room it may be best during the day for the patient to have his or her back to the window. Any people in the room would then be seen in good light, not silhouetted against the bright window.

Physical factors

Visually impaired people often suffer from other disabilities. Hearing loss often coexists with vision loss leading to social isolation with the patient becoming insular and withdrawn. Tremor or loss of grip can make it difficult for patients to handle magnifiers and limit the range of low vision aids that can be prescribed.

Psychological factors

Loss of sight can cause emotional distress to patients, similar to bereavement. The emotional state of each patient needs to be considered because it can act as a barrier to their rehabilitation and acceptance of low vision aids, especially if the patient is expressing denial.

Visual acuity

To measure visual acuity a logMAR or Bailey–Lovie chart is recommended. Adopting a 3-m viewing distance allows many patients to read some of the top lines of letters on the chart rather than the single 6/60 optotype presented by the conventional Snellen chart. This improves patients' confidence and does not intimate 'failure' that having difficulty reading only a single letter on the Snellen chart might imply.

Reading acuity can also be assessed on charts based on the logMAR principle. These charts only have a limited number of words to read, which patients can easily learn and do not represent the types of print that patients are likely to encounter. Functional reading, the ability to read script, instructions, and bills in everyday life, are perhaps the most useful tests of reading ability. A range of books, magazines, letters, and bills are useful additions to a low vision clinic.

Retinoscopy

Many elderly people with failing vision have some degree of cataract or age-related media changes. These will reduce the clarity of the media and may make retinoscopy difficult. It is not unusual to find cylindrical or myopic shifts in refraction due to media changes. To increase the brightness of the retinoscopic reflex the examiner can:

1. Move closer to the patient, remembering to make the correct spherical power adjustment for the shorter working distance (for distance (d) measured in metres, power adjustment $= -1/d$)

2. Focus the retinoscopy beam closer to the patient, thereby reducing its divergence.

Both of these techniques reduce accuracy but may allow the examiner to obtain a result from which to proceed.

Keratometry

When high cylinders are suspected but retinoscopy is not possible (e.g. in cases of corneal disease or following corneal graft) keratometry can be used to estimate the corneal cylinder and its axis. Some keratometers give corneal power along the power axes, for example 46.00 dioptres along 30 or 41.50 dioptres along 120. In this case a cylinder of −4.50 at axis 30 could be inserted into the trial frame or refractor head. Spherical lenses can then be added to the cylinder in an attempt to find the best spherocylindrical combination. To convert a keratometer reading from radius (mm) to dioptres (F), $F = 337.5/\text{radius}$ (mm).

Refraction

The usual techniques of fan and block or cross cylinder can be modified for visually impaired patients. 'Bracketing techniques' are particularly useful.

Bracketing requires a 'no preference' response from patients for equal amounts of blur. Blur is achieved by showing the patient plus and minus lenses of equal but opposite powers which they are asked to contrast. If they have a preference half of the amount of preferred spherical power is added to the prescription in the trial frame and the test repeated. The power of the spherical lenses being shown to the patient are reduced if the vision improves. The process continues until the patient is describing each additional plus and minus lens as equally blurred. Occasionally it is difficult to obtain a clear endpoint—if in doubt give the maximum plus power in the spectacle lens as this will assist intermediate vision and the patient will be slightly over prescribed. The amount of blurring obtained from the lenses must be enough for the patient to recognize a spherical lens producing about 50 to 75 per cent of the theoretical blur being required (1.00 dioptre blur will produce a visual acuity of approximately 6/18 or 20/60).

Contrast sensitivity

Visually impaired people often have poor contrast sensitivity. A reserve of about 10× contrast threshold is required to read comfortably, so it is valuable to record the contrast sensitivity monocularly and binocularly. Do not assume that the eye with the best distance acuity will have the best contrast sensitivity. Eyes with poor visual acuity or contrast sensitivity may interfere with the vision in the better eye and patients may prefer to close or cover an interfering eye.

A wide range of magnifying devices are available for reading and other near vision tasks, varying from reading glasses and hand magnifiers through to more complex telescopic aids. A smaller range of binoculars and monocular telescopes are available to assist distance and intermediate vision.

Optical devices for near vision

Reading is the task most mentioned as a problem by people with failing sight. The importance of the best reading glasses as a near vision aid should not be overlooked. About 10 to 20 per cent of patients attending low vision clinics are assisted by a change of reading correction and in about half of these cases no further help is necessary. Reading additions up to +3.00, if sufficient, work very well; beyond +4.00 many patients complain that the working distance is too short. Elderly people often reject shorter working distances because more shadows are cast over the page, thereby reducing contrast. Also, restricted joint and limb movements cause discomfort and they find themselves unable to adapt to the new reading techniques that they must adopt.

The advantages and disadvantages of the optical options available to practitioners will be described along with the considerations that need to be given to each type of magnifier.

Reading glasses (additions up to +4.00)

Advantages

- Simple to understand
- easy to obtain
- cosmetically good
- a wide range of lens types, including multifocals, are available
- a normal reading posture is adopted by the patient.

Disadvantage to visually impaired people

Reading glasses are not strong enough on their own.

Considerations

- Might be useful for larger prints and everyday tasks (e.g preparing food)
- might work well with a magnifier.

Higher power reading additions (above +4.00)

Advantages

- The patient is able to read smaller print (appears larger because held closer)
- cosmetically acceptable

- bifocal additions available up to +20.00
- both hands free to do tasks
- good field of vision.

Disadvantages

- Short working distance (focal length of reading addition)
- local 'task' lighting usually required. Elderly patients need more light to be able to read. The shorter the working distance the more difficult it is to provide lighting that does not cast shadows.

Considerations

- Patients may need to have one eye occluded if it interferes with binocular vision
- binocular additions (single vision or Franklin split bifocals recommended) may improve reading vision because one eye 'fills in' areas of macular loss in the other. Prisms are recommended to assist convergence: 1 prism dioptre base in per dioptre of addition in each lens for additions +5.00 to a maximum of +12.00.

Reading additions and magnification

Magnification (M) is often specified as a formula $M = F/4$ where F is the the dioptric power of the magnifying system. A comfortable reading distance was considered to be 25 cm and the number 4 is derived from the dioptric power of that focal length. A reading addition (or accommodation) of +4.00 would therefore give unit (one times) magnification and an addition of +14.00 (working distance 7.1 cm) 3.5× magnification. The formula is simple to apply to reading lenses that are used alone but requires modification when more than one lens is involved (see below).

Note: when a reading addition is specified zero accommodation is assumed. Since most low vision patients are elderly this assumption is acceptable.

Hand magnifiers

Advantages

- Patients recognize them and therefore are less suspicious of them compared to other devices
- relatively inexpensive
- easy to transport
- cosmetically reasonable
- can be used with either distance or reading corrections
- the patient is able to adjust the magnifier for most comfortable working distance and best field of view consistent with adequate magnification.

Disadvantages

- Cast shadows over the page thereby further reducing available contrast

- restricted field of view in higher powers, especially over 5 to 6×

- large, low power magnifiers tend to be bulky and heavy

- only one hand is available to undertake tasks unless a double-ended clamp is used (e.g. Eschenbach clamp no.1600)

- of limited use to patients with tremor and poor grip

- magnification specified by the manufacturer is the maximum available

- magnification and field of view vary depending upon the reading addition and distance magnifier held from the spectacles.

Considerations

- Need to estimate the true level of magnification being used by the patient because it may be possible to provide this more efficiently by using other types of magnifier

- the reading addition may need to be changed to achieve the most effective magnification and field of vision through the magnifier.

Optics of hand magnifiers

Hand magnifiers tend to be used in conjunction with reading glasses or multifocal lenses. The patient adjusts the distance of the magnifier to a comfortable position from the page and then proceeds to read. Magnifiers are specified by 'trade magnification' using the formula $M = (F/4) + 1$. This formula makes two major assumptions:

1. That the magnifier is held in contact with the spectacle lens

2. That the spectacle lens incorporates a reading addition of +4.00.

However, very few patients using magnifiers fit the specifications above. Most patients have a reading addition of less than 4.00 dioptres and separate the magnifier from the reading lens by a distance (d); this distance varying from patient to patient. If d is specified in metres the equivalent power of the lens system can be calculated. The equivalent power of a lens system may be thought of as the power of a single, thin lens that would replace the system of lenses.

Note: the equivalent power of the system (F_E) is given by the equation

$$F_E = F_m + F_a - (dF_mF_a)$$

where F_m = the power of the magnifier; F_a = the reading addition; and d = distance of magnifier from glasses (in metres).

To be accurate the power of the magnifier should be the equivalent power of the lens (F_e) but calculating this is time consuming. Most low vision practitioners would be willing to accept back vertex power (measured on a focimeter or by neutralization) as a proxy for equivalent power. This rarely overestimates the equivalent power of the lens by more than 10 per cent.

Note: $F_e = F_1 + F_2 - ((t/n)F_1F_2)$

where F_1 = dioptric power of the front surface of the lens; F_2 = dioptric power of the back surface of the lens; t = central lens thickness (in metres); and n = refractive index.

Example: patient 1 has a +12.00 hand magnifier (e.g. Combined Optical Industries Ltd. magnifier 5204) held at 10 cm and bifocals with a reading addition of +3.00.

$$F_E = F_m + F_a - (dF_mF_a)$$
$$F_E = +12 + 3 - (0.10 \times 12 \times 3)$$
$$F_E = +11.4 \text{ dioptres}$$
$$M = F_E/4$$
$$= 11.4/4$$
$$= 3.8\times.$$

Holding the magnifier closer to the glasses increases the magnification. Maximum magnification is reached when the magnifier is in contact with the glasses and $d = 0$. F_E now equals $F_m + F_a$. Zero magnification occurs if the magnifier is held at the focal length of the reading lens; the magnifier would now be in contact with the page, if it was not the print would appear blurred to the observer. F_E now equals F_a alone.

Some patients elect to use a magnifier with their distance glasses. In such cases F_a is zero and F_E is now equal to F_m alone. F_E does not vary with distance, but the field of view gets smaller as the patient moves the magnifier further away.

Note: field of view (W) through a magnifier is governed by a more complex formula

$$W = a/(dF_E)$$

where a = aperture size of magnifier (mm); d = distance of magnifier from glasses (in metres); and F_E = the equivalent power of the lens system.

If a magnifier is held at a distance from the patient that is less than its focal length then the field of view (W) will be greater than the aperture size (a) of the magnifier; at its focal length W is the same as a; and at distances greater the focal length W is less than a. This effect is independent of reading addition.

Stand magnifiers

Advantages

- Both hands free if necessary

- can be manipulated by some patients who have tremor and poor grip

- the optical system is fixed by the stand height. The level of magnification will not therefore vary between that found in the consulting room and elsewhere

- some are designed so that patients can write beneath them.

Disadvantages

- Cast more shadows than hand magnifiers, therefore even greater reduction in contrast

- can be very bulky in lower powers.

Considerations

Stand magnifiers present three problems to the prescriber.

1. Should a reading or a distance prescription be used?

2. At what distance should the magnifier be held from the spectacles?

3. What is the true level of magnification produced by the system?

Literature from the manufacturers can be misleading and it is recommended that practitioners assess the optical properties of the magnifiers they are prescribing.

Optics of stand magnifiers

All stand magnifiers are set at a height from the page that is within the focal length of the lens. The vergence of rays from the object of regard on the observer's side of the magnifier (L') varies not only between manufacturers but very often within a series of magnifiers produced by the same manufacturer.

A simple test to determine the maximum reading addition that could be used with stand magnifiers and thereby neutralize L' is to interpose trial case lenses between the observer and the stand magnifier (Figs 1, 2) the observer trying hard not to accommodate. If observer accommodation is a problem a 3× telescope focused for infinity can be interposed between the observer and the trial lens. More accurate methods of deter-

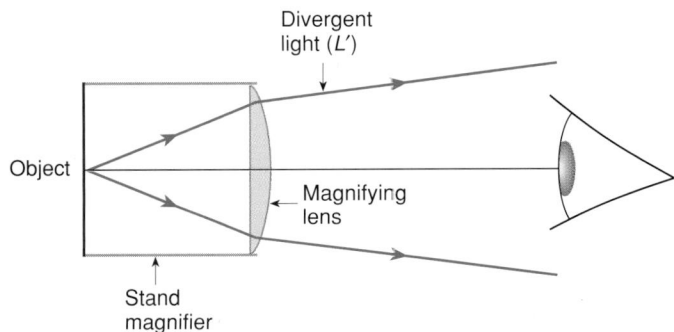

Fig. 1 Stand magnifier: divergent light entering observer's eye. Observer needs to accommodate to view object.

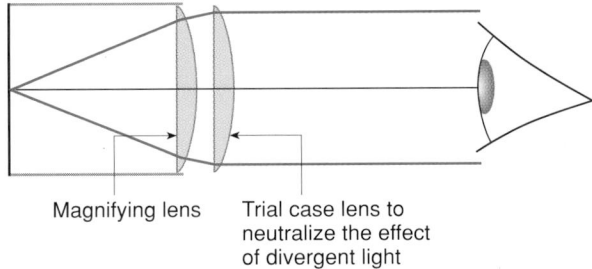

Fig. 2 Stand magnifier: divergent light (L') neutralized by positive power lenses. Parallel light now enters observer's eye.

mining L' are available but are not easily undertaken in a busy low vision clinic.

Note: by knowing the vergence of light (L') the ideal distance (d) at which the patient should use the magnifier can be determined. This is given by $f_a + l'$ where f_a is the focal length of the reading addition and l' the focal length of the emergent light from the stand magnifier.

Example: +6.00 required to neutralize divergent light at the surface of the magnifying lens on the observer's side of the system (therefore $L' = -6.00$ and $l' = -0.1667$ m) and the patient has a reading addition of +4.00 ($f_a = 0.25$ m):

$$d = f_a + l'$$

$$d = 0.25 + (-0.167)$$

$$= 0.083 \text{ m}.$$

F_m may be determined by focimetry or neutralization and the formula $F_E = F_m + F_a - (dF_mF_a)$ can again be used to determine the equivalent power of the system. Magnification can be determined by using the formula $M = F_e/4$ and field of view by the method outlined for hand magnifiers.

For patients requiring magnifiers rated at 7× and above the optical considerations are often of theoretical interest only because they do not notice the induced blur because of their poor vision. The small aperture size and high magnification of these magnifiers means that they have to be held close to the eye or spectacles to achieve a useful field of view.

Illuminated magnifiers

Illuminated magnifiers have one major advantage—they greatly improve contrast. This assists many patients, especially those who are elderly and have macular disease. This improvement in contrast is usually not outweighed by their disadvantages:

- more bulky than other magnifiers

- they use batteries which need to be replaced; this might be difficult for patients with poor grip

- mains operated types are relatively expensive to buy

- many are poorly designed for writing.

Reading telescopes

Advantages

- Increased working distance compared to high power reading spectacles with the same nominal magnification

- both hands free

- may be used for writing and undertaking near tasks

- binocular prescriptions up to 5× magnification possible.

Disadvantages

- Reduced field of view compared to high power reading spectacles of the same magnification. The field of view decreases when the magnification or working distance is increased

- very accurate focusing required on the object of regard; very little depth of field

- skilful fitting required, especially for binocular types

- relatively expensive

- very poor cosmetically.

Consideration

Reading telescopes can be very useful for younger patients, especially those in work who may have specific visual requirements. The optics of reading telescopes are considered below along with those of distance telescopes.

Vision aids for distance

Many visually impaired patients complain that they are unable to see objects clearly at a distance. This often demonstrates itself as an inability to recognize people across the road and to read text on the television. In theory a telescopic device should help but many patients find them frustrating, unacceptable, and difficult to use because of their limited field of view. Moving closer to the television is often a more acceptable solution.

All distance vision aids work upon telescopic principles. In their simplest form they are composed of two separated lenses, a positive powered objective lens, and either a positive powered eyepiece (Keplerian, astronomical, and terrestrial telescopes), or a negative powered eyepiece (Galilean telescopes). Spectacle mounted binocular aids can be used for television (they tend to be limited to 4× power because of limited field of view and weight) and hand-held telescopic aids (up to 10× power) are useful as a mobility aid to allow patients to read signs, notices, and bus numbers. Some patients use telescopes to help them with their outside interests, especially for watching sport or at the theatre.

Telescopes

Telescopic devices demand a basic two–part lens system, one lens (or a compound series of lenses) acting as an objective and another lens (or lens series) acting as an eyepiece. All telescopes have the following optical characteristics.

The magnification produced by the telescope when focused at infinity is given by $M = -F_{eye}/F_{obj}$ where F_{eye} and F_{obj} are the equivalent power of the eyepiece and objective, respectively. Note the minus sign in front of F_{eye}. A positive eyepiece produces a negative number; this shows the image to be inverted and reversed (astronomical telescopes) unless prisms are used to erect and correct the image (terrestrial telescopes). This makes the construction of terrestrial telescopes more complex, and they are more vulnerable to damage, more expensive, and heavier than Galilean types. However, terrestrial telescopes produce better quality images when powers beyond 4 to 6× magnification are being considered.

For an image to be produced that is focused at infinity the separation of the lenses (*s*) equals the sum of their focal lengths (i.e. $s = F_{obj} + F_{eye}$).

Terrestrial (astronomical, Keplerian) (Fig. 3) Terrestrial telescopic systems consist of two positive power lens systems. The image quality of terrestrial systems tends to be better than those of Galilean construction because they produce a real image and have an exit pupil on the observer's side of the system rather than a virtual image and exit pupil within the system. The exit pupil acts as a portal through which the observer looks, the closer he can get to it the wider his field of vision and the better the illumination of the object of regard will be. In a Galilean system the virtual exit pupil is inside the system and is therefore always some distance from the observer's eye. consist of a positive objective and a negative eyepiece. The construction is simple and the telescopes are more robust. Galilean telescopes are preferred for low power (2 to 3×) systems. In the lower power ranges the virtual exit pupil is not a significant problem.

Distance telescopes can be adapted to become reading telescopes in three ways. First, by making them adjustable so that the separation between the objective and eyepiece lenses can be increased beyond the sum of their focal lengths. Increasing the separation brings closer objects into focus. Second, by adding

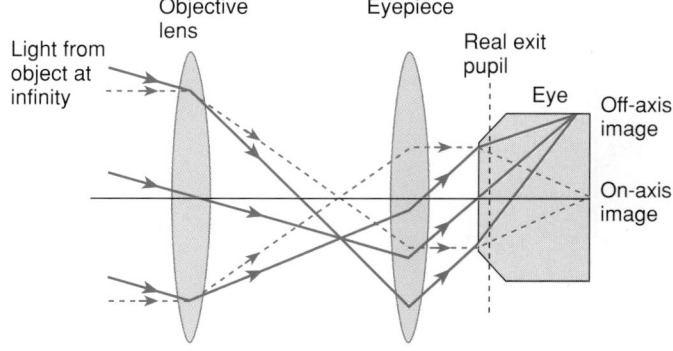

Fig. 3 Astronomical telescope: construction and exit pupil.

a lens of the focal length of the working distance required on to the objective lens of an afocal telescope, for example a working distance of 1 m requires a cap of +1.00; 40 cm of +2.50. A cap is required even for working distances as long as 2 to 4 m. This is because afocal telescopes amplify the divergence of any light that enters them. The amplification effect is approximately equal to the square of the magnification of the telescope (M^2). Light from an object 1 m from a 3× afocal telescope will be −1.00 dioptre divergent at the objective and about −9.00 dioptre (3^2) at the eyepiece. This would demand the exertion of 9.00 dioptre of accommodation to view the object at 1 m.

The third method of adapting distance to become reading telescopes is by adding extra power to the objective lens of an afocal telescope. The principle is very similar to that of the lens cap. For example a 2× afocal telescopic system might consist of a +25.00 objective and a −50.00 eyepiece separated by 2 cm.

If the separation of 2 cm is retained and the objective replaced by a +37.00 lens (a +25.00 lens with a +12.00 addition) the telescope will give a near vision point of 8.3 cm (focal length of a +12.00 lens) and produce a magnification of 6× (3× from the +12.00 addition multiplied by 2× through the telescope).

Further reading

Cole, R.G. (1996). *Remediation and management of low vision*, p. 296. Mosby, St Louis.

Corn, A.L. and Koenig, A.J. (ed.) (1996). *Foundations of low vision: clinical and functional perspectives*, p. 474. Association for the Blind Press, New York.

Farrall, H. (1991). *Optometric management of visual handicap*, p. 241. Blackwell Science, Oxford.

Nowakowski, R. (1994). *Primary low vision care*, p. 374. Appleton & Lange, Stamford.

Rosenthal, B.P. and Cole, R.G. (1996). *Functional assessment of low vision*, p. 164. Mosby, St Louis.

2.4 External eye disease

2.4.1 External eye: anatomy and physiology, examination, and investigation

Stuart D. Cook

The scope of the external eye is vast including the lids; the lashes; the grey line where skin meets mucous membrane; and the conjunctiva which covers the palpebral surface of the lid and is then reflected on to the bulbar surface of the globe where it meets corneal epithelium at the limbus. The mucous membranes are moistened by secretions from the lacrimal gland and adnexal glands present within the external eye. The composition of the tear film itself is complex. A better understanding of the anatomy and physiology of the external eye are important in determining how pathological processes arise. Latterly, attention will be given to methods of examination of the external eye and tear film.

Anatomy of the external eye

The external eye simplistically consists of the lids, conjunctiva, and cornea. The anatomy and physiology of the cornea are described in Chapter 2.6.1. The eyelid consists of skin and its associated appendages. The skin is particularly thin and only attached firmly to the medial and lateral palpebral ligaments. Underlying the skin is a striated muscle layer, the orbicularis oculi muscle. The fibrous orbital septum, Müller's muscle, and the levator palpebrae superioris all insert into the tarsal plate which is a cartilaginous structure. This is covered posteriorly by conjunctiva. Surgically, the lid can be divided into an anterior portion (skin and muscle) and a posterior portion (tarsal plate and conjunctiva) by the grey line. Further details of the structure and function of lid are available in Chapter 2.5.1. The eyelashes rise from follicles approximately 2 mm from the lid margin. They lie on the anterior surface of the tarsal plate. They are therefore in the anterior lamella of the lid, anterior to the grey line. There are two to three rows of lashes and approximately 30 to 40 lashes in each lid. The conjunctival epithelium extends from the epidermis at the lid margin to the corneal epithelium at the limbus and in between

it is reflected into the conjunctival sac. There are therefore two transitional zones, the first at the lid margin and the second at the limbus.

The tarsal conjunctiva consists of two to three layers of cells. There is a basal layer of cuboidal cells and a more superficial layer of cylindrical cells. By contrast the bulbar conjunctiva gradually transforms to the five-layered non-keratinized squamous epithelium of the cornea. Histologically and biochemically conjunctival epithelium is distinct from corneal epithelium. The conjunctiva has a loose stroma with a network of elastic fibres which allow movement against the eyeball and eyelids. Within the specialized epithelium of the conjunctiva are other subpopulations of cells with distinct functions. These include Langerhans' cells (a modified macrophage) and T and B lymphocytes. The conjunctiva has its own lymphatic drainage system. Mucin-producing goblet cells are also dispersed throughout the conjunctiva. Goblet cells comprise 5 to 10 per cent of cells on the ocular surface. Other cell types, including corneal and conjunctival epithelial cells and the lacrimal glands may also contribute to the production of mucin. Goblet cells are most numerous around the caruncle and plica semilunaris, they are also more numerous in the inferior fornix than on the bulbar conjunctiva (Fig. 1). The presence of goblet cells on the cornea is an indication that conjunctival epithelium is present. This can occur in squamous metaplasia when keratinization also occurs.

Three distinct populations of glandular cells can also be identified in the lids and conjunctiva. These are the meibomian glands; and the glands of Moll and the glands of Zeis. In addition, two populations of accessory lacrimal glands are found within the conjunctiva. These are the glands of Krause and Wolfring (Fig. 2). The meibomian glands are sebaceous glands found in the tarsal plate. The distal portion of the meibomian duct is surrounded by muscle bundles (Riolan's muscle) which aid in the secretion of the lipid material on to the lid margin. The lipid ultimately forms the most anterior layer of the tear film. There are approximately 25 meibomian glands in each upper lid and 20 in each lower lid. The glands of Moll are essentially specialized sweat glands, situated anterior to the lashes. In addition, they produce some lipoprotein. The glands of Zeis are rudimentary sebaceous glands located close to the lid margin. The accessory lacrimal glands of Krause are located deep in the subconjunctival connective tissue and the accessory glands of Wolfring are located at the upper border of the tarsal plate. Approximately two or three glands of Wolfring are found in each upper and lower lid. The accessory lacrimal glands in

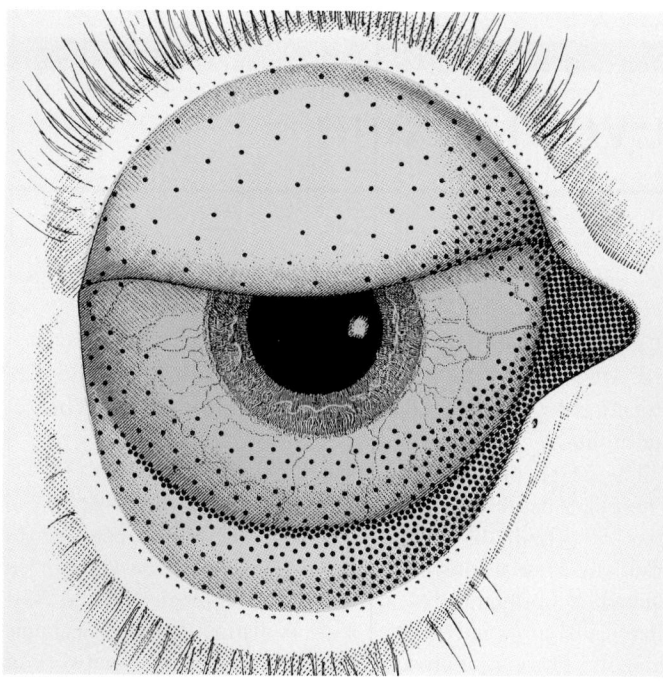

Fig. 1 The external eye showing the distribution of goblet cells; goblet cells are most numerous around the caruncle and plica semilunaris.

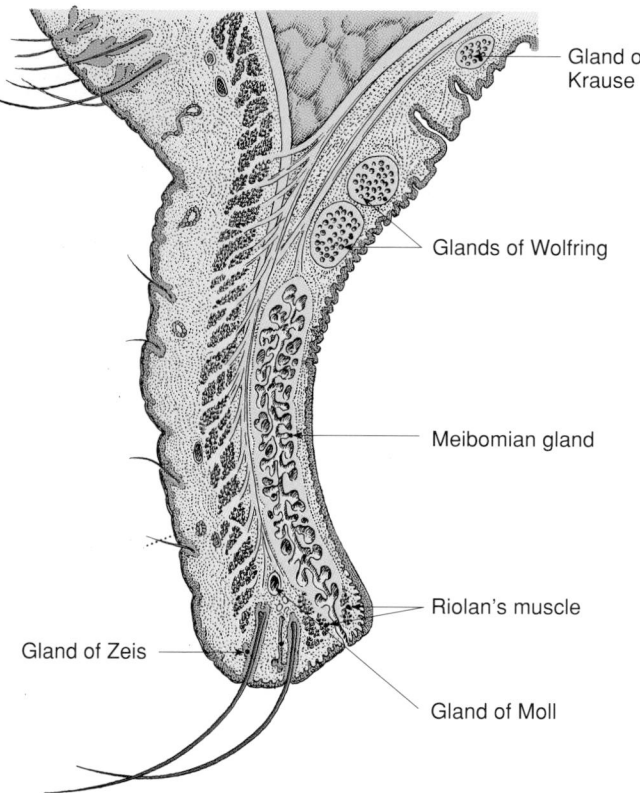

Gland of Krause

Glands of Wolfring

Meibomian gland

Riolan's muscle

Gland of Zeis

Gland of Moll

Fig. 2 Glands of the lid and conjunctiva.

total account for around 10 per cent of the weight of the main lacrimal gland. The histological structure of the accessory glands is essentially the same as the principal lacrimal gland.

The ocular surface epithelium (conjunctiva plus corneal epithelium) acts as a strong barrier against permeation by various molecules. The corneal epithelium has a barrier function approximately 10 times stronger than that of the conjunctival epithelium. Breach of the epithelium allows potentially toxic substances to invade deeper into the cornea. Recent studies have also shown that epidermal growth factor and fibroblast growth factor secreted by the lacrimal gland are present in the tear film. Receptors for these growth factors are also produced within the lacrimal gland. These suggest that the growth factors have autocrine or paracrine function in the lacrimal tissue. Similarly hepatocyte growth factor, keratocyte growth factor, and fibroblast growth factor and their receptors have been identified in primary cultures of human corneal epithelial stromal fibroblast and endothelial cells. Other cytokines such as the interleukins and vascular endothelial growth factor are also produced by ocular surface cells. The interaction between the cytokines, growth factors, and their receptors contribute to the normal maintenance of the ocular surface, wound healing, and the pathophysiology of external eye disease. These mechanisms are also of direct relevance to epithelial wound healing.

Tear film

The tear film until recently was described as a three-layered structure of between 4 and 10 μm in thickness. However, recent work in animals and humans using the techniques of laser interferometry and confocal microscopy suggest that the tear film in man is approximately 40 μm (Fig. 3). The thickness of the tear film decreases when the eyelids are open due to evaporation. The volume of the tear film diminishes with age or if the conjunctiva and cornea are anaesthetized. The functions of the tear film are considerably more complex than its relatively simple structure would suggest. The air–tear interface is the principal refracting surface of the eye. The tear film supplies oxygen and carbon dioxide to the cornea along with other nutrients. The tear film is responsible for the removal of particulate debris from the eye. The tear film importantly acts as a lubricant and prevents adhesions between the tarsal and bulbar conjunctiva. In addition, the tear film prevents drying of the external eye and lastly lysozyme, β-lysin, lactoferrin, and white blood cells are all present in the tear film thus conveying an important antibacterial role to the tear film. Recent studies have also shown that epidermal growth factor secreted by the lacrimal gland is present in the tear film. The principal components of the tear film are listed in Table 1.

The anterior lipid layer of the tear film is around 0.1 μm thick. It is secreted by the meibomian glands. The lipid material contains hydrocarbons, sterol esters, wax esters, triglycerols, free cholesterol, free fatty acids, and polar lipids. The glands of Zeis and Moll also produce some lipid. The hydrophilic terminal chains of the hydrocarbons allows the lipid to form a monolayer on the aqueous component of the tear film. During a blink, closure of the eyelids spreads the aqueous film

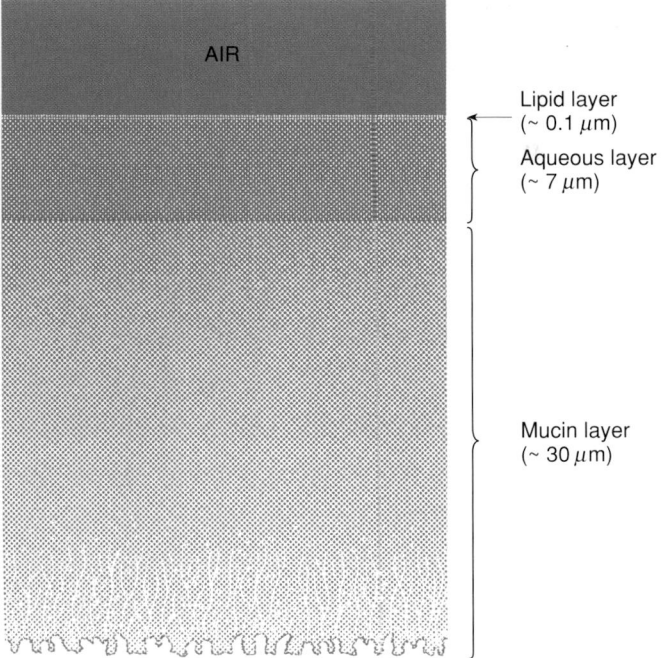

AIR

Lipid layer
(~ 0.1 μm)
Aqueous layer
(~ 7 μm)

Mucin layer
(~ 30 μm)

Fig. 3 The tear film; the tear film is approximately 40 μm in thickness. The mucin layer is densest next to the epithelial villi and gradually reduces in density mixing with the aqueous layer. The lipid layer is the most superior layer of the tear film.

Table 1 Components of the tear film

Electrolytes (mmol/l)	Immunoglobulins (mg 100 ml)	Proteins
Na⁺ 130–170	IgG 14	Prealbumin
K⁺ 26–42	IgA 17	Lactoferrin
Ca²⁺ 0.5	IgM <5	Lysozyme
Mg²⁺ 0.3–0.6	IgD <1	β-lysin
Cl⁻ 120–135	IgE 250 ng/ml	Proteases
HCO₃⁻ 26		Plasminogen activators

over the cornea and conjunctiva. Debris and mucins are removed from the anterior surface and secretions are expressed from the meibomian glands. When the eyelids open, the lipid secretions are spread upwards over the aqueous layer. This process stabilizes the tear film. The aqueous layer of the tear film is approximately 7 μm in thickness. It represents around 20 per cent of the thickness of the tear film. The basal rate of tear secretion occurs in the absence of any stimulation. The rate of tear production is around 1.2 μl/min (the range is 0.5 to 2.2 μl/min). If the production of tears is stimulated this rate of flow can be increased by up to 100 times. The main lacrimal gland secretes up to 95 per cent of the aqueous layer. The balance is made up by secretions from the accessory lacrimal glands of Krause and Wolfring. The mucin layer was previously thought to be only 0.05 μm in thickness. However, recent work suggests that the thickness of the tear film may be as great as 40 μm with the bulk of the thickness consisting of mucin or a partial mucin layer. It has also been suggested that

the mucin although increased basally may be spread through the aqueous layer. The conjunctival goblet cells, the lacrimal glands, and corneal and conjunctival epithelial cells may all contribute to the production of mucin. The mucins consist of glycoproteins.

The main lacrimal gland is found just within the margin of the orbit in the lacrimal fossa to the medial side of the zygomatic process of the frontal bone. The gland consists of two parts separated by the lateral expansion of the levator aponeurosis. The smaller palpebral part can be inspected when the upper lid is everted by looking in the superolateral conjunctival fornix. The excretory ducts from the larger portion of the lacrimal gland traverse the palpebral portion before discharging. The lacrimal gland is a tubuloacinar exocrine gland. Two principal cell types are present; acinar cells which line the lumen of the gland, these cells compose about 80 per cent of the glandular mass; and myoepithelial cells which surround the acini squeezing out the secreted fluid. The lacrimal gland is supplied by the lacrimal artery, which is a branch of the ophthalmic artery.

Examination of the external eye

Ophthalmologists are often guilty of viewing the eye in isolation. The body is not 'a support system for the eye' and many systemic diseases have ocular manifestations. The examination of the patient begins when the patient walks into the consulting room and casual inspection of the patient's face may reveal eczema, acne rosacea, or the butterfly rash of systemic lupus erythematosus. The important signs of many other systemic diseases will often be detected by an intuitive clinician. Similarly a quick look at the patient's hands or gait may reveal signs of rheumatoid arthritis.

Ophthalmologists again may neglect aspects of the patient's history because the clinical signs are most often readily available for the clinician. Ophthalmologists are fortunate in this respect that pathology is often visible. A careful history, however, will often given the diagnosis of a recurrent erosion when clinical signs are absent. Vision improving as the day progresses is a symptom of Fuchs' endothelial dystrophy. The importance of thorough history cannot be overstressed in regard to traumatic injuries, particularly in the case of young children.

The slit lamp is an indispensable aid to examination of the external eye. A comprehensive outline covering the techniques of slit lamp examination is beyond the scope of this chapter but briefly the following techniques are used in everyday practice: indirect lighting, retrograde lighting, specular reflection, and sclerotic scatter. An optical pachymeter can also be used to measure the thickness of the cornea accurately. The slit lamp allows the clinician to examine magnified images of the external eye. An experienced clinician will do much of an ocular examination subconsciously. It is important in training to have a repeatable method that permits systematic examination of the external eye so that no ocular sign is missed. Examination of the lids starts with an assessment of the skin looking for infection, inflammation and tumours most of which would be obvious. The lid position is also important and a clinician should be

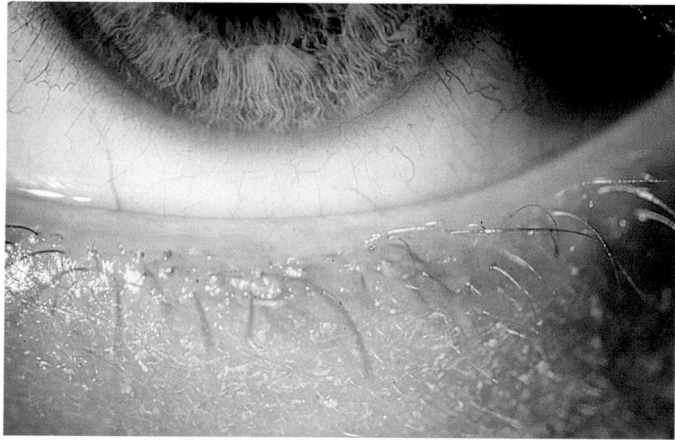

Fig. 4 The lid margin showing broken lashes and crusts between the lashes attributable to blepharitis.

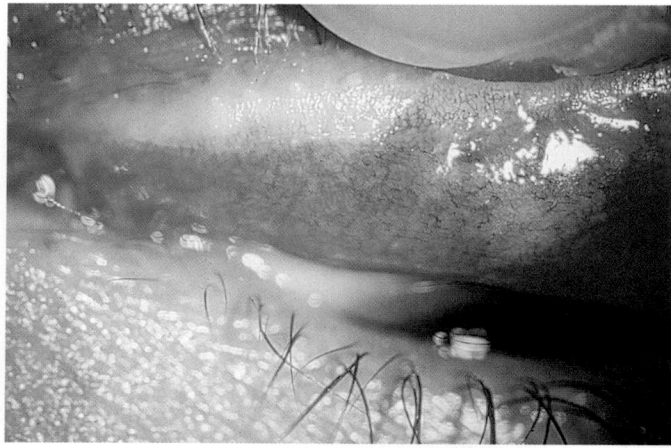

Fig. 5 An everted upper lid; keratin is present at the medial aspect of the upper lid as a consequence of a Stevens–Johnson syndrome.

assessing for any sign of ptosis, ectropion, or entropion, all of which may contribute to external eye disease. A full exposition of the techniques of lid assessment is beyond the scope of this chapter. Attention is then directed to the lashes: is their position anatomically correct or are they inverted? The number of lashes is quickly compared to the norm. Lashes may be broken and this may be a sign of self-induced disease. Crusting in the lash margins may be a sign of a conjunctivitis or evidence of blepharitis (Fig. 4). Occasionally, pubic lice are discovered among the lashes. Infections of the lash follicles may also exist. These are known as styes or external hordeolum. An internal hordeolum (a meibomian cyst or chalazion) can also exist within the tarsal plate and this may be either acute or chronic. The lid margin should be inspected and the meibomian orifices assessed. Most commonly they are not prominent but occasionally lipid secretions can be seen coming from pouting glands; froth occasionally is present on the lid margin as well. These are both signs of meibomian gland dysfunction. Keratin may be present on the lid margin and this may be a manifestation of mucous membrane disorders such as the Stevens–Johnson syndrome or ocular mucous membrane pemphigoid (Fig. 5). The lower lid is pulled down to reveal the tarsal and bulbar conjunctiva. Shortening of the fornices is usually indicative of autoimmune disorders such as ocular mucous membrane pemphigoid (Fig. 6) but can also occur following chemical trauma or toxicity attributable to chronic overuse of ocular medications. Examination of the tarsal and bulbar conjunctiva will also reveal follicles and papillae. Failure to evert the upper lid will often result in missed ocular signs such as subtarsal foreign bodies and large cobble-stone papillae (Fig. 7). The upper lid can also be double everted to reveal the smaller palpebral portion of the lacrimal gland. Inspection of the vasculature of the conjunctiva is important. Disruption of the limbal arcade is often a sign of a previous scleritic process. Telangiectasia may be a sign of a tumour. A large sentinel vessel on the conjunctiva may indicate an underlying uveal melanoma or it may be a sign of vascular malformation.

The systematic examination of the external eye then moves

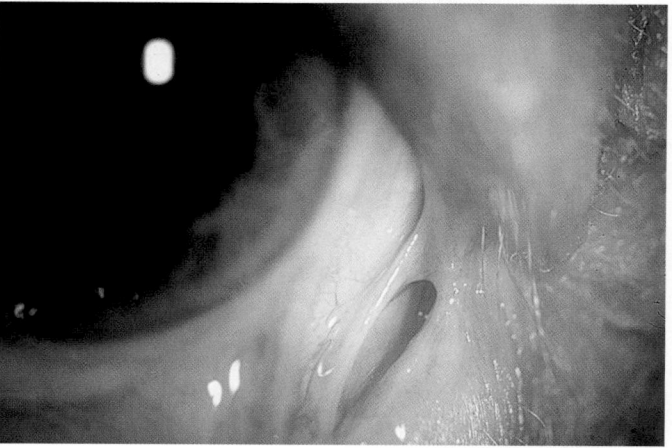

Fig. 6 Symblepharon caused by ocular mucous membrane pemphigoid.

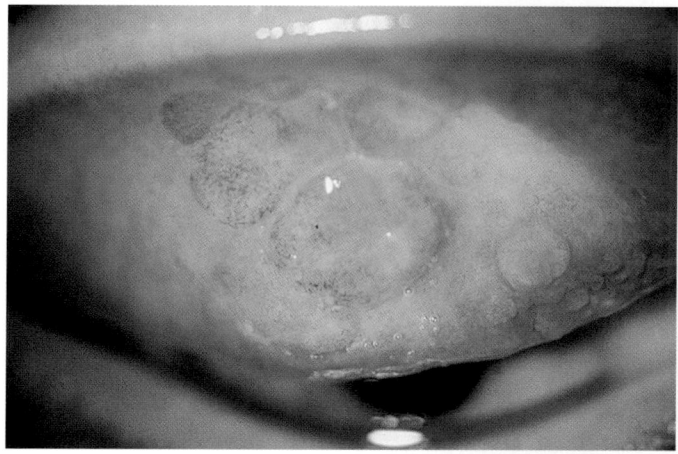

Fig. 7 An everted upper lid showing large papillae in vernal conjunctivitis.

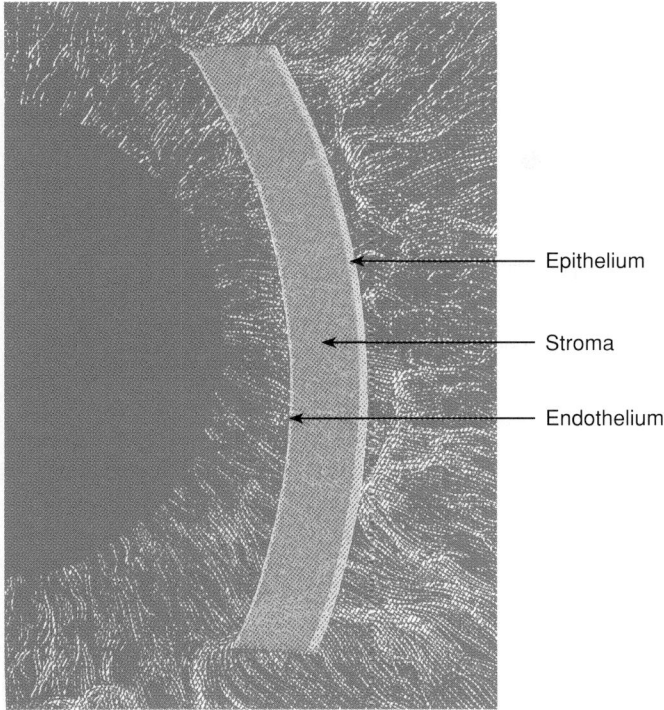

Fig. 8 A slit beam section of the cornea revealing the three layers, the epithelium, stroma, and endothelium. The iris and pupil are visible posteriorly.

to the cornea. The three distinct layers of the cornea should be assessed and these are the epithelium, stroma, and endothelium (Fig. 8). The epithelium may be oedematous or it may be ulcerated. There may be evidence of dysplasia. There may be overgrowth of elastotic tissue from the neighbouring conjunctiva (pterygium) (Fig. 9). It is a mistake for the clinician to stain the cornea early in the clinical examination as this can mask important physical signs. The thickness of the cornea can be assessed clinically. Simplistically if the cornea is thickened it is usually a sign of endothelial dysfunction or inflammation. A thickened cornea is a poor refractive medium. Corneal nerves

enter the stroma radially. These generally will be undetected unless the clinician is searching for them. They are much more prominent in acanthamoeba keratitis where the radial keratoneuritis is an important clinical sign of infection. Lastly, attention is directed to the endothelium. Guttata (Hassle–Henle) bodies are evidence of endothelial cell dysfunction and may predate the development of Fuchs' endothelial dystrophy. Keratic precipitates can also be found on the corneal endothelium. They are often described as mutton fat keratic precipitates in granulomatous uveitis. Signs of corneal graft rejection can occur in an isolated fashion in the three corneal layers: Krachmer's spots in the epithelium, oedema in the stroma, and a Khodadoust's line in the endothelium; or as a mixture of signs amongst the three corneal layers. Peripheral anterior synechiae suggest previous intraocular inflammation or perhaps congenital anomalies in the anterior chamber angle.

Documenting clinical signs is as important as observing them. They will provide a record of either worsening or improvement in the clinical condition. The medicolegal importance of accurate records cannot be overemphasized. Labelled diagrams are a simple way of recording information. Photography is also a useful technique, although its use is not advocated as a substitute for good documentation of physical findings.

Ancillary tests

Stains

The most commonly used technique is to place a drop of diluted fluorescein in the inferior fornix and ask the patient to blink. Fluorescein shows defects in the epithelial cell layer by penetrating into the intercellular space (Fig. 10). However, it must be stressed that much information can be gained by examination alone without recourse to stains. In the author's view 2 per cent fluorescein should only be used when looking for aqueous leaks (the Siedel test). In the Siedel test aqueous from the anterior chamber dilutes the 2 per cent fluorescein and a

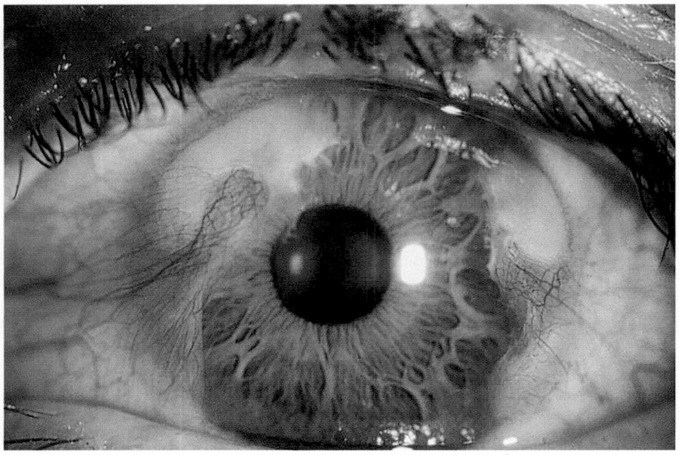

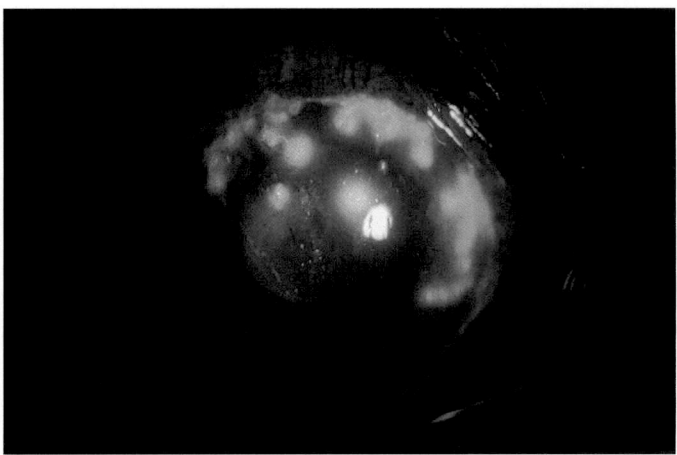

Fig. 9 The external eye showing medial and lateral pterygia. Salzman's nodular degeneration is also present in two sites superiorly.

Fig. 10 The cornea stained with fluorescein. The dendritic pattern of the epithelial defect is characteristic of a herpes simplex virus recrudescence.

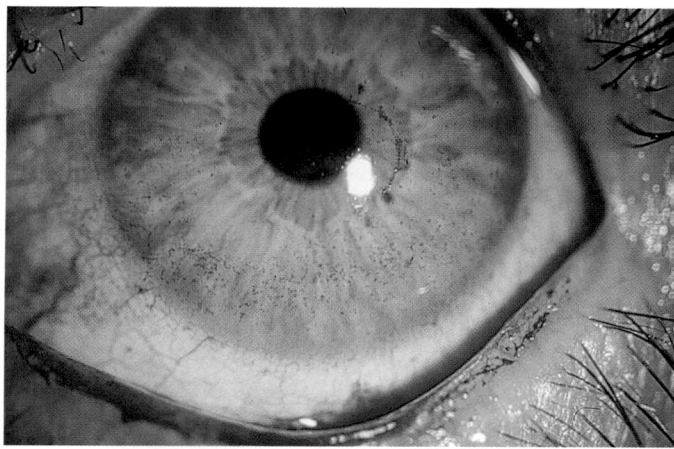

Fig. 11 The cornea stained with Rose Bengal. Epithelium and mucus strands are stained pink.

rivulet of diluted fluorescein can be seen descending from the site of communication with the anterior chamber. This usually occurs as a consequence of a penetrating injury or perhaps leakage from a trabeculectomy bleb. The use of 2 per cent fluorescein in other circumstances tends to mask detail. In patients with normal corneal epithelium a few spots of punctate staining are often evident. This is more noticeable in contact lens wearers. Fluorescein is used in conjunction with the cobalt blue filter on the slit lamp.

Rose Bengal stain is used to stain dead or desiccated epithelial cells. It also stains mucus and is of value in assessing the dry eye (Fig. 11). It is also said to be of use in ascertaining cells infected by virus in herpes simplex keratitis. Rose Bengal is an unpleasant drop and causes acute discomfort lasting a short time. This stain is used in conjunction with the green light on the slit lamp.

Lissamine green is another stain for desiccated or dead cells which can be used in a similar manner to Rose Bengal.

Schirmer's tear test

The Schirmer's tear test is an assessment of tear production per unit of time. In this test a standardized strip of filter paper (Whatman's no. 41) is inserted into the lateral third of the lower conjunctival fornix. The patient closes his eyes for 5 min and the number of millimetres of wetting from the fold in the filter paper is then measured. The Schirmer's test can be done either with or without anaesthesia. The results of this test can be variable as the filter paper may itself induce reflex tearing. A normal value for tear production over a 5-min period is generally 10 mm or more. However, tear production does diminish with age.

Tear film break-up time

The tear film break-up time is a measure of the time elapsed from a blink until the first gap in the precorneal film occurs. The break-up time is influenced by a number of factors, including the composition of the tear film (the mucus, lipid, and aqueous components); the viscosity of the tear film and any epithelial irregularities present. In the test a drop of diluted fluorescein is placed in the inferior fornix and the patient is asked to blink a few times. The test is performed at the slit lamp. The observer should not touch the patient's eyelids. After a blink the patient is asked to keep his eyes open. The observer studies the precorneal film to detect a black gap (a dry spot) appearing. The elapsed time is noted immediately the gap increases in size. The test is quick and two or three measurements can be made and averaged. A normal break-up time is regarded as 10 s or more. The break-up time is reduced in conditions associated with a dry eye.

Mucus tests

Mucus can be demonstrated easily with Rose Bengal stain (Fig. 11). It is important to remember that Rose Bengal also stains dead or desiccated cells. The cells, however, are generally fixed in location, whereas mucus strands can be seen collecting in the inferior fornix, the lid margin, and generally moving over the precorneal tear film. A mucus thread exists as a normal finding in the inferior fornix. It represents an accumulation of detached mucus during the blinking process. The threads move medially during blinking towards the inner canthus and characteristically collect as 'sleep or matter'. Mucus flow can be measured and mucus itself can be subjected to biochemical analysis. With biochemical tests in an appropriately equipped laboratory, almost any component of the tear film can be analysed and measured. As in any clinical investigation, it is necessary for the clinician to know why the test is being requested and how the result of the investigation will alter the management of a clinical situation.

Biopsies

The external eye can easily be biopsied in an attempt to aid diagnosis. This applies to the lids, conjunctiva, and even the cornea. Bacteriological, biochemical, and histological samples can all be obtained. In order to obtain maximal information from any clinical specimen, the clinician should liaise with the laboratory scientist giving accurate information concerning the specimen and details of investigations that would be of value. A diagram will often be of immense use to the scientist.

Microscopy

The external eye lends itself easily to microscopy. The use of the slit lamp has been described, corneal thickness can be determined using an optical pachymeter, and the thickness of the cornea can also be ascertained using ultrasound.

Specular microscopes have become increasingly sophisticated and can give useful information regarding the quality and quantity of endothelial cells.

Lastly, the confocal microscope allows clinicians to observe histological detail in the living cornea.

Further reading

Driver, P.J. and Lemp, M.D. (1996). Major review. Meibomian gland dysfunction. *Survey of Ophthalmology*, **40**, 343–67.

Jackson, W.B. (1993). Differentiating conjunctivitis of diverse origins. *Survey of Ophthalmology*, **38** (suppl), 91–104.

Lemp, M.A. and Marquardt, R. (1992). *The dry eye. a comprehensive guide*. Springer-Verlag, Berlin.

Prydal, J.I. and Campbell, F.W. (1992). Study of precorneal tear film thickness and structure by interferometry and confocal microscopy. *Investigative Ophthalmology and Visual Science*, **33**, 1996–2005.

Prydal, J.I., Artal, P., Hong, W., and Campbell, F.W. (1992). Study of human precorneal tear film thickness and structure using laser interferometry. *Investigative Ophthalmology and Visual Science*, **33**, 2006–11.

Smolin, G. and Friedlaender, M.H. (1994). *International ophthalmology clinics. Dry eye*, Vol. 34, No 1. Little, Brown, Boston.

Sullivan, D.A. (1994). *Lacrimal gland, tear film, and dry eye syndromes. Basic science and clinical relevance*. Plenum Press, New York.

Wilson, S.E. (1991). Lacrimal gland epidermal growth factor production and the ocular surface. *American Journal of Ophthalmology*, **111**, 763–5.

Wilson, S.E., Lloyd, S.A., and Kennedy, R.H. (1993a). Fibroblast growth factor receptor-1, interleukin-1 receptor, and glucocorticoid receptor messenger RNA production in the human lacrimal gland. *Investigative Ophthalmology and Visual Science*, **34**, 1977–82.

Wilson, S.E., Walker, J.W., Chwang, E.L., and Yu-Guang, H. (1993b). Hepatocyte growth factor, keratinocyte growth factor, their receptors, fibroblast growth factor receptor-2, and the cells of the cornea. *Investigative Ophthalmology and Visual Science*, **34**, 2544–61.

2.4.2 Infectious conjunctivitis—a clinical approach

William G. Hodge and Gilbert Smolin

Overview

Infectious conjunctivitis is one of the most common ocular disorders faced by family doctors, paediatricians, and ophthalmologists alike. The range of severity is great. Hyperacute conjunctivitis is an ocular emergency and typically heralds a significant systemic infection as well. At the other extreme of severity, most cases of acute conjunctivitis are self-limited; however, on a public health scale, they can cause significant suffering and a large number of lost work days.

Infectious conjunctivitis can be classified in three main ways based on aetiological agent, time course of signs and symptoms, or clinical findings. The aetiological agent is typically broken down into viral, bacterial, fungal, and miscellaneous causes. The time course can be hyperacute, acute, subacute, or chronic. The clinical findings that can be helpful include the presence of preauricular adenopathy, follicles, membranes, or haemorrhage. In this chapter infectious conjunctivitis is classified based on a combination of the latter two since this gives the clinician a better framework to approach this entity (Table 1).

Not all cases of conjunctivitis are infectious in origin. However, the clinical sign that heralds an infection as the basis of the conjunctivitis is discharge which can be hyperpurulent,

Table 1 Classification of infectious conjunctivitis

Hyperacute

Acute
  with follicles
  without follicles
  haemorrhagic conjunctivitis

Chronic
  with follicles
  without follicles

Membranous and cicatrizing conjunctivitis

purulent, or watery. The type of discharge can often aid in narrowing the differential diagnosis. Hyperpurulent or purulent green or yellow discharge almost certainly indicates a bacterial infection. A watery, clear serous discharge typifies viral infections. *Chlamydia* infections can present with either purulent or watery discharge but never with a hyperpurulent discharge. A mucoid discharge is an exception to the rule that discharge signifies infection. This white stringy discharge is typically found in cases of allergic conjunctivitis.

Epidemiology

Infectious conjunctivitis is ubiquitous in humans but its incidence, prevalence, natural history, and response to treatment is greatly influenced by age, seasonal variation, hygienic conditions, nature of the pathogen, and the individual's immune response. Among bacterial pathogens, staphylococcal species have no seasonal variation and can cause infection in all climates and age groups. Streptococcal species are more commonly seen in cooler climates. *Haemophilus influenza* is also more typically found in cooler climates and is one of the most common causes of conjunctivitis among children. Meanwhile *Haemophilus aegyptius* is almost exclusively found in warmer climates.

Among viral infections, adenovirus and herpes simplex are the most frequent pathogens causing infectious conjunctivitis. A multitude of strains of adenovirus can cause conjunctivitis but the strain most often responsible for epidemic keratoconjunctivitis has been the most studied and is the best understood. Adenovirus 8 was first isolated in 1955. It is a highly contagious pathogen. Transmission in the health-care provider's office has been well documented on numerous occasions. Both hand-to-eye and instrument-to-eye transmission has been reported. Adenovirus transmission by fomite spread is a serious concern as prolonged survival on plastic surfaces has been shown. In the United States there is a very low prevalence of adenovirus 8 antibodies in the general population at less than 5 per cent; hence most people are susceptible to infection by this agent. It may also be possible for selected mutations to occur in the virus allowing it to escape the immune surveillance of the host.

Herpes simplex virus type I is also an important cause of viral conjunctivitis. Unlike adenovirus, prevalence of neutralizing antibody to herpes simplex virus is very high even at a young age. Among 25 year olds, 70 to 80 per cent of people are seropositive and this rises to 97 per cent by age 60. Autopsy studies have cultured this virus from 50 per cent of trigeminal ganglia. Hence factors that affect activation of this virus are more important than those that affect transmissibility in the epidemiology of this infection.

Pathogenesis

Understanding the pathogenesis of bacterial conjunctivitis begins with knowledge of the normal bacterial flora of the conjunctiva. Table 2 summarizes this for both children and adults. As can be seen staphylococcal species and diphtheroids dominate the list. While staphylococcal species can be pathogenic, diphtheroids are probably not. It is rarer for streptococcal species, *Haemophilus* species or Gram-negative coliforms to be isolated from healthy conjunctiva; hence these organisms should always be considered pathogenic when isolated from a patient with suspected infectious conjunctivitis.

The protective mechanisms of the eye that operate to limit the colonization and invasion of bacteria are numerous. The lids provide an anatomical barrier and the blink reflex is important in limiting colonization. The lids also spread the tear film evenly. The tears themselves provide protection by their mechanical flushing effect as well as by their antibacterial contents: lysozyme, β-lysin, and lactoferrin. The tears are also replete with immunoglobulin G and secretory immunoglobulin A. The conjunctiva itself provides a mechanical barrier and contains conjunctival associated lymphoid tissue.

The pathogenesis of bacterial conjunctivitis largely depends on the pathogen involved. *Neisseria* species are Gram-negative diplococci that are able to penetrate intact conjunctiva (and cornea) and virulence appears largely dependent on the presence of pili which allow for stable attachment to mucous membrane surfaces. They also have an outer membrane protein called protein 2 which further enhances attachment. *Neisseria gonorrhoeae, N. meningitidis* along with *Corynebacterium diphtheriae, Listeria monocytogenes*, and *Haemophilus aegyptius* are the only organisms capable of invading intact cornea epithelium.

Staphylococcal infection has been extensively studied but a clear paradigm for pathogenesis is still obscure. *Staphylococcus aureus* releases over 30 active toxins including α-toxin (dermonecrotic), β-toxin (which degrades membranes), and exfoliative toxin (thought to be important in the genesis of toxic epidermal necrolysis). Extensive research has been done on the mechanism of staphylococcal hypersensitivity reactions often focusing on protein A and ribotol teichoic acid. Whether mannitol fermentation is a marker of staphylococcal virulence is unclear. *Pseudomonas* species produce a carbohydrate-binding protein called adhesin which promotes the organism to stick to mucous membrane surfaces. A complete envelope of adhesin and other glycoproteins forms a glycocalyx or slime envelope which not only increases adherence but also inhibits phagocytosis. This organism releases exotoxin A which inhibits protein synthesis, kills macrophages, and is toxic to epithelial cells. The endotoxins released alter the complement pathway and other proteolytic enzymes. Finally, this organism is extremely mobile on wet mounts.

Adenoviral infection disrupts normal cellular physiology at many different levels. The disruption of host DNA synthesis and transcription due to viral DNA is incompatible with survival. Furthermore, part of the structural component of the virus, the penton, is directly toxic to host epithelial cells. This results in epithelial cell death and lysis releasing a million progeny per virus-infected cell. This lytic cycle is responsible for the vast majority of symptoms and signs associated with adenoviral infection.

Herpes simplex virus pathogenesis involves three levels of viral activity: the initial infection, latency, and a recrudescent period. The initial infection and recrudescent period are dynamic periods of viral replication and transcription. In the latent period a limited (if any) form of herpes simplex virus genomic replication and transcription occurs. Latency-associated transcripts may be involved in maintaining the latent state. Reactivation of the latent genome is dependent on many variables, some of which are felt to be stress, trauma, corticosteroid usage, and ultraviolet light. The risk factors involved in herpes simplex virus reactivation are presently being addressed in a multicentre clinical trial.

Clinical syndromes and their management

Hyperacute conjunctivitis (Fig. 1)

Hyperacute conjunctivitis is so named because of its abrupt onset, severe pain, copious discharge, and massive conjunctival and lid swelling. The discharge is so abundant that it characteristically reaccumulates in seconds when wiped away. In addition, preauricular adenopathy may be found (a very rare finding in non-viral conjunctivitis). The palpable lymph nodes are usually very tender. Inflammatory membranes are common in this disorder. Hyperacute conjunctivitis is a very rare entity in industrialized nations but when it presents, it is an ophthalmic emergency. This is because the most common pathogens involved can penetrate intact conjunctival and corneal epithelium and may ultimately even lead to ocular perforation. The typical pathogens are listed in Table 3. The most important

Table 2 Normal conjunctival flora in adults and children

Children	Adults
Staphylococcus epidermidis 36%	*Staphylococcus epidermis* 40%
Diphtheroids 30%	Diphtheroids 30%
Streptococcal species 13%	*Propionibacterium acnes* 21%
Propionibacterium acnes 11%	*Staphylococcus aureus* 15%
Staphylococcus aureus 6%	*Corynebacterium* species 5%
Corynebacterium species 2%	*Haemophilus influenza* 2%
Bacillus subtilis 2%	*Micrococcus* 1%
Sterile eyes 23%	Sterile eyes 21%

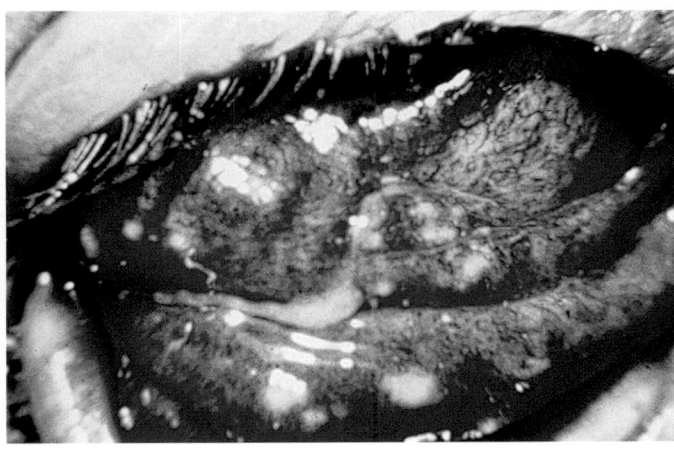

Fig. 1 Hyperacute conjunctivitis caused by *Neisseria gonorrhoeae*.

Table 3 Causes of hyperacute conjunctivitis

Most common
    Neisseria gonorrhoeae
    Neisseria meningitidis

Less common
    Staphylococcus aureus
    Streptococcus species especially β-haemolytic *Streptococcus*
    Haemophilus aegyptius
    Enteric Gram-negative bacilli

pathogens causing this clinical syndrome are the *Neisseria* species.

Neisseria gonorrhoeae is the most common cause of hyperacute conjunctivitis. It is found as a pathogen in neonates and sexually active adults. A careful history of sexual activity typically reveals concurrent urethritis, vaginitis, or proctitis. The conjunctivitis is typically unilateral at presentation. If left untreated the purulent conjunctivitis usually progresses to involve the cornea as a diffuse haze followed by a peripheral gutter infiltrate which progresses both circumferentially and centrally. A corneal abscess followed by perforation is a typical scenario. Laboratory investigation is mandatory when this entity is suspected. Simply performing a Gram stain will usually lead to the diagnosis. On Gram stain, numerous neutrophils will be seen as well as Gram-negative intracellular diplococci. Culture should be performed on chocolate agar enriched with carbon dioxide. Definitive identification involves carbohydrate fermentation. *Neisseria gonorrhoeae* ferments glucose only. Systemic treatment is mandatory. Present recommendations for *Neisseria* conjunctivitis includes a single dose of ceftriaxone 1 g intramuscularly; if the patient is penicillin allergic, a single dose of spectinomycin 2 g intramuscularly must be employed. For patients with concurrent keratitis, a stay in hospital is required and ceftriaxone 1.0 g intravenously every 12 h for 3 days should be used. For penicillin-allergic individuals, spectinomycin 2.0 g intramuscular every 12 h for 2 days is used. Concurrent treatment with tetracycline for *Chlamydia*

should be undertaken. Locally, frequent saline lavages and topical erythromycin ointment four times a day should be used as adjuvant treatment. Infectious disease consultation is mandatory.

Neisseria meningitidis produces a hyperacute conjunctivitis that is clinically very similar to *Neisseria gonorrhoeae*. This organism is transmitted by inhalation of respiratory secretions. It is more common in children than adults. The conjunctivitis may present bilaterally. It may precede meningococcaemia and meningitis; hence early diagnosis and treatment is very important. Cultures of the conjunctiva are again mandatory. Gram stain and culture results will be identical to those for *Neisseria meningitidis*. One of the definitive ways to diagnose this entity is with fermentation studies. In contrast to *Neisseria gonorrhoeae*, *Neisseria meningitidis* ferments both glucose and maltose. Treatment is with intravenous penicillin G as well as topical penicillin 100 000 U/ml hourly. Blood and cerebrospinal fluid cultures are also needed and consultation with the infectious disease service is mandatory.

Acute follicular conjunctivitis (Fig. 2)

An acute conjunctivitis is one that lasts 3 weeks or less. Follicles are avascular oval elevations 0.2 to 2.0 mm in diameter. They are flesh coloured and are usually partially translucent. Blood vessels may sweep over their convexities but never arise from the lower apex of the follicle to travel up its centre. A follicle represents a lymphocytic response with an active germinal centre. The closer the follicles are to the lashes on the palpebral conjunctiva, the more significant they become. When follicles are seen on examination, the differential diagnosis is limited. Table 4 summarizes the differential diagnosis of acute follicular conjunctivitis. By far the most important pathogens are the viruses adenovirus and herpes simplex type I.

Over 40 serotypes of human adenovirus have been distinguished. A range of clinical spectra characterize adenovirus infection but two distinct syndromes span this range. Epidemic keratoconjunctivitis is typically caused by serotypes 8, 19, and 37 and its hallmark is a conjunctivitis and corneal involvement with no systemic complaints. The incubation period is between

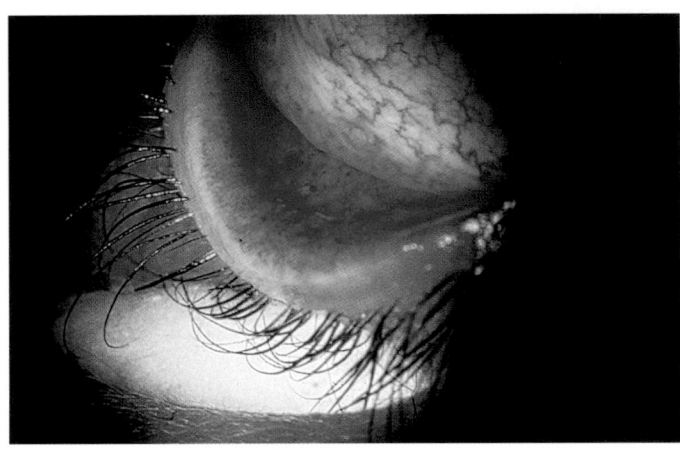

Fig. 2 Acute follicular conjunctivitis caused by adenovirus serotype 8.

Table 4 Causes of acute follicular conjunctivitis

Common
  adenovirus
  herpes simplex
  enterovirus 70
  Coxsackie A24

Rare
  Newcastle's disease
  herpes zoster
  rubella
  Epstein–Barr virus

5 and 10 days. Transmission most commonly occurs through direct contact by contaminated fingers and instruments. Epidemic patterns often occur in communities and not uncommonly the source case comes from the ophthalmologist's office. The clinical course is characterized initially by an intense inflammation of the plica semilunaris and medial bulbar conjunctiva. Soon after the patient complains of red watery eyes with foreign body sensation and occasionally periorbital pain. By this time follicles are easily apparent and are more evident inferiorly than superiorly. Tender non-visible preauricular adenopathy is present. Haemorrhages and pseudomembranes are possible and in very severe cases symblepharons can also form. The conjunctivitis is unilateral at onset but often becomes bilateral after a few days. It is usually less severe in the second eye. Keratitis often complicates the clinical course and has a characteristic appearance and time frame. From day 1 to 7, a diffuse epithelial keratitis is seen that will stain with fluorescein. From day 7 to 30, a focal superficial keratitis occcurs (that also stains with fluorescein) . Finally, from day 11 onward (and sometimes lasting for years), subepithelial opacities form. These are a collection of lymphocytes in the superficial stroma that are triggered by viral antigens.

Patients with epidemic keratoconjunctivitis are infectious for at least the first 14 days of disease. For the individual, treatment is mainly supportive consisting of cool compresses and artificial tears. If subepithelial opacities persist, low dose mild corticosteroids may be of benefit. However, some clinicians have observed a quick rebound and return of the opacities upon discontinuation of the steroids. The most important form of treatment is 'preventive community treatment' consisting of decreasing transmission to others by hand washing between patients, cleaning instruments with a mild bleach, and examining red eye patients in an isolated room.

Pharyngoconjunctival fever is the other end of the adenoviral spectrum of conjunctivitis. In this entity, keratitis is usually mild or absent but systemic symptoms are common. Adenovirus serotype 3 is the most common cause but many other serotypes have also been implicated. The disease is typically found in children and young adults. It has a 5- to 7-day incubation period. The typical triad consists of fever, pharyngitis, and follicular conjunctivitis. Associated symptoms may include malaise, myalgia, and even abdominal discomfort. A small non-visible slightly tender preauricular node may be present. The discharge is watery. The disease is often unilateral and if it becomes bilateral it is typically asymmetrical. The usual method of spread is by upper respiratory droplets though transmission has been reported via contaminated swimming pools. Unlike epidemic keratoconjunctivitis, keratitis is rarely a problem so topical steroid use is never indicated. Symptomatic measures and community prevention are the mainstay of treatment.

Herpes simplex virus type I is most studied as a result of its effect on the cornea. However, this virus can also cause a conjunctivitis without corneal involvement. A follicular conjunctivitis is typically seen as a manifestation of primary infection. However, it is also possible to develop follicles as a result of recurrent infection. Associated findings include eyelid oedema, skin vesicles, and non-visible, slightly tender preauricular adenopathy. A membranous conjunctivitis is also a possible sequelae. Epithelial keratitis can occur in up to two-thirds of cases; it may be classically dendritic or less diagnostic. Treatment for herpes simplex conjunctivitis is controversial but there is biological plausibility in using a 10-day course of oral antivirals in an attempt to reduce future incidence of keratitis and/or lessen its severity. Some clinicians feel there is also a role for a short course of topical antivirals as well.

Acute non-follicular conjunctivitis

Acute non-follicular conjunctivitis is usually accompanied by an inflamed conjunctiva with mild mucopurulent discharge. The patient often complains of unilateral tearing and a foreign body sensation. The second eye often becomes involved within 24 to 48 h. Preauricular adenopathy is not present. A fine punctate epithelial keratitis is occasionally present. The typical causative agent is bacterial and the most common ones are species of *Streptococcus* and *Haemophilus*. Less commonly *Staphylococcus* or Gram-negative bacilli are the cause.

The clinical course of acute non-follicular conjunctivitis is usually self-limited. Nevertheless treatment is usually recommended to shorten the course of the disease, for patient comfort, to prevent chronic conjunctivitis, to decrease transmission to others, and occasionally to prevent spread to other organ systems (otitis media, pharyngitis). Topical therapy is sufficient except for cases of diphtheria (very rarely seen today) or *Haemophilus* influenza in children less than 5 years old (because of the high incidence of concurrent systemic infections such as the otitis–conjunctivitis syndrome).

The choice of antibiotic is based on several considerations. The first is whether culture is necessary. In external eye infections culture is mandatory for sight-threatening infections such as hyperacute conjunctivitis, ophthalmia neonatorum, and central infectious keratitis. Cultures are recommended but not mandatory in cases of membranous conjunctivitis, chronic conjunctivitis, and chronic blepharitis. In other clinical situations such as acute non-follicular conjunctivitis, cultures are usually not required but may be useful in selected subjects such as severe cases, cases unresponsive to therapy, recurrent cases, or atypical cases (e.g. membranous conjunctivitis). The second consideration is whether treatment should be empiric or specific. Empiric therapy is employed when the microbial cause of the infection has not been definitively identified. Selection of therapy should be based on the most likely cause in a given clinical situation. A common reason to employ empiric therapy is for mild infections when culturing has a low cost to benefit ratio. For empiric therapy of mild infections such as acute non-follicular conjunctivitis, the preference is to select a more established antibiotic or antibiotic combination that covers the majority of selected pathogens and possesses a low potential for toxicity. Either bacteriostatic or bactericidal antimicrobials may be appropriate in these circumstances. Newer broad-spectrum antibiotics such as the fluoroquinolones should be reserved for recalcitrant cases, since their overuse may contribute to the emergence of resistant strains. A third consideration is whether to use a single agent or an antibiotic combination. Combinations of antibiotics are indicated in five settings, the most important of which is synergism. When antibiotics act synergistically, their combined effects are greater than the sum of their parts as measured by time–kill curves. Examples of synergistic combinations include the use of oxacillin and an aminoglycoside for staphylococcal infections. By disrupting the cell wall barrier, oxacillin enhances the uptake of the aminoglycoside. A similar mechanism is involved with the use of extended generation penicillins such as ticarcillin and the aminoglycosides in the treatment of infections by *Pseudomonas aeruginosa*. Finally, sulphonamides act synergistically with trimethoprim by inhibiting different steps in folic acid metabolism. The most common indication for use of antimicrobial combinations is for empiric broad-spectrum therapy of serious infections. Though uncommon in ophthalmology, another reason to use antibiotic combinations is for polymicrobial infections. Decreased toxicity is another indication to implement antimicrobial combinations since the dose and frequency of each drug may be reduced when used together. A final reason would be to prevent the emergence of resistant organisms.

The final consideration in choosing an antibiotic or antibiotic combination is the duration and frequency of use. The duration and frequency of antibiotic use depend on three major factors: the concentration of antibiotic necessary, the potential for and justification of toxicity, and the possibility of emergence of resistant organisms.

For antimicrobial therapy to be effective, an adequate concentration of the drug must be delivered to the site of the infection. In general, it is hoped that the local concentration of the drug should equal or exceed the minimum inhibitory concentration and preferably the minimum bacteriocidal concentration of the infecting organism. However, in some situations including intraocular infections, this may not be possible to achieve solely with topical agents and therefore subconjunctival injection should also be performed.

Host factors also influence the efficacy of antibiotics and thus the dose scheduling. For example, higher concentrations of antibiotic must be delivered to the involved tissue in immuno-compromised patients.

The potential for toxicity is an important consideration that underlies the duration and frequency of administration of antibiotics. Many topical antibiotics are toxic to the cornea and frequent concentrated doses must be justified in the clinical situation. Hence hourly use of an aminoglycoside would not be appropriate in most cases of acute non-follicular conjunctivitis even though multiple minimum inhibitory concentrations would be reached. This is because of the well-known epithelial toxicity of these agents.

The introduction of a novel antibiotic for general clinical use is almost invariably followed by the emergence of resistant strains. In order to delay the onset and magnitude of this phenomenon, new antibiotics should only be used for serious infections. Furthermore, concentrations of the antibiotic greater than the minimum inhibitory concentration of the organism are necessary. For example, once daily administration of ciprofloxacin would be an inappropriate choice of antibiotic for acute non-follicular conjunctivitis. Furthermore, this dosage would allow the concentration of the antibiotic to drop well below the minimum inhibitory concentration of the infecting species and encourage the emergence of resistant strains.

Taking all these considerations into account, a rational set of guidelines for antibiotic dosing frequency can be offered. For acute non-follicular conjunctivitis, a solution used four to six times daily for 5 to 7 days would be the appropriate regimen. Although several antibiotics could be justified, one excellent choice for uncomplicated cases is trimethoprim/polymyxin B (Polytrim), a relatively non-toxic combination of established antibiotics. For severe or complicated cases, cultures should be performed and a fluoroquinolone should be used as initial therapy. After results of culture have been obtained, specific therapy can be instituted.

Acute haemorrhagic conjunctivitis (Fig. 3)

Acute conjunctivitis accompanied by either small petechial or diffuse subconjunctival haemorrhage has a limited differential diagnosis and therefore making this diagnosis is very useful.

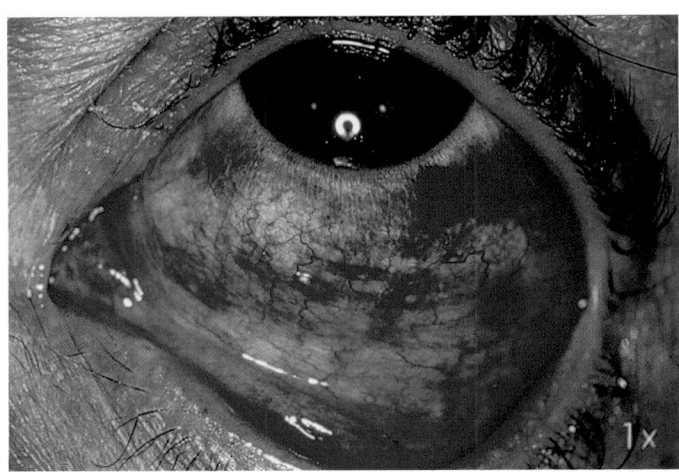

Fig. 3 Acute haemorrhagic conjunctivitis caused by *Streptococcus pneumoniae*.

Table 5 Differential diagnosis of acute haemorrhagic conjunctivitis

Adenovirus
Enterovirus 70
Coxsackie A24
Streptococcus pneumoniae
Haemophilus aegyptius
β-Haemolytic *streptococcus*

Table 7 MacCallan classification of trachoma

Stage 0	No signs of trachoma
Stage I	Immature follicles present on upper tarsus
Stage IIa	Mature follicles present on the upper tarsus with moderate papillary hypertrophy
Stage IIb	Marked papillary hypertrophy of the upper tarsus
Stage III	Mild scarring of the upper tarsus
Stage IV	Marked scarring of the upper tarsus

Table 5 summarizes the differential diagnosis of this entity. Because the causal organisms have already been discussed under previous sections of this review, we will not discuss them further here.

Chronic follicular conjunctivitis

Chronic follicular conjunctivitis is a conjunctivitis that lasts longer than 3 weeks. This is a very important clinical entity in ophthalmology. The differential diagnosis is summarized in Table 6. The most important infectious cause in this category worldwide is trachoma, caused by *Chlamydia trachomatis* serotypes A to C. In the active early stages of trachoma, follicles are common especially on the upper tarsus. This is the only condition that can cause a greater follicular response on the upper rather than lower palpebral conjunctiva. Epithelial keratitis develops especially on the upper half of the cornea. Inflammatory infiltrates and follicles can form at the limbus. With progression of the disease, a papillary reaction dominates and eventually scarring, tear deficiency, entropion, and bacterial superinfection occur. Diagnosis of trachoma is established if any two of the following are present: (a) upper tarsal follicles, (b) linear conjunctival scarring of the upper tarsus, (c) superior pannus, or (d) limbal follicles or their sequelae Herbert's pits. The MacCallan classification of trachoma is presented in Table 7. Treatment of trachoma in the active early stages includes a full 3-week course or tetracycline or doxycycline. In advanced stages of the disease tear substitutes and lid surgery are usually required.

Inclusion conjunctivitis is a sexually transmitted disease caused by *Chlamydia trachomatis* serotypes D to K. After an incubation period of 4 to 12 days, it appears as an acute follic-

Table 6 Differential diagnosis of chronic follicular conjunctivitis

Chlamydia trachoma
Inclusion conjunctivitis
Chlamydia zoonoses
Toxic conjunctivitis including *Molluscum contagiosum*
Parinaud's oculoglandular syndrome
Moraxella conjunctivitis
Nasolacrimal duct observation ('infection in the sac' mainly from *Haemophilus* and streptococcal species)
Staphylococcal blepharitis
Lyme conjunctivitis
Axenfeld and Thygeson's conjunctivitis (historical interest)

ular reaction with a mucopurulent discharge. Because of the density of follicles on the upper lid, the patient may present with ptosis. Corneal findings include punctate epithelial erosions, superficial punctate keratitis, and even epidemic keratoconjunctivitis like subepithelial infiltrates. A micropannus may be seen superiorly. Although preauricular adenopathy is usually present, it is typically non-tender. Diagnosis of inclusion conjunctivitis can be made on cell culture (slow) or by immunofluorescent staining of conjunctival smears (Microtrak). Treatment consists of oral tetracycline (500 mg by mouth four times a day) for 3 weeks. Both the patient and sexual partner should be treated and gynaecological/urological consultation is recommended. Rarely cases of follicular conjunctivitis have been observed in people exposed to chlamydial agents that are usually animal pathogens. The psittacosis agent has as its host many bird species and feline pneumonitis is transmitted from the house cat. A separate Microtrak smear is recommended when these agents are suspected. Treatment is again with tetracycline 500 mg by mouth four times a day for 3 weeks.

Although not an infectious cause of conjunctivitis, it would be remiss to discuss chronic follicular conjunctivitis without mentioning toxic aetiologies. Toxic causes of chronic follicular conjunctivitis are the most common causes of this entity in industrialized nations. The most important toxins are overused topical preparations, both prescription drops as well as over-the-counter remedies. Molluscum lid nodules, eye make-up, lid verrucae, and lid lice may also be the underlying aetiologies.

Parinaud's oculoglandular syndrome is characterized by a granulomatous lesion on the conjunctiva surrounded by follicles and accompanied by a visible, very large preauricular node. There is frequently a history of contact with animals especially cats or rabbits. The aetiology is protean including tuberculosis, leprosy, tularaemia, syphilis, lymphogranuloma venereum, leptotrichosis, and cat scratch disease. Cat scratch disease is probably the most common cause and the small pleomorphic Gram-negative bacillus has now been identified as *Bartonella henselae*. This condition is often protracted (2 to 3 months or longer) though there are almost never long-term sequelae.

Other important infectious causes of chronic follicular conjunctivitis include *Moraxella* as well as bacteria that may reside in an obstructed lacrimal system. Occasionally the aetiology of a chronic follicular conjunctivitis only correlates with the presence of staphylococcal blepharitis. This is especially so in children.

Chronic non-follicular conjunctivitis

The most important infectious agent in this category is *Staphylococcus aureus*. Concurrent lid disease is almost always present. Treating the lid disease aggressively with lid scrubs, topical bacitracin or erythromycin ointment, and occasionally systemic cloxacillin and rifampin is recommended. Other causes of chronic non-follicular conjunctivitis include a retained foreign body, masquerade syndromes, dural sinus fistula, superior limbic keratoconjunctivitis, dry eye, allergic conjunctivitis, floppy eyelid syndrome, lid imbrication syndrome, ligenous conjunctivitis, and factitious conjunctivitis.

Membranous and cicatrizing conjunctivitis (Fig. 4)

Infectious causes of membranous and cicatrizing conjunctivitis are listed in Table 8. As these entities have already been discussed under other headings, they will not be elaborated on further.

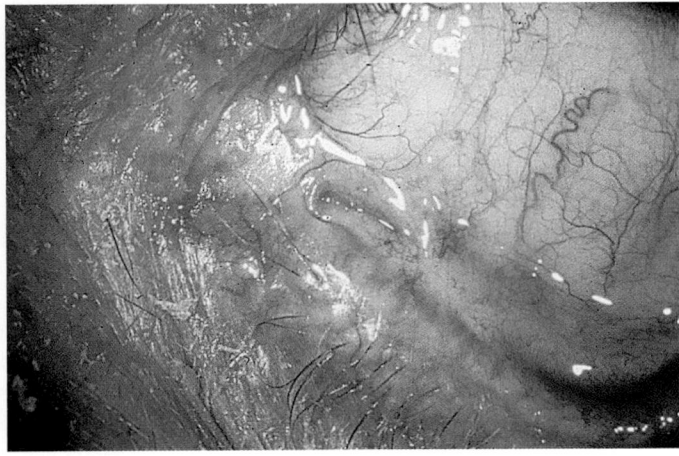

Fig. 4 β-Haemolytic streptococcal infection in a middle-aged male causing cicatrization.

Table 8 Differential diagnosis of membranous and cicatrizing conjunctivitis

Infectious
  adenovirus
  herpes simplex
  β-haemolytic *Streptococcus*
  Neisseria gonorrhoea
  trachoma

Non-infectious
  Stevens–Johnson syndrome
  ocular cicatricial pemphigoid
  atopic keratoconjunctivitis
  radiation injury
  surgery
  chemical burns

Summary

Infectious conjunctivitis is a common ophthalmic condition with a long differential diagnosis. However, by taking a careful history and performing a thorough clinical examination, each case can usually be categorized into a more well-defined heading. This chapter reviews infectious conjunctivitis under headings which aid the clinician's approach to, and management of, this entity.

Further reading

Barquet, N., *et al.* (1990). Primary meningococcal conjunctivitis: report of 21 patients and review. *Review of Infectious Diseases*, **12**, 838.

Bell, D.M., *et al.* (1982). Herpes simplex keratitis: epidemiologic aspects. *Annals of Ophthalmology*, **14**, 421.

Brechner, R.J., West, S., and Lynch, M. (1992). Trachoma and flies: individual vs environmental risk factors. *Archives of Ophthalmology*, **110**, 687–9.

Buehler, J.W., Finton, R.J., Goodman, R.A., *et al.* (1984). Epidemic keratoconjunctivitis: report of an outbreak in an ophthalmology practice and recommendations for prevention. *Infection Control*, **5**, 390–4.

Dawson, C.R., *et al.* (1970). Adenovirus type 8 keratoconjunctivitis in the United States. *American Journal of Ophthalmology*, **69**, 473–80.

Dawson, C.R., Juster, R., Marx, R. *et al.* (1989). Limbal disease in trachoma and other ocular chlamydial infections: risk fctors for corneal vascularization. *Eye*, **3**, 204–9.

Editorial (1977). Adenovirus keratoconjunctivitis. *British Journal of Ophthalmology*, **61**, 73–5.

Fitch, C.P., Rapoza, P.A., Owens, S., *et al.* (1989). Epidemiology and diagnosis of acute conjunctivitis at an inner-city hospital. *Ophthalmology*, **96**, 1215.

Ford, E., Nelson, K.E., and Warren, D. (1987). Epidemiology of epidemic keratoconjunctivitis. *Epidemiology Review*, **9**, 244–61.

Hara, J., Okamoto, S., Minekawa, Y., *et al.* (1990). Survival and disinfection of adenovirus type 19 and enterovirus 70 in ophthalmic practice. *Japanese Journal of Ophthalmology*, **34**, 421–7.

Kemp, M.C. and Hierholzer, J.C. (1986). Three adenovirus type 8 genome types defined by restriction enzymes: prototype stability in geographically separated populations. *Journal of Clinical Microbiology*, **23**, 469–74.

Laibson, P.R. (1984). Ocular adenoviral infections. *International Ophthalmology Clinics*, **24**, 49–64.

Liesegang, T.J., *et al.* (1987). Epidemiology of ocular herpes simplex. Incidence in Rochester, Minnesota, 1950–1982. *Archives of Ophthalmology*, **107**, 1155–9.

McGill, J., *et al.* (1992). Pathophysiology of bacterial infection in the external eye. *Transactions of the Ophthalmology Society UK*, **102**, 7.

McNatt, J., *et al.* (1978). Anaerobic flora of the normal human conjunctival sac. *Archives of Ophthalmology*, **96**, 1448.

Nakhla, L.S., Al-Hussaini, M.K., and Shokeir, A.A.W. (1970). Acute bacterial conjunctivitis in Assiout, upper Egypt. *British Journal of Ophthalmology*, **43**, 540.

Nicas, T.I. and Iglewski, B.H. (1986). Toxins and virulence factors of *Pseudomonas aeruginosa*. In *The bacteria*, (ed. J.R. Sokatch) Vol. X. *The biology of Pseudomonas*. Academic Press, New York.

Pellitteri, O.J. and Fried, J.J. (1950). Epidemic keratoconjunctivitis: report of a small office outbreak. *American Journal of Ophthalmology*, **33**, 1596–9.

Pepose, J.S., Holland, G., and Wilhelmus, K.R. (ed.) (1966). *Ocular infection and immunity*. Mosby, St Louis, MO.

Perkins, R.E., *et al.* (1975). Bacteriology of normal and infected conjunctiva. *Journal of Clinical Microbiology*, **1**, 147.

Rivadeneira, E.D. and Henshaw, N.G. (1992). Adenoviruses and adeno-associated viruses. In *Zinsser microbiology*, (ed. W.K. Hoklik, H.P. Willet, D.B. Amos, and C.M. Wilfert) pp. 968–74. Appleton & Lange, Norwalk.

Thygeson, P. (1948). The epidemiology of epidemic keratoconjunctivits. *Transactions of the American Ophthalmology Society*, **46**, 366–85.

Ullman, S., Roussel, T.J., Culbertson, W.W., *et al.* (1987). *Neisseria gonorrhoeae* keratoconjunctivitis. *Ophthalmology*, **94**, 525.

West, S., Munoz, B., Bobo, L., *et al.* (1993). Nonocular *Chlamydia* infection and risk of ocular reinfection after mass treatment in a trachoma hyperendemic area. *Investigative Ophthalmology and Visual Science*, **34**, 3194–8.

Wildy, P., Field, H.J., and Nash, A.A. (1982). Classical herpes latency revisited. In *Virus persistence*, (ed. B.W.J. Mahy, A.C. Minson, and G.K. Darby). Cambridge University Press, Cambridge.

2.4.3 Immunological, neoplastic, and degenerative diseases of the conjunctiva

D.F.P. Larkin

Immunological diseases

Disease conditions of the conjunctiva which have an immunological aetiology are very common. The allergic group of disorders is most prevalent, some having isolated conjunctival disease and others having associated active allergic disease of the skin, airways, or other tissues. The diseases which result in conjunctival cicatrization as the principal manifestation are much less common. In cicatrizing conjunctival inflammation there is frequently simultaneous involvement of skin or other mucous membranes.

Allergic conjunctivitis

This group of inflammatory disorders have in common the presenting features of itching, mucous discharge, and a papillary conjunctival response. Each have an association with atopy.

Seasonal allergic (hay fever) conjunctivitis and perennial allergic conjunctivitis

Seasonal is much more common than perennial allergic conjunctivitis. Both conditions typically occur in atopes, with onset in childhood or early adulthood. Seasonal allergic conjunctivitis is a hypersensitivity response to seasonal allergens like airborne pollens, whereas perennial allergic conjunctivitis is a response to perennial allergens like house dust mite. These are the only true immediate hypersensitivity diseases of the conjunctiva. The typical clinical presentation is conjunctival injection, chemosis, watering, and mucus discharge. There are no limbal or corneal signs. Diagnosis is usually easily made on the basis of the history of allergen exposure, rhinitis, wheeze, and clinical abnormalities of the conjunctiva.

The mechanism by which an exposure to allergen results in inflammation of the exposed tissue is categorized as a type I hypersensitivity response. The initial event is binding of allergen particles to immunoglobulin E molecules which are attached to tissue mast cells or basophils by their crystallizable (Fc) fragments; following this extracellular molecular interaction, prostaglandins and leukotrienes are formed within the inflammatory cell, degranulation occurs, and chemotactic factors and vasoactive amines such as histamine are released into tissue. Mast cells and eosinophils are found in biopsies of the conjunctiva and upper respiratory mucosa. Eosinophils and immunoglobulin E are found in the tears. Management is avoidance where practicable of allergen, and treatment with topical mast cell stabilizing agents (e.g. disodium cromoglycate or lodoxamide) and antihistamines (e.g. levocabastine). Adjuvant treatment of the upper respiratory mucosa is often helpful for symptom relief. Topical steroid is occasionally necessary in severe attacks.

Vernal keratoconjunctivitis

Onset of vernal keratoconjunctivitis is almost always between 5 and 10 years, and usually in males. It is a self-limiting disease lasting up to 10 years and it usually subsides before the age of 20 years. Pathogenesis of this disease is poorly understood. There is much less information on specific allergens associated with vernal keratoconjunctivitis than seasonal allergic conjunctivitis. Seasonal exacerbations are usual. On conjunctival biopsy, mast cells, eosinophils, and CD4$^+$ T lymphocytes are present in the epithelium. Histamine is the inflammatory mediator of greatest importance in vernal keratoconjunctivitis. It is known to provoke vasodilation, mucus production, and fibroblast production of collagen. Elevated levels of tear histamine are assumed to originate from mast cell and basophil degranulation in the conjunctiva.

Differentiation between vernal keratoconjunctivitis and other allergic or infective disorders can usually easily be made on the basis of characteristic clinical signs. The disease takes slightly different forms in different parts of the world, the palpebral form being more common in developed countries and limbal or mixed forms in warmer latitudes. Itching, mucus discharge, and photophobia are the main symptoms indicating vernal keratoconjunctivitis activity. In the palpebral form, upper tarsal giant (greater than 1 mm diameter) flat-topped papillae give a characteristic cobblestone appearance. In active disease, the papillae are swollen and tightly packed (Fig. 1(a)), and there may be superior corneal punctate erosions. An uncommon complication is formation of an ulcer in the centre of the superior cornea, on the base of which mucus and inflammatory debris become adherent. Vernal ulcer may persist for weeks with minimal symptoms and heals with scarring of Bowman's zone. Occasionally in young patients a characteristic pale grey plaque forms in the floor of the ulcer (Fig. 1(b)). In these ulcers, re-epithelialization may take months. Limbal vernal keratoconjunctivitis is characterized by oedema, extension of gelatinous limbal tissue on to the peripheral cornea, formation of limbal papillae, and whitish Trantas dots (aggregates of eosinophils) (Fig. 2). Epithelial keratopathy may also occur in active limbal disease.

The mainstay of therapy is prophylactic topical disodium cromoglycate four times daily, but only mild forms of vernal keratoconjunctivitis can be controlled by cromoglycate alone. The minimum necessary dose of topical steroid is used to control exacerbations: steroid hypertensive response is more

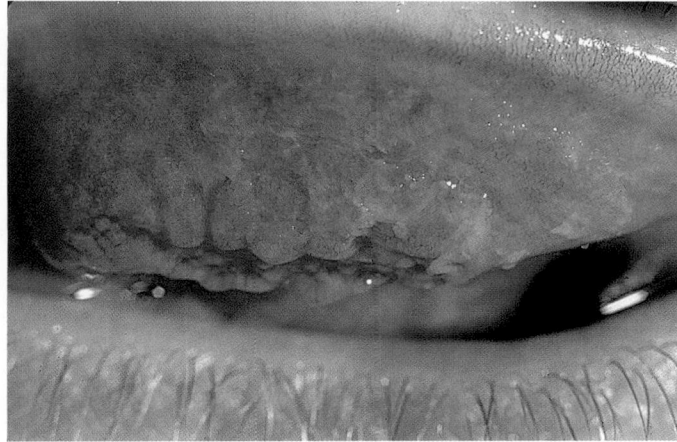

(a)

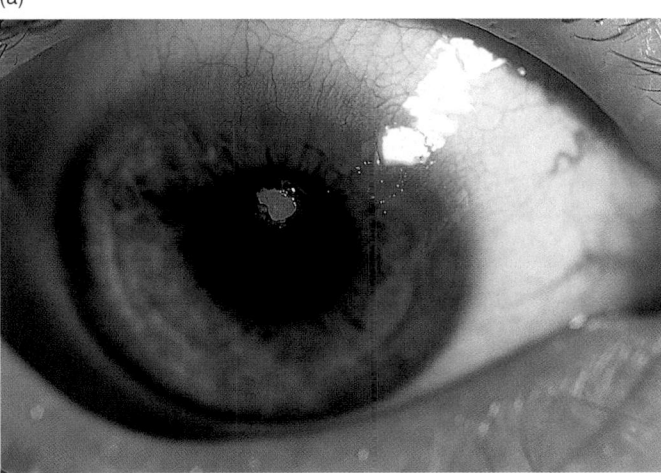

(b)

Fig. 1 (a) Active palpebral vernal conjunctivitis with oedematous giant papillae and mucus discharge. (b) Vernal ulcer and plaque in the superior cornea of the same patient.

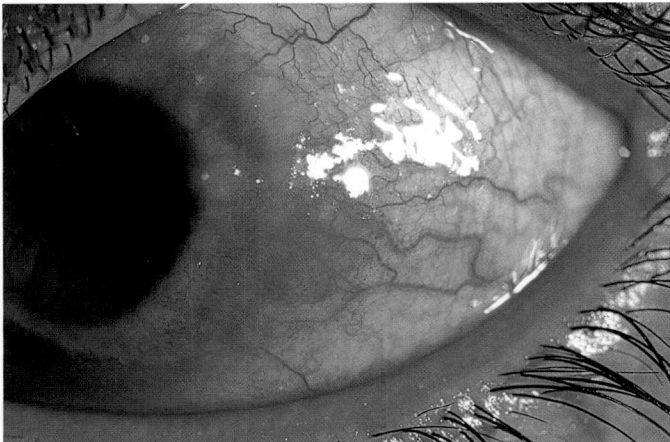

Fig. 2 Active limbal vernal keratoconjunctivitis: limbal oedema, nodules, white (Trantas) dots, and well-demarcated extension of limbal tissue on to the cornea.

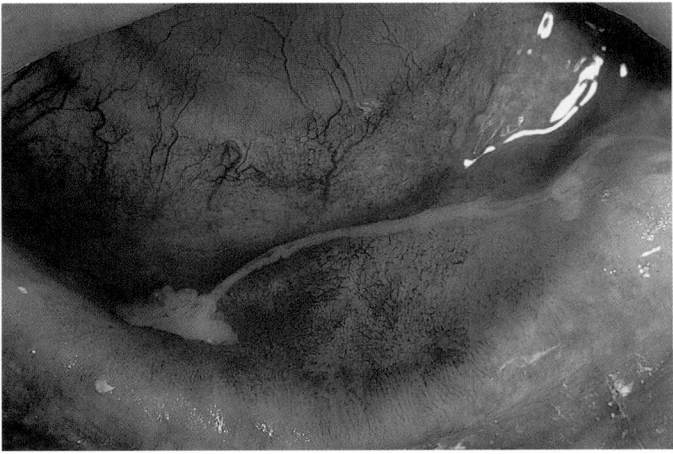

Fig. 3 Long-standing atopic keratoconjunctivitis: conjunctival scarring, forniceal shortening, and corneal vascularization. This patient had very high serum immunoglobulin E levels and a predominantly eosinophil infiltrate on conjunctival cytology and biopsy.

common in vernal keratoconjunctivitis than other allergic diseases because of the longer duration of therapy required. Mucolytic agents can be helpful in vernal keratitis. Vernal plaque can be removed by very superficial keratectomy when disease is in remission.

Atopic keratoconjunctivitis

Onset is usually in young adults (in whom it may develop from vernal keratoconjunctivitis), most often in males. Atopic conjunctivitis is a chronic papillary disease associated with photophobia and blurred vision if keratitis supervenes. Signs are often mild. Many patients have atopic eczema involving lid skin, often associated with coagulase-positive staphylococcal lid margin infection. Tarsal conjunctiva shows hyperaemia, cellular infiltration, and scarring with forniceal shortening (Fig. 3). Typical signs of corneal involvement are inferior punctate epithelial erosions, pannus, erosions, and herpes simplex keratitis. Keratoconus and cataract are associated. In addition to mast cells and eosinophils, CD4+ T lymphocytes are found in the conjunctival epithelium. Treatment of dermatitis and lid margin disease with topical steroid and antibiotics is helpful. Conjunctivitis often responds badly to topical mast cell stabilizers and steroids. Systemic steroids may be required in severe exacerbations to bring disease under control, followed by intensive topical steroid and disodium cromoglycate. Tear supplements and antiviral agents are also required in some patients.

Giant papillary conjunctivitis

This condition is a localized hypersensitivity response to a rough or deposited foreign body surface. It was first observed in contact lens wearers and an association with ocular prostheses and protruding nylon or silk sutures was later recognized. Soft contact lenses are the type most commonly associated with giant papillary conjunctivitis. Giant papillary conjunctivitis is caused by mechanical disturbance, probably in addition to a response to the lens material itself, deposits on

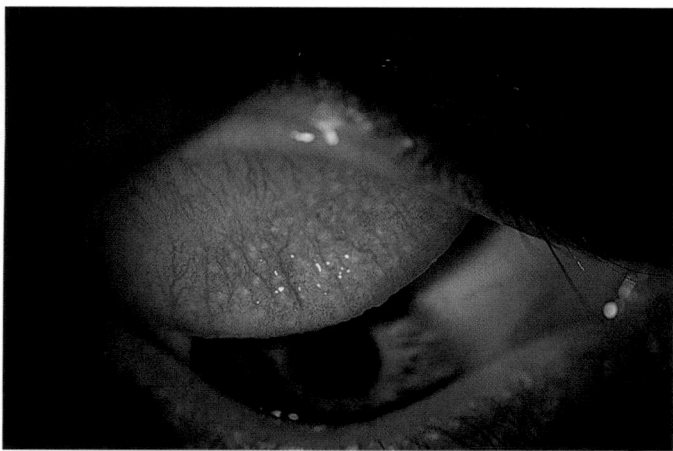

Fig. 4 Mild giant papillary conjunctivitis in a soft contact lens wearer.

the lens surface, or preservatives contained in the disinfecting or cleaning solutions. Atopy is not strongly associated.

Symptoms of itching on contact lens removal and mucus discharge gradually worsen. With advancing disease lens wearers become increasingly intolerant of their lenses and the lens position becomes unstable, interfering with vision. While early giant papillary conjunctivitis is associated with symptoms and minimal signs, eventually hyperaemia and hypertrophic papillae (greater than 1 mm) are seen, initially at the upper border of the superior tarsal plate and later involving tarsal conjunctiva towards the superior lid margin (Fig. 4). Signs may be unilateral or asymmetrical. The bulbar conjunctiva, inferior fornix, and cornea remain normal. Although the conjunctival signs may be similar to those in vernal keratoconjunctivitis, the conditions can be distinguished by history. Chronic papillary conjunctivitis in the presence of a foreign body strongly suggests a diagnosis of giant papillary conjunctivitis. Vernal keratoconjunctivitis usually affects a much younger age group than giant papillary conjunctivitis.

In mild contact lens-related giant papillary conjunctivitis, proper lens hygiene should be reviewed with the patient and wearing time reduced. Consideration should be given to changing from soft to a rigid lens material. If necessary, lens wear can be discontinued, whereupon symptoms resolve quickly and papillae disappear over a few months. Sutures inducing giant papillary conjunctivitis should be removed. Prostheses causing giant papillary conjunctivitis should be polished or replaced. Topical cromoglycate four times daily brings symptoms under control in some patients. Steroids should not be used except in prosthesis cases.

Cicatrizing conjunctivitis

Cicatrizing change in the conjunctiva destroys important epithelial constituents such as goblet cells and causes subsequent abnormalities in the cornea and eyelid. In many patients, scarring is the result of infection or injury by topical medication, irradiation, or chemical burns. In another group, the disease

has a primary immunological basis, usually as a component of an oculocutaneous syndrome in which skin, eye, and other mucous membranes are involved. In this short review, two of the causes with best characterized pathogenesis will be described.

Ocular cicatricial pemphigoid

Cicatricial pemphigoid is a systemic autoimmune disease, the initiating factor of which is unknown. Mucous membrane inflammation results in bulla formation (related to loss of adhesion of basal cells to the basement membrane) and subsequent cicatrization of squamous epithelia. Conjunctiva is involved in the majority of patients, in whom the disease is designated ocular cicatricial pemphigoid. In some patients, ocular involvement may be asymptomatic. Progressive subepithelial fibrosis leads to forniceal shortening, symblepharon, trichiasis, ocular surface keratinization, and blindness. Ocular cicatricial pemphigoid usually affects middle-aged and elderly people. Most cases become bilateral. While onset may be insidious in many, with non-specific signs of inflammation, acute ocular cicatricial pemphigoid is characterized by conjunctival ulceration, hyperaemia, oedema, forniceal shortening, and symblepharon formation (Fig. 5(a)). Eventually the cornea becomes involved, with peripheral vascularization and pannus formation (Figs 5(b) and 5(c)). Patients with chronic ocular cicatricial pemphigoid have no ulceration and minimal signs of inflammation. At the time of presentation with eye disease, most patients have extraocular disease, typically involving the oropharynx, oesophagus, and genital mucous membranes. Histopathological features vary with conjunctival disease activity. Ocular cicatricial pemphigoid is diagnosed on biopsy by identification of immunoglobulin G and/or A, and/or complement deposition on the basement membrane. The epithelial and subepithelial inflammatory cell infiltrate in acutely involved tissue usually comprises a mixed population, with predominant neutrophils and macrophages. In subacute and chronic ocular cicatricial pemphigoid, higher proportions of T lymphocytes are seen.

Acute conjunctival disease may respond to intensive topical steroid, but arrest of the disease requires systemic immunosuppression. Cyclophosphamide is the current agent of choice, in combination with prednisolone. Once clinical response is evident, the cyclophosphamide is gradually reduced to a maintenance dose and the prednisolone rapidly tapered and discontinued once disease is stable. Maintenance dosage of cyclophosphamide is continued for at least 6 months. Myelosuppression, as an extension of its pharmacological effect, is the principal adverse effect of cyclophosphamide. Patients require frequent blood counts in case the dose needs to be temporarily withheld and reintroduced when leucocyte and platelet counts return to normal levels.

For treatment of aqueous tear insufficiency, artificial tears should be used and unscarred puncta occluded. In advanced disease with trichiasis, to protect the cornea, aberrant lashes should be treated as promptly as possible with epilation or cryotherapy. Silicone rubber contact lenses may be used to protect the cornea, but only as a short-term measure. If surgery is

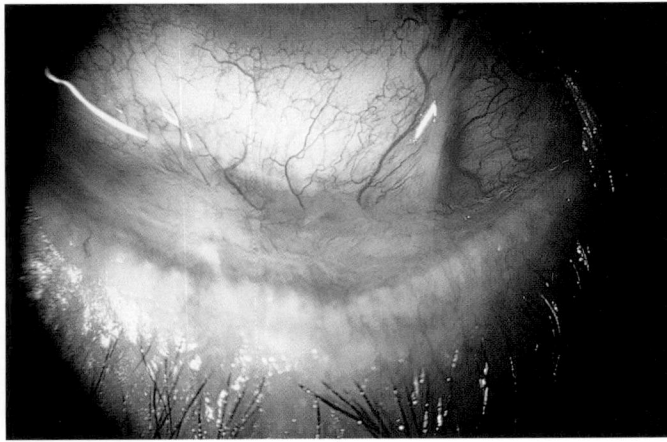

(a)

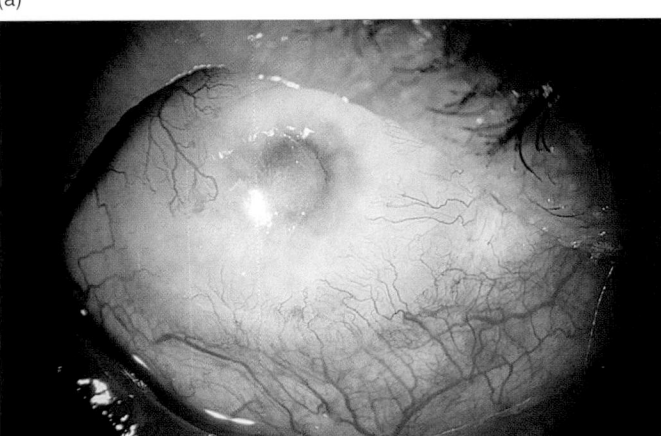

(b)

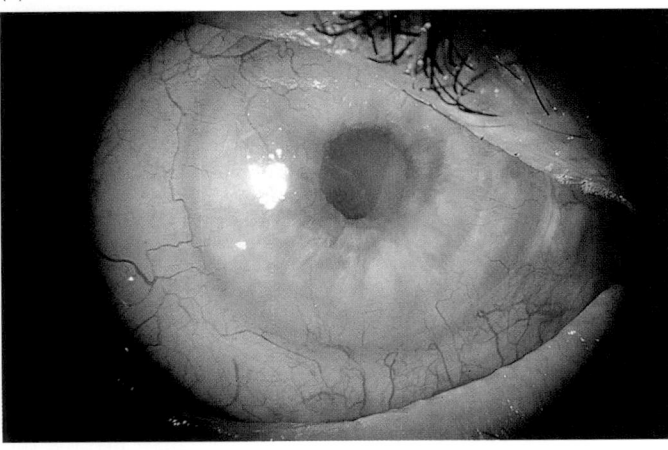

(c)

Fig. 5 (a) Conjunctival scarring in ocular cicatricial pemphigoid 2 weeks after acute onset of bilateral disease: forniceal shortening and symblepharon. The cornea was normal in this left eye. (b) Peripheral corneal vascularization in the right eye at the same time, prior to treatment. (c) Regression of corneal vascularization and pannus formation in the same eye after treatment for 4 weeks with systemic cyclophosphamide and prednisolone.

required to correct cicatricial entropion, it should only be undertaken when the disease is controlled and procedures involving the conjunctiva should be avoided. A lid retractor plication is usually satisfactory.

Erythema multiforme

Stevens–Johnson syndrome and toxic epidermal necrolysis are variants of erythema multiforme, in which acute vasculitis results in erosions of the mucous membranes and epidermis, and severe constitutional symptoms. When there is extensive skin detachment, there is a poor prognosis (mortality rates of 30–40 per cent) and the condition is called toxic epidermal necrolysis. Milder forms are known as Stevens–Johnson syndrome. Both variants are consequences of drug hypersensitivity, infection, or both and occur in previously healthy subjects. The drugs most consistently associated with the conditions are sulphonamides, anticonvulsants, and allopurinol. Acute onset systemic illness, skin rash and haemorrhagic inflammation of two or more mucous membranes may last for up to 6 weeks. In the acute phase of ocular disease, conjunctival involvement may range from papillary conjunctivitis, proceeding to focal infarction, to pseudomembranous conjunctivitis. Conjunctival cicatrization together with lid and lash abnormality develop as late sequelae, although in some patients with initial mild conjunctival involvement, further fibrosis does not occur after the acute illness (Figs 6(a) and 6(b)).

In the acute phase of disease, potentially responsible systemic drugs are discontinued and general supportive management provided. Despite the immunological nature of the condition, the role of systemic immunosuppression is not established. Involved conjunctiva should be treated with topical antibiotic if infection is suspected. Topical steroid and lysing of symblepharon may be helpful but their benefit is not established. Supportive management of those with scarring of the ocular surface is as described for ocular cicatricial pemphigoid. In addition to cryotherapy for trichiasis, patients with cicatricial entropion following erythema multiforme can be managed with a lamellar lid split procedure. Cicatricial conjunctiva can be divided or replaced by a mucous membrane graft.

Neoplastic diseases

The comparative rarity of conjunctival tumours has resulted in insufficient data to allow definitive statements on management. Squamous malignancies are most common, followed by melanomas and lymphoid tumours in that order. In this review, conjunctival tumours are divided into non-pigmented and pigmented.

Non-pigmented tumours

Conjunctival intraepithelial neoplasia (carcinoma *in situ*)

Intraepithelial neoplasia presents as a slightly elevated confluent gelatinous area. It usually begins at the limbus and spreads to involve the fornices and the cornea (Fig. 7), where fimbriated

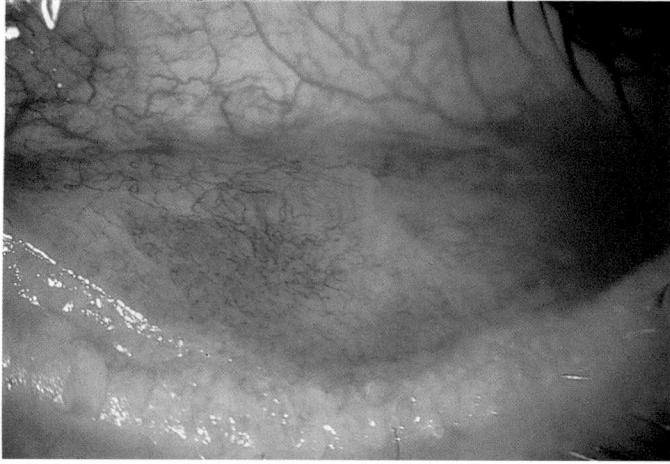

(a)

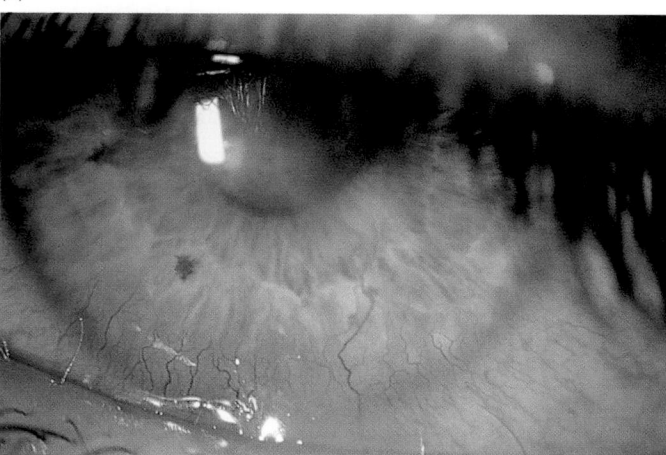

(b)

Fig. 6 (a) Long-standing conjunctival cicatrization 10 years after onset of Stevens–Johnson syndrome. The acute illness was associated with sulphonamide, and conjunctival involvement was mild. (b) Corneal vascularization and metaplastic eyelashes in the same patient. The metaplastic lashes (fine, non-pigmented) are located at the meibomian orifices and treated by cryotherapy.

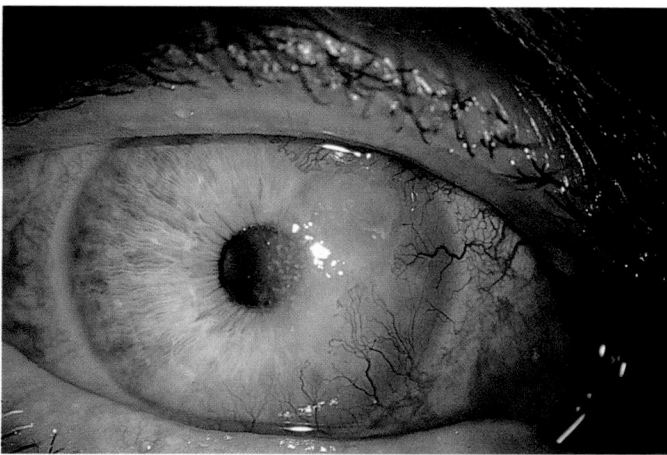

Fig. 7 Conjunctival intraepithelial neoplasia with corneal extension to the visual axis.

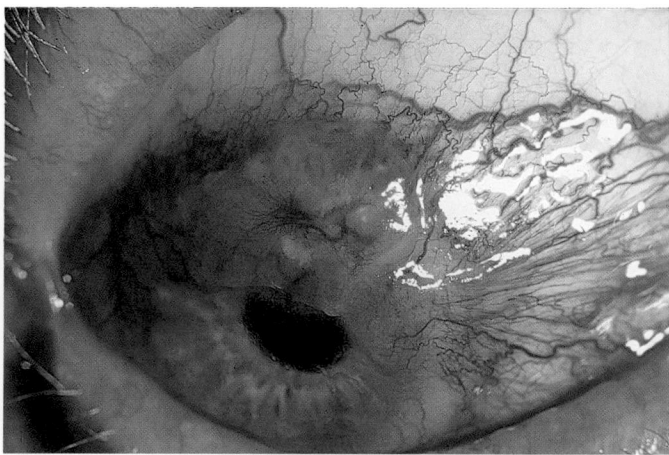

Fig. 8 Conjunctival squamous cell carcinoma arising at the limbus.

demarcated edges are usually seen. This is a premalignant lesion, which is characterized clinically and pathologically by involvement of tissue superficial to the epithelial basement membrane only. Involved conjunctiva is not fixed to the underlying episclera. However, intraepithelial and invasive neoplasia can be difficult to distinguish clinically and the diagnosis must be established by biopsy or excision. While involved conjunctiva can be treated by cryotherapy alone, involvement of limbus or cornea requires surgical excision with adjuvant cryotherapy to surrounding conjunctiva. Most cases of intraepithelial neoplasia do not invade the basement membrane and thus do not progress to invasive squamous cell carcinoma.

Squamous cell carcinoma

Although the most common malignant conjunctival tumour, conjunctival squamous cell carcinoma is rare in temperate latitudes, and involves older patients. While the precise pathogenesis is not known, risk factors such as ultraviolet B light exposure and infection by human papillomavirus have been established. Conjunctival squamous cell carcinoma is much more prevalent in central Africa, associated with the epidemic of human immunodeficiency virus infection and involves younger patients. In a patient with refractory chronic unilateral keratoconjunctivitis, conjunctival squamous cell carcinoma should be suspected. It is characterized by deep invasion of the conjunctival stroma by malignant cells with fixation to underlying tissues (Fig. 8). It spreads locally and may involve the globe. Gonioscopy is important to identify early anterior chamber invasion. While metastatic spread is rare, recurrence rates are very high following incomplete excision, most within the first 2 years. Treatment is complete excision with 2 to 3 mm tumour-free margins, usually including lamellar dissection of the sclera. Extensive limbus resection may require transplantation of limbal tissue from the other eye. Enucleation or anterior exenteration may rarely be necessary in cases of intraocular or intraorbital extension.

Lymphoid tumours

The conjunctiva can be involved in a number of benign and malignant lymphoid diseases. These are usually considered in conjunction with orbital and eyelid lymphomas. Few studies have detailed the histopathological features, management, and prognosis of conjunctival lymphoma. Most conjunctival lymphomas are classified as extranodal non-Hodgkin's lymphoma. They are often bilateral, presenting as pink subepithelial masses, usually arising in the fornix and freely mobile over the episclera. Patients may be asymptomatic. To confirm the diagnosis, patients should initially undergo incisional biopsy. Orbital lymphoma can extend anteriorly beneath the conjunctiva and for this reason orbital computed tomography (CT) scans and systemic examination should be performed on all patients with suspected lymphoma. Systemic survey for lymphoma should include examination for lymphadenopathy and enlargement of liver or spleen, CT scan of abdomen and pelvis, full blood count, protein electrophoresis, and marrow aspirate.

Lesions that are localized and fully accessible to surgery can be excised; other lesions can be treated by local radiotherapy, or cryotherapy with a liquid nitrogen spray. Differentiation of benign and malignant lymphomas is often not possible. If non-Hodgkin's lymphoma is bilateral it implies systemic spread and a poorer prognosis. However, in general conjunctival lymphoma has a good prognosis in respect of recurrence and dissemination, and particularly lymphoma arising in mucosal-associated lymphoid tissue (MALT). These 'MALTomas' can be bilateral without implying systemic spread. Following histopathological diagnosis they can be simply followed up without treatment if minimally symptomatic, or treated with radiotherapy.

Pigmented tumours

Conjunctival melanoma

Primary malignant melanoma of the conjunctiva accounts for less than 2 per cent of ocular melanomas and mainly affects middle-aged adults. It is of epithelial origin. Conjunctival melanoma can arise *de novo* from a naevus, or most commonly from malignant change in a primary acquired melanosis. Conjunctival melanoma usually arises in the limbus or bulbar conjunctiva (Fig. 9). Conjunctival melanomas may be variably pigmented: melanoma *sine pigmento* is well recognized and suspicious lesions should be biopsied. It can extend to the cornea, fornix, lid, or nasolacrimal system and metastasizes by lymphatic or haematogenous routes to local lymph nodes, liver, or other sites. Melanomas located in the fornix or palpebral conjunctiva and thicker tumours have the worst prognosis.

Melanocytes in primary acquired melanosis proliferate within the epithelial layer (Fig. 10). Subepithelial invasion is malignant change, indicated by a localized nodular mass in a previously flat diffuse area of conjunctival pigmentation, change in pigmentation, and tethering of conjunctiva to underlying episclera. Conjunctival melanoma which arises in primary acquired melanosis tends to be multifocal and diffuse, in contrast to that which arises *de novo* or from a naevus. As up to 50 per cent of lesions showing primary acquired melanosis eventually evolve into melanoma (and in most lesions if there

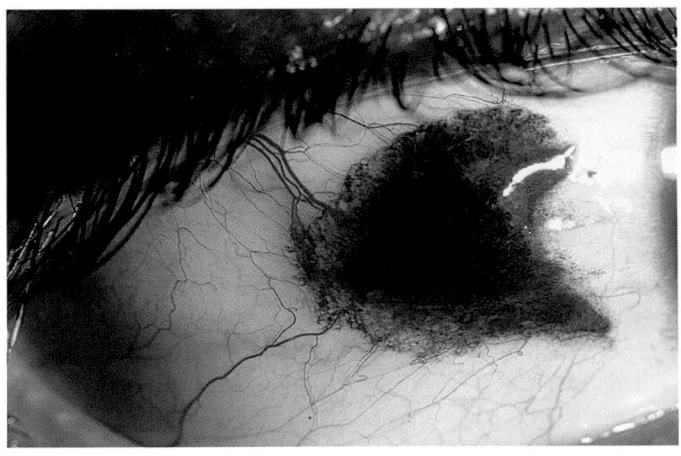

Fig. 9 Circumscribed malignant melanoma which developed in a naevus in interpalpebral bulbar conjunctiva.

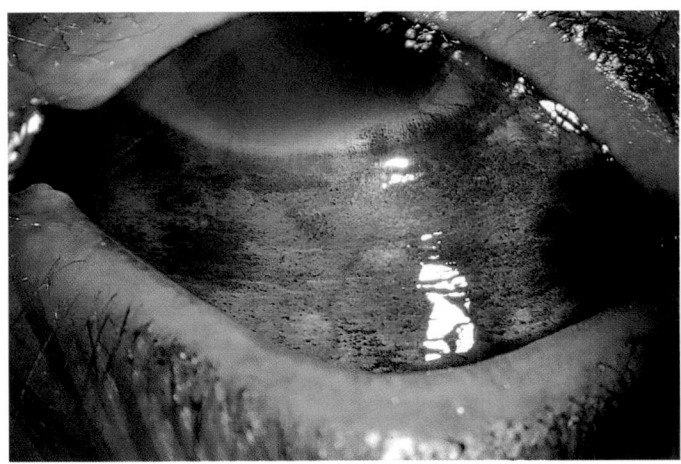

Fig. 10 Primary acquired melanosis.

are atypical cells on biopsy), long-term follow-up of these patients is required.

Wide excision combined with adjunctive double freeze–thaw cryotherapy at –20°C to surrounding conjunctival margins is used in management of circumscribed bulbar conjunctival melanoma. Subconjunctival injection of lignocaine is useful in cryotherapy of bulbar tissue because it 'balloons' the conjunctiva off from the eye wall and minimizes cryoinjury to intraocular structures. Application of the cryoprobe for up to 20 s is necessary to form an ice-ball. The biological basis for cryotherapy is that malignant conjunctival intraepithelial melanocytes are more sensitive than surrounding squamous cells to cryoinjury. Lamellar superficial scleral or corneal dissection may be required for excision of invasive melanoma. Adjunctive β-irradiation is administered to incompletely excised or recurrent tumours. Exenteration is necessary for melanomas which are unresectable due to extensive conjunctival involvement, intraocular, lid, or orbital spread, most of which arise in primary acquired melanosis. Full systemic investigation should be performed in such patients. Patients must be followed up for recurrence following surgical excision. Most deaths from metastases occur within 5 years, with a reported incidence of tumour-related death at 5 years of 13 per cent.

Degenerative diseases

Pinguecula

A pinguecula (Latin: *pinguis*, fat) is a small yellow triangular elevated patch situated in the interpalpebral bulbar conjunctiva on either side of the cornea (Fig. 11). It is most commonly seen in the middle-aged and elderly population, and remains stationary at a small size. Histopathological features are similar to those of pterygium. Elastotic degeneration of collagen in the subepithelial conjunctiva is seen. Excision is rarely necessary.

Pterygium

A pterygium (Greek: wing) is an extension of fibrovascular tissue on to the cornea, arising usually at the nasal interpalpebral limbus. Environmental factors contribute to development of this lesion. It is most prevalent in populations with high exposure to ultraviolet light, particularly exposure in the second or third decade. Little is known of the pathogenesis of pterygium and the way in which ultraviolet wavelengths interact with the limbal conjunctiva. The greater propensity for pterygia to develop on the nasal side is not understood. Histopathological features are non-specific: hyaline degeneration and low grade lymphocytic infiltration with destruction of Bowman's zone. Electron microscopic studies show excessive accumulation of extracellular matrix. Large numbers of proliferating cells and frank neoplastic features are not seen, either in primary or recurrent pterygia.

Pterygia slowly extend horizontally on the cornea and fully developed primary pterygia rarely involve more than half of the cornea. Some pterygia remain stationary for decades, so that excision should not be performed unless growth is confirmed. They have a blunt apex, often preceded by haemosiderin deposition (Stocker's line), and may be inflamed when active and growing. Excision is indicated if the visual axis is

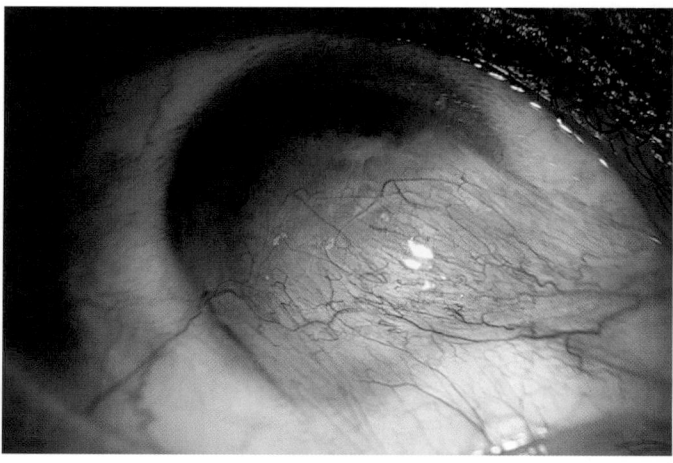

Fig. 12 Recurrent pterygium prior to excision, conjunctival autograft and lamellar keratoplasty.

threatened or if causing marked discomfort. Commencing at the head of the pterygium, lamellar dissection of the lesion and involved superficial cornea is followed by excision of the remaining conjunctival component of the pterygium and any scar tissue. When the sclera is left exposed following pterygium excision, up to 40 to 50 per cent recur within 1 year, most of these occur within 2 months of surgery. Recurrent pterygia are themselves more troublesome in regard to symptoms and management: accelerated growth, increased conjunctival inflammation, and eventually mechanical restriction of horizontal eye movements (Fig. 12). For this reason, excision is combined with various forms of autogenous repair or topical antimitotic therapy. The adjunctive surgical technique in widest use is autotransplantation of a thin layer of normal superior bulbar conjunctiva to resurface the exposed sclera (Fig. 13). A number of antimitotic therapies have been advocated for prevention of recurrence following primary pterygium excision, particularly β-irradiation, topical thiotepa, or mitomycin C (either as a single intraoperative application or drops

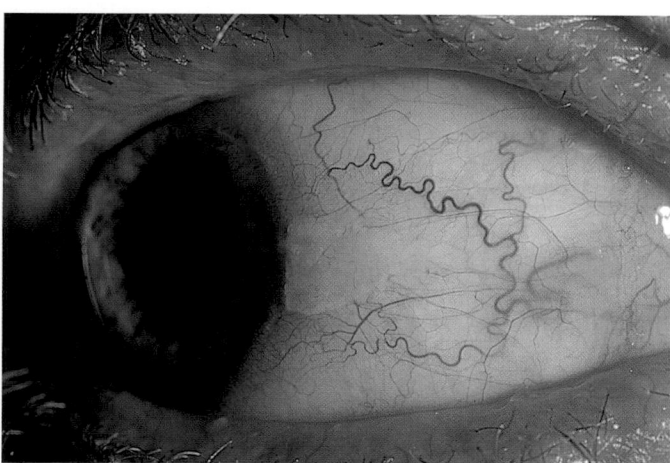

Fig. 11 Pinguecula.

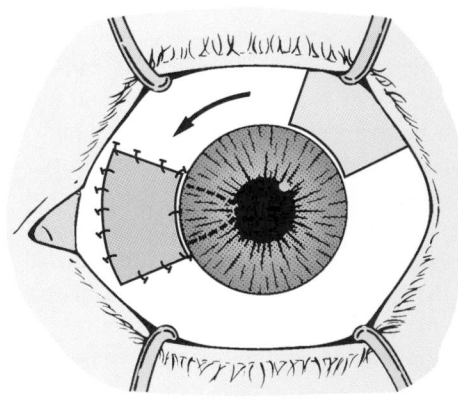

Fig. 13 Conjunctival autograft. Following excision of pterygium from the cornea and sclera, normal bulbar conjunctiva is transposed to the pterygium bed. (Reproduced with permission from *Current Ophthalmic Surgery*, Baillière Tindall, 1990.)

following surgery). While there are low recurrence rates following such regimens, scleral necrosis and infection may complicate their use at a long interval after application. Furthermore, the lack of pathological evidence of cellular proliferation in pterygium does not support the use of antimitotic agents. It is likely that the reported success of procedures in which normal conjunctiva is grafted to the scleral bed is due to replacement of tissue that has been subject to actinic degeneration with healthy tissue in which cell differentiation and extracellular matrix production is normal.

Those patients with axial corneal involvement by pterygium are best initially managed by excision and conjunctival autotransplantation to the scleral bed. This surgery may be combined with lamellar keratoplasty as a combined procedure; alternatively keratoplasty can be undertaken later, when axial scarring and the necessity for keratoplasty can be assessed following initial corneal re-epithelialization.

Further reading

Abelson, M.B. and Allansmith, M.R. (1987). Ocular allergies. In *The cornea. Scientific foundations and clinical practice*. (ed. G. Smolin and R.A. Thoft), pp. 307–21. Little, Brown, Boston.

Cameron, J.A. (1995). Shield ulcers and plaques of the cornea in vernal keratoconjunctivitis. *Ophthalmology*, **102**, 985–93.

Char, D.H. (1989). Conjunctival malignancies: diagnosis and management. In *Clinical ocular oncology*, pp. 63–87. Churchill Livingstone, Edinburgh.

Erie, J.C., Campbell, R.J., and Liesegang, T.J. (1986). Conjunctival and corneal intraepithelial and invasive neoplasia. *Ophthalmology*, **93**, 176–83.

Hungerford, J.L. (1995). Management of ocular melanoma. *British Medical Bulletin*, **51**, 694–716.

Knowles, D.M., Jakobiec, F.A., McNally, L., and Burke, J.S. (1990). Lymphoid hyperplasia and malignant lymphoma occurring in the ocular adnexa (orbit, conjunctiva, and eyelids). *Human Pathology*, **21**, 959–73.

Lee, G.A. and Hirst, L.W. (1995). Ocular surface squamous neoplasia. *Survey of Ophthalmology*, **39**, 429–50.

Lommatzsch, P.K., Lomm, R.E., Kirsch, I., and Fuhrmann, P. (1990). Therapeutic outcome of patients suffering from malignant melanomas of the conjunctiva. *British Journal of Ophthalmology*, **74**, 615–19.

Mondino, B.J. (1990). Cicatricial pemphigoid and erythema multiforme. *Ophthalmology*, **97**, 939–52.

Tuft, S.J., *et al.* (1991). Clinical features of atopic keratoconjunctivitis. *Ophthalmology*, **98**, 150–8.

Wright, P. (1986). Cicatrizing conjunctivitis. *Transactions of the Ophthalmological Societies of the United Kingdom*, **105**, 1–17.

these conditions is important because they follow different courses, they need different treatments, and they have different prognoses. Several classifications have been proposed on the basis of clinical, clinicopathological, and aetiological aspects. The most frequently used was proposed by Watson and Hayreh in their excellent episcleritis and scleritis survey and treatise performed at Moorfields Eye Hospital in London in 1976 (Table 1). This classification is based on the anatomical site of the inflammation and on the clinical appearance of the disease at presentation and it has proved to be useful because the majority of the patients remain in the same clinical type throughout the course of their disease. Two main categories can be differentiated: episcleritis and scleritis. Episcleritis is an acute, benign, recurrent disease, infrequently linked with systemic diseases, whereas scleritis is a chronic, painful, potentially blinding, destructive recurrent disease, commonly associated with potentially lethal systemic diseases (Table 2). It is therefore vital that the correct diagnosis is made and that subsequent adequate treatment be given as early as possible in the course of the disease.

Episcleritis

Episcleritis is a benign inflammatory disease that is characterized by oedema and cellular infiltration of the episclera, the highly vascular, connective tissue, sandwiched between the superficial Tenon capsule and the deep sclera.

Patient characteristics

Episcleritis occurs in young adults, usually females, with a peak incidence in the fourth decade. Although episcleritis may occur in all parts of the world, there are no studies on racial predilection or genetic association.

Clinical manifestations

Episcleritis is abrupt in onset, mild in intensity, and recurrent in nature. The main symptom is mild discomfort, which can be described as a feeling of burning or irritation. Pain is uncommon, but if present, it is usually described as a slight ache localized to the eye (unlike scleritis, where it is usually referred to the forehead, jaw, or sinuses). Other symptoms include tearing (never true discharge) and mild photophobia. Unlike scler-

2.4.4 Scleritis and episcleritis

Maite Sainz de la Maza and C. Stephen Foster

Inflammation of the wall of the eyeball includes a spectrum of conditions, ranging from trivial and self-limiting episodes to severe and uncontrolled processes. Clinical differentiation of

Table 1 Clinical classification of episcleral and scleral inflammation (from Watson and Hayreh 1976)

Episcleritis
Simple
Nodular
Scleritis
Anterior scleritis
diffuse scleritis
nodular scleritis
necrotizing scleritis
with inflammation
without inflammation (scleromalacia perforans)
Posterior scleritis

Table 2 Associated diseases in episcleritis and scleritis

Non-infectious
Connective tissue diseases and other inflammatory conditions
  rheumatoid arthritis
  systemic lupus erythematosus
  ankylosing spondylitis
  Reiter's syndrome
  psoriatic arthritis
  arthritis and inflammatory bowel disease
  relapsing polychondritis

Vasculitis diseases
  polyarteritis nodosa
  allergic angiitis of Churg–Strauss
  Wegener's granulomatosis
  Behçet's disease
  giant cell arteritis
  Cogan's syndrome
  associated with connective tissue diseases and other inflammatory
    conditions

Miscellaneous
  atopy
  rosacea
  gout
  foreign body granuloma
  chemical injury

Infectious
Bacteria
Fungi
Viruses
Parasites

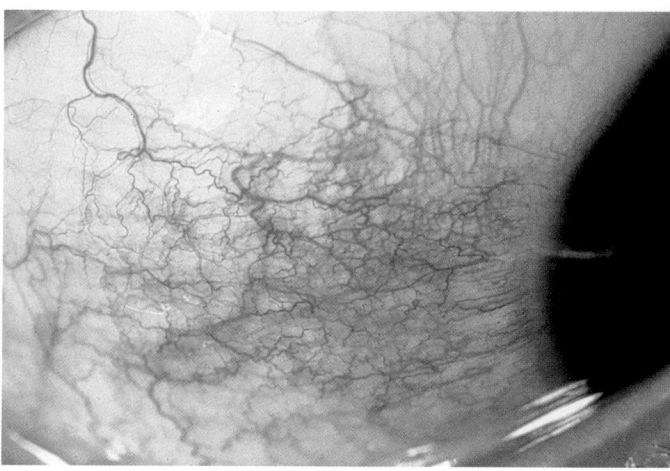

Fig. 1 Episcleritis. Note the vascular dilation of conjunctival vessels and superficial episcleral vessels. There is no underlying scleral oedema. The eye appears bright red.

itis, there is no tenderness to globe palpation. The main sign in episcleritis is redness, which may range from a mild red flush to fiery red, and can be localized in one sector or can involve the whole episclera.

In the authors' experience, episcleritis is bilateral in about 35 per cent of cases. Whether treated or not, the condition is self-limited after a few days or weeks. Recurrences are very frequent over a period of years, but the episodes become less frequent after the first 3 to 4 years until the problem no longer recurs. In spite of these recurrences, episcleritis neither involves sclera nor leaves any residual tissue damage.

Episcleritis rarely causes loss of vision; extension of the inflammatory process to adjacent ocular structures (leading to keratitis, uveitis, glaucoma, cataract, or fundus abnormalities) is very uncommon.

Ocular examination

Two vascular networks can be distinguished in the episclera: the superficial episcleral plexus and the deep episcleral plexus. In episcleritis, maximum congestion is in the superficial episcleral plexus, with no changes in the deep episcleral network. The oedema is localized in the episcleral tissue; the superficial episcleral plexus is displaced forward because of underlying episcleral oedema and the deep episcleral network remains flat

against the sclera. Episcleritis never develops into scleritis. Ocular examination in scleral diseases must include an episcleral and scleral examination and a general eye examination. Episcleral and scleral examination should be in daylight and with the slit lamp; slit lamp light includes the white diffuse light, white beam, and green diffuse light.

Episcleral examination in daylight

External evaluation of the eye in daylight is sometimes the only way to distinguish episcleritis from scleritis because slit lamp light does not disclose subtle colour differences. In episcleritis, the eye appears from mild pink to intense bright red (Fig. 1); there is no bluish discoloration as is observed in scleritis. The congested area may be diffuse, involving the entire globe, or localized and sectorial.

Episcleral examination with the slit lamp

White diffuse illumination by the slit lamp helps to detect the oedema of the episclera and vasodilatation of the superficial episcleral plexus; any localized areas or nodules are mobile over the sclera. In episcleritis, congested vessels follow the usual radial pattern unlike in scleritis, where this pattern is altered and new, abnormal non-radial vessels may be formed. The topical application of a vasoconstrictor such as 10 per cent phenylephrine makes detection of the congested episcleral plexus easier; because the vasoconstrictor blanches the superficial plexus without significant effect on the deep plexus, the eye will appear white in episcleritis (Figs 2, 3).

Slit lamp white beam illumination serves mainly to reveal the depth of inflammation. Since in episcleritis, the vascular congestion is in the superficial episcleral plexus, the anterior edge of the slit lamp beam is displaced forward because of underlying episcleral oedema; the posterior edge of the slit lamp beam remains flat against the sclera, in its normal position.

Green diffuse illumination helps determine with certainty

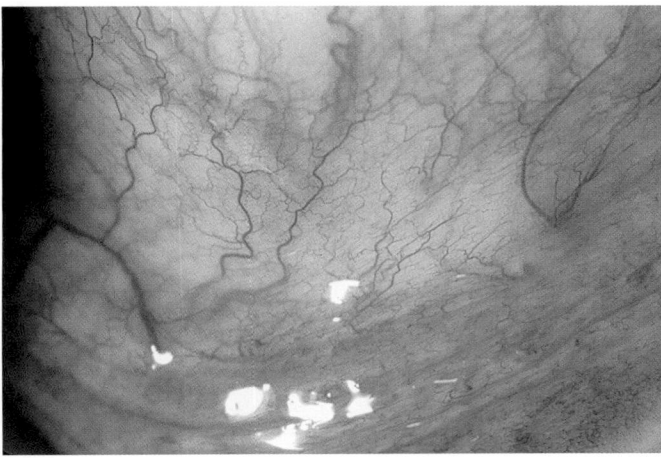

Fig. 2 Episcleritis prior to instillation of 10 per cent phenylephrine drops. Maximum congestion is in the superficial episcleral plexus with no changes in the deep episcleral plexus.

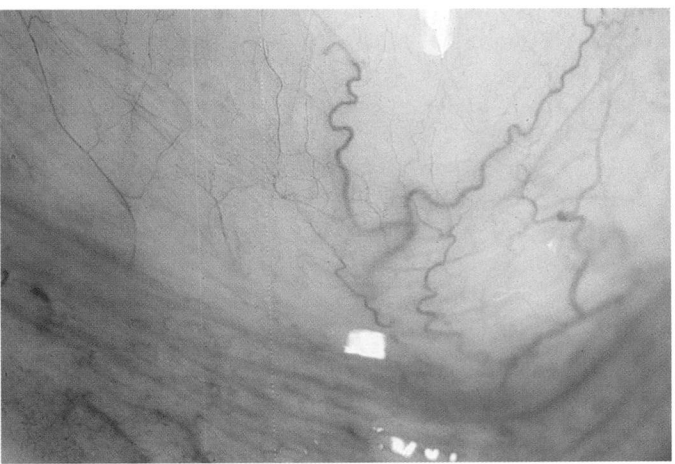

Fig. 3 Same eye as in Fig. 2 after the instillation of 10 per cent phenylephrine drops. Because the vasoconstrictor blanches the superficial plexus without significant effect on the deep plexus, the eye will appear white in episcleritis.

areas with maximum vascular congestion. It is also useful for further study of the areas of lymphocytic infiltration of the episcleral tissue, manifested as yellow spots; because these areas are found in episcleritis, their detection makes differentiation between episcleritis and scleritis easier.

General eye examination

In episcleritis vision is usually not affected. Mild peripheral corneal changes such as superficial and midstromal inflammatory cell infiltration may occasionally be observed in the area adjacent to the episcleral oedema, but these infiltrates never progress to corneal ulceration and usually resolve without any sequelae. Cells in the anterior chamber and aqueous flare may rarely appear, but these are never severe. Glaucoma and cataract are not directly attributed to the episcleral inflammation;

more often they are related to inappropriate topical steroid treatment.

Classification

Episcleritis may be divided into the subcategories of simple and nodular (see Table 1). Both have the same characteristics described above but they differ in onset of the signs and symptoms, in localization of the inflammation, and in clinical course.

Simple episcleritis

Simple episcleritis is more common than nodular episcleritis. The diffusely congested and oedematous area appears abruptly after the symptoms appear, reaching its peak in a few hours, and gradually subsiding over a period usually between 5 and 10 days. Each attack is self-limited, even without treatment, and usually clear without sequelae. Recurrence in the same or opposite eye, involving the same or different areas, may occur. There is a specific subgroup of episcleritis patients with a few prolonged episodes instead of multiple evanescent ones; these patients most often have some associated disease.

Nodular episcleritis

In nodular episcleritis, the inflammation is confined to a well-defined area, forming a red nodule, from 2 to 6 mm or larger in size, with little surrounding congestion. The nodule appears over a period of 2 to 3 days, gradually subsiding over a period of 4 to 6 weeks, without sequelae. Recurrence in the same or opposite eye, involving the same or different areas, may occur, sometimes with more than one nodule at a time. The overlying conjunctiva can be moved over the nodule, and the nodule can be moved over the underlying sclera; that helps to differentiate nodular episcleritis from conjunctival phlyctenule and from nodular scleritis.

Pathology

Light and electron microscopic studies of simple and nodular episcleritis show chronic, non-granulomatous inflammation with lymphocytes and plasma cells, vascular dilatation, and oedema.

Associated diseases

The majority of patients with episcleritis have idiopathic disease; the ones who have any associated disease, usually have connective tissue or vasculitic diseases, spondyloarthropathies, infections, rosacea, gout, or atopy. In our experience, 68 per cent of the patients with episcleritis were ascribed to the idiopathic group, 13 per cent had a connective tissue or vasculitic disease or an spondyloarthropathy, 2 per cent had a herpes zoster or herpes simplex infection, and 17 per cent had either rosacea, gout, or atopy.

Diagnostic evaluation

If the episcleritis attack is the first and evanescent one it is unnecessary to obtain complementary studies. If it is recurrent or persistent, a careful past history, review of the different systems of the body following a questionnaire, and an examination of the head and the extremities should be covered and, depending on the possibilities raised, diagnostic tests should be selected for confirming or rejecting those preliminary diagnoses. It is important to emphasize that, unless the cause is infectious, diagnostic tests alone will rarely establish a systemic diagnosis; rather they will confirm it in the context of the clinical characteristics discovered in the review of systems.

Therapy

Since episcleritis is a benign, episodic, self-limiting process, it may be left untreated except for comfort and supportive therapy, such as cold compresses and iced artificial tears. It appears that, on the basis of the results of a randomized double-masked placebo-controlled clinical trial, topical non-steroidal anti-inflammatory drugs are not effective. Topical steroids may speed the resolution, but they must be tapered slowly to prevent the recrudescence of the condition which occurs if they are stopped suddenly (rebound effect); steroid glaucoma is a danger in susceptible individuals and should always be looked for in patients on this therapy.

If episcleritis becomes persistent, or the frequency of recurrences is so numerous that the patient becomes incapacitated, systemic non-steroidal anti-inflammatory drugs (for example indomethacin, naproxen, diflunisal, flurbiprofen) should be considered. It has been shown that systemic non-steroidal anti-inflammatory drugs are equally as effective as systemic steroids, but beneficial effect is maintained with systemic non-steroidal anti-inflammatory drugs whereas patients treated with systemic steroids tend to deteriorate once treatment is withdrawn (rebound effect). Patients with episcleritis associated with rosacea, atopy, gout, or herpes also require specific therapy for each disease.

Scleritis

Scleritis is a severe inflammatory condition that is characterized by oedema and cellular infiltration of the sclera, the avascular connective tissue, sandwiched between the superficial episclera and the deep choroid. The condition not only may be progressively sight-threatening and destructive, but also may be associated with potentially lethal systemic diseases. Because medical intervention can halt the progression of both ocular and systemic destructive processes, early detection may improve the ocular and systemic prognoses.

Patient characteristics

Scleritis is most common in middle-aged and elderly individuals, usually females, with a peak incidence in the fifth decade. In our experience, the age range of patients is from 22 to 87 years with a mean age of onset of about 52 years, and the female to male ratio is about 1.5 to 1. There is no known geographical or racial predisposition or genetic association.

Clinical manifestations

Scleritis is insidious in onset, moderate to severe in intensity, and recurrent in nature. The main symptom is pain, which

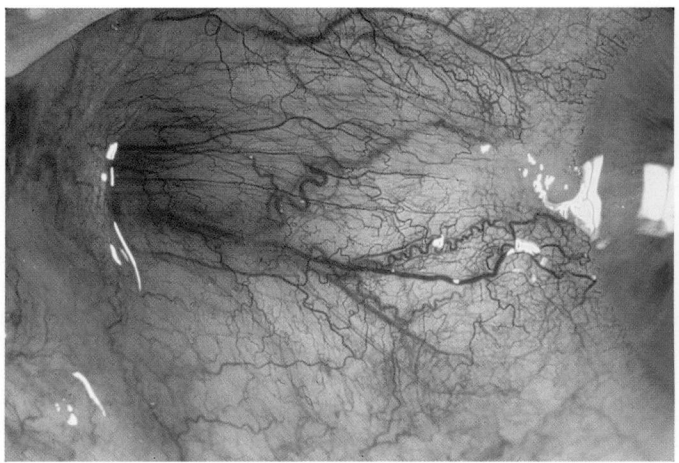

Fig. 4 Scleritis. Note the bluish-red appearance of the inflamed eye, owing to the loss of some of the scleral fibres under the conjunctiva and episcleral tissue.

is moderate to severe and penetrating in character, sometimes localized to the eye, but more frequently referred to the forehead, jaw, or sinuses. This pain may sometimes recrudesce with violent paroxysms triggered by touching the eye or the periocular structures, leading to constant anxiety, depression, and insomnia. Other symptoms include tearing (never true discharge) and mild to moderate photophobia. Patients with scleritis (unlike those with episcleritis) experience tenderness to globe palpation. The main sign is redness which has a bluish-red tinge in appearance and can be localized to one sector, most frequently to the interpalpebral area (followed by the superior quadrants), or may involve the whole sclera (Fig. 4). In the authors' experience, it may be bilateral in about 34 per cent of cases.

Scleritis may recur involving the same or different eyes at different times, or both eyes at the same time. Recurrences may be frequent over a period of many years but the episodes become less frequent after the first 3 to 6 years until the problem no longer recurs.

Scleritis may cause loss of vision through the complications it produces. The main causes of loss of vision are keratitis, uveitis, glaucoma, cataract, exudative retinal detachment, and macular oedema.

Ocular examination

In scleritis, maximum congestion is in the deep episcleral plexus, with also some congestion in the superficial episcleral plexus. The oedema is localized to the scleral and episcleral tissues; both the deep and superficial episcleral plexuses are displayed forward because of underlying scleral and episcleral oedema.

Scleral examination in daylight

In scleritis, the eye has a diffuse, greyish blue tinge; this is because after several attacks of scleral inflammation, the sclera becomes more translucent, and sometimes thinner, allowing the dark uvea to show through. The congested area may be diffuse, involving the entire globe, or localized and sectorial.

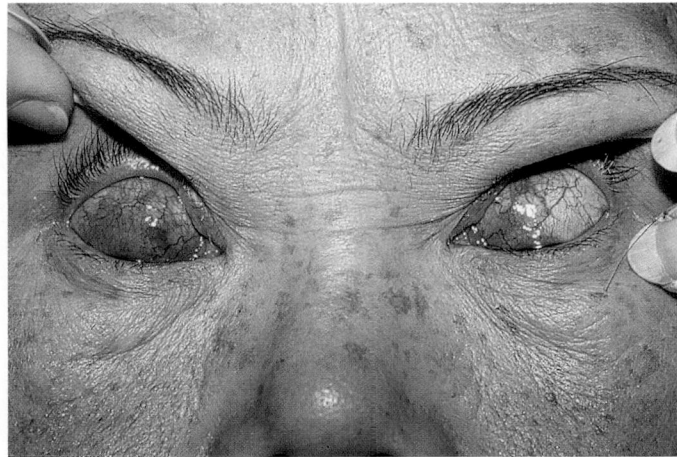

Fig. 5 A dark brown or black tinged area surrounded by active scleral inflammation indicates that a necrotic process is taking place.

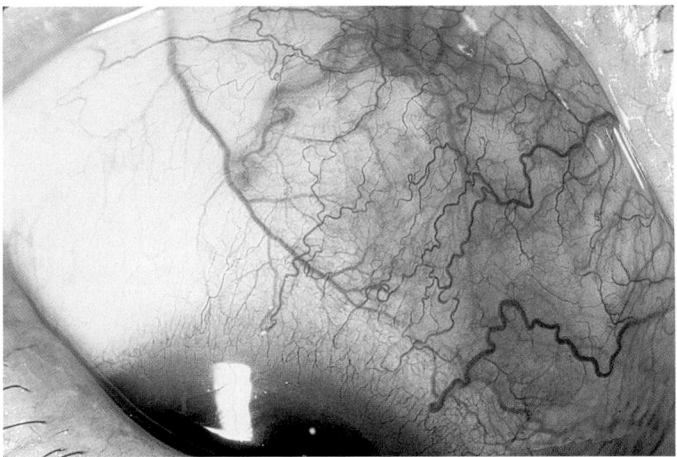

Fig. 6 Scleritis prior to instillation of 10 per cent phenylephrine drops. Maximum congestion is in the deep episcleral plexus with some congestion in the superficial episcleral plexus.

A dark brown or black tinged area surrounded by active scleral inflammation indicates that a necrotic process is taking place (Fig. 5). If tissue necrosis progresses, the scleral area can become avascular, producing a white sequestrum in the centre surrounded by a well-defined dark brown or black circle. The slough may be gradually removed by granulation tissue, leaving the underlying uvea bare or covered only by a thin layer of conjunctiva.

Episcleral examination with the slit lamp

White diffuse illumination by the slit lamp confirms the macroscopic impression of avascular areas with sequestra or uveal show. It also helps to detect new abnormal vessels, usually following an anarchic configuration. The topical application of a vasoconstrictor such as 10 per cent phenylephrine makes differentiation between scleritis and episcleritis easier; because the vasoconstrictor blanches the superficial plexus without significant effect on the deep plexus, the eye will remain congested in scleritis (Figs 6, 7).

Slit lamp white beam illumination serves mainly to reveal the depth of inflammation. Since in scleritis, the vascular congestion is mainly in the deep episcleral plexus with some congestion in the superficial episcleral plexus, both the posterior and the anterior edges of the slit lamp beam are displaced forward because of underlying scleral and episcleral oedema.

Green diffuse illumination helps determine with certainty areas with maximum vascular congestion, areas of new vascular channels, and areas completely avascular.

General eye examination

Scleritis may cause loss of vision because extension of the inflammatory process to adjacent ocular structures (leading to keratitis, uveitis, glaucoma, cataract, or fundus abnormalities) is common.

Classification

Scleritis may be classified as anterior and posterior (see Table 1); anterior scleritis is further classified as diffuse, nodu-

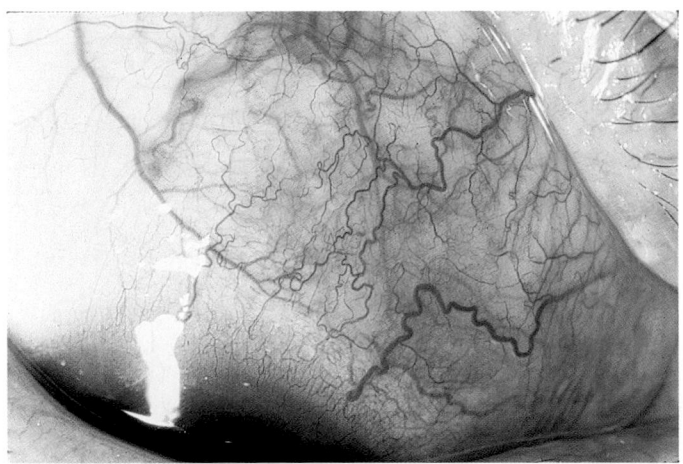

Fig. 7 Same eye as in Fig. 6, after the instillation of 10 per cent phenylephrine drops. Because the vasoconstrictor blanches the superficial plexus without significant effect on the deep plexus, the eye will remain congested in scleritis.

lar, necrotizing with inflammation, and necrotizing without inflammation (scleromalacia perforans).

Diffuse anterior scleritis

The generalized congested and oedematous area appears insidiously after the symptoms appear, reaching its peak in 5 to 10 days (Fig. 8). Without treatment, it may last several months. Although most of the patients diagnosed with diffuse scleritis maintain this category throughout the course of their scleral disease, a few may progress to the more severe category, nodular scleritis, or even to the most severe category, necrotizing scleritis.

Nodular anterior scleritis

In nodular scleritis, the inflammation is confined to a well-defined area, forming a violaceous scleral nodule (or nodules) which is immobile and firm to the touch (Fig. 9). Symptoms

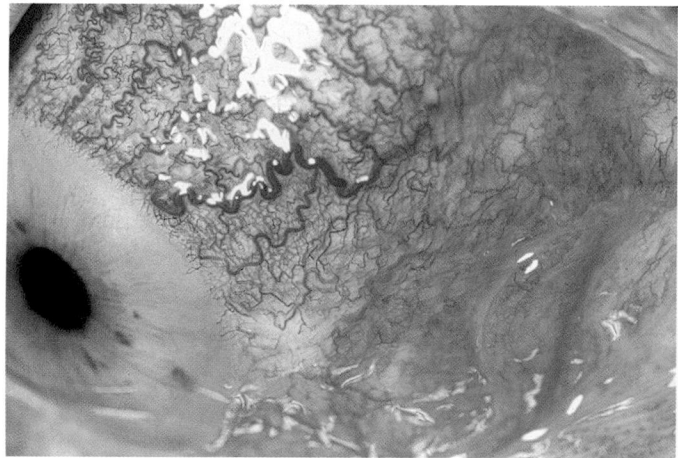

Fig. 8 Diffuse scleritis. Note the generalized congested and oedematous area.

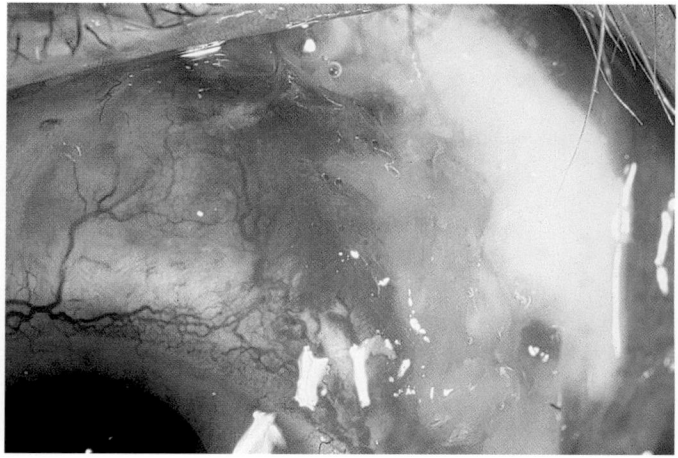

Fig. 10 Necrotizing scleritis. Note the white avascular area surrounded by active scleral inflammation. The damaged sclera becomes translucent and shows the brown colour of the underlying uvea.

The main characteristic determined by ocular examination is the presence of white avascular areas surrounded by swelling of the sclera and acute congestion of anarchically configured neovessels. The damaged sclera becomes translucent and shows the brown colour of the underlying uvea (Fig. 10). Without treatment, the area becomes avascular and may detach from the wall of the globe (sequestra), leaving the uvea bare or covered only by conjunctiva.

Necrotizing anterior scleritis without inflammation (scleromalacia perforans)

Scleromalacia perforans is characterized by the appearance of yellow or greyish anterior scleral nodules that gradually develop a necrotic slough or sequestrum without surrounding inflammation (Fig. 11). This sequestrum may detach from the wall of the globe leaving the uvea bare or covered only by conjunctiva. The uvea does not bulge through these areas unless the intraocular pressure rises. Although spontaneous perforation is

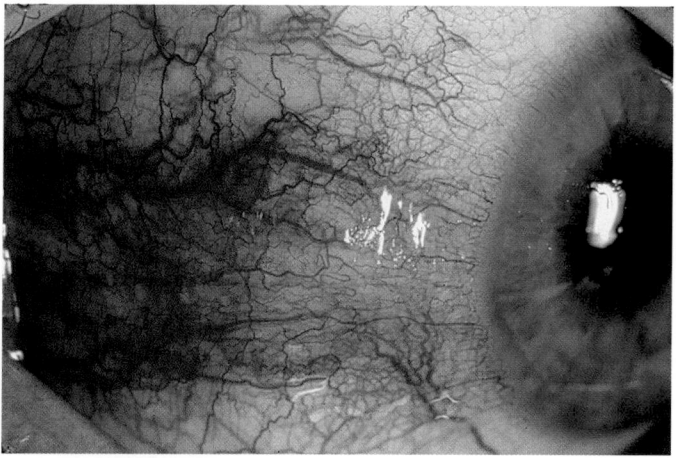

Fig. 9 Nodular scleritis. The inflammation is confined to a well-defined area forming a scleral nodule. As part of the sclera, the nodule is immobile as one tries to palpate and move it.

and signs appear insidiously, reaching its peak in 5 to 10 days, and without treatment, they may last for several months. The nodule is usually localized in the interpalpebral region close to the limbus. Although most of the patients diagnosed with nodular scleritis maintain this category throughout the course of their scleral disease, a few may progress to the most severe category, necrotizing scleritis.

Necrotizing anterior scleritis with inflammation (necrotizing scleritis)

Necrotizing scleritis is the most severe and destructive form of scleritis, sometimes leading to loss of the eye from multiple ocular complications, or even occasionally perforation of the globe. The onset of pain and redness usually is insidious, reaching its peak in 3 or 4 days. The pain, always present without adequate medication, may be so intense and provoked by minimal touch to the scalp that it sometimes seems out of proportion to the ocular findings. It usually worsens at night, keeping the patient awake and very anxious and distressed.

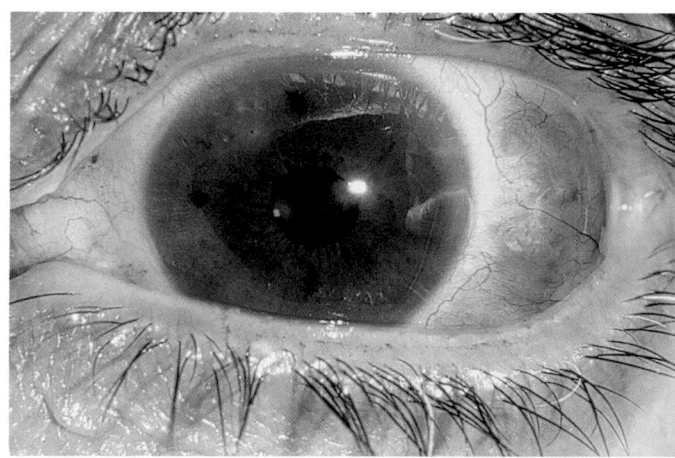

Fig. 11 Scleromalacia perforans. Note the degree of scleral loss of uveal bulge under the stretched conjunctiva. There is no active scleral inflammation.

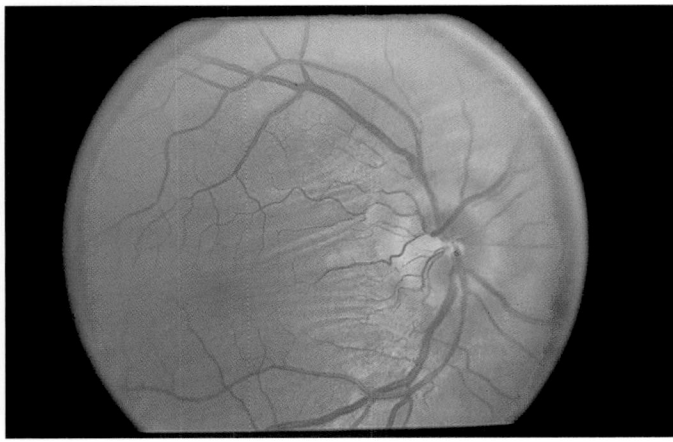

Fig. 12 Posterior scleritis. Note the choroidal folds, as shown by the alternating light and dark lines.

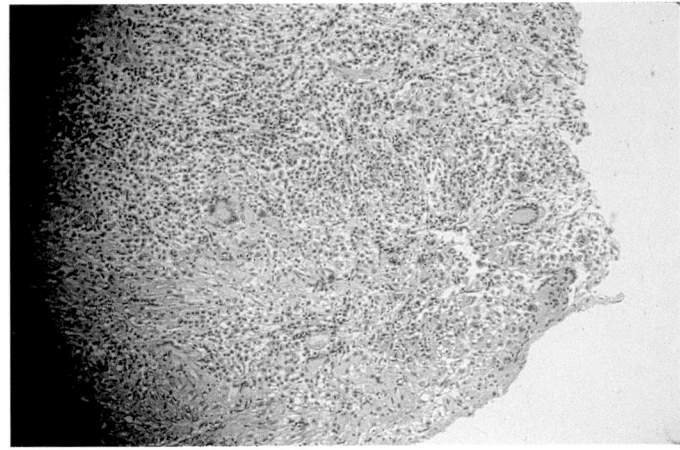

Fig. 13 Scleral biopsy from a patient with necrotizing scleritis. Note the granulomatous inflammation with multinucleated giant cells, lymphocytes, and plasma cells.

rare, traumatic perforation may easily occur. The condition has an insidious onset, slow progression, and absence of symptoms such as pain or tenderness to the touch; therefore, it may often be detected by the patient while looking in the mirror, by the patient's family, or by the rheumatologist. Scleromalacia perforans usually appears in association with severe, progressive, long-standing rheumatoid arthritis with extra-articular manifestations.

Posterior scleritis

Posterior scleritis accounts for the inflammation of the sclera posterior to the ora serrata, which may spread to the posterior segment of the eye, involving choroid, retina, and optic nerve. Posterior scleritis alone can be a difficult diagnosis to establish, and if associated with anterior scleritis, it may be overlooked. Therefore, posterior scleritis is a more common condition than is realized, and the diagnosis is often missed or delayed.

The most common presenting symptoms of posterior scleritis are loss of vision and pain, although diplopia, photopsias, and tenderness may also be present. Some decrease of visual acuity is almost always present in patients with posterior scleritis, and its type and severity depends on the site, type, and degree of complications associated. The pain varies from mild to severe and often is referred to the brow, temple, face, or jaw. The most common presenting sign is redness, if there is anterior scleritis; conjunctival chemosis, proptosis, lid swelling, lid retraction, and limitation of ocular movements may also be detected.

The most common fundus findings are choroidal folds (Fig. 12), subretinal mass, disc oedema, and macular oedema. Annular ciliochoroidal detachment, serous retinal detachment, intraretinal deposits, and retinal striae may also appear.

Ultrasonography is the most useful test in the diagnosis of posterior scleritis, because it shows the thickening of the retinochoroid layers and the presence of oedema in Tenon's space.

Pathology

The sclera in scleritis, either diffuse or nodular, usually shows a non-granulomatous inflammatory reaction characterized by infiltration of mononuclear cells such as lymphocytes, plasma cells, and macrophages. In some cases, however, especially in the most severe ones, mononuclear cells organize into granulomatous lesions. There is also a fibroblast and vascular proliferations.

The sclera in necrotizing scleritis reveals a granulomatous inflammatory reaction characterized by epithelioid cells, multinucleated giant cells, lymphocytes, plasma cells, and less often neutrophils (Fig. 13). There is also an inflammatory microangiopathy (Fig. 14) and extracellular matrix degradation.

Associated diseases

Connective tissue and vasculitic diseases are the main entities to be considered in the differential diagnosis of scleritis (see Table 2). Other diseases that should also be considered are the infections, atopy, rosacea, and gout. In our experience, 57 per cent of patients with scleritis have an associated disease, includ-

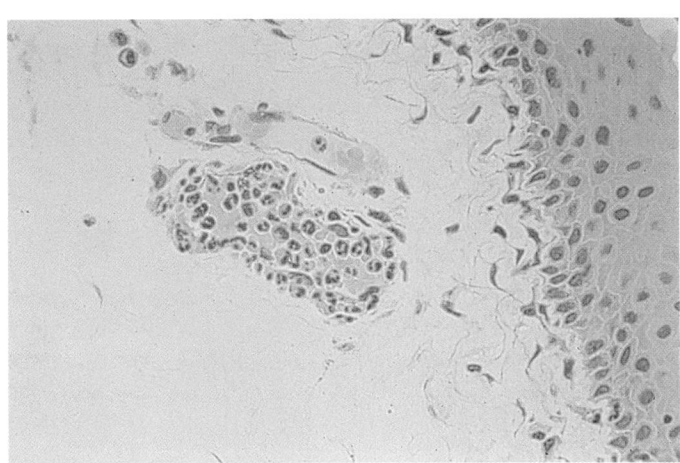

Fig. 14 Scleral biopsy from a patient with necrotizing scleritis. Note the inflammatory microangiopathy characterized by neutrophil infiltration in and around the wall of the vessel.

ing 48 per cent with a connective tissue or vasculitic disease, 7 per cent with an infectious cause, and 2 per cent with atopy, rosacea, or gout. The specific diseases most commonly associated with scleritis are rheumatoid arthritis, Wegener's granulomatosis, relapsing polychondritis, and systemic lupus erythematosus.

The detection of a connective tissue or vasculitic disease in a patient with scleritis is a sign of poor general prognosis because it indicates potentially systemic complications which may be lethal unless managed with prompt and aggressive therapy. The detection of a connective tissue or vasculitic disease in a patient with scleritis also is a sign of poor ocular prognosis, since patients with these diseases frequently have more necrotizing scleritis, peripheral ulcerative keratitis, or reduction in vision than do patients without these diseases. Furthermore, the ocular prognosis of scleritis associated with a connective tissue or vasculitic disease varies depending on the specific disease:

- scleritis associated either with systemic lupus erythematosus or spondyloarthropathies is usually a condition not associated with ocular complications, whereas scleritis in Wegener's granulomatosis is a severe disease that can lead to permanent blindness

- scleritis in rheumatoid arthritis or relapsing polychondritis is a disease of intermediate potential severity, which should be monitored closely for the development of ocular complications.

Diagnostic evaluation

The detection of scleritis (even if the attack is the first one) requires complementary studies. These include a past history, a careful review of the different systems of the body following a questionnaire, and a systemic examination of the head and the extremities. Depending on the possibilities raised, diagnostic tests should be requested for pursuing the suspected causes. Sometimes, one series of diagnostic studies may be insufficient and regular reinvestigations may be necessary to discover the diagnosis.

Therapy

Topical non-steroidal or steroidal drugs are routinely insufficient treatment for scleritis. In the authors' opinion, in patients with diffuse and nodular scleritis, systemic non-steroidal anti-inflammatory drugs (for example indomethacin, naproxen, diflunisal, flurbiprofen) should be the initial choice; in case of therapeutic failure, systemic steroids should be added or substituted as second-line therapy, tapering and discontinuing them as soon as possible while maintaining remission with continued non-steroidal anti-inflammatory drugs; in case of therapeutic failure, immunosuppressive drugs may be added or substituted

as third-line therapy. In patients with necrotizing scleritis, immunosuppressive drugs should be the initial choice. We would caution, as always, that immunosuppressive drugs should be administered by a clinician, either ophthalmologist or chemotherapist, specifically trained in the early recognition and management of drug-induced complications of such treatment.

Surgical repair is rarely necessary in the care of patients with scleritis. There are, however, some patients with large areas of scleral or corneal stromal loss who require tectonic grafting with fresh or preserved donor sclera or lamellar cornea to prevent perforation until immunosuppressive drugs becomes effective (which may take from 4 to 8 weeks).

Surgical intervention may be necessary for patients with scleritis with cataract or glaucoma. This surgery should only be performed once the scleritis is under successful control; perioperative systemic steroids are indicated to minimize the risk of a recurrence precipitated by the surgical procedure.

Further reading

Benson, W.E. (1988). Posterior scleritis. *Survey of Ophthalmology*, **32**, 297–316.

Calthorpe, C.M., Watson, P.G., and McCartney, A.C.E. (1988). Posterior scleritis: a clinical and histological survey. *Eye*, **2**, 267–77.

Fong, L.P., Sainz de la Maza, M., Rice, B.A., *et al.* (1991). Immunopathology of scleritis. *Ophthalmology*, **98**, 472–9.

Foster, C.S. and Sainz de la Maza, M. (1994). *The sclera*. Springer-Verlag, New York.

Lyons, C.J., Hakin, K.N., and Watson, P.G. (1990). Topical flurbiprofen: an effective treatment for episcleritis? *Eye*, **4**, 521–25.

McGavin, D.D., Williamson, J., Forrester, J.V., and Foulds, W.S. (1976). Episcleritis and scleritis: a study of their clinical manifestations and association with rheumatoid arthritis. *British Journal of Ophthalmology*, **60**, 192–226.

Raizman, M.B., Sainz de la Maza, M., and Foster, C.S. (1991). Tectonic keratoplasty for peripheral ulcerative keratitis. *Cornea*, **10**, 312–16.

Sainz de la Maza, M., Tauber, J., and Foster, C.S. (1989). Scleral grafting for necrotizing scleritis. *Ophthalmology*, **96**, 306–10.

Sainz de la Maza, M., Jabbur, N.S., and Foster, C.S. (1993). An analysis of therapeutic decision for scleritis. *Ophthalmology*, **100**, 1372–6.

Sainz de la Maza, M., Foster, C.S., and Jabbur, N.S. (1994*a*). Scleritis associated with rheumatoid arthritis and with other systemic immune-mediated diseases. *Ophthalmology*, **101**, 1281–8.

Sainz de la Maza, M., Jabbur, N.S., and Foster, C.S. (1994*b*). Severity of scleritis and episcleritis. *Ophthalmology*, **101**, 389–96.

Sainz de la Maza, M., Foster, C.S., and Jabbur, N.S. (1995). Scleritis associated with systemic vasculitic diseases. *Ophthalmology*, **102**, 687–92.

Tuft, S.J. and Watson, P.G. (1991). Progression of scleral disease. *Ophthalmology*, **98**, 467–71.

van der Hoeve, J. (1931). Scleromalacia perforans. *Nederlands Tijdschrift voor Geneeskunde*, **75**, 4733–36.

Watson, P. (1992). Diseases of the sclera and episclera. In *Duane's clinical ophthalmology*, vol. 4, pp. 8–23. (ed. W. Tasman E.A. Jaeger), (revised edn). Lippincott, Philadelphia.

Watson, P.G. and Hayreh, S.S. (1976). Scleritis and episcleritis. *British Journal of Ophthalmology*, **60**, 163–91.

Watson, P.G., Lobascher, D., and Sabiston, D. (1966). Double-blind trial of the treatment of episcleritis–scleritis with oxyphenbutazone or prednisolone. *British Journal of Ophthalmology*, **50**, 463.

2.5　The eyelids

2.5.1 Anatomy, physiology, and malformations of the eyelids

A. Jane Dickinson

The eyelids are of immense importance to the visual system, both physically and physiologically. They protect the eyeball from injury, and protect the visual system by regulating the amount of light entering the eye. They provide continual replenishment and distribution of tears, which are then actively removed via the lacrimal pump mechanism.

Anatomy

The eyelids extend from the eyebrows to the nasojugal and malar furrows, enclosing the palpebral fissure. Each is divided into orbital and tarsal portions by a horizontal skin crease, less visible in the lower lid. Differing racial characteristics are apparent as follows. The upper eyelid crease is created by anterior insertions of the levator aponeurosis, and lies 6 to 11 mm above the lid margin in the occidental eye. As the superior orbital septum inserts lower in oriental people, orbital fat may obliterate this crease. The lateral canthus is 2 mm higher than the medial in occidental people, and 5 mm higher in oriental people. The widest point of the palpebral fissure (10–12 mm) is in the medial third of the occidental eye, but at the mid-point of the oriental eye. Finally, a curved fold of skin called the epicanthus is fairly common in young occidental children, but generally disappears by school age. In the oriental population, however, it persists throughout life.

The free margins of the adult eyelid are 2 mm thick and 30 mm long. In the eyelash-bearing portion (ciliary), the margin is square in cross-section, whilst in its medial one-sixth (lacrimal portion) it is rounded. The boundary between these is marked by the papilla lacrimalis, with its central punctum lacrimale which drains the tears. Wedged in the medial canthus lies the caruncle, a triangular fold of hairy, gland-bearing skin, and the vestigial 'third eyelid' (plica semilunaris). Between these structures and the posterior lid margin lies the lacus lacrimalis where tears accumulate prior to drainage.

Each eyelid has distinct anatomical layers (Fig. 1). In tarsal cross-section these comprise skin, subcutaneous tissue, orbicu-

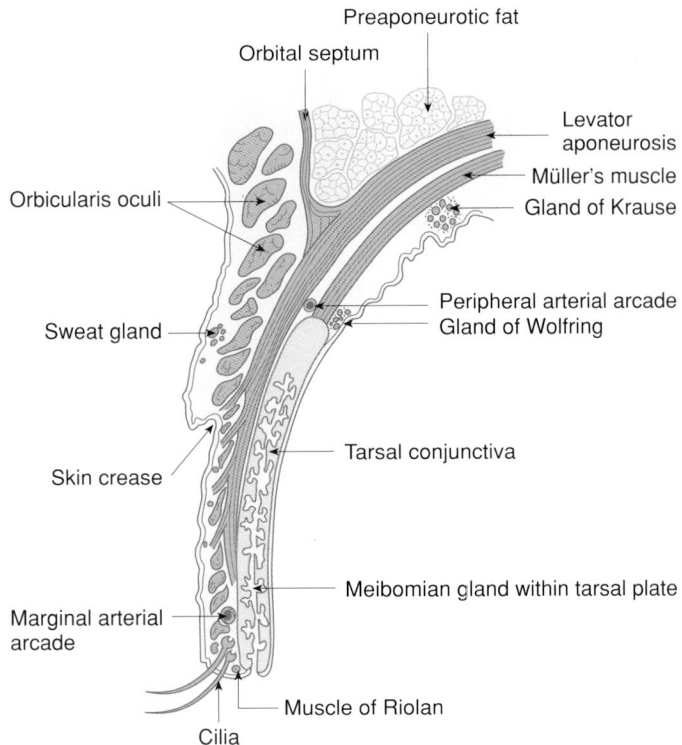

Fig. 1 Cross-section of the upper eyelid.

Preaponeurotic fat
Orbital septum
Levator aponeurosis
Müller's muscle
Gland of Krause
Orbicularis oculi
Peripheral arterial arcade
Gland of Wolfring
Sweat gland
Tarsal conjunctiva
Skin crease
Meibomian gland within tarsal plate
Marginal arterial arcade
Muscle of Riolan
Cilia

laris muscle, tarsal plate, and conjunctiva. In the orbital portion, however, the layers posterior to orbicularis comprise orbital septum, preaponeurotic fat pad, levator aponeurosis insertion, smooth muscle of Müller, and conjunctiva. These layers are mirrored in the lower eyelid, excepting the levator aponeurosis, which is 'replaced' by the lower lid retractor, a fascial expansion of the inferior rectus sheath containing some smooth muscle fibres. It merges with the orbital septum to insert into the tarsal plate. Medially and laterally lie the medial and lateral canthal ligaments, securing the respective canthi.

Eyelid skin is extremely thin and devoid of subcutaneous fat, but has a loose connective tissue base, hence the propensity of the eyelids to swell. Its marked elasticity, however, allows rapid recovery. In addition to the upper lid crease, there are deep attachments to medial and lateral canthal ligaments and the orbital margins, which become apparent when the lids are swollen. The skin contains eccrine sweat glands, and sebaceous glands associated with numerous fine hairs. The latter are largely absent nasally, where the skin is more shiny due to unicellular sebaceous glands. Eyelid skin also contains abundant mobile pigment cells which confer its changing coloration.

The eyelashes (cilia) are 200 to 300 cylindrical hairs arranged in two or three rows along the eyelid margins, two-thirds in the upper. Their follicles have no associated arrector muscle, but several rudimentary sebaceous glands (Zeis). Some, particularly in the lower lid, also have a ciliary apocrine sweat gland (Moll). They are replaced two or three times annually, but if cut, grow rapidly back to size. Eyelashes help prevent foreign bodies from impinging on the globe. Light touch initiates reflex lid closure, mediated by the rich nerve plexus surrounding each lash follicle, with its low threshold of excitation. The other important hair-bearing area, the eyebrow, rests on a very mobile fat and muscle pad overlying the superior orbital rim. Its mobility is of great expressive importance, but it also protects the eye from both light and sweat.

The striated orbicularis muscle effects eyelid closure. Innervated by the facial nerve, it is notionally divided into three concentric zones: pretarsal, preseptal, and orbital. The pretarsal and preseptal fibres arise from superficial and deep heads, the former around the medial canthal ligament, and the latter from the posterior lacrimal crest and lacrimal sac fascia (Horner's muscle). They pass laterally, and around the lateral canthus as the lateral palpebral raphe, with some deep pretarsal fibres also inserting into Whitnall's tubercle. The orbital fibres arise from bone, above and below the anterior limb of the medial canthal ligament. They enclose the preseptal fibres, and interdigitate superiorly with procerus, corrugator supercilii, and frontalis. In contrast to the rest of orbicularis, pretarsal fibres are firmly adherent to underlying tissue, tarsus, and around the eyelid margin form the muscle of Riolan.

The tarsal plate of each eyelid confers shape and stability to the palpebral aperture. Each is 25 mm long and 1 mm thick, with a maximum height of 11 mm in the upper eyelid, and 4 mm in the lower. They comprise dense fibrous tissue surrounding 20 to 30 sebaceous glands. These tarsal (meibomian) glands have 10 to 15 acini surrounding a central vertical duct, often visible through conjunctiva. They secrete lipid into the tears via separate ostia along the mucocutaneous junction of the eyelid margin. This lipid helps stabilize the tear film and reduces evaporation. Each tarsal plate is in vertical continuity with a thinner fibrous layer, the orbital septum, which in turn inserts into the orbital margin. Horizontally, the tarsal plates are anchored to the orbital margins by strong, fibrous canthal ligaments. The lateral canthal ligament is simply a condensation of connective tissue deep to the lateral palpebral raphe. It is 7 mm long and 2.5 mm broad and is attached to the orbital tubercle (Whitnall's tubercle) on the zygomatic bone. The medial canthal ligament, by contrast, is a discreet band with two limbs, and forms a prominence under the skin at the medial canthus. The anterior limb is much more defined. It arises from the anterior lacrimal crest and adjacent maxilla, and passes anterior to the lacrimal fossa to divide and attach to the medial extremities of both tarsal plates. The posterior limb arises from the posterior lacrimal crest and passes anterolaterally, merging with sac fascia, to insert into the back of the anterior limb.

Beneath these structures lie the 8 mm horizontal portions of the canaliculi which generally merge to a common canaliculus before entering the lacrimal sac. Each canaliculus also has a 2 mm vertical portion adjacent to its punctum, and a wider ampulla where the two portions meet.

Eyelid opening is primarily due to the striated muscle, levator palpebrae superioris, innervated by oculomotor fibres, although the sympathetically innervated smooth muscle of Müller also contributes. The levator arises from the orbital apex, above the annulus of Zinn, and passes forwards beneath the orbital roof, sharing fascial connections with the adjacent superior rectus. The superior transverse ligament of Whitnall is a dense fascial condensation bridging the superior orbit between the trochlea and superior orbital notch medially, and the lacrimal gland fascia laterally. It causes the levator muscle to change direction 15 to 20 mm above the tarsal plate, shortly before it thins to become an aponeurosis. Müller's muscle originates from the underside of levator at this level. The horizontal attachments of the aponeurosis consist of medial and lateral horns, which insert into the respective canthal ligaments and adjacent orbital walls. The lateral horn also divides the lacrimal gland into orbital and palpebral lobes. The anterior border of the aponeurosis merges with the orbital septum, and sends fibres through to fuse with pretarsal orbicularis and the anterior surface of the tarsus. The skin crease is created by these attachments in an area where orbicularis and skin are more firmly attached.

The eyelids are lined by mucous membrane, the palpebral conjunctiva, which is in continuity with the bulbar conjunctiva via the fornices. It contains numerous goblet cells, secreting mucous into the tear film, and also contains around 50 accessory lacrimal glands distributed over the tarsi (Henle), at the attached tarsal borders (Wolfring), and in the fornices (Krause). Its substantia propria contains lymphoid follicles, and numerous lymphocytes, histiocytes, and mast cells, of great immunological importance.

Two divisions of the trigeminal nerve supply sensation to the eyelids. Most of the lower lid is supplied by the infraorbital nerve (maxillary division), although the infratrochlear nerve (ophthalmic division) supplies the medial canthus. Other branches of the ophthalmic division, the supratrochlear, supraorbital, and lacrimal nerves, supply the rest of the upper lid (Fig. 2).

The ophthalmic artery supplies blood to the lids via the medial and lateral palpebral arteries, the latter a branch of the lacrimal. Each palpebral artery gives rise to one inferior and two superior branches, which anastamose in the respective lids. The marginal arcade of the upper lid lies 2 mm above the eyelid margin; that in the lower lid is 4 mm below the margin. The other upper lid branch, the peripheral arcade, lies above the tarsal plate anterior to Müller's muscle (see Figs 1, 2). Numerous anastomoses between adjacent arteries connect the internal and external carotid systems. Diffuse eyelid veins also connect the internal and external systems by linking the facial and orbital veins, and hence the cavernous sinus. The main drainage is to the angular and ophthalmic veins medially, and the superficial temporal vein laterally.

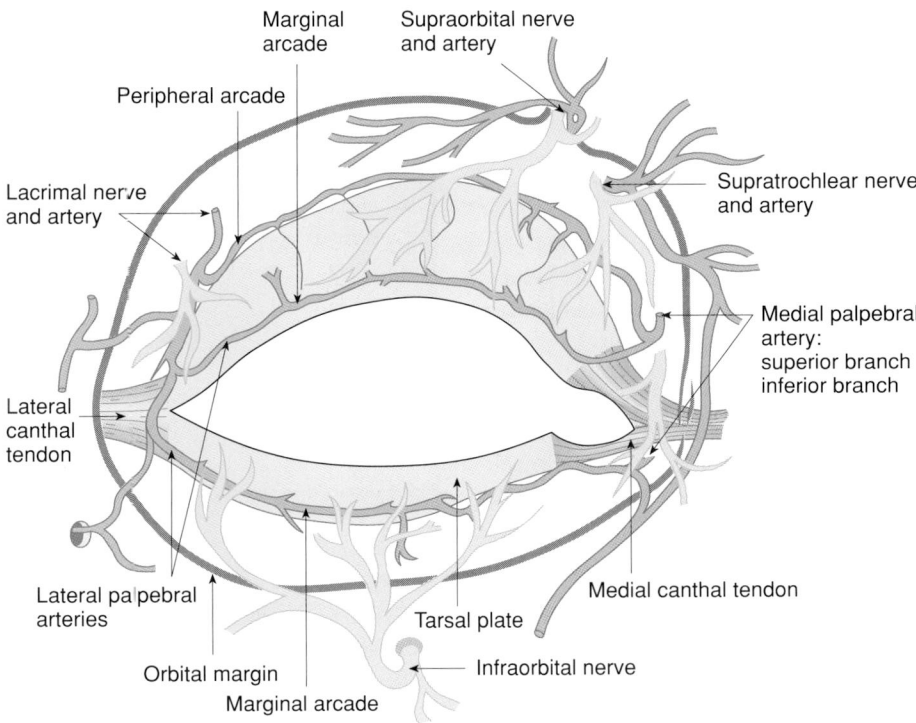

Fig. 2 Sensory nerves and arterial supply of the eyelids.

Lymphatics drain the conjunctiva and tarsal plate to the post-tarsal plexus, and the skin and orbicularis to the pretarsal plexus. The medial canthus and lower lid then drain to the submandibular nodes, whilst the lateral canthus and upper lid drain to the parotid and preauricular nodes.

Physiology

Eyelid movement

Eyelid movements may be involuntary or voluntary. They are not only vital for eyeball protection and for the elimination of tears, but contribute enormously to facial expression.

Closure takes several forms, effected by functionally different groups of motor units of orbicularis oculi. Reflex blinking is a protective mechanism initiated by tactile, visual, or auditory stimuli. Hence the afferent pathway may be the trigeminal nerve (e.g. the corneal reflex, or the glabellar tap), the optic nerve (e.g. the 'menace' reflex), or the acoustic nerve. The efferent arc stimulates the palpebral portion of orbicularis bilaterally. Spontaneous blinking, by contrast, occurs regularly without obvious stimuli, after the first few months of life; however, its frequency may vary from 2 to 30 times/min. It involves simultaneous bilateral contraction of the upper lid palpebral orbicularis preceded by relaxation of the levator, and lasts less than 0.4 s. Visual sensation appears continuous during this period, despite occlusion of the visual axes and simultaneous upward rotation of the globes. Blinking serves to replenish the precorneal tear film and to eliminate excess tears. A wink is a voluntary unilateral closure which interrupts vision. It involves both the palpebral and orbital parts of the orbicularis, if not also brow and cheek muscles. Forced eyelid closure or blepharospasm may be unilateral or bilateral. Whilst often voluntary, it may be involuntary in essential blepharospasm, or in association with inflammation of the anterior segment of the eye. The whole orbicularis is involved, the brows draw downwards, and surrounding muscle groups may also contract. Automatic eyelid closure during sleep involves tonic stimulation of the orbicularis, whilst levator relaxes and the eyes turn upwards. This protective up turning, Bell's phenomenon, is present during all forms of eyelid closure in 90 per cent of individuals, and may be present despite loss of voluntary upgaze in supranuclear palsy.

Eyelid opening is discussed above. The two levator muscles act as yoke muscles, thus Herring's law of equal innervation applies. There is also synergism with the vertical recti, such that the upper eyelid falls on downgaze and rises in upgaze. In extreme upgaze, frontalis also contracts, raising the eyebrows.

Precorneal tear film

The eyelids make a vital contribution to the composition and stability of tears, and by blinking, they resurface the precorneal tear film and propel the tears nasally. This movement relies on the relatively fixed medial canthus, and on eyelid closure beginning laterally. Contraction of orbicularis fibres around the punctum and vertical canaliculus draw these nasally, increasing pressure in the ampulla. Meanwhile, pressure in the lacrimal sac is reduced by contraction of the fibres inserted into its lateral wall. Together with capillary attraction forces, this draws tears into the lacrimal sac.

Embryology

Eyelids originate in ectoderm and mesoderm. Although the plica semilunaris begins to develop from the conjunctival ectoderm in the fifth week, the true eyelid folds only appear around the seventh week. The frontonasal and maxillary mesodermal processes, sandwiched by two ectodermal layers, grow inwards to form the upper and lower lids respectively. These fuse around week 9. Fusion allows differentiation of the margin, with ectoderm moving inwards to form glands and cilia, whilst mesenchyme condenses around the developing meibomian glands forming tarsal plates. Other special structures develop during this period, including orbicularis oculi (second visceral arch mesenchyme), tarsal conjunctiva, puncti, and canaliculi. The latter develop from a core of buried surface ectoderm between the lateral nasal and maxillary processes which itself becomes the lacrimal sac. Between the fifth and seventh months there is keratinization and degeneration of the epithelium between the fused eyelids, and separation occurs.

Malformation of the eyelids

Failure of normal development at a number of embryonic stages results in a variety of congenital malformations.

Cryptophthalmos (Fig. 3)

If lid folds fail to form, the ectoderm surfacing the eyeball remains in continuity with that of surrounding skin. Although rare, it is often bilateral, may be familial, and associated anomalies are common. Treatment is difficult, and although cosmetic improvement may be possible, the visual prognosis is poor.

Coloboma (Fig. 4)

Full-thickness defects arise from either maldevelopment of the encroaching lid folds, failure of eyelid fusion, or from amniotic band damage. Although most common in the upper medial eyelid, they occur anywhere and may be multiple. Whilst often isolated, they occur with mandibulofacial dysostoses.

Ankyloblepharon

This denotes partial or total eyelid fusion, with two main types. Medial canthal fusion, external ankyloblepharon, is more

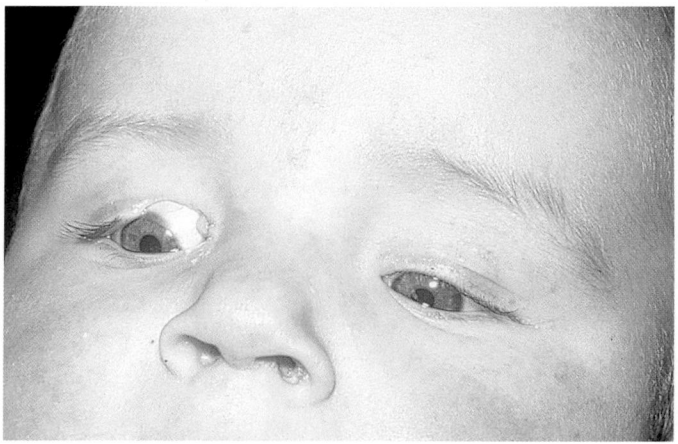

Fig. 4 Upper lid coloboma. (By courtesy of Mr M.P. Clarke.)

common, and occurs in isolation or with other ectodermal facial defects. It may show autosomal dominant inheritance. Ankyloblepharon filiforme adnatum denotes one or more other areas of fusion. Simple division is generally effective.

Dystichiasis

An aberrant row of lashes, usually in the lower eyelid, although occasionally just a small ectopic bunch. It is generally an isolated anomaly, and may show autosomal dominant inheritance.

Euryblepharon (Fig. 5)

This describes a large palpebral aperture, particularly laterally, with downward lateral canthal displacement, and a tendency to lateral ectropion. It occurs with Treacher Collins syndrome or as an autosomal dominant trait.

Epiblepharon (Fig. 6)

An abnormal horizontal lower eyelid fold may push lashes against the eye. It is common, especially in oriental people, but rarely symptomatic, and generally resolves with facial growth.

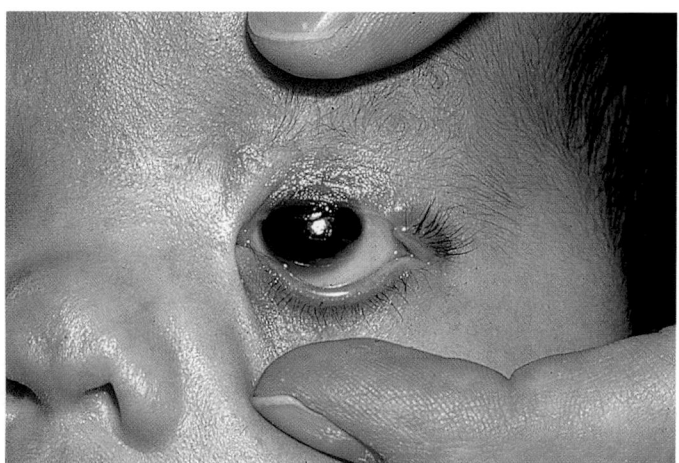

Fig. 3 Cryptophthalmos. (By courtesy of Mr M.P. Clarke.)

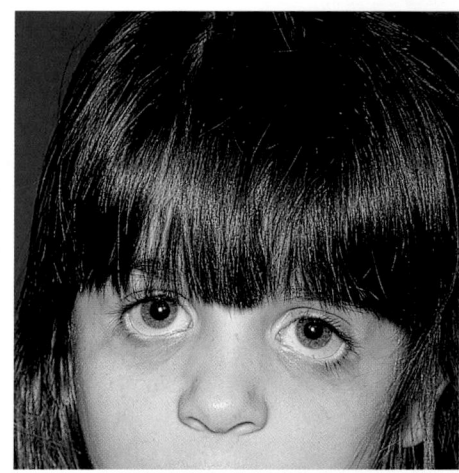

Fig. 5 Euryblepharon. (By courtesy of Mr M.P. Clarke.)

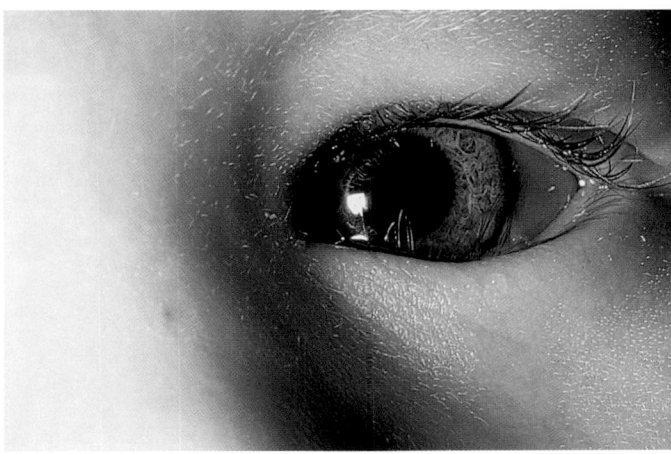

Fig. 6 Epiblepharon. (By courtesy of Mr M.P. Clarke.)

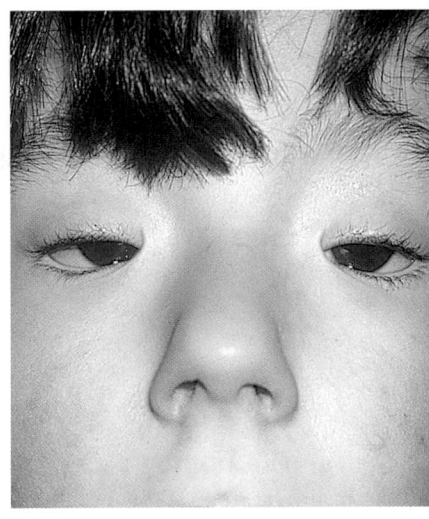

Fig. 7 Blepharophimosis syndrome. (By courtesy of Mr J. Sandford Smith.)

Entropion

Several factors may cause inward rotation of the entire eyelid margin: hypertrophy of marginal orbicularis, tarsal agenesis, tarsal kinks, defects in the lower lid retractors, or lack of posterior support as in microphthalmos or enophthalmos. Although the first two account for isolated entropion of either the lower or upper lid, lower lid entropion secondary to epiblepharon or epicanthus is much more common. Treatment with tape or sutures is often sufficient, but occasionally excision of an ellipse of skin and muscle is required.

Ectropion

This is rare, but can occur with other lid anomalies, for example blepharophimosis syndrome. Babies with Down's syndrome, however, can develop eversion of the lids with crying. Simple repositioning and taping often help.

Telecanthus

With telecanthus, the interpupillary distance is normal, but the medial canthi are widely spaced (compare with hypertelorism— an increased interpupillary distance). Although generally isolated, it occurs in blepharophimosis syndrome.

Epicanthus

An extra fold of skin in the medial canthal region with four common patterns, of which epicanthus tarsalis is typical of the oriental face. In the occidental population, epicanthus palpebralis is present in 20 per cent of normal infants but generally resolves. Epicanthus inversus occurs in Down's syndrome, in blepharophimosis syndrome, or as an isolated abnormality.

Blepharophimosis syndrome (Fig. 7)

This refers to a constellation of associated abnormalities including marked telecanthus, flattening of the supraorbital ridges, epicanthus inversus, ptosis, and small eyelids with a narrow palpebral aperture. Nystagmus, strabismus, and female infertility have been described, and occasional abnormalities of 6q and 10p noted, although chromosomes are generally normal. Sur-

gical correction is often staged, with the telecanthus and epicanthus corrected before ptosis surgery.

Ptosis

Congenital ptosis refers to a developmental dystrophy of the levator muscle or aponeurosis, and is the most common congenital eyelid anomaly. It may be unilateral or bilateral, of variable severity, and does not improve with age. Ptosis at birth due to other causes (e.g. Horner's syndrome, myasthenia, third nerve palsies, or brain abnormalities) is far less common and generally excluded from this term. Congenital ptosis is frequently associated with weakness of the ipsilateral superior rectus; however, it also occurs in isolation or in association with other ocular and non-ocular defects. The ptosis can cause amblyopia, although this is more commonly a consequence of associated anisometropia or strabismus. Unless the visual axis is completely occluded, amblyopia is generally treated first, and ptosis correction deferred until 2 to 4 years. This allows more accurate measurement of both the degree of ptosis and the levator function, enabling the most appropriate procedure to be performed.

Marcus Gunn jaw–winking accounts for 5 per cent of congenital ptosis. It is a paradoxical movement caused by innervation of the levator muscle by trigeminal nerve fibres. The ipsilateral superior rectus is commonly weak. Opening of the mouth with contralateral movement of the mandible cause temporary elevation of the ptotic lid, although occasionally the lid closes instead (inverse Marcus Gunn). Authorities are divided as to whether or not it improves with age, but surgical correction is not generally recommended unless very severe.

Further reading

Anderson, R.L. and Beard, C. (1997). The levator aponeurosis. *Archives of Ophthalmology*, **95**, 1437–41.

Bosniak, S. (ed.) (1996). *Principles and practice of ophthalmic plastic and reconstructive surgery*. Saunders, Philadelphia.

Robinson, R.J. and Stranc, M.F. (1970). The anatomy of the medial canthal ligament. *British Journal of Plastic Surgery*, **23**, 1–7.

2.5.2 Inflammatory lid diseases and degenerative processes of the lids

Stephen J. Ohlrich and Richard Downes

Degenerative processes of the lids

The ageing process is characterized by loss of tone and tissue bulk in the lid proper and its adnexal tissues. The skin becomes redundant and wrinkled due to atrophy and fragmentation of the collagen framework of the dermis. The disruption of dermal collagen is accelerated by sun exposure. The orbital septum weakens and this may be associated with prolapse of orbital fat. Paradoxically, there is absorption of orbital fat with age that causes a relative enophthalmos. There is progressive, generalized horizontal laxity of the lid with relaxation of the canthal tendons. This laxity results in loss of the firm apposition of the lids against the globe and shortening of the horizontal palpebral aperture. Attenuation of the muscular and tendinous supports of the lids further contributes to their involutional changes. Weakening of frontalis and disinsertion of the epicranial aponeurosis leads to brow ptosis. Loss of attachments of the levator aponeurosis produces a high skin crease and blepharoptosis. Disinsertion of the retractors of the lower lid contributes to involutional entropion. Drop-out and depigmentation of the lashes completes the picture of the senescent eyelid (Fig. 1).

The degenerative processes contribute to the malpositions and cosmetic abnormalities of the lids that dominate the practice of ophthalmic plastic surgery. Lid malpositions, including entropion, ectropion, and blepharoptosis, are of functional and cosmetic significance. Brow ptosis, lash ptosis, and dermatochalasis complete the spectrum of degenerative lid disease.

Entropion

Acquired inversion of the upper or lower eyelids resulting in contact between cilia and the globe causes pain and contributes to disease of the ocular surface. The severity of the sequelae at the ocular surface depends, in addition, on the adequacy of the tear film, Bell's phenomenon, and corneal sensation (Fig. 2).

Classification

1. Involutional
2. Cicatricial

Pathogenesis

Involutional entropion is due to weakness or disinsertion of the lower-lid retractors, horizontal lid laxity, and preseptal orbicularis overriding pretarsal orbicularis. Cicatricial entropion is due to contraction of the posterior lid lamella secondary to localized traumatic scarring or a generalized inflammatory process (discussed under 'Inflammatory lid disease' below).

Assessment and management

Management is surgical and depends on assessment as follows. When the normal person looks downward from the primary position the lower eyelid retracts by approximately two-thirds (3–4 mm) of the distance that the globe rotates. This is an assessment of the integrity of attachment of the lower-lid retractors to the lower border of the tarsal plate. In involutional entropion the eyelid has little or no retraction. If the entropion eyelid does retract normally on down-gaze, the diagnosis is cicatricial entropion. Horizontal laxity of the lid is determined by pulling down the lower eyelid and observing the elasticity of return of its margin to the inferior limbus. If the lid can be pulled more than 6 mm away from the globe, the lid is lax. Traction on the medial and lateral canthal tendons can then determine their individual contribution to the overall horizontal laxity of the lid.

The primary pathology of involutional entropion without horizontal laxity is disinsertion of the lower-lid retractors from the lower border of the tarsal plate. This can be corrected by a

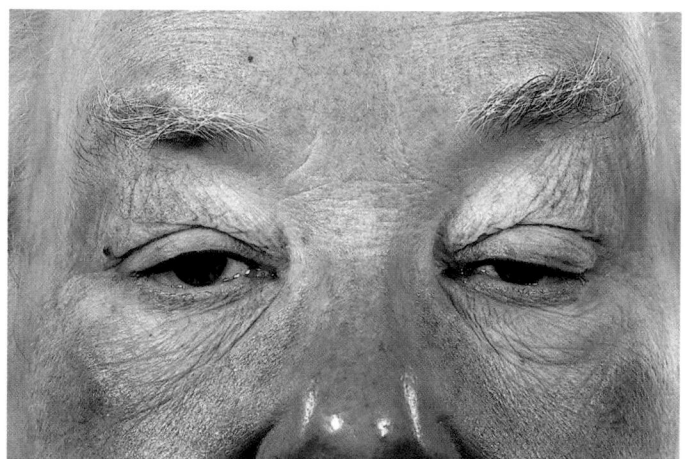

Fig. 1 Senescence of the eyelids.

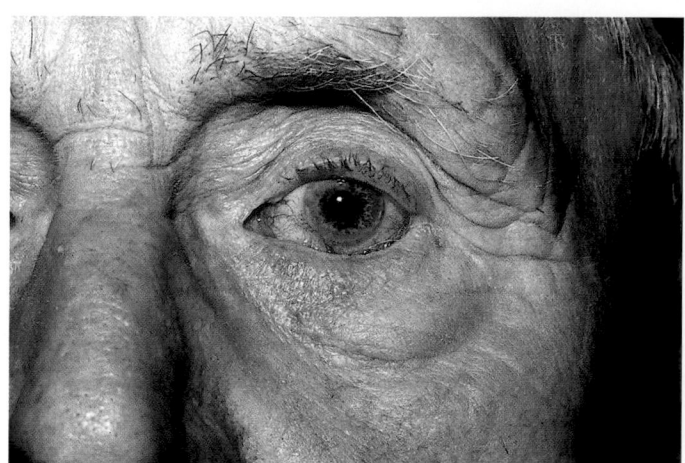

Fig. 2 Involutional entropion.

Jones' plication or often simply by reattachment of the retractors to the lower border of the tarsal plate as a primary procedure. If accompanied by horizontal laxity this component can be corrected by combination with a lateral canthal sling procedure. This modification of the more classical approach as outlined by Collin has the advantage of addressing the primary pathology without introducing the anatomically destructive elements of pentagonal resection and the transverse lid split.

Ectropion

Acquired eversion of the lower lid produces epiphora, ocular irritation, and cosmetic deformity (Figs 3 and 4).

Classification

1. Involutional

2. Cicatricial

3. Paralytic

4. Mechanical

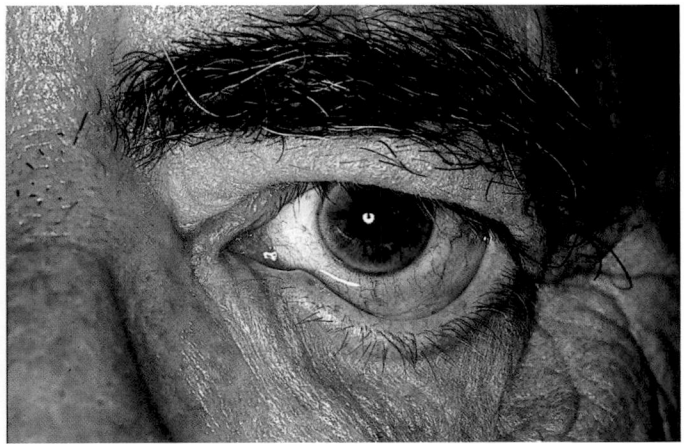

Fig. 3 Involutional ectropion.

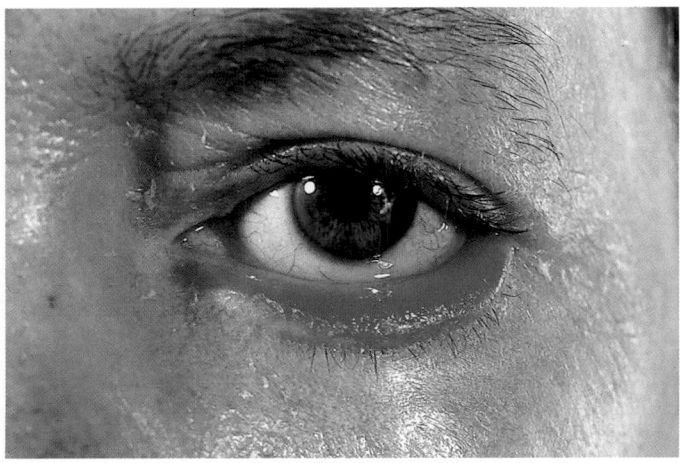

Fig. 4 Cicatricial ectropion.

Pathogenesis

Involutional ectropion is due to weakness of the pretarsal orbicularis, horizontal lid laxity, and relaxation of the medial and lateral canthal tendons. The lower-lid retractors and gravity overcome the weakened orbicularis muscle, which normally pulls the eyelid up tightly against the globe. Chronicity of ectropion or extensive sun exposure add a generalized cicatricial component to the anterior lamella, produce squamous metaplasia of the palpebral conjunctiva, and may lead to punctal stenosis.

Assessment and management

Horizontal laxity of the lid is determined as for involutional entropion. A cicatricial component is recognized by the presence of inferior scleral 'show' and if by grasping the lid margin and pulling it superiorly, it does not reach 2 mm above the inferior limbus.

Management is surgical. The lateral canthal sling procedure may be used to correct horizontal laxity of the lid at any site with preservation of the integrity of the lid margin. It may be coupled with excision of a diamond of tarsoconjunctiva for significant punctal eversion or plication of the medial canthal tendon when there is significant laxity of that structure. The lateral canthal sling procedure readily combines with a blepharoplasty if there is excess skin and is a useful alternative to the classical approach to surgery for involutional ectropion of the lower lid advocated by Collin.

Blepharoptosis (brow ptosis, lash ptosis, and dermatochalasis)

Acquired involutional depression of the upper eyelid relative to the globe is due to dehiscence of the levator palpebrae aponeurosis or its disinsertion from the tarsal plate. It is a frequent postoperative sequela, occurring in up to 5 per cent of cases of intraocular surgery.

Clinical findings

Aponeurotic blepharoptosis is characterized by a decreased vertical palpebral aperture with good levator function (> 12 mm). There is a high or absent skin crease with supratarsal thinning. This may be purely a senescent change, or precipitating factors such as trauma, eyelid oedema, ocular surgery or patching may be identified.

Other degenerative lid sequelae such as brow ptosis, dermatochalasis, and lash ptosis are frequent accompaniments of aponeurotic blepharoptosis. Brow ptosis is a depression of the eyebrow due to weakening of the frontalis muscle or a relative disinsertion of frontalis from the epicranial aponeurosis. Dermatochalasis is characterized by redundant skin of the upper lid, prolapse of fat through a weak orbital septum, and an indistinct skin crease. The loss of firm adhesion between the skin and orbicularis and the underlying tarsal plate allows a drooping of the lashes relative to the lid margin or lash ptosis. Lash ptosis may be primarily involutional or a complication of ptosis surgery.

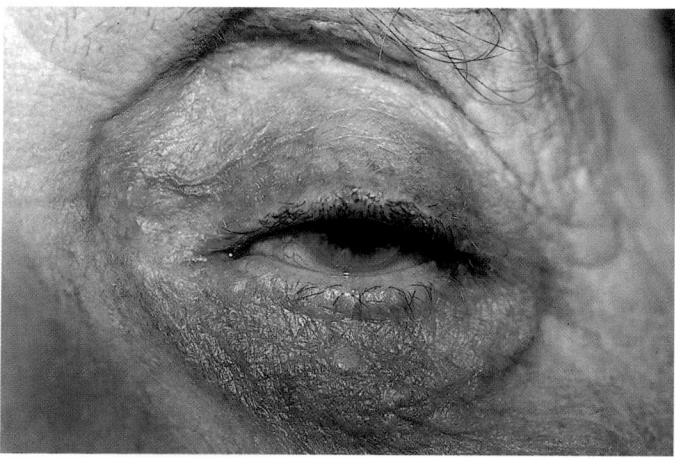

Fig. 5 Aponeurotic ptosis.

Table 1 Classification of inflammatory lid diseases
Anterior lamella skin/appendages
Bacterial: Staphylococcal, streptococcal, *P. acnes*
Viral: Herpes, pox, papilloma
Atypical bacteria, fungal and parasitic infestations
Hypersensitivity reactions
Bullous skin disorders
Posterior lamella
Tarsus/meibomian glands:
Chronic meibomitis and seborrhoeic blepharitis
Conjunctiva:
Infectious
Allergic
Cicatrizing mucous-membrane disorders:
ocular cicatricial pemphigoid, linear IgA disease
Stevens–Johnson syndrome
trachoma
alkali burns
vitamin A deficiency

Classification–acquired blepharoptosis

1. Aponeurotic—involutional (Fig. 5)

2. Myogenic

3. Neurogenic

4. Mechanical

5. Pseudoptosis

Management

Surgical correction with reattachment of the distal edge of the dehisced aponeurosis to the tarsus is the mainstay of the repair of aponeurotic ptosis. In the presence of attenuation, not disinsertion, of the levator aponeurosis, a small resection of the levator may be required.

The frequent concomitants of brow ptosis, lash ptosis, and dermatochalasis may be managed by brow plasty, anterior lamellar reposition, and blepharoplasty, respectively.

Inflammatory lid disease

The pathological process of inflammation is classically characterized by pain, redness, swelling. heat, and loss of function. In the discussion of inflammatory lid disease there is inevitably considerable overlap with conjunctival and external eye disease as well as with the systemic disorders affecting skin and mucous membranes. The following anatomical classification has blurred boundaries but should direct the reader to the appropriate areas of this text for further discussion of the lid inflammations.

Classification and description

A classification of inflammatory lid disease is shown in Table 1; descriptions follow.

Bacterial eyelid infections

Bacterial infections of the lids are caused by normal lid commensals, principally *Staphylococcus* (*aureus* and *epidermidis*), streptococci, and, more rarely, *Propionibacterium acnes* and *mor-axella*. The manifestations include marginal and angular blepharitis, internal and external hordeola, preseptal cellulitis, and impetigo.

External hordeolum

An external hordeolum (stye) is a small abscess localized to a lash follicle and its associated glands of Zeiss and Moll. Spontaneous resolution is aided by the application of warm compresses. Oral systemic antibiotics, such as flucloxacillin, are only required if complicated by preseptal cellulitis.

Internal hordeoleum

An internal hordeoleum (meibomian cyst) is a small, painful abscess within the meibomian glands of the tarsal plate. Management is similar to that for a stye. Incision and curettage are required if large in the acute phase or persistent as in the chronic granulomatous inflammation of a chalazion. Intralesional injection of corticosteroid, such as triamcinolone acetonide, is a useful alternative in the treatment of chalazia (Fig. 6).

Preseptal cellulitis

Preseptal cellulitis is a diffuse, deep infection of the eyelid tissues localized anterior to the orbital septum. Infection by the normal lid flora follows trauma, often minimal, or pre-existing hordeola. In contrast to orbital cellulitis there is no proptosis, restriction of ocular movements, relative afferent pupillary defects, or impairment of visual acuity. Treatment in the adult requires oral antibiotics such as amoxycillin and flucloxacillin. Parenteral administration of antibiotics should be used in the child of 18 months or less or in any age group where constitutional symptoms or toxic signs suggest bacteraemia. In the child of less than 7 years, additional cover for infection by *Haemophilus influenzae* is required; therefore amoxycillin should be replaced by cefotaxime or co-amoxiclav. Impetigo and necrotizing fasciitis associated with a group A streptococcal infection respond to systemic penicillin or erythromycin.

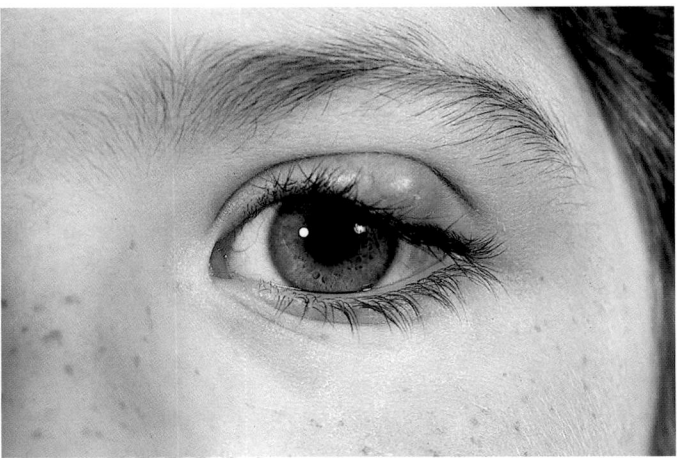

Fig. 6 Chalazion.

Viral eyelid infections

Viral infections of the eyelids often manifest as superficial vesicles and erythema of the eyelid skin. Involvement of the lid margins is frequently accompanied by follicular conjunctivitis and keratitis, but characteristic ocular involvement may be delayed by as long as 10 days following the skin eruption. Principal aetiological agents are the herpesviruses (herpes simplex and varicella zoster) and the poxviruses (variola, vaccinia, and molluscum contagiosum) (Figs 7 and 8).

Herpes simplex and zoster

Differentiation between herpes simplex and the eruption of herpes zoster may be easy with a history of exposure to cold sore, a non-dermatomal distribution, and an absence of pre-eruption paraesthesiae and pain. The pathognomonic dermatomal rash of zoster passes through phases of erythema, clear vesicles, pustules, and crusting. However, in atypical cases, viral culture obtained from clear vesicular fluid may be required for definitive diagnosis. The herpetic rashes are self-limiting, prone to reactivation after sequestration of the virus in the

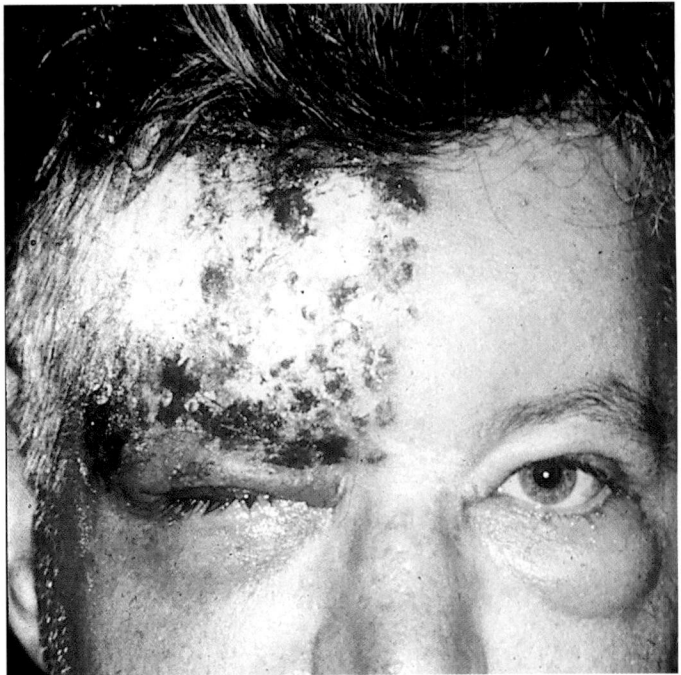

Fig. 8 Herpes zoster—ophthalmic division (illustration by courtesy of Mr A. Zaman).

sensory ganglia, and require symptomatic treatment only. Prophylactic treatment for the ocular complications is, however, necessary. Herpes simplex disease with involvement of the lid margins requires topical antivirals (e.g. acyclovir 0.3 per cent, five times/day). Herpes zoster with involvement of the upper lid requires oral acyclovir in five divided doses, effective if given within 72 h of the onset of the rash. Zoster, in contrast to simplex, may lead to cicatrizing lid changes and trichiasis due to dermal involvement in the inflammatory process.

Molluscum contagiosum

Molluscum contagiosum typically shows numerous pale, waxy, umbilicated nodules. The infection is self-limiting over a period of 18 months. Diagnosis may be confirmed histologically. Treatment is accomplished by curettage, cautery, or shave excision (Fig. 9).

Differential diagnosis

The differential diagnosis of vesiculobullous lesions of the eyelids includes generalized disorders of skin and mucous membrane. These may be idiopathic (pemphigus vulgaris, bullous pemphigoid), autoimmune (ocular cicatricial pemphigoid) or hypersensitivity reactions (erythema multiforme, Stevens–Johnson syndrome, toxic epidermal necrolysis).

Chronic meibomitis and seborrhoeic blepharitis

These represent chronic inflammation of the lid margins characterized by seborrhoeic scales adherent to the sides of the eyelashes (scurf), dilated, inspissated orifices of the meibomian glands, and meibomian froth (many tiny bubbles in the tear meniscus). Patients present with a chronic history of irritation of the ocular surface, worse upon waking in the morning.

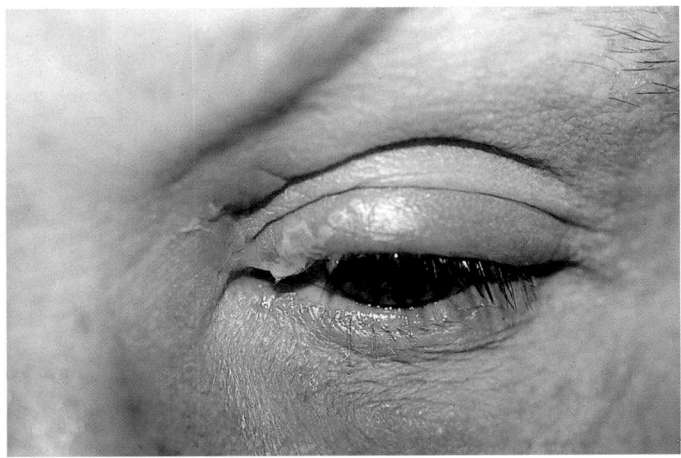

Fig. 7 Primary herpes simplex infection.

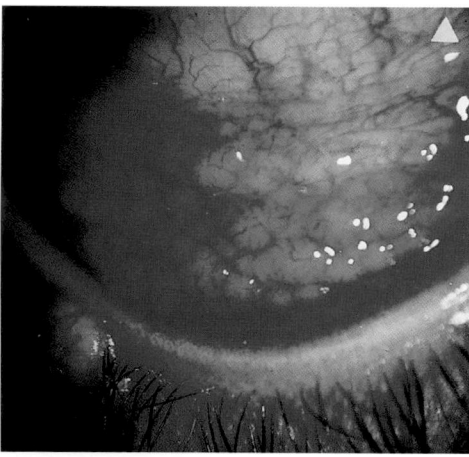

Fig. 9 Molluscum contagiosum with follicular conjunctivitis (illustration by courtesy of Professor H. Dua).

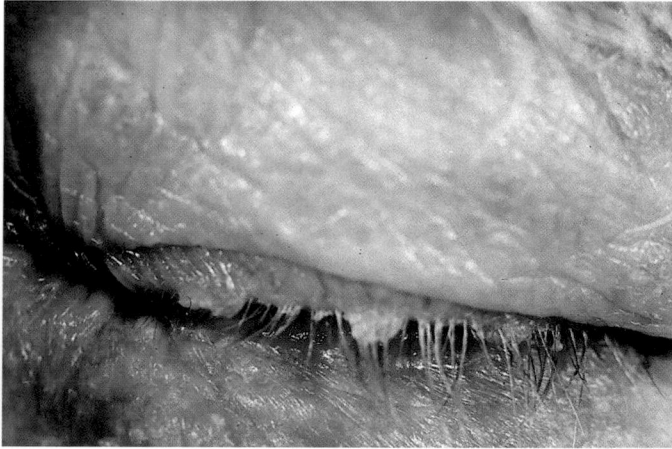

(a)

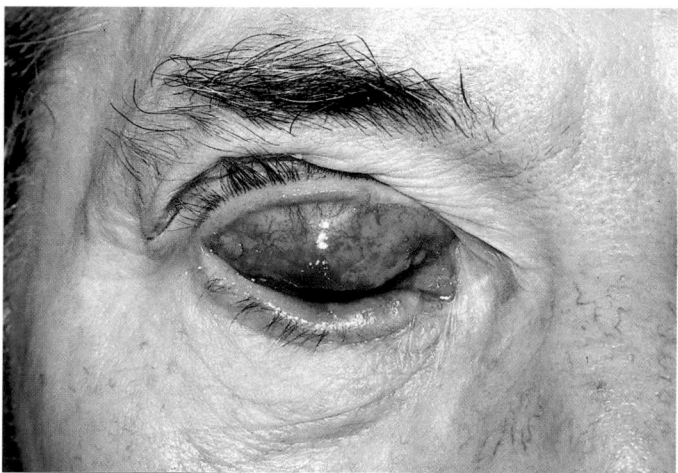

(b)

Fig. 10 (a) and (b). Sebaceous-cell carcinoma of the eyelid, masquerading as chronic seborrhoeic blepharitis.

Recurrent acute internal and external hordeola, superimposed chronic staphylococcal infection of marginal and angular blepharitis, and chronic granulomatous inflammation of the lid chalazion are common. Examination may reveal coexistent greasy scaling of seborrhoeic dermatitis on the scalp, forehead and brows, or the pustules, telangiectasia and erythema of the brow and malar region characteristic of acne rosacea. Secondary phenomena of chronic follicular conjunctivitis, recurrent corneal erosions, marginal keratitis, trichiasis (acquired posterior misdirection of previously nominal lashes), and upper-lid entropion may occur. A high index of suspicion for sebaceous-cell carcinoma should be maintained in all cases of chronic unilateral blepharitis and recurrent chalazia. Eversion of the eyelid is therefore mandatory in this clinical setting.

Pathogenesis

There is probably a primary abnormality in the pilosebaceous unit, producing disturbances of the secretions of the meibomian glands and subsequent obstruction of their orifices. Superimposed chronic infection of the glands by bacteria (staphylococci, *P. acnes*) and parasites (*Demodex folliculorum* and *brevis*) is common. The degradation of meibomian lipids into free fatty acids by the normal eyelid flora may account for the toxic symptoms and signs of meibomitis (Figs 10 and 11).

Assessment and management

Stepwise approach   A systematic, stepwise approach to the management of blepharitis/meibomitis and allied conditions is shown in Table 2.

Hypersensitivity reactions of the eyelids

Urticaria and angioedema

These are acute inflammatory reactions of the superficial epidermis and dermis (urticaria) or deeper subcutaneous tissues (angioedema) due to a type I hypersensitivity reaction. Sensit-

ized individuals upon re-exposure to a specific antigen (inhaled, ingested, parenterally administered, or insect venom) develop a localized cutaneous reaction. Itching and burning are accompanied by oedema of the skin, either discrete, elevated wheals or deeper, diffuse angioedema. The processes are of rapid onset with spontaneous resolution over 48 h and no tissue destruction, and they may be part of a generalized cutaneous or systemic reaction. Treatment includes avoidance of the antigen, cold compresses for local relief of symptoms, and adrenaline, corticosteroids and antihistamines for serious systemic anaphylaxis. Recurrent angioedema, less commonly, may be induced by exercise or exposure to cold or light and there is an inherited form (autosomal-dominant).

Blepharochalasis

Blepharochalasis, characterized by recurrent episodes of painless lid oedema, is caused by a developmental deficiency in the elastic tissue of the eyelids. Both autosomal-dominant and sporadic forms present in the second decade and persist throughout life.

Recurrent attacks of eyelid oedema produce progressive per-

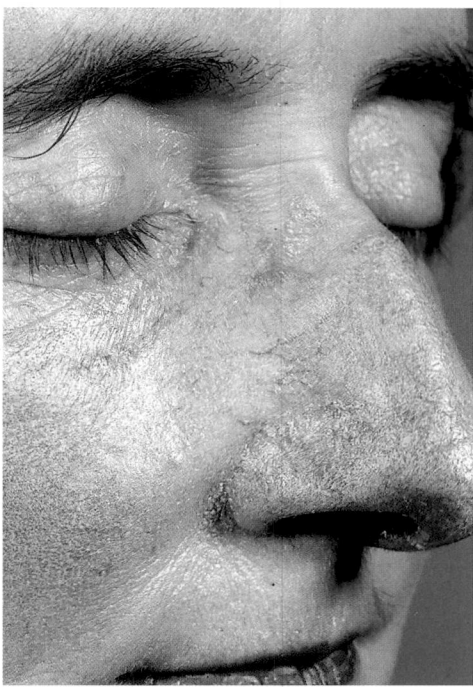

Fig. 11 Acne rosaceae (illustration by courtesy of Mr J. Sloper).

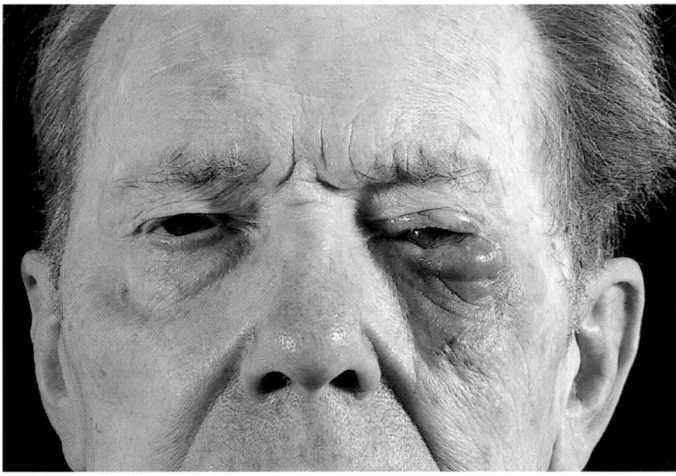

Fig. 12 Allergic contact dermatitis—tobramycin eyedrops.

Table 2 Management of blepharitis/meibomitis

Clinical findings	Management
Seborrhoeic blepharitis Marginal and angular blepharitis	Lid hygiene—lid scrubs twice daily with dilute baby shampoo applied with a cotton-wool bud; warm compresses are used to loosen inspissated meibomian secretions Antiseborrhoeic shampoo to affected scalp and eyebrows Hydrocortisone 0.1 per cent and tetracycline 1 per cent ointment twice daily on initiation of treatment for 2 weeks
Meibomitis/acne rosaceae	Add tetracycline orally four times a day for 1 month, then long-term maintenance at reduced dosage
Trichiasis	Cryotherapy—double freeze-thaw to −20°
Upper-lid entropion	Anterior lamellar reposition; without lash–cornea touch Add lid margin split/wedge resection: with lash–cornea touch

manent changes including excess skin of the upper lid and thickened subcutaneous tissues requiring blepharoplasty and excision of redundant tissue.

Allergic contact eczematous dermatitis

This common, type IV hypersensitivity reaction is precipitated by contact exposure to an allergen. Principal allergens include

ophthalmic drops and ointments, and locally applied cosmetics. Clinically it is characterized by prominent itching, erythema, and oedema of the eyelid skin progressing to the formation of vesicles and bullae. The initial sensitization process can present from 5 days to several years but re-exposure will illicit a response within 24 to 72 h. Treatment includes removal of the offending allergen and cool compresses for symptomatic relief (Fig. 12).

Further reading

Bosniak, S. L. (1987). Ectropion. In *Ophthalmic plastic and reconstructive surgery*, Vol. 1 (ed. B. C. Smith), pp. 562–79. Mosby, St Louis.

Collin, J. R. O. (1989). *A manual of systematic eyelid surgery* (2nd edn). Churchill Livingstone, Edinburgh.

Schaefer, A. J. (1987). Involutional entropion. In *Ophthalmic plastic and reconstructive surgery*, Vol. 1 (ed. B. C. Smith), pp. 546–55. Mosby, St Louis.

Starr, M. B. (1987). Infection and hypersensitivity of the eyelids. In *Ophthalmic plastic and reconstructive surgery*, Vol. 1 (ed. B. C. Smith), pp. 283–307. Mosby, St Louis.

Survey of Ophthalmology (1993) Vol. 38. [An excellent review of inflammatory conjunctival disease with specific reference to allergic conjunctivitis.]

2.5.3 Tumours of the eyelid

Raf Ghabrial and M. J. Potts

In this chapter we discuss the clinical features of neoplasms of the eyelids, classified by their tissues of origin, as distinct from inflammatory or degenerative tumours discussed elsewhere. A list of benign, premalignant and malignant tumours is found in Table 1. Surgical treatment of these tumours and eyelid reconstruction is also discussed elsewhere in this text.

Table 1 Tumours of the eyelid, classified by growth potential and tissue of origin

Benign	Premalignant	Malignant
Papilloma	Actinic keratosis	Squamous cell carcinoma
Seborrhoeic keratosis	Bowen's disease	Basal cell carcinoma
Keratoacanthoma	Radiation dermatosis	Melanoma
Naevus	Lentigo maligna	Sebaceous carcinoma
Sweat gland		Sweat gland
apocrine		apocrine
eccrine		eccrine
Hair follicle		Secondary
Vascular		distant
Capillary		contiguous
haemangioma		
Naevus flammeus		
Kaposi's sarcoma		
Neural		
Neurofibroma		
Fibroma molluscum		

The eyelids are highly specialized structures covered by skin, from whence most neoplasia originates. Adnexal structures include the Meibomian and Zeis' sebaceous glands, Moll's apocrine and other eccrine sweat glands, and follicles of the cilia. There is also a variable amount of lymphoid, neural, and vascular tissue within the preseptal tissues of the eyelid, from which tumours may originate. Optimal treatment of patients with eyelid tumours commences with accurate diagnosis.

Diagnosis

History

Rapidity of growth is a key to diagnosis of any skin tumours. In general, a lesion that has not enlarged over years is benign whereas malignant skin tumours usually develop over months. The characteristic rapid growth (over weeks) of a keratoacanthoma may be the only distinguishing feature from a squamous cell carcinoma on partial biopsy, even in the presence of an experienced histopathologist. The patient should be questioned about any change involving the lesion, including associated bleeding, pruritis, and any change in colour or sensation, any of which may signify recent malignant change. Finally, up to 60 per cent of patients with malignant skin tumours will have a history of similar lesions elsewhere.

Examination

Observation of the lesion should enable accurate recording of the size, colour, associated loss of eyelashes, or ulceration. Palpation reveals the level of fixation of the lesion, as well as any associated preauricular, submandibular, or cervical lymphadenopathy. The Valsalva manoeuvre may reveal engorgement of a vascular tumour. Ideally, any suspicious eyelid lesion should be photographed prior to biopsy and subsequent management.

Investigations

Biopsy for histopathological examination is the gold standard in the diagnosis of eyelid tumours. Small lesions may be easily excised *in toto* and sent for microscopic evaluation. Incisional biopsy may be performed in a representative wedge of a larger tumour, taking care to include adjacent clinically normal tissue. The specimen should be orientated (by diagram or suture fixation) and placed in formalin for histopathological examination. Prior discussion with an experienced ocular or dermatological histopathologist may be required and fresh tissue (for immunohistochemistry), gluteraldehyde (for electron microscopy), or other other fixatives may be appropriate. Radiological studies such as computed tomography (CT) or magnetic resonance imaging (MRI) scans may be indicated for patients with clinically deep or fixed eyelid tumours, especially in the presence of recurrence or medial canthal involvement, although they are often unhelpful. Referral for systemic investigation is appropriate for all malignant melanomas, lymphomas, and other selected cases.

Epidermal-derived neoplasia

Papilloma

Papillomas represent the most common benign neoplasm occurring on the eyelids, originating usually at the eyelid margin, more frequently from a pedunculated than a sessile base (Fig. 1). Molluscum contagiosum and verrucae vulgaris are not frank neoplasms, but are tumours caused by viruses and may be distinguished from squamous cell papillomas by electron microscopy and a variable level of associated inflammation.

Seborrhoeic keratosis

Seborrhoeic keratosis (basal cell papilloma) is a common benign eyelid tumour, typically warty and pigmented in appearance and greasy to palpation. Histologically, seborrhoeic keratoses are benign tumours originating in the deeper layers of the epidermis (basal cells).

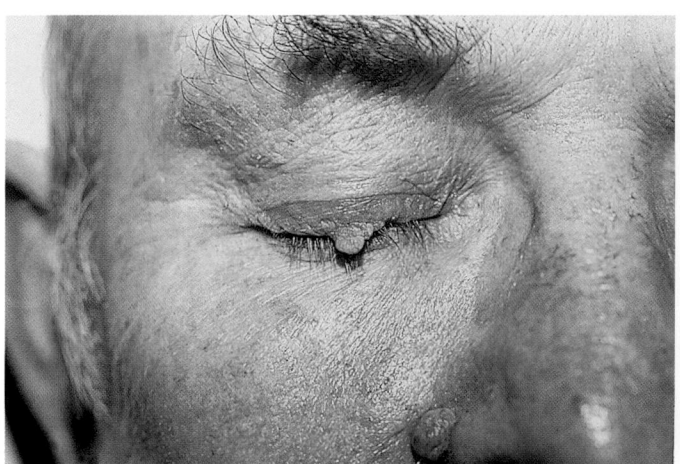

Fig. 1 Squamous papilloma of left upper eyelid.

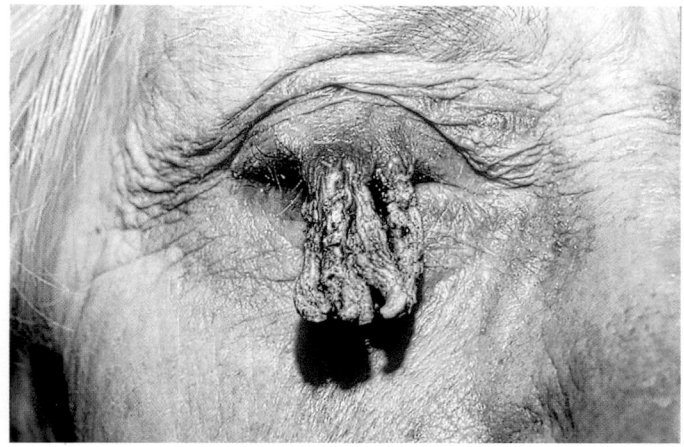

Fig. 2 Atypical keratoacanthoma with cutaneous horn. Keratoacanthomas are typically dome-shaped, but cutaneous horns may occur with keratoacanthomas, solar keratoses, squamous cell carcinoma, or verruca vulgaris.

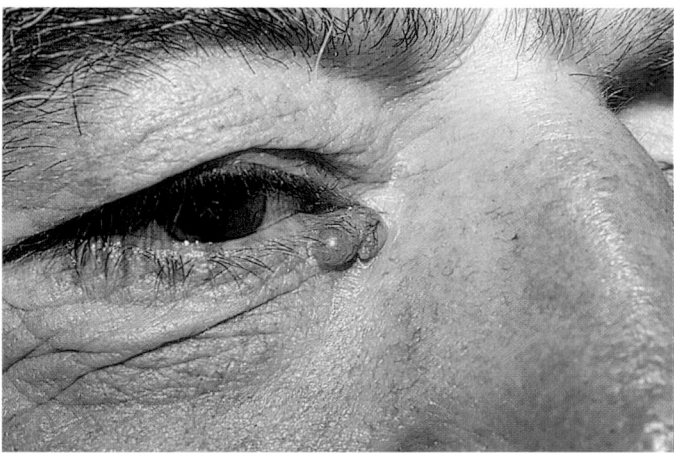

Fig. 3 Nodular basal cell carcinoma of right medial canthus.

Keratoacanthoma

Keratoacanthomas typically appear as rapidly growing crusty outgrowths with a central keratin-filled crater, and can be impossible to distinguish clinically from squamous cell carcinoma (Fig. 2). Although benign, these tumours may have histological features of malignancy, and may be distinguished only by careful histopathological examination of the base, combined with an accurate history.

Actinic keratosis

Actinic (solar or senile) keratosis is a premalignant proliferation of the superficial layers of the epidermis secondary to chronic sun exposure in fair-skinned individuals. Actinic keratoses are typically pale to erythematous, and flat to elevated lesions with a crusty surface, until malignant transformation (to squamous cell carcinoma) occurs.

Basal cell carcinoma

Basal cell carcinoma accounts for 90 per cent of malignant tumours of the eyelids. In over 70 per cent of cases the lower eyelids are primarily involved, followed in frequency by the medial canthus, upper eyelid, and lateral canthus. Older persons are primarily affected following sun exposure. An unusual and aggressive variant is found in a rare autosomal dominant dermatosis, the basal cell naevus (Gorlin–Goltz) syndrome with associated skeletal, neural, and endocrine anomalies.

Basal cell carcinoma appears as a firm upraised nodule typically with raised, rolled, pearly borders and fine telangiectatic vessels, at which stage it is usually described as nodular (Fig. 3). Variants of such a lesion include variable pigmentation and a cystic (centrally necrotic) variety (Fig. 4). Surface ulceration or umbilication leads to the classical 'rodent ulcer' (Fig. 5).

Morpheiform (sclerosing or fibrosing) basal cell carcinoma has a less typical surface appearance with indistinct margins, and spreads radially beneath the epidermis, thus avoiding recognition. Clinical examination is an unreliable method of determining the extent of these lesions, and histological control

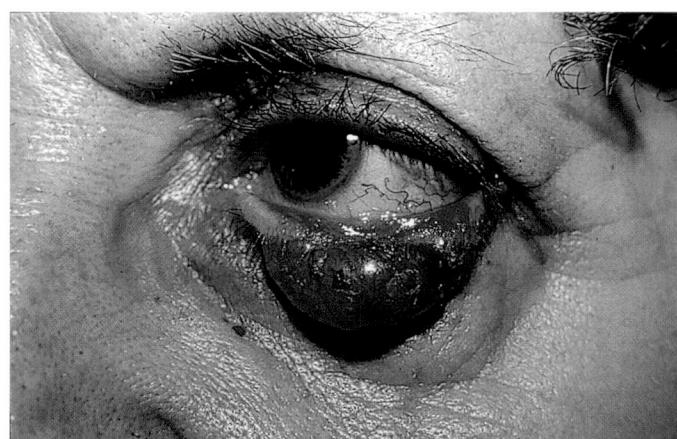

Fig. 4 Massive cystic basal cell carcinoma of left lower eyelid with associated pigmentation.

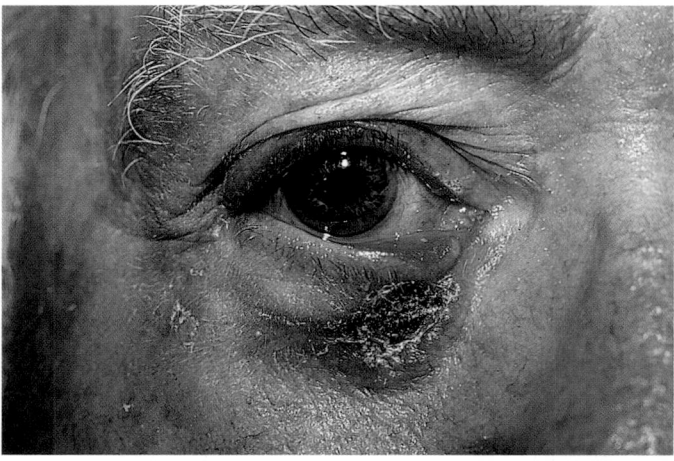

Fig. 5 Ulcerative basal cell carcinoma with associated cicatricial medial ectropion causing epiphora.

(either by frozen section control or Moh's micrographic surgery) is the only definitive method of surgically clearing such tumours.

Local invasion of a basal cell carcinoma can be devastating, especially with a morpheiform tumour at the medial canthus, but distant metastases are extremely rare. Surgical excision of these tumours should include a 3–4 mm margin of macroscopically normal tissue, allowing a more generous margin in clinically aggressive tumours such as morpheiform or medial canthal tumours. Histological confirmation of complete tumour excision is advisable in all cases.

Squamous cell carcinoma

Squamous cell carcinoma accounts for 2 to 5 per cent of eyelid malignancies. It occurs with slightly greater frequency in the lower than the upper eyelids, typically in older patients after prolonged sun exposure. Squamous cell carcinomas may arise from a premalignant lesion such as actinic keratosis, Bowen's disease of the skin (squamous cell carcinoma *in situ*), or areas of chronic irritation (e.g. irradiation or recurrent trauma). Patients with xeroderma pigmentosum are at high risk of developing multiple squamous cell carcinomas at a much earlier age.

Clinically, squamous cell carcinoma may mimic basal cell carcinoma, but is typically more keratinized as a result of the keratin-forming surface squamous cells from which they originate (Fig. 6), often with some level of ulceration. Local invasion occurs, and perineural spread is not uncommon. The potential for distant metastases to regional lymph nodes is well recognized, and visceral spread may occur. Surgical excision of these lesions requires a tumour-free margin of 3 to 4 mm, due to the aggressive nature of these tumours. Lymph node dissection is required if the regional lymph nodes are clinically involved.

Pigmented lesions

Naevi

Cutaneous naevi of the eyelids are classified as for naevi arising elsewhere.

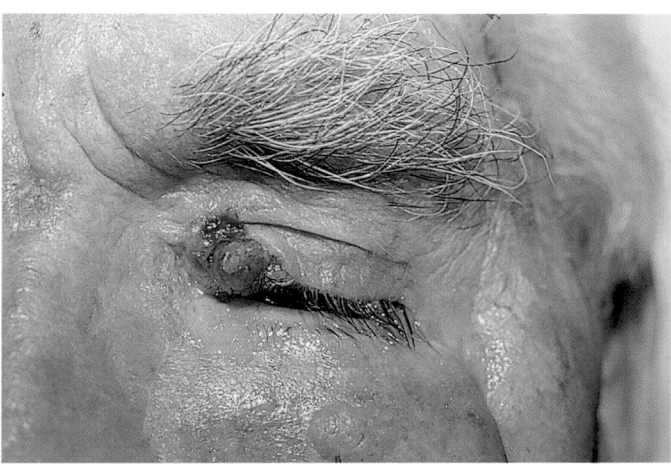

Fig. 6 Squamous cell carcinoma of the left upper eyelid. After primary removal, recurrence and perineural spread necessitated partial exenteration of the left orbit.

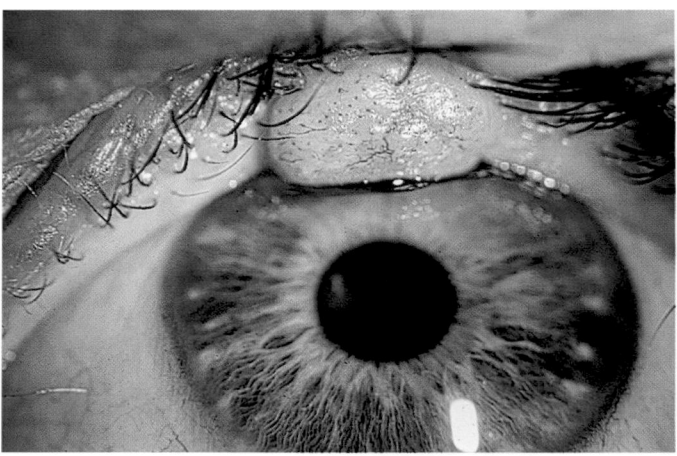

Fig. 7 Benign intradermal naevus.

Junctional naevi

Junctional naevi are flat, and consist of a proliferation of naevus cells at the junction of the epidermis and the dermis. Malignant transformation is rare in junctional naevi.

Compound naevi

Compound naevi are slightly elevated, and microscopic examination reveals some extension of naevus cells into the dermis.

Dermal naevi

Dermal naevi are characterized by extension of epithelial naevocytes into the dermis, clinically evidenced by elevation of the skin surface and involvement of the cilia if marginal (Fig. 7). Deeper naevi have less potential for malignant change to malignant melanoma than superficial naevi. Blue naevi and naevus of Ota (congenital oculodermal melanocytosis) arise primarily from dermal, rather than migrated epidermal melanocytes.

Malignant melanoma

Primary cutaneous malignant melanoma of the eyelid is extremely rare, accounting for less than 1 per cent of all malignant eyelid lesions. None the less, a high index of suspicion needs to be maintained when assessing pigmented lesions of the lids, due to the potential aggressive nature of these tumours. Clinically, there are three distinct forms.

Lentigo maligna melanoma

Lentigo maligna melanoma commences as a flat macular pigmented non-palpable lesion (Fig. 8) with geographic borders (lentigo maligna or Hutchinson's melanotic freckle), and histopathologically represents purely intraepithelial melanocytes. At this stage, the lesion is premalignant. Deeper invasion to the dermis signifies the transformation to frank melanoma, and results in elevation of the lesion. This is the most common variety of melanoma, and carries a good prognosis, with greater than 90 per cent 5-year survival.

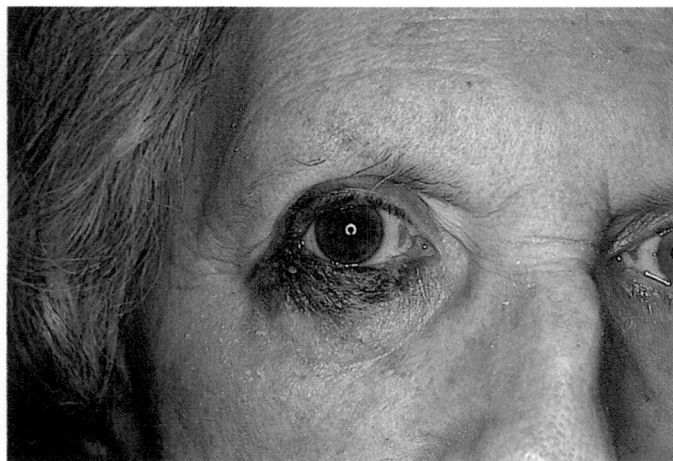

(a)

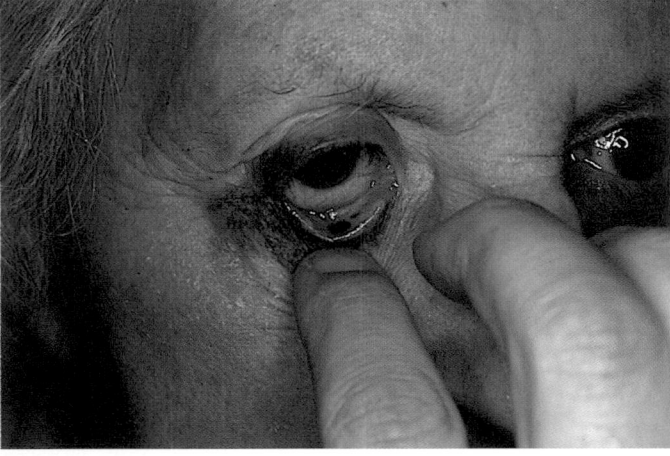

(b)

Fig. 8 (a) Hutchinson's melanotic freckle of right lower eyelid. (b) Eyelid eversion reveals extension of melanocytes into tarsal conjunctiva.

Superficial spreading melanoma

Superficial spreading melanoma appears as a macular lesion with heterogeneous surface pigmentation. Prognosis is intermediate between lentigo malignant melanoma and nodular melanoma.

Nodular melanoma

Nodular melanomas are placoid or nodular, and deeply pigmented, often with a blue–grey hue. Occasionally, they may be amelanotic and mimic any other eyelid lesion. Nodular melanomas are thankfully the least frequently occurring variety of melanoma, and carry a grave prognosis (less than 50 per cent 5-year survival).

The type of melanoma is determined histopathologically after biopsy of the lesion. Prognosis further depends upon the depth of invasion; Breslow found that lesions measuring 0.76 mm or less carried a 100 per cent 5-year survival, whereas those deeper than 1.5 mm had a 50 to 60 per cent 5-year survival rate.

Any patient with biopsy-proven malignant melanoma requires systemic evaluation. Surgical excision with at least 5

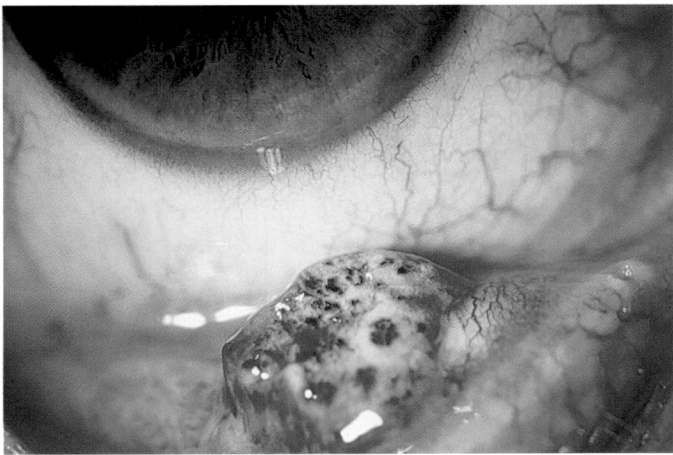

Fig. 9 Nodular sebaceous cell carcinoma.

to 10 mm margins is required to clear cutaneous melanoma safely. Frozen section control is notoriously misleading and is to be avoided in the case of cutaneous melanoma. Melanomas spread relatively early to the regional lymph nodes and viscera. At this stage there is insufficient data to support exenteration in the case of orbital invasion or regional lymph node dissection in the case of associated involvement.

Adnexal tumours

Sebaceous carcinoma

Sebaceous carcinomas arise from the meibomian glands, glands of Zeis, sebaceous glands of the eyebrows, and rarely the caruncle. Sebaceous cell carcinoma accounts for 0.5 to 2 per cent of all malignant eyelid neoplasms. These occur more frequently in ocular adnexal tissues than elsewhere, and more commonly in the upper than the lower eyelid, probably due to the greater number of meibomian glands present. Sebaceous carcinomas occur in older individuals, and may appear as nodular (Fig. 9), a diffuse erythematous area or an area of ulceration. Thus these lesions can mimic chalazia or chronic blepharoconjunctivitis ('masquerade syndrome'), thereby necessitating a high index of suspicion in recurrent chalazia or non-resolving inflammation, and histopathological examination.

Although sebaceous carcinoma is usually slow growing, these tumours may be lethal (overall mortality 10 per cent) with mortality approaching 70 per cent for poorly differentiated anaplastic tumours and 90 per cent if both eyelids are involved. Lesions greater than 10 mm in diameter or those present for more than 6 months duration carry a worse prognosis. Spread to regional lymph nodes occurs much earlier than with basal or squamous cell carcinoma.

Full thickness lid biopsy allows the optimum chance of diagnosis, and the histopathologist should be notified of the suspected diagnosis to allow appropriate fat (oil red O) stains to be performed, as routine fixation with haematoxylin and eosin removes fat from the tissues during alcohol immersion. Biopsy-proven sebaceous carcinoma requires preoperative systemic workup followed, if appropriate, by excision with histological confirmation of tumour clearance, with or without regional lymph node dissection.

Sweat gland tumours

There is a great variety of sweat gland tumours described, and it is often clinically impossible to distinguish these from each other and other tumours. Immunohistochemical and ultrastructural examination is usually necessary to determine the tissue of origin.

Eccrine

Syringoma
A syringoma is a relatively common benign tumour of the sweat gland duct, and usually appears as multiple waxy yellow nodules, occurring more frequently in patients with Down's syndrome.

Chrondoid syringoma
Chrondoid syringoma (pleiomorphic adenoma) is also a benign tumour of the eccrine sweat glands, and is histopathologically indistinguishable from the same tumour of the lacrimal gland.

Eccrine acrospiroma
Eccrine acrospiroma (clear cell hidradenoma) is a benign tumour originating from secretory elements of the eccrine glands, and appears as a smooth firm pink nodule on the skin surface.

Mucinous eccrine adenocarcinoma
Mucinous eccrine adenocarcinoma (adenocyctic carcinoma) is a rare malignant tumour of the eccrine sweat gland with a predilection for periorbital tissues, especially the eyelid. Mucinous eccrine carcinoma typically presents as a smooth firm pink–red nodule.

Apocrine
Tumours originating in the apocrine sweat glands (glands of Moll) are rare and occur on the eyelid margin with nodulocystic consistency and a bluish subcutaneous hue, resulting in the frequent misdiagnosis as haemangiomas or melanotic lesions. The benign form of apocrine neoplasia is named cystadenoma (or hydrocystoma) whereas the malignant variety is called apocrine adenocarcinoma.

Hair follicle tumours

Trichoepithelioma
Trichoepitheliomas are rare small pink–yellow benign tumours with follicular differentiation, and may be difficult to distinguish clinically and histologically from basal cell carcinoma, which may actually arise from trichoepitheliomas. Trichoepithelioma is referred to as Brook's tumour when they are inherited as multiple cystic lesions.

Pilomatrixoma
Pilomatrixoma (calcifying epithelioma of Malherbe) is a rare malignant tumour of hair matrix origin occurring most commonly on the head and neck, with some predilection for the upper eyelid and eyebrow. Clinically pilomatrixomas appear as pink–purple freely mobile nodules, and may mimic basal cell carcinoma clinically and histologically, especially on partial biopsy (when the pathognomonic clear cells may be missed).

Tricholemmoma
Ticholemmoma is a rare benign tumour of the hair follicle arising from the outer hair sheath (tricholemmoma), and is clinically indistinguishable from other adnexal tumours of the eyelid, thus necessitating biopsy.

Vascular tumours

Capillary haemangioma
Capillary haemangiomas (strawberry naevi) usually present prior to six months of age and may be superficial or have a deep connection with the orbit. Clinically, they appear as red flat or elevated lesions (Fig. 10), and typically enlarge up to the age of 12 months. Thereafter, spontaneous involution is the rule by 5 to 7 years of age, although resolution is hastened by treatment with intralesional corticosteroids.

Naevus flammeus
Naevus flammeus (port-wine stain) rarely change in size unless treated. Typically they are flat pink (due to the dermal location of the abnormal vasculature) lesions involving divisions of the trigeminal (fifth cranial) nerve. In 5 to 10 per cent of cases, Sturge–Weber syndrome is associated.

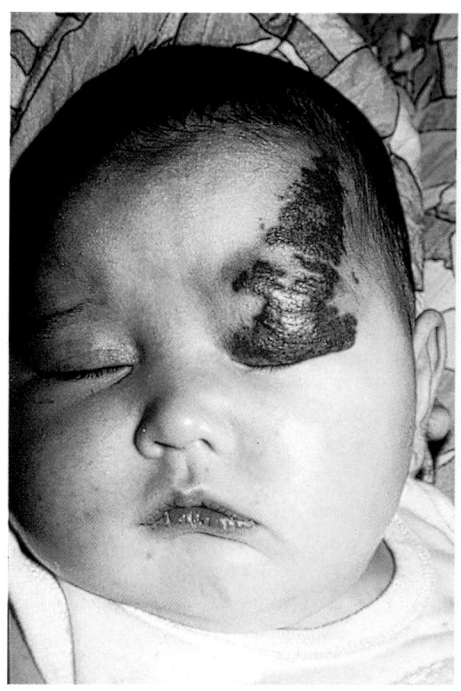

Fig. 10 Capillary haemangioma of the left periorbital tissue.

Kaposi's sarcoma

Kaposi's sarcoma is a purple–red lesion and is frequently associated with the acquired immunodeficiency syndrome. It may arise in the skin or conjunctiva, and in 70 to 80 per cent of patients, there is evidence of similar lesions elsewhere (especially on the hard palate).

Pyogenic granuloma

A pyogenic granuloma may be thought of as a haemangioma with associated granulation tissue secondary to trauma or inflammation. Although often classified as such, it is not strictly speaking a form of frank neoplasia but is reactive in origin.

Neural tissue

Neurofibromatosis

Plexiform neurofibroma

Neurofibromas of the eyelid classically follow an S-shaped contour of the outer half of the upper eyelid. Plexiform neurofibromas are typically associated with neurofibromatosis type I (von Recklinghausen's disease) and other stigmas of this disease must be searched for in the presence of a typical lesion. Even though malignant transformation occurs only rarely, neurofibromas are notoriously difficult to excise completely.

Fibroma molluscum

Also associated with neurofibromatosis type I are fibroma molluscum which appear as multiple small pedunculated proliferations of fibrous tissue.

Secondary malignant neoplasia

Distant metastatic eyelid carcinoma

Metastatic eyelid carcinoma is exceedingly rare but may actually be the presenting sign of carcinoma, most frequently originating from the breast, followed by the lung and the stomach. Clinically, metastatic eyelid carcinoma may present as a nodular or ulcerative, or as diffuse induration. There is orbital involvement in up to a fifth of cases. Incisional or excisional biopsy indicates the diagnosis. As two-thirds of patients with metastatic eyelid carcinoma have a known primary tumour, we cannot emphasize strongly enough the importance of a thorough history. As a similar proportion of these patients have associated visceral metastases, decisions about surgical excision as a treatment option in these patients need to be tailored individually.

Adjacent orbital involvement

The preseptal tissues of the eyelids may be involved with any orbital disorder occurring behind the orbital septum. Lymphoid tumours may originate in the eyelid, but more commonly affect the lid by contiguous spread.

Benign reactive lymphoid hyperplasia, atypical lymphoid

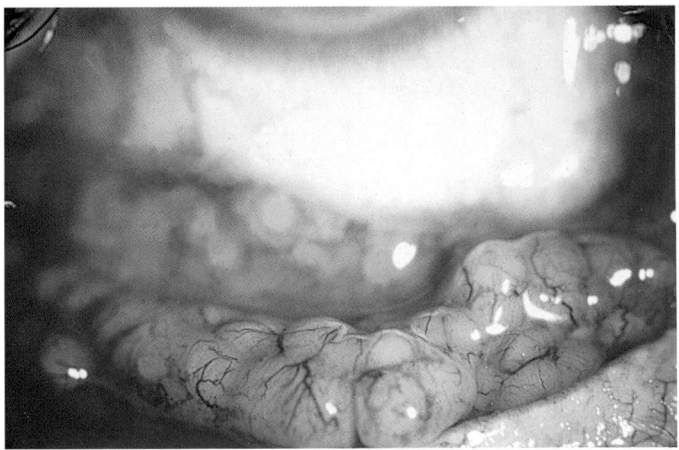

Fig. 11 Malignant lymphoma of entire left lower eyelid, appearing as a conjunctival 'salmon patch'.

hyperplasia, and malignant lymphoma (Fig. 11) represent a spectrum of disease, but are distinguishable only by biopsy and subsequent histopathological (formalin fixative) and immunohistochemical (fresh specimen) examination.

Other tumours originating in the conjunctiva, lacrimal gland, adjacent air sinuses, or nasopharynx may grow to involve the eyelids. In children, spread of adjacent skeletal muscle neoplasia (rhabdomyosarcoma) or leukaemic infiltration (granulocytic sarcoma or 'chloroma') can be confirmed by clinical examination and biopsy. These tumours are described elsewhere in greater detail.

Others

Merkel cell carcinoma

Merkel cell carcinoma is a highly malignant distinct tumour thought to originate in neuroendocrine tissue at the base of hair follicles. Clinically the rapid growth of a non-tender violaceous exophytic lesion should alert the clinician to the possibility of this distinctly rare lesion. Histopathological examination after diagnostic biopsy reveals highly malignant cells which may be misdiagnosed as lymphoma in the absense of diagnostic immunohistochemical markers. After diagnostic biopsy, wide excision of these tumours is indicated with histological control of tumour margin clearance.

Further reading

Arnold, A.C., Bullock, J.D., and Foos, R.Y. (1985). Metastatic eyelid carcinoma. *Ophthalmology*, **92**, 114–19.

Aurora, A.L. and Blodi, F.C. (1970). Lesions of the eyelids: a clinicopathological study. *Survey of Ophthalmology*, **15**, 94–104.

Boynton, J.R. (1991). Eyelid tumours and reconstructive surgery. In *Textbook of ophthalmology* (ed. S.M. Podos and M. Yanoff), pp. 6.1–6.24. Raven Press, New York.

Font, R.L. (1985) Eyelids and lacrimal drainage system. In *Ophthalmic pathology* (ed. W.H. Spencer), pp. 2149–248. Saunders, Philadelphia, PA.

Grossniklaus, H.E. and McLean, I.W. (1991). Cutaneous melanoma of the eyelid: clinicopathologic features. *Ophthalmology*, **98**, 1867–73.

Kass, L.G. and Hornblass, A (1989). Sebaceous carcinoma of the ocular adnexa. *Survey of Ophthalmology*, **33**, 477–90.

Kivela, T. and Tarkkanen, A. (1990). The Merkel and associated neoplasms in the eyelids and periocular tissue. *American Journal of Ophthalmology*, **113**, 674–80.

Rodrigues-Sains, R.S. and Jakobiec, F.A. (1987). Eyelid and conjunctival neo-plasms. In *Ophthalmic plastic and reconstructive surgery* (ed. R.C. Della Rocca, F.A. Nesi, and R.D. Lisman), pp. 759–70. Mosby, St Louis, MO.

Tanenbaum, M., Grove, A.S., and McCord, C.D. (1995). Eyelid tumours: diagnosis and management. In *Oculoplastic surgery* (ed. C.D. McCord, M. Tanenbaum and W.R. Nunery), pp. 145–75. Raven Press, New York.

2.6 Cornea

2.6.1 Anatomy and physiology of the cornea

W.J. Armitage

The cornea is the major refractive component of the eye, contributing approximately 70 per cent of total dioptric power; yet it also serves as a strong barrier protecting the inner structures of the eye against infection and trauma. These unique optical and mechanical properties are consequences of the structure and shape of the cornea, the intraocular pressure, and maintenance of transparency through active control of hydration. The greater part of the cornea consists of a collagenous stroma, which is bounded on its outer surface by a multilayered epithelium with its associated basement membrane, and on its inner surface by Descemet's membrane and a monolayer of endothelial cells (Fig. 1). In primates and a few other vertebrate species, the anterior stroma beneath the epithelial basement membrane is modified to form Bowman's layer. The epithelial cells are derived from the ectoderm during embryological development and they lay down the primary stroma, whereas the endothelium and stromal keratocytes are of mesenchymal origin.

The human cornea is 0.52 mm (SD 0.04 mm) thick at its centre, increasing to 0.66 mm (SD 0.08 mm) at the periphery, and the anterior surface has a radius of curvature of 7.68 mm (SD 0.26 mm). Viewed from the outside the cornea is slightly elliptical (horizontal axis, 11.7 mm; vertical axis, 10.6 mm), while the inner aspect is circular with a diameter of 11.7 mm. There is no difference in corneal thickness between males and females, but the other corneal dimensions are slightly less in females.

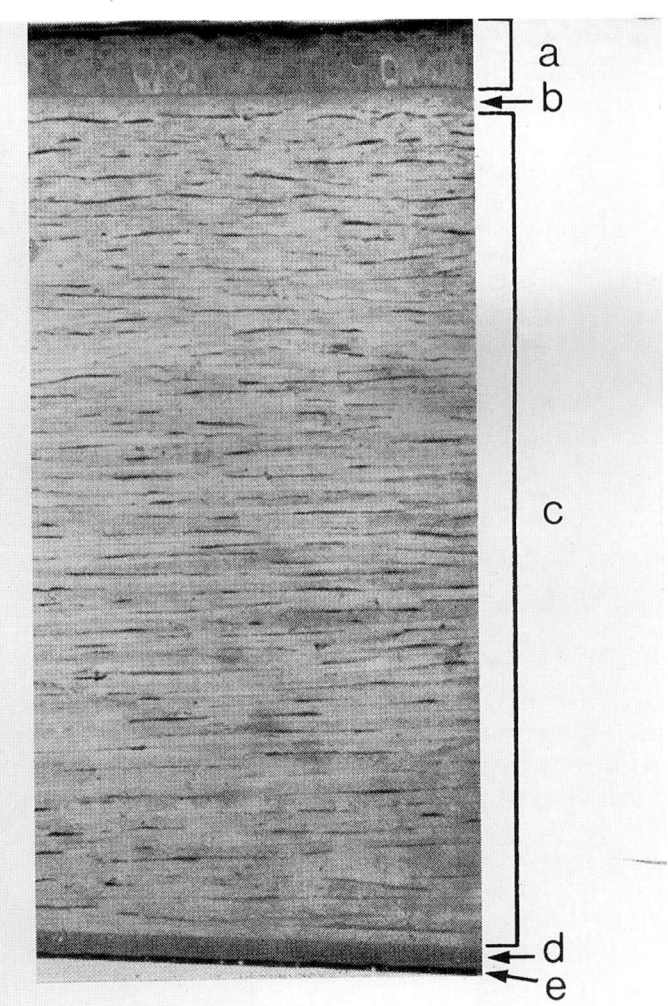

Fig. 1 Transverse section of human cornea: (a) epithelium, (b) Bowman's layer, (c) stroma, (d) Descemet's membrane, (e) endothelium. (Reproduced from Hogan *et al.* 1971, with permission.)

Epithelium

The anterior surface of the cornea consists of a non-keratinized, stratified squamous epithelium, which is five to seven cells thick in the central region (more at the periphery) and accounts for approximately 10 per cent of the thickness of the cornea (Fig. 2). The columnar basal cells, adjacent to Bowman's layer, are about 18 μm high and 10 μm in diameter with a flat basal surface and rounded apical surface. They have a slightly oval nucleus of about 5.7 μm in diameter, and the cytoplasm con-

tains relatively few organelles. The two outermost cell layers consist of highly flattened squamous cells that are only 4 μm thick and up to 45 μm across. Between these superficial cells and the basal cells lie two to three layers of polygonal, wing-shaped cells. Thus, moving anteriorly, the epithelial cells become progressively more flattened, the Golgi complex becomes more prominent, and there are more membrane-bound vesicles. There is also an increase in numbers of desmo-

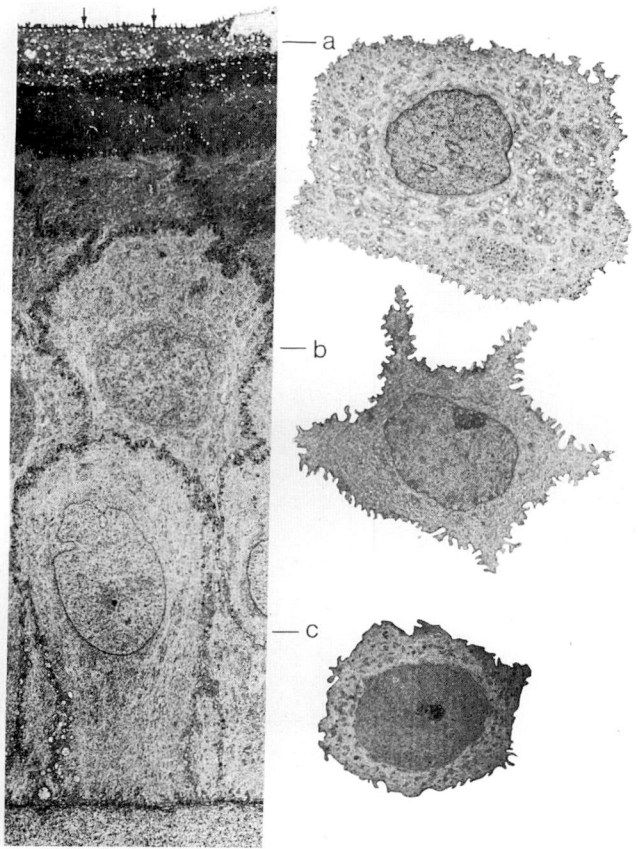

Fig. 2 Transverse section of epithelium with cross-sections of (a) a superficial cell, (b) a wing cell, and (c) a basal cell. (Reproduced from Hogan *et al.* 1971, with permission.)

somal attachments between cells, and tight junctions are present between the superficial cells giving a high paracellular electrical resistance. The position of these apical tight junctions correlates with the distribution of ZO-1, a tight junction protein: ZO-1 is absent in the basal cells but becomes increasingly apparent towards the superficial cell layers. Conversely, uvomorulin (E-cadhedrin), an adhesion molecule associated with the junctional complex, is uniformly distributed along the borders between cells at all layers of the corneal epithelium.

Basement membrane zone

The basement membrane zone is a complex interface between the basal cells of the epithelium and the underlying Bowman's layer. Intermediate filaments (keratin) of the basal cell cytoskeleton are linked to the basal lamina via hemidesmosomes and anchoring filaments. On the stromal side of the basal lamina, anchoring fibrils of type VII collagen, terminating in anchoring plaques, secure the basal lamina to Bowman's layer. The basal lamina itself is composed of type IV collagen, the glycoproteins laminin and entactin/nidogen, and heparan sulphate proteoglycan (perlecan).

The integrins, one of the four cell adhesion molecule superfamilies (the others being the selectins, the cadhedrins, and the

immunoglobulins), are important for interactions between cells, between cells and the extracellular matrix, and for signal transduction. They are glycoproteins consisting of two non-covalently bound α- and β-subunits that have intracellular, transmembrane, and extracellular domains. Integrin subunits α_2, α_3, α_6, β_1, and β_4 have been localized to the interface between basal cells and the basal lamina. The ligands for the integrin heterodimers $\alpha_2\beta_1$ and $\alpha_3\beta_1$ include collagen type IV, laminin, entactin/nidogen, and fibronectin, and $\alpha_6\beta_4$ colocalizes with hemidesmosomes.

The relative composition of the basal lamina and density of hemidesmosomes differs between the cornea and limbus, perhaps reflecting the varying state of differentiation of the epithelial cells in these different regions. These regional variations in the basal lamina also include different isoforms of type IV collagen, which may explain the failure of some to detect type IV collagen in corneal epithelial basement membrane.

Maintenance of epithelium

There is a continual loss of epithelium through desquamation of the superficial cells yet the epithelial cell mass remains constant under normal conditions, which means that there must be an equal replacement of lost epithelial cells through mitotic division. Only the basal cells of the corneal epithelium are capable of division: daughter cells lose their capacity for division as they become detached from the basement membrane, and they become terminally differentiated during migration towards the surface. In addition to this anterior movement of cells from the basal to the superficial layers, migration of basal epithelial cells from the periphery to the central cornea is also observed. An example of this centripetal movement of cells is the complete replacement of donor epithelium in a corneal graft by host epithelial cells over a period of about 1 year. There is not, therefore, a static population of cells permanently resident in the basal layer and the basal cells are thus considered to be transient amplifying cells.

It was originally thought that the primary source of corneal epithelium was from the conjunctiva: ingrowth of conjunctival epithelium on to the cornea has been observed, and these cells do indeed lose some of their conjunctival characteristics; but this conjunctival transdifferentiation is not complete and the cells retain some phenotypic differences from true corneal epithelium. The experimental and clinical evidence currently supports the concept, suggested more than 20 years ago, of a population of epithelial stem cells in the basal layer of the limbal epithelium. All stem cells are characterized by their undifferentiated state, longevity, high potential proliferative capacity, and slow cell cycle. Differences both in the expression of markers of cellular differentiation and in the expression of proteins associated with the various phases of the cell cycle suggest that limbal basal cells are indeed the least differentiated population of epithelial cells, that basal cells of the cornea have a faster cell cycle and only a limited proliferative capacity, and that the suprabasal cells are terminally differentiated and postmitotic (Fig. 3).

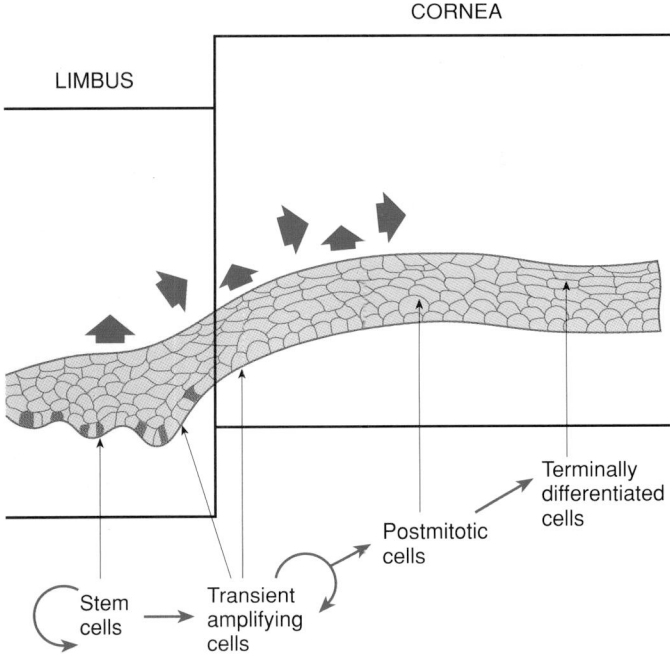

Fig. 3 Limbal and corneal epithelium showing location of the stem cells (blue) and the changing characteristics of cells as they move anteriorly and centrally from the limbus. (Reproduced from Kruse 1994, with permission.)

Small lesions in the corneal epithelium are repaired initially by the migration of neighbouring cells to cover the defect and then by enhanced cell division of the basal cells to replace the lost cells. There is also increased division of the limbal stem cells. Complete loss of corneal epithelium leads to eventual replacement from the limbus. In the absence of limbal cells, the transient amplifying cells can maintain the epithelial mass for a period, but the ability to repair subsequent wounds is severely compromised. Damage both to limbal and corneal epithelium, for example following chemical or thermal burns, causes recurrent epithelial deficiencies. The integrity of the epithelium may in some of these cases be restored by limbal autografts or allografts.

Langerhans' cells

Langerhans' cells are present in the corneal epithelium. These professional antigen-presenting cells carry both class I and II major histocompatibility antigens. They are typically confined to the peripheral third of the epithelium, but disease, trauma, or chemical stimulation can result in a rapid and substantial recruitment of Langerhans' cells to the central cornea. Corneal graft rejection in rats and mice can be modulated either by stimulating an increase or by depletion of Langerhans' cells in donor corneas prior to grafting, thus demonstrating the capacity of Langerhans' cells to present alloantigen directly to host alloreactive T cells. The role of Langerhans' cells in the mechanisms of recognition and rejection of human corneal grafts, however, is unresolved because it is highly unlikely that significant numbers of donor Langerhans' cells would be transferred

on a graft owing to their usual restriction to the corneal periphery and to their depletion during corneal preservation.

Stroma

The stroma consists of 78 per cent water, 20 per cent protein, 1 per cent glycosaminoglycan, and 1 per cent salts. By far the major constituent protein is collagen, which forms 71 per cent of the dry weight of the cornea, and types I, IV, V, and VI have all been identified in human stroma. The first three are striated fibrillar collagens and type VI is a filamentous collagen. The glycosaminoglycans, chondroitin/dermatan sulphate, and keratan sulphate, are covalently linked to proteins to form the proteoglycans decorin and lumican, respectively. The ratio of keratan sulphate to chondroitin/dermatan sulphate increases towards the endothelium suggesting an alteration in hydration properties from the anterior to the posterior stroma.

Bowman's layer

Bowman's layer in human corneas is a modified region of the stroma immediately beneath the epithelial basement membrane. It appears as a rather amorphous region in the light microscope. Electron microscopy reveals a disorganized arrangement of collagen fibrils that are somewhat thinner than those in the rest of the stroma.

Stromal structure

The bulk of the stroma comprises several hundred sheets of collagen fibrils, the lamellae, lying parallel to the epithelial and endothelial surfaces of the cornea (Fig. 4). Each lamella is approximately 2 μm thick and adjacent lamellae lie at large angles to each other. Within each lamella, the collagen fibrils, which are of uniform thickness, all run parallel to one another. The collagen fibrils are approximately 30 nm in diameter and they are spaced approximately 60 nm apart. At the limbus, there is an increase in mean thickness of the collagen fibrils from 30 to over 100 nm and the coefficient of variation of fibril diameter increases from less than 10 per cent in the stroma to about 40 per cent in the sclera.

The uniform diameter and quasi-regular spacing of the fibrils are the result of colocalization of different collagen types in the fibrils and of interactions between collagen and the proteoglycans. Proteoglycan molecules are polyanionic and form hydrated gels that occupy a large volume relative to their size. The protein core binds to specific sites along the collagen fibrils, and the glycosaminoglycan side chains separate adjacent fibrils. Fibrillogenesis studies carried out *in vitro* with mixtures of collagen types I and V show that the presence of type V collagen reduces fibril diameter and that decorin and lumican both slow the rate of fibrillogenesis. There is less type V collagen in sclera than in stroma, which is consistent with the greater fibril diameter observed in the former.

Keratocytes

Scattered throughout the stroma and lying between the lamellae are the fibroblastic-like keratocytes. These highly flattened

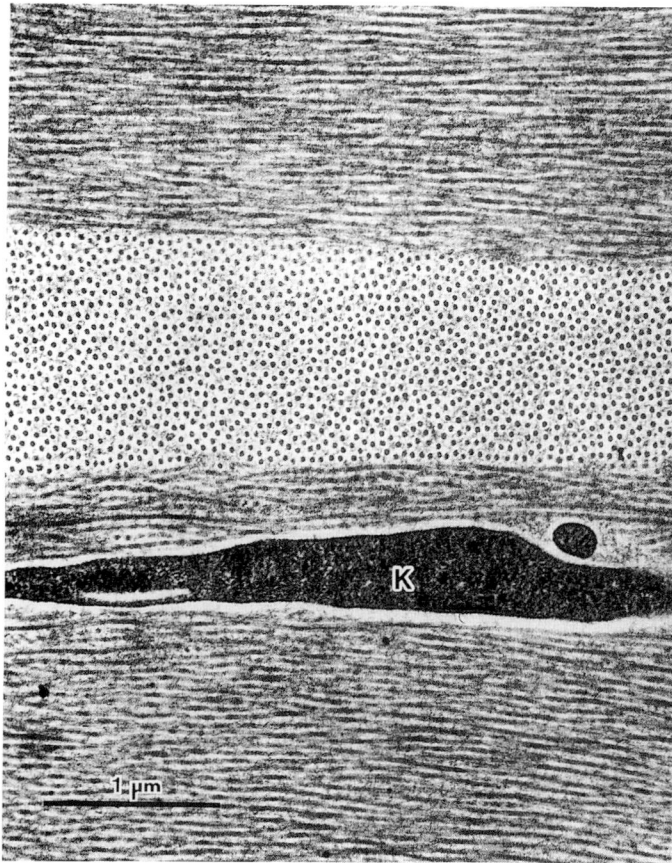

Fig. 4 Transmission electron micrograph of human corneal stroma showing collagen fibrils running parallel to each other within each lamella. The uniform diameter and quasi-regular arrangement of the fibrils is evident from the cut ends of the fibrils in the central lamella. A keratocyte (K) is also present. (Reproduced from Komai and Ulshiki 1991, with permission.)

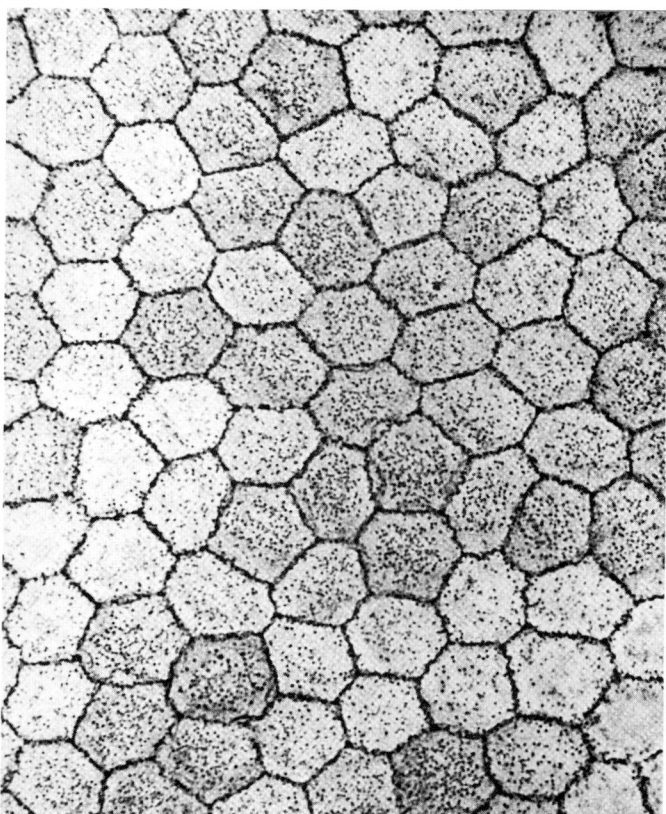

Fig. 5 A phase-contrast micrograph of human endothelium showing the predominantly hexagonal shape and close apposition of the cells. (Reproduced from Hogan *et al.* 1971, with permission.)

cells are only 2 μm at their thickest part around the nucleus. Based on measurements of stromal DNA content in human corneas, it has been estimated that there are approximately 2.5 × 10⁶ keratocytes in the stroma. There is qualitative clinical evidence in human corneas of an anterioposterior decrease in keratocyte density that has been confirmed by quantitative measurements in rabbit corneas. Keratocytes secrete components of the stroma and are thus important both for maintenance and in wound repair, which may involve interaction with the epithelium.

Keratocytes are connected to each other via long cytoplasmic extensions terminating in gap junctions, which have been identified morphologically, immunohistochemically (using an antibody to connexin 43, a gap junction protein), and by the spread of fluorescent dye between neighbouring cells. Cells both within the same lamellar plane and between different lamellae are coupled, though the links are more extensive in the former case.

Endothelium

The endothelium comprises a monolayer of mostly hexagonal cells that forms a continuous mosaic completely covering the posterior surface of the cornea (Fig. 5). The cells contain an oval nucleus and a very large number of mitochondria, consistent with a high energy demand for cellular processes such as active ion transport. The cell borders between adjacent cells are convoluted and they are joined by apical focal tight junctions (i.e. maculae, rather than zonulae, occludentes). The tight junction protein, ZO-1, does not form a continuous band around the apical border between neighbouring cells, which means that the paracellular pathway has a low electrical resistance (73 Ω cm²), unlike that of the superficial cells of the epithelium (1.6–9.1 kΩ cm²). Gaps are also observed in the adherens junctions associated with the apical circumferential belt of actin filaments. The gaps in the tight and adherens junctions are especially prominent at the 'Y' intersections between three neighbouring cells where they may be 1 to 2 μm wide, which suggests that the apical junctional complex is incomplete in this region. Desmosomes are lacking, but endothelial cells do possess gap junctions. Integrins of the β₁ family are also strongly associated with endothelial cells.

In humans, corneal endothelial cells only rarely undergo mitotic division and, based on the pattern of distribution of proteins associated with different phases of the cell cycle, the cells appear to be arrested in the G1 phase. There is little increase in cell numbers from the third trimester of gestation and cell density then falls rapidly over the first 2 postnatal years mainly owing to the growth of the cornea and its consequent increase in area. Thereafter, the loss of cells is compensated by the migration and spreading of neighbouring cells, and there is a continuous decline in cell density with increasing age from approximately 3500 cells/mm^2 in 10 to 19 year olds to 2300 cells/mm^2 in 80 to 89 year olds, which is equivalent to a 1.5-fold increase in cell area. Within a given age group, however, there is a marked variation in cell density, and this variability also increases with age.

Descemet's membrane

Descemet's membrane is the endothelial basement membrane. It is composed of collagen types IV, V, VI, and VIIII, as well as laminin, fibronectin, perlecan, and entactin/nidogen. It is an atypical basement membrane because of its thickness and because type VIII collagen is a major component. At birth, Descemet's membrane is 3 to 4 μm thick and fine collagen filaments form a regular lattice with thickened nodes at the intersections. The membrane is thicker in adults (10–12 μm) and the lattice appearance is confined to the anterior region of the membrane. There is also spatial organization in the chemical composition of Descemet's membrane, which is marked by differences between the stromal and endothelial faces of the membrane: both have type IV collagen (though different isoforms) and fibronectin, but the stromal face lacks laminin, perlecan, and entactin/nidogen.

Transparency

The amount of visible light transmitted by human cornea varies with wavelength from 86 per cent at 400 nm to 94 per cent at 600 nm: there is little change with increasing age. Hardly any light in the visible spectrum is absorbed and there is minimal light scattering; but shorter wavelengths in the ultraviolet range are strongly absorbed. If the collagen fibrils in the stroma all acted independently, more than 90 per cent of incident light would be scattered and the cornea would be opaque. The observed lack of scattering could be explained by a uniformity of refractive index throughout the stroma, achieved through hydration of the collagen fibrils to reduce their refractive index from 1.55 (dry collagen) to that of the ground substance (1.354); but this is evidently not the case since the ratio of the refractive indexes of the fibrils and the ground substance has been measured to be between 1.05 and 1.10.

Alternatively, Maurice proposed that the collagen fibrils were arranged in a crystalline lattice with perfectly regular spacing between the fibrils; thus, the scattered light would interfere destructively in all directions except in the direction of the incident light. Such strict long-range ordering of the fibrils is not apparent either ultrastructurally or from X-ray diffraction studies. It has been shown theoretically, however, that transparency is still possible with at least a degree of short-range ordering.

When stroma becomes oedematous and swells, transparency is lost. The fibril diameter remains constant but the spacing between the fibrils is altered. The increase in light scattering that accompanies a net influx of water is not thought to be caused by a simple disordering of all of the fibrils, rather it is the result of the appearance of random areas apparently devoid of fibrils (so-called 'lakes'), which can be seen quite clearly by electron microscopy.

Swelling pressure

The stroma has a tendency to imbibe water and solutes and removal of either of the bounding cell layers causes the cornea to swell. The stroma appears to behave as a polyelectrolyte gel with a measured swelling pressure at normal hydration (3.2 g H_2O/g dry wt) of approximately 8 kPa. A Donnan effect resulting from the fixed negative charge in the stroma of approximately 40 mmol/l (at normal hydration in 154 mmol/l saline) is the most likely explanation for the origin of the swelling pressure. Early observations that removal of the polyanionic proteoglycans from stroma reduced the tendency to swell supported this hypothesis.

The observed inverse relation between stromal hydration and swelling pressure could be calculated with good agreement from Donnan theory; but there were two experimental observations that, at least initially, appeared to be at odds with a Donnan effect. First, that swelling pressure was inversely related to temperature, whereas a positive temperature coefficient would be expected from theory; and, second, that the actual swelling rates of corneas in hypertonic and hypotonic salt solutions were, respectively, higher and lower than predicted. The apparently anomalous temperature coefficient has since been shown, at least theoretically, to be consistent with a Donnan effect provided that stromal charge is allowed to change with temperature. The second contradiction is resolved by not assuming that the only source of fixed negative charge is the dissociation of the carboxylic and sulphonic acid groups of the stromal glycosaminoglycans, but that there is a significant contribution from the binding of diffusable chloride ions within the stroma, which, in turn, would depend on the concentration of free chloride ions in the bathing medium. There is evidence for such chloride ion binding both from bovine and human cornea.

Maintenance of transparency

The endothelium is a leaky cell layer with a three-fold higher water permeability than the epithelium, and the stromal swelling pressure induces a continuous influx of ions, small molecules, and water across the endothelium from the aqueous humour into the stroma. This is necessary, in the absence of a blood supply, for the nutrition of stromal and epithelial cells because diffusion from the limbal vessels would be insufficient to meet the demands of the cells in the central cornea. The excess water must, however, be removed otherwise the stroma would swell, causing disruption of the regular arrangement of collagen fibrils, and the cornea would lose transparency. The passive permeability of the endothelium does restrict the influx of solute and water to a certain extent because disruption of this endothelial barrier (for example, by the removal of calcium ions, which causes dissociation of intercellular junctions) results in stromal oedema.

That the maintenance of corneal transparency is actually an active process requiring metabolic energy can be demonstrated by 'temperature-reversal' experiments, first described in the 1950s. A reduction in temperature lowers the rate of chemical reactions according to the Arrhenius relation, and biological reactions are typically slowed two- to three-fold for every 10°C fall in temperature. Cooling cells and tissues to, say, 4°C suppresses metabolism to the extent that there is insufficient generation of adenosine triphosphate to maintain energy-dependent processes such as ion transport. Thus, when eyes are placed at 4°C for several hours, the corneas begin to swell and lose clarity owing to the unopposed uptake of water and solute from the aqueous humour; restoration of normal metabolic activity on return to normothermia results in corneal thinning and transparency is regained. Metabolic inhibitors or hypoxia, however, prevent this reversal. It was subsequently shown that the presence of the endothelium but not the epithelium was necessary for this reversal of oedema to occur. The epithelium contributes little to the active control of stromal hydration: the swelling that follows removal of epithelium is mainly a consequence of the loss of the tight permeability barrier that normally prevents influx of water and solute across the anterior corneal surface. The endothelium, therefore, in some way actively extrudes water from the stroma to balance the inward leak from the aqueous humour, thus controlling stromal hydration and corneal thickness and maintaining transparency—the so-called 'pump-leak' hypothesis of corneal transparency.

The unidirectional transfer of water across cell layers is driven by the active transport of ions, although the precise mechanism that actually couples the solute and water fluxes is yet to be resolved. Various hypotheses have been proposed, such as Curran's double membrane hypothesis and Diamond and Bossert's standing gradient osmotic flow hypothesis, but as yet none is without significant objections. The main focus in cornea has been to identify the ion fluxes, in particular in the endothelium, that appear to be linked to water transfer. Although the corneal epithelium does actively secrete chloride ions, the potential water transport capacity of this ion flux is small compared with the leak of water into the stroma from the aqueous, hence the emphasis on the endothelium.

Extensive studies with isolated, perfused corneas have demonstrated that the endothelium is capable of transferring water from its basal to apical surface against a pressure gradient equivalent to intraocular pressure and at rates (i.e. 5 to 6.5 µl/cm^2 per h) sufficient to account for the rate of thinning of corneas during temperature reversal. There is a low transendothelial potential, apical side negative, of 0.5 to 1.3 mV that is directly proportional to this fluid flow. Both the rate of fluid flow and the transendothelial potential decrease with falling Na$^+$ concentration below 40 mmol/l, and the potential is abolished by ouabain, which inhibits Na$^+$/K$^+$-adenosine triphosphatase. But the potential is unlikely to be a direct result of electrogenic Na$^+$ transport across the endothelium for two reasons: first, the polarity of the transendothelial potential would require the net movement of Na$^+$ from the aqueous into the stroma, which would be in the wrong direction to induce a coupled osmotic flow of water out of the stroma; and, second, a net flux of Na$^+$

across the endothelium under short-circuit conditions, which would be expected if Na$^+$ were being actively transported against an electrochemical gradient, has not been consistently observed. A net flux of anions from stroma to aqueous would produce both a movement of solute in the right direction and a potential of the correct polarity. Measurements of the fluxes of chloride and bicarbonate ions in both directions across the endothelium show that the opposite fluxes of chloride are similar but that there is a net flux of bicarbonate from the stroma to the aqueous side. Early experiments showed that the water flux was also dependent on exogenous bicarbonate, but a bicarbonate-dependent adenosine triphosphatase has not been identified in corneal endothelium, suggesting that HCO$_3^-$ is moved by a secondary rather than a primary active transport mechanism: the movement of water from the stroma to the aqueous is thus likely to be a consequence of the coupled transport of sodium and bicarbonate.

A number of models of endothelial ion transport have been proposed to account for the observed physiological characteristics of the endothelial fluid pump (e.g. Fig. 6). The models include a Na$^+$/K$^+$-adenosine triphosphatase pump located on the basolateral membrane, which ultimately provides the energy needed to drive the various coupled ion fluxes because inhibition of this pump by ouabain stops fluid transfer and causes stromal swelling. Since Na$^+$ is not actively transported across the endothelium, Na$^+$ must re-enter endothelial cells via the basolateral membrane rather than the apical membrane. The re-entry of Na$^+$ down its electrochemical gradient would, however, drive the cotransport or exchange of other ions. A basolateral Na$^+$/H$^+$ exchanger, driven by this inward flux of Na$^+$ and inhibited by amiloride, not only provides a route for Na$^+$ re-entry but also removes excess protons, thus controlling intracellular pH.

The source of HCO$_3^-$ is not agreed. Simple diffusion of CO$_2$ across the basolateral membrane into the cell is one possibility, with HCO$_3^-$ and H$^+$ being generated in a reaction of CO$_2$ with water catalysed by carbonic anhydrase. It has also been proposed that sufficient HCO$_3^-$ could be generated by the same reaction but using only metabolically derived CO$_2$, which implies that there is actually no need for an exogenous source of HCO$_3^-$. Conflicting results concerning the source or even the need for HCO$_3^-$ are partly due to differing experimental methodologies, but the need for an exogenous source of HCO$_3^-$ is generally supported. Inhibitors of carbonic anhydrase, such as acetazolamide, only partially inhibit the short-circuit current, which is normally close to the HCO$_3^-$ flux, implying that CO$_2$ diffusion is not the only source of HCO$_3^-$, but that HCO$_3^-$ also crosses endothelial cell membranes as the ion. There is evidence for inward HCO$_3^-$/Na$^+$ cotransport from electrophysiological studies of the effects of anion transport inhibitors, the stilbene derivatives 4-acetoamido-4'-isothiocyanatostilbene-2,2'-disulphonic acid (SITS) and 4,4'-diisothiocyanoatostilbene-2,2'-disulphonic acid (DIDS), in bovine endothelial cell cultures. Another option would be entry of Na$^+$/K$^+$/2Cl$^-$ via a cotransporter coupled with HCO$_3^-$/Cl$^-$ exchange to provide both re-entry of Na$^+$ and the required influx of HCO$_3^-$.

So far as HCO$_3^-$ efflux at the apical membrane is concerned,

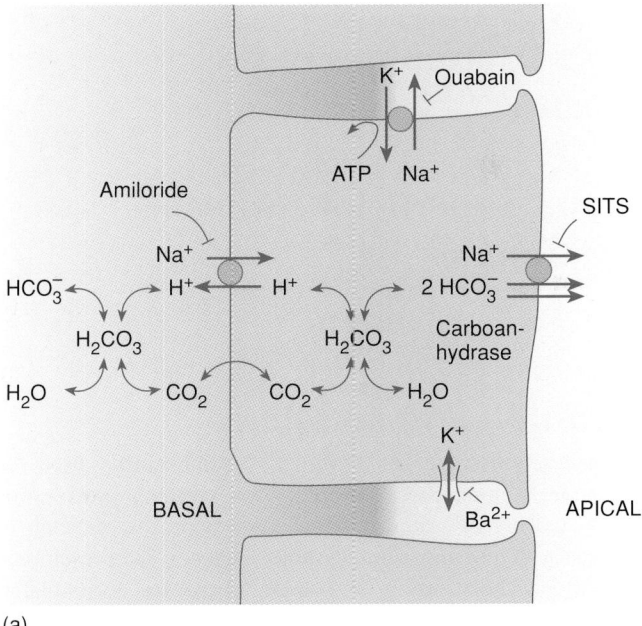

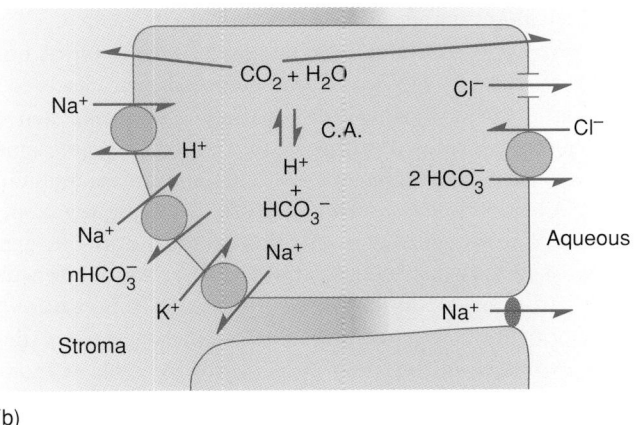

Fig. 6 Two models of ion transport across the endothelium. Both share a basolateral Na^+/K^+ pump and a Na^+/H^+ exchanger, but the modes of HCO_3^- entry and exit differ in the two models: in (a), CO_2 diffuses across the basolateral membrane and HCO_3^- leaves across the apical membrane by a Na^+/HCO_3^- cotransporter; whereas in (b), HCO_3^- enters via a basolateral $Na^+:nHCO_3^-$ cotransporter and leaves via apical HCO_3^-/Cl^- exchange. (Reproduced from (a) Jentsch *et al.* 1985 and (b) Bonanno and Giasson 1992, with permission.)

an uncoupled flux has been proposed as well as HCO_3^-/Na^+ cotransport and HCO_3^-/Cl^- exchange, both of which would be inhibited by DIDS or SITS. A HCO_3^-/Cl^- exchanger has been demonstrated in bovine endothelial cell cultures, which show a DIDS-sensitive uptake of $^{36}Cl^-$ and which would fit in with the apparent requirement for Cl^- for stromal thinning. It should also be noted that not all of the HCO_3^- transport is necessarily associated with water movement.

Since some of these ion transporters are similar to the cell volume regulatory mechanisms found in other cell types, Fischbarg has proposed recently that there is not a steady-state coupling of ion and water fluxes in corneal endothelium, rather that there are transient cell volume changes driven by the various ion transport mechanisms for regulating cell volume. If endo-

thelial cells were polarized such that the ion transporters associated with regulatory volume increases and those associated with regulatory volume decreases were located on, respectively, the basolateral and apical membranes, then it would be possible to induce an overall net efflux of water from the stroma to the aqueous. Such a mechanism would require a transcellular, rather than paracellular, transfer of water across the endothelium. The water channel protein CHIP28 (channel forming integral membrane protein of 28 kDa), a member of the membrane intrinsic protein family, was recently identified in corneal endothelial cells, which not only helps to explain the high water permeability of these cells but could also support the notion of transcellular water transfer. However, the precise mechanism by which the corneal endothelium, or for that matter any other epithelial cell layer, actively transfers water remains to be determined.

Energy metabolism

The main source of energy in the cornea for ion pumping, protein synthesis, and cell division is derived from the metabolism of glucose through glycolysis and oxidative catabolism. Glucose consumption for whole rabbit cornea is approximately $100\ \mu g/cm^2$ per h. The epithelium also contains stores of glycogen that can be broken down to glucose-1-phosphate when the supply of glucose is for some reason insufficient. Oxygen diffuses into the cornea directly from the atmosphere and utilization in rabbit cornea is $10\ \mu l\ cm^{-2}\ h^{-1}$. The relative rates of oxygen consumption by the epithelium, stroma, and endothelium are in the ratio 40 to 39 to 21, respectively. On the basis of consumption per cell, the oxygen uptake by endothelial cells and stromal keratocytes is six-fold that of epithelial cells.

Initial observations showed that intact corneas swelled when made anoxic and that the thinning of swollen corneas was halted in the presence of respiratory inhibitors such as cyanide, antimycin A, or oligomycin. But the rate of swelling induced by cyanide in corneas initially at normal thickness was less than that brought about by ouabain, confirming that there was still some endothelial pump activity even in the absence of respiration. Moreover, swollen, de-epithelialized corneas do thin, despite the presence of respiratory inhibitors, when glucose is present to support increased production of adenosine triphosphate from glycolysis. Anoxia causes a rapid fall in adenosine triphosphate content of the epithelium but, provided glucose is present, adenosine triphosphate levels are maintained in the endothelium at 65 per cent of those under aerobic conditions. Thus, a strong Pasteur effect in the endothelium protects against hypoxia and provides sufficient adenosine triphosphate to maintain the endothelial ion pumps necessary for fluid transport.

The reason for the swelling of anoxic cornea is now known to be the increased production of lactate by the epithelium, rather than failure of the endothelial pump: under anaerobic conditions, the lactate generated in the epithelium as a result of glycolysis passes into the stroma, increasing stromal osmolality and inducing an increased fluid influx. Lactate produced by the endothelium passes directly into the aqueous and does not, therefore, contribute to the increased stromal osmolality.

Further reading

Bonanno, J.A. and Glasson, C. (1992). Intracellular pH regulation in fresh and cultured bovine corneal endothelium. II. Na+:HCO3− cotransport and Cl−/HCO3− exchange. *Investigative Ophthalmology and Visual Science*, **33**, 3068–79.

Cox, S., Aoki, T., Seki, J., Moroyama, Y., and Yoshida, K. (1994). The pharmacology of the integrins. *Medicinal Research Reviews*, **14**, 195–228.

Fischbarg, J. (1997). Mechanism of fluid transport across corneal endothelium and other epithelial layers: a possible explanation based on cyclic cell volume regulatory changes. *British Journal of Ophthalmology*, **81**, 85–9.

Fischbarg, J., Hernandez, J., Liebovitch, L.S., and Koniarek, J.P. (1985). The mechanism of fluid and electrolyte transport across corneal endothelium: critical revision and update of a model. *Current Eye Research*, **4**, 351–60.

Hodson, S.A., Kaila, D., Hammond, S., Revello, G., and Al-Omari, Y. (1992). Transient chloride binding as a contributory factor to corneal stromal swelling in the ox. *Journal of Physiology*, **450**, 89–103.

Hogan, M.J., Alvarado, J.A., and Weddell, J.E. (1971). *Histology of the human eye*. Saunders, Philadelphia.

Jentsch, T.J., Keller, S.K., and Wiederholt, M. (1985). Ion transport mechanisms in cultured bovine corneal endothelial cells. *Current Eye Research*, **4**, 361–9.

Joyce, N.C., Meklir, B., Joyce, J.J., and Zieske, J.D. (1996). Cell cycle protein expression and proliferative status in human corneal cells. *Investigative Ophthalmology and Visual Science*, **37**, 645–55.

Komai, Y. and Ulshiki, T. (1991). The three-dimensional organization of collagen fibrils in the human cornea and sclera. *Investigative Ophthalmology and Visual Science*, **32**, 2244–58.

Kruse, F.E. (1994). Stem cells and corneal epithelial regeneration. *Eye*, **8**, 170–83.

Kwok, L.S. and Klyce, S.D. (1990). Theoretical basis for an anomalous temperature coefficient in swelling pressure of rabbit corneal stroma. *Biophysical Journal*, **57**, 657–62.

Ljubimov, A.V., Burgeson, R.E., Butkowski, R.J., Michael, A.F., Sun, T.T., and Kenney, M.C. (1995). Human corneal basement membrane heterogeneity: topographical differences in the expression of type IV collagen and laminin isoforms. *Laboratory Investigation*, **72**, 461–73.

Marshall, G.E., Konstas, A.G.P., and Lee, W.R. (1993). Collagens in ocular tissues. *British Journal of Ophthalmology*, **77**, 515–24.

Maurice, D.M. (1984). The cornea and sclera. In *The Eye*, (3rd edn), Vol. 1b, (ed. H. Davson), pp. 1–158. Academic Press, London.

McCally, R.L. and Farrell, R.A. (1990). Light scattering from cornea and corneal transparency. In *Noninvasive diagnostic techniques in ophthalmology* (ed. B.R. Masters), pp. 189–210. Springer-Verlag, New York.

Riley, M.V. and Winkler, B.S. (1990). Strong Pasteur effect in rabbit corneal endothelium preserves fluid transport under anaerobic conditions. *Journal of Physiology*, **426**, 81–93.

Riley, M.V., Winkler, B.S., Czajkowski, C.A., and Peters, M.I. (1995). The roles of bicarbonate and CO2 in transendothelial fluid movement and control of corneal thickness. *Investigative Ophthalmology and Visual Science*, **36**, 103–12.

Sharina, A. and Coles, W.H. (1989). Kinetics of corneal epithelial maintenance and graft loss. A population balance model. *Investigative Ophthalmology and Visual Science*, **30**, 1962–71.

2.6.2 Dystrophies of the cornea

2.6.2.1 Superficial corneal dystrophies

Gordon K. Klintworth

Definition and aetiology

The designation 'corneal dystrophy' is traditionally used for spontaneously appearing bilateral, stationary, or slowly progressive, usually inherited, corneal alterations that develop in the absence of inflammation without systemic manifestations. The term has shortcomings and as knowledge has accumulated the weaknesses in this definition have become increasingly apparent. For example, systemic abnormalities have been found in an increasing number of these conditions.

The primary defect in all inherited corneal dystrophies, presumably residues in DNA and the abnormal gene, leads to a disordered chain of biochemical reactions. The major step of mapping some corneal dystrophies to a specific chromosomal locus has been achieved, but the relevant gene and its mutation has been identified in very few conditions involving the cornea (Table 1). The sequence of events that follow the specific genetic mutations vary considerably, but characteristic abnormalities of a particular condition eventually develop. The nature of the abnormality varies considerably. Abnormal genes that become expressed during early corneal growth result in anomalous development (dysgenesis). From a taxonomical standpoint the time is ripe to replace the obsolete designation 'dystrophy' by the more meaningful aetiological denomination 'inherited or genetically determined disorders'. Non-inherited idiopathic and non-specific spontaneously occuring corneal disorders are probably better designated by the non-committal word keratopathy.

Considerable confusion exists concerning inherited disorders that involve Bowman's layer and the anterior corneal stroma (Reis–Bücklers' dystrophy, Thiel–Behnke dystrophy, Waardenburg–Jonkers dystrophy, Grayson–Wilbrandt dystrophy, and superficial granular dystrophy), largely because of their overlapping features. These conditions usually become symptomatic during childhood with painful recurrent corneal erosions and some of their attributes are non-specific results of recurrent epithelial breakdown. Recent follow-up histopathological studies of the original pedigrees and molecular genetic investigations have clarified the subject somewhat.

Based on characteristic deposits in the cornea two distinct autosomal dominant entities, which cannot be differentiated from each other clinically, are recognized: one is a superficial variant of granular corneal dystrophy (Reis–Bücklers' dystrophy); the other has characteristic curly fibres when examined by transmission electron microscopy (Thiel–Behnke

Table 1 Inherited predominantly superficial corneal dystrophies

Dystrophy	Inheritance	Gene locus
Fabry's disease (angiokeratoma corporis diffusum)	XR	Xq22
Recurrent erosions, familial	AD	Unknown
Reis–Bücklers' dystrophy (see granular dystrophy)	AD	5q31
Familial subepithelial amyloidosis	AR	Unknown
Grayson–Wilbrandt dystrophy*	AD	Unknown
Keratosis follicularis spinulosa decalvans	AR	Unknown
Meesmann's dystrophy	AD	12q and 17q
Stocker–Holt dystrophy†	AD	Unknown
Subepithelial mucinous dystrophy	AD	Unknown
Thiel–Behnke dystrophy	AD	5q31
Waardenburg–Jonkers' dystrophy (see Thiel–Behnke dystrophy)	AD	

*Uncertain which superficial dystrophy this represents.
†May be same as Meesmann's dystrophy.
AD, autosomal dominant; AR, autosomal recessive; XR, X-linked recessive.

dystrophy). These two disorders seem to result from different mutations in the β*ig-h3* (keratoepithelin) gene, but more than one gene may also be involved.

Grayson and Wilbrandt documented a familial inherited anterior corneal dystrophy (Grayson–Wilbrandt dystrophy) in which discrete grey–white macular opacities were distributed axially and para-axially in individuals with normal corneal sensation and visual acuity and with infrequent epithelial erosions. An elderly patient with these features had a thickened basement membrane and fibrocellular accumulations over an intact Bowman's layer. The precise nosological identity of this condition remains to be determined.

Recurrent corneal erosions

Definition and aetiology

The term recurrent corneal erosions refers to recurrent episodes in which the corneal epithelium becomes desquamated. It is not a distinct entity, but can follow traumatic abrasions, dry eyes, keratitis due to herpes simplex or herpes zoster, bullous keratopathy, and chemical injuries. The erosions may begin one to two decades after exposure to nitrogen mustard (dichlorodiethylsulphide). Also, recurrent bilateral corneal erosions can occur in Meesmann's dystrophy, Reis–Bücklers' dystrophy, Thiel–Behnke dystrophy, Fuchs' dystrophy, lattice corneal dystrophy types I and IIIA, granular corneal dystrophy, subepithelial mucinous dystrophym, and other disorders of the cornea. In addition they may form spontaneously in the absence of a predisposing factor in individuals with an autosomal dominant condition (primary familial corneal erosions).

Meibomian gland dysfunction is present in some patients with recalcitrant recurrent corneal erosions, and facial telangiectasia, rhinophyma, and acne rosacea are present in a high percentage of such patients.

Pathophysiology and biochemistry

Subepithelial cellular debris and fibrous tissue containing disoriented collagen fibres often replaces Bowman's layer. After recurrent epithelial erosions the features of fingerprint and microcystic keratopathy commonly develop.

Epithelial erosions presumably recur because the epithelium is unable to form appropriate adhesions to its basement membrane with hemidesmosomes or anchoring fibrils. The epithelium separates from the underlying basement membrane and fractures form within the displaced epithelium.

Clinical features

Corneal erosions may begin at any age and have been noted by the age of 5 years. Irrespective of their cause dot-like opacities (intraepithelial cysts; Cogan's microcystic 'dystrophy'), as well as fingerprint, linear, map-like, and other opacities (map–dot–fingerprint corneal 'dystrophy') commonly follow recurrent corneal erosions.

Microcystic, map–dot–fingerprint, and epithelial basement membrane corneal 'dystrophy'

Definition and aetiology

In 1950 Guerry reported extremely fine fingerprint-like wavy lines in the corneal epithelium of two patients. One individual had early bilateral cornea guttata; the other subsequently developed recurrent herpetic keratitis. More than a decade later Cogan and colleagues drew attention to relatively nonprogressive small pleomorphic lardaceous-appearing greyish-white opacities in the corneal epithelium. Terms applied to these related entities include: map–dot–fingerprint dystrophy, Cogan–Guerry microcystic epithelial dystrophy, and epithelial basement membrane dystrophy. Because this disorder is heterogeneous in origin and usually not inherited, the designation 'keratopathy' seems more appropriate than 'dystrophy' in nonfamilial cases because of implications inherent in the latter label.

Affected individuals often have antecedent dry eyes, trauma, bullous keratopathy, herpes simplex or herpes zoster keratitis, or recurrent epithelial erosions. Fingerprint lines form in the superior cornea following cataract extraction. A high percentage of normal individuals develop map–dot–fingerprint dystrophy spontaneously. Relatives of patients with recurrent epithelial erosions may have asymptomatic map–dot–fingerprint changes in the cornea and sometimes the condition is familial. Family studies indicate a probable dominant inheritance with variable penetrance in some instances.

Pathophysiology and biochemistry

The intraepithelial microcysts, which form at various depths in the corneal epithelium are lined by flattened squamous epithelium and contain degenerating and necrotic cellular debris. The cysts form within the epithelium posterior to an insinuation of basement membrane (Figs 1 and 2). Intraepithelial ectopic extensions of basement membrane as well as ridges of subepithelial discontinuous multilaminar thickened basement membrane that contain collagen fibrils and cellular debris account for the fingerprint or map-like patterns observed clinically. Rarely multinucleated cells are present. The space between adjacent epithelial cells may be widened.

Aberrant intraepithelial basement membrane blocks the normal migration of epithelial cells towards the surface. This causes maturing epithelial cells to degenerate and become encysted with collections of debris.

Clinical features

This highly prevalent keratopathy mainly affects middle-aged or elderly individuals and sometimes children, but the severity of the disorder does not correlate with age (Fig. 3). The abnormalities occur predominantly in the lower cornea overlying the pupil. The small fat-like opacities come and go without apparent cause and are typically bilateral, although not necessarily symmetrical. When unilateral the fellow eye may be affected subtly. The opacities vary in shape over time as they become displaced externally by the maturing underlying epithelial cells or as they coalesce with other cysts before eventually bursting through the surface to discharge their contents. The alterations

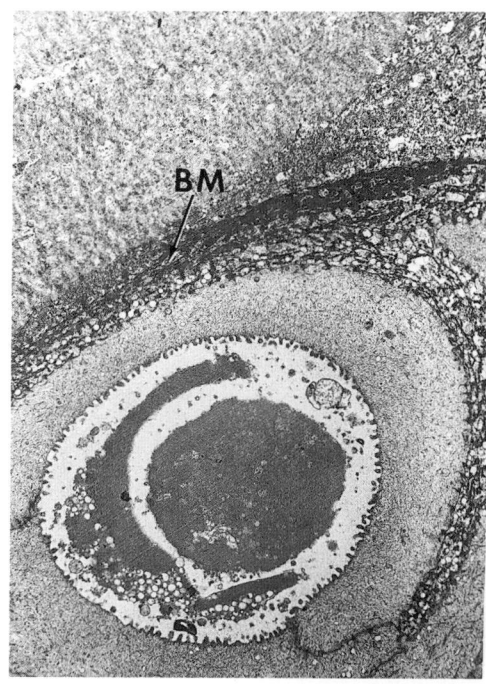

Fig. 2 Transmission electron micrograph illustrating an intraepithelial cyst posterior to aberrant basement membrane (BM). The cyst contains cellular debris and is bordered by an intact cell having villous processes, × 5550. (Reproduced with permission from Cogan *et al.* 1974.)

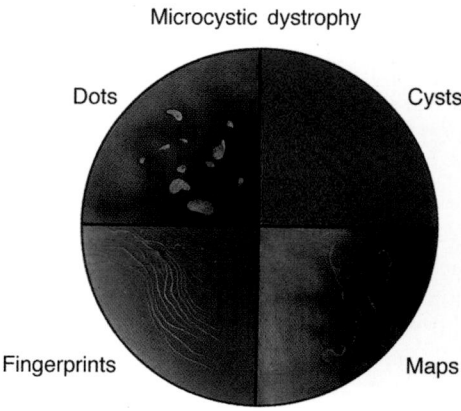

Fig. 3 Microcystic 'corneal dystrophy'. (By courtesy of Jack Kanski and Buttterworths.)

are frequently asymptomatic and discovered fortuitously, but slight blurring of vision, a mild early morning irritation, a foreign body sensation, or prominent painful erosive episodes are common. Irregular corneal astigmatism with complaints of distorted or ghost images occasionally develop. Symptoms may follow minor trauma.

In asymptomatic persons as well as in those with a history of recurrent epithelial erosions, fibrillogranular material may form mounds between the basement membrane and Bowman's zone giving the clinical appearance of a subepithelial bleb. This abnormality, which has been observed in men and women

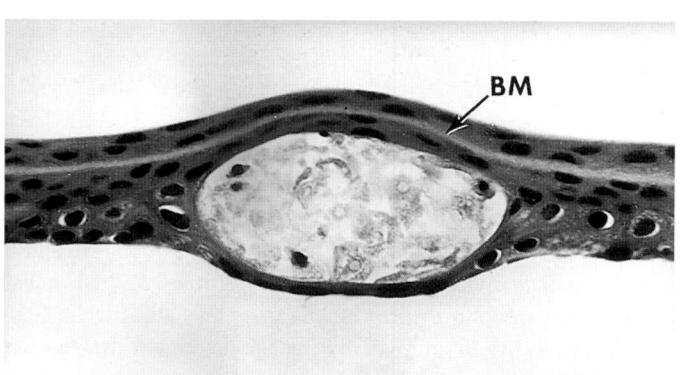

Fig. 1 Microcystic 'corneal dystrophy'. Microcyst within corneal epithelium posterior to ectopic basement membrane (BM). Haematoxylin and eosin, × 227. (Reproduced with permission from Cogan *et al.* 1974.)

between 39 and 81 years of age, has been designated bleb-like or bleb dystrophy.

Primary familial subepithelial corneal amyloidosis

Definition and aetiology

The designation primary familial subepithelial corneal amyloidosis is recommended for a specific inherited type of corneal amyloidosis, which involves mainly the subepithelial area and Bowman's layer. The condition is also termed gelatinous drop-like corneal dystrophy. The latter term, unfortunately has also been used for chronic actinic keratopathy (climatic droplet keratopathy). The mode of inheritance is considered to be autosomal recessive, but apparent sporadic cases have been documented.

Basic epidemiology

Primary familial subepithelial amyloidosis has been detected in many parts of the world, but most reports are from Japan, where the condition was first described.

Pathophysiology and biochemistry

Mounds of amyloid accumulate primarily in the central cornea between the epithelium and Bowman's layer (Fig. 4), but fusiform deposits of amyloid similar to those in lattice dystrophy may form in the deeper stroma (see above). The amyloid contains abundant lactoferrin.

Clinical features

During the first two decades of life amyloid begins to accumulate beneath the epithelium of both corneas producing multiple prominent milky-white gelatinous nodules that resemble a mulberry in shape (Fig. 5). Other features are severe photophobia,

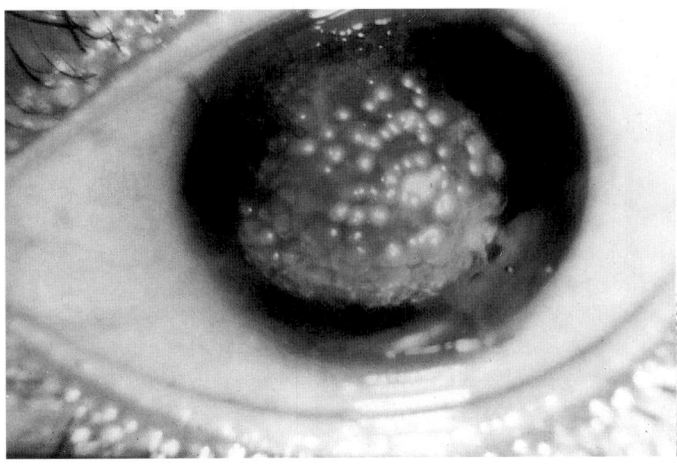

Fig. 5 Familial subepithelial corneal amyloidosis. Clinical photograph of nodular deposits of amyloid in cornea. (Reproduced with permission from Klintworth 1980.)

tearing, a corneal foreign body sensation, and a severe progressive loss of vision.

Cornea verticillata and Fabry's disease

Definition and aetiology

The designation vortex corneal dystrophy (cornea verticillata) was applied to innumerable minute brown spots arranged in curved lines in the superficial cornea in a whirlpool-like pattern. Initially an autosomal dominant mode of transmission was suspected, but subsequently it became apparent that these cases were affected hemizygous males and asymptomatic female carriers of an X-linked systemic metabolic disease caused by a deficiency of α–galactosidase (Fabry's disease). Fabry's disease, due to mutations in the GLA gene, is located on the long arm of the human X chromosome (Xq22). Non-familial whorl-like corneal opacities also form in individuals on chloroquine, amiodarone, phenothiazines, or indomethacin therapy and striate melanokeratosis.

Basic epidemiology

Fabry's disease has been detected in individuals from many ethnic groups, but most cases have involved Caucasians.

Pathophysiology and biochemistry

The corneal epithelium contains numerous intracytoplasmic bodies, which are lamellar and osmiophilic when examined by transmission electron microscopy. Similar structures are also evident within keratocytes in the corneal stroma. The characteristic whorl-like corneal changes involve virtually all affected males and may result from a series of subepithelial ridges or duplications of the basement membrane of the corneal epithelium. Fabry's disease results from a genetically determined deficiency of the lysosomal enzyme α–galactosidase. This defect

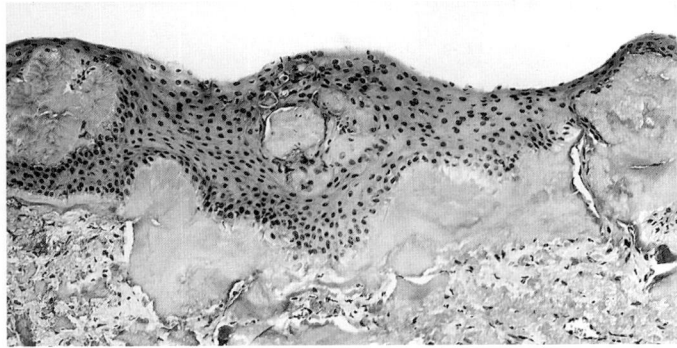

Fig. 4 Familial subepithelial corneal amyloidosis. Histological appearance of amyloid deposits in superficial cornea. Haematoxylin and eosin, × 76. (Reproduced with permission from Klintworth 1980.)

prevents the breakdown of glycophospholipids in all tissues of the body.

Clinical features

The cutaneous manifestations are a striking feature of Fabry's disease in males. These include angiokeratomas which gradually develop from early in life as dark red to blue–black punctate spots in the superficial skin of the abdomen. Other features include burning pains in the extremities, fever, and renal dysfunction. Eventually death results from renal or cardiac failure. Whirl-like opacities form in the cornea and star-shaped opacities form in the posterior part of the crystalline cornea. Hemizygous females are only mildly affected and develop the cornea verticillata.

Meesmann's dystrophy (juvenile familial epithelial dystrophy)

Definition and aetiology

Although first reported clinically in 1935 by Pameijer of The Netherlands this dystrophy of the corneal epithelium became well documented as a distinct entity by Meesmann.

Stocker and Holt described grey, punctate, scattered corneal opacities in descendants of Moravians from near Dresden in Saxony, Germany between the ages of 7 months to 70 years. The epithelial basement membrane was thickened and sometimes produced an irregular epithelial surface, but Bowman's layer appeared normal. Stocker–Holt dystrophy may be related to Meesmann's dystrophy, but the same genetic mutation is not present and the peculiar substance characteristic of the latter entity has not been identified in affected corneas.

Basic epidemiology

Meesmann's dystrophy has been detected in Germany and several other countries. A large pedigree (761 persons in 12 generations) has been traced to Schleswig–Holstein in 1620.

Pathophysiology and biochemistry

The thickness of the corneal epithelium is irregular and the cells often lack normal stratification. Numerous intraepithelial cysts contain degenerated cellular debris, which stains with periodic acid–Schiff and Hale's colloidal iron technique. It manifests autofluorescence in ultraviolet light. The contents of the cysts are resistant to diastase and neuraminidase digestion. The corneal epithelium also contains intracytoplasmic pathognomonic aggregations of cytokeratin ('peculiar substance') that is only detectable by transmission electron microscopy (Fig. 6).

The corneal epithelium, but not the cysts, sometimes contains abundant glycogen granules which dissolve during histological preparation forming vacuoles. Mitoses are often evident within young active epithelial cells. The epithelial basement membrane is thickened and has irregular excrescences, which may extend into the overlying epithelium. Bowman's layer and the corneal stroma and corneal endothelium are unremarkable.

Despite abundant glycogen within some epithelial cells

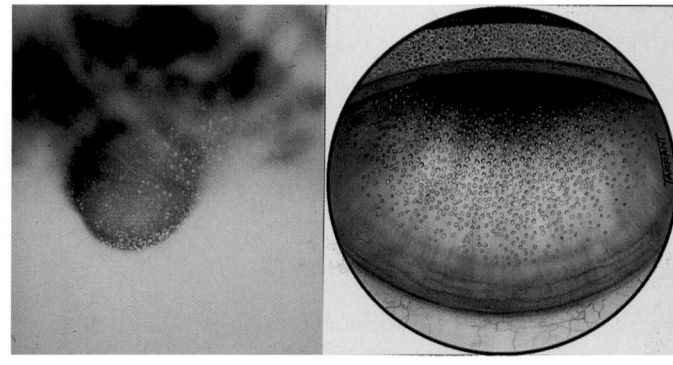

(a)

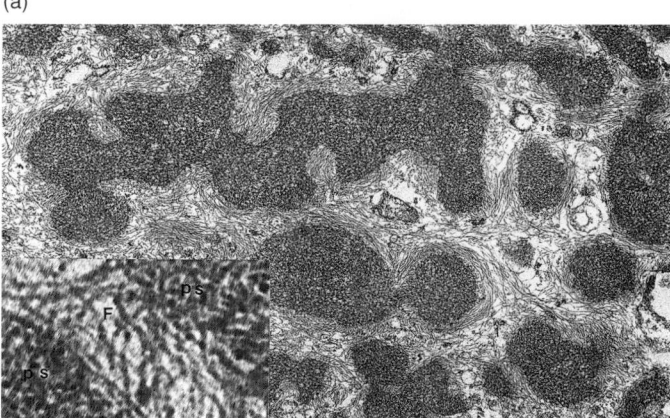

(b)

Fig. 6 (a) Meesmann's corneal dystrophy. (By courtesy of Jack Kanski and Butterworths.) (b) Transmission electron micrograph of cornea with Meesmann's corneal dystrophy illustrating the characteristic 'peculiar substance' that accumulates within the cytoplasm of some corneal cells. in the superficial corneal stroma, ×20 400. Insert shows cytoplasmic filaments (F) closely connected to adjacent fibrillogranular 'peculiar substance' (ps), ×72 600. (Reproduced with permission from Fine *et al.* 1977.)

Meesmann's dystrophy is not a disorder of glycogen metabolism. The glycogen accumulation reflects a rapid turnover of epithelial cells. Normal regenerating corneal epithelium has a comparable glycogen content. The primary defect in Meesmann's corneal dystrophy is a mutation in the genes for the cornea-specific cytokeratin K3 or K12.

Clinical features

Numerous small clear or whitish-grey, closely packed punctate opacities within the epithelium are usually discernible on slit lamp biomicroscopy, especially in the interpalpebral zone, but not with the naked eye. The corneal spots, which are caused by microcysts, are uniform in size and shape and occasionally only involve the lower cornea. The abnormalities are usually bilaterally symmetrical and most often become apparent during the first 2 years of life, but sometimes not until puberty. In neonates asymptomatic epithelial opacities can be detected in affected family members. Under reflected light, the nontransparent spots resemble vesicles and droplets, and are sharply demarcated from the unaffected areas. In advanced cases the opacities, which sometimes stain with topically applied fluorescein form whorls and garlands. Initially vision is normal, but by the end of the first decade of life visual impairment, as well as episodic photophobia and lacrimation may develop. Older individuals complain of a foreign body sensation and mildly decreased visual acuity. Repeated attacks of keratitis may cause central subepithelial corneal scarring and impair vision severely enough to warrant keratoplasty.

Thiel–Behnke dystrophy (Waardenburg–Jonkers dystrophy)

Definition and aetiology

In 1967 Thiel and Behnke documented a dystrophy of the anterior cornea affecting 234 members of an 11-generation family. Honeycomb-like opacities at the level of Bowman's layer were accompanied by recurrent erosions and a moderately decreased visual acuity.

Waardenburg and Jonkers documented a family with a thin superficial stromal haze made up of snowflake-like opacities with some resemblance to granular corneal dystrophy, but with an earlier onset and an absence of radial lines and dots in the initial stage. A subsequent follow-up of the pedigree disclosed that the affected corneas contained the typical curly fibres of Thiel–Behnke dystrophy.

Pathophysiology and biochemistry

Perry, Fine, and Caldwell drew attention to characteristic curled filaments in a superficial corneal dystrophy designated Reis–Bücklers' dystrophy. These short yet to be characterized curled filaments, are interspersed among normal collagen fibrils in Bowman's zone and the contiguous structures (Fig. 7). However, a detailed study of the original pedigree described by Reis and Bücklers had rod-shaped bodies identical to those in granular corneal dystrophy, whereas electron microscopic evaluations of the family reported by Thiel and Behnke indicated that 'curly' fibres were a feature of that dystrophy. Lami-

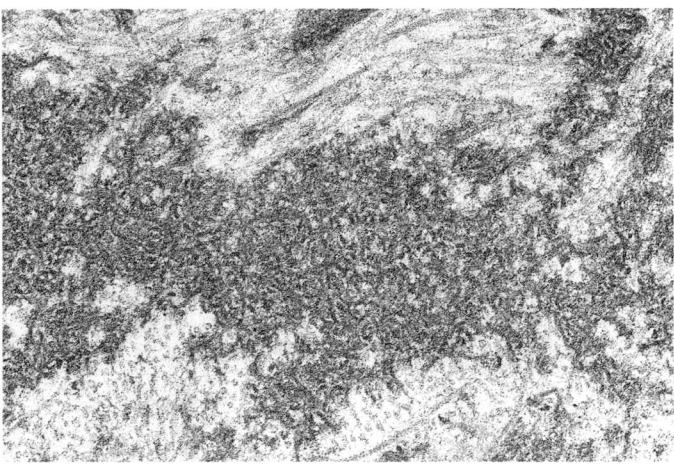

Fig. 7 Thiel–Behnke dystrophy. Transmission electron micrograph of cornea with Thiel–Behnke dystrophy illustrating the characteristic curly fibrils in the superficial corneal stroma, ×57 000. (Reproduced with permission from Klintworth 1980.)

nin and bullous pemphigoid antigen have been localized in a piebald mosaic distribution through the aberrant subepithelial fibrous tissue suggesting primarily an epithelial disease with the peculiar curly material paralleling the distribution of attachment proteins. The disease has been linked to chromosome 5 and a mutation in the $\beta ig\text{-}h3$ (keratoepithelin) gene has been identified.

Clinical features

Onset occurs during childhood with painful corneal erosions. The clinical features of Thiel–Behnke dystrophy overlap with those of Reis–Bücklers' dystrophy and the two conditions cannot be distinguished purely on clinical grounds. However, the opacification in the superficial cornea often resembles a honeycomb rather than confluent geographical opacities and visual loss tends to be less pronounced. Recurrences following keratoplasty or keratectomy seem to be later and less pronounced than in Reis–Bücklers' dystrophy.

Reis–Bücklers' corneal dystrophy

Definition and aetiology

A bilateral symmetrical dystrophy of the superficial cornea was described by Reis in 1917. Three decades later pedigree studies by Bücklers' demonstrated the condition in two to four successive generations, indicating an autosomal dominant mode of inheritance.

Pathophysiology and biochemistry

The literature on Reis–Bücklers' dystrophy is confusing because this designation has been used for at least two distinct entities. Many histopathological reports on Reis–Bücklers' dystrophy have in reality been on what is now called Thiel–Behnke dystrophy. The characteristic 'rod-shaped' bodies that accumulate within the cornea in Reis–Bücklers' dystrophy are identical to those in granular corneal dystrophy and Reis–Bücklers' dystrophy is a phenotypical variant of granular corneal dystrophy and it results from a mutation in th $\beta ig\text{-}h3$ (keratoepithelin) gene on chromosome 5 (see below). The specific deposits are located mainly in Bowman's layer and immediately beneath the corneal epithelium, which is often irregular in thickness and rests on an apparently normal basement membrane. The epithelium, particularly its basal portion, frequently manifests non-specific degenerative changes.

Clinical features

During the first or second decades of life patients usually become symptomatic with bilateral recurrent epithelial erosions. These episodes often last several weeks at a time, are precipitated by minor trauma, smoke, or dust and result in conjunctival hyperaemia, photophobia, and severe ocular pain. The epithelial erosions usually become arrested by the end of the second decade of life, sometimes only to recur again after 40 years of age. The anterior cornea becomes scarred and acquires an uneven, irregular, and roughened surface. Superficial opacities of varying sizes are associated with areas of epithelial desquamation. Despite a ground-glass like cloudiness the cornea regains its transparency. Corneal sensitivity is nearly always diminished, sometimes absent, and, rarely normal. The deep corneal stroma and endothelium as well as Descemet's membrane are not affected. Visual acuity gradually deteriorates due to diffuse, asymmetric corneal opacification and the irregular astigmatism. Rings and disc-shaped opacities form within the superficial cornea and stellate figures spread into the deeper stroma. At about 4 to 5 years of age a reticulated opacity appears in Bowman's zone of the axial cornea and progressively evolves into a central ring or geographical-shaped pattern. When viewed with the slit lamp, innumerable delicate, cotton-like strands are seen in the superficial cornea. The opacification eventually extends into the midperiphery of the cornea with a thinly distributed external stromal haze. In some cases the clinical appearance lacks these characteristics. Reis–Bücklers' dystrophy becomes symptomatic earlier and with a higher frequency of recurrent erosions than most cases of granular corneal dystrophy. In common with granular corneal dystrophy the clinical picture of Reis–Bücklers' dystrophy has also been documented in association with lattice corneal dystrophy.

Subepithelial mucinous corneal dystrophy

Definition and aetiology

The term subepithelial mucinous corneal dystrophy was coined by Feder *et al.* for a unique autosomal dominant anterior corneal dystrophy in which subepithelial mucinous material accumulates in the cornea.

Basic epidemiology

The only documented family was of Slovak descent.

Pathophysiology and biochemistry

A band of periodic acid–Schiff positive material deposits between the corneal epithelium and Bowman's layer. The accumulation stains with alcian blue (pH 1.4), is sensitive to digestion by testicular hyaluronidase, and reacts with a monoclonal antibody that recognizes 4-sulphate disaccharides of chondroitin and dermatan sulphate. When viewed by transmission electron microscopy fine fibrillar material is evident in the abnormal zone.

Based on its histochemical and immunohistochemical attributes the aberrant subepithelial accumulations contain chondroitin-4-sulphate and dermatan sulphate.

Clinical features

Frequent recurrent corneal erosions develop during the first decade of life. Bilateral subepithelial opacities and a haze involve the entire cornea, but it is most dense centrally. The clinical features resemble those of Grayson–Wilbrandt dystrophy, but the conditions differ histochemically.

Keratosis follicularis spinulosa decalvans

Definition and aetiology

Keratosis follicularis spinulosa decalvans is a rare inherited X-linked disorder that was first described by Siemens in 1926.

Basic epidemiology

All cases have been found in The Netherlands.

Pathophysiology and biochemistry

The histopathology of the condition has not been well characterized.

Clinical features

Keratosis follicularis spinulosa decalvans is characterized by cutaneous follicular papules and loss of hair (especially on scalp, eyebrows, and eyelashes). Numerous yet to be identified punctate opacities are found beneath the corneal epithelium. Marked photophobia is common. Female carriers may manifest the disorder usually in a mild form.

Principles of treatment

Recurrent corneal erosions

Initial conventional treatment is with lubricants, hypertonic saline ointment, patching, or a bandage soft contact lens. Alternative approaches are debridement of severely aberrant epithelium or superficial keratectomy to remove subepithelial debris. Eyelid hygiene and oral oxytetracycline with or without topical prednisolone is beneficial in the management of recalcitrant recurrent corneal erosions. Phototherapeutic keratectomy is promising for recurrent corneal erosions resistant to conservative conventional therapy.

Meesmann's dystrophy

Simple removal of the abnormal corneal epithelium is not effective, and the original abnormality recurs in the regenerated epithelium.

Reis–Bücklers', Thiel–Behnke, and other superficial corneal dystrophies

When visual acuity is significantly diminished the pathological tissue can be excised by superficial keratectomy, lamellar keratoplasty, or pentrating keratoplasty. However, phototherapeutic keratectomy using an argon–fluoride 193-nm excimer laser has significant advantages over other more invasive and aggressive surgery in the treatment of anterior corneal dystrophies and makes it possible to postpone corneal grafting or even makes it unnecessary. Phototherapeutic keratectomy is now the procedure of choice when intervention is required. While visual acuity often improves following phototherapeutic keratectomy a mild hyperopic shift and a haze may develop during the first few months after surgery. Unfortunately phototherapeutic keratectomy destroys the pathological tissue making it impossible to establish a tissue diagnosis.

Both penetrating and lamellar keratoplasty have yielded poor long-term results in Reis–Bücklers' and Thiel–Behnke dystrophies, because these dystrophies may recur in the graft.

Primary familial subepithelial amyloidosis

The response to both lamellar and penetrating keratoplasty as well as superficial keratectomy is unsatisfactory as amyloid recurs in the graft within about 5 years.

Further reading

Behnke, H. and Thiel, H.-J. (1965). Über die hereditäre Epitheldystrophie der Hornhaut (typ Meesmann-Wilke) in Schleswig-Holstein. *Klinische Monatsblatter fur Augenheilkunde*, **147**, 662–72.

Bücklers, M. (1949). Ueber eine Weitere familiäre Hornhautdystrophie (Reis). *Klinische Monatsblatter fur Augenheilkunde*, **114**, 386–97.

Cogan, D.G., Kuwabara, T., Donaldson, D.D. *et al.* (1974). Microcystic dystrophy of the cornea. A partial explanation for its pathogenesis. *Archives of Ophthalmology*, **92**, 470–4.

Feder, R.S., Jay, M., Yue, B.Y., *et al.* (1993). Subepithelial mucinous corneal dystrophy. Clinical and pathological correlations. *Archives of Ophthalmology*, **111**, 1106–14.

Fine, B.S., Yanoff, M. Pitts, E. and Slaughter, F.D. (1977). Meesmann's epithelial dystrophy of the cornea. *American Journal of Ophthalmology*, **83**, 633–42.

Franceschetti, A.T. (1968). La cornea verticillata (Gruber) et ses relations avec la maladie de Fabry (Angiokeratoma corporis diffusum). *Ophthalmologica*, **156**, 232–8.

Grayson, M. and Wilbrandt, H. (1966). Dystrophy of the anterior limiting membrane of the cornea (Reis–Buckler type). *American Journal of Ophthalmology*, **61**, 345–9.

Guerry, D. (1965). Observations on Cogan's microcystic dystrophy of the corneal epithelium. *Transactions of the American Ophthalmological Society*, **63**, 320–34.

Hope-Ross, M.W., Chell, P.B., Kervick, G.N., *et al.* (1994). Recurrent corneal erosion: clinical features. *Eye*, **8**, 373–7.

Irvine, A.D., Corden, L.D., Swnsson, O., *et al.* (1997). Mutations in cornea-specific keratin K3 or K12 genes cause Meesmann's corneal dystrophy. *Nature Genetics*, **16**, 184–7.

Klintworth, G.K. (1980). Corneal dystrophies. In *Ocular pathology update* (ed. D.H. Nicholson), pp. 23–54. Masson, New York.

Klintworth, G.K. and Damms, T. (1995). Corneal dystrophies and keratoconus. *Current Opinion in Ophthalmology*, **6**, 44–56.

Klintworth, G.K., Valnickova, Z., Kielar, R.A., *et al.* (1997). Familial subepithelial corneal amyloidosis a lactoferrin related amyloidosis. *Investigative Ophthalmology and Visual Science*, **38**, 2756–63.

Kuchle, M., Green, W.R., Volcker, H.E.. *et al.* (1995). Re-evaluation of corneal dystrophies of Bowman's layer and the anterior stroma (Reis–Bücklers and Thiel–Behnke types): a light and electron microscopic study of eight corneas and a review of the literature. *Cornea*, **14**, 333–54.

Meesmann, A. and Wilke, F. (1939). Klinische und anatomische Untersuchungen über eine bisher unbekannte, dominant vererbte Epitheldystrophie der Hornhaut. *Klinische Monatsblatter für Augenheilkunde*, **103**, 361.

Munier, F.L., Korvatska, E., Djemai, A., *et al.* (1997). Kerato-epithelin mutations in four 5q 31-linked corneal dystrophies. *Nature Genetics*, **15**, 247–51.

Pameijer, J.K. (1935). Ueber eine fremdartige familiäre oberflächliche Hornhautveranderung. *Klinische Monatsblatter für Augenheilkunde*, **95**, 516–17.

Perry, H.D., Fine, B.S., and Caldwell, D.R. (1979). Reis–Bücklers dystrophy: a study of eight cases. *Archives of Ophthalmology*, **97**, 664–70.

Reis, W. (1917). Familiare, fleckige Hornhauteartung. *Deutsche Tierarztliche Wochenschrift*, **43**, 575.

Rubinfeld, R.S. (1995). Recurrent corneal erosion. In *Master techniques in ophthalmic surgery* (ed. R. Rubinfeld). Williams & Wilkins, Washington DC.

Siemens, H.W. (1926). Keratosis follicular spinulosa decalvans. *Archives of Dermatological Syphilology*, **151**, 384–7.

Small, K.W., Mullen, L., Bartletta, J., *et al.* (1996). Mapping of Reis–Bücklers corneal dystrophy to chromosome 5q. *American Journal of Ophthalmology*, **121**, 384–90.

Stocker, F.W. and Holt, L.B. (1955). Rare form of hereditary epithelial dystrophy: genetic, clinical and pathologic study. *Archives of Ophthalmology*, **53**, 536–41.

Thiel, H.J. and Behnke, H. (1967). Ein bisher unbekannte subepitheliale hereditare Hornhautdystrophie. *Klinische Monatsblatter fur Augenheilkunde*, **150**, 862–74.

Waardenburg, P.J. and Jonkers, G.H. (1961). A specific type of dominant progressive dystrophy of the cornea, developing after birth. *Acta Ophthalmologica*, **39**, 919–23.

2.6.2.2 Predominantly stromal dystrophies

Gordon K. Klintworth

Granular corneal dystrophy

Definition and aetiology

A corneal dystrophy characterized by discrete granular white spots in the superficial corneal stroma was initially designated 'noduli corneae' by Groenouw, but subsequently became designated granular corneal dystrophy. This autosomal dominant condition has a mutation rate of about 0.3/1000 000. In some families penetrance is 100 per cent; in others it is incomplete.

Basic epidemiology

Granular corneal dystrophy is particularly common in Denmark, where the largest pedigree has been published.

Pathophysiology and biochemistry

Eosinophilic irregularly lobulated granules are located within the superficial central corneal stroma and occasionally between or within basal epithelial cells (Fig. 1). Sometimes the deposits are limited to the subepithelial region or the epithelium (superficial granular dystrophy). The deep and peripheral stroma as well as parts between the deposits is unremarkable, and so is Descemet's membrane and the corneal endothelium.

Masson's trichrome stain discolours the deposits red and Wilder's reticulin stain discloses tangles of argyrophilic fibres within the characteristic lesions. By transmission electron microscopy they appear as discrete, rod-shaped or trapezoid bodies with discrete borders (Fig. 2). Some appear homogeneous without a discernible inner structure; others are composed of an orderly array of closely packed filaments. Additional deposits appear moth-eaten.

Corneas with granular dystrophy contain an abundance of β_{ig}-h3 and histochemical procedures indicate that the accumu-

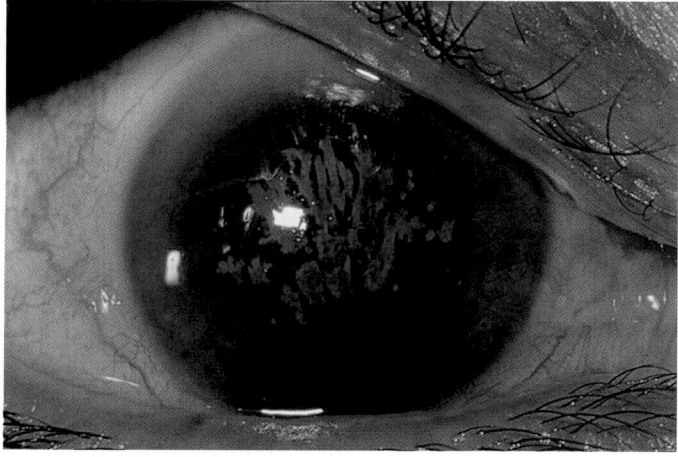

(a)

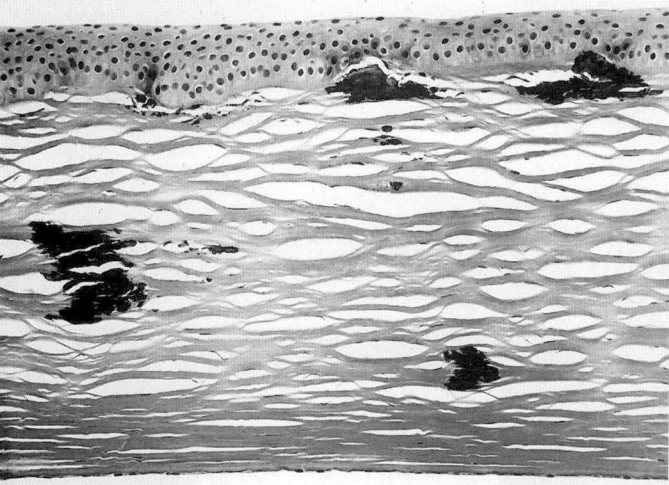

(b)

Fig. 1 (a) Granular corneal dystrophy. (b) Light microscopic appearance of stromal deposits. Masson's trichrome, ×130. (Reproduced from Klintworth 1980, with permission.)

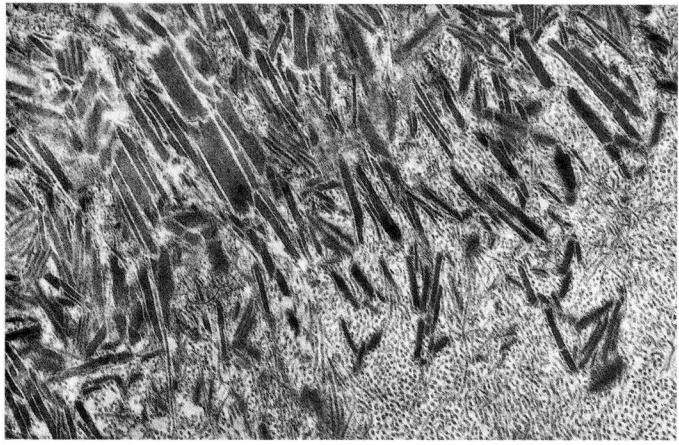

Fig. 2 Granular corneal dystrophy. Transmission electron micrograph of cornea with granular corneal dysrophy illustrating the characteristic rod-shaped bodies, ×14 820. (Reproduced from Klintworth 1980, with permission.)

lations in granular corneal dystrophy consist predominantly of protein and that they react with antibodies to the β_{ig}-h3 protein. An increased content of every phospholipid class and alterations in the fatty acid profile of phospholipids has been reported.

Sometimes amyloid is present within the corneal stroma in granular corneal dystrophy and lattice corneal dystrophy type I has been associated, initially in persons whose ancestry was traced from the Avellino region of Italy (Avellino dystrophy). The genes for granular corneal dystrophy, Avellino dystrophy, and lattice corneal dystrophy type I have been mapped to the same region of chromosome 5 (5q22–q32) (Table 1) and these dystrophies, together with Reis–Bücklers dystrophy and Thiel–Benke dystrophy result from different mutations in the β_{ig}-h3 gene.

Clinical features

Initially small white sharply demarcated ground-glass spots that resemble bread crumbs or snowflakes appear in the cornea beneath Bowman's zone within the first decade of life (Fig. 3). Sometimes they accumulate beneath, or within, the corneal epithelium. By 20 years of age many opaque spots are apparent particularly in the central and superficial cornea and rarely in the deep stroma. They eventually extend throughout almost

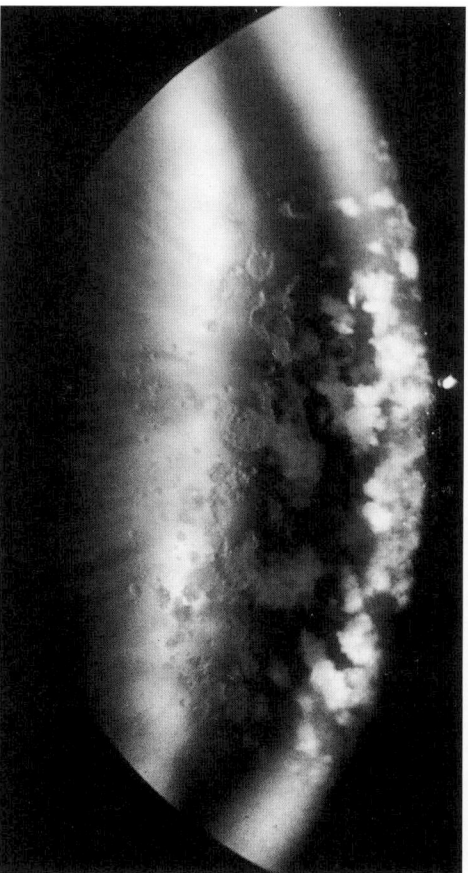

Fig. 3 Granular corneal dystrophy. Slit lamp appearance of variable shaped stromal opacities. (By courtesy of Dr G.N. Foulks.)

Table 1 Classification of stromal dystrophies

Dystrophy	Inheritance	Gene locus
Bietti's marginal crystalline dystrophy	AR	Unknown
Congenital hereditary stromal dystrophy	AD	Unknown
Familial chronic actinic keratopathy	?	Unknown
Central cloudy dystrophy	AD	Unknown
Central crystalline dystrophy (Schnyder's dystrophy)	AD	1p34.1–p.36
Fleck dystrophy	AD	Unknown
Granular dystrophy	AD	5q22–q32
Lattice dystrophy		
type I	AD	5q22–q32
type II	AD	9q34
type III	?AR	Unknown
type IIIA	AD	Unknown
Macular dystrophy		
type I	AR	16q21
type II	AR	?16q21
Posterior amorphous stromal dystrophy	AD	Unknown

AD, autosomal dominant; AR, autosomal recessive.

two-thirds of the corneal diameter. Tissue between the opacities as well as a peripheral rim of cornea remains clear. The intrafamilial variation in the appearance of the cornea may be considerable. Individuals homozygous for the granular corneal dystrophy gene may develop unusually severe granular corneal dystrophy with an earlier onset.

Vision often remains reasonable, but when the visual axis is involved eyesight becomes impaired usually after the age of 40 years. In some families vision is markedly diminished by the third decade. Recurrent epithelial erosions with episodic photophobia, conjunctival hyperaemia and ocular pain may follow a diffuse superficial corneal haze. In some families, all affected individuals develop painful episodes.

Macular corneal dystrophy

Definition and aetiology

Macular corneal dystrophy is an autosomal recessive disorder characterized by bilateral diffuse clouding of the corneal stroma and aggregations of irregular shaped greyish-white spots, especially in the superficial cornea. A gene for macular corneal dystrophy is located on chromosome 16 (16q22.1).

Basic epidemiology

The prevalence of macular corneal dystrophies varies considerably throughout the world. It is common in some inbred regions of the United States and India. In Saudi Arabia and Iceland macular corneal dystrophy is the most frequent corneal dystrophy requiring penetrating keratoplasty. In Iceland it is the main indication for a corneal graft.

Pathophysiology and biochemistry

Material that stains with histochemical methods for glycosaminoglycans accumulates within the cytoplasm of keratocytes and extracellularly within the corneal stroma, in Bowman's zone, and in Descemet's membrane (Fig. 4). Some corneal endothelial cells are affected (Fig. 5), but the corneal epithelium is not. When viewed by transmission electron microscopy involved corneal cells contain delicate fibrillogranular material within intracytoplasmic vacuoles (Fig. 6). The rough-surfaced endoplasmic reticulum is dilated within keratocytes and certain corneal endothelial cells. The stroma of macular corneal dystrophy corneas contains numerous randomly distributed electron-transparent lacunas and aggregations of filaments amongst collagen fibrils of normal diameter, but with diminished interfibrillar spacing. This close-packing of collagen fibrils may account for the reduced corneal thickness in macular corneal dystrophy.

Descemet's membrane contains electron-lucent vacuoles (presumably from pockets of extracellular glycosaminoglycans) as well as focal thickenings (cornea guttata). Deposits comparable to those in the cornea do not occur in cartilage or other non-corneal tissues.

Macular corneal dystrophy is not a lysosomal storage disease due to a defective enzyme involved in the degradation of certain corneal glycosaminoglycans. Three immunophenotypes are recognized: the more common variety (macular corneal dystrophy type I) has no detectable antigenic keratan sulphate in the serum or cornea; macular corneal dystrophy type II has normal amounts of antigenic keratan sulphate in the serum and cornea and the abnormal corneal accumulations in this variant react with antikeratan sulphate antibody. Corneas with macular corneal dystrophy types I and II synthesize dissimilar proteoglycans and lactosaminoglycan–glycoproteins. Macular corneal dystrophy type I corneas synthesize considerably less keratan sulphate and lumican than normal corneas presumably because of defective sulphation of lactosaminoglycans, but serum from patients with macular corneal dystrophy has normal sulphotransferase activity. In macular corneal dystrophy type I the

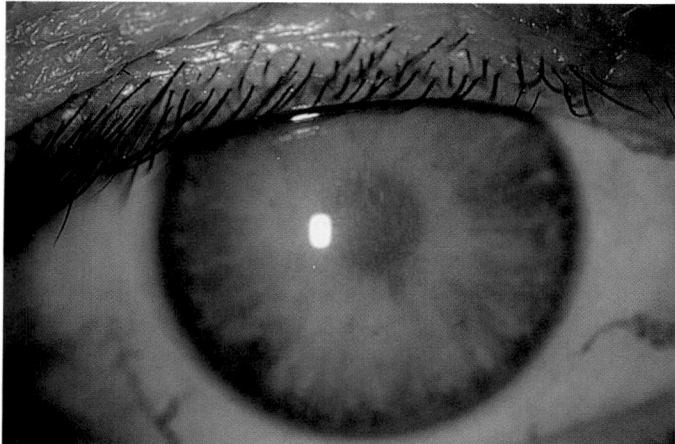

(a)

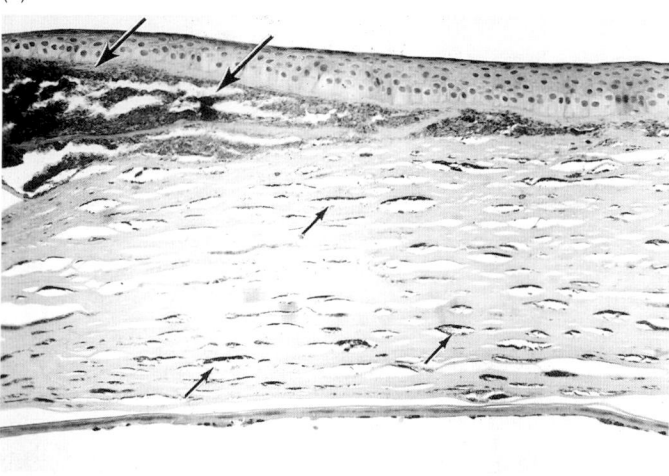

(b)

Fig. 4 (a) Macular corneal dystrophy. (b) An extracellular deposit of abnormal glycosaminoglycans is located beneath the epithelium (*large arrows*). Individual keratocytes also contain a similar substance. Hale's colloidal iron technique, ×127. (Reproduced from Klintworth 1980, with permission.)

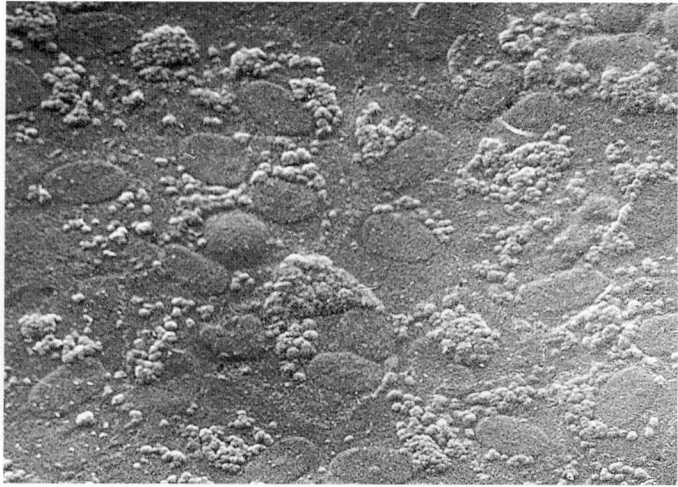

Fig. 5 Macular corneal dystrophy. Scanning electron micrograph of corneal endothelium in macular corneal dystrophy showing profiles of intracytoplasmic storage vacuoles, ×722. (Reproduced from Klintworth 1980, with permission.)

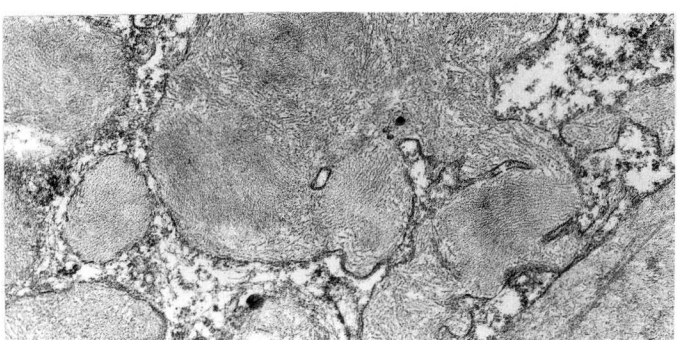

Fig. 6 Macular corneal dystrophy. Appearance of intracytoplasmic stored fibrillary material within single membrane delimited vacuoles, ×28 215. (Reproduced from Klintworth 1980, with permission.)

antigenic keratan sulphate content of nasal cartilage is at least 800 times lower than normal. A metabolic defect in macular corneal dystrophy type I presumably involves the sulphation of keratan sulphate in lumican and other keratan sulphate containing proteoglycans.

Clinical features

Ill-defined grey–white cloudy regions with indistinct edges usually first appear within a hazy stroma of both corneas during adolescence, but may become apparent in early infancy or even after the fifth decade of life. The opacities progressively merge over time as the entire corneal stroma gradually becomes cloudy causing severe visual impairment usually before the fifth decade.

Initially the central superficial stroma is mainly affected, but ultimately the opacities involve the peripheral cornea and the entire thickness of the corneal stroma. The endothelium is affected and Descemet's membrane develops guttata. In addi-

tion the cornea is often thinner than normal. In keeping with its autosomal recessive mode of inheritance parental consanguinity is frequent.

Fleck dystrophy

Definition and aetiology

In 1956, François and Neetens described two different autosomal dominant dystrophies involving the corneal stroma which came to be known by several names, including fleck and central cloudy dystrophy. Fleck dystrophy is characterized by multiple, non-progressive symmetric asymptomatic minute opacities disseminated throughout the corneal stroma. In central cloudy dystrophy asymptomatic opacities resembling clouds are found predominantly in the posterior axial corneal stroma, which is otherwise clear. Both phenotypes have been detected in the same family and even in the same individual and are almost certainly expressions of a single genetic mutation.

Basic epidemiology

This disorder appears to be uncommon worldwide.

Pathophysiology and biochemistry

In fleck dystrophy some corneal fibroblasts contain fibrillo-granular material within intracytoplasmic vacuoles or pleomorphic electron-dense and membranous intracytoplasmic inclusions. The stored material has the histochemical attributes of glycosaminoglycans and lipids and a storage disease involving these compounds is suspected. Extracellular alterations are rare, but foci of broad spaced collagen have been observed. Comparable abnormalities have not been found in other tissues.

The histopathology and biochemistry of the central cloudy phenotype is unknown.

Clinical features

The opacities are scattered symmetrically throughout a clear stroma usually in both corneas, but unilateral cases have been reported. One type of opacity consists of numerous small oval, round, wreath-like or semicircular-shaped flattened greyish particles with distinct borders ('flecks'); others that resemble clouds or snowflakes are small and greyish with ill-defined margins and are most numerous in the central third of the cornea and are occasionally most dense in the vicinity of Descemet's membrane. The disorder affects males and females equally and has been observed throughout life and even in children as young as 2 years of age. Vision is minimally affected and corneal sensation is usually normal. Rarely mild photophobia is present.

Lattice corneal dystrophies

Definition and aetiology

Lattice corneal dystrophy, a disorder of the corneal stroma with a lattice pattern of linear opacities, was first described by Biber. Its dominant inheritance was later established by Haab and Dimmer. Other types of lattice corneal dystrophy were subsequently discovered. One variety has systemic amyloidosis—lattice corneal dystrophy type II, familial amyloid polyneuropathy type IV (Finnish or Meretoja type). Another variant of lattice corneal dystrophy (type III) with an apparent autosomal recessive mode of inheritance has thick corneal lines, an older age of onset than types I and II, and an absence of recurrent corneal erosions. An additional form of lattice corneal dystrophy has thick corneal lines and a late onset equivalent to type III, but an autosomal dominant inheritance (type IIIA).

Pathophysiology and biochemistry

In all of the lattice corneal dystrophies, eosinophilic deposits have an affinity for Congo red and other dyes for amyloid and possess characteristic randomly dispersed electron-dense fibrils (80 to 100 Å in diameter) (Fig. 7). The amyloid in lattice corneal dystrophy type I is related to a mutant of β_{ig}-h3 protein; in lattice dystrophy type II (see below) it is a portion of mutated

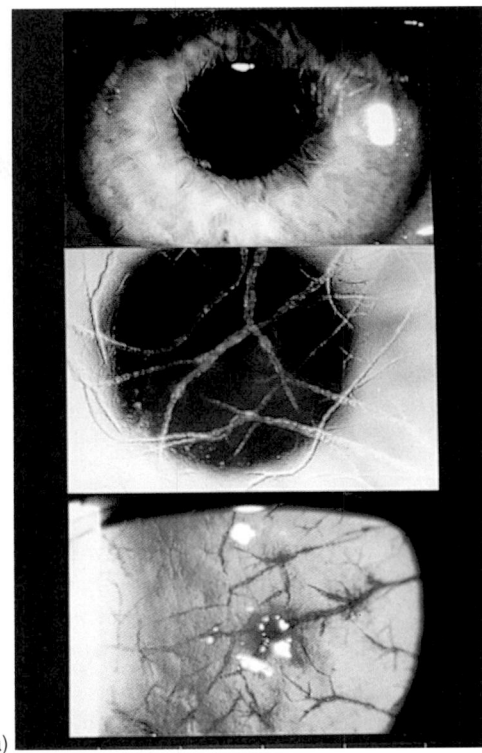

(a)

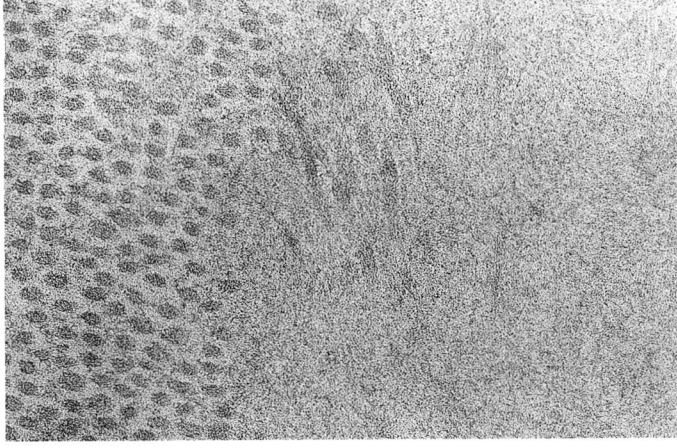

(b)

Fig. 7 (a) Lattice corneal dystrophy type I. (By courtesy of Jack Kanski and Butterworths.) (b) Transmission electron micrograph of amyloid fibrils with collagen fibres (left side), ×57 000. (Reproduced from Klintworth 1980, with permission.)

gelsolin. The nature of the amyloid in the other lattice dystrophies remains unknown. Attempts to identify it have relied on immunohistochemical analyses using antibodies to a few selected known amyloid proteins without appropriate controls and usually without adequate tissue preparation.

Lattice dystrophy type I

In lattice corneal dystrophy type I the foci of amyloid are scattered throughout the corneal stroma and sometimes immediately beneath the epithelium (Fig. 8). They are argyrophilic, but nerves are not related to the deposits. The corneal endothe-

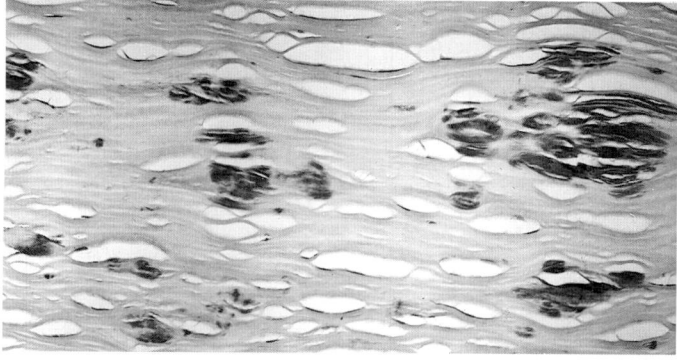

Fig. 8 Lattice corneal dystrophy type I. Light microscopic appearance of amyloid in corneal stroma. Congo red, ×130. (Reproduced with permission from Klintworth 1980.)

lium and Descemet's membrane are not involved. Amyloid has not been detected in non-corneal tissues. Lattice corneal dystrophy type I is the only inherited amyloidosis known to map to chromosome 5, suggesting that it is different from other identified amyloid proteins.

Lattice dystrophy type II

Amyloid accumulates in the corneal stroma and between the epithelium and Bowman's layer (Fig. 9). It also deposits asymptomatically in scleral, choroidal, and adnexal blood vessels as well as in the lacrimal gland and perineurium of ciliary nerves. Furthermore, amyloid accumulates in the heart, kidney, skin, nerves, wall of arteries, and other tissues. In contrast to other corneal amyloidoses the amyloid in lattice corneal dystrophy type II reacts with the antigelsolin antibody.

The amyloid in lattice corneal dystrophy type II is composed of a 71 amino acid long fragment of the actin-modulating protein gelsolin with an amino acid substitution. The responsible gene has been mapped to the long arm of chromosome 9 (9q34). The mutation in many families involves a G to A substitution

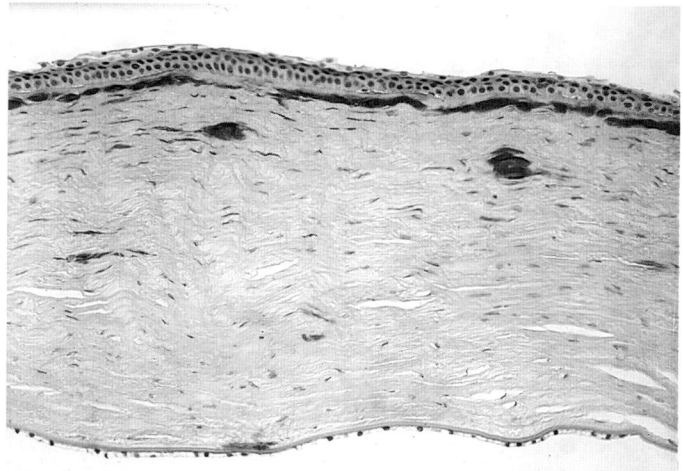

Fig. 9 Lattice corneal dystrophy type II. Light microscopic appearance of amyloid in corneal stroma in lattice corneal dystrophy type II. Congo red, ×115. (Reproduced from Klintworth 1980, with permission.)

at nucleotide 654 (codon 187), resulting in an Asn-187 variant of gelsolin. In one Danish and one Czech family a different mutation has a G to T transversion in position 654 at codon 187 which results in the substitution of tyrosine for aspartic acid (see Fig. 1).

Lattice corneal dystrophy types III and IIIA

In lattice corneal dystrophy types III and IIIA the deposits of amyloid are much thicker than those in types I and II.

Clinical features

Lattice corneal dystrophy type I

A network of delicate interdigitating branching filamentous and other shaped opacities collect particularly within the central corneal stroma, usually in both eyes. The lesions resemble nerves on casual scrutiny and corneal sensation is frequently diminished. The corneas may be asymmetrically involved; sometimes one is clear or has discrete rather than linear opacities. The dystrophy usually begins towards the end of the first decade of life, occasionally in middle life, and rarely by 2 years of age. Progression is slow and substantial discomfort and visual impairment usually ensues before the sixth decade, but the clinical course varies notably in different individuals and even within the same family. A corneal graft is usually not indicated until after the fourth decade, but may be necessary by 20 years of age. Recurrent epithelial erosions are common and as a rule begin during the first decade of life. They may antecede the corneal opacities and in some families recurrent epithelial erosions appear in individuals without stromal disease. A superficial haze of the central corneal stroma develops and becomes markedly opaque while the peripheral cornea remains relatively transparent.

Lattice corneal dystrophy type II

Both corneas contain randomly scattered short fine glassy lines, which are sparse, more delicate and more radially oriented than those in type I disease. In homozygotes it begins earlier. Vision does not usually become significantly impaired before the age of 65 years.

Progressive bilateral cranial (facial, glossopharyngeal, vagal, and hypoglossal) and peripheral nerve palsies, dysarthria, a dry and extremely lax itchy skin with amyloid deposits, a characteristic 'mask-like' facial expression, protruding lips with impaired movement, pendulous ears, and blepharochalasis are prominent (Fig. 10). Open angle glaucoma and pseudoexfoliation of the lens capsule are common.

Lattice corneal dystrophy types III and IIIA

Late in life radially orientated lattice lines much thicker than those in lattice corneal dystrophy types I and II become apparent in the anterior and midstroma in types III and IIIA disease. Usually both eyes are affected, but sporadic unilateral examples of lattice corneal dystrophy type III have been documented. Recurrent epithelial erosions were absent in the first reports of type III disease, but two sporadic cases had them.

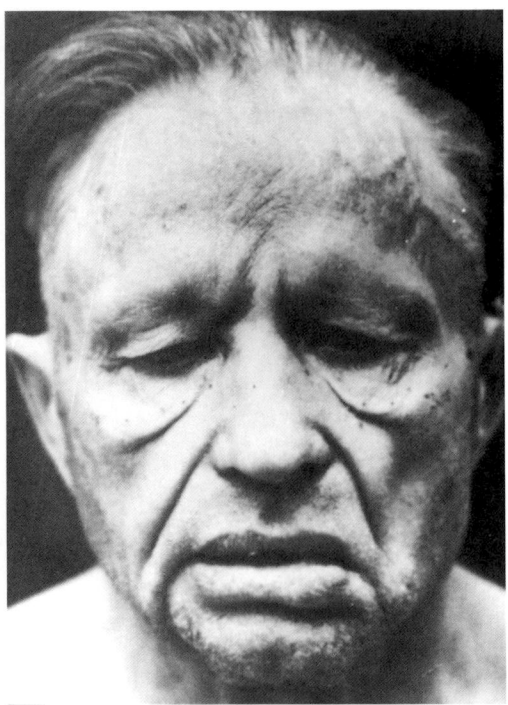

Fig. 10 Lattice corneal dystrophy type II. Facial appearance of patient with lattice corneal dystrophy type II (familial amyloid polyneuropathy type IV). (Reproduced from Meretoja 1969, with permission.)

The differences between the lattice corneal dystrophies are summarized in Table 2.

Central crystalline dystrophy (Schnyder's dystrophy)

Definition and aetiology

Central crystalline dystrophy (Schnyder's dystrophy) is characterized by crystalline opacities in the anterior central portion of both corneas. A crystalline corneal dystrophy in dogs may be the canine counterpart.

Basic epidemiology

The two largest pedigrees discovered in the United States trace their ancestry to towns within a 100 km radius on the Bay of Bothnia on the Southwest coast of Finland.

Pathophysiology and biochemistry

Birefringent cholesterol crystals and associated lipids accumulate within keratocytes and extracellularly. They dissolve during standard tissue processing, but in unfixed frozen tissue neutral fats and cholesterol are detectable histochemically. Sudanophilic neutral lipid is present in Bowman's layer, between the superficial corneal lamellae and dispersed within the stroma midst the collagen fibrils. Lipid-laden macrophages appear in the corneal stroma.

The abnormal corneal lipids, which are predominantly phospholipid and cholesterol (esterified and unesterified), probably reflect defective lipid metabolism. Familial hypercholesterolaemia, dysbetalipoproteinaemia, or hypertriglyceridaemia are sometimes associated.

Clinical features

Typically a ring-shaped yellow–white opacity composed of innumerable fine needle-shaped crystals form in Bowman's layer and the adjacent anterior stroma of the central cornea early in life. It has not been observed at birth, but may be evident by the age of 18 months. While sometimes appearing dull white, the crystals are frequently scintillating with variegated red and green hues. The remaining stroma is unremarkable initially, but with time it may acquire small white opacities and a diffuse haze. The crystals usually remain in the anterior third of the cornea, but with time the cornea usually becomes involved throughout its thickness. Within affected families the opacities manifest considerable intrafamilial variation. Only

Table 2 Comparison of lattice corneal dystrophies

	Type I	Type II	Type III	Type IIIa
Peripheral cornea		Mainly affected		
Central cornea	Mainly affected	Almost spared		
Lattice lines	Prominent	Delicate, sparse	Very thick	
Onset (years)	< 20	> 20	Late in life	
Vision		Usually good		
Keratoplasty	Common	Rare		
Corneal sensation		Normal		
Amorphous deposits	Common	Uncommon		
Nature of amyloid	Unknown	Gelsolin	Unknown	
Inheritance	AD	AD	AR	AD
Recurrent erosions	Common	No	Rare	Yes
Location of gene	5q31	9q34	Unknown	

AD, autosomal dominant; AR, autosomal recessive.

parts of the central corneal opacity may contain crystals, and occasionally, crystals are not detectable clinically. The peripheral cornea may contain a white nasal and temporal arcus and usually a clear zone persists between the corneoscleral limbus and the central corneal opacity. Unlike other lipid keratopathies corneal vascularization is absent. The condition is usually bilateral, but one eye may become affected earlier than the other. Although usually stationary after childhood, the disorder may progress over time as a dense, discoid pattern of corneal crystals along with a bilateral diminution in vision. Visual acuity is usually good, but it may become sufficiently impaired to warrant keratoplasty. The epithelium, Descemet's membrane, and the endothelium are spared.

Genu valgum has been associated, perhaps as a result of non-allelic genes with a relatively low crossover frequency. Some individuals with central crystalline dystrophy have arcus lipoides, xanthelasma, cardiovascular disease, and other manifestations of hypercholesterolaemia.

Posterior amorphous stromal dystrophy

Definition and aetiology

In 1977 Carpel, Sigelman, and Doughman reported a family with irregular symmetric grey–white, sheet-like opacities in the deep central posterior corneal stroma that spread peripherally towards the corneoscleral limbus. They coined the term posterior amorphous stromal dystrophy for this autosomal dominant disorder.

Basic epidemiology

Posterior amorphous stromal dystrophy has apparently only been detected in the United States.

Pathophysiology and biochemistry

A specimen obtained at corneal graft from a 5-year-old child disclosed disorganized posterior stromal collagen, breaks in the posterior stromal collagen lamellae, a thin Descemet's membrane, and focally attenuated endothelial cells.

Clinical features

Transparent stroma may intervene between the corneal opacities, which sometimes indent Descemet's membrane and the endothelium, which may have focal endothelial abnormalities. Both centroperipheral and peripheral forms are recognized. In advanced cases the cornea is thinner than normal. Visual acuity is usually minimally impaired, but may be severe enough to warrant a penetrating keratoplasty. Other ocular features include hyperopia with corneal flattening, iris abnormalities (glassy sheets on the iris surface, corectopia, pseudopolycoria, and iris processes extending to Schwalbe's line).

Bietti's marginal crystalline dystrophy

Definition and aetiology

Bietti's marginal crystalline dystrophy was first recognized in Italy by Bietti. The condition is characterized by delicate crystals in the peripheral cornea and retina.

Basic epidemiology

The disorder, is relatively common in China and most cases reported in the West have been of Oriental extraction.

Pathophysiology and biochemistry

Corneal and conjunctival fibroblasts as well as circulating lymphocytes contain crystals and complex osmiophilic inclusions of uncertain nature. A systemic disorder of lipid metabolism is suspected and affected individuals sometimes have hyperlipoproteinaemia.

Clinical features

Very fine crystals that are difficult to see by slit lamp biomicroscopy gather in the peripheral paralimbal anterior corneal stroma in persons with areas of retinal pigment epithelial atrophy. Similar crystals are present in all layers of the retina, especially at the posterior pole. This rare condition has a slowly progressive loss of visual function. Many cases retain good vision, but become symptomatic because of poor dark adaptation and paracentral scotomas.

Congenital hereditary stromal dystrophy

Definition and aetiology

Congenital hereditary stromal dystrophy is a congenital autosomal dominant non-progressive disorder of the cornea characterized by flaky or feathery clouding of the corneal stroma.

Basic epidemiology

Only one large family with descendants in Germany and France is known.

Pathophysiology and biochemistry

The abnormalities are limited to the corneal stroma and consist of a peculiar arrangement of tightly packed lamellae having highly aligned collagen fibrils of unusually small diameter. Nothing is known about the biochemical alterations, but the abnormally small stromal collagen fibrils and disordered lamellae suggest a disturbance in collagen fibrogenesis.

Clinical features

Flaky or feathery opacities occur particularly in the central corneal stroma, which is of normal thickness. Both Descemet's membrane and the corneal endothelium are relatively normal.

Principles of treatment

Granular dystrophy

Corneal grafting is seldom necessary in granular corneal dystrophy, but when indicated both penetrating and lamellar keratoplasty restore visual acuity with similar success, despite the fact that lamellar keratoplasty does not remove the abnormal accumulations within the deep corneal stroma. In young individuals in whom multiple procedures may be necessary over a lifetime due to recurrent disease lamellar keratoplasty, superficial keratectomy or phototherapeutic keratectomy is preferable to penetrating keratoplasty in managing visually disabling granular corneal dystrophy, especially if the deposits are limited to the superficial cornea. Granular corneal dystrophy may recur after keratoplasty (usually superficial to the donor tissue, or at the host–graft interface). The recurrence is sometimes delayed for 10 to 15 years, but in some families granular corneal dystrophy almost invariably recurs in the graft within 4 years and the recurrence-free interval is independent of the size or type of graft. Recurrences may occur within a year.

Lattice dystrophies

Initial treatment in lattice corneal dystrophy type I is symptomatic and depends on the severity of the visual impairment and discomfort of the patient. Recurrent corneal erosions can be managed as discussed elsewhere. Because the amyloid involves the entire thickness of the cornea penetrating keratoplasty is the procedure of choice when visual acuity is significantly marred. The outcome of penetrating keratoplasty is excellent, but amyloid may deposit in the donor tissue 2 to 14 years later. A corneal graft is rarely indicated in lattice corneal dystrophy type II, but when performed a neurotrophic persistent epithelial defect may develop. Treatment of lattice corneal dystrophy types III and IIIA is the same as for type I.

Macular dystrophy

The treatment for macular corneal dystrophy is penetrating keratoplasty. Rarely macular corneal dystrophy recurs in the graft after many years and this is usually not clinically significant.

Fleck and central cloudy dystrophy

Fleck dystrophy does not require specific treatment, but it did not recur in a corneal graft within 10 years in a patient who underwent a penetrating keratoplasty for an associated keratoconus.

Central crystalline dystrophy (Schnyder's dystrophy)

Because central crystalline dystrophy usually stabilizes with time, only occasional patients with severe visual impairment require corneal grafting. Hyperlipoproteinaemia and its manifestations should be considered and followed by appropriate therapy when indicated.

Further reading

Akova, Y.A., Unlu, N., and Duman, S. (1994). Fleck dystrophy of the cornea; a report of cases from three generations of a family. *European Journal of Ophthalmology*, **4**, 123–5.

Bietti, G. (1937). Ueber familäres Vorkommen von 'Retinitis punctata albescens' (verbunden mit 'Dystrophia marginalis cristallinea cornea'). Glitzern des Glaskörpers und anderen degenerativen Augenveränderungen. *Klinische Monatsblatter fur Augenheilkunde*, **99**, 737–56.

Carpe, E.F., Sigelman, R.J., and Doughman, D.J. (1977). Posterior amorphous corneal dystrophy. *American Journal of Ophthalmology*, **83**, 629–32.

de la Chapelle, A., Kere, J., Sack, G.H. Jr, *et al.* (1992a). Familial amyloidosis, Finnish type: G654—a mutation of the gelsolin gene in Finnish families and an unrelated American family. *Genomics*, **13**, 898–901.

de la Chapelle, A., Tolvanen, R., Boysen, G., *et al.* (1992b). Gelsolin-derived familial amyloidosis caused by asparagine or tyrosine substitution for aspartic acid at residue 187. *Nature Genetics*, **2**, 157–60.

Delleman, J.W. and Winkelman, J.E. (1968). Degeneratio corneae cristallinea hereditaria. A clinical, genetical and histological study. *Ophthalmologica*, **155**, 409–6.

Eiberg, H., Møller, H.U., Berendt, I., *et al.* (1994). Assignment of granular corneal dystrophy Groenouw type I (CDGG1) to chromosome 5q. *European Journal of Human Genetics*, **2**, 32–138.

Folberg, R., Stone, E.M., Sheffield, V.C., *et al.* (1994). The relationship between granular, lattice type 1, and Avellino corneal dystrophies. A histopathologic study. *Archives of Ophthalmology*, **112**, 1080–5.

Johnson, A.T., Folberg, R., Vrabec, M.P., *et al.* (1990). The pathology of posterior amorphous corneal dystrophy. *Ophthalmology*, **97**, 104–9.

Jonasson, F., Oshima, E., Thonar, E.J.-M.A., *et al.* (1996). Macular corneal dystrophy in Iceland: a clinical, genealogical and immunohistochemical study of twenty-eight cases. *Ophthalmology*, **103**, 1111–17.

Klintworth, G.K. (1980). Corneal dystrophies. In *Ocular pathology update*, (ed. D.H. Nicholson), pp. 23–54. Masson, New York.

Klintworth, G.K. (1994a). Proteins in ocular disease. In *Pathobiology of ocular disease: a dynamic approach* (ed. A. Garner and G.K. Klintworth), pp. 973–1032. Dekker, New York.

Klintworth, G.K. (1994b). Disorders of glycosaminoglycans (mucopolysaccharides) and proteoglycans. In *Pathobiology of ocular disease: a dynamic approach* (ed. A. Garner and G.K. Klintworth), pp. 855–92. Dekker, New York.

McCarthy, M., Innis, S., Dubord, P., *et al.* (1994). Panstromal Schnyder corneal dystrophy. A clinical pathologic report with quantitative analysis of corneal lipid composition. *Ophthalmology*, **101**, 895–901.

Meretoja, J. (1969). Familial systemic paramyloidosis with lattice dystrophy of the cornea, progressive cranial neuropathy, skin changes and various internal symptoms. I. A previously unrecognized heritable syndrome. *Annals of Clinical Research*, **1**, 314–24,

Moller, H.U. (1991). Granular corneal dystrophy Groenouw type I. Clinical and genetic aspects. *Acta Ophthalmologica*, **198**, (suppl) 1–40.

Steiner, R.D., Paunio, T., Uemichi, T., *et al.* (1995). Asp187Asn mutation of gelsolin in an American kindred with familial amyloidosis, Finnish type (FAP IV). *Human Genetics*, **95**, 327–30.

Stone, E.M., Mathers, W.D., Rosenwasser, G.O., *et al.* (1994). Three autosomal dominant corneal dystrophies map to chromosome 5q. *Nature Genetics*, **6**, 47–51.

Vance, J.M., Jonasson, F., and Lennon, F., *et al.* (1996). Linkage of a gene for macular corneal dystrophy to chromosome 16. *American Journal Human Genetics*, **58**, 757–62.

Weiss, J.S., Rodrigues, M.M., Kruth, H.S., *et al.* (1992). Panstromal Schnyder's corneal dystrophy. Ultrastructural and histochemical studies. *Ophthalmology*, **99**, 1072–81.

Wilson, D.J., Weleber, R.G., and Klein, M.L. (1989). Bietti's crystalline dystrophy. A clinicopathologic correlative study. *Archives of Ophthalmology*, **107**, 213–21.

Witschel, H., Fine, B.S., Grutzner, P., *et al.* (1978). Congenital hereditary stromal dystrophy of the cornea. *Archives of Ophthalmology*, **96**, 1043–51.

2.6.2.3 Posterior corneal dystrophies

Gordon K. Klintworth

Fuchs dystrophy

Definition and aetiology

Fuchs dystrophy is a bilateral corneal disorder named after the German ophthalmologist, who first described epithelial oedema, stromal clouding, and impaired corneal sensitivity in elderly individuals. Later it became recognized that hyaline excrescences form centrally on Descemet's membrane (cornea guttata) in this condition. Fuchs dystrophy is the commonest posterior corneal dystrophy (Table 1).

Fuchs dystrophy appears to have an inherited predisposition. The condition may involve siblings and affect two or more successive generations, apparently as an autosomal dominant disorder with greater expressivity in the female. Most patients with Fuchs dystrophy lack a positive family history, but blood relatives sometimes manifest cornea guttata.

Rarely cornea guttata have been noted at birth and such non-progressive congenital guttata frequently have an autosomal dominant inheritance. Some acquired cornea guttata have been observed in monozygotic twins, in siblings, and in two or more successive generations. Such observations support an autosomal dominant mode of inheritance of some cornea guttata. Familial cornea guttata may coexist with anterior polar cataracts.

Cornea guttata may also be a sequel to interstitial keratitis, ageing, and macular corneal dystrophy. When secondary to interstitial keratitis, the guttate excrescences tend to be confluent and aligned in a geographical pattern.

Basic epidemiology

Fuchs dystrophy is relatively common in the United States and in certain other countries, but it is extremely rare in Saudi Arabians and the Japanese.

Pathophysiology and biochemistry

In Fuchs dystrophy the corneal endothelium contains intracellular vacuoles of variable size and a dilated intercellular space. This abnormal cellular monolayer is often attenuated and frequently contains intracytoplasmic melanin that is probably derived from the iris (Fig. 1). The corneal endothelial cells may manifest fibroblast-like features.

Numerous prominent anvil- or mushroom-shaped excrescences project from the posterior surface of Descemet's membrane (cornea guttata) (Fig. 2). These manifest a variety of patterns: some are focal thickenings of Descemet's membrane, others are multilayered, and some are encased in multilaminated collagenous tissue. Fissures, which contain attenuated portions of corneal endothelial cells or cellular debris, are prominent within some guttata. These guttata are similar to clinically

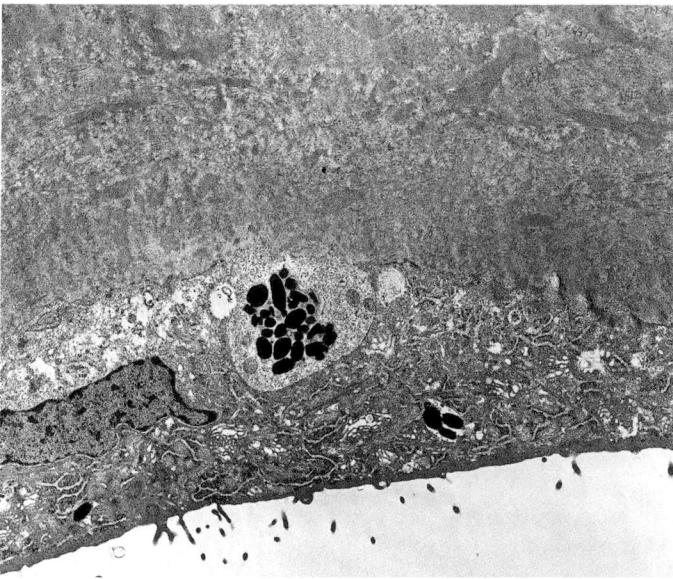

Fig. 1 Fuchs dystrophy. Transmission electron micrograph of corneal endothelial cell and an adjacent collagenous layer containing fibrils running in variable directions. The endothelial cell contains melanosomes, ×6670. (Reproduced from Klintworth 1980, with permission.)

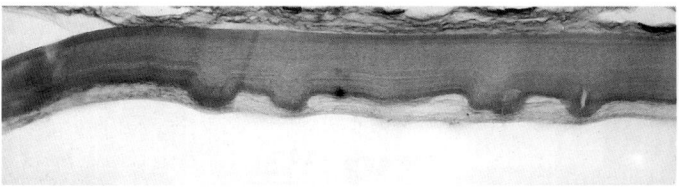

Fig. 2 Fuchs dystrophy. Light microscopic appearance of cornea guttata associated with a delicate collagenous layer. Masson's trichrome, ×300. (Reproduced from Klintworth 1980, with permission.)

Table 1 Classification of posterior corneal dystrophies

Disease	Inheritance	Gene locus
Congenital hereditary dystrophy		
autosomal recessive type	AR	Unknown
autosomal dominant type	AD	20p
Cornea farinata (steroid sulphatase deficiency)	XR	Xp22.32
Deep filiform dystrophy (steroid sulphatase deficiency)	XR	Xp22.32
Fuchs dystrophy	AD	Unknown
Posterior polymorphous dystrophy		
autosomal dominant type	AD	20q12–q13.1
autosomal recessive type	AR	Unknown

AD, autosomal dominant; AR, autosomal recessive; XR, X-linked recessive.

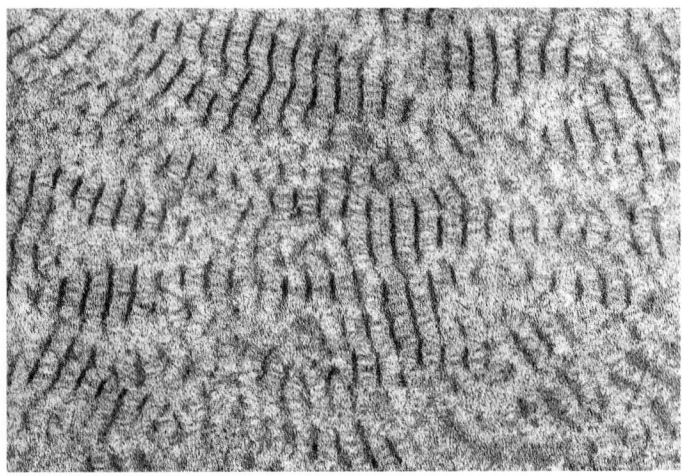

Fig. 3 Fuchs dystrophy. Transmission electron micrograph of malaligned broad-banded collagen in Descemet's membrane, ×22 500. (Reproduced from Klintworth 1980, with permission.)

insignificant excrescences (Hassall–Henle bodies) which form on the peripheral part of Descemet's membrane, but they tend to be larger and cleft formation occurs infrequently. When examined by transmission electron microscopy the cornea guttata resemble the normal anterior banded fetal portion of Descemet's membrane, but the striated bands are haphazardly arranged in cornea guttata, and in the thickened Descemet's membrane (Fig. 3).

Aside from having guttate excrescences Descemet's membrane is multilayered and often irregularly thickened (two to four times normal) due to excessive collagen deposition. The anterior (100–110 nm) banded fetal portion of Descemet's membrane and the contiguous non-banded portion of this structure is normal. An extra layer posterior to Descemet's membrane contains bundles and sheets of fibrous long spacing collagen with a cross-striational macroperiodicity of about 55 to 110 nm and shorter subbands (about 30–40 nm apart). Within this material horizontal fibrils run perpendicular to the vertical bands. A layer containing delicate collagen fibrils is intermingled with homogenous basement membrane-like material on the posterior surface of the cornea in advanced cases and often buries existing guttata. Extracellular material that reacts with antibodies to fibrin and fibrinogen is present in the posterior collagenous layer.

Corneas with Fuchs dystrophy manifest the sequelae of chronic epithelial and stromal oedema. In mild cases the basal epithelium is oedematous, but in advanced examples the epithelial basement membrane adhesion complexes are abnormal and the corneal epithelium is separated from the underlying basement membrane, which is often fragmented and not attached to the basal epithelium by hemidesmosomes. In advanced cases subepithelial collagenous tissue accumulates in the region of bullous oedema. Bowman's layer is usually unremarkable.

The corneal endothelium degenerates prematurely and produces excessive amounts of an abnormal Descemet's membrane

of a type analogous to that assembled *in utero*. As the endothelial cells greatly diminish in number with age without the capacity to undergo cell division the enduring cells spread to provide a complete monolayer that initially remains effective as a barrier and pump in maintaining corneal deturgescence. Simultaneously Descemet's membrane thickens diffusely and develops guttate excrescences. Ultrastructural abnormalities in Descemet's membrane suggest that the endothelial cell function is abnormal prior to 20 years of age.

Sequential observations on numerous patients have disclosed that the endothelial alterations precede the epithelial changes. After remaining sparse in the central cornea for years guttata may become abundant. As endothelial cells progressively degenerate they become ineffective in maintaining corneal hydration so that the corneal stroma and epithelium become oedematous and bullous keratopathy develops. Most individuals with cornea guttata do not manifest epithelial and stromal oedema.

Clinical features

Fuchs dystrophy customarily presents clinically during the fifth or sixth decade of life and seldom at an earlier age. Women are affected much more often than men and comprise about 75 per cent of cases. Asymptomatic guttate excrescences form on the central portion of Descemet's membrane in association with a delicate stippling of bronze pigment in the corneal endothelium. On slit lamp biomicroscopy Descemet's membrane has a beaten metal appearance. Slowly, over one to two decades the cornea guttata become more numerous, and Descemet's membrane gradually thickens. One eye can be involved earlier or more severely than the other, but the dystrophy almost always becomes bilateral. Vision becomes blurred, especially on awakening and symptoms of glare develop. Eventually the corneal stroma becomes oedematous axially and spreads peripherally. With time the epithelium becomes involved and subepithelial bullae form (bullous keratopathy). These blisters frequently rupture causing a foreign body sensation or pain and sometimes secondary infection follows. Ultimately a subepithelial pannus forms and this compromises visual acuity further. Cataract extraction, the implantation of an intraocular prosthetic lens or other intraocular surgery accelerates the progression of the dystrophy by damaging existing endothelial cells.

Posterior polymorphous corneal dystrophy

Definition and aetiology

Posterior polymorphous corneal dystrophy is an inherited disorder in which the corneal endothelium consists of cells with varied appearances. Similar configurations of the posterior surface of the cornea may follow recurrent uveitis and keratitis (posterior polymorphous keratopathy).

Blood relatives of persons with typical posterior polymorphous corneal dystrophy may have autosomal dominant congenital hereditary endothelial dystrophy (hereditary corneal oedema), which is probably a manifestation of the same disorder. A gene for autosomal dominant posterior polymorphous corneal dystrophy has been mapped to the pericentromeric region of human chromosome 20 (20q12–q13.1). A gene for autosomal dominant congenital hereditary endothelial dystrophy is also located in this region supporting the earlier belief that the two disorders may be related.

Pathophysiology and biochemistry

Because posterior polymorphous corneal dystrophy is usually asymptomatic, corneal tissue has only been examined in cases severe enough to require penetrating keratoplasty. Instead of an endothelial monolayer the posterior cornea is lined by variable numbers of stratified squamous epithelial cells having tonofilaments, cytokeratin, and desmosomes (Fig. 4). These cells have numerous microvilli (Fig. 5), but unlike normal corneal epithe-

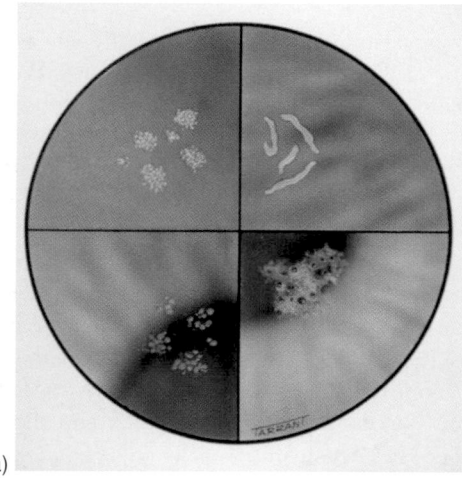

(a)

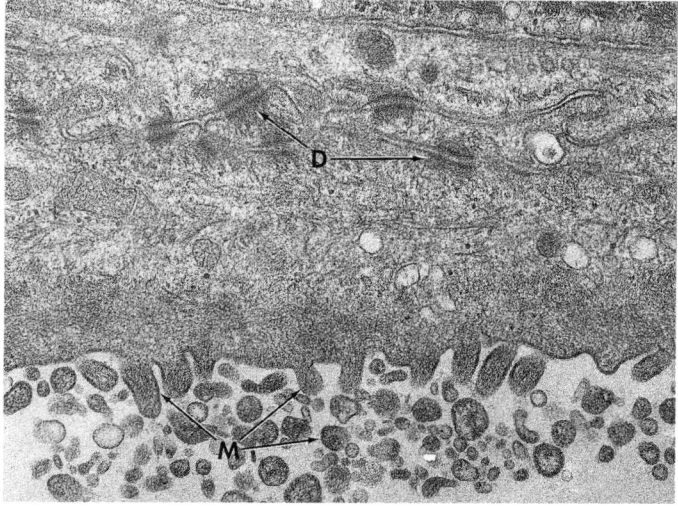

(b)

Fig. 4 (a) Posterior polymorphous dystrophy. (By courtesy of Jack Kanski and Butterworths.) (b) Transmission electron micrograph of epithelial cells lining the posterior corneal surface (D, desmosomes; M, microvilli). (Reproduced from Boruchoff and Kuwabara 1971, with permission.)

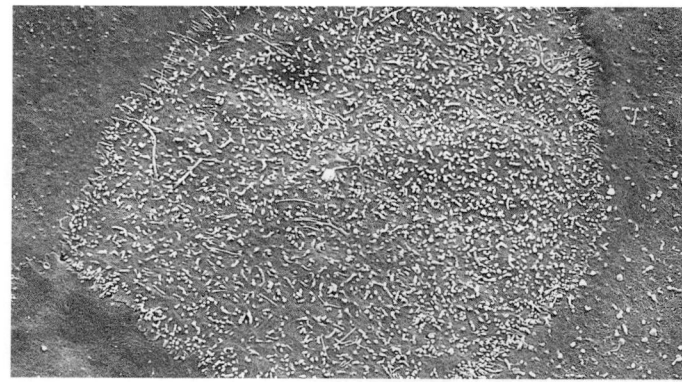

Fig. 5 Posterior polymorphous dystrophy. Scanning electron micrograph showing numerous microvilli on surface of cells covering the posterior cornea, × 855. (Reproduced from Klintworth 1980, with permission.)

lium, microplicae are not a feature. Cells on the posterior corneal surface of Descemet's membrane may also have a fibroblast-like appearance. By transmission electron microscopy the anterior banded fetal layer (110-nm banded layer) of Descemet's membrane is usually unremarkable, but may be thin in the axial cornea in infants. In such instances the paraxial portion of this layer contains defects, and the peripheral cornea lacks Descemet's membrane. Posteriorly, the anterior banded zone is lined by degenerate endothelial cells, fibroblast-like cells and a collagenous layer. Defects in Descemet's membrane contain abnormal keratocytes.

An irregularly thickened, multilaminar Descemet's membrane, occasionally contains focal nodular excrescences, but typical cornea guttata are absent. The normal non-banded portion is thinner than normal and a layer posterior to it contains numerous delicate collagen fibrils (10–20 nm in diameter with a normal cross-striational periodicity) as well as long spacing collagen (with a banding of 55–110 nm) interspersed with fine granular homogeneous basement membrane-like material.

The abnormalities of the corneal endothelium presumably represent anomalous development secondary to a genetic mutation. Failure to produce a continuous anterior banded zone indicates that the cornea is affected before the twelfth week of gestation. In other cases the morphologically unremarkable anterior banded portion of Descemet's membrane indicates that the corneal endothelium synthesizes normal basement membrane until late in gestation. Because posterior polymorphous corneal dystrophy is usually not associated with corneal oedema, the corneal endothelium presumably maintains a normal state of corneal hydration in most affected individuals.

Two possible explanations for the stratified squamous epithelial cells on the posterior surface of the cornea exist. These morphologically abnormal cells may have been displaced during ocular development. Alternatively, they may have undergone metaplasia after lining the posterior surface of the cornea. The latter possibility seems more likely because mesothelial cells in other tissues sometimes acquire epithelial or fibroblastic features under pathological conditions.

Clinical features

In posterior polymorphous corneal dystrophy the posterior surface of the cornea is lined by cells with an extremely variable appearance. Slit lamp biomicroscopy is ordinarily sufficient to substantiate the diagnosis, but specular microscopy helps to distinguish posterior polymorphous corneal dystrophy from other disorders. Both corneas are commonly affected, but sometimes asymmetrically. Most patients are asymptomatic and are discovered incidentally because visual impairment is usually insignificant. Some cases develop oedema of the corneal stroma and epithelium. This is occasionally evident at birth or during infancy. Posterior polymorphous corneal dystrophy may remain stable or gradually progress and lead to keratoplasty by middle age.

Sometimes broad adhesions are present between the iris and the peripheral cornea. Descemet's membrane may extend on to the anterior surface of the iris and obliterate the anterior chamber angle, at times causing glaucoma. In this regard the entity resembles the iridocorneoendothelial syndrome (iris–nevus syndrome, Chandler's syndrome, and essential iris atrophy).

Congenital hereditary endothelial dystrophy

Definition and aetiology

An inherited bilateral congenital relatively non-progressive diffusely symmetrical corneal oedema caused by a disorder of the endothelium has been recognized since the beginning of this century. The entity is now known as congenital hereditary endothelial dystrophy and autosomal dominant and autosomal recessive types are recognized. A gene for autosomal dominant congenital hereditary endothelial dystrophy has been mapped to the same pericentromeric region of human chromosome 20 as autosomal dominant posterior polymorphous corneal dystrophy.

Basic epidemiology

Congenital hereditary endothelial dystrophy is rare in most countries but is the second most frequent corneal dystrophy in Saudi Arabia. In Saudi Arabia recessive congenital hereditary endothelial dystrophy is found, but in the United Kingdom the autosomal dominant type is commoner than the autosomal recessive variety.

Pathophysiology and biochemistry

Only occasional abnormalities are apparent in the corneal endothelium in early childhood, but these cells are sparse and extensively abnormal by the age of 14 years. The remaining endothelial cells are often atrophic and may undergo fibroblastic transformation. Descemet's membrane possesses a normal anterior 110-nm banded portion, but the posterior non-banded region is absent or narrower than normal. In contrast to Fuchs dystrophy guttata are absent. Delicate collagen fibrils (20–40 nm in diameter) and variable quantities of basement membrane-like material may produce a thick collagenous layer behind Descemet's membrane. This band contains collagen types I, III, IV, and V, and an excessive amount of laminin: the latter is also localized to fine-banded and granular material in the posterior non-banded zone. The corneal stroma is markedly oedematous, but unlike other forms of corneal oedema individual collagen fibres within the stroma are considerably thicker than normal (sometimes attaining a diameter of 600 Å).

Non-specific morphological consequences of chronic corneal oedema include swollen basal epithelial cells, a thickened epithelial basement membrane with disruptions, and irregularities of Bowman's layer and pannus formation.

The defective corneal endothelium fails to produce a normal Descemet's membrane and does not maintain the cornea in a deturgescent state. The endothelial abnormalities become manifest *in utero* after the fetal anterior portion of Descemet's membrane is produced. The thickened collagen fibres within the corneal stroma suggests that the stromal opacification is not solely caused by oedema and that defective collagenesis by the corneal fibroblasts occurs.

Clinical features

Autosomal recessive congenital hereditary endothelial dystrophy is evident at or shortly after birth and pursues a non-progressive course, whereas the slowly progressive autosomal dominant type (infantile hereditary endothelial dystrophy) presents during the first 2 years of life with photophobia and tearing. Nystagmus is a feature of autosomal recessive congenital hereditary endothelial dystrophy, but is absent in the dominant variety. Bilateral corneal clouding ranges from a slight haze to a milky, ground-glass opacification. The cornea is two to three times thicker than normal (much thicker than a cornea with diffuse corneal oedema due to posterior polymorphous corneal dystrophy).

Epithelial microbullae may be evident. Despite extreme epithelial and stromal oedema symptoms of discomfort are inconspicuous. Descemet's membrane sometimes appears uniformly thickened, but without guttata.

Deep filiform dystrophy and cornea farinata

The terms deep filiform dystrophy and cornea farinata have been applied to small grey punctate opacities that accumulate in the deep stroma immediately anterior to Descemet's membrane in the central cornea, or in a ring around the middle of the cornea. Deep filiform dystrophy has been noted in association with keratoconus and X-linked ichthyosis (steroid sulphatase deficiency). The opacities in ichthyosis may also have the appearance of cornea farinata.

Pathophysiology and biochemistry

Keratocytes anterior to Descemet's membrane contain membrane-bound intracytoplasmic vacuoles that included fibrillo-granular material and electron-dense lamellar bodies. In

X-linked ichthyosis abnormal depositions of basement membrane protein have been identified in the anterior stroma. Immunoglobulin deposits may generate deep filiform opacities in hypergammaglobulinaemia.

Clinical features

The opacities are of variable shape and may resemble commas, circles, lines, threads (filiform), flour (farina), or dots. Deep filiform dystrophy consists of small multiple thread-like, grey opacities in the pre-Descemet area that affect the entire width of the cornea except for the perilimbal region. In this disorder the corneal subepithelial and anterior stromal layers may contain white–grey granular opacities associated with irregular overlying corneal epithelium and a thickened basement membrane including irregular extensions into Bowman's layer. Small punctate or filiform opacities form in the deep corneal stroma.

The opacities in cornea farinata, which is common in elderly individuals, resemble flour and do not usually reduce visual acuity.

Principles of treatment

Fuchs dystrophy

The symptoms of bullous keratopathy may be relieved by lubricants, a bandage soft contact lens, or cautery of Bowman's layer. Eventually penetrating keratoplasty is required for visual rehabilitation.

Posterior polymorphous corneal dystrophy

Patients with severe endothelial decompensation and impaired vision from stromal oedema require penetrating keratoplasty. Posterior polymorphous dystrophy can recur in the graft following perforating keratoplasty.

Congenital hereditary corneal dystrophy

Penetrating keratoplasty is the only available treatment. Because of possible amblyopia this should be performed early in life and the second cornea needs to be grafted soon after the first one.

Further reading

Adamis, A.P., Filatov, V., Tripathi, B.J., *et al.* (1993). Fuchs' endothelial dystrophy of the cornea. *Survey of Ophthalmology*, **38**, 149–68.

al Faran, M.F. and Tabbara, K.F. (1991). Corneal dystrophies among patients undergoing keratoplasty in Saudi Arabia. *Cornea*, **10**, 13–16.

Boruchoff, S.A. and Kuwabara, T. (1971).Electron microscopy of posterior polymorphous degeneration. *American Journal of Ophthalmology*, **72**, 879–87.

Bourne, W.M., Johnson, D.H., and Campbell, R.J. (1982). The ultrastructure of Descemet's membrane. III. Fuchs' dystrophy. *Archives of Ophthalmology*, **100**, 1952–5.

Brooks, A.M., Grant, G., and Gillies, W.E. (1989). Differentiation of posterior polymorphous dystrophy from other posterior corneal opacities by specular microscopy. *Ophthalmology*, **96**, 1639–45.

Curran, R.E., Kenyon, K.R., and Green, W.R. (1974). Pre-Descemet's membrane corneal dystrophy. *American Journal of Ophthalmology*, **77**, 711–16.

Dohlman, C.H. (1951). Familial congenital cornea guttata in association with anterior polar cataract. *Acta Ophthalmologica (Copenhagen)*, **29**, 445–73.

Grandon, S.C. and Weber, R.A. (1994). Radial keratotomy in patients with atypical inferior steepening. *Journal of Cataract and Refractive Surgery*, **20**, 381–6.

Grayson, M. and Wilbrandt, H. (1967). Pre-Descemet dystrophy. *American Journal of Ophthalmology*, **64**, 276–82.

Heon, E., Mathers, W.D., Alward, W.L., *et al.* (1995). Linkage of posterior polymorphous corneal dystrophy to 20q11. *Human Molecular Genetics*, **4**, 485–8.

Hirst, L.W. and Waring, G.O. (1983). Clinical specular microscopy of posterior polymorphous endothelial dystrophy. *American Journal of Ophthalmology*, **95**, 143–55.

Hogan, M.J., Wood, I., and Fine, M. (1974). Fuchs' endothelial dystrophy of the cornea. 29th Sanford Gifford Memorial lecture. *American Journal of Ophthalmology*, **78**, 363–83.

Iwamoto, T. and DeVoe, A.G. (1971). Electron microscopic studies on Fuchs' combined dystrophy. I. Posterior portion of the cornea. *Investigative Ophthalmology and Visual Science*, **10**, 9–28.

Kanai, A., Waltman, S., Polack, F.M., *et al.* (1971). Electron microscopic study of hereditary corneal edema. *Investigative Ophthalmology*, **10**, 89–99.

Kayes, J. and Holmberg, A. (1964). The fine structure of the cornea in Fuchs' endothelial dystrophy. *Investigative Ophthalmology and Visual Science*, **3**, 47–67.

Klintworth, G.K. (1980). Corneal dystrophies. In *Ocular pathology update*, (ed. D.H. Nicholson), pp. 23–54. Masson, New York.

Kraupa, A. (1934). Ueber Epithel und Endotheldystrophien. *Zeitschrift für Augenheilkunde*, **83**, 179–89.

Laganowski, H.C., Sherrard, E.S., and Muir, M.G. (1991). The posterior corneal surface in posterior polymorphous dystrophy: a specular microscopical study. *Cornea*, **10**, 224–32.

Levenson, J.E., Chandler, J.W., and Kaufman, H.E. (1973). Affected asymptomatic relatives in congenital hereditary endothelial dystrophy. *American Journal of Ophthalmology*, **76**, 967–71.

Liakos, G.M. and Casey, T.A. (1978). Posterior polymorphous keratopathy. *British Journal of Ophthalmology*, **62**, 39–45.

Lorenzetti, D.W.C., Uotila, M.H., Parikh, H. *et al.* (1967). Central cornea guttata. Incidence in general population. *American Journal of Ophthalmology*, **64**, 1155–8.

McTigue, J.W. (1967). The human cornea: a light and electron microscopic study of the normal cornea and its alterations in various dystrophies. *Transactions of the American Ophthalmological Society*, **65**, 591–660.

Maeder, G. and Danis, P. (1947). Sur une nouvelle forme de dystrophie cornéenne (dystrophia filiformis profunda corneae) associée à un kératocône. *Ophthalmologica*, **114**, 246–8.

Miller, K.H., Green, W.R., Stark, W.J., *et al.* (1980). Immunoprotein deposition in the cornea. *Ophthalmology*, **87**, 944–50.

Paufique, L. and Etienne, R. (1950). La 'cornea farinata'. *Bulletin de la Societe d Ophtalmologie*, **50**, 522.

Pippow, G. (1941). Erbbedingheit der Cornea farinata. (Mehlstaubartige Hornhautedegeneration). *Albrecht von Graefes Archives of Ophthalmology*, **144**, 276–9.

Polack, F.M. (1974). The posterior corneal surface in Fuchs' dystrophy. Scanning electron microscope study. *Investigative Ophthalmology*, **13**, 913–22.

Polack, F.M. (1976). Contributions of electron microscopy to the study of corneal pathology. *Survey of Ophthalmology*, **20**, 375–414.

Rosenblum, D., Stark, W.J., Maumenee, I.H., *et al.* (1980). Hereditary Fuchs' dystrophy. *American Journal of Ophthalmology*, **90**, 455–62.

Santo, R.M., Yamaguchi, T., Kanai, A., *et al.* (1995). Clinical and histopathologic features of corneal dystrophies in Japan. *Ophthalmology*, **102**, 557–67.

Sekundo, W., Lee, W.R., Kirkness, C.M., *et al.* (1994). An ultrastructural investigation of an early manifestation of the posterior polymorphous dystrophy of the cornea. *Ophthalmology*, **101**, 1422–31.

Theodore, F.H. (1939). Congenital type of endothelial dystrophy. *Archives of Ophthalmology*, **21**, 626–38.

Toma, N.M.G., Ebenezer, N.D., Inglehearn, C.F., *et al.* (1995). Linkage of congenital hereditary endothelial dystrophy to chromosome 20. *Human Molecular Genetics*, **4**, 2395–8.

Waring, G.O., Bourne, W.M, Edelhauser, H.F., *et al.* (1982). The corneal endothelium. Normal and pathologic structure and function. *Ophthalmology*, **89**, 531–90.

2.6.2.4 Corneal ectasias

Gordon K. Klintworth

Keratoconus

Definition and aetiology

Keratoconus is a progressive, non-inflammatory, axial thinning of the cornea. The condition has a genetic predisposition and mechanical factors are probably involved in its pathogenesis. In numerous cases the inheritance is autosomal dominant or autosomal recessive; in others it is multifactorial. Keratoconus has been reported in monozygotic twins, but also in only one of two identical twin pairs. Affected pedigrees manifest variable expressivity with some blood relatives only developing myopic asymmetrical astigmatism or preconical stages of keratoconus. Corneal abnormalities in some family members requires computer-assisted topographical analysis for detection.

A variety of different conditions may accompany keratoconus (Table 1) and some associations seem to reflect genetic factors. For example, genetic factors rather than excessive eye rubbing caused by poor visual acuity seems to be important for the association with Leber's congenital amaurosis.

Also, the connection between keratoconus and atopy may be genetic. Individuals with atopy frequently have a positive family history of this immunological response and several independent genetic systems along with environmental factors are probably involved in the reaction. Genes influencing atopy include those involved in the immune response, immunoglobulin E production, responses of type 2 helper cells, cytokines, and a putative atopy gene on human chromosome 11 (11q13).

A relationship with entities that predispose to ocular rubbing or pressure implicates a role for excessive eye rubbing or tension in the causation of keratoconus. In keratoconus tears in Bowman's layer and Descemet's membrane suggest corneal stretching. Perhaps mechanical pressure on the eye causes collagen lamellae to slide over each other and become displaced peripherally and so thinning the corneal stroma. Repeated vigorous eye rubbing is characteristic of most patients with keratoconus and of several associated conditions (atopic traits, skin diseases, contact lens wearing, ocular disorders with poor vision, and Down's syndrome and other causes of mental retardation) and this may intensify, hasten, or even cause keratoconus.

Reduced mechanical stability of the cornea is also suspected of producing keratoconus, because the distensibility and elasticity of the corneal tissue may be increased. Ocular rigidity is decreased in some cases of keratoconus. Rigid contact lenses frequently generate photokeratoscopic images that simulate early keratoconus, but the question of whether contact lenses cause keratoconus, or contribute to its expression, in predisposed individuals remains unanswered. Because contact lenses are commonly used to treat myopia, astigmatism, and early keratoconus the association may be coincidental.

Basic epidemiology

Keratoconus is estimated to affect between 50 and 230 persons per 100 000 population and individuals of both sexes are probably affected equally. The overall average annual rate is 2.0 per 100 000 population in one county in the United States (Olmsted County, Minnesota). The overall prevalence rate in that population is 54.5 per 100 000.

Pathophysiology and biochemistry

The corneal epithelium is frequently of irregular thickness with iron in areas corresponding to Fleischer's ring. The epithelial basement membrane may be abnormally thickened, fragmented, or disrupted. Multiple focal prominent fractures of Bowman's zone correspond to the linear and often branching clear spaces which are frequently evident on slit lamp biomicroscopy (Fig. 1). They become filled with keratocytes and collagen (Fig. 2).

The corneal stroma is thinner than usual, especially in the ectatic portion. Synchrotron X-ray diffraction patterns indicate that the corneal stroma is thinner in keratoconus as a result of closer packing of the collagen fibrils. The collagen fibres are of standard diameter and the individual collagen lamellae may be thinner than normal or of usual thickness. Evidence of collagen degeneration as found in corneal ulcers is conspicuously absent. Corneal fibroblasts may manifest ultrastructural abnormalities

Table 1 Conditions associated with keratoconus

Leber's congenital amaurosis
Down's syndrome (trisomy 21)
Atopic disease
    vernal keratoconjunctivitis
    bronchial asthma
    hay fever
    atopic dermatitis (eczema)
Connective tissue disorders
    Ehlers–Danlos syndrome
    other systemic disorders of collagen
Direct mechanical pressure on globe
    floppy eyelid syndrome
    contact lens wear

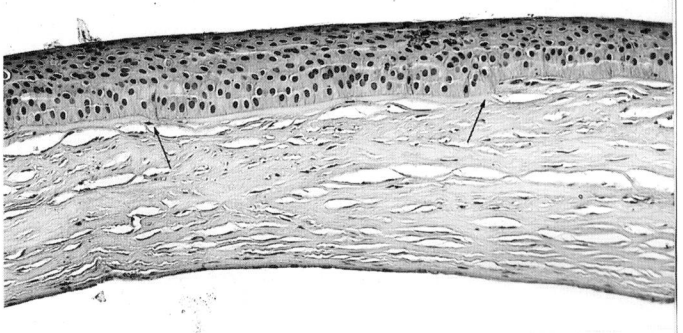

Fig. 1 Light microscopy of cornea with keratoconus illustrating the thinner than normal corneal stroma and fractures in Bowman's layer (arrows). Haematoxylin and eosin, ×114. (Reproduced from Klintworth 1994, with permission.)

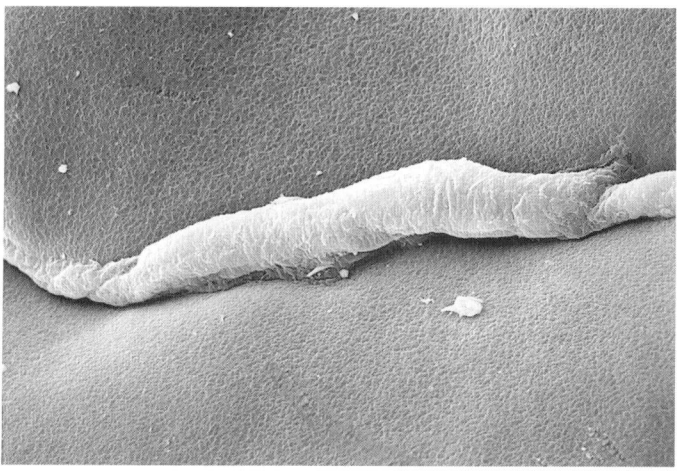

Fig. 2 Scanning electron micrograph of surface of Bowman's layer in keratoconus illustrating the herniation of fibrocollagenous tissue through a defect in Bowman's layer, ×594.

and abundant fibrillogranular material, sometimes surrounds abnormal corneal fibroblasts and separates individual collagen fibres. The corneal stroma occasionally contains amyloid deposits. Late in the course of the disease the stroma may be thickened by oedema following ruptures of Descemet's membrane. After such episodes the torn edges of Descemet's membrane become retracted as scrolls and the corneal endothelium with its contiguous recently formed Descemet's membrane extends over the exposed posterior stroma.

Keratoconus is probably not a discrete disorder, but the final common path of several pathological processes with different causes. The corneal thinning results from the loss of structural components in the stroma, while stretching of the cornea increases its curvature. Little is known about the fundamental defect(s) that lead to the corneal thinning or why keratoconus becomes arrested as an abortive form in certain members of affected families, but this could occur because of fewer collagen lamellae, less collagen fibrils per lamella, closer packing of collagen fibrils, or combinations of these possibilities. These abnormalities could follow defective formation of the corneal extracellular matrix, a destruction of previously formed components of the cornea (from digestion by increased levels of proteolytic and other enzymes) or decreased levels of protease inhibitors (such as α_1-antitrypsin, α_2-macroglobulin), an increased distensibility of corneal tissue with sliding of the collagen fibres and/or collagen lamellae, or combinations of these mechanisms.

Evidence in favour of a loss of corneal stroma by enzymatic digestion caused by a disturbance in the balance between proteases and their inhibitors is supported by biochemical and immunohistochemical studies. One notable observation is the increased collagenolytic activity in corneas with keratoconus, as well as in the medium surrounding organ cultures or corneal fibroblast cultures from affected corneas. However, against collagenolysis being the basis of corneal thinning in keratoconus is the lack of expected morphological features of stromal destruction from excessive enzymatic digestion of collagen. Both the corneal epithelium and stroma have been proposed as

the source of proteolytic activity. The corneal epithelium is suspected because of an apparent increase in lysosomal acid hydrolase activity, and this possibility finds support in the weaker than normal immunohistochemical staining of the epithelial basement membrane using antibodies to fibrin or fibrinogen in keratoconus corneas. However, if an initial digestion from an epithelial source did take place one would expect the initial defect to be digestion of the underlying basement membrane. Evidence for this is lacking.

Because the mechanical strength of the cornea depends primarily on collagen, and especially its cross-links, much attention has been devoted to corneal collagen in keratoconus. In most studies collagen synthesis, structure, or composition has been normal. Except for osteogenesis imperfecta type I, the collagen in keratoconus corneas has been normal. With the exception of scar tissue in the superficial cornea collagen types I, III, IV, V, VI, and VII have a normal distribution in corneas with keratoconus. One study found prolyl-4-hydroxylase activity to be elevated in keratoconus corneas, suggesting that the synthesis of collagen by such tissue may be enhanced.

Research on keratoconus has been severely hampered by several factors: (a) difficulties in defining the early stages of keratoconus; (b) all tissue studies have occurred late in the course of the disorder when scarring, prior treatment, and other secondary effects complicate interpretations; (c) investigations have usually failed to consider potentially important associations; and (d) an acceptable experimental model of keratoconus has not yet been identified. A major difficulty in understanding keratoconus stems from the fact that many observations have not been confirmed and investigators who have carried out apparently comparable studies have made conflicting observations. Explanations for contradictory reports include the almost certain heterogeneity of keratoconus, the vagaries of cell culture systems, different states of activation of cultured corneal fibroblasts, and associated corneal scarring.

Clinical features

Keratoconus usually becomes apparent in one eye during adolescence and in about a quarter of the cases, the condition slowly progresses, particularly during the second decade, before eventually stabilizing (Fig. 3). In up to 90 per cent of cases both corneas eventually become affected. Sometimes one eye appears to be spared, but in such cases the conical deformity is often mild in the other cornea and accompanied by asymmetric astigmatism.

The initial clinical manifestation is frequently a minimal irregular astigmatism detectable using the placido disc, retinoscope, keratometer, keratoscope, or computer-assisted videokeratography (Fig. 4). Sophisticated instrumentation allows the course of keratoconus to be followed objectively. The distinction between contact lens induced corneal warpage and early keratoconus may be difficult, but automated computer-assisted videokeratoscopy can differentiate keratoconus patterns from other conditions. Computer-assisted photokeratoscopy can detect a slightly relucent anterior corneal stroma in early keratoconus before slit lamp biomicroscopy.

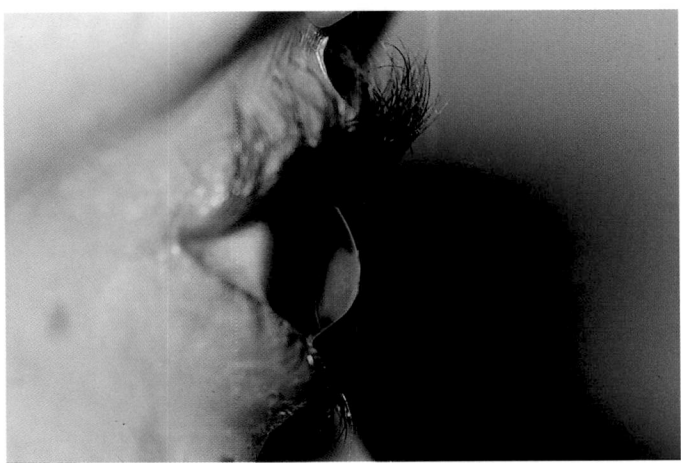

Fig. 3 Clinical photograph of cornea with keratoconus. (By courtesy of Dr Alan Carson.)

Videokeratography has led to the recognition of a clinical entity designated keratoconus suspect. It has been detected in more than 10 per cent of eyes screened for refractive surgery. The earliest physical sign of keratoconus is a steepening of the corneal curvature. At an early stage the entire cornea becomes thinner than normal, especially at the cone, as its apex protrudes forward. The ectasia most often involves the inferotemporal paracentral cornea and the cone extends towards the corneoscleral limbus. The cone may have a well-demarcated round nipple-shape usually with a slightly inferonasal apex. It may also be oval shaped and sagging and this tends to be closer to the corneoscleral limbus and displaced inferotemporally. The cone rarely affects the entire corneal surface. Some central conical corneas resemble a bow-tie as in astigmatism, but in contrast to the latter the gradient of cones is usually asymmetric. In downgaze the cone distorts the lower eyelid producing a V-shaped configuration (Munson's sign) (Fig. 5). Irregular superficial linear and branching defects are frequently evident in Bowman's layer at the conical apex and opaque subepithelial scars frequently follow them. In long-standing cases, a prominent yellow or olive-green arc or ring (Fleischer's ring) often forms in the epithelium at the base of the cone.

Progressive visual impairment follows the irregular myopic astigmatism and opacification of the cone. Corneal opacities may also result from amyloid deposition. In advanced keratoconus lateral illumination of the cornea sharply focuses light near the nasal part of the corneoscleral limbus (Rizzuti's sign).

In keratoconus corneal hypoaesthesia is most marked in the inferior cornea coinciding with the area of pronounced protru-

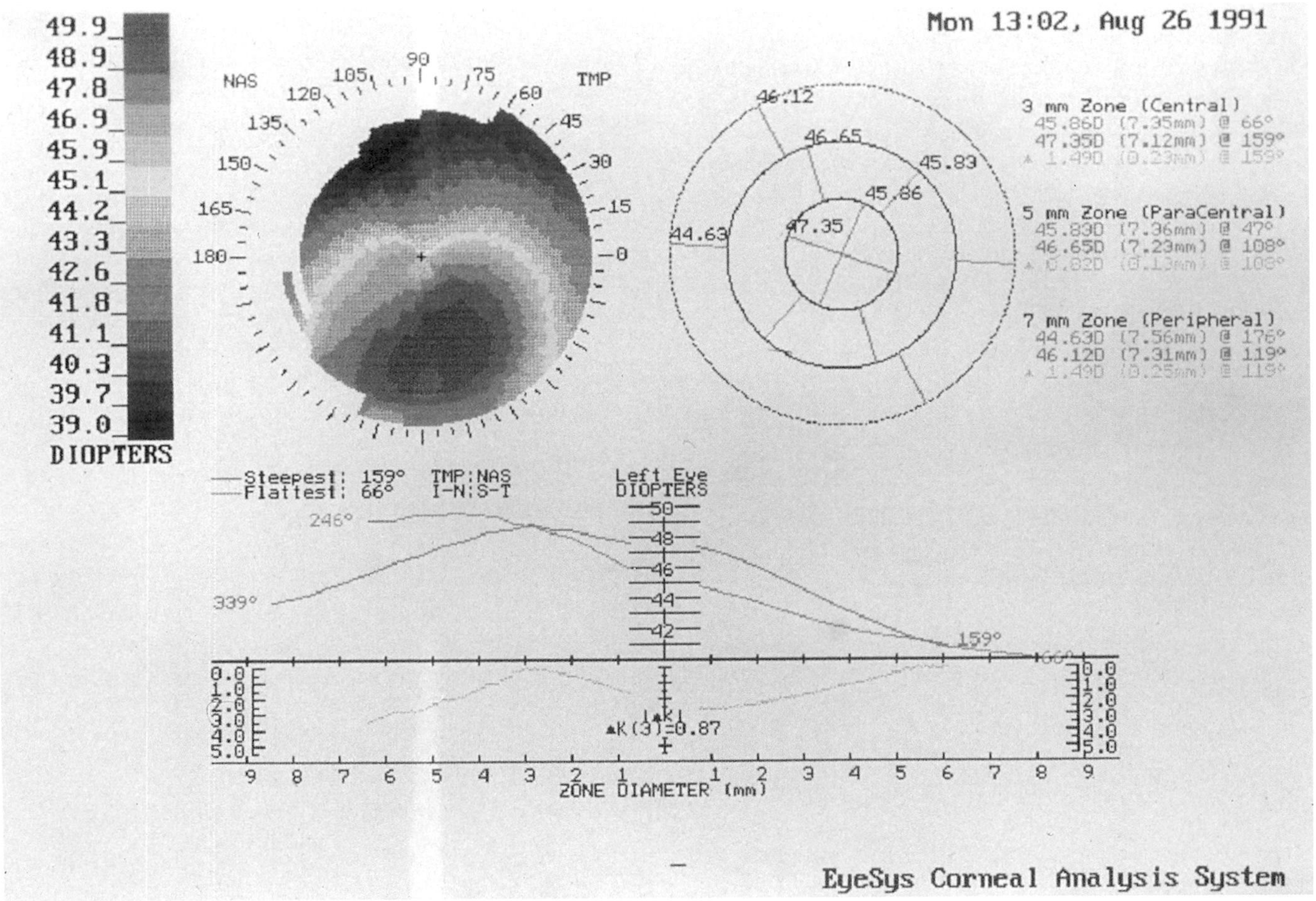

Fig. 4 Videokeratograph of normal cornea with keratoconus. (By courtesy of Dr Alan Carson.)

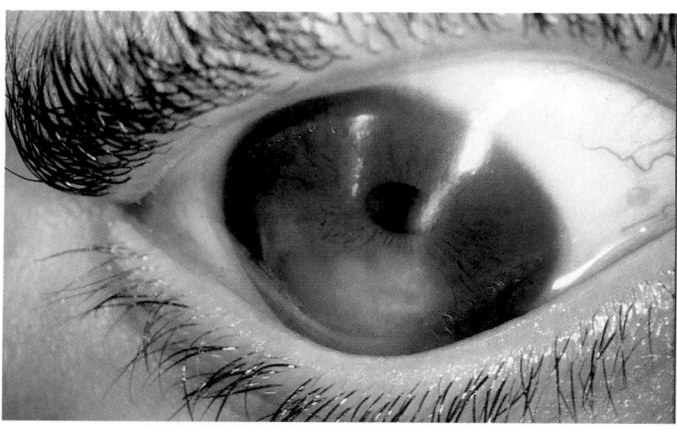

Fig. 5 Keratoconus demonstrating a positive Munson's sign. (By courtesy of Dr Alan Carson.)

sion. The corneal nerves in keratoconus do not differ from controls despite previous claims that they become more prominent than usual.

Deep within the posterior stroma and Descemet's membrane vertical striations are frequently detected (Vogt's striae). Descemet's membrane and the endothelium may crack and produce an abrupt turbid swelling of the central corneal stroma in the region of the cone (acute hydrops). This sometimes follows vigorous eye rubbing and is particularly common in Down's syndrome and other causes of mental retardation. Following acute hydrops the cornea can regain its transparency, while the defects in Descemet's membrane become scarred. Rarely, a stromal pseudocyst in continuity with the anterior chamber develops through breaks in Descemet's membrane and simulates severe corneal ectasia. Corneal perforation is extremely rare.

Endothelial cells elongate with their long axes parallel to the lines of stress, with increased variation in area (polymegathism) and shape (pleomorphism) and a decreased number of hexagonal cells. This may be due to contact lens wear.

Keratoglobus

Definition and aetiology
Keratoglobus is a bilateral non-progressive disorder in which the corneal tissue is uniformly thinned. The condition may be related to keratoconus as both entities have been noted in some families. Special cases are associated with Ehlers–Danlos syndrome, the blue sclera syndrome or Leber's congenital amaurosis, but not with megalocornea or congenital glaucoma.

Basic epidemiology
Keratoglobus is extremely rare worldwide.

Pathophysiology and biochemistry
Tissue has been examined rarely. Features have included an absence of Bowman's layer and a markedly thin corneal stroma, which is sometimes scarred. A variably thickened corneal epi-

thelium as well as breaks in Bowman's layer and Descemet's membrane may be present.

Clinical features
The cornea is transparent with a globoid ectasia. Its diameter is normal or somewhat increased. Keratoglobus is almost always present at birth, but may apparently start during adolescence or in later life. Occasionally Descemet's membrane ruptures.

Posterior keratoconus

Definition and aetiology
Posterior keratoconus is a non-progressive non-inflammatory disorder in which the posterior corneal surface has a focal (keratoconus posticus circumscriptus) or diffuse concavity, whereas the anterior surface of the cornea has a normal curvature. Most cases occur sporadically; some are familial.

Basic epidemiology
Posterior keratoconus is rare worldwide.

Pathophysiology and biochemistry
The steepening of the posterior corneal curvature results from a loss of the adjacent stroma. Bowman's layer is absent centrally and the stromal lamellae anterior to the concavity are irregular in thickness and in organization. In contrast to Peters' anomaly Descemet's membrane and the corneal endothelium are intact. Excrescences may be present on Descemet's membrane, which is occasionally thickened around the depression.

Clinical features
Posterior keratoconus is usually an isolated unilateral congenital anomaly, but some cases are associated with other ocular abnormalities, such as an anterior polar cataract, lenticonus, ectopia lentis, or posterior polymorphous dystrophy with iris adhesion. The lens is extremely close to the posterior surface of the cornea. Systemic abnormalities found in some cases include short stature, hypertelorism, a flat nose, a webbed neck, and an abnormal gait.

Terrien's disease

Definition and aetiology
Terrien's disease (marginal degeneration, Terrien's disease, senile marginal degeneration, Fuchs' degeneration) is a rare idiopathic bilateral symmetric non-inflammatory marginal corneal thinning.

Basic epidemiology
This disorder affects males more often than females.

Pathophysiology and biochemistry
Bowman's layer and the peripheral superficial stroma are destroyed in the involved thin region. The affected area may

be replaced with vascularized fibrocollagenous tissue. A thin fibrovascular layer may extend between the epithelium and Descemet's membrane in the site of degenerated collagen lamellae. A leucocytic infiltrate is evident initially but is not a major component.

Clinical features

This painless condition usually becomes evident after 50 years of age, but may occur over a wide age range (10–70 years). The malady begins in the upper peripheral cornea as a marginal opacification and can extend towards the central cornea. A non-inflamed opaque zone and an indentation parallel to the corneo-scleral limbus form and slowly develop into a gutter-like furrow, while the overlying epithelium remains intact. The thin base eventually bulges forwards and the iris may prolapse into the ectasia in late cases. Irregular astigmatism caused by the altered corneal curvature at the site of the corneal thinning can be significant clinically.

Principles of treatment

Keratoconus

Treatment initially depends on the severity of the irregular astigmatism and includes the use of glasses and rigid contact lenses. In advanced cases surgical correction needs a lamellar or penetrating keratoplasty, epikeratoplasty, thermokerato-plasty, or wedge resection of the cornea.

Contact lenses

Severe astigmatism can be corrected with a rigid contact lens. In people who cannot tolerate this, an oxygen permeable hard contact lens 'piggybacked' on a soft lens may be successful. Failures may result from giant papillary conjunctivitis, difficulty in lens handling, lack of motivation, and severe defects in corneal curvature. Striae and an enhanced visibility of them may develop after placing rigid gas permeable contact lenses on corneas with early keratoconus. In contrast to irregular astigmatism they subside in keratoconus upon removal of the rigid lens.

Thermokeratoplasty

Thermokeratoplasty is sometimes a permissible temporary procedure, but is usually followed by resteepening, scarring, or persistent epithelial defects.

Epikeratoplasty

Epikeratoplasty can flatten the cornea in keratoconus but is unsatisfactory for correcting refractive errors. This procedure may be useful in individuals in whom apical scarring does not encompass the visual axis. Radial and astigmatic keratotomy are unpredictable in keratoconus, but can be performed after a previous epikeratoplasty. Experience with more patients is needed to determine if the combination of epikeratoplasty and refractive keratotomy can be advocated in the treatment of keratoconus.

Excimer laser superficial keratectomy

In selected cases excimer laser superficial keratectomy can smooth the corneal surface and reduce the steepness of the cone. Ablation of prominent central corneal opacifications with phototherapeutic keratectomy enables patients to be fitted with a contact lens and thereby obtain good visual acuity. Patients do not experience pain during the procedure and report minimal discomfort postoperatively. The opacification may recur but can be retreated successfully.

Keratoplasty

In advanced keratoconus after visual loss is no longer correctable with glasses or contact lenses penetrating keratoplasty provides a long-term successful visual restoration. Even in Down's syndrome corneal transplantation may improve the quality of life, but some cases fail because of postoperative trauma and/or infection. The visual results of lamellar kerato-plasty in keratoconus corneas with contact lens intolerance or marked corneal scarring over the visual axis compare favourably with penetrating keratoplasty. Despite the fact that the donor material is usually thicker than the adjacent recipient tissue the success rate of corneal grafting is high (> 80 per cent). Most rejections are reversible with steroid treatment and some have survived up to 10 years.

A suction-guided trephine or intraoperative keratometry can potentially reduce trephination errors and astigmatism after suture removal. After penetrating keratoplasty the graft steadily becomes thinner reaching a subnormal thickness about 6 months postoperatively, but the grafted tissue then gradually thickens and attains a normal compactness within 6 years of corneal grafting. The axial length of the eye shortens after penetrating keratoplasty if the donor tissue has a diameter 0.3 mm less than the excised recipient cornea and is a major determinant of postoperative refractive error. Keratoconus sometimes recurs in the graft after many years.

Posterior keratoconus

When indicated penetrating keratoplasty may be necessary, but the other associated ocular abnormalities hinder its success rate.

Keratoglobus

Therapy is difficult and contact lenses are dangerous because of the high risk of perforation. The diffuse thinness of the cornea and sclera makes penetrating keroplasty problematic. Epikerophakia has been advocated.

Terrien's disease

Therapy mainly focuses on grafts that prevent and patch perforations of the thin ectatic regions.

Further reading

Bechrakis, N., Blom, M.L., Stark, W.J., et al. (1994). Recurrent keratoconus. Cornea, 13, 73–7.

Crews, M.J., Driebe, W.T. Jr, and Stern, G.A. (1994). The clinical management of keratoconus: a 6-year retrospective study. CLAO Journal, 20, 194–7.

Elder, M.J. (1994). Leber congenital amaurosis and its association with keratoconus and keratoglobus. *Journal of Pediatric Ophthalmology and Strabismus*, 31, 38–40.

Kenney, M.C., Chwa, M., Opbroek, A.J., *et al.* (1994). Increased gelatinolytic activity in keratoconus keratocyte cultures. A correlation to an altered matrix metalloproteinase-2/tissue inhibitor of metalloproteinase ratio. *Cornea*, 13, 114–24.

Klintworth, G.K. (1994). Degenerations, depositions and miscellaneous reactions of the ocular anterior segment. In *Pathobiology of ocular disease: a dynamic approach*, (2nd edn), (ed. A. Garner and G.K. Klintworth), pp. 743–94. Dekker, New York.

Klintworth, G.K. and Damms, T. (1995). Corneal dystrophies and keratoconus. *Current Opinion in Ophthalmology*, 6, 44–56.

Kremer, I. (1991). Terrien's marginal degeneration associated with vernal conjunctivitis. *American Journal of Ophthalmology*, 111, 517–18 (letter).

Kwitko, I.L., Justo, D.M., Putz, C., and Kwitko, S. (1994). Intraocular lens implantation in Terrien's marginal corneal degeneration. *Journal of Cataract and Refractive Surgery*, 20, 78–9.

Lembach, R.G. (1991). Keratoconus. *International Ophthalmology Clinics*, 31, 71–82.

Marsh, D.G. (1995). Genetics of atopy and IgE. In *Samter's immunologic diseases* (ed. M.M. Frank, K.F. Austin, H.N. Charman, and E.R. Unanue), pp. 1257–72. Little, Brown, Boston.

Mortensen, J. and Ohrstrom, A. (1994). Excimer laser photorefractive keratectomy for treatment of keratoconus. *Journal of Refractive and Corneal Surgery*, 10, 368–72.

Rabinowitz, Y.S. (1998). Keratoconus. *Survey of Ophthalmology*, 42, 297–319.

2.6.3 Corneal infectious disease

Gavin W. Marsh and David L. Easty

Infections of the cornea can be caused by a vast number of diverse organisms that may be difficult to differentiate solely by their clinical features. Indeed, different groups of organisms may cause infection in similar circumstances as a result of common predisposing factors. Thus accurate diagnosis may be difficult and must be approached systematically. Decisions on management must rely on careful analysis and good judgement, and particularly in the case of infectious disease, on whether there is quiescent or active inflammation. Understanding how to determine this is important, and can only be gained by clinical experience.

Corneal inflammation

Inflammatory disease of the cornea, whether caused by microbial agents or immunological processes, requires a full examination of the external eye. This detailed examination can easily be neglected in busy clinics, but careful observation avoids mistakes in diagnosis and treatment. Always examine the lids and lid margins for subtle signs of blepharitis, meibomitis, and tri-

We would like to acknowledge Dr John Leeming of the Department of Microbiology, University of Bristol, for his help in the preparation of this manuscript

chiasis; palpate for a preauricular gland, check the tarsal plates, tear film, and marginal strip, and examine for limbal pathology, which can be subtle. The manifestations of corneal disease are commonplace, but can direct attention to the cause in many conditions. Inflammatory disease of the cornea is peripheral and/or central, and epithelial, stromal or both.

Corneal inflammatory disease can effect the three main corneal layers individually or in combination. Damage to the epithelium commonly presents as superficial keratitis, whereas stromal disease manifests as interstitial keratitis.

Superficial keratitis

In superficial keratitis the inflammatory process is affecting the corneal epithelium and superficial stromal lamellae. Many diverse conditions may produce superficial corneal disease, which may be manifest as punctate epithelial erosions, or punctate epithelial or subepithelial keratitis. In many instances they may coexist and diagnosis of the underlying cause is often based on the distribution and exact nature of the corneal abnormality, the staining characteristics with vital dyes, and associated generalized and, in particular ocular adnexal, findings.

Punctate epithelial erosions

These are minute areas of focal epithelial loss, transparent under normal illumination and requiring demonstration with stains such as fluorescein. They are non-specific and may accompany almost any kind of keratitis—traumatic, toxic, or inflammatory. Although such lesions appear negligible, they can induce marked symptoms of foreign-body sensation, photophobia, tearing, and blepharospasm. Their treatment must depend upon the original cause. Table 1 lists the common causes. An uncommon cause is known as superior limbic keratoconjunctivitis, where there is hyperaemia and oedema of the upper limbus, with punctate staining of the conjunctival surface extending on to the upper part of the cornea (Fig. 1).

The distribution of punctate epithelial erosions is helpful in differential diagnosis. Generalized lesions occur in drug toxicity, and in early bacterial and viral infections. Lesions confined to the upper cornea suggest superior limbic keratoconjunctivitis, chlamydial infection, or vernal disease. An interpalpebral distribution may occur in exposure, damage caused by ultraviolet light, dry eye, or, if centrally located, excessive wearing of contact lenses. Inferior corneal lesions suggest staphylococcal blepharoconjunctivitis or abnormalities of the lower lid such as lagophthalmos, trichiasis, or entropion. Localized linear lesions should prompt a search for sources of mechanical damage such as a subtarsal foreign body or conjunctival concretion. In factitious, self-inflicted injury in malingerers or psychologically disturbed patients, linear plus punctate erosions can be seen, particularly in the lower nasal quadrant of the cornea, often extending on to the conjunctiva. In the recurrent erosion syndrome, signs suggestive of an epithelial dystrophy may be evident (see Section 2.6.2).

Punctate epithelial keratitis

This is characterized by white or opaque lesions that are visible without the aid of a stain. They represent focal accumulations

Table 1 Causes of punctate epithelial erosions in the cornea

Toxicity:
Medications
Contact lens solutions

Trauma:
Direct
Contact lens wear
Dry eye
Exposure keratopathy
Ultraviolet light exposure

Lid disease:
Entropion
Trichiasis
Warts
Molluscum bodies
Trapped subtarsal foreign body
Blepharoconjunctivitis

Conjunctival disease:
Vernal disease
Mucous membrane pemphigoid
Erythema multiforme
Reiter's disease

Infections:
Herpes simplex
Varicella zoster
Trachoma
Inclusion conjunctivitis (TRIC)
Bacterial

Others:
Superior limbic keratoconjunctivitis
Recurrent erosion syndrome
Rosacea
Neuroparalytic keratopathy

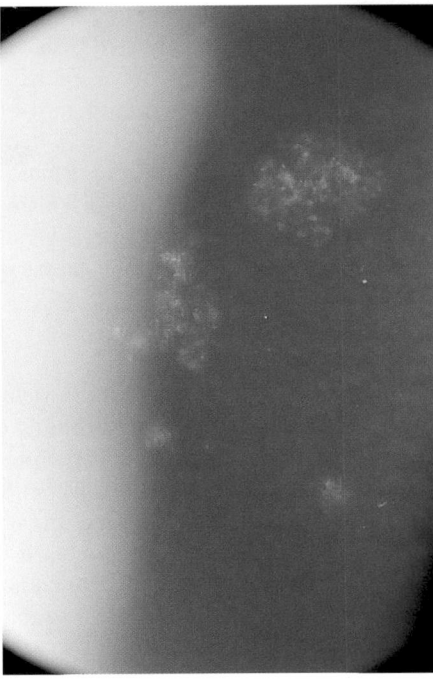

Fig. 2 Thygeson's punctate epithelial keratitis (illustration by courtesy of Nicholas Brown).

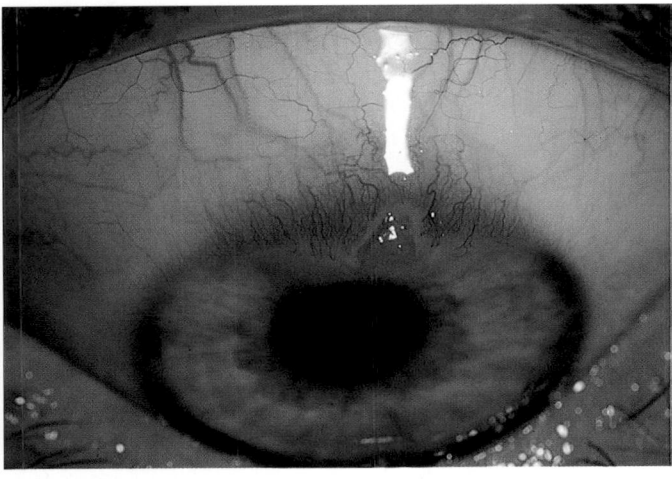

Fig. 1 Punctate corneal erosions in the upper third of the cornea in superior limbic keratitis.

of epithelial cells and adjacent inflammatory cells that characteristically stain a brilliant red with rose bengal, though they may also take up fluorescein if associated with an epithelial erosion. These lesions may be fine, when they are only visible under slit-lamp examination, or coarse, when they may be visible with the naked eye. Fine lesions are most commonly associated with viral infections, typically adenovirus but also in such as molluscum contagiosum or herpes simplex keratitis. A similar appearance may be seen in staphylococcal blepharoconjunctivitis, allergic keratoconjunctivitis, trachoma and inclusion conjunctivitis, keratitis sicca, rosacea keratitis, and, rarely, with vaccinia or Reiter's syndrome. Coarse lesions are typical of late adenoviral disase and Thygeson's superficial punctate keratitis (Fig. 2), though they may occur in drug reactions, usually in association with widespread, punctate epithelial erosions.

Combined epithelial and subepithelial keratitis

This occurs commonly with late-stage adenovirus infections: fine lesions are typical of types 3, 4, and 7, and coarse lesions of type 8 infection, for example (Fig. 2). Similar lesions are seen in herpes simplex, staphylococcal blepharoconjunctivitis, inclusion conjunctivitis, trachoma, vaccinia, Reiter's disease, and rosacea. In many instances the epithelial keratitis resolves leaving a non-staining, subepithelial keratitis that may persist.

Associated ocular findings

The presence of other ocular findings may give a clue to the cause of the superfical corneal disturbance. Examination of the lids may reveal molluscum, vesicles consistent with herpetic infection, or staphylococcal blepharitis. The presence of a follicular conjunctivitis may indicate viral or chlamydial infection, or drug toxicity. Preauricular lymphadenopathy is commonly associated with adenovirus infection and is also found with chlamydia. The presence of filaments or mucous plaques may indicate a dry eye or superior limbic keratoconjunctivitis, a condition of middle-aged females characterized by bilateral, punctate staining of the upper third of the cornea and adjacent bulbar conjunctiva with associated hyperaemia, and, in the later stages, keratinization of the limbal and palpebral conjunctiva (Fig. 1). Micropannus is often present in superior limbic keratoconjunctivitis, but may also be associated with chlamydial infection, rosacea, vernal catarrh, or staphylococcal keratoconjunctivitis. Reduced corneal sensation may indicate herpes simplex, herpes zoster, or neurotrophic keratitis.

Superficial punctate keratitis

This term should be specifically reserved for the condition, first described by Thygeson, characterized by diffusely distributed, coarse epithelial lesions with normal intervening epithelium that comprise a collection of minute white dots with an irregular edge, with or without minimal opacity in the superficial stroma (Fig. 2). They can sometimes be confused with herpes simplex keratitis, though ocular adnexal examination is otherwise normal. They are extremely responsive to topical steroid therapy.

Interstitial keratitis

Stromal opacity without ulceration was designated by Hutchinson (1858) as interstitial keratitis to describe the ground-glass appearance of the cornea in patients with syphilis. However, although the term interstitial keratitis is frequently used specifically in this context, there are many other causes (Table 2).

Table 2 Aetiology of interstitial keratitis

Viral diseases:
Herpes simplex virus type I and II
Varicella zoster virus
Epstein–Barr virus
Adenovirus
Mumps virus
Rubella virus

Bacterial infections:
Congenital or acquired syphilis
Tuberculosis
Leprosy
Lymphogranuloma venereum
Lyme disease

Parasitic diseases:
Leishmaniasis
Trypansomiasis
Malaria
Cysticercosis
Onchocerciasis
Acanthamoeba keratitis

Keratitis of unknown cause:
Sarcoidosis
Cogan's syndrome
Mycosis fungoides
Incontinentia pigmenti

Table 3 Early manifestations of congenital syphilis

Stillbirth
Failure to thrive
Rhinitis
Osteochondritis
Pneumonia
Hepatosplenomegaly
Periostitis
Nephrosis/nephritis
Cutaneous eruptions—mucous patches:
  Vesicular
  Bullous
  Papulosquamous

Common causes of interstitial keratitis are herpes simplex keratitis, onchocerciasis, and, in previous times, syphilis. Tuberculosis is a common cause in the developing world.

Syphilitic interstitial keratitis

Syphilitic interstitial keratitis is caused by *Treponema pallidum* and is usually reported in the congenital form (90 per cent of cases). Although congenital syphilis is now much less common, there is evidence that there was an increase in incidence the United States during the years 1960 to 1970. It is contracted when the spirochaete invades the fetus from the infected mother. Early manifestations of general disease occur either during the first 2 years of life (Table 3), or as late disease after the first 2 years, which does not involve live organisms.

Interstitial keratitis is a late manifestation. Other manifestations include dental deformities, sabre shins, frontal bossing, saddle nose, palatal perforation, hydroarthrosis, nerve deafness, rhagades, mental retardation, and degenerative disease of the central nervous system. Interstitial keratitis, deafness, and Hutchinson's teeth are known as Hutchinson's triad. Interstitial keratitis occurs predominantly in females (sex ratio of 5:1) between the ages of 5 and 20 years. In congenital disease, the keratitis is bilateral: it is unilateral in acquired disease and is one of the most common features of eye involvement.

Clinical features

There are three stages to the disease: progressive, florid, and retrogressive. Focal opacities coalesce to form diffuse stromal haze, with epithelial oedema and keratic precipitates. At first the appearance can be sectoral, with the ingress of deep blood vessels that spread centrally over a period of weeks or months. The entire cornea may become involved, with dense neovascularization. This stage can be associated with iridocyclitis, though this may be difficult to identify through an opaque cornea. In the florid stage the cornea becomes vascularized such that it appears pink; this represents the climax of the inflammatory response, and it is then that the stage of retrogression begins. Eventually, scarring and ghost vessels result (Fig. 3). Sometimes, in the burnt-out state, band-like thickening is seen in Descemet's membrane. Other conditions of the eye that may be seen with interstitial keratitis include chorio-

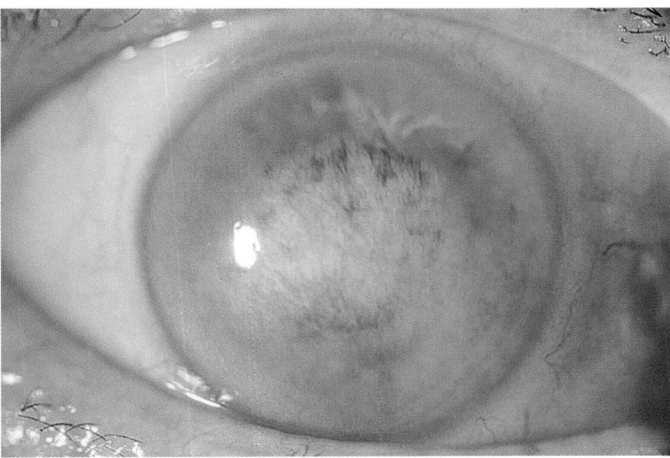

Fig. 3 Inactive interstitial keratitis in an elderly patient.

retinitis, retinal vasculitis, papillitis, iris nodules, episcleritis, scleritis, and retinal detachment. Features of eye involvement in various stages of syphilis are listed in Table 4.

Pathology
The pathogenesis appears to be a delayed hypersensitivity response to direct infection by *T. pallidum*, but humoral immune responses are undoubtedly also involved. There is a mucopolysacharride component that protects against the effect of specific antibodies, and there is a second mucopolysaccharide that enables the organism to adhere to host cells.

Investigation
Spirochaetes are identifiable in tissue fluids by dark-field microscopy in the primary infection. Serological screening tests using the Venereal Disease Research Laboratory (VDRL) and the rapid plasma reagin test (RPR) are preferred, however, although false-positive reactions occur in patients with lupus erythematosus or leprosy. More specific are the fluorescent treponemal antibody absorption (FTA-Abs) test and the microhaemagglutination assay (TPHA).

Treatment
Treatment of infants with congenital syphilis is with benzathine penicillin for up to 10 days. Interstitial keratitis is treated with potent topical corticosteroid two-hourly for the first 48 h and then tapering off gradually.

Corneal infections
Infections of the cornea are contracted by a number of mechanisms. In bacterial and mycotic infection there is often an easily recognizable fault in the anatomical, physiological, or immunological mechanisms of ocular protection (Table 5). Careful examination of the external eye as well as the cornea itself is therefore necessary when evaluating infectious keratitis.

Bacterial keratitis
Infectious corneal ulcers are common conditions presenting to ophthalmic emergency departments. They can be difficult to

Table 4 Ocular manifestations of syphilis

Primary
Chancre

Secondary
Blepharitis
Madarosis
Conjunctivitis
Dacryocystitis
Dacryoadenitis
Keratitis
Iris nodules
Iridocyclitis
Episcleritis
Scleritis
Chorioretinitis
Vitritis
Neuroretinitis
Disc oedema
Exudative retinal detachment
Perivasculitis

Tertiary
Gummas in lids
Unilateral interstitial keratitis
Punctate stromal keratitis
Bilateral periostitis of orbital bones
Episcleritis
Scleritis
Anterior and posterior uveitis
Chorioretinitis
Vasculitis
Venous and arterial occlusive disease
Exudative detachment
Macular oedema and neuroretinitis
Vitritis
Pseudoretinitis pigmentosa
Chorioretinal neovascular membrane
Lens dislocation
Argyll Robertson pupil
Oculomotor palsies

diagnose accurately and treat, and are time-consuming and costly to manage. In addition, they may, if inappropriately treated, result in visual loss, and even sometimes in loss of the eye.

Pathogenesis
Infectious corneal ulcers usually occur where the protective mechanisms of blinking, tear dynamics, and epithelial integrity are compromised. Under normal circumstances the corneal epithelium provides an excellent physical barrier to microbial invasion and infections are relatively rare. Occasionally, epithelial damage may allow pathogenic organisms to breach the epithelial surface and subsequent elaboration of specific toxins may facilitate entry into the stroma. Once an organism has invaded the corneal stroma an inflammatory reaction is set up, with locally elaborated chemotactic factors attracting polymorphonuclear leucocytes to the site (Fig. 4). The release of bacterial and leucocyte enzymes is poorly tolerated by the stroma, and

Table 5 Mechanisms for corneal protection

Anatomical/physiological
Full lid closure
Good resting blink reflex
Normal Bell's phenomenon
Normal corneal sensation
Good tear flow
Maintenance of the epithelial barrier

Immunological
Lactoferrin
Lysozyme
Betalysin
Mucus
Secretary IgA
IgG
Immunocompetent T and B cells in limbal, bulbar, and tarsal
  conjunctiva
Normal systemic and local immune response mechanisms (humoral
  and cellular)
Presence of specific IgG within the corneal stroma
Normal cytokine production by corneal and inflammatory cells

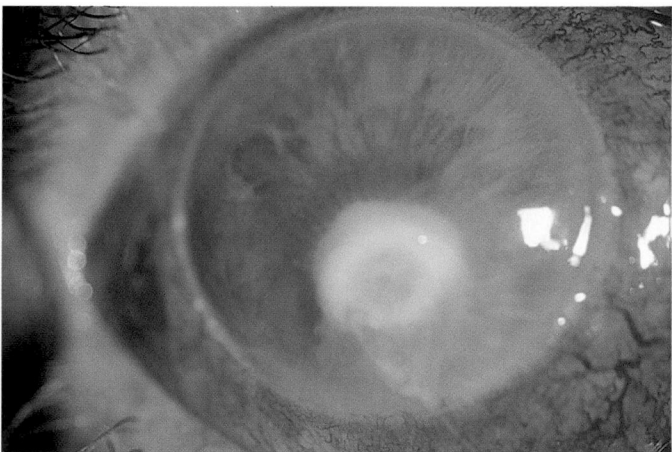

Fig. 5 *Staphyloccus aureus* keratitis.

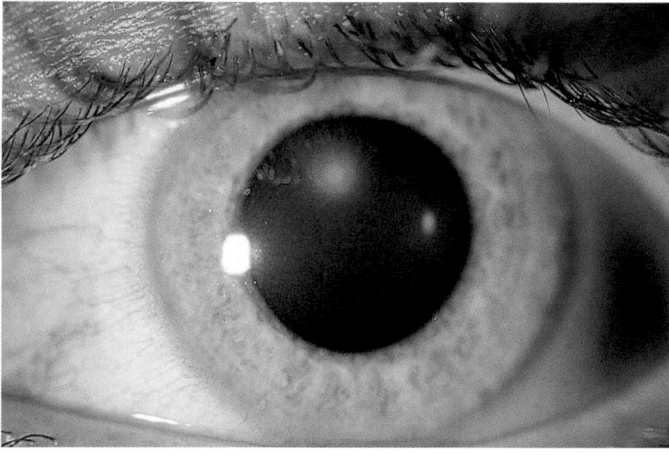

Fig. 4 Early bacterial keratitis.

various degrees of corneal melting and scarring may occur. Some bacteria, such as *Neisseria gonorrhoeae*, listeria, corynebacteria, and *Haemophilus* spp., may cause infection in the absence of epithelial damage by adhering to and penetrating intact epithelium. The most common bacteria isolated from cases of bacterial keratitis are staphylocci, streptococci, and *Pseudomonas* spp. Some of the more common bacteria causing infectious keratitis and their pathogenic and clinical features are listed in Table 6.

Gram-positive organisms often produce toxins and enzymes that either cause damage directly, stimulate host cells to release enzymes, or produce a damaging hypersensitivity reaction. *Staphylococcus aureus* produces various haemolysins that are cytolytic (Fig. 5); the sterile infiltrates found in marginal keratitis are thought to caused by a hypersensitivity reaction to toxin. Coagulase-negative staphylococci such as *S. epidermidis* may

also produce toxins, but these are generally much less damaging and cause a less marked keratitis. *Streptococcus pneumoniae* produces pneumolysin, which is chemotactic and cytotoxic for neutrophils, and induces collagenase production by corneal fibroblasts, promoting corneal ulceration. *Streptococcus viridans* keratitis is associated with infectious crystalline keratopathy, a slowly progressive stromal deposition of crystalline infiltrates that may particularly occur after penetrating keratoplasty associated with corneal oedema and chronic steroid treatment (Fig. 6). *Streptococcus pyogenes* may cause marginal ulceration associated with dacrocystitis. *Bacillus cereus* is often associated with soil-contaminated trauma and must also be considered in intravenous drug users.

Gram-negative organisms are important causes of infectious keratitis. A common example is *Pseudomonas aeruginosa*, which produces a proteoglycanase responsible for stromal melting, and an exotoxin that inhibits protein synthesis and causes loss of epithelial and stromal cells (Fig. 7). Rapid progression of the ulcer can result in corneal perforation or less frequently involve the sclera. *Proteus* is a rare cause of Gram-negative ker-

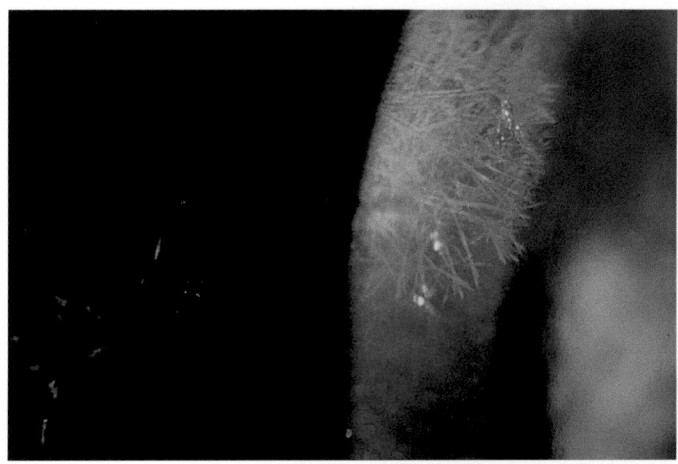

Fig. 6 Arborescent bacterial keratopathy (infectious crystalline keratopathy) (illustration by courtesy of M. G. Kerr-Muir and A. B. Tullo).

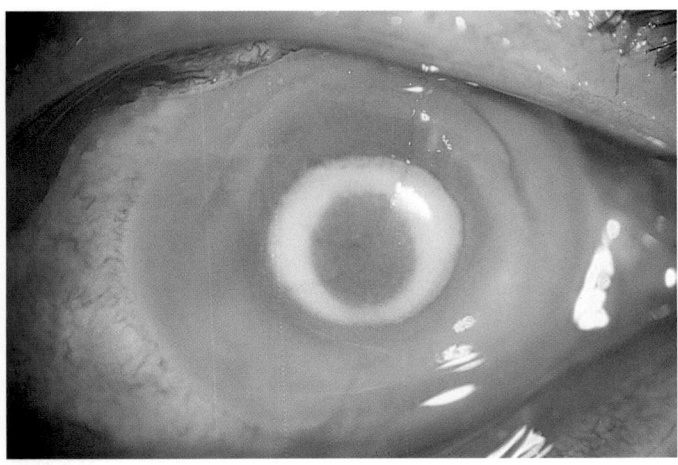

Fig. 7 Ring infiltrate in *Pseudomonas* ulcer secondary to wearing contact lenses.

atitis, and produces endotoxins and numerous degradative enzymes that are involved in the pathogenesis. *Moraxella* spp. may cause infection in alcoholic and debilitated patients; this produces dense stromal infiltration and abscess formation secondary to damage caused by proteases, and the organisms possibly produce endotoxins. It is associated with hypopyon and less commonly hyphaema formation. Niesseriae often produce an intense conjunctival reaction with purulent discharge and chemosis. Other rare organisms such as mycobacteria and *Nocardia* spp. may not be identified in the initial work-up because they do not stain well with conventional methods or grow well on conventional media, and they are therefore likely to be missed if not actively considered.

Various predisposing factors increase the chances of infection; these may be amenable to treatment, and therefore must be identified and managed correctly. If this is neglected, resolution may not occur or may be needlessly prolonged, resulting in a poor result for vision. The use of contact lenses and the associated complexity of regimens asssociated with wearing

Table 6 Organisms giving rise to bacterial keratitis

Organisms	Pathogenesis	Clinical features and characteristics
Staphylococcus aureus	Extracellular toxins and enzymes	Indolent, central, yellow-white ulcer under epithelial defect with minimal anterior-chamber reaction May produce marginal sterile ulcer
Staphylococcus epidermidis	Possible toxin production	Similar to above but less severe Especially in compromised corneas
Streptococcus pneumoniae	Polysaccharide capsule increases virulence Rapid pneumolysin exotoxin production leads to corneal melt	Grey-yellow infiltrate creeps towards corneal centre with an overhanging advancing edge; rapidly perforates Hypopyon common Important in paediatric infections
α-Haemolytic *Streptococcus* (*viridans*)	Low-grade pathogenicity but can cause corneal ulcers if local immunosuppression	Indolent grey-white ulcer under epithelial defect May be associated with crystalline keratopathy
β-Haemolytic *Streptococcus* (*pyogenes*)	Similar to *Strep.viridans*	Uncommon; associated with dacrocystitis
Streptococcus faecalis	Impaired host resistance	Usually occurs following prior epithelial injury or immunosuppression
Pseudomonas spp.	Requires epithelial breakdown Proteoglycanase production leads to breakdown of corneal matrix Adheres to contact lens via a glycocalyx	Contact lens wearers, especially the elderly Central grey infiltrate with yellow discharge Ring abscess formation associated corneal oedema and sterile hypopyon frequent
Bacillus proteus	Endotoxin and multiple degradative enzyme production	Rare, dense infiltrate may lead to perforation
Moraxella spp.	Protease, endotoxin production	Dense infiltrate leads to stromal abscess often painless Hypopyon and less often hyphema occurs
Klebsiella spp.	Affects normal eyes	Rare
Neisseria gonorrhoeae	Binds to intact epithelium and penetrates it	Profuse purulent discharge and intense conjunctival inflammation and chemosis
Corynebacterium diphtheriae	Penetrates intact epithelium diphtheria endotoxin probably causes corneal melt	Rarely complicates conjunctivitis; rapidly perforates
Listeria spp.	Penetrates intact epithelium	Rare, may get brown hypopyon
Haemophilus spp.	Penetrates intact epithelium	Important in paediatric infections
Bacillus cereus	Many factors produced including lecithinase, which may play a major part in pathogenesis	Usually harmless but can cause endophthalmitis following soil contaminated trauma or in intravenous drug users

lenses have resulted in an increased incidence of corneal infections and are now the major risk factor in bacterial keratitis. This is thought to occur as a result of a combination of lens-induced epithelial trauma, physiological stress, pathogenic bacteria colonizing the lens surface, and decreased clearance of organisms due to alteration in tear flow and blinking mechanisms. Extended wearing, particularly overnight, is more likely to lead to infections, especially if lens hygiene is poor. The risk with extended wearing may be as much as 15 times that of daily wearing, and the chance of infection increases proportionately with length of lens wear, poor cleaning, and inadequate disinfection. Gram-negative keratitis, particularly *Ps. aeruginosa*, is most often associated with using contact lenses. It is extremely important to rule this out in any contact lens-related corneal infection. Ocular abrasions, lacerations or penetration following occupational or recreational injuries are an important cause of infectious keratitis, especially in younger age groups and males. In-turning eyelashes or conjunctival concretions may abrade the epithelium, allowing organisms to enter. Decompensated corneal grafts, especially for herpetic disease or previous microbial keratitis, compromise the epithelial barrier. Loose sutures following any form of anterior-segment surgery may act as the focus for mucous adherence with subsequent colonization providing a direct route of infection to the stroma (Fig. 8). In older age groups, pre-existing external eye diseases such as dry eye syndromes damage the integrity of the epithelium, reduce periocular, antibacterial tear factors, and result in poor clearance of organisms. The cornea can be jeopardized in bullous, exposure, or neurotrophic keratopathies, in which poor healing follows minor injury. Herpes simplex infection is an important risk factor for subsequent infectious keratitis, especially with recurrent ulcerative disease. General debility associated with age, chronic illness, immunodeficiency or immunosupression may lead to corneal infection due impaired host response. Prolonged local steroid or antibiotic treatment can lead to altered adnexal flora and host defence mechanisms, resulting in corneal infection. In less developed countries, vitamin A deficiency produces corneal drying, leading to corneal ulceration and subsequent infection. The main risk factors for bacterial keratitis are summarized in Table 7.

Clinical features

Bacterial keratitis typically presents with redness, decreased visual acuity, photophobia, purulent discharge, and epiphora. Examination shows a central epithelial defect with underlying corneal infiltration and an adherent mucous or purulent exudate. Underlying reactive uveitis with aqueous flare, keratitic precipitates, and pupillary constriction are seen; in severe cases, fibrin exudation and hypopyon occur (Fig. 9). Associated corneal changes include stromal and epithelial oedema, and Descemet's folds. Important signs found in infectious keratitis and their response to treatment are shown in Table 8. One should try to differentiate between infectious corneal infiltrates and those that are sterile. The latter are often seen in contact lens wearers or associated with staphylococcal lid disease, and are generally peripheral, circumscribed subepithelial opacities with little or no fluorescein staining (Fig. 10). Distinction is difficult

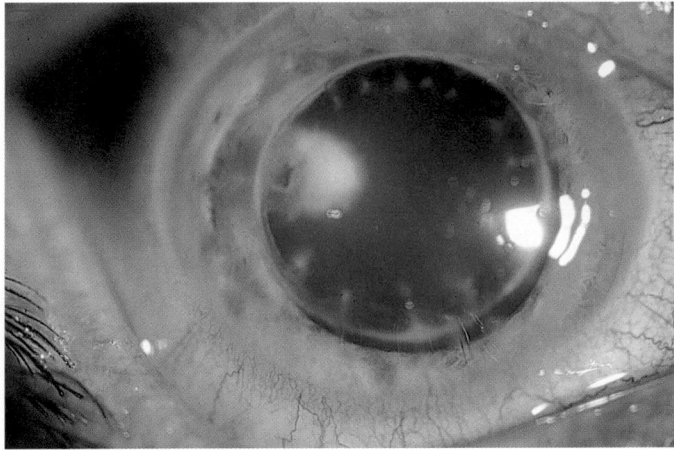

(a)

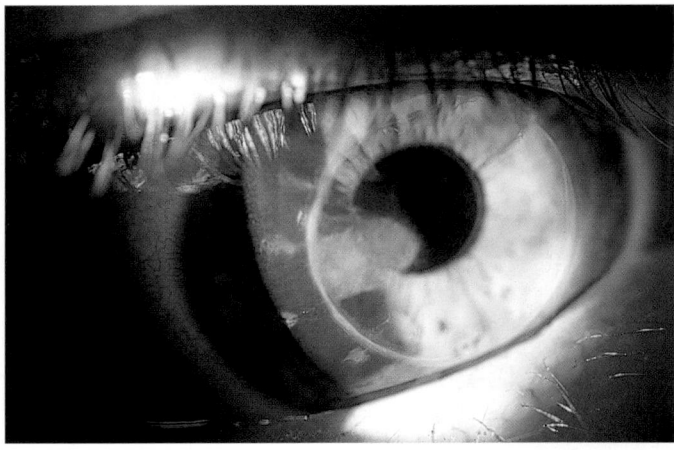

(b)

Fig. 8 (a) Suture-related bacterial corneal abcess following keratoplasty; (b) scarring after resolution.

and in cases of doubt the management should be that of infectious keratitis until proved otherwise.

The differential diagnosis of bacterial keratitis includes herpes simplex virus, fungal, acanthamoebal, and mycobacterial infections, many of which can coexist. A methodical and comprehensive approach, as indicated below, must be applied in each case to prevent diagnostic confusion and ensure a complete recovery.

Investigation

Diagnostic tests must be made promptly after diagnosis, and broad-spectrum topical antibiotic therapy instituted. Most individuals may be managed effectively as outpatients, with follow-up at regular intervals. Severe cases, or those where there is diagnostic uncertainty, questionable compliance or poor response to treatment, should be admitted to hospital. Alternative diagnostic tests should be considered where treatment response is poor, as rare organisms must be identified. The following steps should be taken in all cases of suspected microbial keratitis.

1. Instil preservative-free anaesthetic and take a corneal

Table 7 Predisposing factors for microbial keratitis

Predisposing factor	Example	Comments
Trauma	Contact lenses	Especially extended wear regimens and poor hygiene
	Direct	Corneal abrasions, ingrowing lashes, conjunctival concretions
		Loose sutures, e.g. post-keratoplasty
	Surgery	All the above result in disruption of the corneal epithelium
Pre-existing eye disease	Dry eye syndrome	Leads to reduced antibacterial factors and compromised epithelial surface
	Bullous keratopathy	Chronic epithelial and stromal oedema leads to corneal compromise
	Exposure keratopathy	Poor lid closure results in recurrent minor trauma and surface drying
	Herpes simplex keratitis	Recurrent disease leads to damaged epithelium
	Neurotrophic keratitis	Corneal anaesthesia and trophic factors
	Peripheral ulcerative keratitis	Epithelial defects promote stromal invasion by organisms
	Atopic eye disease	Increases risk of bacterial infection due to epithelial compromise
	Lacrimal obstruction	Leads to poor tear drainage and clearance of organisms
	Chronic eyelid infection	Provides reservoir of bacteria and causes surface erosions
Systemic factors	Ageing	General impaired host defences increase risk of infection and alter host
	Immunosuppression	response to it
	Diabetic mellitus	
	Rheumatoid arthritis	
	Debility	
	Vitamin A deficiency	In underdeveloped countries, vitamin A deficiency often leads to corneal drying and ulceration
Drugs	Systemic or local steroid treatment	Altered immune responses
	Immunosuppressants	
	Chronic topical antibiotic treatment	Encourages development of resistant organisms

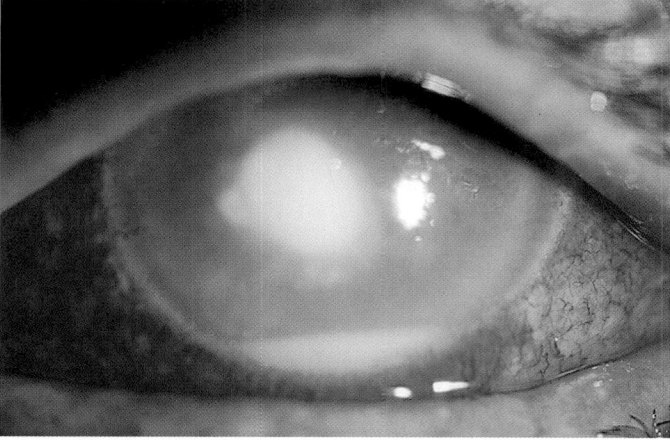

Fig. 9 Densely infiltrated, central, bacterial corneal ulcer with hypopyon following corneal foreign body; pneumococci were grown.

scrape with a sterile needle from the advancing edges and base of the ulcer. Scraping is therapeutically beneficial by debridement of necrotic material and enhances corneal penetration of antibiotics.

2. Place the material obtained first on to various culture media, and then on to two glass slides for microscopy, as outlined in Figs 11 and 12. Communication with the microbiologist is paramount to ensure that specimens are processed correctly and promptly in order to maximize yield. Some studies have shown positive Gram staining in 75 per cent of ulcers thought to be

Table 8 Signs of microbial keratitis and response to treatment

Signs of infective keratitis	Response to treatment
Conjunctival injection	Becomes less marked and disappears with treatment
Corneal epithelial defect	Reduces in size with complete re-epithelialization occurring in most cases
	May be persistent if continuing inflammation or untreated external eye disease present
Stromal infiltrate	Reduces in size and density in the stroma adjacent to ulcer and usually clears completely
	Careful steroid treatment may be required to clear up any residual inflammation
Stromal oedema	Resolution of oedema in transition zone adjacent to ulcer unless persistent inflammation or endothelial compromise
Anterior uveitis; keratic precipitates, anterior chamber cells, flare, fibrin, hypopyon	Usually settles with improvement in keratitis
	Worsening uveitis may indicate early secondary endophthalmitis

infected, but this percentage varies according to practice and may be considerably less in many instances. Reincubation of the initial plates and either restaining

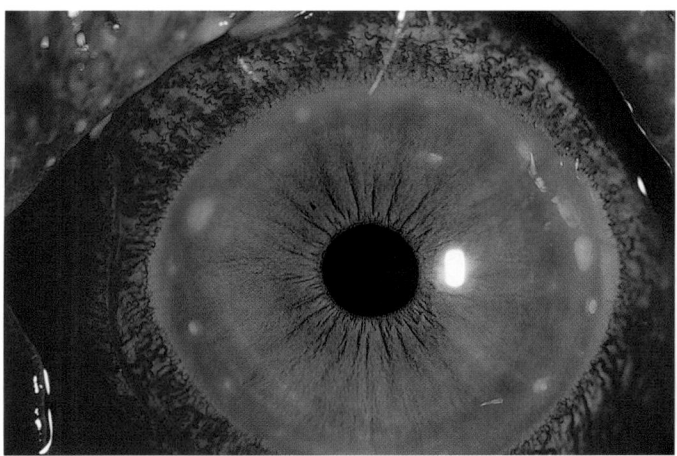

Fig. 10 Multiple, sterile, peripheral marginal infiltrates associated with blepharitis.

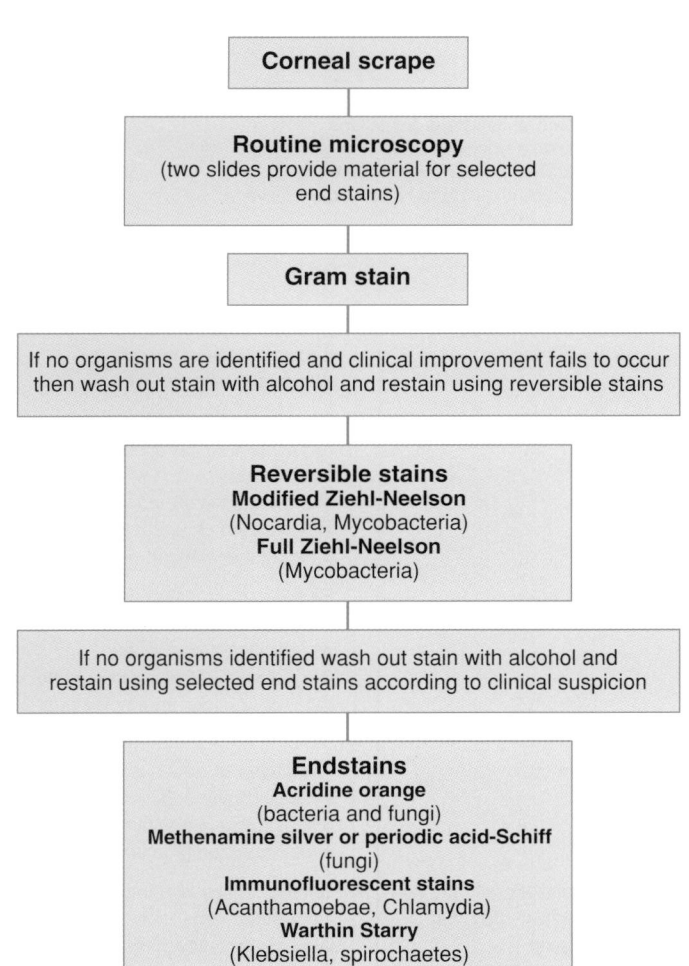

Fig. 11 Microscopy in bacterial keratitis (adapted from L. Flicker).

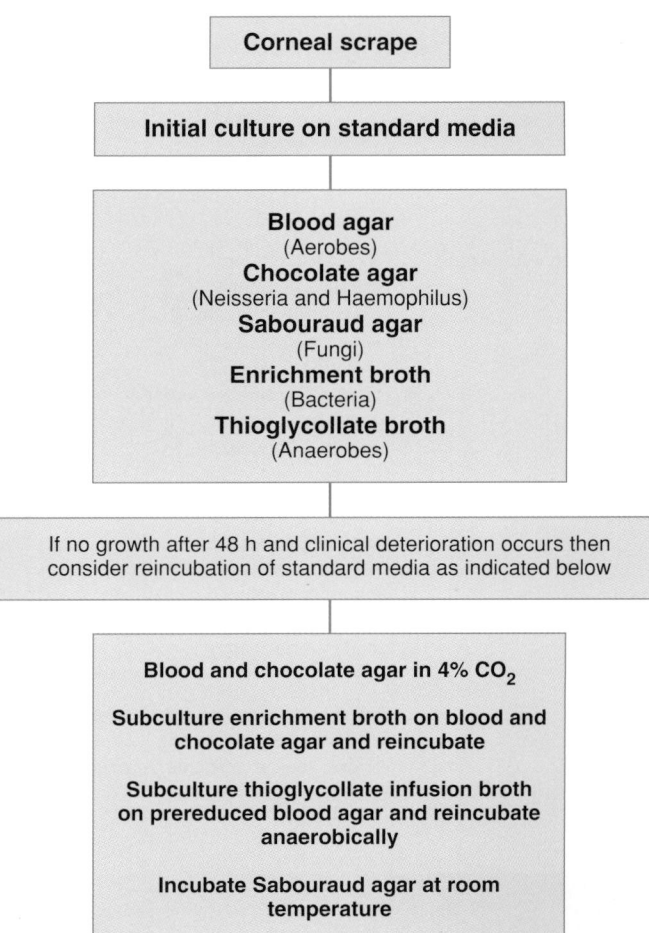

Fig. 12 Standard culture media for investigation of bacterial keratitis (adapted from L. Flicker).

of the original slides if available, or rescraping, should be considered in cases not responding to treatment (Figs 11 and 12)

3. Obtain contact lenses, cases, and solutions for culture in severe cases associated with contact lens wear and inform the patient that these will be destroyed.

4. Make a good-quality drawing in the notes after the corneal scrape. The size and shape of the epithelial defect and infiltrate, and the presence of associated complications such as corneal thinning, uveitis and hypopyon should be noted. Figure 13 shows a simple scheme for recording the various signs associated with microbial keratitis that should be used to monitor recovery or deterioration. An example of the scheme applied to a case is shown in Fig. 14.

5. Identify predisposing factors and treat them.

Treatment

The aim is first to sterilize the cornea with intensive antibiotic treatment and then to prevent subsequent superinfection whilst healing occurs. Broad-spectrum, topical antibiotics are chosen

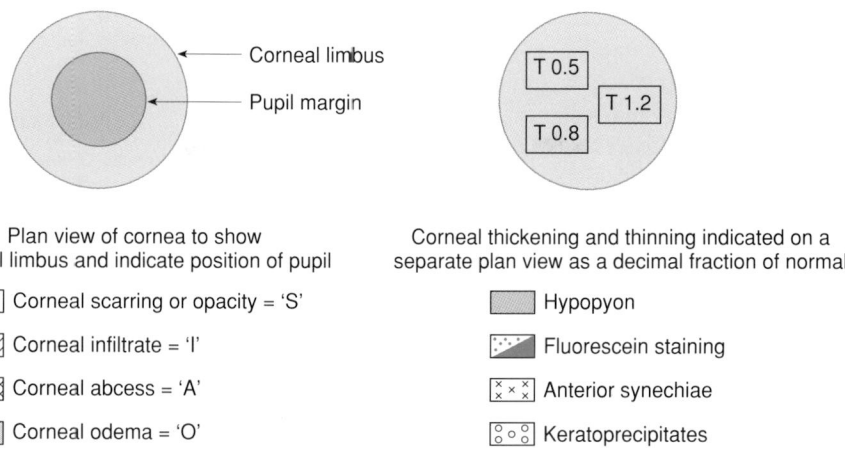

Plan view of cornea to show
corneal limbus and indicate position of pupil

⊞ Corneal scarring or opacity = 'S'

⊞ Corneal infiltrate = 'I'

⊞ Corneal abcess = 'A'

▢ Corneal odema = 'O'

⊠ Superficial vascularization

Corneal thickening and thinning indicated on a
separate plan view as a decimal fraction of normal

▢ Hypopyon

▢ Fluorescein staining

⊞ Anterior synechiae

⊞ Keratoprecipitates

⊠ Deep vascularization

Fig. 13 Scheme for documentation of features of microbial keratitis, useful for corneal signs in corneal disease. In microbial keratitis it is particularly useful for monitoring response to treatment and for decision-making on deterioration requiring active intervention. In plan view, the corneal limbus is represented by a solid circle and the pupil by a dashed line. Deep vascularization is indicated by red lines drawn from within the corneal limbus, and superficial vascularization by blue lines beginning outside the corneal limbus. An area of corneal oedema is indicated by grey pencil shading and labelled 'O', infiltration by oblique single hatching and labelled 'I ', scarring by vertical hatching and represented by the letter 'S', and a corneal abcess by oblique double hatching and the letter 'A'. The depth of these lesions is shown on a cross-section of cornea taken through a point indicated on the plan diagram by an arrow (see Fig. 10). Hypopon is represented by a yellow level. An area of epithelial defect staining with flourescein is indicated in green, and punctate staining by green dots. Similarly, rose bengal staining may be shown in red, and punctate staining in red dots. Keratic precipitates are shown by small circles at the appropriate site on the endothelium and anterior synechiae by a cross or row of crosses. The dimensions of the lesions can be indicated in millimetres as measured by the slit lamp. In addition, relative quantification of the severity of any individual lesion can be indicated by a scale of 1 to 4 and thus allows comparison over time: 1 = minimal change; 2 = mild change; 3 = moderate change; 4 = severe change. A record of relative corneal thickening and thinning can be kept as a separate plan diagram, thus reducing confusion due to overcomplexity. An example of the scheme as applied to a case of microbial keratitis is shown in Fig. 10. (Adapted from A. Bron.)

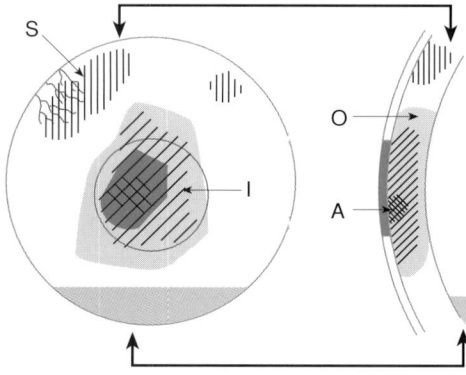

Fig. 14 Example of a documentation scheme applied to microbial keratitis. The diagram shows a central corneal abcess with an overlying epithelial defect and surrounding infiltrate, and corneal oedema. An associated hypopyon is shown. There are two areas of scarring present in the peripheral cornea, one of which has deep stromal vascularization related to it. The diagram on the left shows a cross-section of the cornea at the point indicated by the vertical arrows on the plan view. Dimensions in millimetres can be added and allow monitoring of progress. (Taken from Bron, A.J. (1973). A simple schema for documenting corneal disease, *British Journal of Ophthalmology*, **57**, 629–34.)

Table 9 Initial antibiotic choice in bacterial keratitis

Topical antibiotic choice	Mechanism of action
Cefuroxime fortified 5.0% (50 mg/ml) and	Bactericidal Inhibit cell-wall synthesis
gentamicin fortified 1.4% (14 mg/ml)	Bactericidal Inhibit protein synthesis via interaction with ribosomes
or	
Ciprofloxacin (0.3%)	Bactericidal Inhibits DNA replication via inhibition of bacteria-specific DNA gyrase

a specific diagnosis. A treatment regimen must be instituted immediately after specimen collection (Table 9). A combination of a topical aminoglycoside (e.g. gentamicin, 14 mg/ml) and a second-generation cephalosporin (e.g. cefuroxime, 50 mg/ml) is usually chosen. This combination is usually adequate to cover staphylococci, streptococci, *Pseudomonas*, and the enterobacteraciae that cause the vast majority of cases of bacterial keratitis. An alternative is monotherapy with a fluoroquinolone (e.g. ciprofloxacin), which may cause less epi-

initially, irrespective of the Gram–stain result, polymicrobial infections being frequent. A negative Gram stain does not exclude bacterial infection, and clinical features rarely signify thelial toxicity. The use of multiple medications must be avoided in outpatients because of poor compliance, increased toxicity, dilution effects, the risk of superinfection, and the possibility of diagnostic confusion. The ultimate choice of antibiotic treatment is governed by sensitivity testing, clinical response, and discussion with a microbiologist, with whom close contact should be maintained throughout. Topical treatment is instilled hourly between 6 a.m. and 12 midnight for outpatients, with appropriate antibiotic ointment applied before sleep. In severe cases, hourly treatment overnight is required and admission is indicated. Subconjunctival antibiotics offer no benefit over intensive topical therapy and should be avoided. Symptomatic relief with mydriatics (e.g. cyclopentolate, 1 per cent three times a day or atropine, 1 per cent twice daily) is usually necessary, will ease discomfort, and prevent secondary complications such as posterior synechiae and secondary glaucoma. Oral analgesics should be used for pain relief as necessary.

The patient should be assessed at 48 h to determine the response to treatment and review the results of culture and sensitivities. A deterioration must prompt admission to hospital to ensure compliance, and the initial choice of treatment should be continued unless sensitivities indicate possible resistance. Complete resolution of signs in the cornea and anterior chamber may be expected in most cases. Topical corticosteroid treatment is generally unnecessary but can be considered in cases of culture-positive bacterial keratitis that have not completely healed after adequate antibiotic treatment where persistent inflammation may be a factor. Steroid treatment, however, should be started from the outset in cases of bacterial keratitis in patients with corneal grafts to reduce the risk of a rejection episode, which may be triggered under these circumstances.

Management of complications (Table 10)

A persistent epithelial defect after adequate intensive therapy should be encouraged to heal by reducing the frequency of instillations and eliminating unnecessary treatments. Sometimes the use of preservative-free drops, correction of tear deficiency, reducing corneal exposure, and treatment of associated lid disease can all help speedy resolution. Taping the eyelid closed may allow re-epithelialization and a careful trial of bandage contact-lens use may be required. Ultimately, debridement of necrotic cornea with lamellar keratoplasty, or a temporary tarsorraphy, can be valuable. Penetrating keratoplasty may be necessary to reduce morbidity and hasten resolution. When the condition remains static or deteriorates and no specific organism has been identified on culture or microscopy, an unanticipated bacterial, viral, fungal or amoebic should be suspected and specialist advice must be sought.

In an indolent (static) keratitis, where no improvement has occurred despite intensive treatment and measures to promote healing, the initial slides should be restained with other stains as indicated in Fig. 11. Reversible stains, such as the modified or full Ziehl–Neelsen stain for mycobacteria and nocardia, should be applied in the first instance. These can be washed off with alcohol and the slide restained with specific, irreversible stains to identify uncommon groups of organisms, the

Table 10 Complications of microbial keratitis and their management

Complications	Management
Persistent epithelial defects	Preservative-free treatment Reduced frequency of treatment Treat associated external eye disease Lid taping Consider trial of therapeutic contact lens
Indolent keratitis	Seek specialist advice Consider stopping treatment for 24 h and repeating corneal scrape
Progressive keratitis	Seek specialist advice Stop treatment for 24 h and perform corneal biopsy
Corneal perforation	Seek specialist advice Add systemic antibiotics Bandage contact lens Cyanoacrylate glue Emergency penetrating keratoplasty if above measures fail
Endophthalmitis	Diagnostic vitrectomy and intraocular antibiotics
Residual scarring	Elective lamellar or penetrating keratoplasty for visual improvement

choice of these being determined by clinical suspicion. This recycling of stained preparations prevents unnecessary biopsies and therefore limits corneal damage. If the initial scrape specimen is inadequate or unavailable, however, treatment should be stopped for 24 h and the corneal scrape repeated.

Similarly, if no organisms are grown on routine culture media, then reincubation of the initial plates or subculture of the infusion broth on various media, as indicated in Fig. 12, should be done to identify fastidious organisms. In the event of persistent culture-negative keratitis, more specific culture media may be employed (Fig. 15).

Progressive keratitis in the presence of negative cultures is an indication for corneal biopsy. This should be done with preservative-free topical anaesthesia under the operating microscope, and provides a relatively large specimen for culture and microscopic analysis. It also removes necrotic tissue, which may be a barrier to healing. Light microscopy with sequential staining may identify bacterial, fungal, and protozoal infections; immunohistochemical analysis may identify herpes simplex. These techniques enable identification of less common organisms with a high degree of accuracy and speed, and may offer a greater diagnostic yield than subsequent cultures. Consultation with a histopathologist is essential to enable optimal preparation and processing. Failure to identify a causative organism may suggest an alternative diagnosis such as autoimmune disease or other causes of sterile keratitis, and these should be considered in the differential diagnosis.

Marked corneal thinning with imminent or actual perforation should receive specialist referral (Fig. 16). Periodic Seidel

> **Withhold treatment for 24 h, rescrape and inoculate standard media plus special media as indicated below**
>
> **Reduce blood agar anaerobically**
> (anaerobes)
> **Lowenstein-Jensen**
> (Mycobacteria)
> **Non-nutrient, *E. coli* seeded agar**
> (Acanthamobae)
> **Chlamydia and virus transport media**
> (Chlamydia and Herpes simplex)
>
> **If no growth after 1 week's incubation consider corneal biopsy or lamellar or penetrating keratoplasty and culture of specimen on standard and special media**

Fig. 15 Special culture media for persistent culture negative keratitis (adapted from L. Flicker).

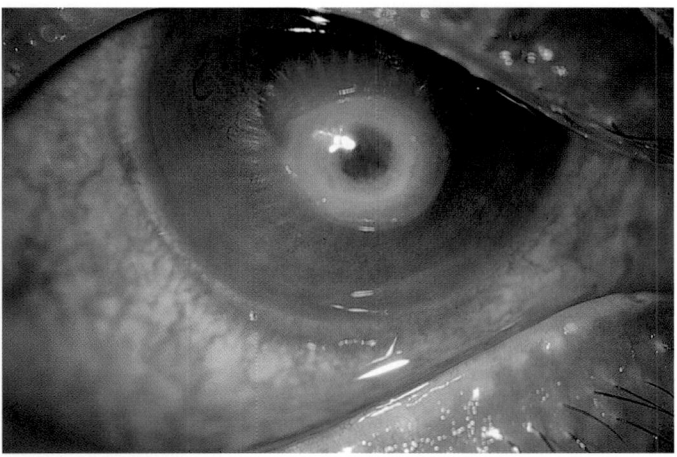

Fig. 16 Perforation in bacterial keratitis is heralded by iris prolapse and radial folds in Descemet's membrane.

testing and close observation of the depth of the anterior chamber will identify perforation, which is an indication for a trial of therapeutic contact lenses in an attempt at reformation. In this instance, start systemic antibiotics, for example ciprofloxacin. Where the anterior chamber does not reform, cyanoacrylate glueing can be done. This is a temporizing measure to enable continuation of medical treatment before elective penetrating keratoplasty at a later date when the eye is quiet. However, emergency penetrating keratoplasty may be required. Remember that the infected recipient button should be examined microbiologically so that appropriate postoperative antibiotics can be used. Endophthalmitis is a rare complication and should be managed by diagnostic vitrectomy and intravitreal antibiotics. Residual scarring after an episode of microbial keratitis may lead to reduced visual acuity. Superficial lesions may

be treated effectively by lamellar keratectomy in the absence of endothelial decompensation; however, deep stromal scarring may require full-thickness corneal grafting.

Mycotic keratitis

Fungi are often spore-forming, eukaryotic organisms, classified into filamentous fungi (moulds), diphasic fungi, and yeasts. They are distinguished according to their geographic distribution, clinical disease, laboratory diagnosis, and response to treatment. A simple classification of the various pathogenic fungi indicating the main sites of ocular infection is shown in Table 11. Septate filamentous fungi, so called because their hyphae are partitioned by cross walls, together with yeasts, cause infection in the cornea. Non-septate filamentous fungi are most conmmonly associated with aggressive orbital and sinus infections. Dimorphic fungi, which may exist in yeast and filamentous forms and are responsible for systemic mycoses, rarely infect the cornea.

Fungal keratitis is an uncommon clinical problem in northern climates, accounting for about 2 per cent of corneal infections. Widespread use of broad-spectrum antibiotics and steroid treatments, together with improved data collection, may account for the apparent increased frequency of diagnosis. The type of fungus found depends largely on geographic distribution. In the United Kingdom, *Aspergillus* and *Candida* spp. are the most common, whereas in the United States *Fusarium* is more frequently isolated. Fungal keratitis is frequently initiated by exogenous organisms in association with corneal epithelial trauma involving vegetable matter in farm workers and enthusiastic gardeners. The use of nylon-line lawn trimmers has been associated with the corneal inoculation of organisms in gardeners.

Pathogenesis

Although fungi are present in the normal flora of the conjunctival sac, they are unable to penetrate intact corneal epithelium. Corneal decompensation or epithelial damage associated with trauma or contact lens wear, particularly in hot, humid climates, may permit most fungi to become pathogenic. The filamentous fungi are plant pathogens and produce a variety of mycotoxins and proteolytic enzymes that enable them to penetrate deep into corneal tissue in man. Their pathogenicity relates, in part, to their large hyphae, which are resistant to ingestion by neutrophils. In contrast, *Candida*, commonly found as a commensal, is opportunistic, becoming pathogenic in conditions of altered host defence such as in predisposing corneal disease, diabetes, or immunosuppression. Transformation from spore to pseudohyphal phases, together with the production of proteolytic enzymes, are important in causing infection. Mixed fungal infection is uncommon because of the different conditions under which the various fungi are pathogenic. Candidal infection may, however, coexist with bacterial keratitis as the predisposing factors are similar. Therapeutic and extended-wear contact lens increase the risk of infection, owing to local trauma and colonization of lenses and cases by

Table 11 Classification and behaviour of important fungi in ocular infections

Fungal type	Microscopic behaviour and appearance	Specific examples	Site of infection
Filamentous	Multicellular, produce long branching hyphae	Septate: *Aspergillus* *Fusarium* *Penicillium* *Acremonium* *Curvalaria*	Corneal infection particularly associated with trauma
		Non-septate: *Mucor*	Aggressive orbital and paranasal infections with high mortality in diabetics, malignancy and immunosuppression
Yeasts	Unicellular, oval or round; reproduce by budding pseudohyphae	*Candida* spp.	Infection of compromised corneas
Diphasic	Exist in filamentous and yeast forms	*Blastomyces* *Coccidioides* *Histoplasma*	Systemic mycoses rarely affect cornea

fungal organisms. Topical steroid treatment, by suppressing the immune response, allows replication of filamentous fungi, potentiating infection.

Clinical features

The classical clinical features of filamentous fungal keratitis include a mild, grey–white corneal infiltrate with feathery edges, corresponding to fungal hyphal elements, manifesting within 24 to 48 h after trauma. In the early stages (Fig. 17(a), a mild cellular infiltrate is seen and satellite lesions indicating multiple inoculation may be found. Small microabscesses and immune rings may be seen but are less specific. Hypopyon and endothelial plaque formation related to anterior uveitis and fungal replication may occur. There is marked variation in virulence between the filamentous fungi, with organisms such as *F. solani* and some species of aspergillus producing dense, necrotic inflammation, and others, such as *Curvularia*, producing focal, non-necrotizing keratitis. *Candida* spp., in the early stages, produce an epithelial defect with necrotizing stromal infiltration and oedema, and a brisk uveitis similar to bacterial keratitis. No hyphae are seen. Both filamentous fungi and yeasts may produce a picture resembling bacterial keratitis in the later stages, with dense suppurative necrosis of the stroma and full-thickness corneal oedema, ultimately leading to perforation and the risk of endophthalmitis if not adequately treated. In addition, fungi may grow in the anterior chamber and, together with inflammatory exudate, may cause the iris to adhere to the lens and lead to a build up of aqueous behind the lens, with subsequent shallowing of the anterior chamber and so-called fungal malignant glaucoma. Fortunately this is rare nowadays, owing to improved recognition and early treatment of fungal keratitis.

Investigation

A corneal scrape and staining are done as shown in Fig. 18. Under ultraviolet illumination, acridine orange, a sensitive reagent for fungal hyphae, which stain yellow–orange or green, and yeasts, which stain brilliant orange, is used initially; this

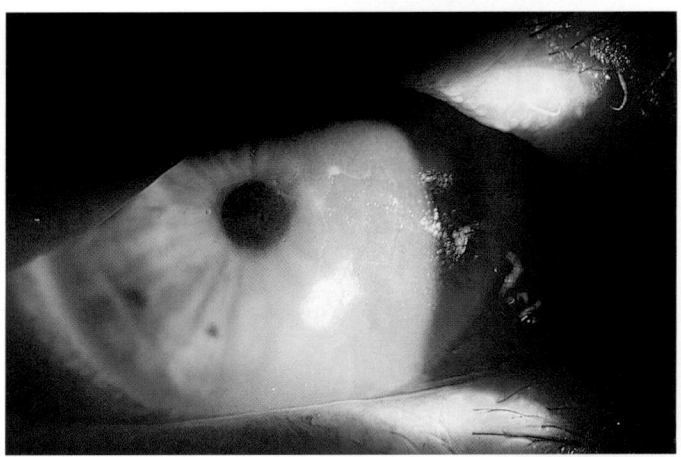

(a)

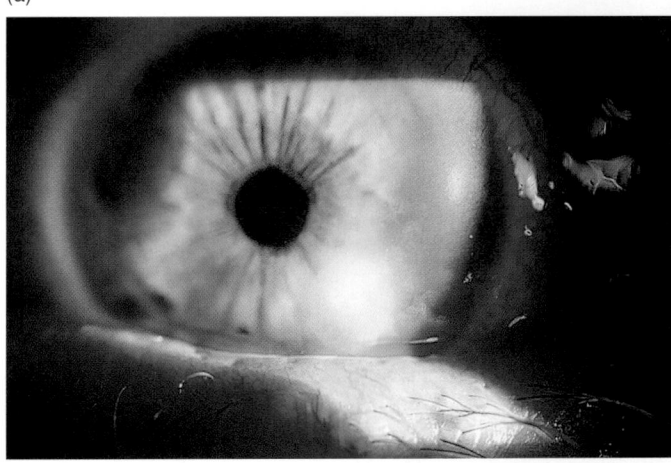

(b)

Fig. 17 Fungal keratitis: (a) an epithelial defect with underlying discrete infiltrate mimicks bacterial keratitis; (b) following inappropriate antibacterial treatment the keratitis becomes progressive.

method requires a fluorescence microscope, and when this is not available, Giemsa stain, though not as sensitive, colours

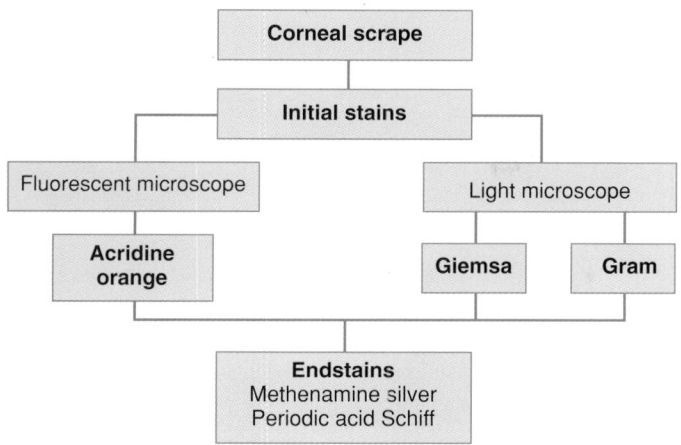

Fig. 18 Stains used in the investigation of fungal keratitis.

fungal fragments dark blue or purple. If initial stains are negative and the diagnosis is strongly suspected, then specimens should be restained with more specific, irreversible reagents such as methenamine silver (which stains fungal walls black) or periodic acid–Schiff (which stains hyphae red). Fungi often appear indistinct on Gram staining, which is therefore not a very satisfactory method for their visualization.

Material obtained from the initial scrape should be inoculated on to culture media as indicated in Fig. 12. In most cases, results may be obtained within 72 h. However, when an early identification is not obtained, cultures should be maintained, as growth may take up to 3 weeks. No single growth medium will support the growth of all fungi but Sabouraud's agar supplemented with chloramphenicol, incubated at 30°C, is a reasonable choice for primary cultures. If no growth is obtained, then further incubation in Sabouraud's medium at room temperature may encourage it.

After the organism has been isolated, cultures should be kept to allow sensitivity testing if standard treatment regimens fail. Where there is a suspicion of fungal keratitis despite negative stains and cultures, and where a broad-spectrum antibacterial treatment fails to induce improvement, then a corneal biopsy

must be performed. Paracentesis of the anterior chamber may be indicated if the above interventions fail to isolate an organism and a hypopyon is present. Ultimately, excision of a corneal button during penetrating keratoplasty may be the only measure that confirms the diagnosis.

Treatment

Choice and route of administration of an antimycotic agent are guided by the organism identified, its known sensitivities, and the depth of stromal involvement. In many cases the clinical course is indolent and treatment should not be instigated without confirmation of the diagnosis. Topical treatment is used for superficial infections and the agent is instilled hourly until a clinical response is noted and then four times daily for up to 2 to 3 months. This must be combined with systemic treatment in deep-seated, severe infections or peripheral corneal infections where scleral involvement is a risk. With the exception of natamycin, which is commercially available in the United States, antifungal agents are not available as proprietary preparations and therefore must be formulated in local pharmacies. The suggested choice of antimycotic agents is indicated in Table 12.

Antifungal treatment should be continued for a minimum of 3 months in most cases, especially if associated with deep corneal infection. Because of the risk of disease progression even low-dose steroid treatment is contraindicated (Fig. 17(b)). Complications associated with fungal keratitis reflect those of microbial keratitis in general: the risk of fungal endophthalmitis, which may occur, without perforation or limbal or scleral involvement, secondarily to progressive keratitis, necessitates close follow-up and early penetrating keratoplasty, with excision of at least 1 mm of clear cornea to remove viable organisms and prevent loss of the eye.

Parasitic infections

Onchocerciasis

Clinical features

Onchocerciasis is discussed in Section 2.15. Microfilariae can be seen in the anterior chamber, but are difficult to identify

Table 12 Drug choice in the main keratomycoses

Organism	Superficial infections	Deep infections
Aspergillus	Clotrimazole or econazole 1% drops	Add oral ketoconazole 400 mg daily or consider intravenous miconazole
Fusarium	Natamycin 5% drops	Add oral ketoconazole 400 mg daily and consider intravenous miconazole
Candida	Flucytosine 1% drops ± amphotericin B 0.15% or miconazole 1% drops	Add oral flucytosine 100–150 mg/kg and consider intravenous miconazole
Other fungi infections	Econazole or miconazole 1% drops	Add oral ketoconazole 400 mg daily and consider intravenous miconazole
Blind treatment of mycotic keratitis while awaiting culture results	Natamycin 5%	Oral ketoconazole and consider intravenous miconazole

within the cornea, although they can be picked up on retroillumination with the slit lamp. They are tolerated well while live, but when they die they produce a local inflammatory response that causes two types of keratitis, punctate and sclerosing. The punctate opacities are faint, and about 0.5 mm in diameter. They are termed snowflake, fluffy, or cracked ice and tend to disappear without scarring. Sclerosing keratitis occurs after prolonged infection. The location is peripheral and interpalpebral, but may rarely spread across the visual axis. In addition, secondary glaucoma, optic neuritis, and chorioretinitis occur. Results of corneal grafting are unsatisfactory due to concurrent involvement of the rest of the eye.

Pathology
Microfilariae become surrounded by a plasma-cell and lymphocytic infiltration in the corneal stroma. Investigation is by microscopy for microfilariae in biopsies taken from skin nodules in the periorbital cutaneous tissue.

Treatment
Treatment in the past involved drug regimens that kill microfilariae, but the dilemma was that it is the dead rather than live organisms that excite an immune response and tissue damage. Diethylcarbamazine was used, but has now been superseded by ivermectin, a compound that acts to reduce the numbers of microfilariae gradually over a few months, resulting in little inflammatory response. It is prescribed once yearly in endemic regions.

Acanthamoeba keratitis
Acanthamoebae were first identified as pathogenic by Culbertson in 1959 in mice and non-human primates. Before that they were considered harmless organisms. It then became apparent that they can cause keratitis and granulomatous encephalitis in man; the encephalitis remains rare but the keratitis is becoming increasingly common.

Acanthamoebae exist in two forms, either motile trophozoites or highly resistant cysts (Fig. 19). The cysts allow the organisms to survive in unfavourable environments. They are widely distributed, free-living organisms, having been identified in soil, air, and fresh and polluted waters from rivers, lakes, ponds, the sea, and reservoirs. The causative agents of human disease are either *Acanthamoeba polyphagia*, or *A. castellani*. To date, there appears to be no reliable evidence that there are significant differences in virulence amongst strains isolated from different sites, either corneal or environmental. The prognosis is reasonably good provided that appropriate therapy is instituted early in the disease. There appear to be no true incidence studies. Whilst the cornea is the predominant site of ocular infection, acanthamoeba uveitis and optic neuritis have been described.

Pathogenesis
The pathogenesis of acanthamoeba infection is described in detail in Chapter 1.2.2.

Clinical features
The first documented cases with keratitis occurred with the use of soft contact lens, and there appears to be no evidence of

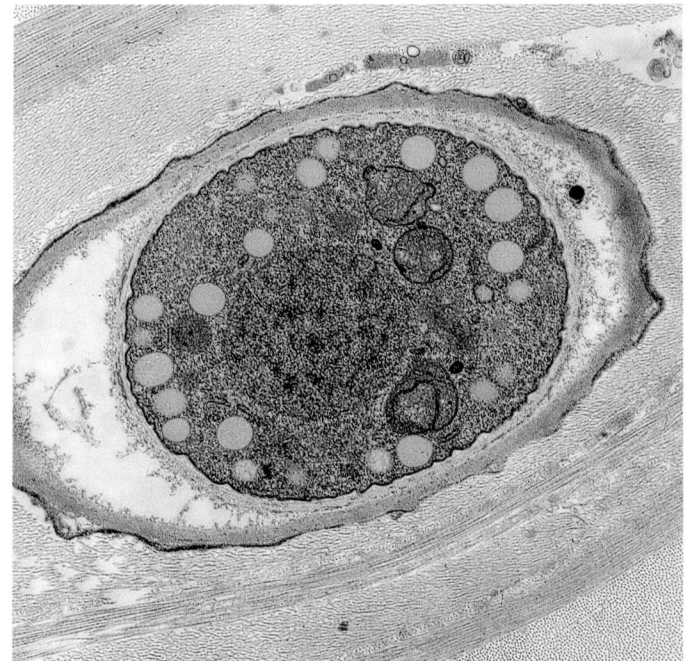

(a)

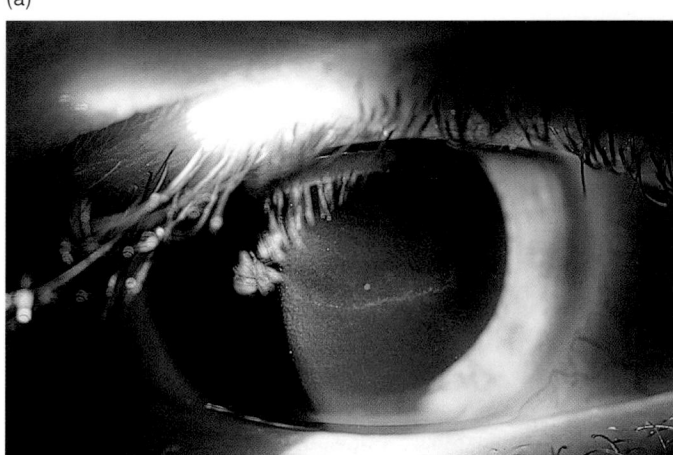

(b)

Fig. 19 (a) Electron micrograph of an encysted acanthamoeba. (b) Grade I acanthamoeba keratitis: the linear appearance of the infiltrate may be confused with herpetic infection; assessment of corneal sensation may aid diagnosis.

acanthamoeba keratitis before this time. The disease undergoes exacerbation and remission, probably due to the activation of encysted to active protozoal forms. There is evidence that chlorine-based cleaning and sterilizing solutions for contact lenses do not inhibit acanthamoebae, and there is often a history of inadequate lens hygiene by the patient. Table 13 illustrates the symptoms and signs that characterize the infection. There is frequently a history of wearing soft contact lens, with inadeqate attention to hygienic care of the lenses or their containers. The condition is usually unilateral but occasionally bilateral. Persistent pain, irritation, and watery discharge are presenting symptoms, with blurring of vision. The early lesion imitates a dendritic ulcer of herpes simplex virus without the typical end bulbs (Fig. 19(a)). The distribution of epithelial

Table 13 Symptoms and signs in acanthamoeba keratitis

Symptoms and signs	Comments
Watering, photophobia, soreness and pain, blurred vision Conjunctival hyperaemia Lid swelling, follicular conjunctivitis Palpable preauricular lymph node	Outstanding symptom is pain
Grade I keratitis; epithelial and subepithelial infiltration, with fluorescein staining	Can masquerade as herpes simplex keratitis
Grade II keratitis; discrete subepithelial opacities	Can masquerade as adenoviral keratitis
Grade III keratitis; interstitial or disciform keratitis—often without vascularization Ring infiltrates Infiltration around corneal nerves	Mimicks herpes simplex keratitis Useful specific sign Useful specific sign in making diagnosis
Grade IV keratitis; suppurative keratitis, scleritis, ulceration	
Grade V keratitis; descemetocele or perforation	May require emergency penetrating keratoplasty
Permanent scarring	May indicate elective penetrating keratoplasty, once fully controlled by treatment

lesions may vary between observations, which is uncharacteristic of ulcerative herpetic keratitis. Diagnosis at this stage has become much more frequent with increasing awareness of the condition. Untreated cases then develop stromal lesions, first as nummular lesions, subepithelial opacities (Fig. 20), with developing satellite lesions. Disciform oedema, immune rings (Fig. 21), perineural infiltrates, persistent epithelial deficits, stromal thinning (Fig. 22), and descemetocele can all occur. Corneal perforation is possible. Untreated disease in the long term is associated with pronounced conjunctival and scleral hyperaemia, which probably indicates spread of the organism further afield.

Investigation

Investigation must include culture of corneal epithelial scrapings, contact lenses, and lens cases on a lawn of *Escherichia coli*

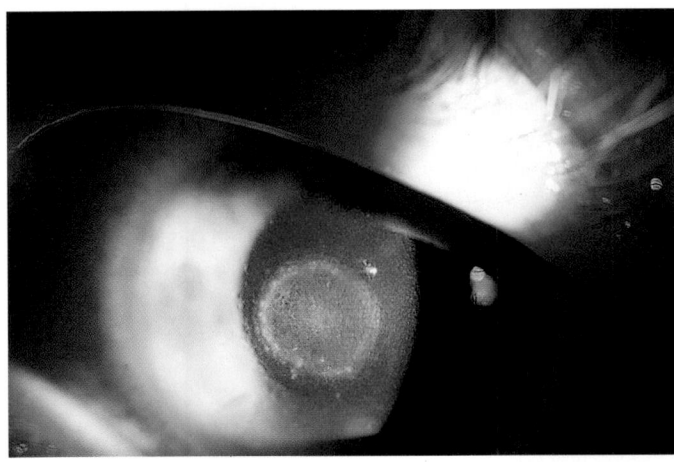

Fig. 21 Grade III acanthamoeba keratitis; interstitial disease with ring infiltration.

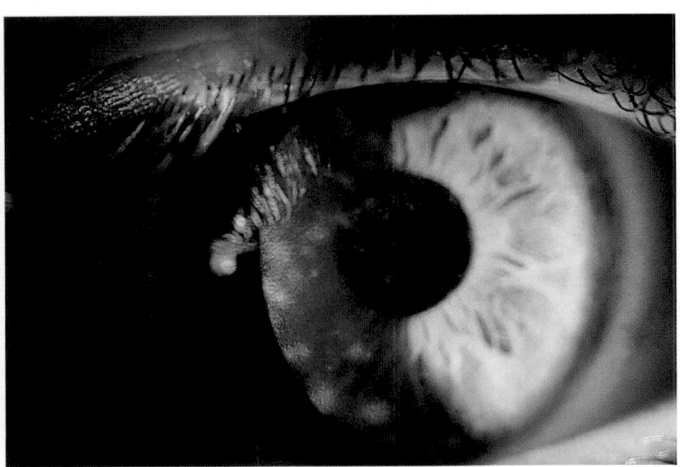

Fig. 20 Grade II acanthamoeba keratitis; discrete subepithelial opacities may resemble adenoviral keratitis.

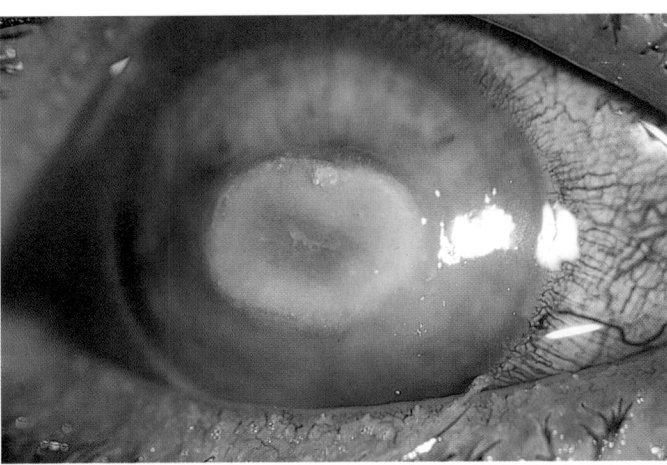

Fig. 22 Grade IV acanthamoeba keratitis; dense, suppurative infection with central thinning.

Table 14 Investigations in acanthamoeba keratitis

1. Take scraping (try to obtain an epithelial sheet), or biopsy from cornea, and take cultures from contact lens as well as the container
2. Culture for acanthamoeba on *E. coli* 'lawn' on non-nutrient agar
3. Do not forget to take bacterial cultures
4. Stain scraping or biopsy with calcafluor white
5. Consider immune peroxidase staining with polyclonal antibody
6. PCR, nested PCR and *in situ* PCR (only available in specialized microbiology units) may be required

PCR, polymerase chain reaction.

on non-nutrient agar gel. If the cultures are initially negative and the diagnosis strongly suspected , a biopsy should then be taken with a microtrephine 1 to 2 mm in diameter. Bacterial cultures should not be neglected. Specific staining with calcafluor white and immunofluorescent reagents may be necessary. If facilities are available, assay by polymerase chain reaction may clinch the diagnosis. Table 14 lists the investigations of use in acanthamoeba keratitis.

Treatment

Treatment is best instituted early after cultures have been taken to isolate the organism; Table 15 lists the medical and surgical management. It should be kept in mind that response to therapy is not always immediate, particularly in grade III or more severe disease. Sometimes, on beginning topical treatment, the symptoms and signs may worsen, perhaps because steroid medication has been stopped but probably more often due to killing

Table 15 Medical and surgical treatment in acanthamoeba keratitis

Therapeutic agent	Comments
Brolene (propamidine)	Does not provide complete response
Polyhexamethylbiguanide (PHMB)	Demonstrates good clinical efficacy with low toxicity; is still an experimental compound
Chlorohexidine	Demonstrates good clinical efficacy
Antibiotics	Secondary bacterial infection is common
Corticosteroids	Should be employed once the clinical signs improve as a response to therapy
Elective penetrating keratoplasty in quiescent disease	Best results obtained when the condition has been controlled by medical therapy; requires continuation of amoebicidal therapy
Emergency penetrating keratoplasty for perforation, or threatened perforation	Postoperative course stormy, and increased risk of recurrence and graft rejection. Requires continuation of topical amoebicidal compounds

of trophozoites, which thereby become more immunogenic. Utimately, where treatment is effective, the corneal inflammation dies down, the limbal hyperaemia reduces, and the symptoms regress. Treatment can be successfully achieved when it is applied early in the disease process. Propamidine isethionate 0.1 per cent was shown to be effective by Wright in 1985, but it was unsuccessful in some patients. Combinations of propamidine with miconazole, clotrimazole, and oral itraconazole with topical miconazole were reportedly effective in small numbers of patients. An advance was made in the 1990s when *in vitro* sensitivity studies showed that the cationic disinfectant polyhexamethylene biguanide was highly effective, and its successful clinical use at a concentration of 0.02 per cent was reported by Larkin in 1992. The advantage over other compounds lies in its consistently high cysticidal activity. There does not as yet appear to be any problem of toxicity associated with polyhexamethylene biguanide, in contrast to propamidine (Brolene). Experience has shown that polyhexamethylene biguanide is successful provided it is used early enough in the course of the disease, in which case penetrating keratoplasty is unlikely to be necessary. Treatment with polyhexamethylene biguanide must be begun either hourly or two-hourly, and continued at this frequency until improvement occurs, after which the drops can be used four times a day. Treatment must be continued for at least 4 months after resolution of inflammation. This is because late reactivation is possible. Polyhexamethylene biguanide can be combined with propamidine isethionate, although care is required to avoid toxicity of the propamidine. Recently the use of the diamidine derivative hexamidine, which also has cysticidal activity, has been reported. The use of chlorhexidine (0.02 per cent) as an alternative to polyhexamethylene biguanide has been reported in a number of patients. The main difficulty is that many of the compounds which have been used are not licensed for topical use in the eye. Brolene is available in the United Kingdom, but not in the United States, and polyhexamethylene biguanide must be prepared from commercial disinfectant. Clorhexidine must be specially prepared. Where no clear recommendation has been made by a professional or regulatory body based upon the results of a clinical trial, a physician must make a balanced judgement as to the most appropriate therapy to recommend.

Cycloplegic drops such as cyclopentolate or atropine are usually applied daily, and topical steroid may be required to depress inflammation after amoebicidal drops have taken effect. In advanced cases, corneal transplantation may be necessary. This is usually successful in uninflamed eyes but failures have been reported where inflammation has not been controlled. Owing to the improved efficacy of antiamoebal agents, penetrating keratoplasty is now usually unnecessary in the acute phase, except in cases where the corneal has become thin and perforation is threatened. Currently, the common indication is to improve vision in scarred corneas.

Avoidance

The wearers of contact lenses must be warned about risk factors, and advised to comply with instructions for lens-care solutions. Tap water should not be used to make up saline solutions with salt tablets. It is advisable to use thermal methods for sterilization, at temperatures of 70 to 80°C . Solutions containing hydrogen peroxide are valuable, but require 2 to 3 h to produce a reliable effect. Chloride-containing solutions are not so effective against acanthamoeba. Contact lenses must not be worn when swimming in baths or in sea water.

Viral keratitis

Viruses may invade the eye by two routes. The local route, whereby virus replication occurs on the ocular surface and the adjacent tissues, will concern this section. The alternative is by generalized infection, in which the eye is only one of several organs in which the virus replicates. The viruses that may involve the cornea (as well as the external eye) are listed in Table 16.

Herpesviruses

Herpes simplex virus

Herpes simplex virus (HSV) is one of the most common and most successful infections in man. There are two distinct serotypes, which are usually transmitted by different routes. HSV-I is transmitted by contact between skin or mucosal surfaces involving areas above the waist. HSV-II is transmitted by venereal routes, or via maternal genital infection to the newborn. In young adults, HSV-II primarily infects the genitalia. HSV-I is one of the more common causes of ocular infection in Western communities. It has been estimated that probably 500 patients with dendritic ulceration are seen per year per million population. The maximum incidence occurs between 40 and 50 years of age, with greater numbers of males than females affected. Associated recurrent herpes of the lips is reported in about 50 per cent of patients. Ocular recurrence occurs in 61 per cent, while the average number of attacks is 3.4. Primary attacks occur in 5 per cent of new cases. Neonatal infection of the skin, eyes or mouth, or as disseminated disease, occurs following primary infection close to birth. It is now occurring in about 1 in 3500 to 5000 births in the United States. Similar to other target organs, infection of the eye by HSV-II results in more serious disease than with HSV-I.

Pathogenesis In primary infection the virus multiplies in epithelial cells, reaching peak titres 3 to 4 days after infection. Active disease ceases within 2 weeks. Predictably, disease severity is related to the dose and the virulence of the virus.

Although cell-mediated responses clear the infection at the peripheral site, the virus is able to spread within the sensory nervous system and establish a latent infection in the related sensory ganglion very soon after the primary infection. In laboratory studies, virus introduced into the lip spread via the mandibular or maxillary divisions of the trigeminal nerve to the brainstem and then out via the ophthalmic division to reach the trigeminal ganglion. Further studies have shown that latency, identified by the presence of virus in the supernatant medium following culture of neuronal tissue, or by *in situ* hybridization of latency-associated transcripts, occurs within each compartment of the trigeminal ganglion. It is therefore probable that, following the establishment of latent virus within the ophthalmic part of the trigeminal ganglion, viral reactivation and neuronal spread to the cornea via the sensory nerve may lead to clinical disease under appropriate circumstances. This does not exclude direct inoculation as the mode of infection and the evidence, though not convincing, indicates that 5 per cent of all cases of ulcerative corneal disease represent primary disease. Reactivation and recurrence of disease in the eye are thought to be triggered by a number of factors that include sunlight, pyrexia, menses, and trauma. Ultraviolet irradiation triggered recrudescence in laboratory experiments. HSV has also been identified in corneal tissue taken from patients who have undergone transplantation for stromal herpes simplex keratitis in the absence of clinical evidence of active inflammatory disease (Fig. 23); here the precise form of the virus remains uncertain.

Histologically, epithelial disease in the form of dendritic keratitis is associated with the formation of multinucleated giant cells and intranuclear inclusion bodies. Necrosis of epithelial cells alongside the area of ulceration is accompanied by neutrophil infiltration of the underlying stroma.. In stromal keratitis, in addition to the influx of neutrophils, lymphocytes are present and are critical in the cascade of events that predisposes to chronic inflammatory sequelae. Granulomatous reactions can be seen at the level of Descemet's membrane, the mid-stroma, and Bowman's layer. Using immunoperoxidase techniques, herpes simplex antigens can be detected in keratocytes, endothelial cells and epithelioid histiocytes, together with multinucleated giant cells in necrotizing stromal keratitis, in contrast to inactive disease where viral antigen is not apparent, although it can be identified by coculture of corneal material taken from graft recipients for periods of up to 12 days. This suggests that the virus exists in either a latent or persistent form rather than as whole virus.

Table 16 Major groups of viruses that infect the eye

Family	Nucleic acid	Viruses that infect the eye
Herpetoviridae	DNA	Herpes simplex, varicella zoster, cytomegalovirus, Epstein–Barr
Adenoviridae	DNA	Adenovirus serotypes 3,4,7,8,10,12,14,15,19,21
Poxviridae	RNA	Molluscum contagiosum
Papoviridae	DNA	Wart virus
Picornaviridae	RNA	Coxsackie A24, enterovirus type 70
Togaviridae	RNA	Rubella
Bunyaviridae	RNA	Sandfly fever, Rift valley fever
Paramyxoviridae	RNA	Newcastle disease, mumps, measles

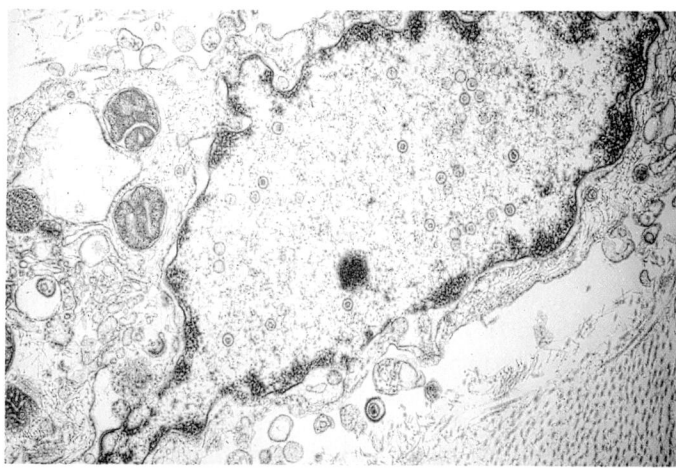

Fig. 23 Electron micrograph of herpes simplex virus in stroma; virus was isolated in the corneal button taken from a recipient with inactive central scarring. The tissue was organ-cultured for several days before sectioning for electron microscopy.

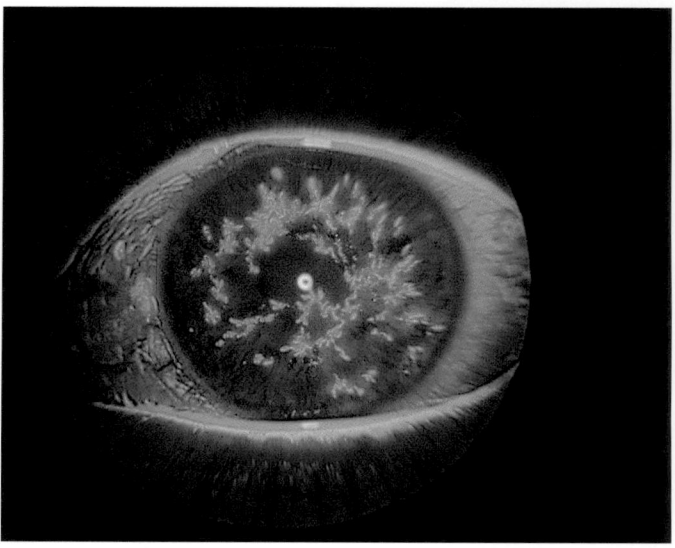

Fig. 25 Fluorescein staining of dendritic ulcer.

Clinical features Primary or recurrent disease can occur in the eye, usually affecting the cornea or the anterior uvea. Primary disease is rare, and involves the skin and lid margins as small vesicles (Fig. 24), the conjunctiva as a follicular inflammatory response, and the cornea as a single, often large, dendritic ulcer. Occasionally there may be many small ulcers extending on to the conjunctiva. Involvement of the deeper corneal tissue (the stroma) does not generally occur in primary disease.

In recurrent disease there is dendritic ulceration but the corneal stroma can also be involved, producing severe inflammation. At the tips of the branches of the ulcer, bulbs of opacity occur in the stroma. Iritis is a commonly associated feature.

The epithelial disease causes severe pain, watering, and photophobia. The infection is generally unilateral. Dendritic ulcers are the common feature of the ulcerative disease. The ulcer has an irregular zigzag configuration, with side branches forming a complex arborescence, and stains after the instillation of dilute fluorescein drops (Fig. 25). The surrounding epithelium becomes loose, and can be easily debrided with a cotton-wool applicator, a feature that in the past was used for treatment. The margin is vertical, where cells are opaque, laden with virus, and stain brilliantly with rose bengal. The ulcer usually heals in 5 to 12 days in the untreated state. Epithelial deficits or ulcers may remain for longer and can cause concern, but they probably represent poor epithelial regeneration rather than viral persistence. Table 17 presents manifestations of epithelial disease associated with HSV infection. Trophic ulcers, which differ from dendritic ulcers in having a rolled edge, are occasionally seen and are thought to be due to the corneal anaesthesia that is caused by HSV infection. They may be maintained in a chronic state by prolonged used of topical antivirals, which

Table 17 Disease of the corneal epithelium in herpes simplex keratitis

Primary disease	Punctate epithelial keratitis, necrotic plaques, areolar dendritic figure, multiple dendrites
Recurrent dendritic ulcers	Usually single figure, sharp edge
Resolving dendritic ulcer	Localized punctate keratitis
Ulcerative disease following topical steroid, or in immunodeficiency	Geographic keratitis (extends on to conjunctiva), increased frequency of attacks of dendritic ulceration
Trophic corneal ulceration	Persistent ulceration, rolled edge
Dendritic ulcer leading to secondary bacterial infection	Bacterial corneal ulcer in a patient with history of recurrent dendritic ulceration
Antiviral toxicity	Diffuse punctate keratitis extending to conjunctiva (first-generation antivirals), persistence of epithelial ulceration

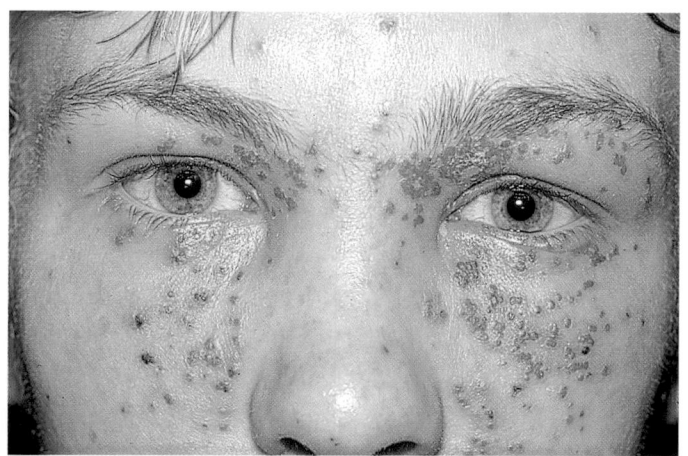

Fig. 24 Primary cutaneous herpes simplex in an atopic child.

in the past have been rather toxic. Since the advent of topical acyclovir ointment, chronic trophic ulcers are seen less frequently.

Investigation   Ulcerative keratitis is diagnosed by viral culture or immunofluorescent techniques. Enzyme-linked immunosorbent assays have proved useful, and they remain positive for viral antigen after treatment when culture has become negative. These enzyme assays are rapid and their results correlate with those from culture.

Stromal disease   Involvement of the stroma is the common sight-threatening manifestation of HSV infection. The manifestations of stromal disease are varied, and produce a number of clinical changes. In approx. 30 per cent of all patients experiencing ulcerative disease, the virus or its antigens can spread into the corneal stroma inducing various clinical appearances (Table 18).

Ghosting of dendritic figures occurs in the stroma underlying the previous ulcer, initially as a branched area of stromal oedema, and then persisting as a scar that may slowly disappear over many months or even years. When situated over the visual axis, vision will be affected (Fig. 26).

Superficial stromal punctate keratitis occurs on occasions, persisting for many months. The opacities are distributed mainly in the superficial stroma, and are variable in position, size, and shape (Fig. 27).

In disciform keratitis there is diffuse stromal oedema, infiltration with inflammatory cells, and other signs of active inflammation. There are folds in the deep layers such as Descemet's membrane, and keratoprecipitates; a mild iritis is charac-

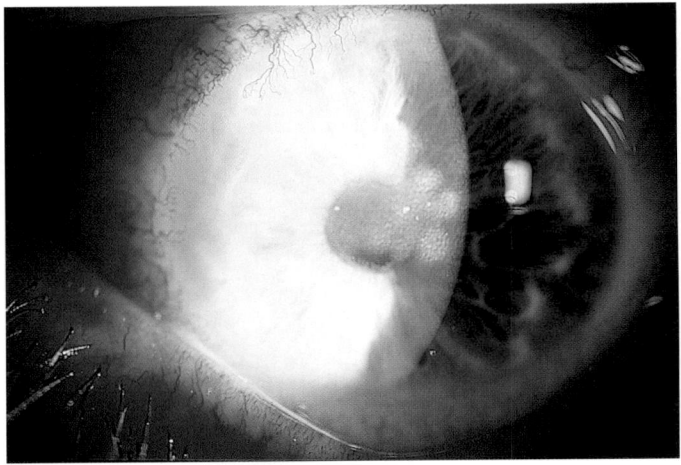

Fig. 26 Herpes simplex keratitis: ghosting of dendritic endbulbs.

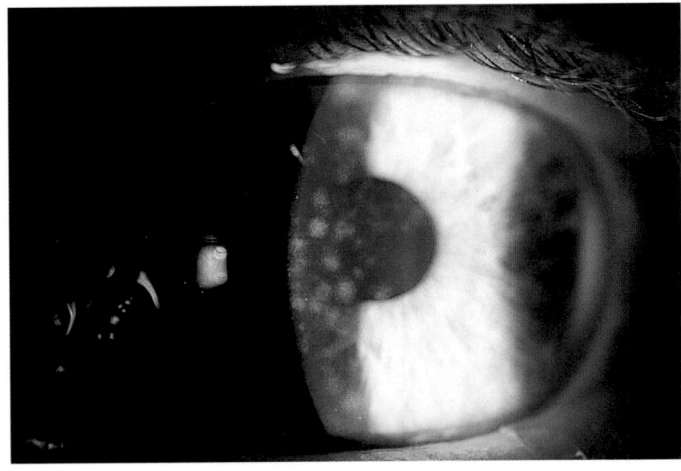

Fig. 27 Stromal punctate keratitis.

teristic. There are no blood vessels in the stroma, but there is limbal hyperaemia.

The formation of 'immune rings' can occasionally be seen, attributable to the deposition of antibody–antigen complexes within the stromal compartment attracting inflammatory cells (Fig. 28).

Peripheral (limbal) keratitis is characterized by a prolonged inflammatory response, vascularization by superficial and deep blood vessels, and often a persistent epithelial deficit. It may be slow to respond to treatment (Fig. 28).

Necrotizing stromal keratitis is a persistent form associated with foci of cellular infiltration, white or yellowish in colour, that fail to respond to anti-inflammatory treatment (Fig. 29).

Keratouveitis occurs when, in addition to corneal involvement, there is inflammation arising in the iris, with flare and cells within the anterior chamber, and large keratic precipitates.

Stromal keratitis (Fig. 30) with thinning or perforation can be seen in neglected cases.

Permanent stromal scarring generally follows stromal inflammation (Fig. 31). This may not be enough to cause per-

Table 18 Manifestations of stromal keratitis due to herpes simplex virus

Ghost of dendrite	Mild stromal oedema and subepithelial infiltrates closely resemble stromal reaction to previous dendrite
Superficial stromal punctate keratitis	Isolated punctate opacities irregular in size and shape
Disciform keratitis	Central corneal oedema and infiltration
Immune (Wessely) ring	Ring of inflammatory cells due to immune-complex formation
Peripheral keratitis	Persistent limbal keratitis, with vascularization and infiltration
Necrotizing keratitis	Severe stromal disease with focal collections of inflammatory cells
Keratouveitis	Diffuse keratitis with uveitis and large keratic precipitates
Stromal keratitis with thinning	May occur if treatment is neglected or inadequate
Inactive stromal scarring—central or peripheral	Absent oedema, infiltration and vascular hyperaemia

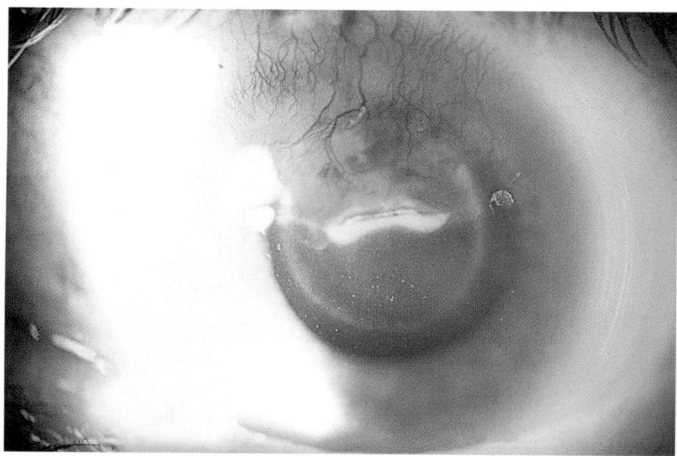

Fig. 28 Herpes simplex keratitis: immune ring formation; lipid deposition at the leading edge of the vascularized cornea is shown. (Slit lamp photograph using limbal scatter technique of illumination.)

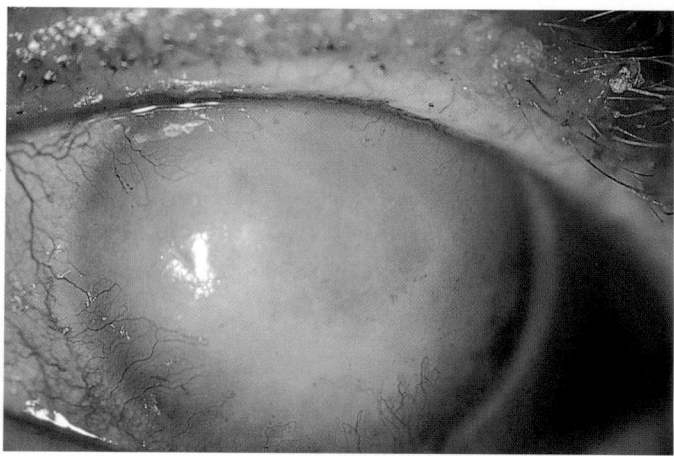

Fig. 31 Permanent stromal scarring involving the visual axis in herpetic keratitis.

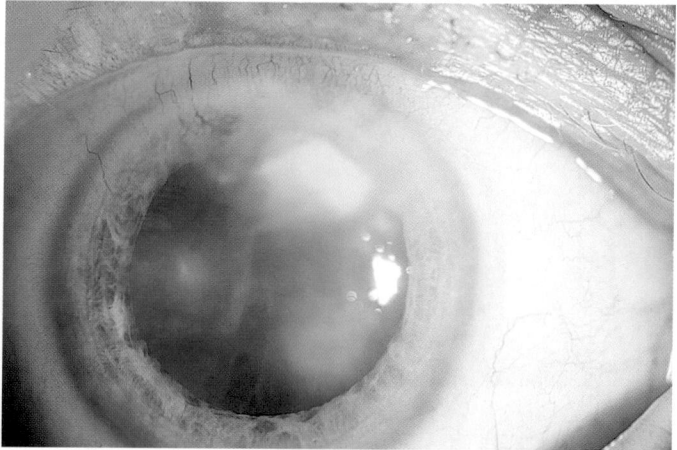

Fig. 29 Necrotizing stromal herpes simplex keratitis.

manent visual handicap, although keratoplasty is a common therapeutic outcome.

The corneal manifestations of neonatal infection take the form of diffuse stromal infiltration and oedema, with early vascularization.

Treatment The objective of treatment is to inhibit viral replication and at the same time reduce the inflammatory and immune reaction in the stroma, which, if ignored can lead to lasting damage to stromal collagen fibrils. Topical corticosteroid should never be used to treat dendritic ulcers because the virus can replicate freely in the presence of steroid-induced local immunosuppression, leading to enlargement of the ulcer. Such ulcers are known as amoeboid or geographic because of diffuse viral spread both within the epithelium and to the stroma (Fig. 32).

Choice of drug Certain analogues of purine and pyrimidine nucleosides are valuable in the treatment of infection due to HSV, where they act by competition with the nucleosides

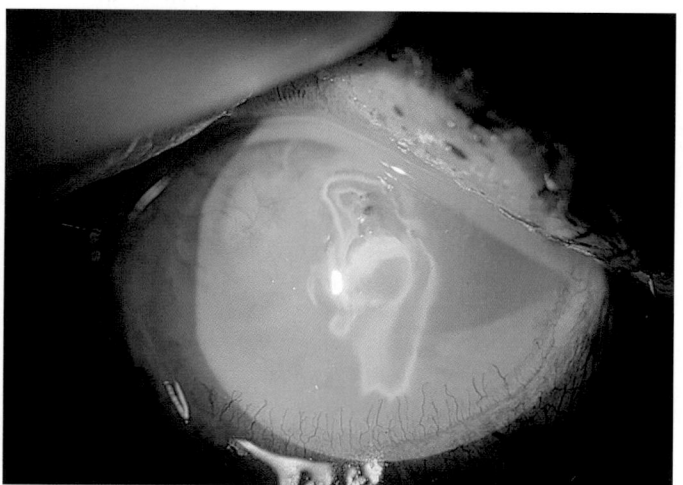

Fig. 30 Perforation following herpes simplex keratitis, with a positive Seidal test.

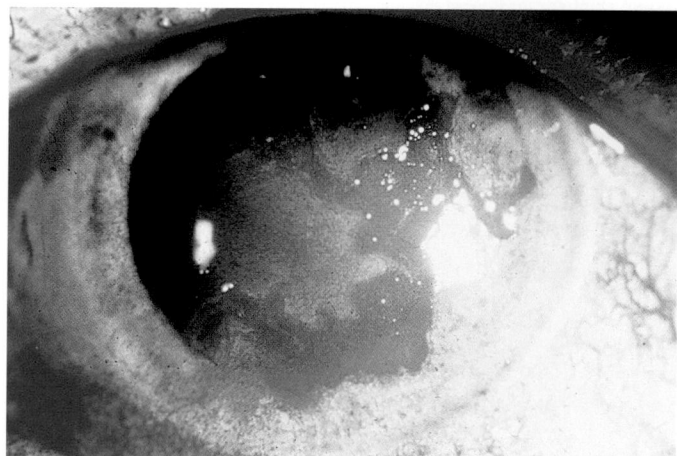

Fig. 32 Geographic ulceration in herpes simplex induced by topical steroid medication.

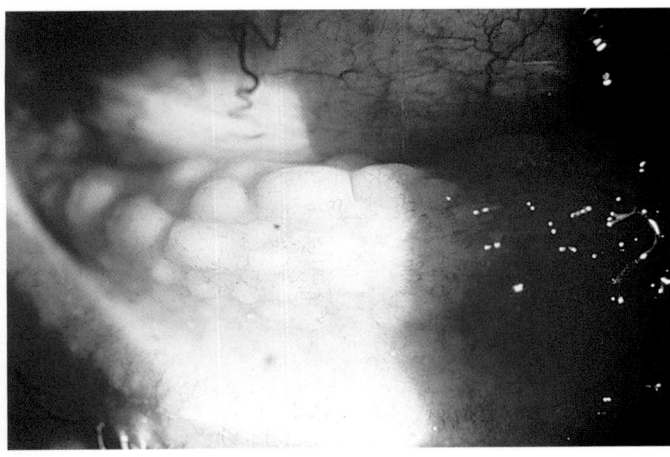

Fig. 33 Follicles in the lower fornix induced by prolong medication with iododexyuridine.

required for synthesis of the viral DNA. The rationale for their use depends on the slower proliferation of target cells than viral-infected cells, and therefore their toxic effects are minimal. Iodoxyuridine is a thymidine analogue that can be phosphorylated and incorporated into DNA. It was synthesized in 1959, following which it was found to inhibit plaque formation by HSV in culture. Kaufman first reported the activity of iodoxyuridine against ocular HSV infection *in vivo* in laboratory experiments and then in man in 1962. A number of groups subsequently reported therapeutic efficacy in herpes simplex keratitis. Adenine arabinoside acts by incorporation into viral DNA and inhibition of DNA polymerase. It has a similar effect to iodoxyuridine. The low solubility of iodoxyuridine and adenine arabinoside prevents good penetration into the stroma, limiting their effectiveness. Trifluorothymidine, however, is 10 times more soluble in water than iodoxyuridine, and does not produce toxic effects to such a high degree.

Acycloguanosine (acyclovir; Zovirax) is the generic term for 9-(2-hydroxyethoxymethyl)guanine. This is a prodrug, being converted *in vivo* by virus-specific thymidine kinase to the active form. The major advantage of this drug is its ability to penetrate the epithelial barrier of the cornea to reach the stroma and anterior chamber in therapeutic quantities. Plaque inhibition assays have shown that acyclovir is more active than iodoxyuridine, trifluorothymidine, and adenine arabinoside. Introduction of the drug as a therapeutic agent in patients with systemic herpes simplex infection in a dosage of 5 mg per kg 8-hourly demonstrated minimal toxicity with good efficacy. A number of investigators have reported a therapeutic effect of systemic acyclovir with topical corticosteroid in the treatment of stromal keratouveitis in uncontrolled studies.

Antiviral toxicity Toxicity occurs with the original antivirals after prolonged usage but is rarely a problem with short-term use as in the treatment of recurrent ulcerative disease. Toxic effects include follicular conjunctivitis (Fig. 33), bulbar conjunctival chemosis and hyperaemia, constriction of the puncti of canaliculi, punctate epithelial keratopathy, chronic epithelial deficits, reduction of tear secretion, and keratinization of the tarsal plates. Toxic changes are generally not seen with acyclovir, although after prolonged use punctate epithelial keratopathy occurs.

Systemic acyclovir may cause renal insufficiency, gastrointestinal distress, and headache. Less common side-effects are encephalopathy, nausea and vomiting, rash, urticaria, and phlebitis.

Indications for antiviral use Antivirals must be used in the treatment of primary herpes simplex keratitis, in association with systemic acyclovir where there is a significant mucocutaneous or facial eruption. As dendritic ulceration may act as a portal of entry for bacteria and not uncommonly cause a secondary bacterial abcesss, an adjunctive topical antibiotic is advisable.

In recurrent disease, antivirals should be used prophylactically where the trigger factors are known. Patients with frequent recurrences should have a topical antiviral available to instil immediately they become symptomatic, and should be advised to seek medical advice as soon as possible.

Treatment of stromal disease requires careful management. The presence of active inflammation must be recognized and documented. Do not use potent steroids in the treatment of stromal disease if possible; instead try to use the minimal dosage of steroid that will achieve control of the inflammation. Always taper down a potent steroid through lesser dilutions to avoid rebound of inflammation. Where full-strength, or dilutions of, topical corticosteroid are applied, an antiviral 'umbrella' should be used simultaneously. Since this may be for long periods, antivirals with low toxicity should be employed. A summary of treatment recomendations in stromal disease is given in Table 19.

Corneal grafting in herpes simplex keratitis Corneal grafting should be done only when there is a significant visual deficit. The main indication is for inactive corneal scarring, or for active disease where a corneal perforation has occurred. It is judicious to cover the use of topical steroids with a non-toxic antiviral to prevent recurrences during the postoperative period. Since surgical manipulation can induce viral shedding, many physicians use oral acyclovir for 10 days perioperatively as additional prophylaxis.

Varicella zoster virus
Varicella and zoster have very different clinical manifestations though caused by the same virus. The primary infection by varicella zoster virus results in chickenpox; approximately 3 000 000 cases per year occur in the United States, peaking in the spring. A benign condition in general, it carries significant morbidity in adults, immunosuppressed children, and in the unborn when contracted late in pregnancy. In the United States over 90 per cent of adults have serological evidence of previous infection by varicella zoster virus. It is estimated that up to 20 per cent of individuals will undergo reactivation of varicella zoster virus at some time during their life. Risk factors for an attack of zoster are advanced age, previous history of

Table 19 Treatment recommendations in stromal keratitis due to herpes simplex virus

Stromal keratitis in presence of dendrite or epithelial deficit	Avoid steroid until epithelium healed
Active stromal keratitis	(i) Use minimal concentration of steroid to achieve therapeutic effect (ii) Use antiviral cover (avoid first-generation antivirals for long-term use because of their toxicity) (iii) Dilate pupil with short-acting mydriatic
Resolved stromal keratitis	(i) Taper topical steroid through reducing dilution (prednisolone drops 0.5, 0.25, 0.125%) (ii) Continue to use antiviral cover
Inactive corneal scarring reducing vision to dishabilitating levels	Penetrating keratoplasty, requires: (i) initial intensive topical steroid medication (ii) antiviral cover: (a) topical (long-term) (b) systemic (e.g. 7–14 day course, acyclovir 200 mg four times a day)

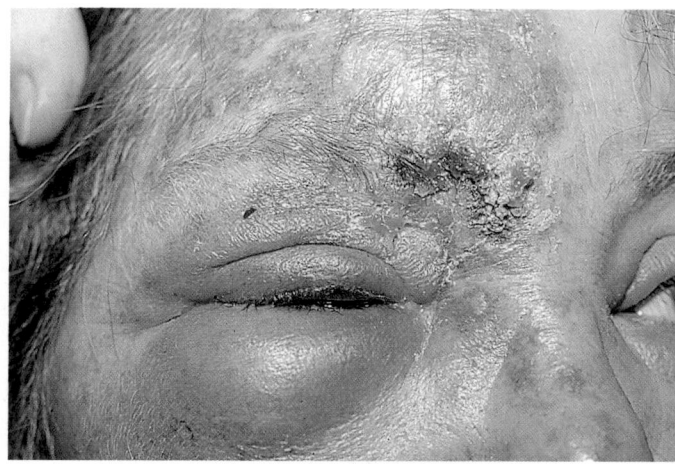

Fig. 34 Herpes zoster ophthalmicus.

cancer, anticancer therapy, bone marrow transplantation, surgery, and trauma. Immunosuppressive treatment and immunodeficiency, particularly the acquired immune deficiency syndrome, are important risk factors.

Pathogenesis For many years, zoster was believed to represent reactivation of latent varicella, but it was only recently that epidemiological, immunological, and molecular biological data have confirmed that the same virus is implicated in primary varicella infection and reactivated zoster in the same patient. The viral genome is thought to exist in a latent form in satellite cells of the neurone, and on reactivation, replication occurs in these cells with subsequent spread to the neurone and to a peripheral site. Corneal complications of herpes zoster ophthalmicus result from a combination of factors. These include presumed replication of the virus, limbal vasculitis, abnormal tear film, hypaesthesia, neurotrophic damage, and exposure, together with the vascular and inflammatory responses to all these factors.

Clinical features Herpes zoster ophthalmicus involves the first division of the trigeminal nerve, the rash extending from the eye to the vertex of the skull, without crossing the midline. The eruption is preceded by dermal hyperaemia and is at first vesicular, becoming pustular or haemorrhagic by day 3 to 4, and then drying with scab formation occuring at 7 to 10 days, leaving pitted scars in the long term (Fig. 34). The nasociliary nerve becomes involved in about 30 per cent of patients, but

ocular involvement may be seen in up to 50 per cent. Associated systemic features include headache, fever, and malaise. Prolonged and severe postherpetic neuralgia may occur. Herpes zoster is seen in patients infected with the human immunodeficiency virus, warranting consideration in patients who may be in a recognized risk group.

Involvement of the eye and surrounding tissue may take many forms (Tables 20 and 21). Corneal and scleral inflammation can be severe, and may occur many weeks after the eruption has healed. The corneal complications of varicella zoster infection include punctate epithelial keratitis, pseudodendrites (Fig. 35), anterior stromal infiltrates, sclerokeratitis, keratouveitis, serpiginous ulceration, mucous plaque formation, disciform keratitis, exposure keratitis, and neurotrophic keratitis. Occasionally the keratitis can be very severe and debilitating, particularly when associated with postherpetic neuralgia and severe lid disease. The acute phase may last for about 4 weeks, and in many cases may completely resolve. A chronic relapsing phase is also recognized. Corneal involvement is thought to be due to viral replication or the persistence of viral antigen in the deep tissue. However, other manifestations of corneal disease are caused by severe damage to the lid margins and tarsal plates, poor lid closure, limbal vasculitis (Fig. 36), neurotrophic damage, and recurrent variation in the host response.

Punctate epithelial keratitis occurs at an early stage; it is situated in the periphery of the cornea, and can lead to the appearance of microdendrites, which are well stained with rose bengal. It is thought that the lesion may be due to active viral replication, as virus has occasionally be isolated at this stage. Lesions may form filaments, when cores of epithelial cells become coated with mucus. Stromal infiltrates are seen in about 40 per cent of cases. Scleritis or episcleritis are often seen, and may be associated with sclerokeratitis. Lipid deposition is commonly seen in corneal lesions, particularly at the periphery of vascularized scars (Fig. 37). Uveitis is frequently concurrent, particularly when there is a disciform reponse, and is generally associated with vasculitis leading to sectors of iris atrophy, which is

Table 20 Non-corneal complications of herpes zoster ophthalmicus

Cutaneous eruption	Overlies V1 division of trigeminal nerve; rarely associated with simultaneous involvement of other dermotomes of Vth nerve; does not cross midline; nasociliary involvement implies ocular disease
Central nervous system	Delayed contralateral hemiplegia due to necrotizing angiitis of cerebral vessels
Cranial nerves	Transient oculomotor and facial nerve palsies
Sensory nervous system	Postherpetic neuralgia
Orbit	Proptosis, ptosis, myositis
Sclera	Episcleritis or scleritis—delayed for many months
Conjunctiva	Hyperaemia, haemorrhages, follicles, occasional vesicles or membranous conjunctivitis
Lids	Necrosis, scarring, notching, damage to lash follicles and meibomian glands, cicatricial entropion or ectropion
Uvea	Uveitis due to ischaemic vasculitis, with sectoral atrophy
Trabecular meshwork	Trabeculitis may cause elevated intraocular pressure
Retina and optic nerve	Retinal vasculitis, ischaemic optic neuropathy, retinal artery or vein occlusion, acute retinal necrosis syndrome

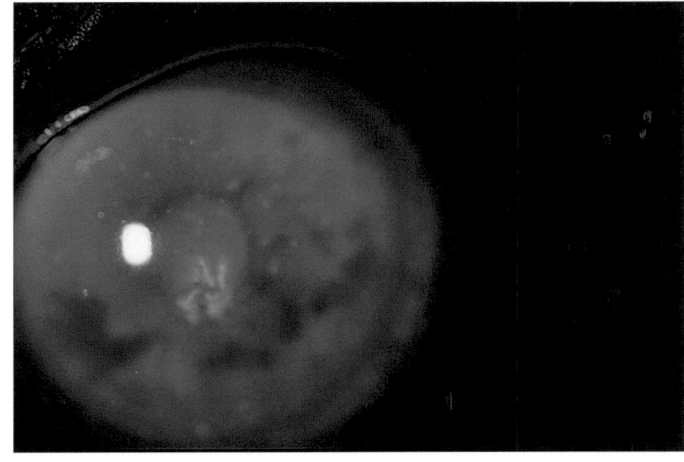

Fig. 35 Dendritiform ulceration in early herpes zoster ophthalmicus (illustration by courtesy of Ron Marsh).

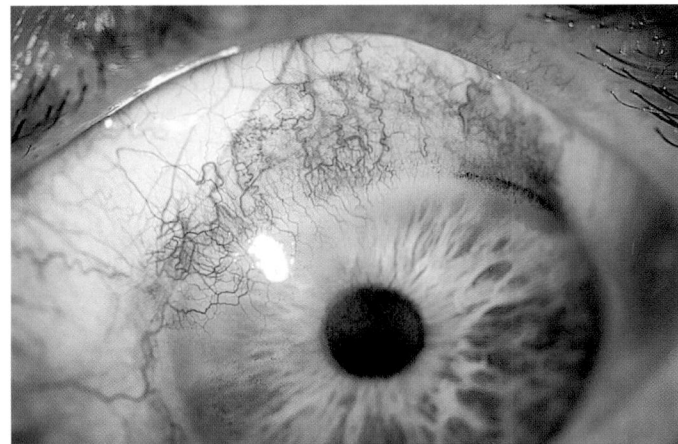

Fig. 36 Herpes zoster limbal vasculitis.

Table 21 Corneal complications of herpes zoster ophthalmicus

Epithelial	Puncutate epithelial keratitis Pseudodrendite Mucous plaque
Stromal	Limbal keratitis Cellular infiltration and oedema with subsequent vascularization, scarring, lipid deposition
Endothelial	Decompensation, and even detachment rarely
Limbal	Vasculitis associated with nodular scleritis
Exposure	Punctate keratitis, ulceration, vascularization, keratinisation, secondary bacterial infection
Neurotrophic	Persistent epithelial deficit, threatened corneal perforation
Secondary to treatment	Severe exacerbation of stromal keratitis on sudden cessation of topical steroid

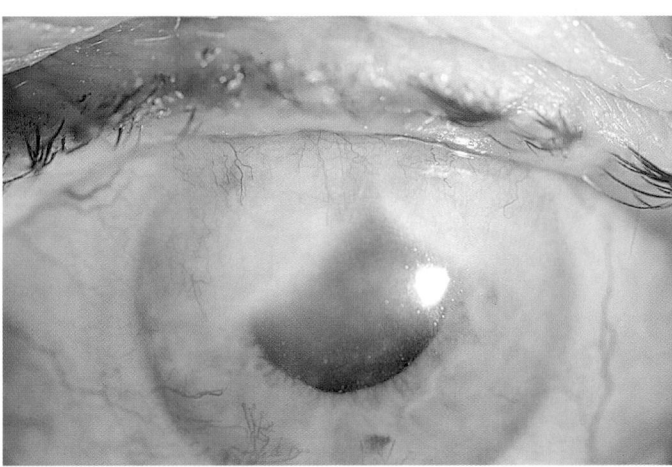

Fig. 37 Old limbal keratitis in herpes zoster; there is lipid deposition in the scars.

a typical sign easily demonstrated by coaxial illumination through the pupil with a narrow slit-lamp beam, highlighting the atrophic region by retroillumination. Serpiginous ulceration can be seen between 2 to 20 weeks after the original attack, and can be associated with mucous plaques. These plaques are white or grey lesions that are attached to swollen epithelial cells and stain with rose bengal. Neurotrophic or exposure keratitis occur somewhat later. Neurotrophic keratitis is seen in about 25 per cent of patients, and is associated with decreased corneal sensation. Disciform keratitis occurs in 20 per cent of patients with herpes zoster ophthalmicus, and in 78 per cent of patients in whom previous epithelial disease has occurred, often about 3 to 4 months after the original infection.

Investigation   The diagnosis of herpes zoster ophthalmicus is clear in the majority of cases, and laboratory tests are not usually necessary. However, on occasions HSV can present a zosteriform eruption. Other conditions that can resemble herpes zoster ophthalmicus include dermatitis, burns, and impetigo. A rapid diagnosis may be necessary where the skin eruption is atypical, and there is some urgency in prescribing the correct treatment. The simplest procedure is to stain material from a vesicle with haematoxylin and eosin, or Giemsa, to demonstrate multinucleated giant cells, abnormal nuclear chromatin, and acidophilic intranuclear inclusion bodies. Alternative, more specific methods are electron microscopy using immunogold techniques, immunoperoxidase staining or enzyme-linked immunosorbent assay of viral cultures, and DNA hybridization.

Treatment   Antiviral therapy in the past included idoxyuridine, cytosine arabinoside, and adenine arabinoside. Although there were therapeutic advantages demonstrable at the time, the discovery of acyclovir has rendered previous therapeutic modes obsolete. Intravenous acyclovir was first shown to be effective in placebo-controlled trials, demonstrating that outcome was improved in terms of duration of new lesion formation, time to loss of vesicles, and time to full crusting. Eventually is was determined that oral acyclovir was as equally effective as intravenous infusion. A number of clinical trials have been conducted, and these support the findings of the original intravenous study. However, there seems to be little effect on the severity and frequency of postherpetic neuralgia. It is important that acyclovir be administered within 72 h of the onset of the rash, and when it remains vesicular and not crusted. It has been shown repeatedly that oral acyclovir reduces late ocular complications. In one study, there were complications in 50 per cent of placebo-controlled patients and 29 per cent of acyclovir-treated patients. However, in a retrospective, case-controlled study over 5 years, no difference was indentified in the incidence of complications. Topical acyclovir ointment was found to be efficaceous when compared to topical steroid treatment, although it was uncertain whether topical steroid had a deleterious effect or whether there was a genuine advantage obtained with acyclovir. In immunocompetent patients the acute eruption should be treated with oral acyclovir tablets five times daily for 10 days, within 72 h of the first appearance of the rash. In immunodeficiency or immunosuppr-

ession, intravenous acyclovir is used. In addition, supportive treatment with analgesia and fluids is recommended.

Inflammation of the anterior segment in herpes zoster ophthalmicus must be treated conservatively. Where there is corneal involvement, with a stromal lesion interfering with vision, topical steroid is indicated in low dosage, using the minimal amount that achieves a clinical response. This is because it is not known whether topical steroid excites increased viral replication. Therefore use it sparingly, with a careful, tapering regimen on resolution to avoid rebound inflammation and severe recrudescence. Systemic steroid therapy does not seem to have a role in treatment, although it was once considered to be effective.

Other measures that may be necessary in severe disease include lateral or central tarsorrhaphy, corrective lid surgery, lid taping for exposure keratitis, and antibiotics to avoid secondary infectious keratitis; attention must also be paid to disease of the lid margin such as trichiasis and ectropion or entropion.

Stromal scarring can be treated by penetrating keratoplasty, although this can be hazardous where there is severe anaesthesia. However, where perforation is threatened there will little alternative to therapeutic keratoplasty. Visual results are considered satisfactory when patients are carefully selected to exclude those with severe corneal anaesthesia.

Epstein–Barr virus

Epstein–Barr virus was found during attempts to identify the cause of a lymphoma described by Burkitt in 1958 in East Africa. In 1962, Burkitt suggested that the lymphoma might be due to a virus because the geographical distribution was similar to that of yellow fever across equatorial Africa. In 1964, Epstein and Barr established continuous cell lines of lymphoblastoid cells, and virus particles that were morphologically similar to herpesvirus group were subsequently identified in sections of those cells. Corresponding viral particles were then recognized in patients with various malignancies and infectious mononucleosis.

Pathogenesis   The main portal of entry is the oropharynx, the virus replicating in the epithelia of the parotid and other salivary gland ducts and then involving B cells. The virus can be demonstrated in resting B cells of all Epstein–Barr virus-seropositive individuals in a latent state, and as a result probably escapes the immune surveillance of the host. In common with other members of the herpesviruses, Epstein–Barr virus is associated with symptomatic or asymptomatic primary infection. Thereafter the virus can persist for the remainder of the life of the host.

Clinical features   Most primary infections are acquired early in life and may be asymptomatic or provide non-specific symptoms, or cause an upper respiratory-tract infection. The oncogenic effects of the virus in the form of Burkitt lymphoma are now accepted, while B-cell lymphomas occur in organ-transplanted patients undergoing immunosuppression, patients with human immunodeficiency virus infections, and certain congenital immunodeficiency syndromes.

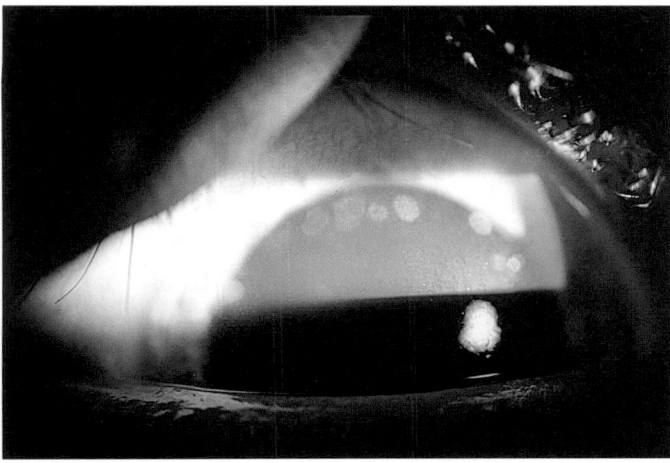

Fig. 38 Superficial stromal keratitis following Epstein–Barr virus infection.

Clinical disease of the eye is rare, and because of this is not easily recognized. Direct involvement of the eye or its adnexa has been recorded. Conjunctivitis with a follicular response in the tarsal plates and associated white spots, which are probably collections of inflammatory cells, can occur. Host membranous conjunctivitis is rare, as is keratitis. The keratitis may be sectoral or take the form of initial punctate erosions, with the development of stromal disease in the underlying regions. These are discrete, sharply demarcated, multifocal, pleomorphic or ring-shaped, and granular (Fig. 38), with normal intervening stroma, seemingly distinct from adenoviral or herpes simplex stromal keratitis. Other stromal manifestations resemble syphilitic keratitis. Nummular keratitis may be associated with infectious mononucleosis. Dacryoadenitis with periorbital oedema, episcleritis, uveitis, optic neuritis, and retinal vasculitis have been reported, but conjunctivitis is thought to be the most common ocular manifestation.

Investigation The diagnosis is suggested by detection of circulating autoantibodies induced during infectious mononucleosis, the classical one being the Paul–Bunnell heterophile antibody, which is directed against antigens on the surface of sheep erythrocytes. Serological testing is done to identify IgG to capsid antigen, indicating past infection and some degree of immunity. IgM anticapsid antibody indicates a current infection. A rising antibody titre to one of the capsid antigens indicates primary infection. Diagnosis rests on the demonstration of the virus, viral antigen, or viral DNA. Biologically active virus can be isolated from saliva, peripheral blood, or lymphoid tissue by means of its ability to immortalize cultured human lymphocytes. Epstein–Barr virus is demonstrated in pathological material by nucleic acid hybridization using southern blotting or *in situ* hybridization to identify the viral DNA.

Treatment Treatment of the keratitis is by careful use of topical steroid. The nummular lesions may remain in the long term.

Adenovirus

Virology

The adenoviruses are a large group of viruses that may cause inflammatory disease in other species as well as in man. There are now 41 serotypes recognized in man. The virus is composed of a central core of double-stranded DNA of between 35 000 to 40 000 bp surrounded by a capsid composed of 240 capsomeres that form a icosahedron . The 12 capsomeres at the apex of the icosahedron are known as pentons. At each vertex, there is an elongated glycoprotein structure that consists of a base and a fibre. Viral strains are identifiable by DNA mapping, although this seemingly bears little relation to virulence and pathogenicity.

Clinical features

Adenoviruses cause two types of conjunctivitis: epidemic keratoconjunctivitis associated usually with stroma punctate keratitis (Fig. 39), and pharyngoconjunctival fever, which is not associated with significant corneal pathology. Epidemic keratoconjunctivitis has been reported following infections by adenovirus 3, 4, 5, 7, 9, 11, 19, 21, and 10/19. Adenoviral conjunctivitis is discussed in Chapter 2.4.2. Transmission may often occcur through direct contact in hospitals, large institutions, physicians' offices, but community-based infections also occur. Contaminated fomites, such as applanators, solutions and fingers, are particularly liable to spread infectious virus. Hands must be washed between patients to reduce such risks.

Epidemic keratoconjunctivitis presents with follicular conjunctivitis and ipsilateral preauricular lymphadenopathy. The conjunctivitis can be both follicular and papillary, and is associated with subconjunctival haemorrhages. Involvement of the caruncle and semilunar fold is a pointer to diagnosis both in epidemic keratoconjunctivitis and pharyngoconjunctival fever. There is a watery or mucopurulent discharge, and sometimes a pseudomembrane may form, occasionally leading to scarring. A superficial punctate intraepithelial keratitis occurs, followed by focal epithelial keratitis, leading to lesions in Bowman's

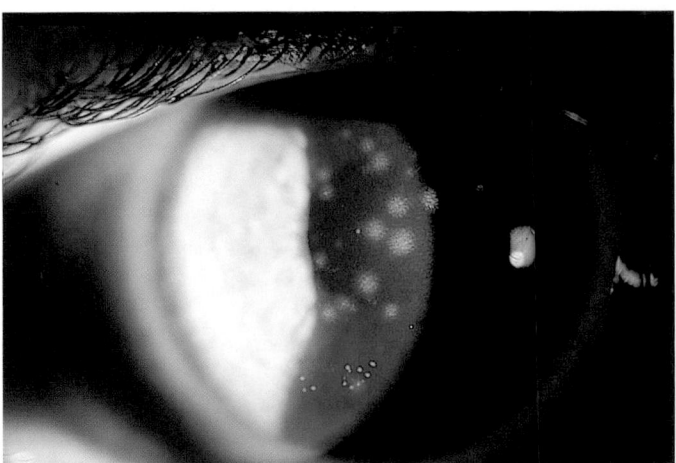

Fig. 39 Superficial punctate stromal keratitis following epidemic keratoconjunctivitis.

membrane and the anterior corneal stroma (Fig. 39). The stromal lesions are circular, and best demonstrated by limbal scatter using the slit-lamp beam. After a few days the epithelial lesions disappear, but the stromal lesions may persist, although they eventually regress. It during the stage of epithelial disease that the virus can be indentified by culture. It is speculated that the stromal lesions represent an immunological response to persistent viral antigen. When the centre of the cornea is involved, the vision is adversely effected. Epidemic keratoconjunctivitis should be differentiated from Thygeson's superficial punctate keratitis, which is epithelial, characterized by clusters of small dots, and lacking generally in a stromal component. It rapidly disappears after treatment by topical steroid, but generally recurs after cessation of treatment.

Pharyngoconjunctival fever is highly infectious and associated with follicular conjunctivitis, occasionally haemorrhagic, and enlargement of regional lymph nodes. Non-specific follicular conjunctivitis due to adenoviral infection may occur in children or adults, and is caused by a number of other serotypes without corneal involvement. On occasions, adenovirus can be isolated in cases of chronic papillary conjunctivitis after several weeks after infection.

Investigation
In the first few days of infection, paired blood samples may be taken to demonstrate a rising titre of antibody. The first should be taken at 7 days, and the second 2 to 3 weeks later. There should be a fourfold rise in complement-fixing antibody. Other tests include immunofluorescence and enzyme-linked immunosorbent assays. Scrapings demonstrate a mixed lymphocytic reaction and neutrophil infiltrates with degenerate epithelial cells.

Treatment
At present there is no appropriate antiviral for adenoviral conjunctivitis or keratitis, although there is the promise of suitable agents becoming available in the future. The treatment of superficial stromal punctate keratitis with dilute topical corticosteroid to relieve symptoms and infiltrates temporarily has been controversial for many years. It is considered that, although steroid drops help to reduce stromal opacities, their use may induce persistence and recurrence when the dose is tapered down. On the whole it is prudent to avoid topical steroid, only using it when there is visual impairment. Topical antibiotic should be used particularly where there is membrane formation. Isolation facilities should be used in clinics during epidemics, while hygienic measures must be used by medical and nursing staff to avoid hospital-based spread of infection.

Molluscum contagiosum
The molluscum agent is a DNA virus of the pox group. Attempts to culture the virus have not been successful, and humans are the only known host. It is more commonly found in children up to the age of 10. It is also seen in immunodeficiency such as in acquired immunodeficiency syndrome. Spread is by direct contact and the incubation period is up to 6 months.

Clinical features
Molluscum contagiosum is occasionally found in the skin of the lids as discrete nodules, 2 to 5 mm in diameter, limited to the epidermis. The lesions are white, painless, and umbilicated; at their top is a small white core. Viral shedding causes secondary conjunctivitis with a follicular reaction in the fornices and tarsal plates. The conjunctivitis may persist for at least 2 years. In severe cases, punctate epithelial keratitis, occasionally with filamentary keratitis, can occur. Superficial vascularization can be seen. The keratitis occurs in the upper part of the cornea at the superior limbus. It disappears once the nodules have been removed.

Pathology
The nodules are cup-shaped and the hyperplastic epidermis contains hyaline, acidophilic, cytoplasmic masses called molluscum bodies, which are eosinophilic at first and then become basophilic. These bodies are divided into cavities in which are clustered masses of viral particles that have a similar brick shape to that of the vaccinia virus. Investigation is by microscopy of curretted lesions using Giemsa stain, which reveals the molluscum bodies. Scrapings from the conjunctiva may also be investigated in the same way.

Treatment
The molluscum is easily removed in total. In addition it can be treated by cryothermy, but remember that this results in depigmentation, which can be unacceptable in black subjects. In acquired immune deficiency syndrome the infection is severe and is not self-limiting.

Human papillomavirus (HPV)
Papillomas may arise in the conjunctiva and are pedunculated or sessile, with a fibrovascular core covered by acanthotic squamous epithelium. Bilateral cases occur, and may be associated with HPV-6, -9 or -11. Lesions may spread to the tarsal conjunctiva, and keratinization can occur.

Intraepithelial dysplasia is thought to be related to HPV infection, originating in the conjunctiva as a barely visible thickening that is demonstrated 2 to 3 min after the instillation of fluorescein dye, when the extent of abnormal cellular proliferation is clearly demarcated by faint, punctate staining, visible with a blue filter. Like the conjunctival papillomas themselves, the appearance of this proliferation varies from that of a gelatinous mass to merely an isolated island of dysplastic cells. Once the lesions have invaded the corneal epithelium, their appearance becomes easily defined by islands of grey cells with a fimbriated edge, often in continuity with a conjunctival lesion (Fig. 40). Conjunctival lesions are associated with increased vascularization, but vessels invade corneal lesions at a late stage. Various other terms have been used to describe these lesions including intraepithelial epithelioma, Bowen's disease, precancerous epithelioma, or conjunctival intraepithelial neoplasm.

Histology
There is now evidence that HPV may be involved in conjunctival papillomas, intraepithelial dysplasia, and conjunctival car-

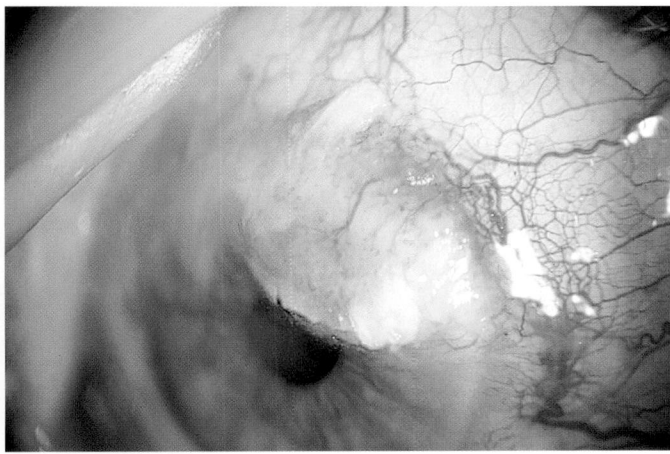

(a)

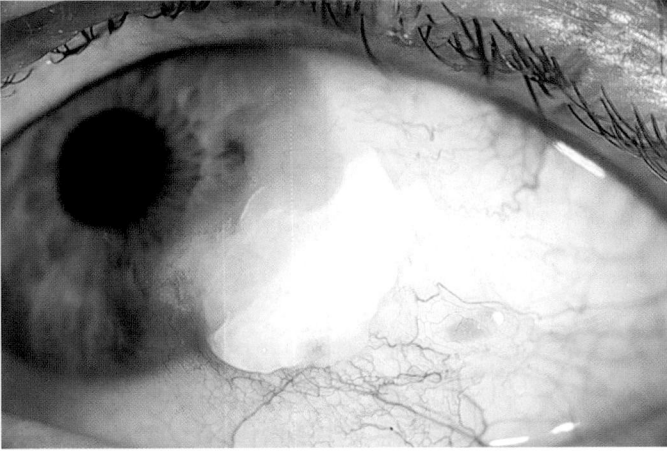

(b)

Fig. 40 (a) and (b) Two examples of corneal intraepithelial dysplasia.

cinoma. This is based on the high prevalence of HPV DNA, as identified by the polymerase chain reaction, in conjunctival papillomas and intraepithelial dysplasia. HPV-16 and -18 have been found in association with mucosal dysplasias, including the conjunctiva. Histologically the various clinical manifestations of HPV in the conjunctiva resemble the epithelial lesions of the uterine cervix. Koilocytosis (cells with shrunken, hyperchromatic nuclei and cytoplasmic clearing), which is associated with HPV infection of other mucosae, has been identified in these conjunctival and corneal lesions. Dependent on the position of mitotic figures (basal, half-thickness, and full-thickness), lesions are described as mild, moderate, and severe.

Treatment

Treatment of intraepithelial dysplasia is by surgical excision, although this is followed by recurrence in many cases. Operative removal is assisted by cryotherapy, and β-irradiation.

References

Abbott, R. L., Kremer, P. A., and Abrams, M. A. (1994). Bacterial corneal ulcers. In *Duane's clinical ophthalmology* (ed. Tasman, W. and Jaeger, E.A.), Vol. 14, Chapters 18, 18A. Lippincott–Raven, Philadelphia.

Alizadeh, H., Niederkorn, J. Y., and McCulley, J. P. (1996). Acanthamoebic keratitis. In *Ocular infection and immunity* (ed. J. S. Pepose, G. N. Holland, and K. R. Wilhelmus), pp.1062–71. Mosby, St Louis.

Allan, B. D. S. and Dart, J. K. G. (1995). Strategies for the management of microbial keratitis. *British Journal of Ophthalmology*, **79**, 777–86.

Bron, A. J. (1973). A simple schema for documenting corneal disease. *British Journal of Ophthalmology*, **57**, 629–34.

Duke, B. O. L. *et al.* (1990). Effects of multiple monthly doses of ivermectin on adult *Onchocerca volvulus*. *American Journal of Tropical Medcine and Hygiene*, **43**, 657–64.

Duke, B. O. L. *et al.* (1991). Viability of adult *Onchocerca volvulus* after six two weekly doses of ivermectin. *Bulletin of the World Health Organization*, **69**, 163–8.

Easty, D. L. *et al.* (1987). Herpes simplex virus isolation in chronic stromal keratitis. Human and laboratory studies. *Current Eye Research*, **6**, 69.

Ficker, L., Kirkness, C., McCartney, A., and Seal, D. (1991). Microbial keratitis—the false negative. *Eye*, **5**, 549–59.

Foster, C. S. (1992). Fungal keratitis. *Infectious Disease Clinics of North America*, **6** (4).

Jones, B. R. (1975). Principles in the management of oculomycosis. *American Journal of Ophthalmology*, **79**, 719–51.

Jones, D. B. (1981). Decision making in the management of microbial keratitis. *Ophthalmology*, **88**, 814–20.

Garner, A. (1976). Pathology of ocular onchocerciasis, human and experimental. *Transactions of the Royal Society of Tropical Medicine and Hygiene*, **70**, 374–7.

Hay, J., Kirkness, C. M., Seal, D. V., and Wright, P. (1994). Drug resistance and *Acanthamoeba* keratitis, the quest for alternative antiprotozoal chemotherapy. *Eye*, **8**, 555–63.

Hyndiuk, R. and Glasser, D. (1986). Herpes simplex keratitis. In *Infections of the eye* (ed. K. F. Tabbara and R. Hindiuk), p. 343. Little Brown, Boston.

Larkin, D. F. P. (1992). Treatment of *Acanthamoeba* keratitis with polybexamethylene biguanide. *Ophthalmology*, **99**, 185.

Larkin, D. F. P. and Easty, D. L. (1991). Experimental *Acanthamoeba* keratitis, immunohistochemical evaluation. *British Journal of Ophthalmology*, **75**, 421.

Leisegang, T. (1985). Corneal complications from herpes zoster ophthalmicus. *Ophthalmology*, **92**, 316

Liesengang, T. *et al.* (1989). Epidemiology of ocular herpes simplex. Incidence in Rochester, Minnesota (1950 through 1982). *Archives of Ophthalmology*, **107**, 1155.

Matoba, A., Wilhelmus, K., and Jones, D. (1986). Epstein Barr viral stromal keratitis. *Ophthalmology*, **93**, 746.

Pavan-Langston, D. (1990). Major ocular viral infections. In *Antiviral agents and viral diseases in man* (3rd edn) (ed. G. Galasso, R. Whitley, and T. Merrigan), p. 183. Raven, New York.

Pavan-Langston, D. (1994). Viral disease in the cornea and external eye. In *Principles and practice of ophthalmology* (ed. D. M. Albert and F. A. Jacobiec), pp. 117–61. Saunders, Philadelphia.

Stehr-Green, J. K., Bailey, T. M., and Visvesvara, G. S. (1989). The epidemiology of *Acanthamoeba* keratitis in the United States. *American Journal of Ophthalmology*, **107**, 331.

Taylor, H. R. and Nutman, T. B. (1996). Onchocerciasis. In *Ocular infection and immunity* (ed. J. S. Pepose, G. N. Holland, and K. R. Wilhelmus), pp. 1481–504. Mosby, St Louis.

Watson, A. P., Tullo, A. B., and Kerr-Muir, M. G. (1988). Arborescent bacterial keratopathy (infectious crystalline keratopathy). *Eye*, **2**, 517.

Wilson, R., II. (1986). Varicella and herpes zoster ophthalmicus. In *Ocular infection* (ed. K. Tabbara and R. Hyndiuk), p. 369. Little Brown, Boston.

2.6.4 The cornea in immunological, degenerative, and metabolic disease

Gavin W. Marsh and David L. Easty

Immunological disease

The cornea is affected by a number of immunological diseases including peripheral ulcerative keratitis, Mooren's ulcer, rosacea keratitis, phlyctenular keratitis, Cogan's syndrome, and corneal graft rejection. Immunological diseases of the conjunctiva or sclera lead to secondary disease of the cornea, as in Stevens–Johnson syndrome, cicatricial mucous membrane pemphigoid, pseudomucous membrane pemphigoid (associated with topical therapies such as sympathomimetic agents used in the treatment of glaucoma), Sjögren's syndrome, graft-versus-host disease following marrow transplantation, and various forms of scleritis.

It is the anatomical features of the corneal periphery that seem to lead to an added risk of immunologically based inflammatory disease. For example the end capillaries of the vascular system and the lymphatic drainage begins at the limbus. There are a number of specialist cells, in greater profusion than elsewhere, such as Langerhan's cells, and mast cells. Other features of the limbus that make it susceptible to disease are indicated in Table 1.

There are many conditions that can be encountered at the corneal periphery, for example limbal vernal catarrh, peripheral ulcerative keratitis, and staphylococcal infiltrates (Table 2). In addition degenerative and certain metabolic disorders demonstrate peripheral corneal changes.

Peripheral ulcerative keratitis

This is one of the most severe management problems that a clinician will encounter. It is thought to be the ocular counterpart of a systemic disorder involving the immune system because of the association with a number of connective tissue disorders such as rheumatoid arthritis (Table 3). Sometimes

Table 1 Features of the corneal limbus

Contains arcades of end vessels	Watershed for immune responses
Lymphatics originate	Drain to the preauricular and submandibular lymphatic nodes
Mast cells present in greater numbers	Account for limbal acute allergic response
Rapid inflammatory and immune response	Immediate response to corneal insults
Langerhan's cells present	Process central corneal antigen
Stem cells	Source for epithelial replication

Table 2 Peripheral corneal disease

Peripheral corneal infiltrates	Associated with *Staphylococcus aureus* in lids
Rosacea keratitis	Look for cutaneous signs
Trachomatous pannus	Do full external eye examination
Peripheral ulcerative keratitis	Eliminate systemic disease
Herpes simplex keratitis	Check for keratic precipitates and iris atrophy
Phlyctenular keratitis	Check family history for tuberculosis
Limbal vernal disease	Classical appearance of follicles
Mooren's ulcer	Not associated with systemic disease
Pelucid marginal degeneration	Inferior corneal thinning (beer belly appearance)
Keratoglobus	Globoid protrusion of thin cornea
Terrien's ulceration	Usually begins upper limbus — with stromal opacity
Arcus senilis	Band of grey–white deposit separated from limbus by translucent zone

Table 3 Systemic conditions seen in association with peripheral ulcerative keratitis

Condition	Comments
Rheumatoid arthritis	General endstage arthritis
Wegener's granulomatosis	May be a presenting manifestation
Polyarteritis nodosa	Comparatively rare cause
Scleroderma	Multisystem disease; skin thickened, + Raynaud's phenomenon
Systemic lupus erythematosus	Multisystem disorder, with arthritis, skin, haematological, pulmonary, cardiovascular, and neurological disorders
Relapsing polychondritis	Inflammation in cartilagenous tissues
Giant cell arteritis	Rare; can be associated with scleritis
Psoriasis	Plaque keratotic skin lesions

sterile peripheral ulcerative keratitis presents before a systemic disease, and so in every case, a full set of investigations for connective tissue disorders should be performed. The commonest disease association is rheumatoid arthritis, which is also associated with keratoconjunctivitis sicca, episcleritis, scleritis, peripheral and central corneal ulceration, and sclerokeratitis. In sclerokeratitis there is inflammatory infiltration of the peripheral cornea with vascularization and without thinning. There may be crystalline stromal opacities due to lipid deposition (Fig. 1). Occasionally stromal ulceration occurs.

Peripheral ulcerative keratitis is difficult to manage when associated with rheumatoid arthritis (Fig. 2). Usually the arthritis is advanced with considerable deformity in the hands and feet. Nevertheless it is not clinically active. Sometimes it is associated with scleritis, but at other times, it can be seen with minimal scleral or limbal inflammation. Rarely peripheral

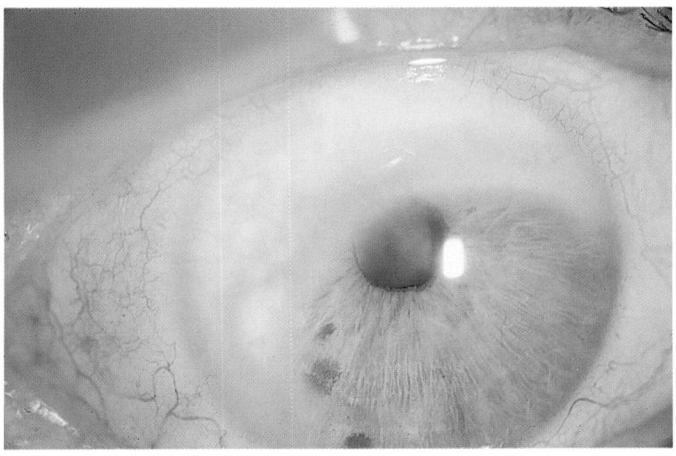

Fig. 1 Lipid keratopathy associated with recurrent attacks of scleritis.

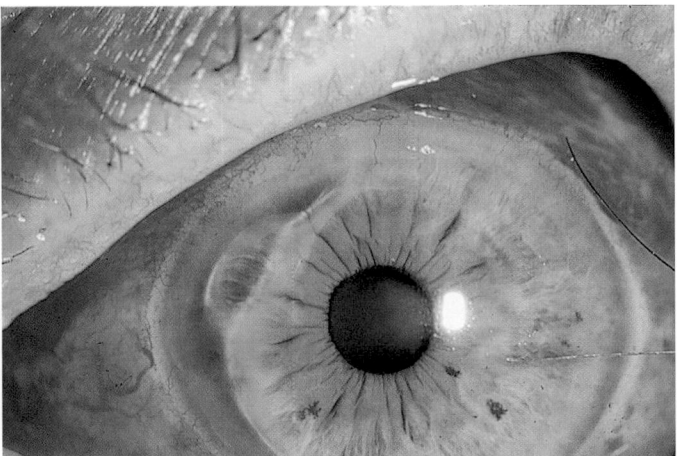

Fig. 2 Peripheral ulcerative keratitis associated with rheumatoid arthritis.

ulcerative keratitis is activated in rheumatoid patients undergoing cataract extraction, or as a result of an apparent marginal ulcer due to staphylococcal blepharitis. There is occasionally evidence of conjunctival shrinkage with shallow conjunctival fornices, and there is commonly advanced Sjögren's syndrome.

Pathogenesis

The systemic disorders that are associated with peripheral ulcerative keratitis may be characterized by a vasculitic component, but it is not always possible to identify this fundamental immunological response in biopsy material which is not frequently available. It is the inflammatory reaction at the limbus that is held to be the cause of the ulcer by the production of destructive enzymes in the tissue leading to loss of basement membrane (type IV collagen), particularly induced by specific matrix metalloproteases. The limbal infiltrate is composed of an array of different cell types, but predominance of granulocytes leads to excess enzyme production and tissue damage.

Table 4 Clinical features of peripheral ulcerative keratitis

Feature	Comments
Epithelial deficit inside limbus	Sign of activity
Stromal thinning	Generated by locally produced matrix metalloproteases
Limbal hyperaemia	May not be pronounced
Elevated limbal conjunctiva	Sign of activity
Descemetocele and threatened perforation	Perforation often the indication for surgical intervention

Clinical features

The clinical features are shown in Table 4. In peripheral ulcerative keratitis there is a varying amount of peripheral ulceration, with sometimes no infiltration or vascularization (Fig. 2). There may be a descemetocele formation leading to perforation (Fig. 3). The signs of active disease are crucial, and include limbal hyperaemia, although it is unusual to see active vascularization of ulcerated areas. The elevated or rolled edge to the limbal conjunctiva is a key sign of active inflammation, and until this has disappeared, the disease is probably not fully controlled by treatment. Table 5 indicates the signs of resolving disease and a case of resolved peripheral ulcerative keratitis is

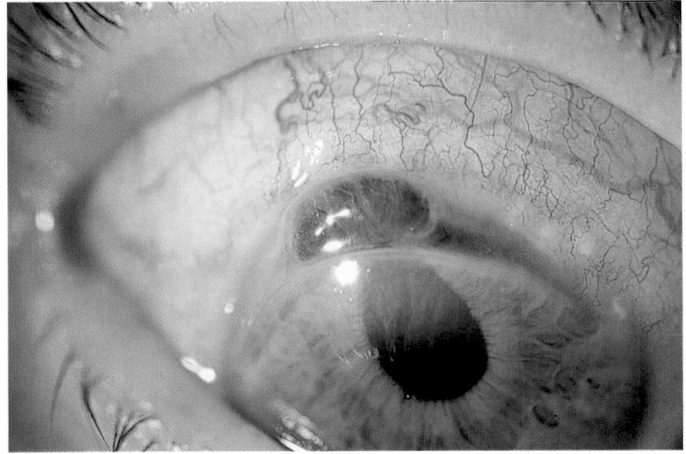

Fig. 3 Descemetocele formation resulting in perforation in peripheral ulcerative keratitis.

Table 5 Signs of resolution of peripheral ulcerative keratitis

Resolution of epithelial deficit
Resolution of limbal hyperaemia
Vascularization of ulcerated area
Faint superficial scarring of ulcer
Flattening of elevated limbal conjunctiva
Stromal thinning persists but does not progress

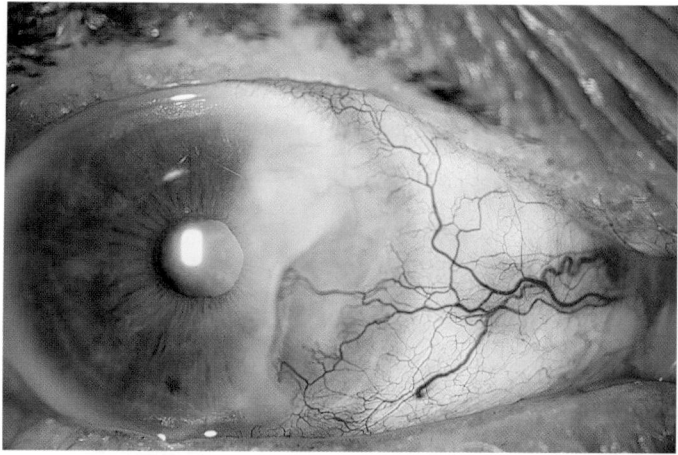

Fig. 4 Inactive peripheral ulcerative keratitis—resolution of limbal hyperaemia is accompanied by vascularization and scarring in the thinned cornea.

Table 6 Outcomes following various treatment modes in peripheral ulcerative keratitis

Topical antibiotics, steroids and tear substitutes	Be careful of toxicity induced by multiple therapy. Steroids may enhance melting process
Bandage contact lens	May increase risk of infection in a dry eye
Permanent occlusion of lacrimal canaliculi	Important to consider as severe sicca syndrome is common. Important after keratoplasty for corneal perforation
Histoacryl glue for perforation	A useful aid to preserve ocular integrity, prior to control by systemic treatment, and prior to keratoplasty
Resection of, or cryotherapy to limbal conjunctiva	Has not proved effective in the experience of many
Conjunctival flap	Partial flap may induce further melt alongside
Lamellar overlay graft in perforation	Can be useful as a temporary procedure
Peripheral circumferential keratoplasty	A difficult procedure, and compromises vision
Large eccentric penetrating keratoplasty	Should be performed following control of the peripheral melt with systemic therapy
Systemic immunosuppression corticosteroids azathioprine cyclosporin A	Takes time to control. Monitor for side-effects. Taper therapy down once the disease is controlled. Use in conjunction with a clinical immunologist

shown in Fig. 4. It is necessary to recognize the difference between active and inactive disease to obviate placing the patient on treatment when it is not necessary.

In contrast to peripheral ulcerative keratitis which is associated with systemic disease, Mooren's ulcer occurs in the absence of any apparent systemic manifestations. The condition which is idiopathic appears at the corneal periphery and progresses centrally and circumferentially. There is cellular infiltration at the centre which is undermined. This eventually may encroach on the corneal centre, which eventually may slough away, leaving a thinned and vascularized layer. It is because of the similarity of the disease to peripheral ulcerative keratitis that the condition is included in this chapter. There is limited evidence for circulating immune complexes and circulating corneal antibodies according to a number of reports. A severe form of Mooren's ulcer can occur in healthy black males. The condition is bilateral and unremitting. It is thought to be related to helminthiasis in Nigerian patients.

Treatment

Peripheral ulcerative keratitis is a rare form of corneal disease, and must be treated by a corneal specialist. Try to control the condition using topical steroid, although be careful, as it may worsen the process of stromal melting, and hasten perforation. Since the condition seems generally to be associated with a systemic immunological disorder, treatment with immunosuppressive regimes, in association with a clinical immunologist, should be considered although the complications of must be borne in mind and monitored regularly. Such treatment does not produce an immediate clinical response, and so surgical intervention must be delayed until the process becomes inactive. Where there is a risk of perforation, avoid surgical treatment as long as possible as the result can be significant loss of vision. Table 6 outlines various treatments that can be employed, and comments on their relative value according to personal experience. It is because the precise mechanisms involved are not understood that specific treatment has yet to be identified.

Rosacea keratitis

Rosacea is a chronic disorder of the skin of the face, with primary involvement of the sebaceous glands. Chronic meibomitis can be associated, with secondary corneal disease. Patients are aged between 40 and 60 years. Blepharitis is associated with a thickened and irregular lid margin. Orifices of the meibomian ducts are wide open, with cloudy secretion, or alternatively they consist of a semi-solid plug of keratinized epithelial cells. Change then occurs in the ocular surface, with conjunctival hyperaemia and punctate epithelial erosions in the interpalpebral zone. In severe disease, the cornea becomes ulcerated and infiltrated with inflammatory cells in the lower nasal and temporal quadrants, with occasionally chronic thinning and the threat of perforation (Fig. 5).

Treatment

Therapy consists of management of meibomian gland malfunction, by eyelid hygiene employing lid scrubs with baby shampoo. Treatment of lid margins with antibiotic ointments such as bacitracin or erythromycin. It is unwise to employ topical steroid for long-term use for lid margin disease because of

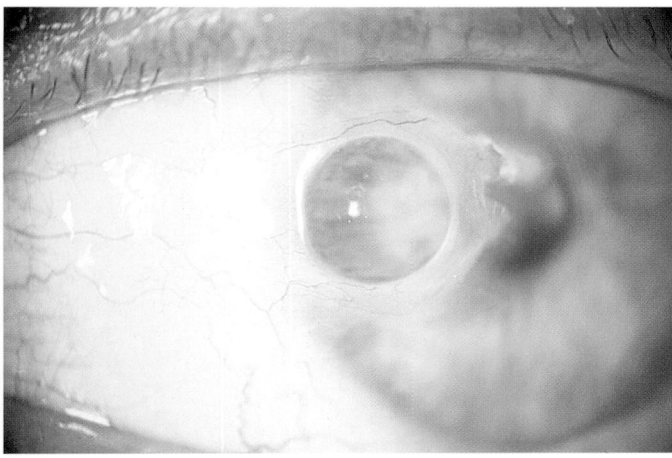

Fig. 5 Descemetocele due to rosacea keratitis. The eventual perforation was treated by penetrating keratoplasty.

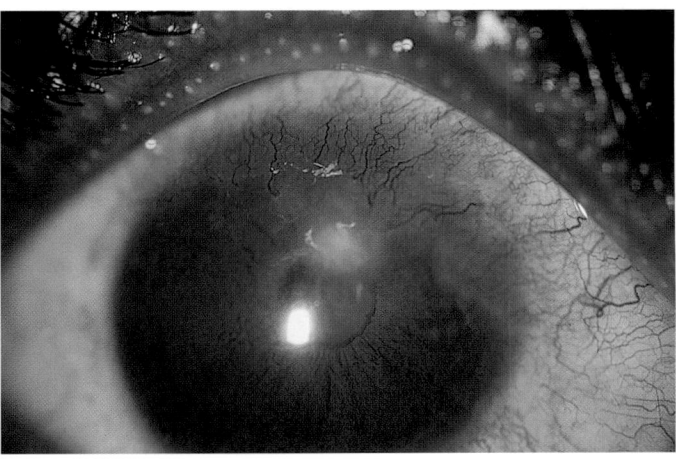

Fig. 6 Phlyctenular keratitis—note the characteristic grey–white nodules associated with superficial vascularization.

dependence. Rosacea keratitis may require the sparing use of topical steroid, although once again dependence becomes a problem. Occasionally peripheral corneal thinning may lead to perforation requiring penetration keratoplasty. Preservative-free artificial tear preparations may be considered where there is reduced tear secretion. In the presence of active blepharitis or meibomitis, treatment with systemic tetracycline or Minocin for a up to 6 weeks will help to control the condition. Systemic tetracycline can be used for persistent lid margin inflammation.

Phlyctenular disease

Phlyctenular conjunctivitis or keratitis are manifestations of similar immunological processes, involving type IV hypersensitivity, where the causal antigen is thought to be either the bacterial proteins of *Mycobacterium tuberculosis* or *Staphylococcus aureus*. Other causal antigens that are recognized include fungi such as *Candida albicans*, gonococcal antigens, *Lymphogranuloma venereum*, adenovirus, and leishmaniasis. The disease is rare in Western communities, but is seen more commonly in developing countries, particularly the African continent.

Pathogenesis

Partial support for the immunopathogenesis has been shown by immunizing rabbits with *Staphylococcus aureus*, and then injecting a cell wall antigen, ribitol teichoic acid, into the stroma. The infiltration is composed of lymphocytes at the level of Bowman's membrane, such that the epithelium becomes elevated, similar to the clinical condition in the human.

Clinical features

The clinical disease may be either predominantly conjunctival, or corneal, or both. There are symptoms of soreness and, in particular, severe photophobia. Single or multiple elevated grey–white nodules occur at or within the limbus, composed of infiltrations of lymphocytes, and associated with superficial vascularization (Fig. 6). Sometimes they may proceed towards the centre of the cornea, leaving a residual scar following res-

olution. Occasionally there is diffuse punctate epithelial keratitis.

Treatment

The lesions respond rapidly to topical corticosteroid. Attention should be focused on the causal infection, keeping in mind the possibility that tuberculosis might be present in the patient, or within the family.

Marginal corneal infiltrates

Marginal infiltrates are commonly seen in the accident rooms of eye departments in Western communities. The infiltrates are single, but less frequently are multiple, and sometimes are extensive (Fig. 7). There is a higher prevalence of associated blepharitis and meibomitis, and *Staphylococcus aureus* infection, although the ulcers are sterile on culture.

There are symptoms of photophobia and soreness, the infiltrates occurring just inside the limbus with a clear area of

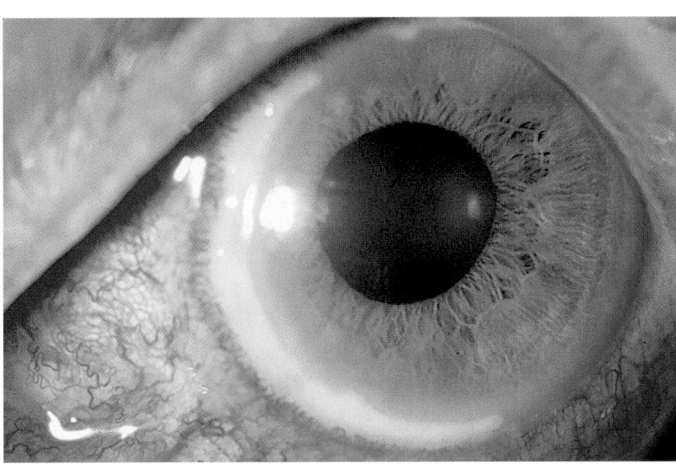

Fig. 7 Extensive confluent marginal ulceration.

cornea at the outer margin. There is local hyperaemia but little tendency for vascularization. The ulcer stains with fluorescein, although the epithelium remains intact.

Treatment

Blepharitis must be controlled, and topical antibiotic used, with introduction of topical steroid at 48 h. The response to this therapy is almost immediate.

Cogan's syndrome

Cogan's syndrome is uncommon, there being a comparatively small number of reports in the literature. It is considered to be an autoimmune disease, causing inflammation in the eye, ear, and blood vessels which responds to immunosuppressive regimes. It begins in adult life, with 50 per cent presenting with ocular disease. In addition there are vestibuloauditory problems, interstitial keratitis, conjunctivitis, iritis, scleritis, corneal ulceration, and posterior segment inflammation. There is a patchy corneal infiltrate, in the deep stroma, with eventual vascularization. Peripheral subepithelial infiltrates are seen that mimic adenoviral infection, but which responds to topical steroid.

A small proportion of patients develop large vessel vasculitis, including aortitis, against a background of systemic symptoms and signs such as fatigue, fever, arthralgia and arthritis, lymphadenopathy, hepatomegaly, splenomegaly, or gastrointestinal bleeds.

Keratitis-associated conjunctival shrinkage disorders

There are a large number of disorders that cause conjunctival scarring and shrinkage. These diseases have secondary effects on the cornea, that result from reduced tear secretion, entropion, and trichiasis. The cornea displays punctate epithelial keratitis caused by reduced secretion of tears, scarring or keratinization of tarsal plates, or entropion and trichiasis. More extensive epithelial deficits lead to loss of the barrier function of the epithelium, and risk of secondary infection. In severe disease, particularly in mucous membrane pemphigoid and Stevens–Johnson syndrome, keratinization of the corneal surface occurs (Fig. 8). Superficial vascularization is common, and deep vascularization occurs following microbial disease, which in advanced disease leads to perforation.

Treatment

Avoidance of advanced disease of this kind depends on early recognition and treatment, sometimes by the use of immunosuppressive regimes in autoimmune diseases such as mucous membrane pemphigoid. Because of the risk of corneal infection, it is wise to assess bacteriology by regular culture of conjunctival swabs. Where there is keratinization of the tarsal plate, removal by gentle scraping can ease discomfort and reduce corneal epithelial disease. In the presence of dry eye, bandage contact lenses increase the risk of corneal infection and must be avoided. Treatment depends upon tear replacement, topical low strength corticosteroid used sparingly, and lid hygiene. Lid

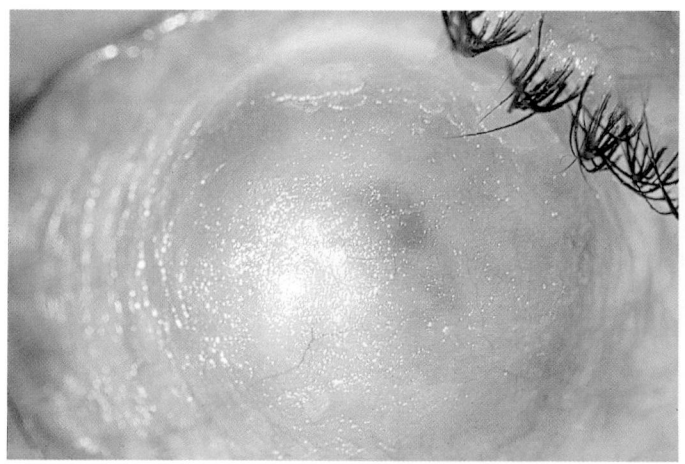

Fig. 8 Corneal keratinization in mucous membrane pemphigoid.

surgery is tempting but only performed when other measures fail.

Vernal catarrh and atopic conjunctivitis

Vernal catarrh and atopic conjunctivitis are two conditions that are predominantly seen associated with atopic disease in general, and in part are the ocular manifestations of immediate or type I hypersensitivity, although type IV hypersensitivity undoubtedly plays a role as well. These entities are discussed in Chapter 00. The cornea displays features when the disease is active, and in atopic conjunctivitis, the adult counterpart of childhood vernal catarrh, there is thought to be a specific keratitis in association. The corneal manifestations are shown in Table 7. Limbal vernal catarrh is seen in endemic regions of the world (Fig. 9(a)). Occasionally papillae encroach on to the corneal surface (Fig. 9(b)).

In vernal catarrh, it is the punctate epithelial keratitis

Table 7 The corneal manifestations in vernal and atopic conjunctivitis

Vernal keratoconjunctivitis	
Pannus	Commonly seen
Gerontoxin	Uncommon — persists long term
Punctate epithelial keratitis	Useful clinical sign of active disease
Large epithelial deficit	Indicates urgent treatment required
Corneal plaque formation	May need surgical removal
Secondary infectious keratitis	Easy to miss where strong +ve Bell's
Permanent scarring	Ring scars occur following removal of plaque
Atopic keratoconjunctivitis	
Punctate epithelial keratitis	Sign of active conjunctivitis
Epithelial plaque	Rare complication
Atopic keratitis	Irregular subepithelial scarring
Herpes simplex keratitis	Greater susceptibility in atopic patients
Secondary bacterial/mycotic infection	Increased risk in atopic conjunctivitis

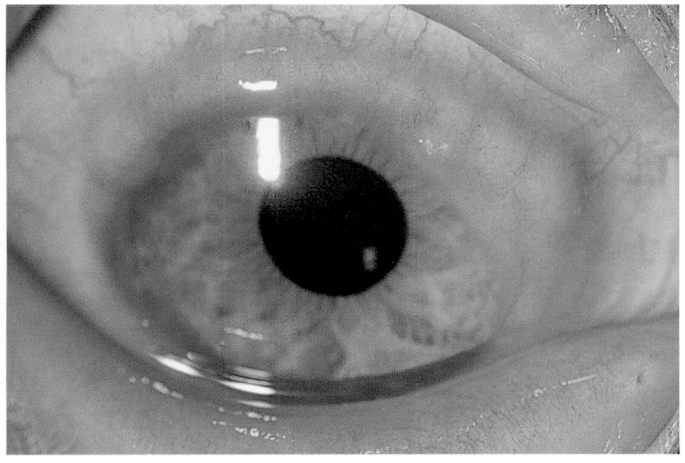

(a)

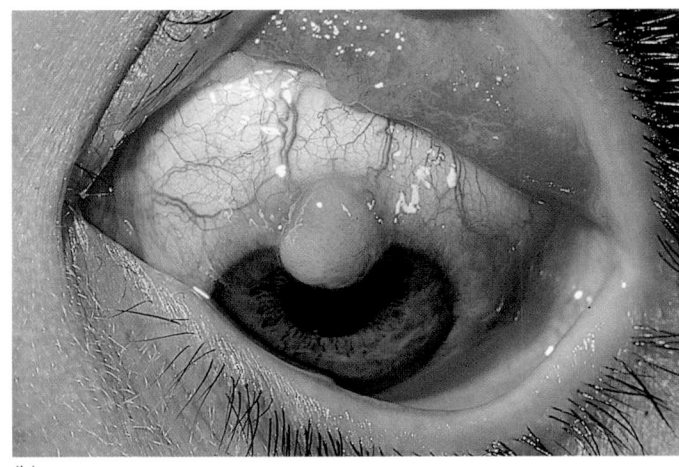

(b)

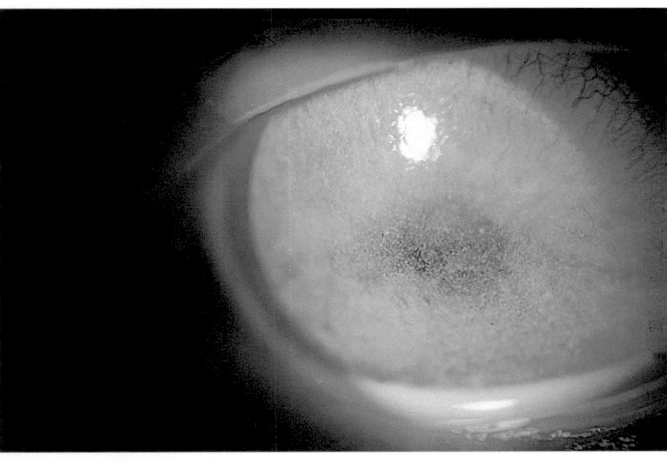

(c)

Fig. 9 (a) Limbal vernal catarrh. (b) Large limbal papillae encroaching on to the cornea. (c) Punctate epithelial keratitis associated with severe active vernal disease. (d) Macro-photograph of punctate keratitis with an extensive epithelial deficit. (By courtesy of Mr Nicholas Brown.)

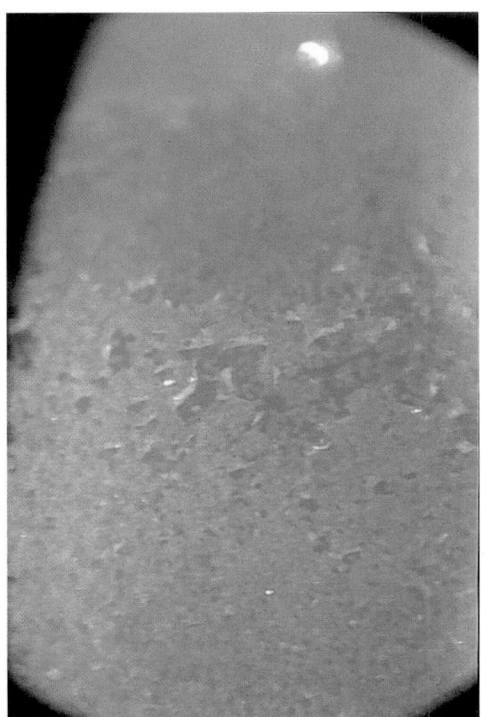

(d)

that causes soreness and photophobia. It indicates that the conjunctivitis is actively responding to a sensitizing allergen. It precedes the persistent plaque formation that becomes the major problem in treatment. The punctate epithelial keratitis is in the upper part of the cornea, but in severe attacks may involve the whole of the surface layer (Fig. 9(c) and (d)). The vernal ulcer follows the punctate keratitis, and once the mucous plaque has formed it becomes chronic with severe pain, photophobia, and blepharospasm. The symptoms can be so severe that it becomes impossible to examine a child mainly because of the positive Bell's phenomenon that prevents useful viewing of the cornea. Vernal ulcers may be missed for this reason and may indicate an examination under anaesthetic. It is thought that the pathogenesis involves the laying down of altered mucus, that occurs during active inflammation, in layers, such that the epithelium is unable to regenerate and resurface the cornea (Fig. 10).

Vernal catarrh and atopic conjunctivitis are often associated with eczema, allergic asthma, and rhinitis. These patients have increased susceptibility to infection by viruses, and in particular they can contract ocular herpes simplex infection. It is worth keeping in mind that recurrent disease of the cornea can sometimes be due to recurrent herpetic keratitis, that may be atypical, but which responds well to antiviral therapy.

Investigation

The investigation of vernal catarrh and atopic conjunctivitis is outlined elsewhere in this textbook. Occasionally when you observe corneal disease that cannot be explained, it is worth exploring the tarsal conjunctiva for signs of previous signs of vernal disease. Typically there may be lace-like scarring of either the upper or lower tarsi, which is unique to these diseases (Fig. 11). Where there are suggestive signs of this kind, then further investigation using skin prick testing for immediate hypersensitivity to common allergen, serum immunoglobulin E, and radioallergosorbent test is useful.

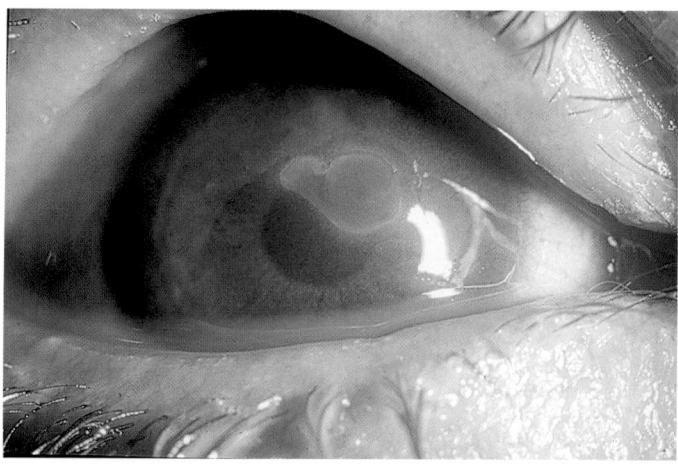

Fig. 10 Vernal keratitis—failure of re-epithelialization with mucous plaque deposition.

Table 8 Treatment of vernal and atopic keratitis

Admission to hospital if active	Avoidance of environmental allergen
Antihistamines (e.g. topical antistan privine)	Moderate effect
Mast cell stabilizers (topical disodium cromoglycate, nedocromil solution, lodoxamide)	Moderate effect
Mucolytic agents (e.g. acetyl cysteine drops)	Valuable in early disease
Topical antibiotic	Reduces risk of bacterial conjunctivitis
Topical corticosteroid	Intensive treatment required for short period. Avoid long-term treatment, and steroid dependence
Operative removal of mucus plaque	Requires general anaesthetic in children

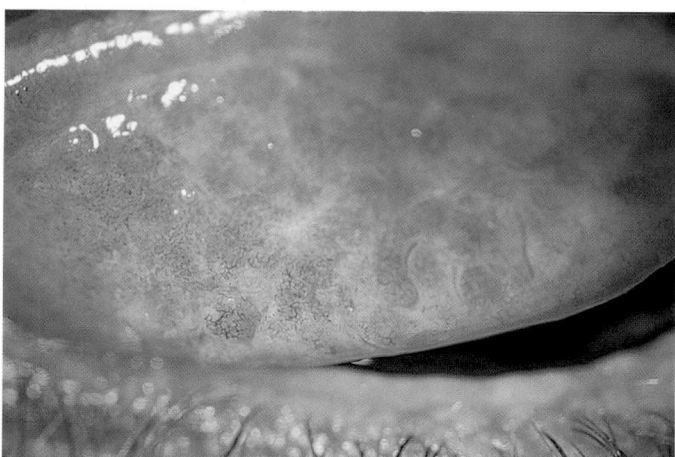

Fig. 11 Fine conjunctival 'lace' scarring in vernal disease—active conjunctivitis is also present.

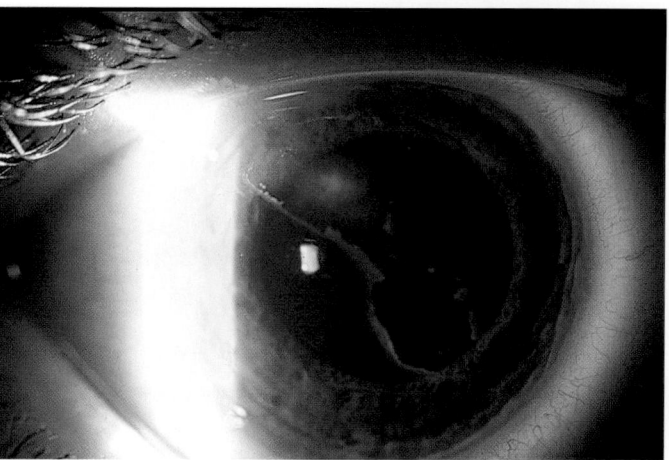

Fig. 12 Vernal keratoconjunctivitis with map-like opacity after plaque removal; demonstrated by the limbal scatter examination technique.

Treatment

Early treatment of punctate epithelial keratitis is essential to avoid the more serious sequelae of corneal plaque and unrecoverable damage. Use intensive topical corticosteroid for 48 h and rapidly taper to four times a day. Always use a topical antibiotic at the same time. The side-effects of steroids can be seen in these conditions mainly because they are so effective, and because they may be available without prescription in some parts of the world. Thus steroid glaucoma and lens opacity is seen and can cause severe visual loss in children and young adults. Parents must be warned of the consequences of long-term treatment. Cases with recurrent keratitis must be monitored regularly to avoid such complications. The different treatment modalities available are indicated in Table 8.

Corneal ulceration due to mucus plaque may require operative removal. Try to control the keratitis and conjunctivitis with topical steroid, and if there is failure to re-epithelialize, then remove the plaque by dissection under general anaesthetic. A ring of superficial stromal opacity may remain after the surface has reformed (Fig. 12). Even then the plaque can recur. In such cases, where there is a risk of steroid complications, low dose systemic steroid (e.g. prednisolone 5 mg every other day) can reduce the requirement for topical steroids, and can produce a valuable remedial effect. Such medication must be used for a short period only. Treatment of cobblestone papillae in the upper tarsal plate by removal, cryothermy, or mucous membrane autotransplant have been unsuccessful.

Corneal graft rejection

Corneal graft rejection remains the most common cause of penetrating allograft failure. It is generally associated with loss of corneal privilege due to vascularization. It is also seen after previous inflammatory disease, and in regrafts. It is much less common in avascular corneas such as in keratoconus or a corneal dystrophy. Any one of the three coneal layers is involved, the endothelium being the most common. Rarely an epithelial rejection line is seen, more easily after staining with fluorescein drops. Stromal rejection presents as punctate keratitis with subepithelial infiltrates somewhat similar to that seen in keratitis due to adenovirus 8, but more diffuse and irregular stromal opacities are probably a manifestation of rejection as well. The most important manifestation is an endothelial rejection line of T cells and macrophages, that causes destruction of the layer, and results in diffuse oedema of the donor cornea if not treated urgently. Allograft rejection may occur any time up to 2 years after a transplant, but frequently happens within the first 6 months. There is increased risk of rejection after suture manipulation or removal. The main features of rejection are that it may begin as early as 3 weeks following the transplant, the inflammation is confined to the donor tissue, and the process begins at the margin of the graft, usually near an area of deep stromal vascularization. If the condition is not treated, then transparency is lost and vision fails to improve. Treatment is by intensive topical corticosteroid. Allograft rejection can be reduced by maintaining topical steroids during the postoperative period, for a variable period depending on the inflammatory response during this time, and the presence of vascularization. Grafts for keratoconus should be treated for 4 to 6 months, in low dosage, but high-risk transplants may need continuous treatment for 12 to 18 months.

Congenital and acquired immunodeficiency disorders

Immunodeficiency diseases are composed of a broad group of disorders that have in common an increased susceptibility to infection that may occasionally involve the cornea and conjunctiva. These disorders are congenital or acquired. Primary immunodeficiencies may be in antibody, cell-mediated, combined antibody and cell-mediated, phagocytic, and in complement-mediated immunity (Table 9). Certain of the primary disorders manifest ocular signs that are not inflammatory, that may be the reason for first clinical presentation

to ophthalmologists rather than to other disciplines. Aquired immunodeficiency occurs in haemopoietic disorders, burns, exudative enteropathy, nephrotic syndrome, sarcoidosis, after splenectomy, uraemia, viral infections, malnutrition, immunosuppression, and the acquired immunodeficiency disorder. Involvement of the cornea in patients with human immunodeficiency virus (HIV) infection seems less common in practice than might be expected.

Primary immunodeficiency

Selective immunoglobulin A deficiency can be associated with an increased risk of infection. Serum immunoglobulin A levels are less than 5 mg/100 ml, but other antibody levels are normal, together with normal cell-mediated immunity. Patients have increased incidence of autoimmune disease, atopic disease, and recurrent infection. The authors have seen patients with selective immunoglobulin A deficiency with vernal catarrh, keratoconus, severe inclusion conjunctivitis (Fig. 13), corneal abscesses, and dacryocystitis.

Highly atopic patients with considerable elevation of serum

Table 9 Classification of primary immunodeficiency disease

Immunodeficiency of prematurity
   transient hypogammaglobulinaemia of infancy
   immunodeficiency of the newborn
Antibody immunodeficiency
   selective immunoglobulin deficiency
Immunodeficiency with thymic hypoplasia
   thymic hypoplasia (Di George syndrome)
   severe combined immunodeficiency (Swiss type)
   autosomal recessive immunodeficiency with lymphopaenia
   immunodeficiency with generalized haemopoietic hypoplasia
Other cellular immunodeficiencies
   with ataxia telangiectasia
   with thrombocytopenia and eczema
Disorders of the phagocytic system
Disorders of the complement system

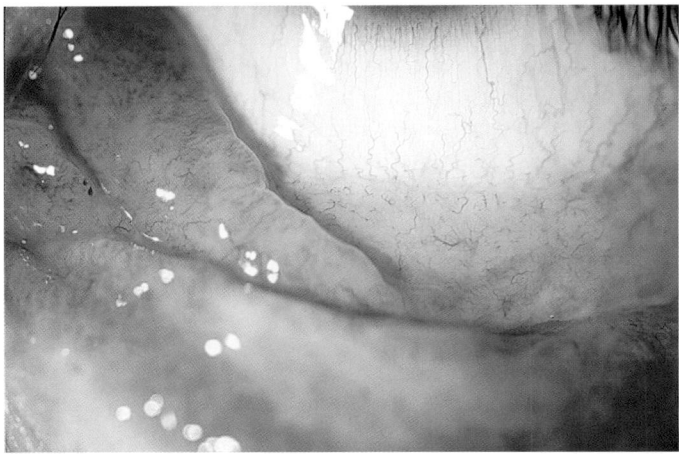

(a)

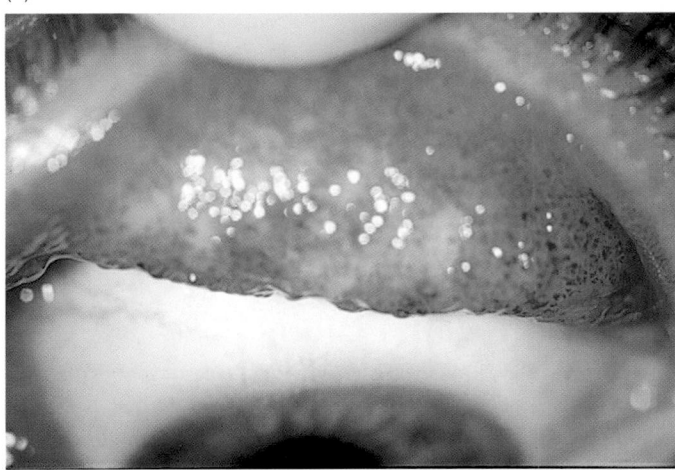

(b)

Fig. 13 Severe inclusion conjunctivitis in an immunoglobulin A deficient teenager. (a) Involvement of the caruncle and semilunar fold. (b) Severe follicular conjunctivitis of upper tarsal plate.

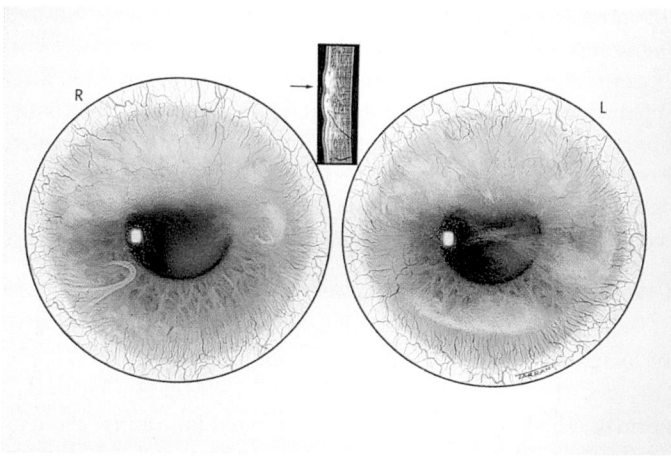

Fig. 14 Punctate keratitis and superficial stromal scarring with pannus in chronic mucocutaneous candidiasis.

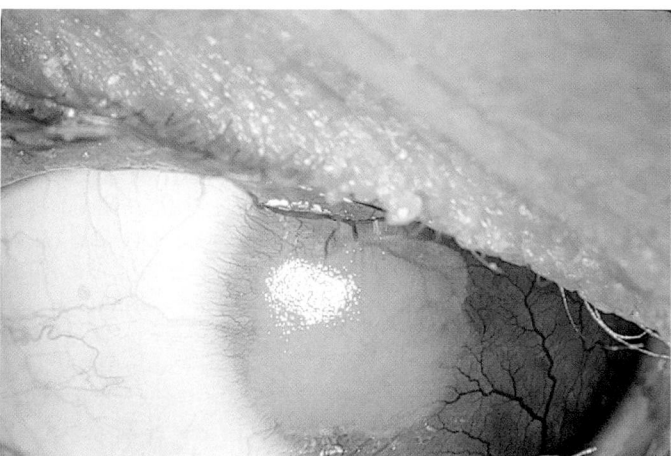

Fig. 15 Corneal epithelial keratinization in the keratitis–icthiosis–deafness syndrome.

immunoglobulin E levels are known to suffer severe corneal and lid infection, in particular severe recurrent herpes simplex keratitis.

There are two examples of cellular immunodeficiencies that have characteristic signs in the external eye. In autosomal recessive ataxia–telangiectasia, there is telangiectasia initially in the conjunctiva, progressive ataxia, and variable immunodeficiency involving either antibody or cellular immune systems, or both. In chronic mucocutaneous candidiasis there is a defect in cell-mediated immunity, endocrinopathy including hypoparathyroidism, steatorrhoea, portal cirrhosis, Addison's disease, tooth hypoplasia, poor growth, and delayed puberty. There may be a rare form of keratitis with punctate epithelial erosions, superficial vascularization, and superficial stromal oedema and scarring (Fig. 14).

An example of phagocytic disorder with associated corneal disease is seen in the keratitis–icthiosis–deafness syndrome characterized by severe infections of the skin and a unique corneal appearances with epithelial hyperplasia and keratinization (Fig. 15). Severe recurrent conjunctivitis, blepharitis, and corneal infection is seen with frequent positive cultures of *Staphylococcus aureus*, *Bacillus proteus*, and *Pseudomonas aeroginosa*.

Awareness of the primary and acquired causes of immunodeficiency may help in the care of a group of patients who are at constant risk of viral or bacterial infection in general, particulary of the cornea and external eye.

Corneal degenerations

Corneal degenerations are a heterogeneous group of disorders which are classified as either primary, where they occur as a result of the normal ageing process, or secondary to another local or systemic pathological process (Table 10). The cause of most of these disorders is unknown and they vary widely in their clinical appearance, production of symptoms, and their requirement for, or response to, treatment. Conjunctival degenerations whilst not strictly arising from the cornea often

Table 10 Classification of corneal degenerations

Primary	Secondary
Iron lines	Pinguecula
White limbal girdle of Vogt	Pterygium
Corneal farinata	Spheroid degeneration
Anterior and posterior crocodile shagreen	Salzmann's nodular degeneration
Corneal arcus (arcus senilis)	Terrien's
Hassal–Henle bodies	Corneal amyloid
	Lipid degeneration
	Coat's white ring
	Band keratopathy
	Neurotrophic keratopathy
	Exposure keratopathy
	Recurrent erosion syndrome

involve it and are therefore included in the following account.

Primary

These are typically common, age-related, bilateral conditions occurring in superficial or deep corneal layers. Rarely they may be unilateral or occur in young patients, when their significance may be of more importance.

Iron lines

These occur due to iron deposition in the corneal epithelium. There are several eponymous types which occur due to different causes. Hudson–Stähli lines are usually horizontal, brown curved lines occurring at the junction of the middle and inferior thirds of the cornea. They increase in prevalence and intensity with age until around the seventh decade when they may begin to decrease. They occur with equal freqency in men and women. They have been demonstrated in young people with normal corneas and may be physiological rather than pathological. The source of the iron is unknown, but is probably

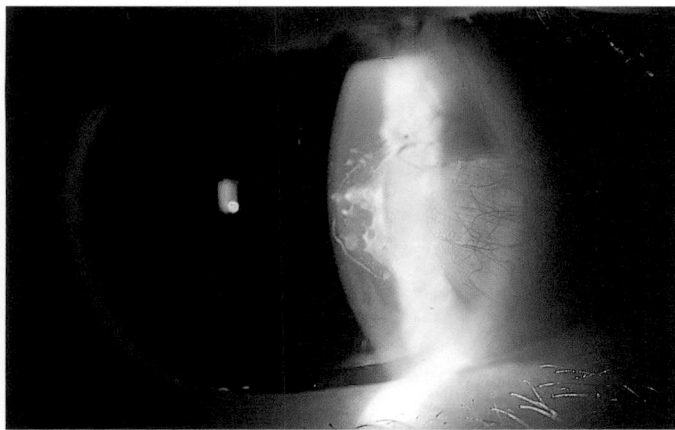

Fig. 16 Stocker line.

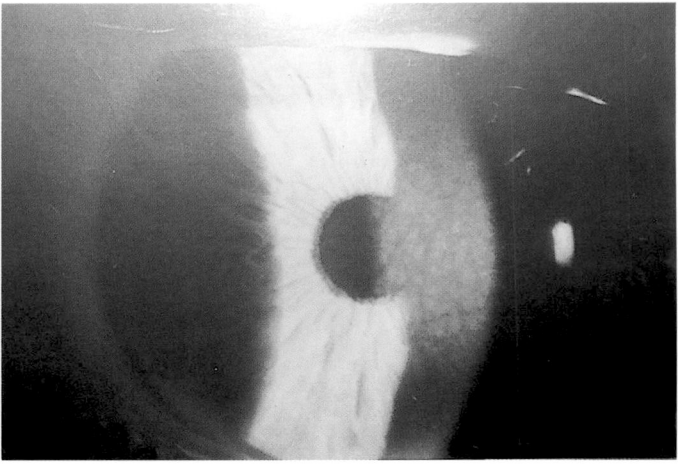

Fig. 18 Crocodile shagreen

derived from the tear film following abnormalities in tear flow. Histologically there is specific staining for iron deposition in the deep epithelium. They are asymptomatic and require no treatment. Iron lines have been reported at the base of the cone in keratoconus (Fleischer ring), around a trabeculectomy filtering bleb (Ferry line), at the head of pterygia (Stocker line, Fig. 16), and associated with nodules in Saltzmann's degeneration. Histologically these are identical to the Hudson–Stähli line.

White limbal girdle of Vogt (Fig. 17)

Vogt's limbal girdle occurs in two forms. They appear as white, crescentic, peripheral corneal opacities occurring in the interpalpebral area. Type 1 is rare and probably represents early band keratopathy and is separated from the limbus by a clear zone. Within the opacity irregular clear holes are found. Type 2 is common, affecting 100 per cent of people over 80 years of age, occurring more commonly at the nasal than temporal limbus with no peripheral clear zone present. Fine white radial lines are seen and histologically consist of subepithelial hyaline

and elastotic changes. It occurs in most people over 40 years, is almost ubiquitous in the elderly and requires no treatment.

Corneal farinata

These occur as minute, grey white opacities resembling flour, located in the deep corneal stroma. They are frequently axial, asymptomatic, and best seen on retroillumination. They are common and associated with increasing age, though familial cases have been reported. They have no clinical significance. Corneal farinata can easily be confused with early guttate endothelial dystrophy.

Anterior and posterior crocodile shagreen (Fig. 18)

Anterior crocodile shagreen occurs in the elderly population and consists of a bilateral mosaic-like pattern of polygonal grey–white opacities seen in the central and peripheral anterior cornea. Histologically, ridging of Bowman's membrane with calcium deposition is seen. Very rarely it may interfere with vision. Posterior crocodile shagreen looks similar in appearance but occurs in the central deep cornea. Histologically irregularity of stromal collagen lamellae is seen.

Hassal–Henle bodies

These represent peripherally located focal thickenings of the posterior, non-banded portion of Descemet's membrane. They are identical to central guttate dystrophy and increase with age. They have no visual significance.

Corneal arcus (arcus senilis) (Fig. 19)

This is a peripheral corneal, extracellular deposition of cholesterol esters, phospholipids, and triglycerides which may occur independently or in association with systemic disorders or abnormalities of lipid metabolism. The sharp peripheral margin is separated from the limbus by a clear zone whilst the diffuse inner margin merges with the cornea. It usually begins in the superior and inferior cornea and gradually spreads circumferentially to involve the whole periphery. The characteristic distribution may be related to temperature-dependent local vari-

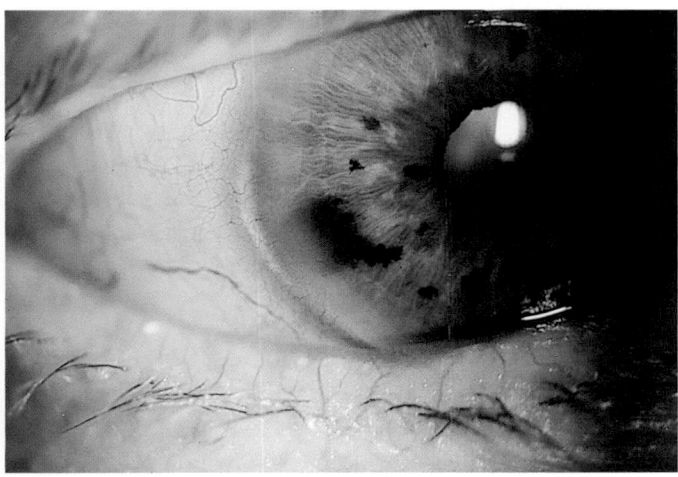

Fig. 17 White limbal girdle. (By courtesy of Jack Kanski and Butterworths.)

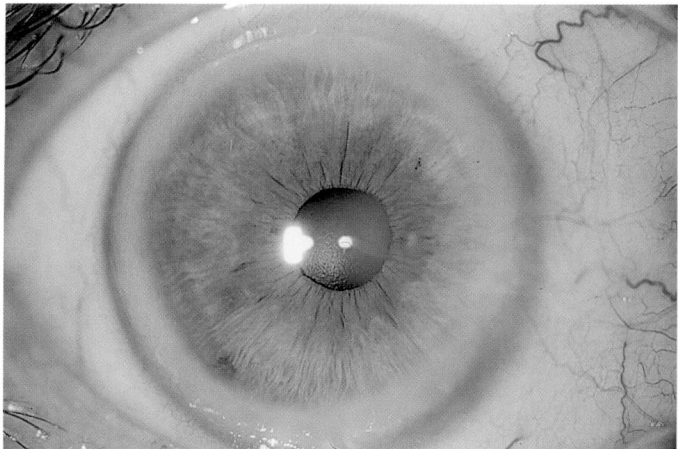

Fig. 19 Corneal arcus.

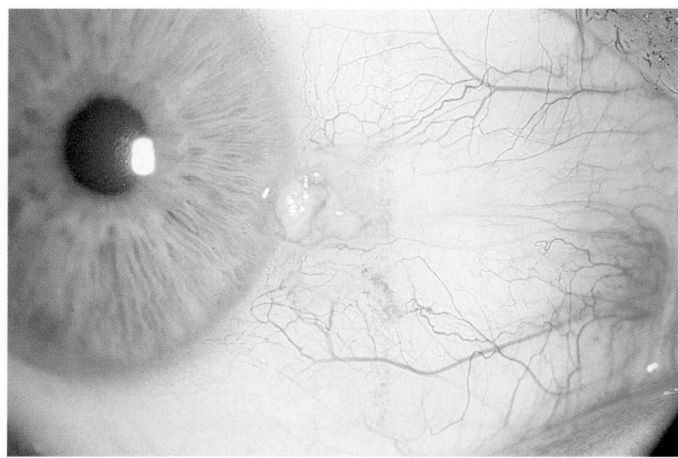

Fig. 20 Pingecula.

ations in vascular permeability. Deposition begins in the deep cornea, just anterior to Descemet's membrane and then at the level of Bowman's membrane where it is most dense, eventually meeting in the central stroma to give an hour glass appearance on histological cross-section.

It affects males more commonly than females and increases with age to become universal in those over 80 years of age. If present under 40 years of age it is a significant risk factor for coronary heart disease and is associated with raised low density lipoproteins predominantly found in familial hypercholesterolaemia and familial hyperbetalipoproteinaemia. Serum lipid analysis is indicated in this instance.

Secondary

These are often related to a local or systemic abnormality and are frequently symptomatic, producing significant reduction in visual acuity due to either induced astigmatism or central corneal opacification.

Degenerations associated with ultraviolet light exposure

Pinguecula (Fig. 20)

Pingueculae are small variably shaped conjunctival thickenings located at the nasal and less frequently the temporal limbus in the interpalpebral area. They are thought to occur secondary to ultraviolet light exposure and are more common with increasing age, in outdoor workers, and in populations near to the equator. They are less translucent than the surrounding normal conjunctiva and their raised opaque appearance may be a cosmetic problem. Histologically they are composed of subepithelial hyalinization, elastotic change and concretions. Rarely they may enlarge and encroach upon the cornea. Usually they are asymptomatic but can be a cosmetic problem requiring excision. Occasionally they may become inflamed and require a course of topical steroid treatment.

Pterygium (Fig. 21)

A pterygium is a grey triangular fibrovascular membrane, which like a pinguecula is located mainly at the nasal interpal-

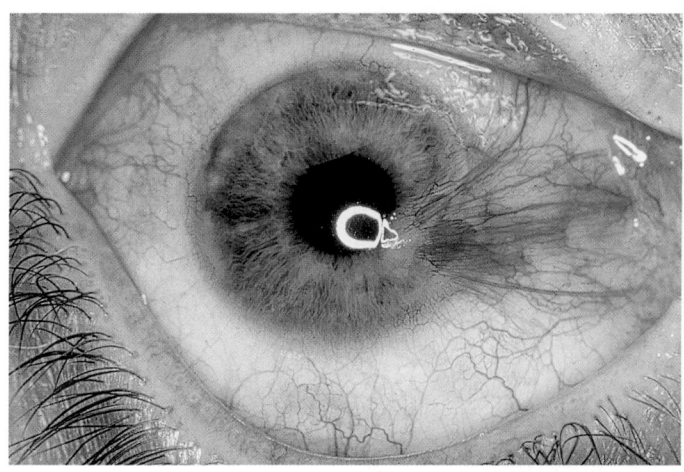

Fig. 21 Pterygium.

pebral limbus. Risk factors are similar and include exposure to sunlight and the elements, and proximity to the equator. There is evidence to suggest that reduced exposure to light is associated with a reduced risk of development of pterygium. Pterygia are identical histologically to pingeculae but unlike pingeculae, invade the cornea and destroy Bowman's membrane. They should be distinguished from pseudopterygia, which are folds of conjunctiva adherent to the cornea but not attached to the corneal limbus. They occur secondary to trauma or inflammation and may occur at sites away from the interpalpebral area. This spread from conjunctiva to cornea may result in reduction of visual acuity due to induced irregular astigmatism or glare or decreased contrast sensitivity due to involvement of the visual axis, which usually takes years but in some cases occurs in a few months. Pterygia may be asymptomatic or become inflamed and give rise to irritation, redness, or lacrimation. Corneal extension may be associated with foreign body sensation. They may also be a significant cosmetic problem. Characteristics of an active pterygium are rapid growth, engorged vessels, a grey leading edge in the cornea, and superficial punctate staining of the surrounding cornea. Occasionally they stop growing spontaneously and stable lesions may be associated with iron deposition in the corneal epithelium (Stocker's line).

Intermittent mild symptoms are often controlled by a short course of topical steroids; however, persistent troublesome symptomatology is an indication for surgical excision. Unfortunately, excision is often complicated by recurrence, a fact reflected by the many varied techniques used to treat them, including simple excision with primary conjunctival closure or bare sclera technique, conjunctival autografting, lamellar keratectomy, and lamellar keratoplasty. In addition these methods have been combined with topical antimetabolites such as mitomycin-C and local β-irradiation delivered perioperatively via a radioactive applicator. These adjunctive therapies are generally associated with a reduced recurrence rate but may lead to unpleasant side-effects.

Climatic droplet keratopathy (labrador keratopathy, Bietti's band-shaped nodular dystrophy, spheroid degeneration) (Fig. 22)

Climatic droplet keratopathy may exist in more than one form, having been described as either a primary age-related corneal degeneration, or a secondary form occurring due to other ocular disease such as traumatic corneal scars, herpetic keratitis, chronic corneal oedema, lattice dystrophy, and chronic open angle glaucoma. A third form described as a predominately conjunctival degeneration, is frequently associated with pingueculae. The prevalence varies widely according to geographical location and males are affected more than females. Although usually bilateral, it may be unilateral if associated with local corneal disease. Clinically, yellow or gold subepithelial droplets, which may initially be clear and subsequently become opaque, advance from the peripheral cornea towards the centre and in the latter stages spread outwards to involve the limbus, eliminating the peripheral clear zone present in the early stages. Symptoms include foreign body sensation, irritation, and gradual decrease in vision to 6/60 Snellen or worse due to build-up of subepithelial material causing formation of large yellow nodules on the visual axis. Histologically, extracellular proteinaceous material is found at the level of Bowman's membrane and the anterior stroma, and is thought either to be deposited via the conjunctival limbal vessels or result from actinic damage to collagen and the extracellular matrix. Lamellar keratectomy or keratoplasty may be needed in the later stages to improve discomfort and improve visual acuity.

Other secondary corneal degenerations

Salzmann's nodular degeneration

This is a slowly developing condition which usually represents the late sequelae of previous corneal inflammation, most frequently phlyctenular keratitis, trachoma, and vernal disease but also less commonly following exposure keratopathy, interstitial keratitis, and other chronic keratitis. Rarely it may be idiopathic (Fig. 23) or occur following contact lens wear or corneal surgery. It mainly affects elderly females but has been seen in children. Clinically grey or grey–blue elevated fibrous nodules are seen in the anterior stroma occurring within, or at the junction of, scarring related to a previous site of inflammation. The nodules themselves are not vascularized, but may be found overlying stromal vascularization or next to an area of pannus.

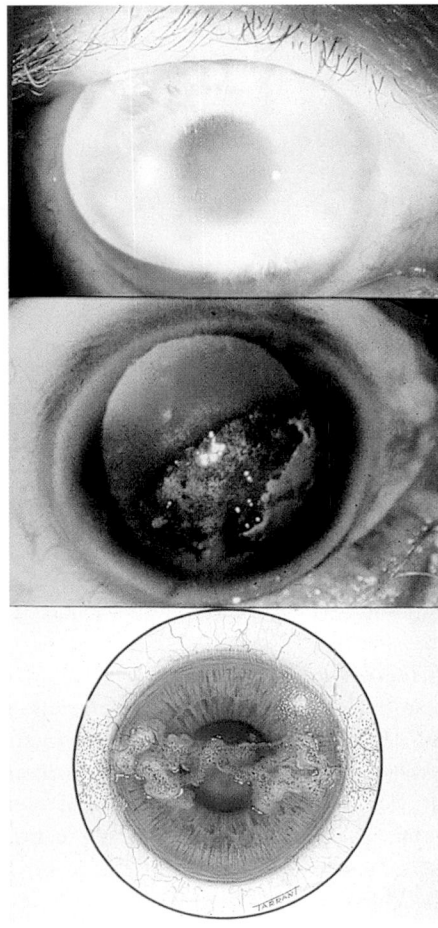

Fig. 22 Climatic droplet dystrophy. (By courtesy of Jack Kanski and Butterworths.)

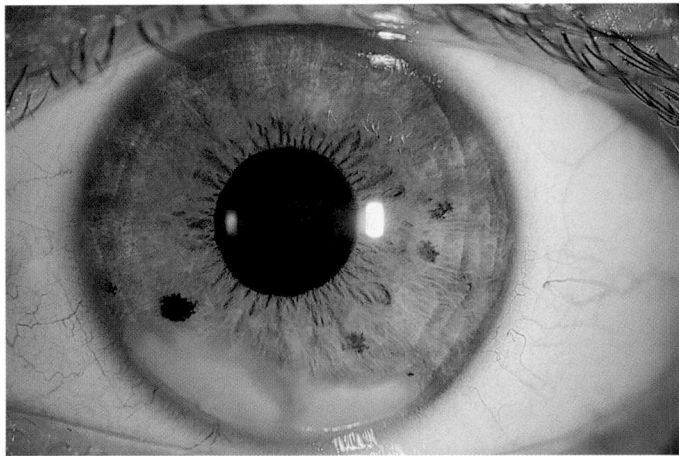

Fig. 23 Idiopathic Salzmann's degeneration. (By courtesy of Stuart Cook.)

Clear areas of cornea may be present between the nodules which may form a circular array. Histologically, thinning of the overlying epithelium and associated basal epithelial cell degeneration is seen with old corneal scarring present beneath the nodules. Bowman's laayer is replaced by eosinophilic material. The nodules may be asymptomatic but can cause discomfort if large and give rise to epithelial breakdown. Central lesions cause glare and reduced acuity which may require lamellar or penetrating keratoplasty. Recurrence in the graft has been reported. More recently excimer laser keratectomy has been used to treat these lesions.

Corneal amyloid

Amyloid is an extracellular deposit of material consisting of delicate fibrils of non-branching protein rods. It may rarely occur in the cornea as either (a) a primary abnormality associated with lattice dystrophy, gelatinous drop-like dystrophy, or polymorphic amyloid degeneration; or (b) secondary to local ocular disorders such as corneal trauma, chronic conditions such as trachoma, uveitis, bullous keratopathy, interstitial keratitis, phlyctenulosis, keratoconus, or leprosy. Very rarely corneal involvement may occur in association with blepharochalasis, facial nerve palsy, and peripheral neuropathy in the autosomal dominant Finnish type familial amyloidosis with corneal lattice dystrophy (lattice dystrophy type II). The clinical picture of corneal amyloid varies considerably from non-specific grey stromal opacities to translucent white, yellow, or pink flat or nodular deposits. Lattice-like corneal deposits occur in familial systemic amyloidosis which is associated with blepharochalasis and cranial nerve palsies. Gelatinous drop-like dystrophy, a recessive corneal dystrophy, demonstrates subepithelial or anterior stromal white raised 'mulberry-like' lesions which may cause irritation, marked photophobia, or visual loss. Polymorphic amyloid degeneration is characterized by bilateral, visually insignificant, posterior stromal filamentous or punctate opacities in the axial cornea with clear intervening stroma and occurs around the fifth decade or later. Clinical diagnosis of amyloid is difficult and ultimately histological evidence of Congo red staining or ripple green dichroism with polarized light, is necessary to confirm the diagnosis. Electron microscopy reveals the characteristic fibrillar pattern. Visual symptoms may be treated by lamellar or penetrating keratoplasty.

Lipid degeneration

Lipid degeneration is the accumulation of deposits of cholesterol and fatty acids in the cornea. It may rarely be primary, where it is usually bilateral and occurs in the absence of stromal vascularization (Fig. 24), or more commonly secondary to leakage from stromal vessels (Fig. 25). It may appear as crystalline or diffuse, yellow or cream, discrete or fan-like deposits around an area of vessels. Often it may appear suddenly from long-standing vascularization and produce a drop in visual acuity. It most commonly occurs following neovascularization from corneal trauma, infectious keratitis due to herpes simplex or zoster and interstitial keratitis. Occasionally it may regress spontaneously. Argon laser to the feeding vessels may promote resolu-

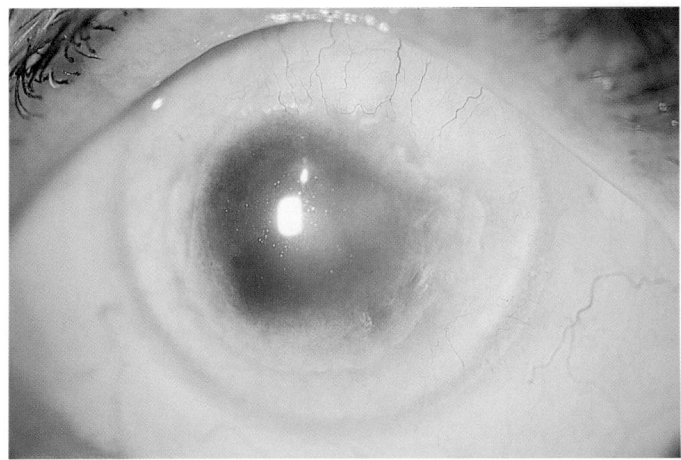

Fig. 24 Primary lipid keratopathy.

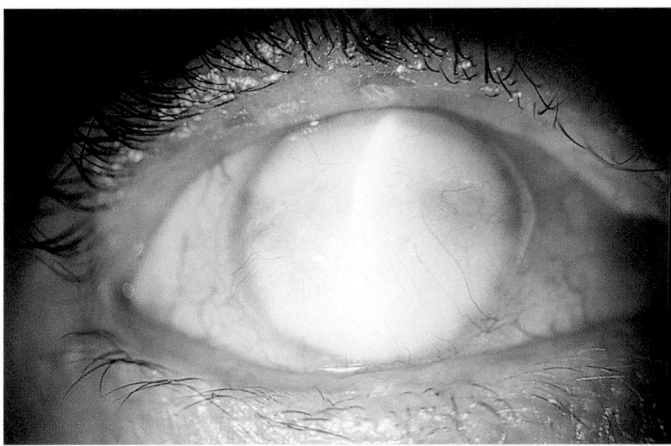

Fig. 25 Secondary lipid keratopathy following herpes zoster keratitis.

tion, but if it interferes significantly with vision then penetrating keratoplasty may be required. Recurrence in the graft may occur.

Coats' white ring

This is due to iron deposition at the level of Bowman's membrane secondary to a corneal foreign body. It is seen as a small oval or circular ring composed of white dots found to be iron on histological examination. No treatment is necessary

Band keratopathy

Band keratopathy is a common secondary corneal degeneration which can be caused by local or systemic factors resulting in calcium phosphate deposition in the anterior cornea. This calcium deposition is found to be intracellular if caused by systemic abnormalities of calcium metabolism and extracellular if caused by local ocular disease. Causes of band keratopathy include local ocular disease, topical medications, and systemic calcium abnormalities and are indicated in Table 11. Clinically, band keratopathy is confined to the interpalpebral fissure, with

Table 11 Causes of band-shaped keratcpathy

Chronic ocular disease
Uveitis
(Juvenile chronic arthritis)
Glaucoma
Corneal oedema
Interstitial keratitis
Phthisis

Ocular trauma
Climatic exposure
Mercurial containing preservatives

Systemic abnormalities
Hypercalcaemia
Hyperphosphataemia

Hereditary
Norrie's disease
Autosomal recessive band keratopathy

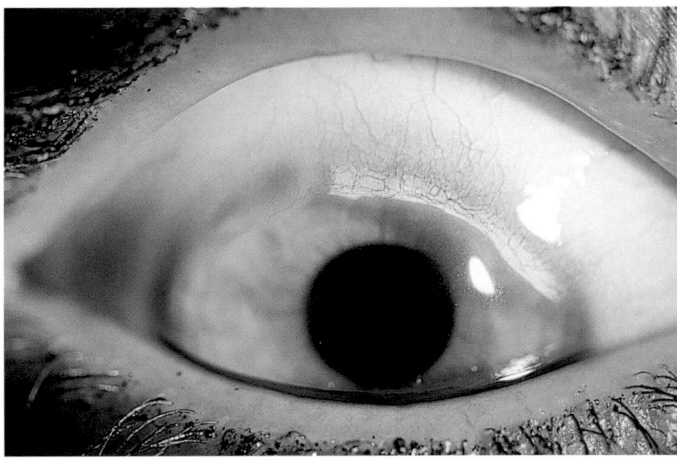

Fig. 27 Terrien's marginal degeneration.

a peripheral clear zone at the limbus and appears as a white band of calcification which begins at the nasal and temporal limbus that slowly migrates centrally. Small clear holes are present within the band giving it a 'Swiss cheese' appearance and may represent gaps through which the corneal nerves perforate Bowman's layer (Fig. 26). Histologically, calcium deposition is indicated by basophilic staining of the epithelial basement membrane, followed by calcium deposition and fragmentation of Bowman's membrane and the anterior stromal lamellae. A fibrous pannus then develops under the epithelium and scarring occurs. A similar band-like picture occurs in urate deposition but is typically a brown colour. Ulceration of the corneal epithelium may cause discomfort and vision may be reduced if the visual axis is involved depending on the underlying visual potential of the eye. Treatment consists of removal of the epithelium and chelation of the calcium salts with disodium ethylenediamine tetra-acetic acid applied repeatedly with a saturated

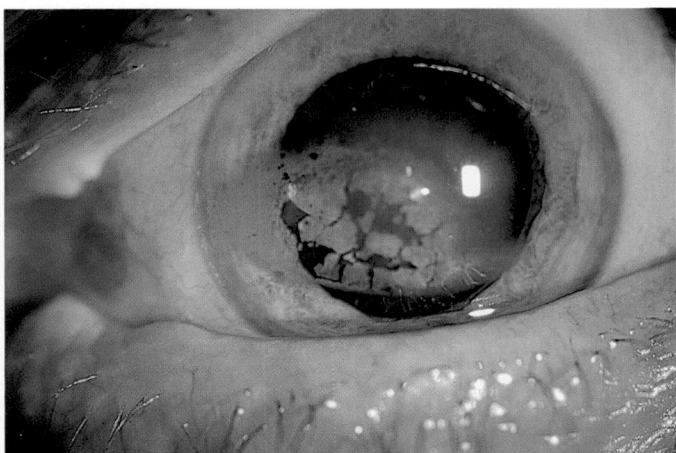

Fig. 26 Band keratopathy.

cellulose sponge followed by mechanical debridement with a blade or burr.

Terrien's marginal degeneration

This is an uncommon ideopathic disorder of the peripheral corneal which predominately affects young males. Manifesting initially as focal corneal opacification and fine vascularization, gradual thinning of the superior cornea occurs and may slowly extend to involve the entire corneal circumference and rarely the central cornea. The thinned area has a gradually sloping leading edge with lipid deposition, and the intact overlying epithelium is associated with superficial vascularization and confluent corneal opacification which is characteristically separated form the limbus by a clear zone (Fig. 27). Usually bilateral it is often asymetric in its severity. The early stages are usually asymptomatic though mild irritation may occur. Corneal thinning occurring in the later stages gives rise to peripheral ectasia leading to induced against-the-rule astigmatism. Rarely this may lead to spontaneous or traumatic corneal rupture. Whilst most cases are non-inflammatory, cases associated with marked corneal and conjunctival vascular congestion have been described. In these cases a mixed lymphocytic and neutrophil reaction in the corneal stroma has been demonstrated. Management of astigmatism is with spectacles or contact lenses depending on severity. Severe astigmatism or thinning at risk of perforation will necessitate surgical repair with either excision of ectatic tissue and direct closure, eccentric penetrating keratoplasty, or crescentic onlay lamellar keratoplasty.

Dellen

These elliptoid ulcerations of the peripheral cornea are caused by local elevation of the adjacent limbal conjunctiva which leads to abnormal wetting of the corneal surface and results in local corneal disturbance. They characteristically have a flat base at the limbus and their rounded margin extends centrally. They are usually confined to the epithelium where focal loss of epithelium is demonstrated by fluorescein staining. They tend to disappear with resolution of the underlying cause but if persist-

Table 12 Causes of neurotrophic keratopathy

Local	Herpes simplex
	Herpes zoster
	Topical anaesthetics
	Lattice dystrophy
	Irradiation
Systemic	Fifth nerve lesion (surgery, tumour, stroke, aneurysm)
	Diabetes mellitus
Congenital syndromes	Riley–Day (familial dysautonomia)
	Goldenhar
	Moebius

ent, may lead to significant corneal thinning which may become scarred resulting in corneal 'facets'. Treatment of non-inflammatory conjunctival elevations with additional pressure dressing is combined with regular ocular lubrication. Patients with dellen occurring in association with inflammatory elevations requiring topical steroid treatment should receive antibiotic cover, and followed closely until resolution because of the risk of superimposed microbial keratitis.

Neurotrophic keratopathy

This condition arises due to loss of corneal and conjunctival sensation due to any lesion affecting the trigeminal nerve. The causes of neurotrophic keratopathy are given in Table 12. The clinical consequences of this are usually mild but severe sequelae occur in approximately 15 per cent of cases. Characteristic features of less severe disease include increased conjunctival mucus production and rose bengal staining of the bulbar conjunctiva, representing increased epithelial cell death and indicating the likely development of keratopathy. Tear film abnormalities and diffuse corneal drying may also occur. Diffuse punctate epitheliopathy is an initial sign; more severe disease such as corneal ulceration may present with a sudden reduction in visual acuity. Stromal melting is the last stage of the disease process. It is important to recognize that keratopathy may occur long after initiation of anaesthesia. Diffuse punctate epithelial erosions may be associated with reduced sensation, and so remember to test both cornea and palpebral conjunctival sensitivity in unexplained situations. If either is present neuroparalytic keratopathy is unlikely to occur. Combined facial and trigeminal nerve palsy can prove to be major management problems. The cornea becomes infiltrated with inflammatory cells, and heavily vascularized. A tarsorrhaphy is the only useful measure in such a case.

Treatment The management of these patients depends on the severity of the clinical picture. Mild punctate epithelial keratopathy often requires no treatment. More severe epitheliopathy requires intermittent or constant lid taping and the use of tear substitutes is recommended to prevent corneal ulceration. The use of bandage contact lenses is best avoided as the risks of secondary microbial keratitis is significant in the age group usually affected. Oral oxytetracycline has been reported to reduce mucous secretion and may be of benefit. Temporary botulinum toxin or surgical tarsorrhaphy may be required for more severe corneal disease when repeated taping is impractical and is usually combined with cycloplegia and topical broad-spectrum antibiotics. Long-term lid closure with surgical central tarsorrhaphy is rarely required but is useful in severe, chronic relapsing disease.

Exposure keratopathy

Corneal exposure due to any cause may give rise to a keratopathy of varying severity. Failure of the normal wetting mechanisms allows superficial drying and damage to the exposed epithelium which may progress from superficial punctate epitheliopathy to diffuse epithelial involvement. More severe or prolonged exposure may result in corneal ulceration leading to perforation in rare instances. If the cause is poor lid closure, as in seventh nerve palsy or lagophthalmos, the inferior cornea is predominately involved. In cases of proptosis the central cornea is typically affected. Rose bengal staining of devitalized cells may identify early cases and allow treatment to prevent more serious complications.

Treatment Treatment to preserve epithelial integrity is similar to that for neurotrophic keratopathy with temporary measures such as artificial tears, lubricant ointment, moisture chamber, and taping used in cases where resolution of the underlying cause is anticipated and more permanent measures such as medial and central tarsorrhaphy reserved for prolonged exposure.

Recurrent erosion syndrome

In the recurrent erosion syndrome, there is exfoliation of the epithelium at intervals causing severe pain, most typically on opening the eyes in the morning. There is often a history of minor trauma to the eye long since forgotten which has resulted in basement membrane damage. On occasions there may be no such history, and there is evidence that the lesions are dystrophic in origin. Loss of epithelium results from an abnormal interaction between the basal epithelium and the basement membrane. Usually by the time that the patient is seen, the abrasion has healed, but there may be evidence of epithelial blebs, cysts, and finger-print lines, suggestive of map dot fingerprint dystrophy, best demonstrated by retroillumination with the slit lamp microscope. These signs will usually be bilateral.

Treatment Treatment should be by taping the lids during sleep, use of artificial tears (for example carboxymethylcellulose 0.5/1.0 per cent, and hydroxypropylcellulose drops, and various white petroleum lubricants) at night before sleep, a bandage contact lens, or excimer laser therapeutic keratectomy that aims to re-establish the basement membrane allowing normal epithelial regeneration and adhesion.

Metabolic disease

The systemic diseases are inherited as autosomal recessive, and usually result from enzyme deficiency that causes accumulation of substrate either locally or via transport through the blood-

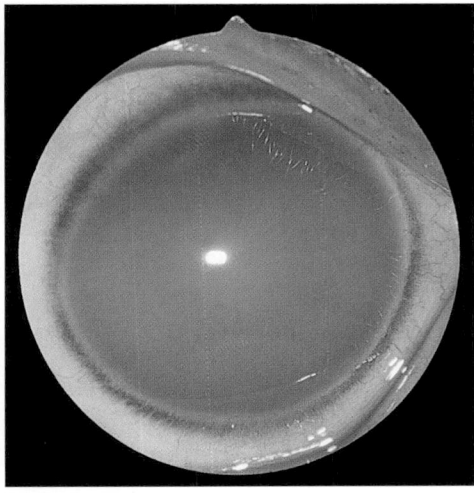

Fig. 28 Corneal clouding in mucopolysaccharidosis type I (Hurler's). (By courtesy of Jack Kanski and Butterworths.)

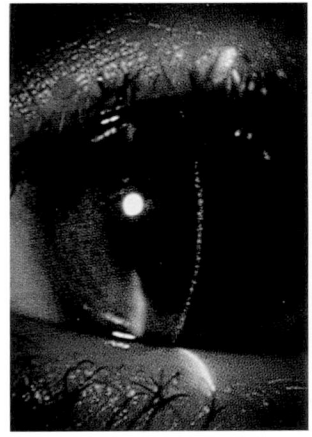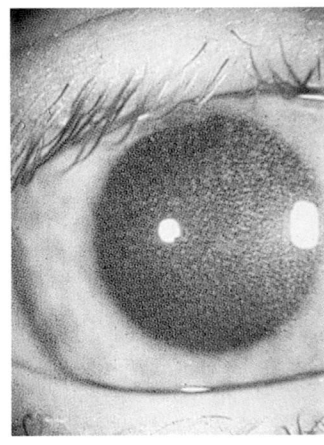

Fig. 29 Crystalline keratopathy in cystinosis. (By courtesy of David Taylor.)

stream. Glycosoaminoglycan is represented in the cornea, and it is not very surprising that mucopolysaccharides are involved in metabolic disease of this tissue, for example in Hurler's disease (Fig. 28), cystinosis, and tyrosinaemia. The corneal signs can be important and helpful in reaching the correct diagnosis.

Disorders of amino acid metabolism

Tyrosinaemia

Tyrosine is a precursor of pathways of amines including thyroid hormones and neurotransmitters such as adrenaline, noradrenaline, dopamine, and tyramine. When there are elevated levels in the serum there can be transient neonatal tyrosinaemia, as well as two recessive conditions (tyrosinaemia type I and II). In type I there is hepatorenal tyrosinaemia and in type II there is oculocutaneous tyrosinaemia. Type I disease is more common, and is associated with acute liver failure, hepatic cirrhosis, hepatocellular carcinoma, Fanconi's syndrome, but corneal changes have not been reported. Type II disease is due to deficiency of tyronsine aminotransferase, normally found in liver, brain, and muscles. Serum levels become elevated, 2.5 to 25 times the normal level. Keratoconjunctivitis with corneal opacities can occur, with superficial crystalline deposits that appear dendritiform on occasions. Spiral deposits have been seen. Skin lesions occur in the palms and soles where tyrosine deposition causes erosions and crusting, and eventually hyperkeratotic lesions. Dietary reduction of phenylalanine and tyrosine can reduce severity of the lesions, if introduced early.

Alcaptonuria

Deficiency of homogentisic acid oxidase causes homogentisic excretion in the urine. Pigmentation (ochronosis) manifests at the end of the second decade, causing pigmentation of cartilage. Generative arthropathy is associated, in the hips, knees, and shoulders. The cornea and sclera become pigmented particularly in the interpalpebral zone, but there is no loss of vision. Fine brown oily droplets occur at the level of Bowman's

membrane. The pigmentation occurs during the third decade of life.

Cystinosis

In this autosomal recessive disease the cystine accumulates intracellularly within lysosomes. Corneal deposition of fine-needle shaped crystals form. The most severe is nephropathic cystinosis. Fanconi's syndrome is established during the first year of life. Dysfunction of proximal renal tubules occurs. Life has been extended by renal transplantation on occasions.

Corneal crystals are not apparent at birth but occur during the first year. They are present in the periphery and anterior stroma. With advancing age the crystals spread posteriorly and centropetally (Fig. 29), and by the age of 7 years, crystals can be found within the endothelium. Corneal thickness is increased, and sensation is reduced. Photophobia is an important symptom. In an intermediate form, occurring between 18 months and teenage years, there are corneal crystals and a variable crystalline retinopathy. In the benign or asymptomatic form seen in adults, there are corneal crystals without a retinopathy or renal dysfunction. There are other causes of apparently crystalline deposits, including multiple myeloma, rheumatoid arthritis, lymphoproliferative disease, and certain monoclonal gammopathies.

Diagnosis of cystinosis requires measurement of free cystine content in leucocytes or cultured cells. Treatment is symptomatic.

Dyslipoproteinaemias

These disorders of lipid metabolism include hypolipoproteinaemia, lecithin hypercholesterol acyltransferase deficiency, Tangier's disease (familial high density lipoprotein deficiency), and fish eye disease. These diseases can be associated with corneal arcus at an early age, and coronary artery disease. In hyperlipoproteinaemia, these proteins are responsible for cholesterol, triglyceride, and phospholipid transport, and may be very low density, low density, and high density.

Where there are abnormal levels of chylomicrons, associated with hepatosplenomegaly, and dysfunction of the central nervous system, pancreatitis, and lipaemia retinalis, there are generally no significant corneal signs. In abnormal elevation of β-lipoprotein and pre-β-lipoprotein (type II hyperlipoproteinaemia) there is corneal arcus associated with cutaneous xanthelasma and conjunctival xanthomas. In familial dys-β-lipoproteinaemia (type III hyperlipoproteinaemia) chylomicrons are not removed due to deficiency of binding proteins. Again there is early corneal arcus, and lipaemia retinalis. In hyperpre-β-lipoproteinaemia (type IV hyperlipoproteinaemia) there is elevation of the very low density lipoproteins, corneal arcus, and xanthelasma. In hyperpre-β-lipoproteinaemia and hyperchylomicronaemia (type V hyperlipoproteinaemia) triglyceride levels are high, but corneal arcus is not seen.

Classically corneal arcus is first seen in the upper and lower quadrants, but eventually the two parts become confluent. Pathologically there is deposition of lipid in the stroma, Descemet's membrane and Bowman's layer. There is generally an intervening space between the limbus and the arcus opacity.

In hypolipoproteinaemia, there is reduction in levels of circulating lipoproteins. In lecithin hypercholesterol acyltransferase deficiency, unesterified cholesterol accumulates in, for example, blood vessels and bone marrow. There is a dense peripheral arcus and a stromal haze, due to fine greyish opacities. In familial high density lipoprotein deficiency (Tangier's disease), there is autosomal recessive inheritance and it is associated with corneal clouding, and irregular pigmentation in the retinal pigment epithelium.

In fish eye disease there is inability to esterify cholesterol

Table 13 Corneal findings in selected metabolic disorders

Metabolic disorder	Enzyme deficiency	Ocular manifestations	Corneal manifestations
Mucolipidoses			
Type I	Glycoprotein	Macular cherry red spot	Nil
Type II	Sialidosis	Spoke lens opacities, cherry red spot, vascular tortuosity in conjunctiva and retina	Fine epithelial and stromal opacities
Type II	Abnormal *N*-acetylglucosamine phosphotransferase	Orbital lymphoma	Megalocornea and clouding
Type III	*N*-acetylglucosamine phosphotransferase	Papilloedema and maculopathy	Stromal opacities
Type IV	Ganglioside transferase		Diffuse clouding first year
Galactosialidoses	Sialidase and β-galactosidase	Macular cherry red spot	Occasional mild clouding
Sphingolipidoses			
Fabry's disease	α-galactosidase A	Turtuosity of retinal and conjunctival vessels	Vortex opacities in epithelium
Multiple sulphatase deficiency	Arylsulphatase A, B, C steroid sulphatase	Macular cherry red spot	Occasional clouding
Mucopolysaccharidoses (MPS)			
Hurler's disease (MPS I–H)	α₁-iduronidase	Retinopathy with hyperpigmentation (bone spicules), optic atrophy	Cloudy at 3 years (Fig. 28)
Scheie's syndrome (MPS V)	α-iduronidase	Optic atrophy and pigmentary retinal degeneration	Clouding
Hurler–Scheie syndrome (MPS I–HS)	α-iduromidase	Glaucoma, optic atrophy, retinal degeneration	Progressive clouding
Hunter's syndrome (MPS II type A and B)	Iduronate sulphatase	Papilloedema, optic atrophy	Mild clouding
Sanfillipo's syndrome (MPS II A–D)	Enzyme deficiencies in heparin sulphate metabolism	Optic atrophy and pigmentary retinopathy	Occasional opacity (faint)
Morgnio's syndrome (MPS IV types A and B)	*N*-acetylgalactosamine-6-sulphatase (A); β-galactosidase (B)		Diffuse clouding
Galactosidosis			
Type I	β-galactosidase	Macular cherry red spot, optic atrophy	Diffuse clouding
Type II	Hexosaminidase A and B	Macular cherry red spot and optic atrophy	Clear

within high density lipoproteins, although there is no deficiency of lecithin hypercholesterol acyltransferase activity. The cornea becomes cloudy due to minute yellow opacities in all layers. The corneal periphery is the more opaque, and there may the appearance of a ring-shaped opacity 1 mm from the limbus.

Lysosomal storage diseases

This group of diseases include the mucolipidoses, the mucopolysaccharidoses, the galactosialidoses, fucosidoses, gangliosidoses, mannosidosis, and sphingolipidoses (Table 13). The main feature of these metabolic disorders is abnormal accumulation of major storage products.

Mucolipidoses

The mucolipidoses are characterized by the accumulation of oligosaccharides. There are deficiencies of hydrolytic enzymes involved in carbohydrate components of glycoproteins and glycolipids.

There are four types of mucolipidosis. In mucolipidosis type I there is deficiency of the α-neuraminidase. In the type I, there is loss of visual acuity, cherry red spots, and punctate corneal opacities. In type II, due to a similar enzyme deficiency, there are abnormal facies with prominent brow, saddle nose, frontal bossing, mental retardation, hearing loss, and neurological decline. There are fine epithelial and stromal opacities in the cornea.

In mucolipidosis type II there is deficiency of lysosomal phosphotransferase. There are fine opacities in the corneal stroma that do not effect vision. Mucolipidosis type III is due to deficiency of lysosomal phosphotransferase; the condition is relatively mild, with a reasonable lifespan. There can be central and peripheral stromal opacities, that do not interfere with vision. In mucolipidosis type IV, resulting from gangliosialidase deficiency, there is prominent and diffuse corneal opacity present at birth. There are vacuoles in the epithelium that contain fibrogranular material suggesting mucopolysaccharide deposition.

Sphingolipidoses

In the sphingolipidoses, which are lipid storage diseases, caused by deficiencies in specific enzymes, there is lipid accumulation in the tissues. All are autosomal recessive, apart from Fabry's disease. In this there is deficiency of α-galactosidase A with accumulation of ceramide trihexoside in lysosomes of blood vessels, and smooth muscle cells. Transmission is X linked. There is renal failure and cardiovascular disease. The cornea presents epithelial changes, with fine opacities best seen by retroillumination, that form a vortex pattern. The centre of the vortex is usually in the inferior third, and similar distribution of opacities are seen following amiodarone toxicity (Fig. 30), phenothiazine toxicity, indomethacin, and chloroquine. In addition there is tortuosity of retinal and conjunctival vessels, with occasional lens opacities. Inclusion bodies are seen within cutaneous, renal, and conjunctival cells. There are characteristic Maltese cross intracelluar inclusions that are birefringent found in affected tissues that can be identified histologically.

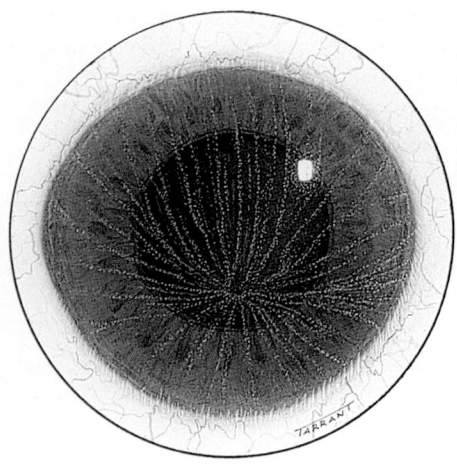

Fig. 30 Cornea verticillas due to systemic treatment with amiodarone. (By courtesy of Ragge and Easty, and Mosby.)

Systemic disease occurs in the form of renal failure and cardiovascular complications. Patients may survive in adulthood. Small punctate skin lesions occur known as angiokeratoma corporis diffusum around the inguinal region and buttocks. The absence of α-galactosidase activity can be identified in males, while in female carriers about 50 per cent have normal levels. There is the possibility of therapeutic intervention by recombinant technology in the future, as the DNA sequence for α-galactosidase has been identified.

Gangliosidoses

Gangliosidoses are inborn errors of sphingolipid metabolism, inherited as autosomal recessive traits. Glycosphingolipids contain sialic acid in oligosaccharide side chains, and occur in many cell types, including brain and the membranes of nerve endings in highest concentration. There are two groups of disorders affected by deposition of GM1 ganglioside (type I, with a defect in β-galactosidase) and GM2 ganglioside (type II, with defect in hexosaminidase A/B). There may be infantile, juvenile and adult forms of type I, and the three variants of type II are Tay–Sachs disease, Sandoff's disease, and GM2 activator deficiency. Ocular disease in type I includes mild corneal clouding, with intracytoplasmic vacuoles within all cells that are seen in histological section. In addition there is the macular cherry red spot, strabismus, optic atrophy, and nystagmus. In type II disorders, there is excessive deposition of gangliosides in neuronal cells resulting from defects in hexosaminidase A or B. In Tay–Sachs disease there is the hallmark of a macular cherry red spot and optic atrophy. There does not seem to be recorded evidence of corneal involvement. In Sandoff's disease, the macular cherry red spot is found, but clinical evidence of corneal disease is not reported.

Metabolic disorders including metals

The main metals that may manifest corneal symptoms and signs are calcium, copper, and iron.

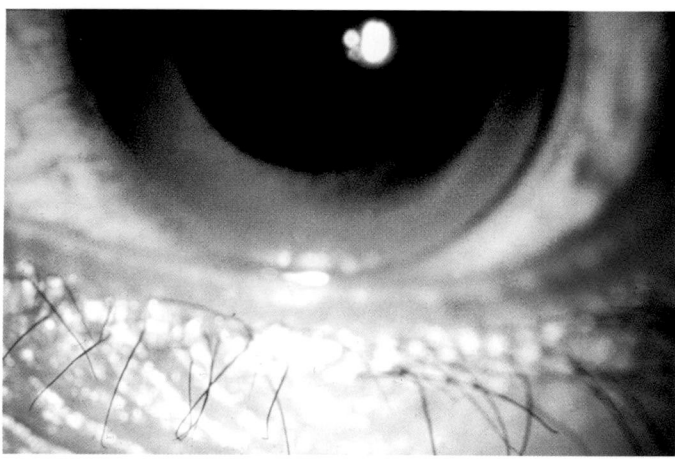

Fig. 31 Kayser–Fleischer ring in Wilson's disease. (By courtesy of Ragge and Easty, and Mosby.)

Hypercalcaemia

Hypercalcaemia is caused by excessive production of parathormone by parathyroid tumour, while secondary hypercalcaemia occurs in hypervitaminosis D, sarcoidosis, multiple myeloma, and selected carcinomas. Corneal and conjunctival calcification can occur. Deposits of hydroxyapatite occur in the interpalpebral zone, at the limbus, and gradually spreads towards the centre. Causes of band-shaped keratopathy are shown in Table 11.

Wilson's disease (hepatolenticular degeneration)

Wilson's disease is an autosomal recessive disorder associated with reduced incorporation of copper in caeruloplasmin and impairment of excretion of copper in the bile. This results in excess copper in the circulation that is loosely bound to albumin, which is readily deposited in certain tissues. The disease occurs after 6 years of age, and may present any time up to 60 years. The copper deposits lead to liver damage, as well as the basal ganglia, causing choreoathetosis and tremor. Brown–yellow deposits occur in the periphery of the cornea and are known as the Kayser–Fleischer ring (Fig. 31). This manifestation occurs early, simultaneous to deposition in basal ganglia. The deposits are in Descemet's membrane in the first instance, particularly in the upper quadrant, followed by the lower quadrant. Diagnosis can be confirmed by liver biopsy to demonstrate marked increase in copper concentration. Treatment of Wilson's disease is by systemic penicillamine which has strong chelating properties. The Kayser–Fleischer ring disappears once treatment has been initiated.

Further reading

Allansmith, M.R., Hahn, G.S., and Simon, M.A. (1976). Tissue, tear and serum IgE concentrations in vernal conjunctivitis. *American Journal of Ophthalmology*, **81**, 417–18.

Barchiesi, B.J., Echel, R.H., and Ellis, P.P. (1991). The cornea and disorders of lipid metabolism. *Survey of Ophthalmology*, **36**, 1–22.

Berman, E.R. (1994). Mucolipidoses. In *Pathobiology of ocular disease—a dynamic approach* (ed. A. Garner and G.K. Klintworth), pp. 923–38. Marcel Decker, New York.

Casey, T.A. and Sharif, K.W. (1991). *A colour atlas of corneal dystrophy and degenerations*. Mosby, St Louis.

Cogan, D.G. and Dickerson, G.R. (1964). Non-syphilitic interstitial keratitis with vestibuloauditory symptoms: a case with fatal aortitis. *Archives of Ophthalmology*, **71**, 172–5.

Jayson, M.I.V. and Easty, D.L. (1977). Ulceration of the cornea in rheumatoid arthritis. *Annals of Rheumatic Disease*, **36**, 428.

Mondino, B.J. (1990). Bullous diseases of the skin and mucous membranes. In *Duane's clinical ophthalmology*, Vol. 4 (ed. W. Tasman and E.A. Jaeger). Philadelphia, Lippincott.

Robin, J.R. and Dugel, R.J. (1988). Immunological disorders of the cornea and conjunctiva. In *The cornea* (ed. H.E. Kaufman, B.A. Barron, M.B. McDonald, and S.R. Waltman). Churchill Livingstone, Edinburgh.

Sugar, A. (1988). Corneal and conjunctival degenerations. In *The cornea* (ed. H.E. Kaufman). Churchill Livingstone, Edinburgh.

Sugar, J. (1988). Metabolic disorders of the cornea. In *The cornea* (ed. H.E. Kaufman, B.A. Barron, M.B. McDonald, and S.R. Waltman), pp. 361–82. Churchill Livingstone, Edinburgh.

2.7 Lens and cataract

2.7.1 Anatomy of the lens

G. A. Shun-Shin

Introduction

The lens is the only organ that grows continually in size throughout life. It provides one-third of the dioptric power of the eye. A knowledge of the anatomy of the lens allows an understanding of how transparency is maintained throughout life and of the pathological mechanisms of cataractogenesis.

The lens consists of an anterior and a posterior surface, which are paraboloids. This is thought to limit spherical aberrations. It is enclosed by a capsule and is attached to the ciliary processes by the lens zonules. The centres of the anterior and posterior surfaces are called the anterior and posterior poles. The axis of the lens joins the anterior to the posterior pole. The circumference of the lens is called the equator. The diameter is between 8.8 and 9.2 mm. Its thickness or anteroposterior length varies with accommodation. The unaccommodated thickness is about 4 mm at birth and does not increase much until adulthood. Thereafter there is a gradual linear increase in thickness at a rate given by $t = 0.026a + 3.35$ (where t is the thickness in millimetres and a is the age of person). At birth, the lens weighs 65 mg, at 20 years 152 mg, and 258 mg at 80 years.

The capsule

The capsule is a particularly thick, transparent basement membrane chiefly consisting of type IV collagen with some contribution from types I and III. Laminin and fibronectin are also present. By electron microscopy it is seen to consist of approx. 40 lamellae. The anterior capsule is formed by the lens epithelium and the posterior capsule by the elongating fibre cells. The anterior capsule thickens during life from 8 μm to 14 mm, whilst the posterior capsule remains at 2 to 3 mm thickness. The anterior capsule is thicker peripherally than centrally. It is inextensible but very flexible. Fincham proposed that the capsule moulded the lens in accommodation, whist Koretz and Handelman propose that it acts as a force distributor. The capsule is permeable to small molecules and protein up to 70 kDa. Unlike the lens, the most superficial part of the capsule is the oldest.

The lens epithelium

Deep to the anterior capsule are the lens epithelial cells, which are of two distinct types: cells of the central zone, which do not undergo mitosis, and cells of the germinative zone, which give rise to the lens fibres (Fig. 1). The lens epithelium is polarized, and, as the lens is formed by an invagination of the lens placode, the apical side faces inwards and the basal end outwards, next to the capsule.

The cells of the central zone are polygonal but cuboidal in cross-section. Macrophotographically, their width has been measured *in vivo* to be 13 μm and their height 5 to 8 μm; their density is of the order of 5000 cells/mm², with men having a lower density than women. These cells contain organelles and cytoskeletal protein. Of particular interest are characteristic polygonal arrays or 'geodomes' of microfilaments, which line the apical end and attach to the lateral membrane, and are thought to help maintain structure during accommodation. The only crystallin present is α-crystallin. Unlike typical epithelial cells, there are no tight junctions or zona occludens between adjacent epithelial cells. These cells are interconnected by gap junctions and desmosomes. Low molecular-weight metabolites and ions can be exchanged.

There are, however, few gap junctions between epithelial cell and lens-fibre cell at the epithelial–fibre cell interface, which is not unexpected as this is an apicoapical junction. Endocytosis

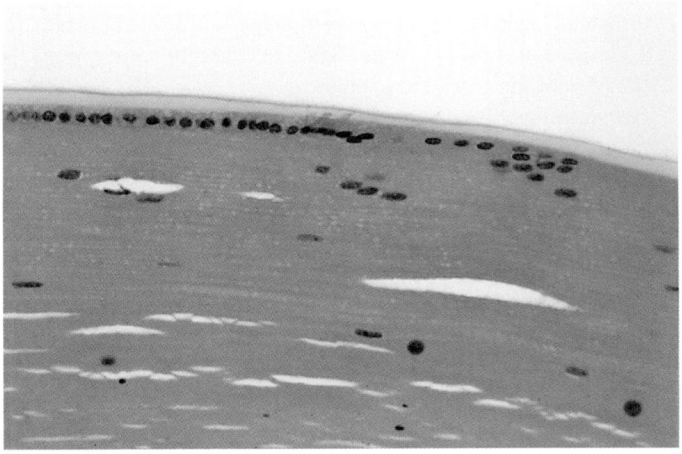

Fig. 1 Light micrograph of the human lens equator showing the lens epithelium maturing into lens fibres. The nuclei lie on a curve, the lens-fibre nuclear bow. (Illustration with thanks to Dr B. MacDonald.)

allows nutrients and receptor-mediated substances across the epithelial–fibre cell interface. Square arrays are present at the interface; these are thought to be important in volume regulation. Na^+K^+ ATP-ase is found in the apicolateral membrane and pumps $3Na^+$ outwards for every $2 K^+$ inwards. A calmodulin-dependent, Ca^{++}-activated ATP-ase is also found in the epithelium. Amino acids are actively transported across the epithelium.

The epithelium modulates the passage of electrolytes, nutrients, and metabolites to the lens fibres. The anterior capsule is produced by these cells. Receptors to insulin and β-adrenergic agonists are present.

The lens fibres

In the pre-equatorial zone are the mitotic lens epithelial cells, which will produce nearly 2 million lens fibres in 80 years. The cells undergo mitosis, elongate, and turn through 180°. The fibre cells retain their polarity, with a basal and apical end. The nuclei of these cells form the lens-fibre nuclear bow. The fibres terminally differentiate with pyknocytosis and loss of the nucleus and cell organelles, which is one of the factors important in achieving lens transparency. The elongating ends lie between the epithelial cells and the earlier lens fibre anteriorly or between the posterior capsule and the earlier lens fibre posteriorly. Thus the youngest fibres are to be found most superficial in the lens. The lens fibres are tightly packed and the total extracellular space is only 1.3 per cent. They are thin, elongated cells measuring up to 10 mm long and only 1.5 to 2 μm wide, and 10 to 12 μm from apex to apex. The posterior half of the lens fibre is thinner than the anterior. The younger fibres are hexagonal in cross-section, with two broad surfaces and four thin. Their ends flare as they meet at the suture. This configuration ensures the tightest packing of fibres. There is a distinct change in morphology as the fibres mature. The superficial lens fibres have 'ball-and-socket junctions' whilst the deeper fibres have grooves and ridges on their surface (Fig. 2). It is thought that this may maintain lens architecture during accommodation.

The lens crystallins make up 90 per cent of the mass of the fibres and provide the high refractive index of the lens. The cytoskeletal proteins maintain cell shape and are important in cell elongation. About 50 per cent of the fibre membrane is MIP, membrane intrinsic protein.

Scheimpflug slit-image studies of human lenses have demonstrated compaction of the fibres as they move centrally. This is mirrored in morphological differences in superficial and deep cortical fibres. The cholesterol:phospholipid ratio is higher in the central 65 per cent of the lens than in the superficial 35 per cent. It suggests that the central fibres have little osmotic activity. The superficial fibres have a high density of intramembrane particles and numerous gap junctions; the deeper fibres are largely free of intramembrane particles but retain gap junctions.

The lens sutures

The embryonic nucleus, which is formed by the primary lens fibres, has no suture. The fetal nucleus has a pair of Y-shaped

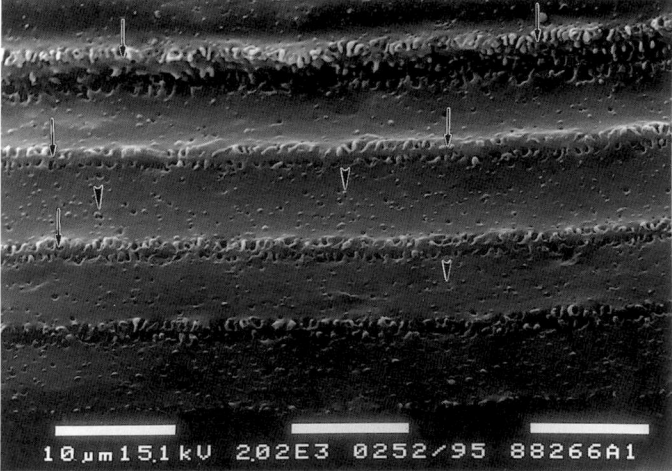

(a)

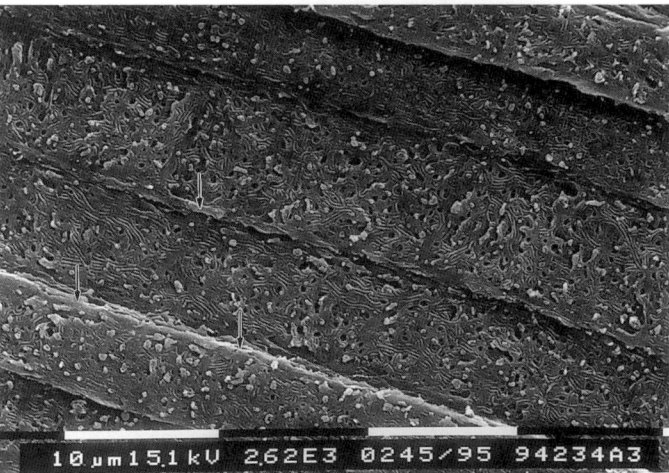

(b)

Fig. 2 (a) Scanning electron micrograph of the superficial human lens cortex showing the 'ball-and-socket' joints. (b) Scanning electron micrograph of the deep human lens cortex showing the tongue and grooves. (Illustration with thanks to Professor G. Vrensen.)

sutures: the anterior is upright and the arms are at 120° to each other; the posterior is inverted. Fetal fibres, from successive shells of growth, are longer but otherwise of the same shape. The suture of each shell is thus in register and the fetal fibre tips all meet on one of six planes. This explains why the fetal suture can be readily seen in the biomicroscope. Postnatally the structure increases in complexity until, in the adult cortex, a suture shaped like a nine-pointed star exists. The anterior and posterior parts are exactly offset. A few straight fibres run exactly in meridian 20° apart whilst the neighbouring fibres have tips that curve and expand before they form the suture. The ends curve in opposite directions as they meet the anterior or posterior suture. At middle age, the suture has 12 branches. It is to be noted that the suture is not a structure as such but an area of discontinuity in the lens where fibre tips meet. These tips are specialized regions with a concentration of organelles and enzymes. They have characteristics of transporting epithe-

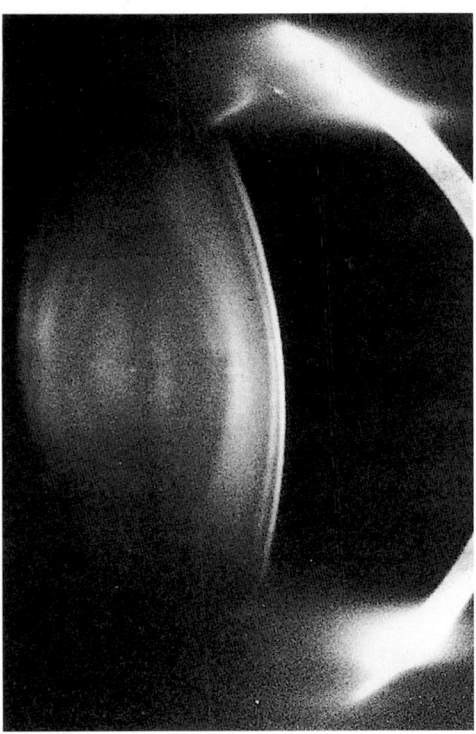

Fig. 3 Scheimpflug slit image of a human lens *in vivo* showing the zones of disjunction. The most superficial bright line is the capsule. The first dark zone is C1α; the next bright zone is C1β; the next zones are C2, C3 and C4.

lia and may be the site of exchange of nutrient, ions, essential metabolites, and receptor-mediated substances.

Nucleus and cortex

The lens is divided into nucleus and cortex. The nucleus consists of all fibres laid down before birth. The embryonic nucleus of primary lens fibres is surrounded by the fetal nucleus. It is to be noted that the entity loosely called 'the nucleus' by the cataract surgeon in fact consists of nucleus and surrounding deep cortex. The cortex consists of alternating zones of light and dark on slit illumination that correspond to areas of greater or lesser scattering of light. This is most easily seen in the biomicroscope in the 50-year-old lens. The first bright line represents the capsule. The first dark zone has been called the anterior clear zone or zone C1α: it measures approximately 150 mm in thickness and represents the youngest, 2- to 3-year-old fibres. Zone C1β appears bright; zones C2, C3, and C4 are alternating dark, bright, and dark zones (Fig. 3). The four zones originate at approximately the ages of 4, 9, 19, and 46 years, respectively. Interestingly, the zones of discontinuity seem to correspond to the formation of increasingly complex lens sutures.

The zonules

The zonules suspend the lens from the ciliary body. They consist of fibrillin, a 350-kDa, cysteine-rich glycoprotein found also in vascular and connective tissue. The zonule consists of microfibrils of about 10 nm in diameter, which form fibres up to 1 mm in diameter. These in turn form bundles up to 60 times this size. The fibres mostly arise from the posterior part of the pars plana. At the pars plicata, this sheet of fibres divides into discrete bundles named zonular plexuses, to pass in the valleys between the ciliary processes. Small strands, or tension fibres, connect to the ciliary processes. At the anterior end of the pars plicata, the plexus divides into three branches, the zonular fork: the pre-equatorial, equatorial, and postequatorial. The pre-equatorial fibres divide further and insert and merge into the

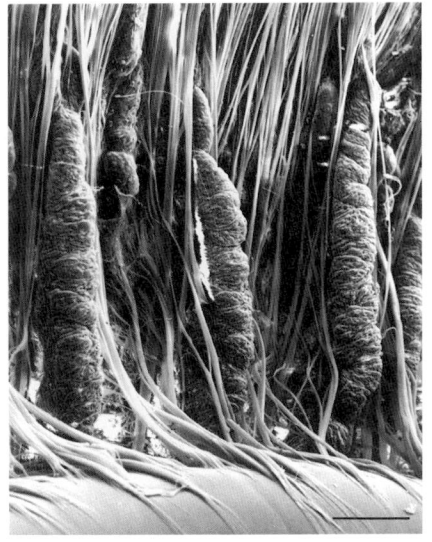

(a)

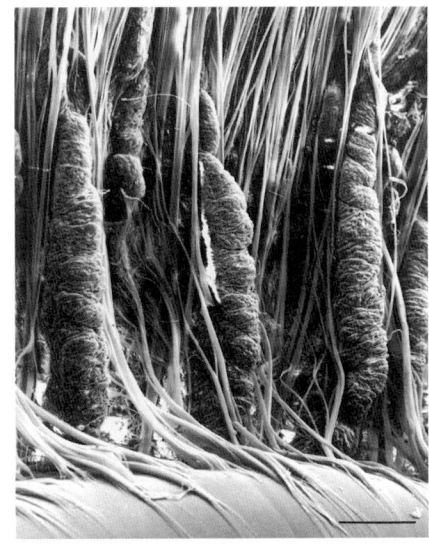

(b)

Fig. 4 (a) and (b) Scanning electron micrographs of zonules passing through the valleys in the pars plicata. The zonule (Z) passes between the ciliary processes (C) and then divides into three main systems at the zonular fork (F) before reaching the surface of the lens (L). At the posterior margin of the ciliary processes the zonular fibres rearrange themselves to form a series of zonular plexuses (P). Bars = 160 μm and 60 μm, respectively. [Reproduced with permission, and with thanks to Professor J. Marshall *et al.*, from Marshall, J., Beaconsfield, M., and Rothery, S. (1982). The anatomy and development of the human lens and zonules. *Transactions of the Ophthalmological Society of the United Kingdom*, **102**, 423–39 (their Fig. 6a,b).]

capsule just anterior to the equator. The equatorial fibres are less well developed (Fig. 4). The postequatorial fibres insert at a variety of levels behind the equator.

References

Borchman, D., Delamere, N., and Patterson, C. A. (1989). Ca^{++}ATP-ase activity in the human lens. *Current Eye Research*, **8**, 1049–54.

Brown, N. A. P. and Bron, A. J. (1987). An estimate of the human lens epithelial cell size *in vivo*. *Experimental Eye Research*, **44**, 899–906.

Fagerholm, P. P. and Philipson, B. T. (1981). Human lens epithelium in normal and cataractous lenses. *Investigative Ophthalmology and Visual Science*, **21**, 408–14.

Gorthy, W. C. and Anderson, J. W. (1980). Special characteristics of the polar regions of the rat lens: morphology and phosphatase histochemistry. *Investigative Ophthalmology and Visual Science*, **19**, 1038–52.

Gorthy, W. C. and Steward, D. R. (1991). Localisation of dipeptyl peptidase II in the rat lens during normal ageing and during formation of an age-related cataract: light and electron microscopic analysis. *Investigative Ophthalmology and Visual Science*, **32**, 2119–29.

Gorthy, W. C., Snavely, M. R., and Gerrong, N. D. (1971). Some aspects of transport and digestion in the lens of the normal young adult rat. *Experimental Eye Research*, **12**, 112–19.

Howcroft, M. J. and Parker, J. N. (1977). Aspheric curvatures for the human lens. *Vision Research*, **17**, 1217–23.

Kinsey, V. E. and Reddy, D. V. N. (1965). Studies in the crystallin lens. *Investigative Ophthalmology and Visual Science*, **4**, 104–16.

Koretz, J. F., Cook, C. A., and Kuszak, J. R. (1994). The zones of discontinuity in the human lens. *Vision Research*, **34**, 2955–62.

Kuszak, J. R. (1995). Embryology and anatomy of the lens. In *Duane's Clinical ophthalmology* (ed. W.Tasman and E.A.Jaeger), Chapter 75a, pp.1–9. Lippincott-Raven, Philadelphia.

Marshall, J., Beaconsfield, M., and Rothery, S. (1982). The anatomy and development of the human lens and zonules. *Transactions of the Ophthalmological Society of the United Kingdom*, **102**, 423–39.

Phelps Brown, N. and Bron, A.J. (1996). *Lens disorders. A clinical manual of cataract diagnosis*. Butterworth Heinemann, Oxford.

Rafferty, N. S. and Scholz, D. L. (1984). Polygonal arrays of microfilaments in epithelial cells of the intact lens. *Current Eye Research*, **3**, 1141–9.

Rafferty, N. S. and Scholz, D. L. (1989). Comparative study of actin filament patterns in lens epithelial cells. Are these determined by the mechanism of lens accommodation. *Current Eye Research*, **8**, 569–79.

Reddy, V. N. (1973). Dynamics of transport systems in the eye. *Investigative Ophthalmology and Visual Science*, **15**, 731–50.

Unakar, N. J. and Tsui, J. Y. (1980). Sodium potassium dependant ATP-ase. *Investigative Ophthalmology and Visual Science*, **19**, 630–41.

Van Marle, J., Vrensen, G., and van Veen, H. Maturing human lens fibre membranes and filipin cytochemistry. Eye lens membranes and ageing. In *Topics in ageing research in Europe*, Vol. 15 (ed. G. Vrensen and J. Clauwaert), pp. 123–34. Eurage, Leiden.

Vrensen, G., Van Marle, J., Van Veen, H., and Willekens, B. (1992). Membrane architecture as a function of lens fibre maturation: a freeze fracture an scanning electron microscopy study in the human lens. *Experimental Eye Research*, **54**, 433–46.

2.7.2 Physiology and biochemistry

Darren W.A. Hook and John J. Harding

Introduction

The primary function of the lens is to ensure the correct focusing of light on to the light-sensitive retina. This requires the lens to neither absorb nor scatter light over a wide range of frequencies in the visible spectrum. To achieve this the genetic machinery and organelles of the lens-fibre cells are degraded, with resultant loss of protein synthesis. Despite this constraint the lens-fibre cells are metabolically active and the lens remains a viable organ for many decades.

Lens development

A single layer of epithelial cells is found immediately beneath the anterior lens capsule (Fig. 1). This layer continuously divides throughout life and its cells migrate towards the equator, undergo elongation losing their organelles, and are eventually overlaid with newly formed layers of fibre cells. During development the oldest lens-fibre cells become increasingly isolated from the periphery and these constitute the lens nucleus.

The crystallins

A high protein content is required in the lens for the correct focusing of light on to the retina. The major proteins of the lens are the crystallins, which are ideally suited to life therein by virtue of their extremely stable structure and their contribution to short-range order within the lens. In the mammalian lens there are principally three types of crystallin: α, β, and γ. Subsets of all three are expressed extralenticularly at low concentrations. In the rat and bovine lens, the differential and developmentally regulated expression of the crystallins contributes towards the increasing protein-concentration gradient

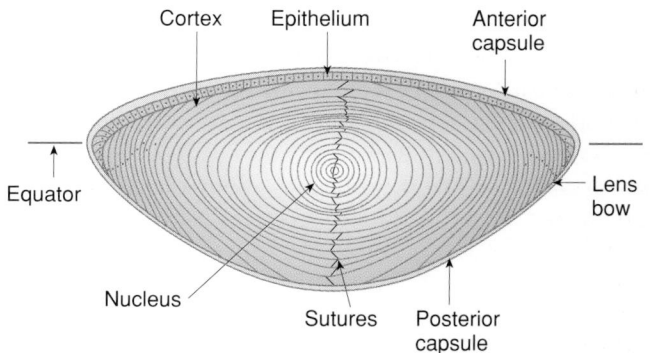

Fig. 1 Schematic transverse section of a human lens (illustration by J. Cronin).

Table 1 Properties of mammalian crystallins

Crystallin	Subunit (kDa)	Aggregate (kDa)	State	Secondary structure	Tertiary structure
α	20	700	Oligomer	Some β	Unknown
β	23–35	40–200	Oligomer	Mostly β	Two separated domains, each consisting of two Greek-key motifs
γ	20	20	Monomer	Mostly β	Two self-associating domains, each consisting of two Greek-key motifs

from the periphery to the nucleus. This difference in concentration results in a differential refractive-index gradient throughout the lens, which provides a more powerful optical lens in these species. By contrast the differential refractive-index gradient between the capsule/epithelium and fibre cells is thought to be responsible for the correct refraction of light in man. Some properties of the crystallins are summarized in Table 1.

A variety of other crystallins collectively termed the enzyme crystallins are found in the lenses of other vertebrates and invertebrates. These have sequence homology with ubiquitous cellular enzymes and may or may not be enzymatically active. δ-Crystallin, which replaces γ-crystallin in avian and reptile lenses, has 60 per cent homology with human arginosuccinate lyase and retains partial enzymatic function in the avian lens. The rich diversity of these crystallins and their subunits discourages self-assembly, which could otherwise lead to light scatter and opacification.

α-Crystallin structure

α-Crystallin is the major protein of the mammalian lens and can contribute more than 40 per cent of its dry weight. It normally consists of an aggregate of up to 40 subunits derived from two gene products, αA and αB. These products are phosphorylated early in development and further post-translational modifications lead to the accumulation of a variety of additional α-crystallin products.

The α-crystallin molecule is heterogeneous in size and can be isolated in aggregates ranging from 350 kDa to several million Da. Although a native form of α-crystallin (M_r approx. 800 kDa) has been isolated at pH 6.9, 37°C, by gel chromatography, the size of the aggregate is sensitive to the temperature, pH, and the ionic strength of the elution buffer. Chemical denaturants such as urea can dissociate α-crystallin into its subunits (M_r approx. 20 kDa). Upon denaturation, reaggregation occurs but is incomplete.

A crystal structure for α-crystallin has yet to be deduced, although circular dichroism spectroscopy shows it is a protein rich in β-sheet structure. Various models have been proposed for α-crystallin based on its native size, electron microscopy, nuclear magnetic-resonance spectroscopy, the susceptibility of its residues to proteolysis/chemical modification, and its *in vitro* activity. Recent models are based on the premise that each subunit can be divided into a core hydrophobic N-terminal

domain and a more hydrophilic C-terminal domain with a flexible C-terminal extension. There is some evidence that α-crystallin may contain a cavity at its centre but this remains open to debate. Models for α-crystallin range from Bindel's original three-layered model, through Augusteyn's micellular arrangement to Carver's double-ring model based on the structure of the chaperone GroEL (chaperenin 60).

α-Crystallin function

In addition to its structural role in the lens, the subunits of α-crystallin, mostly αB, are expressed extralenticularly and amounts of αB are increased in a variety of neurodegenerative diseases.

α-Crystallin has sequence homology with, as well as structural and functional similarities to, the small heat-shock proteins. The initial observation by Horwitz that α-crystallin forms stable complexes with unfolded proteins and prevents their precipitation has led to the acceptance of α-crystallin as a molecular chaperone. Indeed the soluble, high molecular-weight fraction that elutes before α-crystallin upon gel chromatography consists of α-crystallin complexed with β- or γ-crystallins. It is possible that such associations in the lens may prove to be essential in maintaining lens transparency.

βγ-Crystallins

Members of this family can be divided into four subgroups—$β_H$-, $β_L$-, γ- and $γ_s$-crystallins: γ- and $γ_s$-crystallins are monomers of 20 and 21 kDa, respectively; β-crystallins are oligomers with subunit masses of between 23 and 35 kDa (Table 1). More distantly related members of this family include the spore-coat protein S of *Myxococcus xanthus*, human C-*myc* oncogene protein, transducin, desmin, and vimentin. γ-Crystallins are classified in a complicated fashion that varies between species. In the rat the genes and proteins are commonly classified as γA to γF and $γ_s$. Originally $γ_s$ was classified as $β_s$ by virtue of its similarities to β-crystallins, but when its cDNA sequence was deduced, it became clear that it was more closely related to the γ-crystallins.

γ-Crystallins are compact, highly stable proteins, rich in β-sheet structure and devoid of α-helices. The N-terminal amino acid of γ-crystallins, in contrast to α- and β-crystallins, is not acetylated. Bovine γII-crystallin was the first crystallin to have its structure elucidated at high resolution (1.6 Å). The γII polypeptide consists of two domains encoded by separate

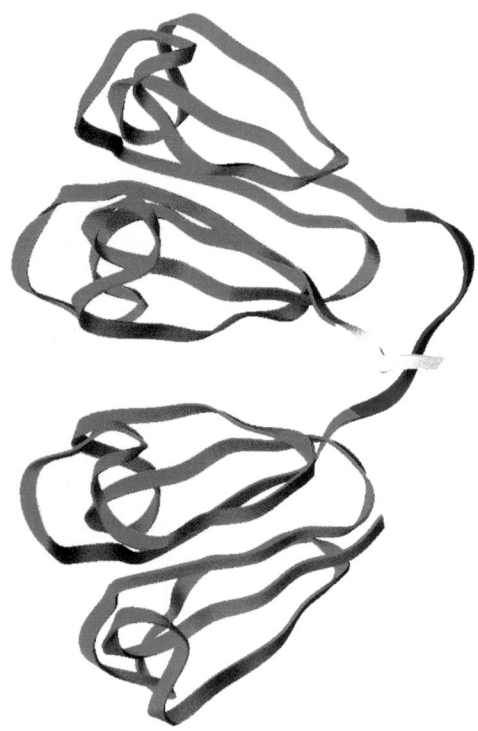

Fig. 2 Structure of γB-crystallin. Ribbon diagram showing folding of the Cα backbone of the polypeptide chain. The protein is formed from colinear Greek-key motifs that fold into two compact domains: motifs 1 and 3 are coloured azure blue and are on the outside of the protein molecule; motifs 2 and 4 are in red and are close together at the interface between the two domains. The domains are covalently joined by a linker coloured in royal blue and the molecule has a short C-terminal extension coloured yellow. Note the great conformational similarity of the four motifs: there is an approximate 2-fold axis relating the paired motifs in each domain and the two domains are related by a further 2-fold axis. (This colour photograph of γB-crystallin was kindly provided by Brian Norledge and Christine Slingsby of Birkbeck College, London.)

exons. Each domain contains two Greek-key motifs of four antiparallel β-strands (Fig. 2). This motif is conserved throughout the βγ superfamily and is stabilized by a folded hairpin structure. In γ-crystallins, both domains are in contact with each other and this arrangement constrains these crystallins to a monomeric form. Critical residues within the folded hairpin are at least semiconserved among the different βγ crystallins. The crystal structures of bovine γIIIb and γIVa have also been resolved and are similar to that of γII. γII-Crystallin contains an elaborate surface-charge network in which most charged ions are found at the surface of the molecule and are paired. This is a property shared by the extremely stable enzymes of the thermophilic bacteria.

Developmentally regulated synthesis of γ-crystallins ensures that they are found in the lens nucleus, a region that is highly dehydrated in some species. Their ion-pairing properties therefore make them especially desirable molecules for life in the nucleus as they have very few free ions that are capable of binding water molecules.

β-crystallins can be divided into two groups, acidic and basic, which are represented by the nomenclature βA and βB, respectively. In common with α-crystallin, βB₂ and βB₃ may be phosphorylated. β-Crystallin polypeptides are also found in

a truncated form as is the case for βB₁, which may lose 11 residues from its N-terminus. Gene sharing is employed, as demonstrated by bovine βA₁ and βA₃, which utilize different start codons to produce near-identical polypeptides of slightly differing lengths.

The solution to the structure of the βB₂-crystallin dimer confirmed the conservation of the Greek-key motif among the β- and γ-crystallins. A key difference between these crystallins, the aggregational properties of the β-crystallins, was explained by the observation that the two domains of a βB₂ polypeptide were not in contact but were widely separated and in contact with complementary domains of another βB₂ polypeptide. βB₂ also forms hetero-oligomers and may participate in stabilizing aggregates of β-crystallins. β-Crystallins are similar to γ-crystallins in their primary structural organization, with the exception that they contain N-terminal extensions. Acidic β-crystallins have insertions whereas basic β-crystallins have C-terminal extensions. The charge networks of β-crystallins are even more extensive than those of γ-crystallins.

γₛ-Crystallin, although classified as a γ-crystallin from its sequence homology and monomeric behaviour, shares structural similarities with the acidic β-crystallins distinct from those of other γ-crystallins. It is relatively flexible and is more readily denatured than the other, more compact γ-crystallins. Like acidic β-crystallins it contains a flexible, 4-amino acid, N-terminal extension and its N-terminal amino acid is acetylated.

Lens metabolism

General

The lens maintains a pH of around 6.9 and a temperature below that of the body core. Glycolysis is the major pathway of energy production in the lens, consistent with the low oxygen tension within the fibre cells. However, carbohydrates can also be metabolized by oxidative phosphorylation (primarily in the lens epithelium), the pentose-phosphate pathway, and the α-glycerophosphate shuttle. Generation of the nucleotide NAD⁺ is required for glycolysis and α-glycerophosphate oxidation whereas the pentose-phosphate pathway is dependent on NADPH metabolism. There is negligible synthesis and degradation of proteins in the centre of the lens. Enzymes of carbohydrate metabolism decrease in activity from the periphery to the lens nucleus. Nevertheless, there is significant metabolism occurring even within the lens nucleus.

Ionic balance

The ionic balance of the lens is controlled by active transport mechanisms including the transmembrane proteins Na, K-ATPase and Ca-ATPase. Na, K-ATPase catalyses the translocation of potassium and sodium ions against the concentration gradients of the lens membrane. Potassium ions are pumped into the cytosol as sodium ions are expelled from lens cells. Both these processes are coordinated by the ATPase activity of the enzyme. Ca-ATPase actively pumps calcium from peripheral lens cells. Na, K-ATPase, although concentrated in epithelial membranes of the lens, is also detectable in the cortex and nucleus. Ca^{2+}-ATPase activity is, however, not found in the lens nucleus. Other ions and small molecules enter the lens and are readily passed between fibre cells throughout the lens.

Carbohydrate metabolism

d-Glucose enters the lens via glucose transporters. Glucose metabolism was monitored by Wolfe, who followed its conversion to other metabolites in homogenates of calf lens by using radiolabelled glucose. Glucose 6-phosphate was the major metabolite and sorbitol was detected as a minor metabolite. Little carbon dioxide was produced, confirming that glycolysis was the major pathway of glucose metabolism in the lens, although the pentose-phosphate pathway can be stimulated if needed.

It has been suggested that the accumulation of sorbitol might be involved in sugar cataract. It is claimed that aldose reductase converts glucose and other sugars to sorbitol. Elevated concentrations of sugars, if rapidly converted to sorbitol and other polyols, could cause an osmotic imbalance leading to swelling and opacification of the lens. Several powerful factors argue against such a scheme for human diabetic cataract. The assay for aldose reductase is based on the metabolism of glyceraldehyde, an unstable substrate that autoxidizes under the assay conditions. Glucose has yet to be shown to be a substrate for aldose reductase. As previously mentioned, sorbitol is only a minor metabolite during glucose oxidation and aldose reductase has comparatively low activity in the human lens.

Aldehyde dehydrogenase can convert a variety of aldehydes to less toxic compounds. Aldehydes derived from lipid peroxidation readily modify lens proteins. It is therefore not surprising that aldehyde dehydrogenase is active throughout the lens.

Protein synthesis

The lens transports the amino acids it needs from the aqueous humour. The majority of protein synthesis is concerned with that of the crystallins and this is developmentally regulated. α-Crystallin is continuously synthesized throughout development in the lens epithelium, although the ratio αA:αB decreases during fetal development until, by 1 year postnatal, a ratio of less than 3 is reached. By contrast, β- and γ-crystallins are synthesized exclusively during or after elongation. γ-Crystallin is synthesized early in fetal development. The cryoproteins γD, γE, and γF are the most abundantly expressed γ-crystallins in the young embryonic rat lens, after which synthesis switches to γA, γB, and γC. Around birth, synthesis of γ-crystallin ceases and there is an explosive and continuous synthesis of $γ_s$. γC and γD are the major γ-crystallins in the young human lens. As for the β-crystallins, they are synthesized in increasing amounts and their subunits are differentially regulated during fetal development.

Genes for α-crystallin subunits are found on different chromosomes and their synthesis is controlled by different regulatory elements. The murine αA promoter contains several cis regulatory elements 5' of its coding sequence. Two such elements bind the ubiquitous transcription factor, Pax6, which stimulates αA promoter activity. In transient transfection assays, αA was also shown to contain negative control sequences further upstream of the promoter. Murine αA regulatory sequences were able to direct transcription in chicken lens cells in cotransfection experiments, suggesting that transcription factors for αA-crystallin may be conserved across these species. The αB promoter is able to function efficiently in lens cells and promoter activity was only weakly augmented in the presence of elements from an upstream enhancer that has been shown to be essential for gene expression in other tissues. Expression of this gene in different tissues is controlled by the differential utilization of shared and tissue-specific regulatory elements. αB has also been shown to contain a putative heat-shock element.

Genes for all six rat γ-crystallins are found on chromosome 9, five of which are clustered. The murine γF-crystallin is found exclusively in the central nuclear fibre cells of the adult lens. A -67/+45 element in the γF gene was enough to produce a low, basal, lens-specific transcriptional activity. This element is conserved among the γ-crystallins. The HMG protein SOX-2 is highly enriched in lens cells and specifically augmented the activities of the mouse γF promoter and the chicken $δ_1$ enhancer in transfection assays. The SOX-binding sequence is highly conserved amongst the mammalian γ-crystallins. Optimum expression of this gene in fibre cells has also been demonstrated when its two enhancer elements and the proximal promoter are present. Continued expression of this gene during late development of the fibre cell was due to the increased strength of the promoter modulated by the action of at least the proximal enhancer.

In cell culture, demethylation of γD sequences preceded promoter occupancy and transcription during basic (**b**) fibroblast growth factor (**FGF**)-induced differentiation of rat lens fibres. There is evidence that the gene has four regulatory regions containing proximal activators and a repressor element responsible for limiting γD expression during the development of fibre cells.

Cell-culture studies have shown that bFGF induces lens differentiation in vitro. FGF also induces differential responses in a concentration-dependent manner and the responsiveness of epithelial cells to FGF was related to both their age and state of differentiation. Insulin augments the inductive action of FGF. Transforming growth factor-β induced cataract in lens culture and cataract-like changes in lens epithelial explants.

Most studies support the widely held view that there is negligible protein synthesis in the lens nucleus This has been demonstrated by incubation of lenses in media containing labelled amino acids, whereby only a negligible proportion of protein-bound radiolabel was found in the nuclear soluble-protein fraction compared to the cortex. However, one study, which used labelled methionine, found a significant amount of label enriched in the nuclear fraction. Methionine is metabolized to cysteine, which is a constituent of the tripeptide glutathione. Glutathione and free cysteine are found at high concentrations throughout the lens and bind non-covalently to lens proteins. Therefore, it seems likely that the contradictory findings of that study may owe more to the promiscuous nature of glutathione and cysteine than to de novo protein synthesis.

Protein breakdown

Many proteins are degraded during lens development and ageing. Peptide fragments accumulate with age and are found at greater concentration in the older nucleus than in the younger cortical tissue. Many products of crystallin cleavage are enriched in the nucleus. Human and bovine αA- and βB$_2$-crystallins lose their C-terminal serine residue progressively with time. αA also loses additional C-terminal residues with increasing age. Of the other crystallins, cleavage products of αB, βA$_1$/A$_3$, γ$_D$, and γ$_s$ have also been isolated in increasing quantities from older lens tissue. Cytoskeletal proteins are also processed in a pattern coincident with fibre differentiation.

No products of the cleavage of lens proteins have unambiguously been identified as the result of endogenous proteolytic action, but the lens does possess a wide range of proteolytic systems. Ubiquitin is a highly conserved proteolytic complex identified throughout the rabbit lens. This protein requires ATP for activation and its conjugation with other polypeptides targets damaged proteins for destruction. Conjugated ubiquitin is found throughout the lens at similiar concentrations whereas free ubiquitin is enriched in the epithelium.

A high molecular-weight, proteolytic enzyme complex of around 650 kDa, consisting of peptides between 22 and 32 kDa, known as the multicatalytic proteinase complex, has been isolated from the bovine lens. Activity of this complex was previously known as neutral proteinase activity. The complex contains at least two enzymes, one of which has properties consistent with those of a serine protease, and the complex may also contain at least one exopeptidase. Other members of this proteasome include the heat-shock proteins hsp90 and α-crystallin. Substrates include all the major bovine crystallins with the exception of γ-crystallin.

Generally, the concentrations of proteolytic enzymes decrease from the epithelium to the nucleus. Serine proteases and calpain are all active within the lens and their concentrations vary between species. The crystallins, especially α-crystallin, and cytoskeletal proteins were targets for these proteases *in vitro*. *In vivo*, proteolytic activity is controlled by the presence of excess inhibitors. Up to three trypsin-like inhibitor activities have been demonstrated within the lens. Their specific activities decrease flom the periphery to the nucleus, although they are most active in an aggregated, water-insoluble form. α-Crystallin also partially inhibits trypsin, although it is itself a substrate and is rapidly degraded by the enzyme *in vitro*. The endogenous inhibitor of calpain II, calpastatin, is also present in the bovine and human lens and is found in excess of calpain throughout the lens.

Peptide products of various proteolytic cycles present substrates for the action of the aminopeptidases, including aminopeptidase III, which has negligible activity in the bovine lens nucleus. An acylpeptide hydrolase activity has been detected in the human, rabbit, and rat lens.

Glutathione and ascorbic acid

The concentration of glutathione decreases from the cortex to the nucleus. Glutathione is a tripeptide that is synthesized sequentially by the enzymes γ-glutamylcysteinyl synthetase and glutathione synthetase. The rate-limiting step of glutathione synthesis is the initial step catalysed by γ-glutamylcysteinyl synthetase, as this enzyme is found at low concentrations in the human lens.

Glutathione reduces a variety of compounds in a reaction that leaves it in an oxidized form (GSSG) which may form mixed disulphides with lens proteins. In one such reaction, glutathione is oxidized and hydrogen peroxides are detoxified. Both processes are catalysed by glutathione peroxidase, a selenium-containing enzyme that may be of particular importance to the human lens where the ubiquitous hydrogen-peroxide scavenger catalase is found at low concentrations. Regeneration of reduced glutathione (GSH) is achieved through the action of glutathione reductase, which is highly active in human lenses. Glutathione S-transferases, along with other helper enzymes, have multiple roles in detoxification. Concentrations of enzymes of glutathione metabolism vary amongst species. Ascorbic acid and glutathione help maintain each other in a reduced state. In such a reaction, ascorbic acid may be oxidized to dehydroascorbic acid. Ascorbic acid is not synthesized in guinea-pigs and primates and must be supplied in the diet of these species.

Other metabolites

cAMP and cGMP are at their highest concentrations in the epithelial cells. Adenylate cyclase is a membrane-bound protein that regulates the metabolism of these nucleotides and is found in significant amounts in the epithelium and cortex. Lenses also synthesize small amounts of prostaglandins. Inositol is found at high concentrations in the lens and the phosphoinositol cycle can be stimulated in the lens by various factors.

Membrane and cytoskeleton

Lens membrane

The lens has a resting potential of approx. 75 mV. The structure of the lens membrane consists of lipids (mostly phospholipids) and proteins, both of which may have carbohydrate moieties. Membranes of the cortex and nucleus contain a variety of fatty acids. Permeation of ions occurs from cell to cell through specific channels. Lens fibres are electrically coupled to each other and directly exchange metabolites. In other tissues this communication is mediated by various channels, including gap junctions, which allow small molecules of less than 1 kDa to pass. The gap junctions between lens-fibre cells are distinct from those found in other cell types. Major constituents of gap junctions are connexins (**Cx**), subtypes of which are differentially distributed amongst lens cell types. Cx43, Cx56, and Cx45.6 are differentially expressed in the chick lens. The lens also contains a unique and differential distribution of integrins. These glycoproteins mediate attachment between the lens and the extracellular matrix.

Membrane proteins

MIP26 and MP70 are membrane-bound proteins that are abundantly and specifically expressed in lens-fibre cells. Both are substrates for phosphorylation. MIP26 is a mainly α-helical protein that transverses the membrane several times. There is some evidence to suggest that MIP26 is a constituent of lens-fibre channels and that the regulation of those channels is controlled through the gated action of its C-terminus, which is exposed to the lens cytoplasm. Calmodulin, which is activated by calcium, interacts with C-terminal residues of MIP26, and regulates channel permeability *in vitro*. MIP22 is a C-terminal truncated product of MIP 26 that has reduced gating properties and increases in proportion to MIP26 in older tissue.

MP70 is a connexin (Cx50) that is a major constituent of lens-fibre gap junctions. It is abundant in the outer cortex whereas its cleavage product, MP38, is abundant in the nucleus. MP17 proteins are specific to lens-fibre cells and are exclusively found in thick junctions. This protein binds calmodulin and is a substrate for cAMP-dependent protein kinase and protein kinase C. The EDTA-extractable proteins include calpactin I, endonexin II, and a homologue of endonexin I. These are a group of proteins of approximately 32 to 35 kDa that are glycosylated and contain phosphotyrosine residues. Binding to the membrane is coordinated through calcium ions and probably involves phospholipids.

Cytoskeletal proteins

The cytoskeleton consists of several networks including microtubules, actin-containing microfilaments, vimentin intermediate filaments, and the beaded intermediate filaments. Components of the cytoskeleton are predominantly found in the outer cortex and sometimes in the epithelial cells but are largely absent from the inner cortex and nucleus.

Intermediate-sized filaments appear to be attached both to the plasma membrane and to actin filaments. Actin, vimentin, and spectrin are all identified in human superficial fibre cells and are lost from deeper cortical regions and the nucleus. Vimentin-type intermediate filaments are found both in the intact lens and in cultured cells. Actin filaments were arranged in polygonal arrays in human lens epithelial cells from 25- to 94-year-old individuals. Plectin is a component of the bovine cytoskeleton that associates with vimentin and is found in both the lens epithelium and cortex.

The beaded filament is a cytoskeletal structure that is unique to the lens-fibre cells. CP49 (phakinin) and filensin are the major components of this structure and are found throughout the lens. *In vitro* the formation of beaded filaments requires the presence of α-crystallin, which might also form the beads *in vivo*. Many membrane and cytoskeletal components can be phosphorylated. Phosphorylation of the CP49 polypeptide of beaded filaments and vimentin was increased by adrenergic agents and this led to a redistribution of CP49 from the cytoplasm to the membrane.

Protein 4.1 is closely associated with the plasma membrane. It binds to lens spectrin and can also bind actin and tubulin. The proportion of protein 4.1 increases after fibre differentiation. Many components of the lens cytoskeleton are homologues of components of the erythrocyte cytoskeleton. These include the membrane-anchoring components of band 3 and ankyrin, as well as spectrin, actin, and protein 4. 1. αA has also been identified as a cytoskeletal protein that specifically binds to the lens plasma membrane and α-crystallin has been shown to associate with actin. It has been suggested that the phosphorylation of α-crystallin may be involved in the assembly of actin/tubulin.

Cataract

Many of the changes that occur within the human lens with age are exacerbated with the onset of cataract. Such changes are also prominent in experimental cataract. The reducing potential of the lens is affected as the concentrations of reduced glutathione and some enzymes of glutathione metabolism are lowered. Concentrations of the antioxidant enzymes catalase and superoxide dismutase are also lowered, as is that of ascorbate. The net effect of these changes contributes towards the increasing oxidation that occurs within the lens. Some investigators have found increased malondialdehyde in nuclear and cortical cataract in the thiobarbituric assay but this method is not, in fact, completely specific for malondialdehyde. An increase in cross-linked proteins and mixed disulphides also occurs, which manifests itself as a decrease in the soluble lens-protein fraction, an increase in the insoluble fraction, and a disruption of the integrity of the lens membranes. The concentrations of enzymes of carbohydrate metabolism are decreased in cataract. Concentrations of nucleotides, including ATP, ADP, and GTP, were decreased in all regions of the lens in some human cataracts.

The ionic balance in the human lens is also compromised with the onset of cataract. A dramatic increase in calcium and a significant increase in sodium ions has been detected. Such changes suggest that the active transport processes of the lens have been altered and indeed Na, K-ATPase activity is reduced in cataract lenses. There is also a net increase in free, but not total, water.

Many risk factors for cataract have been identified. These include diabetes, myopia, glaucoma, glucocorticoid therapy, renal failure, and severe diarrhoea. Diabetic lenses have markedly increased amounts of sugars and sugar phosphates. This is paralleled by an increase in glycated lens proteins. The changes noted above are also seen. Glucocorticoid–protein adducts were found in the lenses of patients that had undergone glucocorticoid therapy. Such modifications disrupt protein structure. These changes implicate post-translational modifications in the progression of a majority of human cataracts, but whether they have a causative role remains to be confirmed. A speculative scheme for some of the pathways leading to human cataract is shown in Fig. 3.

It remains to be elucidated which of the aforementioned changes is the initial causative factor for cataract, although animal models such as the diabetic rat and rabbit have shown that a decrease in glutathione, amino acid metabolism, and inositol alongside an increase in sugar are early changes. A drop

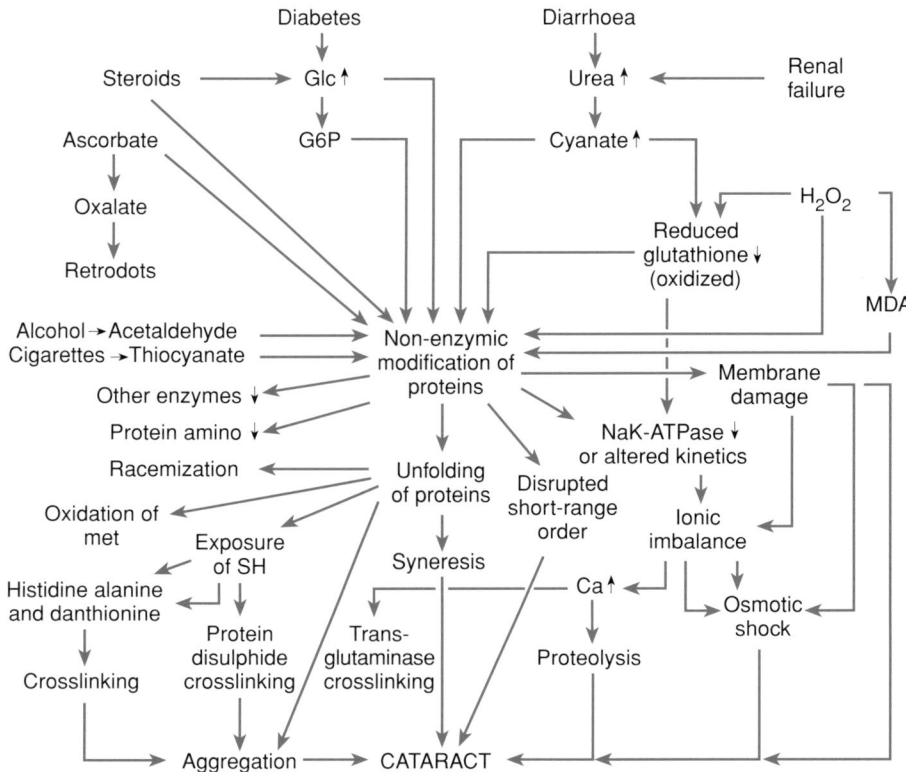

Fig. 3 Possible common pathways in human cataract. G6P, glucose 6-phosphate; MDA, malondialdehyde [flow diagram from Harding (1991) by permission of Chapman & Hall, London].

in NADPH is also seen. Protein thiols are lost, and NADH and sorbitol increase. Concentrations of glucose 6-phosphate dehydrogenase and 6-phosphogluconate dehydrogenase decrease, resulting in a reduction in energy metabolized via the pentose-phosphate pathway and therefore of NADPH. The concentration of ATP decreases, while the glycation and disulphide cross-linking of lens proteins gradually increase. These changes occur before the first opacities are detected and precede the loss of ionic control of the lens.

Similar changes are seen in other experimental cataracts including the X-ray cataract, which has been studied extensively. In human cataract it is difficult to identify early changes but in the slow cataractogenic process, the protein changes seem to be of central importance.

Further reading

Alcala, J. and Maisel, H. (1985). Biochemistry of lens plasma membranes and cytoskeleton. In *The ocular lens: structure, function and pathology* (ed. H. Maisel), pp. 169–222. Dekker, New York.

Bloemendal, H. (1985). Lens research: from protein to gene. *Experimental Eye Research*, **41**, 429–48.

Cheng, H. M. and Chylack, L. T. (1985). Lens metabolism. In *The ocular lens: structure, function and pathology* (ed. H. Maisel), pp. 223–64. Dekker, New York.

Chepelinsky, A. B. *et al.* (1991). Lens protein gene expression: α–crystallins and MIP. *Lens and Eye Toxicology Research*, **8**, 319–44.

Crabbe, M. J. C., Jordan, R. M., Ting, H. H., and Hoe, S. T. (1986). Bovine lens aldehyde dehydrogenase: activity and non-linear steady state kinetics. *Experimental Eye Research*, **43**, 177–84.

David, L. L. and Shearer, T. R. (1989). Role of proteolysis in lenses: a review. *Lens and Eye Toxicology Research*, **6**, 725–47.

de Jong, W. W., Lubsen, N. H., and Kraft, H. J. (1994). Molecular evolution of the eye. *Progress in Retinal Eye Research*, **13**, 392–442.

Dirks, R. P., Klok, E. J., van Genesen, S. T., Schoenmakers, J. G., and Lubsen, N. H. (1996). The sequence of regulatory events controlling the expression of the gamma d-crystallin gene during fibroblast growth factor-mediated rat lens fiber cell differentiation. *Developmental Biology*, **173**, 14–25.

Duncan, G. (1994). Calcium, cell signalling and cataract. *Progress in Retinal Eye Research*, **13**, 623–52.

Duncan, G. and Jacob, T. J. C. (1984). The lens as a physicochemical system. In *The eye*, Vol IB (ed. H. Davson), pp. 159–206. Academic, London.

Gopal-Srivastava, R., Haynes, J. I., and Piatigorsky, J. (1995). Regulation of the murine alpha B-crystallin/small heat shock protein gene in cardiac muscle. *Molecular Cell Biology*, **15**, 7081–90.

Goring, D. R., Bryce, D. M., Tsui, L. C., Breitman, M. L., and Liu, Q. (1993). Developmental regulation of cell type-specific expression of the murine γF gene is mediated through a lens specific element containing the γF-1 binding site. *Developmental Dynamics*, **196**, 143–52.

Hales, A. M., Chamberlain, C. G., and McAvoy, J. W. . (1995). Cataract induction in lenses cultured with transforming growth factor-beta. *Investigative Ophthalmology and Visual Science*, **36**, 1709–13.

Harding, J. J. (1997). The lens. In *Biochemistry of the eye* (ed.Harding, J.J.). Chapman and Hall, London.

Harding, J. J. (1991). *Cataract, biochemistry, epidemiology and pharmacology*. Chapman and Hall, London.

Harding, J. J. and Crabbe, M. J.C. (1984). The lens: development, proteins, metabolism and cataract. In *The eye*, Vol IB (ed. H. Davson), pp. 207–492. Academic, London.

Jaffe, N. S. and Horwitz, J. (1992). *Lens and cataract* (ed. S. M. Podos and M. Yanoff). Gower Medical, London.

Kamachi, Y., Sockanathan, S., Liu, Q., Breitman, M., Lovell Badge, R., and Kondoh, H. (1995). Involvement of SOX proteins in lens-specific activation of crystallin genes. *EMBO Journal*, **14**, 3510–19.

Kistler, J. and Bullivant, S. (1989). Structure and molecular biology of lens membranes. *CRC Critical Reviews of Biochemistry and Molecular Biology*, **24**, 151–81.

Kobayashi, R., Nakayama, R., Ohta, A., Sakai, F., Sakuragi, S., and Tashima, Y. (1990). Identification of the 32 kDa component of bovine lens EDTA extractable protein as endonexins I and II. *Biochemical Journal*, **266**, 505–11.

Kuszak, J. R. (1995). Development of lens sutures. *Progress in Retinal Eye Research*, **14**, 567–91.

Lubsen, N. H., Aarts, H. J. M., and Schoemakers, J. G. G. (1988). The evolution of lenticular proteins: the β and γ-crystallin super gene family. *Progress in Biophysics and Molecular Biology*, **51**, 47–76.

Piatigorsky, J. and Wistow, G. J. (1989). Enzymes/crystallins: gene sharing as an evolutionary strategy. *Cell*, **57**, 197–9.

Rae, J. L. and Mathias, R. T. (1985). The physiology of the lens. In *The ocular lens: structure, function and pathology* (ed. H. Maisel), pp. 93–121. Dekker, New York.

Rafferty, N. S. (1985). Lens morphology. In *The ocular lens: structure, function and pathology* (ed. H. Maisel), pp.1–60. Dekker, New York.

Reddy, V. N. (1990). Glutathione and its function in the lens—an overview. *Experimental Eye Research*, **50**, 771–8.

Richardson, N. A., McAvoy, J. W., and Chamberlain, C. G. (1992). Age of rats affects response of lens epithelial explants to fibroblast growth factor. *Experimental Eye Research*, **55**, 649–56.

Sax, C. M., Ilagan, J. G., and Haynes, J. I. (1996). Lens preferred activity of the –18091/+46 mouse αA-crystallin promoter in stably integrated chromatin. *Biochimica Biophysica Acta*, **1305**, 49–53.

Slingsby, C. (1985). Structural variation in lens crystallins. *Trends in Biochemical Sciences*, **10**, 281–4.

Spector, A. (1985). Aspects of the biochemistry of cataract. In *The ocular lens, structure, function and pathology* (ed. H. Maisel), pp. 405–38. Dekker, New York.

Vrensen, G. F. (1995). Ageing of the human lens—a morphological point of view. *Comparative Biochemistry and Physiology. A. Physiology*, **111**, 519–32.

Wagner, B. J. and Margolis, J. W. (1995). Age dependent association of isolated bovine lens multicatalytic proteinase complex (proteasome) with heat shock protein, an endogenous inhibitor. *Archives of Biochemistry and Biophysics*, **323**, 455–62.

Wannemacher, C. F. and Spector, A. (1968). Protein synthesis in the core of the calf lens. *Experimental Eye Research*, **7**, 623–5.

Wistow, G. J. and Piatigorsky, J. (1988). Lens crystallins: the evolution and expression of proteins for a highly specialised tissue. *Annual Review of Biochemistry*, **57**, 479–504.

Wolfe, J. K., Gillis, M. K., and Chylack, L. T. (1985). Glucose metabolism in the calf lens. *Experimental Eye Research*, **40**, 629–41.

2.7.3 Physical aspects of lens clarity and image degradation

John M. Sparrow and N. Andrew Frost

The primary function of the crystalline lens is participation in the process of assembling incoming light to form a sharp retinal image of the visual environment. Several distinct physical mechanisms can be held responsible for imperfections of retinal image formation.

Light scatter

A number of physical mechanisms can result in light scatter. Mie scatter is produced by relatively larger particles and results in a redirection of scattered photons through multiple angles. Rayleigh scatter is produced by small particles (e.g. in the atmosphere). The criteria for Mie scattering of light in a transmitting medium are met when there exist short-range fluctuations in refractive index. The relevant spatial dimension for particles that can cause Mie scattering relates to the wavelength of the scattered light. For visible wavelengths (400–600 nm) the lower limit for particle size is around 30 to 50 nm and the upper limit around 5 to 10 μm. In the normal crystalline lens, special anatomical and physiological features ensure that there are few opportunities for this type of scatter. These include:

- Narrow fibre membranes: the width of secondary lens-fibre membranes is small and fibre membranes therefore offer little opportunity for scatter.

- Small interfibre spaces: the extracellular compartment of the lens is less than 1 per cent of the volume of the lens.

- High concentration of structural lens proteins (crystallins): adjacent protein molecules are tightly packed with little space between protein molecules and hence an absence of scatter.

- Terminal differentiation of secondary lens fibres with degeneration of the cell nucleus and other potentially scattering intracellular organelles in mature fibres.

- Where there are variations in refractive index these occur across regularly curved zonal boundaries.

In the normal lens, light scatter increases with age (Fig. 1). This increase in scatter is observed locally within various parts of the lens, but in addition, because the lens continues to grow

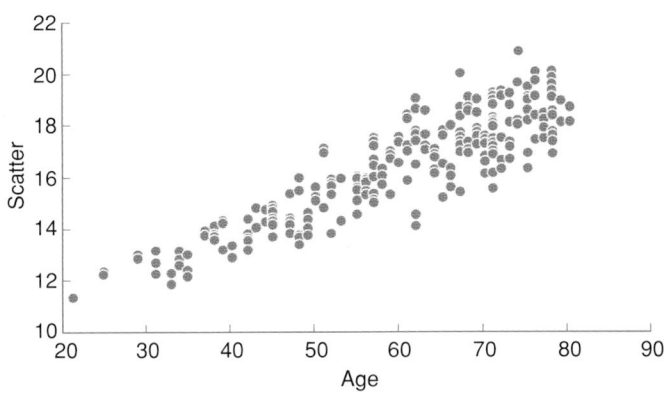

Fig. 1 Central nuclear scatter measured in arbitrary units using Scheimpflug slit-beam photography.

throughout life, its increasing bulk means that the overall increase in scatter for the lens as a whole is considerable. Within the lens nucleus the physiological increase in scatter with increasing age may gradually and imperceptibly merge into the pathological scatter of nuclear cataract. (The earliest sign of nuclear cataract may be a myopic shift. This global rise in the refractive index of the nucleus may herald subsequent visually significant changes that accompany the development of true nuclear cataract.) Nuclear scattering cataract is believed to result from cumulative damage to the long-lived structural lens proteins, the crystallins. Damage to individual protein molecules results in alterations to their surface charge and subsequent unfolding of the tertiary protein structure. Reactive chemical groups normally buried within the tertiary structure become exposed and adjacent unfolded molecules become covalently linked, with a gradual building up of macromolecular complexes. (Interestingly, α-crystallin has a dual role in the lens: not only does it function as a structural lens protein, but it also plays a protective role as a heat-shock protein, limiting damage to and denaturation of the other crystallins.) Once the macromolecular complexes reach appropriate dimensions, short-range fluctuations in refractive index exist, with variations between the macromolecules themselves and the intervening water spaces. Macromolecules thus cause scattering through multiple angles, which results in a veiling luminance being cast over the retina, a reduction of retinal image contrast, and a decrease in the 'signal to noise ratio'. Criteria for Mie scatter are met and typically this manifests as a diffuse increase in the scattering properties of the lens nucleus. Pathological light scatter can occur not only in the lens nucleus: scatter is frequently observed in cortical and (posterior) subcapsular cataracts.

In the normal eye there is small-angle scatter about the direction of the refracted ray. If a localized point-source of light is present in the visual field, a point image on the retina will not be formed. The incident light will spread out on to adjacent retina, the distribution of this light being described by the 'point-spread function'. The point-spread function has a high peak at 0° (the forward direction) and declines rapidly with increasing angle.

Chaotic refraction

Degradation of the retinal image may also occur as a result of 'chaotic refraction' or 'irregular astigmatism'. This occurs when light is refracted in a haphazard manner, being bent within the confines of Snell's law. Chaotic refraction typically occurs in the lens in the presence of a vacuolated posterior subcapsular cataract. The irregular surfaces of the vacuoles refract the light in a chaotic manner and thus break up the image. Although the two frequently coexist in the lens, in a physical sense chaotic refraction is quite distinct from light scatter and these mechanisms should not be confused. Mie-scattered light originates from a scattering point and the direction of a Mie-scattered ray is through any angle. In chaotic refraction the behaviour of an individual ray of light is predetermined and its path depends on the fine morphological detail of the irregularly refracting

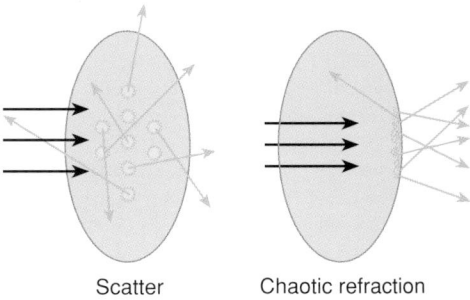

Fig. 2 Random' reorientation of light by Mie scatter (macromolecular protein aggregation with short-range fluctuation in refractive index) and chaotic refraction due to optical imperfections as typically observed in a vacuolated posterior subcapsular cataract (redirection of light within the confines of Snell's law).

interface and the refractive indices on either side of the interface (both mechanisms are illustrated in Fig. 2). The term 'forward scatter' has sometimes been used to describe this phenomenon, but this term does not help to differentiate between 'random' Mie scatter, small-angle scatter, and chaotic refraction. Other imperfections in the refractive capacity of the lens include spherical and chromatic aberrations, each of which will widen the point-spread function.

Diffraction

Diffraction occurs when a portion of the wave front is eliminated by traversing an opaque edge. Thus visual disturbance can be produced by the lens-fibre architecture; an example of this is the well-known entoptic lens halo. Diffraction may occur at the boundaries of discrete lens opacities, but the contribution of this effect to image degradation in cataract is uncertain.

Fluorescence

Fluorescence occurs when an 'unexcited' molecule absorbs a photon (which raises an electron to a higher energy level) and subsequently re-emits a fluorescent photon at a longer wavelength (Fig. 3). Flurophores exist in the human lens and the intensity of lens fluorescence increases with age. Fluorescence of the lens has been observed at a number of different combinations of excitation and emission wavelengths, for example ultraviolet/blue, blue/green, orange/red. The direction of emitted fluorescent photons is entirely random and these emitted photons represent a source of spectrally restricted stray light in the eye.

Absorption due to nuclear pigmentation (brunescence)

As part of the normal ageing process, pigmentation of the lens occurs. In extreme cases the lens nucleus may become heavily pigmented and this is usually observed in association with nuclear cataract (Fig. 4). In slit-beam illumination, pigmentation of the nucleus gives the appearance of an increasing intensity

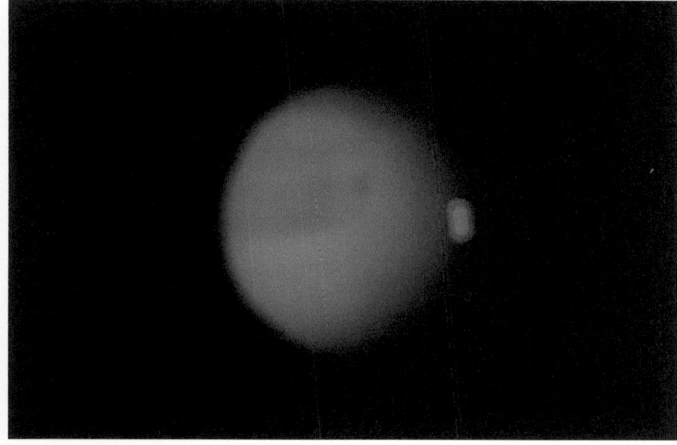

Fig. 3 Blue–green fluorescence of the lens as observed at the slit lamp.

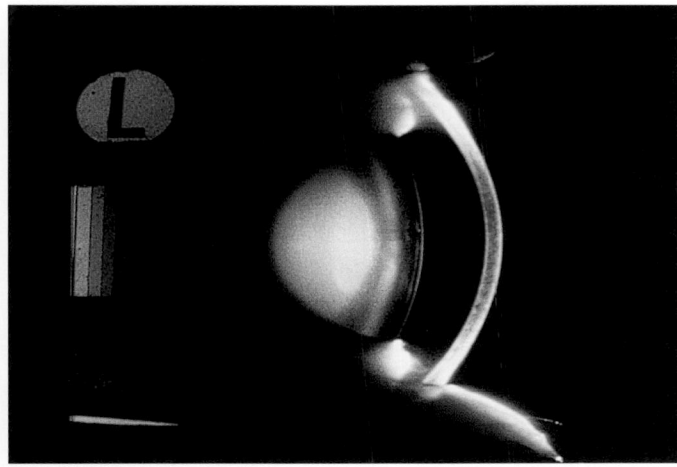

Fig. 4 Nuclear brunescence with pigmentation seen typically in association with scattering nuclear cataract.

of pigment with increased depth within the lens. This appearance is artefactual and is due to the fact that the pigmented nucleus is behaving as a spectrally selective 'thick' filter; thus the greater the light path through the nucleus (once in and once back out to the observer), the greater the opportunity for spectrally selective absorption, and the greater the apparent colour change. Colour vision may be disturbed by spectrally selective absorption and, in extreme examples, absorption of light by pigmented species may cause a noticeable reduction in light transmission. An effect of lens pigment on the results of blue–yellow perimetry has been recognized.

Summary

Image degradation from lens changes can result from a number of different physical mechanisms. 'Random' stray light within the eye produces a 'veiling luminance' with a reduction in the 'signal to noise ratio', and chaotic refraction of light from abnormal refractive interfaces contributes to image break-up.

Further reading

Benedek, G. B. (1971). Theory of transparency of the eye. *Applied Optics*, **10**, 459–73.

Benedek, G. B. (1984). The molecular basis of cataract formation. In *Human cataract formation* (CIBA Foundation Symposium 106) (ed. J. Nugent and J. P. Whelan), pp. 237–47.

Philipson, B. T. and Fagerholm, P. P. (1973). Lens changes responsible for increased light scattering in some types of senile cataract. In *The human lens in relation to cataract* (CIBA Foundation Symposium 19) (ed. K. Elliot and D. W. Fitzsimons), pp. 45–63. Elsevier, Amsterdam, London, New York.

Siew, E. L., Opalecky, D., and Bettelheim, F. A. (1981). Light scattering of normal human lens. II. Age dependence of the light scattering parameters. *Experimental Eye Research*, **33**, 603–14.

Sparrow, J. M., Bron, A. J., Brown, N. A. P., and Neil, H. A. W. (1992). Auto-fluorescence of the crystalline lens in early and late onset diabetes. *British Journal of Ophthalmology*, **76**, 25–31.

Trokel, S. (1962). The physical basis for transparency of the crystalline lens. *Investigative Ophthalmology*, **1**, 493–501.

2.7.4 Ageing changes in the lens

Robert A. Weale

The lens occupies a representative place both in the evolutionary scheme of mammals and in the pattern of human senescence. For example, Tréton and Courtois have demonstrated a significant correlation between the growth time of (mammalian) lenses and the lifespan of their owners.

Growth of the lens

This subject needs to be considered because the growing diameter of the lens has long been held to play a role in the decline of the accommodative amplitude or presbyopia. This is the term used for the progressive diminution in the capacity of the lens to adjust its focus to the distance of the external object which it helps to image on the retina.

The embryonic development of the human eye can be described by logarithmic growth curves, as is true of the corneal diameter, and the transverse lenticular diameter: linearity with log age is observed well into infancy.

The lens grows overall throughout life, but does not, as it were, inflate keeping a constant shape: its sagittal thickness exhibits a greater percentage increase than its transverse diameter. Consequently, the curvature mainly of the anterior surface steepens, increasing the power of the lens. The fact that we do not as a result become normally myopic in old age is due to a change in the gradient of the internal refractive index of the lens which counteracts this by a mechanism as yet unknown.

Lens growth is achieved by cell division in the pre-equatorial anterior lenticular epithelium: the originally tubby cylindrical cells elongate, forming fibres which stretch from suture to suture, which are normal radial discontinuities in the lens matrix formed by the terminations of the fibres. Tréton and Courtois believe that the completion of this process can be deduced for various species from the shape of the growth curve of the lens. It is more likely that it is determined by age-related changes in the pattern of tensile forces in the zonule. This tissue holds the lens in place and attaches it to the ciliary muscle controlling the shape of the lens (see below). At the same time, the similarity of the growth curves for a number of mammalian species, including the human, is consistent with Tréton and Courtois view that a given set of genes is involved in the growth of the lens in the absence of any significant evolutionary influence. It is unlikely that this useful generalization can be extended to the phenomenon of accommodation, which appears to be linked to the evolution of manual dexterity.

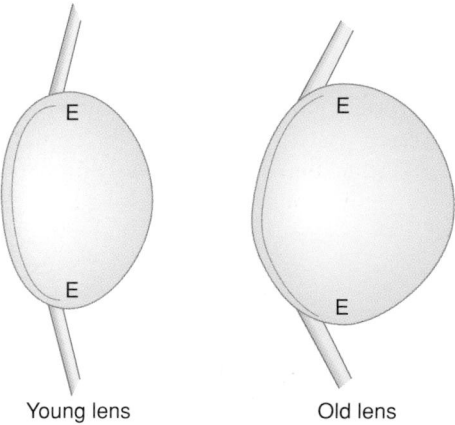

Young lens   Old lens

Fig. 1 Schematic representation of the age-related variation of effective zonular tension and its potential influence on lens shape (not to scale). (By courtesy of Pierscionek and Weale 1995*b*.)

Presbyopia

The above-mentioned ciliary muscle controls not accommodation, as is frequently surmised, but its relaxation. This follows from the fact that the excised lens assumes its accommodated form; indeed, the curvature of its surfaces steepens even more when it is decapsulated, which proves that both the lens matrix and its containing capsule are elastic. Consequently, the suspension of the lens in the eye flattens it, and only when the muscle relaxes its force, thereby moving inward and forward, do the elastic forces of the lens permit it to steepen the curvature predominantly of the anterior surface.

Fisher's painstaking studies of the mechanical properties of the lens showed that they play a dominant role in the development of presbyopia. He demonstrated that both the capsule and the lens matrix were elastic. In the case of the capsule, Young's modulus, a measure of elasticity, decreases with age. The reverse is true of the lens matrix: as time goes on, the lens shape changes progressively less readily. However, the age-related variation of these properties does not completely explain the measured changes in accommodative amplitude, and this may have several causes.

Fisher showed that the shape of the lens plays a crucial role: the more nearly spherical the lens the more energy is needed for its shape to change. We noted in the previous section that ageing is accompanied by a steepening of the curvature of the lens surfaces, which is in keeping with this observation.

The equatorial growth of the lens probably plays only a subsidiary role in the progress of presbyopia even though it must patently lead to a reduction in zonular tension. The iris prevents the reliable measurement of the equatorial lenticular diameter *in vivo* for any accommodative state, let alone for its variation with age. Pierscionek and Augusteyn have shown that, even *in vitro*, it varies much more than expected. At present, the only way of estimating the magnitude of the *in vivo* diameter is by the use of the sagittal (i.e. anteroposterior) thickness, and by making simplifying assumptions about the geometrical shape of the lenticular surfaces. An estimate of the change of sagittal thickness with accommodation is also

required. If all factors other than equatorial diameter remain constant, equatorial growth, between the ages of 20 and 60 years, is unlikely to account for more than about 1 dioptre loss in accommodation owing to the resultant drop in zonular tension. Therefore other factors must be more important.

For example, Farnsworth and Shyne observed an age-related shift of the proximal zonular attachments at the anterior lens face. The epithelial layer remains constant since the positions of the proximal zonular attachments do not change relatively to the anterior pole and remain close to the edge of the epithelial layer. Lens growth results from the differentiation of the epithelial cells and their migration towards the equatorial region. If the distance moved by the migrating epithelial cells before differentiating into fibres is assumed constant—there is no evidence that the epithelial layer increases in area with age—then the position at which fibre cell elongation begins moves forward. This causes an apparently anterior shift of the zonular attachments. In the unaccommodated state, an increased bending moment is therefore applied to the anterior face of the lens, and zonular tension is less reduced in accommodation. Therefore the component of zonular tension keeping the lens flat is reduced, but, at the same time, the anterior surface curvature increased (Fig. 1): both factors impede the older lens from accommodating when the ciliary muscle is activated.

Several observations support this view. First, as mentioned above, the anterior curvature has been found to become more curved with age both *in vivo* and, generally, *in vitro*. The *in vivo* result may follow from the constancy of zonular elasticity with age, and of the ligamental length. Secondly, the anterior capsular face is thicker and stronger and more elastic than the inactive posterior one.

Furthermore, changes in the iris sphincter may affect the action of the physiologically relatively stable ciliary muscle. Miosis assists the accommodative increase in lens curvature. Age-related miosis pulls at the iris root: this is transmitted to the ciliary tissue causing a centripetal migration of the distal zonular anchors. Since the ligamental length remains constant, capsular tension is reduced, and lenticular curvature increased with age. This is consistent with presbyopia occurring earlier in regions where sunlight is intense and hence pupil sizes are smaller, although the effects of higher temperatures on both pupil size and accommodation cannot be ruled out.

The age-related loss of accommodative amplitude occurs faster than any other function, and this is probably due to a multifactorial system of not exclusively senescent features. The following may be relevant.

1. The above changes in the mechanical properties of the lens

2. The changes contingent on the pattern of cellular synthesis and differentiation

3. The constancy of proximal and ciliary zonular insertions, and of their elastic properties

4. Pupillary miosis and its effect on accommodation.

Factors 2 and 3 are unconnected with ageing, which may explain why the accommodative amplitude does not decline typically more slowly. Everything conspires to reduce it with advancing years. Presbyopia does not appear to be a phenomenon of genetically determined ageing, and should be viewed as an interactive consequence of growth, tissue constancy, and ageing—perhaps because accommodation is an evolutionary after-thought.

Coloration

Lenticular yellowing, confined largely to the nucleus, stems from at least two pigments. One is linked to 3-hydroxykynurenine from birth. Its absorbance (maximal at 360 nm in ultraviolet A) tends to rise throughout life. Another chromophore, absorbs maximally at approximately 470 nm, and accumulates after birth, at a rate greater than the former. The log of their absorbance rises linearly with age, which explains why, in the first decade or two, the rise may appear to be non-existent.

The cause of the yellowing has been subject to speculation. Some view it as an adaptive mechanism which has evolved for the retina to be protected from photic insults.

To a Darwinian such a view would appear to be specious, because the retina might well be in need of protection when it is young, and the individual is at the peak of his or her reproductive powers: the yellowing in advanced years might smack of bolting the stable-door after the horse has bolted. That said, it has been found recently in an epidemiological study that the prevalence of age-related maculopathies is reduced amongst those who have been protected from ultraviolet A during the second half of their lives.

There is, indeed, some evidence to suggest that lenticular yellowing may be due to the exposure of the lens to light, notably ultraviolet A radiation. For example the lenses of young Egyptians are darker and yellower than those of coeval Britons; and the average annual irradiation in Egypt is significantly greater than in the United Kingdom. Several authors have irradiated excised human and animal lenses with intense ultraviolet A radiation, and succeeded in demonstrating an increase in absorbance. Such experiments, however, raise the following unanswered questions:

1. Are the results reversible? That is to say, does the absorbance drop when the lenses are put in the dark?

2. Are the results meaningful? For example, if the laboratory irradiation is so high that, if maintained for a few weeks, the absorbance would rise to such an extent as to render the eye blind, it is quite unlikely that the conditions of the experiment replicate physiological conditions.

3. Are repair processes maintained *in vitro*?

The absence of answers to these important questions has led to ingenious studies attempting to provide direct answers. Thus Girgus *et al.* made use of the fact that yellowing of the lens should affect colour vision in general, and the way colours are matched with mixtures of constant spectral stimuli in particular. The idea is that a lens with a young eye will match, say, a field of blue–green light with measurable amounts of a mixture of blue, green, and red light. An older eye needs more of the blue matching stimulus, because more of it is absorbed in the lens in transit to the retina. Girgus *et al.* estimated from answers to questionnaires the cumulative numbers of hours of ultraviolet exposure for each subject, allowing for the absorption by correcting lenses, the time they were worn, and so on. They found no correlation between ultraviolet exposure and lenticular yellowing. The result is not conclusive, however, because the light used had a wavelength of approximately 490 nm, which is not optimal for detecting the effect. Moreover, age was 'held relatively constant', but its potential effect was not controlled.

Fluorescence

This is the term used for the phenomenon which occurs when a chromophore is excited with a quantum usually of a short wavelength, as a result of which one of its electrons is raised to a higher excitation level, and then drops back to its unexcited level while emitting a quantum of a longer wavelength.

Depending on the chromophores involved, lenticular fluorescence is divided into two types, tryptophan and nontryptophan fluorescence. A number of authors have used nontryptophan fluorescence for *in vivo* estimates of human lens transmittance, which may help in the understanding of lenticular yellowing. In such experiments, a short-wavelength exciting pencil of radiation enters the eye as far as possible from the bundle of emergent fluorescent rays. The resulting (longer-wavelength) fluorescence intensity is measured approximately perpendicularly to the entering (exciting) light beam. Traversing the nucleus, the exciting beam is weakened, causing less fluorescence. Since the fluorescent beam has to emerge from the lenticular interior, it too suffers absorption. However, because its wavelength is longer than that of the exciting beam, the fractional loss in intensity is correspondingly smaller.

The technique enables one to build up a fluorescence profile for any given lens: in general this is characterized by two peaks

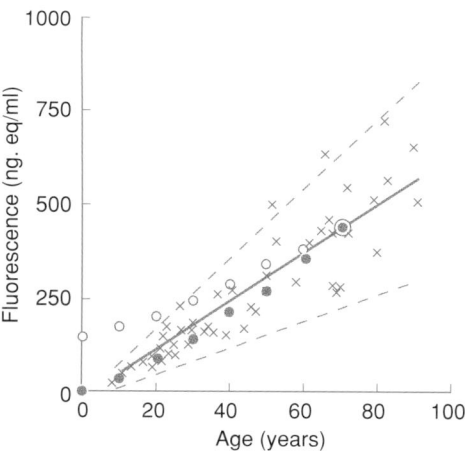

Fig. 2 The age-related variation of human lenticular fluorescence (ng fluorescein/ml; data from Bleeker *et al.* 1986); plots for a constant conversion efficiency of exciting into emitted radiation (open circles); and for one increasing with age (filled circles).

separated by a saddle. The anterior peak is higher than the posterior one, presumably owing to the accentuated absorption suffered by the latter. On the assumption that Beer's and Lambert's laws apply to the lens, Zeimer and Noth have shown that the ratio of the amplitudes of the two peaks provides a measure of lenticular transmissivity. It can be shown that, though the peaks are due to the fluorescent radiation that is emitted, the measurement is, in fact, determined by the wavelength of the exciting radiation.

Bleeker *et al.* determined fluorescence as a function of age. While the difficult problem of contamination of the measuring beam by the exciting beam cannot be entirely ruled out from their study, their measure of the anterior peak leaves little doubt but that fluorescence rises systematically with age (Fig. 2). It has recently been shown that this can be explained in terms of changes in lenticular transmittance if an important assumption is made. This relates to the efficiency with which an exciting radiation leads to emission. If it is assumed to be constant throughout life, the observations would be expected to agree with the course of the empty circles. If, however, the efficiency increases with age somewhat less than exponentially, the data would be expected to agree with the filled circles as, in fact, they do. Bleeker *et al.* are of the opinion that the increase in fluorescence results from the lenticular exposure to light, whence one would conclude that this will also be true of coloration (for effects on vision see Van den Berg 1993).

This view is supported by Lerman's study showing the variation with age in two widely different locations, namely in Oregon and Atlanta. The function giving fluorescence as a function of age for Atlanta was significantly raised with respect to the one for Oregon by amounts, explicable in terms of the relative average annual light intensities in the two cities.

Diabetes

Lerman's important data are, however, potentially vitiated by the fact that no information is given on the number of diabetics,

if any, in the sample population. This would have been important because both Zeimer and Noth and van Best *et al.* have shown that, in diabetic patients, lenticular fluorescence is enhanced in proportion to the duration of the disease. It is almost certain that this cannot be the result of an increased rate of accumulation of the pigment(s) thought to accumulate in the normally ageing lens, but the relatively simple task of determining a few spectral characteristics of the fluorophor associated with diabetes does not seem to have been undertaken so far.

Fluorescence, age, and cataract

Lerman and Borkman have shown that the nucleus fluoresces up to three times more in the cataractous than the coeval normal lens. This becomes understandable on the basis of the ideas put forward above and an additional circumstance.

An increase in fluorescence is associated with the post-translational unfolding of lenticular proteins. If visible or near ultraviolet A radiation can promote the unfolding of lenticular proteins, it is not surprising that they should become more vulnerable to hazards with advancing years. But we can see that Fig. 2 is consistent with an age-related increase in the efficiency with which fluorescent radiation is produced, presumably because the above-mentioned unfolding of proteins facilitates the absorption of, and action by, the exciting quanta.

The increase in fluorescence observed in nuclear, but not cortical, cataract is consistent with the notion that an abnormal unfolding of protein molecules is involved. Hence the tendency for nuclear cataractogenesis would not be due directly to the absorption of radiation, as has often be postulated. The first normal, non-pathological step is molecular unfolding which renders the molecule more sensitive to noxious stimuli. On this view short wavelength radiation may be perceived as a catalyst rather than as an immediate cause of nuclear cataractogenesis.

Further reading

Bito, L.Z., Davson, H., and Snider, N. (1965). The effects of autonomic drugs on mitosis and DNA synthesis in the lens epithelium and on the composition of the aqueous humour. *Experimental Eye Research*, **4**, 64–71.

Bleeker, J.C., van Best, J.A., Vrij, L., van der Velde, E.A., and Oosterhuis, J.A. (1986). Autofluorescence of the lens in diabetic and healthy subjects by fluorophotometry. *Investigative Ophthalmology and Visual Science*, **27**, 791–4.

Collins, W.J. (1906). The crystalline lens in health and in cataract. *Annals of Ophthalmology*, **15**, 39–58.

Farnsworth, P.N. and Shyne, S.E. (1979). Anterior zonular shifts with age. *Experimental Eye Research*, **28**, 291–7.

Fisher, R.F. (1969). Elastic constants of the human lens capsule. *Journal of Physiology*, **201**, 1–19.

Fisher, R.F. (1982). The vitreous and lens in accommodation. *Transactions of the Ophthalmological Society UK*, **102**, 318–22.

Girgus, J.S., Coren, S., and Porac, C. (1977). Independence of *in vivo* human lens pigment from ultraviolet light ecxposure. *Vision Research*, 17, 749–50.

Grover, D. and Zigman, S. (1972). Coloration of human lenses by near ultra-violet photo-oxidized tryptophan. *Experimental Eye Research*, **13**, 70–6.

Lerman, S. (1988). Human lens fluorescence aging index. *Lens Research*, **5**, 23–31.

Lerman, S. and Borkman, R. (1978). Ultraviolet radiation in the aging and cataractous lens. *Acta Ophthalmologica*, **56**, 139–49.

Liang, J.N. (1987). Fluorescence study of the effects of aging and diabetes mellitus on human lens crystallin. *Current Eye Research*, **6**, 351–5.

Niesel, P., Kräuchi, H., and Bachmann, E. (1976). Der Abspaltungsstreifen in der Spaltlampenphotographie der alternden Linse. *Graefes Archiv für Klinische Experimentelle Ophthalmologie*, **199**, 11–20.

Occhipinti, J.R., Mosier, M.A., and Burstein, N.L. (1986). Autofluorescence and light transmission in the aging crystalline lens. *Ophthalmologica*, **192**, 203–9.

Pau, H. (1950). Warum beginnt der Permeabilitätskatarakt die Trübung unter der hinteren Kapsel? *Berichte der Deutschen Ophthalmologischen Gesellschaft*, **56**, 240–1.

Pierscionek, B.K. (1995). Variations in refractive index and absorbance of 670 nm light with age and cataract formation in human lenses. *Experimental Eye Research*, **60**, 407–14.

Pierscionek, B.K. and Augusteyn, R.C. (1991). Shapes and dimensions of *in vitro* human lenses. *Clinical Experimental Optometry*, **74**, 223–8.

Pierscionek, B.K. and Weale, R.A. (1995a). The optics of the eye-lens and lenticular senescence. *Documenta Ophthalmologica*, **89**, 329–35.

Pierscionek, B.K. and Weale, R.A. (1995b). Presbyopia—a maverick of human senescence. *Archives of Gerontology and Geriatrics*, **20**, 229–40.

Said, F.S. and Weale, R.A. (1959). The variation with age of the spectral transmissivity of the living human crystalline lens. *Gerontologia*, **3**, 213–31.

Saladin, J.J. and Stark, L. (1975). Presbyopia: new evidence from impedance cyclography supporting the Hess–Gullstrand theory. *Vision Research*, **15**, 537–41.

Swegmark, G. (1969). Studies with impedance cyclography on human accommodation at different ages. *Acta Ophthalmologica*, **47**, 1186–206.

Tréton, J. and Courtois, Y. (1989). Evidence for a relationship between longevity of mammalian species and a lens growth parameter. *Gerontology*, **35**, 88–94.

Van Alphen, G.W.H.M. and Graebel, W.P. (1991). Elasticity of tissues involved in accommodation. *Vision Research*, **31**, 1417–38.

Van Best, J.A., Tjin, A., Tsoi, E.W.S.J., Boot, J.P., and Oosterhuis, J.A. (1985). *In vivo* assessment of lens transmission for blue–green light by autofluorescence measurement. *Ophthalmic Research*, **17**, 90–5.

Van den Berg, T.J.T.P. (1993). Quantal and visual efficiency of fluorescence in the lens of the human eye. *Investigative Ophthalmology and Visual Science*, **34**, 3566–73.

Weale, R.A. (1962). Presbyopia. *British Journal of Ophthalmology*, **46**, 660–8.

Weale, R.A. (1982). *A biography of the eye—development, growth, age*. H.K. Lewis, London.

Weale, R.A. (1987). Age and the transmittance of the human crystalline lens. *Journal of Physiology*, **395**, 577–87.

Weale, R.A. (1992). *The senescence of human vision*, pp. 82–5. Oxford University Press, Oxford.

Weale, R.A. (1995). Why does the human eye age the way it does? *Experimental Eye Research*, **60**, 49–55.

Weale, R.A. (1996). A theoretical link between lenticular absorbance and fluorescence. *Proceedings of the Royal Society, London B*, **263**, 1111–16.

Zeimer, R.C. and Noth, J.M. (1984). A new method of measuring *in vivo* the lens transmittance, and study of lens scatter, fluorescence and transmittance. *Ophthalmic Research*, **26**, 246–55.

2.7.5 Age-related cataract–epidemiology and risk factors

Sheila West

The epidemiology of cataract is relatively straightforward; age-related cataract is ubiquitous in virtually every population and is one of, if not the, leading cause of visual loss and blindness wherever blindness surveys have been carried out. The World Health Organization (WHO) estimates that 16 million people, or close to 50 per cent of blindness worldwide, is attributable to cataract. The majority of these cases, probably 99 per cent according to the WHO, occur in developing countries. The increase in life expectancy, coupled with the population growth in these countries, guarantees that cataract will continue to be a major public health problem into the next century.

From a public health perspective, there are two major issues to be addressed in the prevention of blindness from cataract. First, health management research is needed on how to provide affordable, safe, and effective sight restoration surgery for the present millions with cataractous blindness, and how to plan for the future increase in demand. The second issue is the development of strategies to prevent or delay the onset of vision-threatening cataracts. However, in order to design preventive strategies, sound epidemiological investigations are needed that identify the risk and protective factors involved in cataractogenesis. Clearly, cataract is a multifactorial condition with several risk factors, some of which may be more or less important in different populations. This chapter reviews some basic epidemiological characteristics of cataract that may provide insight into these factors, and summarizes some of the known associations with cataractogenesis.

The term 'cataract' has been used in a non-specific manner to indicate loss of lens transparency, usually in the context of vision loss. However, from a research perspective, cataract actually covers a number of lens changes, and these deserve clarification and definition (Table 1). Researchers interested in cataract aetiology focus on factors associated with the earliest lens changes because of the temporal relationship to the onset of cataractogenesis. In addition, because different risk factors seem to be associated with different cataract types, lens opacities are typically classified into morphological types, according to anatomical location. The most common types are nuclear, cortical, posterior subcapsular, and mixed opacities. Precise grading schemes for cataract assessment are described more fully elsewhere. Since many of the systems are similar, the creation of some amalgamation that would permit comparisons across studies would be most desirable. The WHO is currently developing a simplified cataract assessment scheme

Table 1 Definitions of lens changes for epidemiological studies

Lens opacity	Loss of transparency in part or all of the ocular lens, without regard to visual or functional consequences. Typically, lens opacities are classified by anatomical location; nuclear, cortical, or posterior subcapsular primary sclerosing cholangitis
Cataract	Lens opacities accompanied by or capable of causing some level of visual loss, usually measured as acuity loss
Functional cataract	Lens opacities causing visual loss sufficient to produce functional disability

Table 2(a) Prevalence (%) of lens opacities and cataract in studies from the United States

Age (years)	NHANES* Lens opacity	NHANES* Cataract	Framingham† Lens opacity	Framingham† Cataract	Maryland Waterman study‡ Lens opacity	Maryland Waterman study‡ Cataract	Beaver Dam§ Lens opacity	Beaver Dam§ Cataract
30–34	—	—	—	—	2	—	—	—
35–44	—	—	—	—	3	—	—	—
45–54	12	3	—	—	6	3	12	2
55–64	28	10	42	4.5	37	5	38	7
65–74	58	29	73	18	72	25	74	20
75–84	—	—	91	46	94	59	89	43

*Cataract is opacity causing vision loss to 6/7.5 or worse (Leske and Sperduto 1983).
†First age group is 52–64 years; cataract is opacity with accompanying vision loss of 20/30 or worse (Leibowitz *et al.* 1980).
‡Cataract in age group 45–54 years is defined the same as NHANES, thereafter, cataract is defined the same as Framingham (Adamsons *et al.* 1991).
§First age group is 43–54 years; cataract is opacity with vision 20/32 or worse; last age group is 75+ (Klein *et al.* 1992).
NHANES, National Health and National Examination Survey.

Table 2(b) Prevalence of lens opacities and cataract in studies from Nepal and India

Nepal* Age (years)	Nepal* Cataract	India† Age (years)	India† Cataract
30–34	0.2	30–39	0.2
35–44	1	40–49	2
45–54	6	50–59	15
55–64	16	60–69	42
65–74	33	70–79	56
75–84	48	80+	88

*Cataract is both early and late cases, diagnosed with ophthalmoscope, in pupils dilated only in presence of vision less than 6/18 (Brilliant *et al.* 1983).
†Cataract is opacity accompanied by visual loss of 6/18 or worse (Chatterjee *et al.* 1982).

that combines features of several systems, and it should prove useful for field studies.

Prevalence

Comparison of prevalence data from different studies must be done cautiously because there is no standard system for the assessment of lens opacities or cataract. The data from six studies is shown in Table 2(a) and (b). The prevalence of cataract in these studies was based on definitions requiring that the lens opacities be accompanied by or cause a reduction in visual acuity. Depending on the visual acuity criterion used, and the differences in the distribution of cataract type in differing populations, the prevalence may vary substantially but not substantively. The four population surveys from the United States include the Framingham Eye Study, the National Health and Nutrition Examination Survey, the Maryland Waterman Study, and the Beaver Dam Eye Study. For comparison, data from population-based surveys done in the Punjab of India,

and in Nepal are also shown. All but the Beaver Dam Study used clinical examinations to detect lens opacities, and the latter used photographic assessment of the lens.

With these caveats, the similarity of data between the four studies carried out in the United States, and the generally lower rates compared to rates from Nepal and India, are noteworthy. The prevalence rates in Nepal for the oldest age groups do not seem to differ markedly from the rates in the American studies, but the visual acuity criterion was much more severe. A population-based study of the incidence of new blinding cataract over a 4-year period was carried out in India based on clinical examinations in 19 communities. For those aged 65 and older, the incidence of new blinding cataract was estimated at 5.8 per 100 persons per year. In the Maryland Waterman Study, the incidence of any opacity, regardless of the impact on vision, for this age group was not even double that rate: 9.4 per 100 persons per year. The seemingly earlier age of onset, and higher prevalence and incidence of cataract in Asian countries compared to other countries, has been noted before and has provided fruitful grounds for investigations into possible reasons for these differences.

Risk factors

In the last 10 years, a number of solid epidemiological investigations have been carried out to elucidate possible factors that may be related to the onset or progression of cataract. In this chapter, the emphasis is placed on the factors which may be modifiable. Risk factors include smoking, alcohol use, diarrhoea, and sunlight exposure, and protective factors include antioxidants and certain drugs.

Smoking

An association between nuclear opacities, and possibly primary sclerosing cholangitis opacities, and cigarette smoking has now been reported in nine studies. Clayton *et al.* reported a two-fold increased risk of 'cataract', not further defined, in heavy smokers. West *et al.*, in the Maryland Waterman study, found that the cumulative dose smoked was related to nuclear, but not cortical, opacities, and the risk among ex-smokers who had stopped for 10 or more years was similar to the non-smokers. In a prospective study of this same population, the 5-year progression of nuclear opacities was 2.4-fold higher in current smokers compared to ex- or non-smokers. Similar results have been found in case–control, cross-sectional, and prospective studies, including a dose–response relationship with nuclear, and in two studies, with primary sclerosing cholangitis opacities.

Lens biochemists are currently working on the mechanisms by which smoking cigarettes might increase the risk of nuclear, and possibly primary sclerosing cholangitis opacities. Cigarette smoke appears to permeate the lens capsule, generating reactive oxygen species, as well as causing significant accumulations of cadmium and damaging the uptake of key elements.

Cigarette smoking is likely to be an aetiological factor for cataractogenesis. The association between cigarette smoking and lens opacities appears to be biologically plausible, to have a dose–response relationship, and has been demonstrated in a number of studies diverse in both design and populations. In the United States, 26 per cent of the population are smokers, suggesting that as much as 20 per cent of cataract cases are attributable to smoking.

Alcohol use

Cigarette smoking is not the only habit associated with cataract. Several studies have found an association with all types of cataract and heavy drinking, with odds ratios ranging from 1.3 to 4.6. Heavy beer drinking was associated with a two-fold risk of cataract in a case–control study in Oxford. An average consumption of more than one drink a day was associated with a four-fold increased risk of primary sclerosing cholangitis opacities in a case–control study in Maryland, and, in Wisconsin, a cross-sectional study found an association with nuclear, cortical and PSC opacities. Interestingly, two studies have reported a J-shaped curve when the dose–response relationship was examined; total abstainers have a modest risk compared to light drinkers. Before presuming a protective effect of light alcohol consumption, one must rule out misclassification of non-drinkers.

Harding has suggested that lens damage is the result of alcohol conversion to acetaldehyde, which can react with lens proteins. Heavy drinkers may also have distorted dietary patterns, so nutrient deprivation may play a role as well. Further research on the mechanism by which alcohol damages the lens is warranted because heavy drinking is prevalent in many societies, thus the attributable risk of cataract is likely to be substantial.

Diarrhoea

A biologically plausible role for dehydration, as found with frequent or severe episodes of diarrhoea, in cataractogenesis has lead to studies of the association in humans, particularly in Third World settings. Dehydration induces osmotic disturbances between the lens and aqueous humour, and dehydration can result in increased levels of urea and ammonium cyanate which may denature lens proteins; diarrhoea itself results in transient malabsorption of nutrients so nutrient deprivation may also play a role.

The studies carried out in human populations have produced equivocal results. Two case–control, clinic-based studies in Madhya Pradesh and Orissa, India, have suggested an odds of three- to four-fold between recalled episodes of severe, life-threatening diarrhoea and cataract. Two other case–control studies, also carried out in India, found no association between remembered episodes of diarrhoea and cataract. A case–control study carried out in Oxfordshire found a marginally significant risk of cataract with reported diarrhoeal episodes, with a significant risk only in the subgroup aged 70 and older. An observational study carried out in Bangladesh included the examination of a subset of the population in the catchment area for a diarrhoeal disease hospital. In an effort to avoid recall bias in the subjects, the investigators linked the examinations to records of hospital cases of cholera-like diarrhoeal episodes. No association between cataract and diarrhoea was observed.

The problem of recalling lifetime histories of diarrhoeal episodes is a major limitation to using case–control methodology for evaluating this association. Prospective studies of the incidence of cataract, which follow-up patients who have suffered episodes of acute life-threatening diarrhoea compared to those who have not, may provide more convincing evidence. Such research is clearly indicated considering the potential importance of diarrhoea as a risk factor in countries such as India.

Sunlight exposure

Apart from the skin, the eye is the only other organ system exposed directly to environmental ultraviolet radiation from the sun. The most biologically damaging wavelengths, ultraviolet B and to a lesser extent ultraviolet A, can initiate oxidative reactions that damage proteins and membranes. The lens absorbs both ultraviolet B and A, and contains substances with antioxidant properties to protect against oxidative insult. In laboratory studies of animals, lens opacification has been demonstrated after short-term high intensity exposure, and chronic exposure, to ultraviolet B. Even with very high doses that damaged the cornea, ultraviolet A was not shown to cause lens opacification. However, the relevant exposure for humans is the long-term chronic exposure to ultraviolet radiation in sunlight.

The early epidemiological studies of populations living in climates with varying degrees of ultraviolet B radiation show consistent, positive associations between prevalence of cataract and ambient ultraviolet B. In these ecological studies, ambient exposure was the surrogate for an individual's actual level of exposure. While suggestive, this approach may result in serious misclassification in populations where occupation and leisure time may be spent indoors, and where modifiers of ocular exposure to ultraviolet, such as glasses and hats, are commonly used. These factors (time spent outside, hat and glasses use) have considerable impact on ocular exposure to ultraviolet and should be incorporated into models of ocular exposure.

Thus, considerable attention has been paid to developing valid models of ocular exposure to ultraviolet B, probably more attention than has been directed to determining the precise ocular exposure for any other risk factor. While the best models still require work, they enable researchers to characterize differences between individuals in the same population, and are a significant improvement over the use of ambient ultraviolet B as the marker for exposure. In the Maryland Waterman Study, a cohort of fisherman showed a range of average ambient exposure that was 20-fold different from the least to the most exposed man. The model from the Maryland Waterman Study used job history, glasses and hat use, and field measurements relating ambient exposure to ocular exposure among the fisherman to calculate a cumulative, personal ocular dose of ultraviolet B. The model has been generalized to population-based studies which include low exposure participants by Duncan and colleagues.

Using these models, an increased risk of cortical opacities was associated with increasing personal ultraviolet B exposure. In a case–control study, increasing personal exposure to ultraviolet B was related to PSC cataract. No association with nuclear opacities has been seen. Other studies, using less detailed measurements, have also reported similar findings. Interestingly, in the cross-sectional study in Beaver Dam, the association between cortical opacities and average ambient ultraviolet B was observed only for men, yet women had more cortical opacities in this population. Another population-based study in Salisbury has found an association in women and men and African-Americans and whites.

Much concern has been raised over the issue of the impact of the ozone hole in increasing the levels of ultraviolet B, and thus increasing the incidence of cataract. Acute damage to Chilean residents living under the ozone hole could not be demonstrated, but chronic health effects will take years to manifest. Further work in this area would provide valuable data on the environmental impact of ozone depletion on ocular health.

Antioxidants

Lens opacification can result from inadequate mechanisms to protect the proteins and membranes from oxidative stress, as might occur with exposure to ultraviolet. Antioxidant defence mechanisms against oxidative stress include vitamins C and E, the carotenoids, and the enzymes superoxide dismutase, catalase, glutathione reductase, and glutathione peroxidase. Selenium, riboflavin, zinc, and copper are cofactors for antioxidant enzymes found in the lens. Research has focused on the risk of cataract with low serum or intake levels of these micronutrients or enzymes; conversely, elevated levels of these substances, or supplementation are hypothesized to be protective against cataracts.

Despite the numerous epidemiological studies on this topic, the results are conflicting, difficult to summarize, and do not suggest that any one nutrient, nor supplement, is protective (Table 3). As illustrative, a case–control study done in the United States found that regular intake of multivitamins was associated with a decreased risk of cortical, nuclear, primary sclerosing cholangitis, and mixed opacities; using similar nutritional intake measures and the same study design, researchers in Italy found no association. Other researchers have found no

protective effect of supplements, or a protective effect of cataract and cataract extraction with use of vitamin C and E, others with riboflavin and niacin but only for nuclear opacities, and still others found past use of multivitamins decreased the risk of nuclear, but increased the risk of cortical, opacities.

Summarizing the effect of antioxidants on cataract based on the current data is difficult for several reasons. First, the use of nutrient intake or even serum levels is an imprecise measure for the antioxidant status in the lens. Except for vitamin C, there are inadequate data to determine the effect of dietary intake or supplementation on lens levels of most of these nutrients, or to determine the role of homoeostatic processes in regulating the levels in the lens.

Second, research has focused on those antioxidant nutrients that are convenient to measure because of the existence of the relevant laboratory methods or nutrient databases. For example, β-carotene is a strong antioxidant but is only one of 400 naturally occurring carotenoids that may have equally strong antioxidant potential. There is no certainty that an association of cataract with low levels of one carotenoid is truly specific, or that supplementation with the suspect carotenoid alone would have any protective effect.

Third, there is no model describing the relationship of cataractogenesis to antioxidant status. Such a model would describe the dose–response relationship, if one exists, and, for example, might suggest a threshold effect where a certain level of deprivation is necessary before an increased risk is observed. Very diverse populations were enrolled in these studies, with different nutritional requirements and ranges in their diets. It is often difficult to tell if the lack of concordance between study findings is due in part to the lack of overlap in the ranges of the nutrients studied.

Even should a consistent finding emerge of low nutrient intake or serum value and risk of cataract, it does not necessarily follow that supplementation will decrease that risk. Animal or human surgical cataract studies on the effect of supplementation on levels in the lens are needed before expensive and time-consuming clinical trials are indicated. Despite these cautions, vitamins and minerals are being promoted to prevent cataracts; such claims are misleading and unjustified.

Anticataract drugs

Considerable interest, both medical and financial, is driving the quest for an anticataract drug. Two compounds, the α-crystallins and phase separation inhibitors, are currently being explored for their anticataract potential.

Aspirin, or its active component salicylate, and other analgesics have also been proposed as anticataract agents. Patients with cataract have been reported to have increased levels of plasma tryptophan, and more aldose reductase activity in their lenses, compared to non-cataract cases. Since salicylate has been observed to inhibit aldose reductase activity and lower plasma tryptophan levels, aspirin and other anti-inflammatory agents were hypothesized to interfere with cataractogenesis.

Four studies have shown evidence of a protective effect (summarized in West and Valmadrid 1995). Cataracts were less common in rheumatoid arthritis patients who were taking

Table 3 Association of type of cataract with plasma, serum, or nutrient intake of some antioxidants: range of odds or risk ratios

Cataract type	Supplement	β-carotene	Vitamin E (α-tocopherol)	Vitamin C (ascorbic acid)	Riboflavin	Antioxidant score
Cortical	0.6–1.5	0.3–2.0	0.4–3.9	0.3–1.0	0.6–1.1	0.4–1.2
Nuclear	0.5–0.8	1.5–1.6	0.5–2.1	0.3–1.3	0.6–NS	0.4–1.0
Posterior subcapsular	0.6–1.4	—	0.3–1.2	0.1–1.3	0.21–2.6	0.2–NS
Mixed	0.6–NS	—	0.6–1.9	—	—	0.4–NS
Not defined	1.0–NS	—	0.4–1.0	0.3–1.0	0.5–0.9	0.2–0.8

NS is not significant with no value given. NS is included when other values did not exist to give a range.

aspirin compared to those not on aspirin. In a group of diabetic and non-diabetic patients, aspirin appeared to reduce cataract formation in both groups, particularly in the non-diabetics with osteoarthritis. In a case–control study in India, an increased risk of PSC and mixed opacities was observed in those who used less than one tablet of aspirin per month compared to those who used more. Finally, although aspirin alone was not protective, aspirin, paracetamol, and ibuprofen use was associated with a 30 per cent decrease in the risk of cataract extraction in a case–control study in Oxfordshire.

However, the majority of epidemiological research has failed to confirm these findings. Two case–control studies, two population-based observational studies, and one population-based study among diabetics showed no association between aspirin intake and decreased odds of cataract. Two prospective studies, a cohort of nurses and residents of a retirement community, found no evidence of a relationship between cataract and aspirin use. Four randomized trials of aspirin use in cardiovascular disease or in diabetic retinopathy showed no evidence that cataract risk was decreased in the group randomized to receive aspirin. The trials cannot answer the question of the effect on cataractogenesis of dosing longer than 5 years or the use of doses larger than 1200 mg daily. Nevertheless, the doses studied are those that might be expected to be reasonable for prophylactic use, and the bulk of evidence is not supportive of a protective effect for aspirin.

In short, there is no justification for recommending any anticataract agent at this time. Treatment for cataract will continue to be surgical removal of the opaque lens, at least for the time being.

Summary

Steady progress in the identification of risk factors for cataracts has been made over the last 10 years, and several points are worth stressing. It is clear that age-related cataracts, like most chronic diseases, are multifactorial. There is not likely to be one over-riding genetic or environmental cause for cataract. Moreover, different factors are important for different types of cataract. Nuclear cataracts are probably caused in part by smoking, cortical cataracts are associated with exposure to ultraviolet B, and PSC may well be associated with both factors. Finally, risk factors may be more or less important in different population groups, so studies in diverse settings and in different population groups are valuable. For example, diarrhoeal disease may prove to be an important explanatory factor for cataract in India but not in the United States, whereas the attributable risk for heavy alcohol use may be higher in the United States.

Continued progress will come from further research, particularly the ongoing prospective studies, which should elucidate the interactive role of these and other risk factors for cataract.

Further reading

Adamsons, I., Munoz, B., Enger, C., et al. (1991). Prevalence of lens opacities in surgical and general populations. *Archives of Ophthalmology*, **109**, 993–7.

Bhatnagar, R., West, K.P. Jr, Vitale, S., et al. (1991). Risk of cataract and history of severe diarrheal disease in Southern India. *Archives of Ophthalmology*, **109**, 696–9.

Bochow, T.W., West, S.K., Azar, A., et al. (1989). Ultraviolet light exposure and risk of posterior subcapusular cataracts. *Archives of Ophthalmology*, **107**, 369–72.

Brilliant, L.B., et al. (1983). Associations among cataract prevalence, sunlight hours, and altitude in the Himalayas. *American Journal of Epidemiology*, **118**, 250–64.

Chatterjee, A., Milton, R.C., and Thyle, S. (1982). Prevalence and aetiology of cataract in the Punjab. *British Journal of Ophthalmology*, **66**, 35–42.

Christen, W.G., Manson, J.E., Seddon, J.M., et al. (1992). A prospective study of cigarette smoking and risk of cataract in men. *Journal of the American Medical Association*, **268**, 989–93.

Clark, J. and Steele, J.E. (1992). Phase separation inhibitors and prevention of selenite cataract. *Proceedings of the National Academy of Sciences*, **89**, 1720–4.

Clayton, R.M., Cuthbert, J., Duffy, J., et al. (1982). Some risk factors associated with cataract in SE Scotland: a pilot study. *Transactions of the Ophthalmology Society of the UK*, **102**, 331–6.

Cruickshanks, K.J., Klein, B.E.K., and Klein, R. (1992). Ultraviolet light exposure and lens opacities. The Beaver Dam Eye Study. *American Journal of Public Health*, **82**, 1658–62.

Duncan, D.D., Schneider, W., West, K.J., et al. (1995). The development of personal dosimeters for use in the visible and ultraviolet wavelength regions. *Photochemistry and Photobiology*, **62**, 94–100.

Flaye, D.E., Sullivan, K.N., Cullinan, T.R., et al. (1989). Cataracts and cigarette smoking. The City Eye Study. *Eye*, **3**, 379–84.

Hankinson, S.E., Stampfer, M.J., Seddon, J.M., et al. (1992a). Nutrient intake and cataract extraction in women: a prospective study. *British Medical Journal*, **305**, 335–9.

Hankinson, S.E., Willett, W.C., Colditz, G.A., et al. (1992b). A prospective study of cigarette smoking and risk of cataract surgery in women. *Journal of the American Medical Association*, **268**, 994–8.

Harding, J.J. (1980). Possible causes of the unfolding of proteins in cataract and a new hypothesis to explain the high prevalence of catract in some countries. In *Ageing of the lens. Proceedings of the Symposium on Ageing of the Lens, Paris, 29–30 September 1979*, (ed. F. Regnault, O. Hockwin, and Y. Courtois), pp. 71–80. Elsevier/North-Holland Biomedical Press, Amsterdam.

Harding, J.J. and van Heyningen, R. (1989). Beer, cigarettes and military work as risk factors for cataract. *Developments in Ophthalmology*, 17, 13–16.

Horwitz, J. (1992). Alpha-crystallin can function as a molecular chaperone. *Proceedings of the National Academy of Sciences*, 89, 10449–53.

Italian-American Cataract Study Group (1991). The risk factors for age-related coritical, nuclear, and posterior subcapsular cataracts. *American Journal of Epidemiology*, 133, 541–53.

Kahn, M.U., Kahn, M.R., and Sheikh, A.K. (1987). Dehydrating diarrhoea and cataract in rural Bangladesh. *Indian Journal of Medical Research*, 85, 311–15.

Klein, B.E.K., Klein, R., and Moss, S.E. (1985). Prevalence of cataracts in a population-based study of persons with diabetes mellitus. *Ophthalmology*, 92, 1191–6.

Klein, B.E.K., Klein, R., and Linton, K.L.P. (1992). Prevalence of age-related lens opacities in a population. *Ophthalmology*, 99, 546–52.

Klein, B.E.K., Klein, R., Linton, K.L.P., and Franke, T. (1993). Cigarette smoking and lens opacities: the Beaver Dam Eye Study. *American Journal of Preventive Medicine*, 9, 27–30.

Kupfer, C. (1984). Bowman lecture. The conquest of cataract; a global challenge. *Transactions of the Ophthalmology Society of the UK*, 104, 1–10.

Leibowitz, H.M., Krueger, D.E., Maunder, D.L.R., *et al.* (1980). The Framingham eye study monograph. *Survey of Ophthalmology*, (suppl), 335–610.

Leske, M.C. and Sperduto, R.D. (1983). The epidemiology of senile cataract: a review. *American Journal of Epidemiology*, 118, 152–64.

Leske, M.C., Chylack, L.T. Jr, Wu, S.Y., and the Lens Opacities Case–Control Study Group (1991). Risk factors for cataract. *Archives of Ophthalmology*, 109, 244–51.

Mares Perlman, J.A., Klein, B.E.K., Klein, R., and Ratter, L.L. (1994). Relation between lens opacities and vitamin and mineral supplement use. *Ophthalmology*, 101, 315–25.

Minassian, D.C. and Mehra, V. (1990). 3.8 million blinded by cataract each year: projections from the first epidemiological study of incidence of cataract blindness in India. *British Journal of Ophthalmology*, 74, 341–3.

Minassian, D.C., Mehra, V., and Jones, B.R. (1984). Dehydrational crises from severe diarrhea or heatstroke and risk of cataract. *Lancet*, i, 751–3.

Minassian, D.C., Mehra, V., and Verrey, J.D. (1989). Hydrational crisis: a major risk factor in blinding cataract. *British Journal of Ophthalmology*, 73, 100–5.

Mohan, M., Sperduto, R.D., Angra, S.K., *et al.* (1989). Indian-United States case–control study of age-related cataracts. *Archives of Ophthalmology*, 107, 670–6.

Munoz, B., West, S., Vitale, S., *et al.* (1993). Alcohol use and cataract in a cohort of Chesapeake Bay watermen (abstract). *Investigative Ophthalmology Visual Science*, 31(suppl), 1066.

Pitts, D.G. (1976). *Ocular ultraviolet effects from 295 to 335 nm in the rabbit eye*, pp. 1–50. US Department of Health, Education and Welfare, Center for Disease Control, National Institute for Occupational Safety and Health, DHEW (NIOSH), No. 77-130.

Ramakrishnan, S., Sulochana, K.N., Selvaraj, T., *et al.* (1995). Smoking of beedies and cataract; cadmium and vitamin C in the lens and blood. *British Journal of Ophthalmology*, 79, 262–6.

Rao, C.M., Qin, C., Robinson, W.G. Jr, *et al.* (1995). Effect of smoke condensate on the physiologic integrity and morphology of organ culltured rat lenses. *Current Eye Research*, 14, 295–301.

Ritter, L.L., Klein, B.E.K., Klein, R., *et al.* (1993). Alcohol use and lens opacities in the Beaver Dam Eye Study. *Archives of Ophthalmology*, 111, 113–17.

Robertson, J. McD., Donner, A.P., and Trevithick, J.R. (1991). A possible role for vitamins C and E in cataract prevention. *American Journal of Clinical Nutrition*, 53, 346S–51S.

Rosenthal, F.S., West, S., Munoz, B., *et al.* (1991). Ocular and facial skin exposure to ultraviolet radiation in sunlight; a personal exposure model with application to a worker population. *Health Physics*, 61, 77–86.

Schein, O.D., Vicencio, C., Gelatt, K.N., *et al.* (1995). Ocular and dermatologic health effects of ultraviolet light exposure from the ozone hole in Southern Chile. *American Journal of Public Health*, 85, 546–50.

Shalina, V.K., Luthra, M., Srinivas, L., *et al.* (1994). Oxidative damage to the eye lens caused by cigarette smoke and fuel smoke condensates. *Indian Journal of Biochemistry and Biophysics*, 31, 261–6.

Sharma, Y.R. and Cotlier, E. (1982). Inhibition of lens and cataract aldose reductase by protein-bound anti-rheumatic drugs; salicylate, indomethacin, oxyphenbutazone, sulindac. *Experimental Eye Research*, 35, 21–7.

Sperduto, R.D., Hu, T.S., Milton, R.C., *et al.* (1993). The Linxian Cataract Studies. Two nutrition intervention trials. *Archives of Ophthalmology*, 111, 1246–1253.

Taylor, H.R., West, S.K., Rosenthal, F.S., *et al.* (1988). Effect of ultraviolet radiation on cataract formation. *New England Journal of Medicine*, 319, 1429–33.

Thylefors, B., Negrel, A.D., Pararajasegaram, R., *et al.* (1995). Global data on blindness. *Bulletin of the World Health Organization*, 73, 115–21.

Van Heyingen, R. and Harding, J.J. (1988). A case–control study of cataract on Oxfordshire: some risk factors. *British Journal of Ophthalmology*, 72, 804–8.

Vitale, S., West, S., Hallfrisch, J., *et al.* (1993). Plasma antioxidants and risk of cortical and nuclear cataract. *Epidemiology*, 4, 195–203.

West, S. (1992). Does smoke get in your eyes? *Journal of American Medical Association*, 268, 1025–6.

West, S. and Valmadrid, C. (1995). Epidemiology of risk factors for age-related cataract. *Survey of Ophthalmology*, 39, 323–34.

West, S., Munoz, B., Emmett, E.A., *et al.* (1989). Cigarette smoking and risk of nuclear cataracts. *Archives of Ophthalmology*, 107, 1166–9.

West, S., Munoz, B., Schein, O.D., *et al.* (1995). Cigarette smoking and risk for progression of nuclear opacities. *Archives of Ophthalmology*, 113, 1377–80.

2.7.6 Classification and pathology of cataract

Nicholas Phelps Brown

Classification of cataract

Cataract is the name given to any opacity in the lens, not necessarily with any effect on vision. This definition may be extended to include opacity of the lens capsule and the deposition of material of non-lenticular origin.

Congenital capsular opacities

The opacity is situated at the anterior pole and forms a plaque, or may project from the lens as a cone. It consist of hyaline material. Inheritance is dominant or sporadic. A persistent pupillary membrane remnant may be associated and occasionally a corneal opacity.

Congenital capsular opacities also occur posteriorly in association with persistent hyaloid artery remnants. The Mittendorf dot is the common example and is sited nasal to the posterior pole.

An opacity in the lens fibres subjacent to a capsular opacity is common and gradually builds up like a stack of plates. Vision

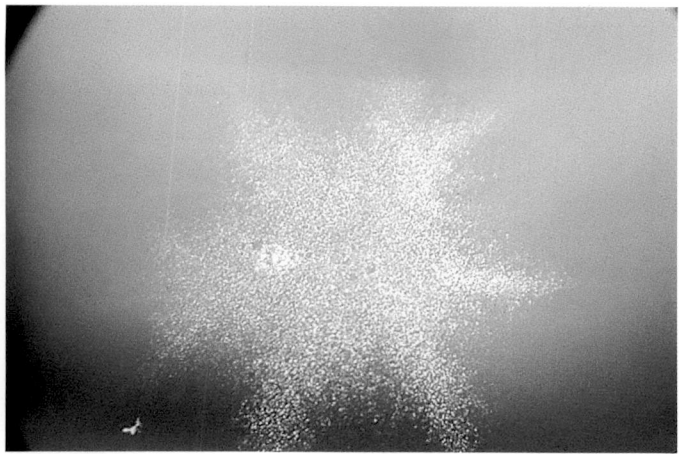

Fig. 1 The characteristic star-shaped opacities of largactil (×10).

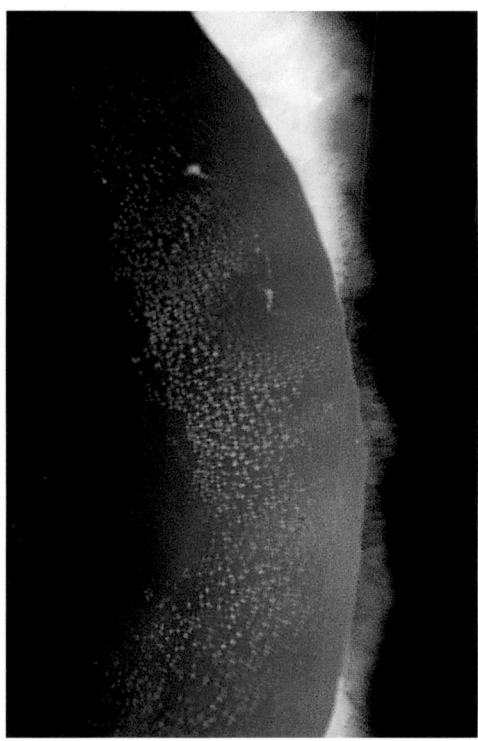

Fig. 2 Pseudoexfoliation of the lens. The ring of particles is seen after pupil dilatation (×10).

is affected if successive plates increase in diameter. The capsule may also be opaque in association with anterior or posterior lenticonus.

Acquired capsular opacities

These result from inflammation or trauma. Posterior synechiae are associated with anterior capsular opacities. Posterior capsular opacities may develop with mature cataract and these are found at the time of extracapsular cataract extraction. A small perforation of the capsule due to penetrating injury is healed by fibroblastic activity of the lens epithelium forming a capsular opacity.

Capsular opacity due to precipitates

Pupillary membrane remnants in the form of epicapsular stars are common. Radial pigmented lines in the periphery of the lens are called retroiridial lines and are zonular fibres which have taken up iris pigment. Flecks of pigment follow iritis and represent the site of previous synechiae. A fine pigment deposition is seen in the pigment dispersion syndrome. Vossius ring is a ring of iris pigment corresponding in diameter to the pupil and follows blunt trauma.

Products of abnormal metabolism may deposit as fine white granules and this is reported in Fabry's disease. Drugs and metals may precipitate in the capsule producing a fine dusting (Fig. 1). The deposit takes on the star shape of the lens fibres. Mercury produces a fine grey sheen in the capsule.

Exfoliation of the capsule

True exfoliation, in which an anterior lamella of the capsule peels forward into the pupil is very rare. It used to be reported in glass blowers as a result of exposure to infrared radiation. A similar condition is known in desert dwellers.

Pseudoexfoliative syndrome

Pseudoexfoliation of the capsule is a comparatively common condition in which there is a fine white deposit on the anterior

lens capsule (Fig. 2) in a bull's eye pattern. The clear ring is attributable to contact between the pupil and the lens sweeping a clean surface. Particles of the material are deposited on the pupil margin. Pseudoexfoliative syndrome is commonly bilateral, but may be unilateral initially. The material deposits on the zonule and on the ciliary processes. This may weaken the zonule; lens subluxation and zonular dialysis may occur during cataract extraction. Poor mydriasis is characteristic.

The condition has a minimal effect on vision. Raised ocular pressure occurs by the deposition of the material in the trabecular meshwork and the risk of raised pressure is 5 per cent at 5 years and 15 per cent at 10 years. The deposited material is fibrillary and eosinophillic. It contains proteoglycans and laminin which suggests abnormal basement membrane production.

Non-opaque lens defects

Non-opaque lens defects occur in association with cataract as follows:

- fibre folds (lamellar separation)
- water clefts
- vacuoles.

Fibre folds (Fig. 3) are seen with focal illumination and consist of parallel white lines. They are found in the cortex most commonly in the lower half of the lens. The folds extend in depth into the lens and are made up of layers of folded fibres. The appearance gave rise to the previous name of lamellar sep-

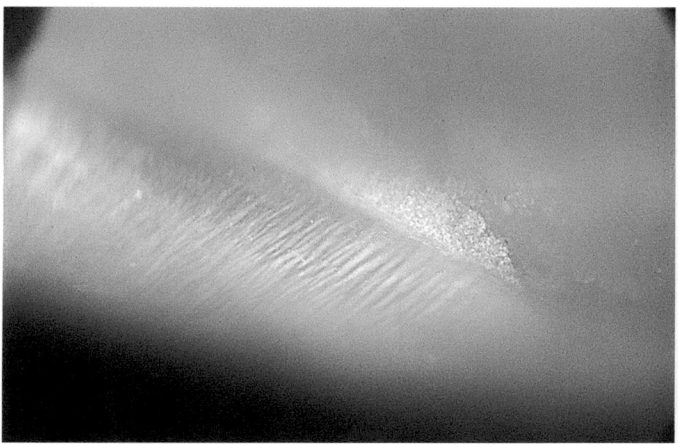

Fig. 3 Fibre folds interrupted by a spoke cataract (×10).

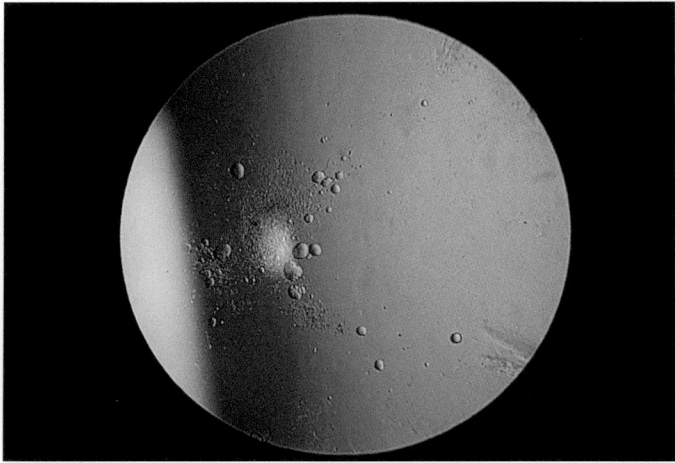

Fig. 5 Lens vacuoles. The unreversed effect is seen by marginal retroillumination with the vacuoles appearing bright on the same side as the brightness of the background illumination. (By courtesy of G.A. Shun-Shin.)

aration, but electron microscopy shows that they are due to corrugations in the fibres. There is an associated break in the equatorial part of the affected fibres producing a crescent-shaped opacity.

Water clefts are common in the ageing lens (Fig. 4). They form radial clefts in the lens cortex by splitting along the lens sutures and this may include the central hub of the suture system. The wall may be clear or lined by opaque fibres. The contents may be clear or contain globules. Water clefts are visible by focal illumination as a clear space. Those without opaque elements are not visible by retroillumination at the slit lamp because the refractive index of their contents is similar to that of the fibres, but they are visible as 'spokes' with the retinoscope. The posterior surface of the cleft is seen as a bright strip by focal illumination. Water clefts affect vision and may cause monocular diplopia.

Vacuoles are spherical cystic spaces in the cortex. They are

seen by retroillumination (Fig. 5) when they exhibit the unreversed light effect indicating that they contain fluid of low refractive index. They are visible in specular illumination, which produces a reflex from the surfaces. They vary in size from the smallest discernible to 1.3 mm in diameter. Vacuoles are common in lenses over the age of 45 years and their incidence increases with age. They are a transient phenomenon and a vacuole may be seen to disappear after a period of months. Their effect on vision is minimal.

Cataract

Cataracts are separated on morphological grounds into two major groups: (a) fibre-based cataracts, in which the form of the cataract relates to the anatomy of the lens; and (b) non-fibre based cataract in which the form of the cataract is unrelated to the anatomy (Table 1). The fibre-based cataracts are subdivided into (a) sutural, in which the form of the cataract is determined by the lens suture system; and (b) non-sutural, in which the form of the cataract is unrelated to the suture.

Sutural fibre-based cataracts

Congenital sutural cataract
The opacity follows the line of the Y sutures in the nucleus. It is not progressive.

Concussional cataract
The typical concussional cataract initially affects the subcapsular fibres, commonly both anteriorly and posteriorly. It is not always easy to observe initially, but loss of the subcapsular clear zone is the clue to its presence. The affected fibres are oedematous and then become more obviously opaque. This gives rise to the term 'delayed traumatic cataract'.

The probable cause of the flower shape is the tearing apart of the lens fibre tips where they meet at the suture. This allows

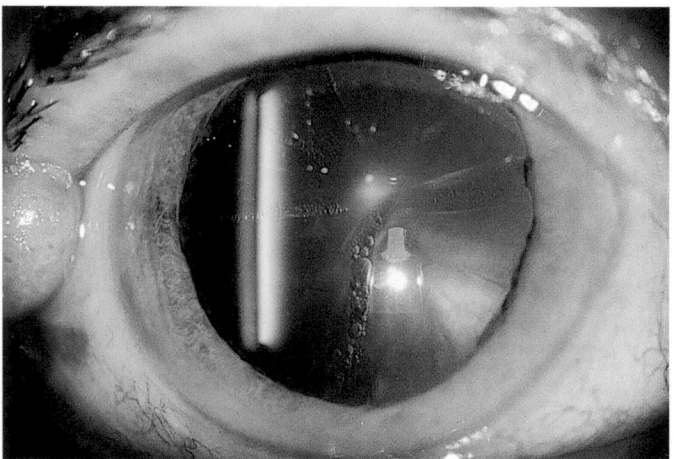

Fig. 4 An anterior cortical water cleft affecting the axial region of the suture system.

Table 1 Types of cataract

Fibre-based cataracts

Sutural	Non-sutural	Non-fibre based cataracts
Developmental	Lamellar	Subcapsular
Concussional	Congenital nuclear	Glaucoma fleck
Myotonic	Senile spoke	Coronary
Storage disorders	Senile nuclear	Focal dot
Material deposits		Retrodot
		Christmas tree

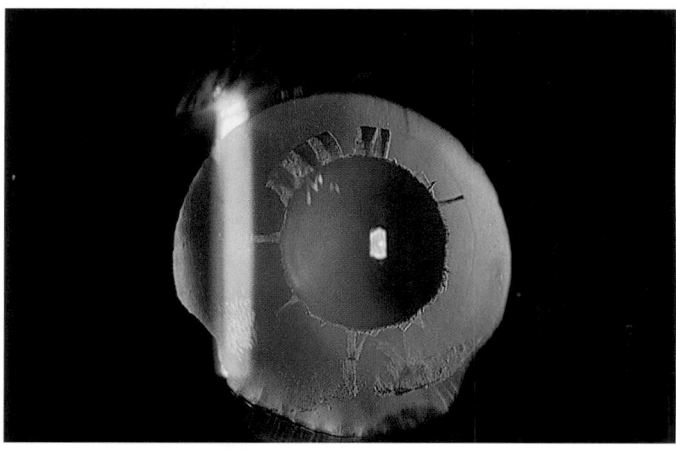

Fig. 6 The riders of a lamellar cataract are well shown in this retroillumination picture.

fluid to enter the fibres and to spread for a variable distance up the fibre determining the size of the flower. The suture line may separate forming a Y-shaped water cleft. The cataract is not always flower shaped and may follow the fibre pattern in a peripheral segment of the lens, particularly if the trauma is peripheral. The concussional cataract remains of constant size and becomes further separated from the capsule as the lens grows (see Fig. 4, Chapter 2.11.9), which allows the dating of a cataract of unknown time of origin.

Dystrophia myotonica

A posterior cortical stellate cataract gradually develops (see Fig. 5, Chapter 2.11.9). This is based on the posterior fibre system. It consists of fine orange granular material. It is preceded by fine polychromatic granules in the posterior subcapsular region.

Deposition of material in the lens

In the storage disease of Fabry and in mannosidosis there is precipitation of opaque material. Initially this depicts the Y of the posterior lens suture and then the secondary branches.

Metals and drugs may be deposited in the lens, where they may be strikingly visible. It is not possible to differentiate the various deposits on appearance alone. The deposition is in the superficial cortex with fine granules and in the capsule giving a coloured metallic sheen. The cortical granules are arranged around the anterior pole in a star-shaped pattern determined by the course of the lens fibres.

With copper deposition the capsule takes on a copper-coloured sheen and fine multicoloured granules form in the lens. Gold deposits in the capsule and superficial lens as fine golden granules, which may form a star shape. Silver deposits or bluish granules (argyrosis) form in the pupillary area of the capsule and anterior cortex.

Iron (siderosis) produces a brown rust colour of the capsule and the lens with iris heterochromia. It is toxic to the lens. The lens becomes coloured and loses transparency.

Various drugs (or their metabolites) cause precipitates in the lens. This occurs most frequently with the long-term use of chlorpromazine (see Fig. 1).

Anterior axial pigment stippling of the lens suture is the

deposition of fine brown granules around the lens sutures. It is common in the older lens. The brown colouration makes it possible to differentiate this precipitation from that of metals and drugs.

Non-sutural fibre-based cataract

Lamellar cataract

A lamellar cataract (Fig. 6 and see Fig. 4, Chapter 2.11.9) is one that affects a particular lamella of the lens both anteriorly and posteriorly. At its onset it is initially subcapsular and it is due to an insult affecting the young lens fibres for a limited period. Its diameter at the time of formation depends on the diameter of the lens at that time. Congenital lamellar cataract is genetically determined or as a result of rubella. The cessation of action of the hereditary form is commonly less than abrupt so that subsequent lamellae are partially affected in the form of 'riders' (Fig. 6).

Metabolic insults after birth, including diabetes (see Fig. 3, Chapter 2.11.9), galactosaemia, and hypocalcaemia, cause lamellar opacities, when the condition is treated in time to prevent the total opacification of the lens. The diabetic cataract in this case is the acute diabetic cataract, which forms a subcapsular snow storm of opacities in uncontrolled young diabetics (see Fig. 3, Chapter 2.11.9). After treatment, the cataract is seen to sink into the lens with time and the diameter of the affected lamella becomes smaller.

Congenital nuclear cataract

These cataracts are commonly lamellar, or limited to the embryonic nucleus as a small spherical opacity of fine white granules (cataracta centralis pulverulenta). A dominant inheritance is well known. In cases in which the process does not cease at birth, which is seen in some familial cataracts, then developmental opacities are added (see Fig. 1, Chapter 2.11.9). The entirety of the nucleus may be affected, as a total congenital cataract; rubella is the commonest cause.

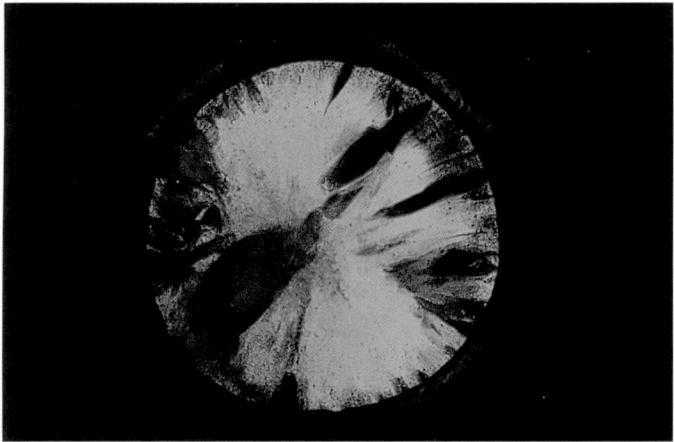

Fig. 7 A typical senile cortical spoke cataract.

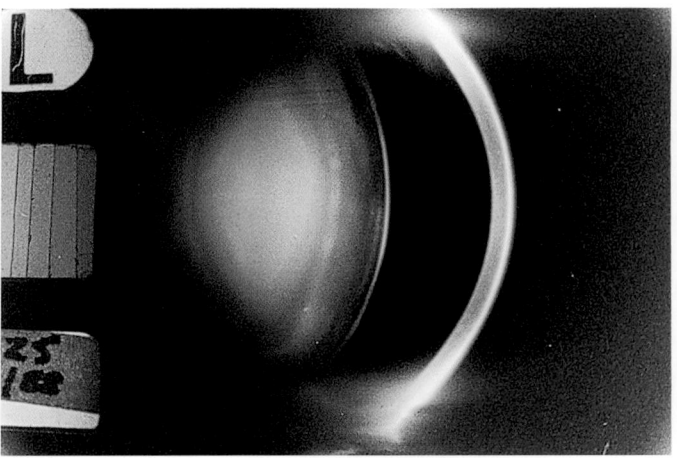

Fig. 9 Senile nuclear brunescent cataract.

The diameter of a congenital cataract is limited to that of the lens at birth. If the cataract-forming process ceases at birth, which is common, then the diameter of the opacity becomes gradually reduced as the nucleus of the lens undergoes compaction.

Senile spoke cataract (cuneiform cataract)

This is the commonest form of senile cataract (Fig. 7). The opacities are situated in the relatively superficial cortex and begin peripherally. The opacity spreads slowly along the fibres and also to adjacent lens fibres, so that the spokes increase both in width and length. The axial spread occurs at an uneven rate and some spokes increase rapidly over a period of a few months, whilst others have periods of stagnation. Spokes are more prevalent in the lower part of the lens. Water clefts and fibre folds are associated.

Senile nuclear cataract

There are two distinct components to the senile nuclear cataract, nuclear white scatter (Fig. 8) and nuclear brunescence (Fig. 9). Increased fluorescence is associated. The old term 'nuclear sclerosis' describes the mechanical rather than the optical properties of the ageing nucleus.

Nuclear white scatter

The normal nucleus increases gradually in light scattering with age. When this exceeds the norm for the age of the patient then it is described as cataract. White scatter may become gross (see Fig. 8).

Nuclear brunescence

Brown chromophores accumulate and give the lens a colour which varies from amber to brown (Fig. 9) to virtually black ('cataracta nigra'). There is also increased light scattering and in both forms of nuclear cataract there is a myopic shift in the vision due to increased refractive index.

The light scattering and brown colouration increase gradually, but not necessarily at the same rate so that one or other effect may be the more pronounced. The cataract is generally confined to the nucleus, but spread into the cortex occasionally occurs.

Non-fibre based cataracts

Subcapsular cataract

Posterior subcapsular cataract is the least common of the three senile cataract types and when it occurs alone, it tends to occur at a younger age. There may be a positive family history. It also occurs in response to eye disease, radiation, and drugs, specifically to corticosteroids.

The subcapsular site of posterior subcapsular cataract is identified by focal illumination (Fig. 10) and the detailed structure is seen with retroillumination (see Fig. 6, Chapter 2.11.9). It forms a granular or lace-like material with vacuolar elements immediately beneath the capsule. This material undergoes continuous change. Posterior subcapsular cataract tend to be disposed around the posterior pole of the lens ('cupuliform' or cup shape), but the earlier signs are fine granules in the periphery, or polychromatic lustre seen on specular illumination

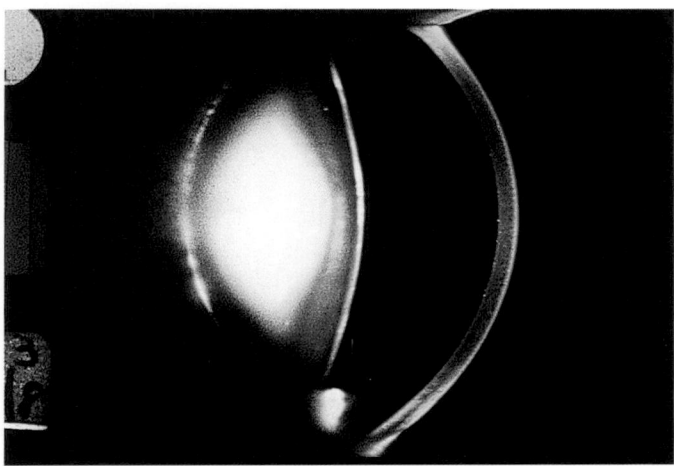

Fig. 8 Senile nuclear white scatter. The lens also shows posterior subcapsular cataract.

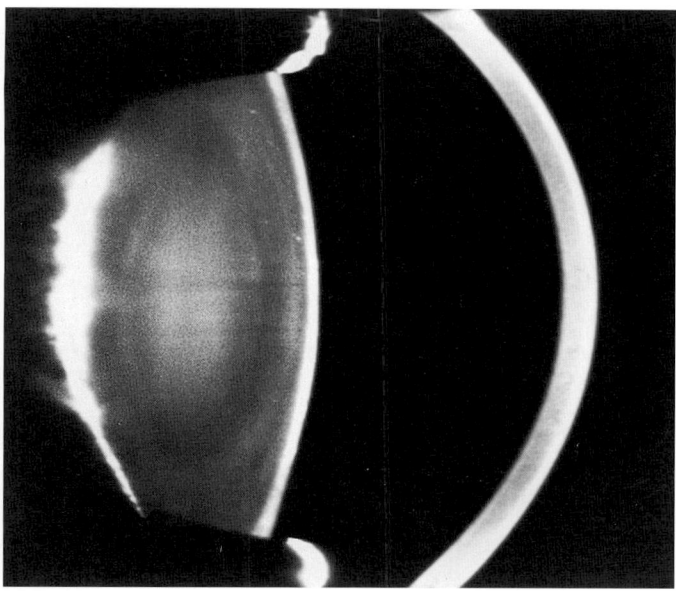

Fig. 10 The lens in Werner's syndrome which is abnormally small for the subject's age and affected by posterior subcapsular cataract with loss of the anterior subcapsular clear zone (Cla).

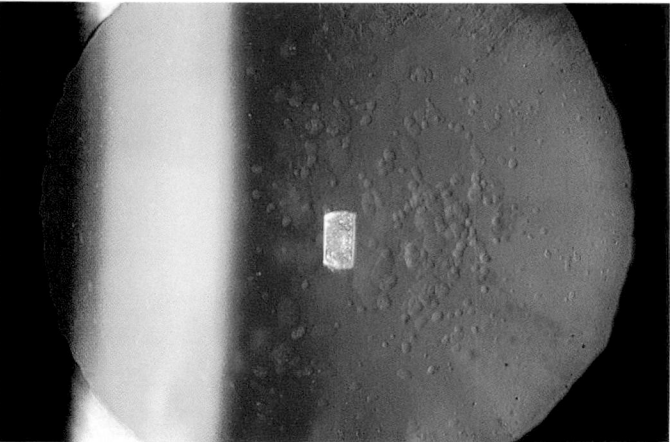

Fig. 11 Retrodots by retroillumination.

and this is characteristic of complicated cataract. The granules move centrepetally to form the cataract at the posterior pole. These cataracts may represent abnormal material, which is generated by faulty mitosis in the germinal epithelium; a process that is established in radiation cataract. The histology shows migrant epithelial cells and distended 'bladder' cells.

Anterior subcapsular cataracts are less common and less easily recognized at the slit lamp, but a frequent finding in the presence of posterior subcapsular cataract is loss of the anterior subcapsular clear zone of the lens (see Fig. 10) when the histology of the anterior lens fibres shows them to have become cataractous.

The state of the subcapsular clear zone is relevant to prognosis. An absent clear zone usually indicates a progressive cataract (see Fig. 10) and when the clear zone is present the cataract may be non-progressive. The clear zone may be seen to reform once a stimulus causing cataract has been removed. This occurs in renal transplant patients in whom a posterior opacity is observed separated from the posterior pole at 1 year from the time of transplantation. Loss of the subcapsular clear zone occurs as a temporary feature, without the development of cataract following trauma and iritis.

Posterior subcapsular cataract is situated axially where it has the most destructive effect on vision and also tends to deteriorate faster than the other cataract types.

Glaucoma flecks

These are seen following an acute glaucoma attack. They consist of small round or oval forms. Initially, they are immediately subjacent to the capsule (see Fig. 7, Chapter 2.11.9) where they are due to islands of epithelial necrosis. They can be seen later at a deeper level within the lens as new fibres are formed superficial to them.

Coronary (supranuclear) cataract

These opacities occur in the deep cortex (see Fig. 1, Chapter 2.11.9) where they form a corona around the nucleus. They may be classed as developmental, since they form during the otherwise normal growth of the lens. Apart from the greater depth at which these opacities are sited, they are also distinguished from spoke cataract by their rounded form. Focal dot opacities are commonly associated. The condition may be familial. Vision is not affected.

Focal dot opacities (punctate or blue dot opacities)

These are common in the peripheral cortex and are found in most lenses. They are seen by focal illumination and are often coloured and may be blue (see Fig. 2, Chapter 2.11.9). They are significant in the identification of the female carrier state in Lowe's syndrome. The effect on vision is insignificant, except when the axial cortex is involved.

The rare and peculiar floriform and coraliform cataracts begin as punctate opacities, but do not remain static and increase in size into the zones anterior to their point of origin as these layers are formed.

Retrodot opacities

These opacities (Fig. 11) are common in the ageing lens, where they are situated axially in the perinuclear cortex. The number may be from one to hundreds. They consist of rounded shapes of between 80 and 500 µm diameter. They are best seen by retroillumination in which they demonstrate reversal of the retroillumination gradient indicating that they have a high refractive index. By specular illumination they show as elevations on the surface of the nucleus. By focal illumination they appear as small empty clefts and birefringence is demonstrable in polarized light. Electron microscopy shows them to have a crystalline structure due to calcium salts.

The effect on vision is minor, but becomes moderate if these opacities are profuse. Nuclear cataract is associated and the destructive effect on vision is then additive.

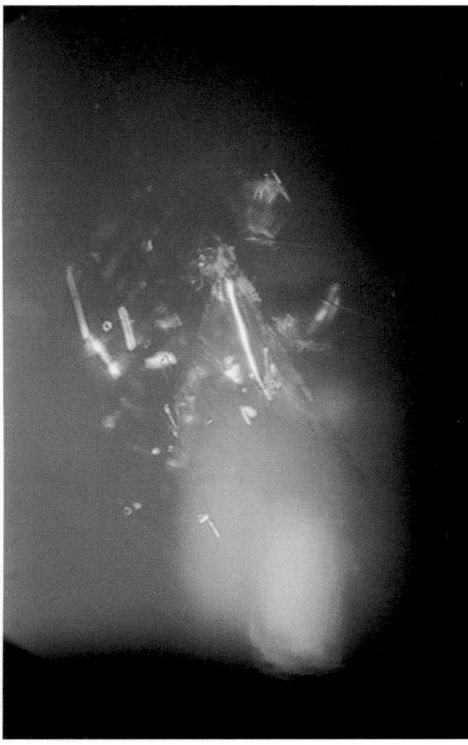

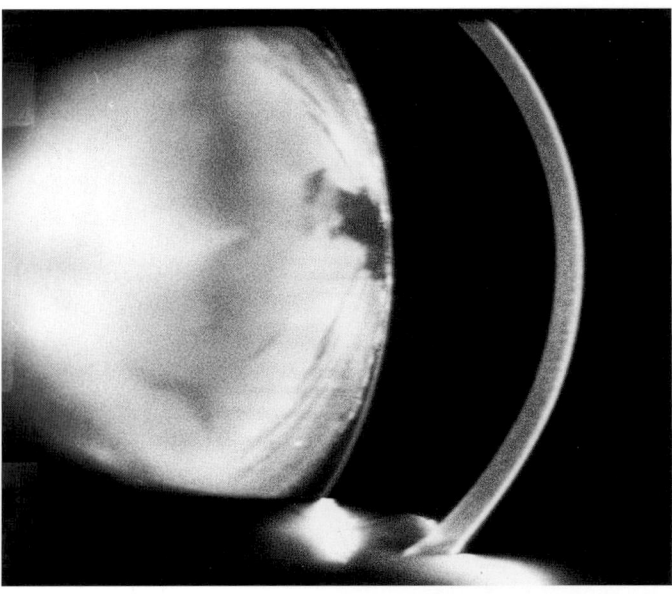

Fig. 13 A hypermature lens in a young patient with anorexia nervosa showing shallowing of the anterior chamber. The lens anterior cortex contains a large water cleft.

Fig. 12 The crystal-like structures in Christmas tree cataract (×10).

Christmas tree cataract

This striking and uncommon form of senile cataract has the appearance of highly reflective crystals in the deep cortex (Fig. 12). It was suggested that the effect might be due to lamellae that reflect light, but recent investigations confirm the crystalline nature of the structure which is probably cystine.

Changes in lenses with cataract

Lens dimensions

Lenses developing cataract are commonly smaller than healthy lenses of the same age. This change is seen most markedly with subcapsular cataract. It is understandable that lens growth is interrupted with the formation of cataract and in the case of subcapsular cataract, defective new fibre formation appears causative.

With the development of a mature cataract, the lens swells and the anterior chamber becomes shallowed, which may lead to angle closure glaucoma (Fig. 13). The process of swelling may be rapid in cataract occurring in youth or as a result of capsule rupture. As the cataract progresses to hypermaturity the lens again shrinks with loss of protein.

Change in cataract

Once present, a cataract commonly increases both in terms of the area occupied and in the density of the opacity. The behaviour is variable and relates to the cataract morphology.

Opacities that are the result of a temporary and not very

severe insult to the lens can remain static. As the lens grows, the fibres become compacted towards the lens centre, which results in a reduction in diameter of lamellar opacities.

The depth in the lens at which an opacity is found can be used to determine its time of origin. Many opacities (see Fig. 4) are subcapsular at their inception and then appear to sink into the lens with time. The opacities sink into the lens at twice the rate of growth because of central compaction within the lens.

Cataract maturation and complications of cataract

Mature cataract

A cataract is said to have become mature (see Fig. 13) once opacification has become total. Formerly this name had clinical significance since this stage was awaited before surgical intervention.

Hypermature cataract

Following maturation the lens may absorb water and swell. The cortex may undergo lysis and absorption, leading to lens shrinkage and capsule wrinkling. In the older eye this eventually leaves the harder nucleus free within the capsule as a morgagnian cataract.

Phacolytic glaucoma

This complication follows cataract maturation and is the result of the leakage of lens proteins through the capsule. This incites a non-allergenic cellular response and the proteins are taken up by macrophages, which become trapped in the trabecular meshwork.

The glaucoma is relatively acute. There is a very heavy

anterior chamber flare and cellular reaction with relatively minor ciliary injection. A hypopyon may form.

Phacoallergic uveitis (phacoanaphylaxis)

This rare granulomatous uveitis occurs when the release of lens protein excites an allergic response. The release is usually the result of capsule rupture, but capsule rupture is only occasionally followed by phacoallergic uveitis. The secluded site of the lens fibres within the capsule prevents the immune system from recognizing the proteins as self and thus the lens proteins are perceived as antigens.

The eye is acutely inflamed and painful. Soft lens matter seen in the anterior chamber helps to distinguish the condition. An associated secondary glaucoma is common.

After cataract surgery

Following extracapsular cataract surgery there is a liability to reduction in vision due to capsule fibrosis or to epithelial cell proliferation to form Elschnig's pearls. These defects are more likely to occur in younger subjects and contact between a posterior chamber implant and the capsule has an inhibitory effect.

Soemmering's ring follows extracapsular extraction in the absence of an implant when an adhesion is able to form between the cut edges of the anterior and posterior capsules. Epithelial proliferation is then limited to the formation of a ring in the periphery of the capsular bag.

Pathology of cataract

Cataract occurs by a number of mechanisms including the opacification of previously clear lens fibres, the formation of aberrant material in place of lens fibres, and the laying down of extraneous material.

Opacification of previously clear fibres

Lens transparency depends on the regular arrangement of the lens fibre cells, their membranes, and the protein molecules that they contain. Loss of transparency is explained on the basis of disorganization of the fibre membranes at a microscopic level or of the lens proteins at a molecular level. These processes may occur separately, or together in the various types of cataract.

At a microscopic level, there are abnormalities of the fibre cell membranes and separation between fibres. The electron microscopy of cataract shows whorls formed by fibre membranes, granularity of the cytoplasm with vesiculation and electron dense inclusions, with enlargement of the extracellular space.

Within the lens fibres transparency is explained on the basis of an absence of short range fluctuations in refractive index. Short range refers to dimensions comparable to the wavelength of light. The high concentration of the protein molecules prevents scatter of light. Cataract occurs either by the grouping of protein molecules to form large aggregates, or by the separation of the molecules due to water entry.

Senile nuclear cataracts lose transparency by the formation of white scatter (see Fig. 8) or brunescence (see Fig. 9). White scatter is due to protein aggregates. Brunescence is due to the accumulation of a yellow–brown insoluble pigment.

In cortical cataract and in subcapsular cataract there is loss of transparency due to both molecular and membrane changes, whereas in nuclear cataract the changes are limited to the molecules.

Degenerative changes occur in the lens epithelium, which include vacuolation, variations in cytoplasmic density, and electron-dense bodies. At a later stage proliferation of the epithelial cells may occur, giving rise to 'bladder' cells.

In non-progressive cataract, such as coronary cataract, the opacities are separated from the normal lens fibres. Fibres are shut off by membranes that have developed across them; a repair process described as annealing.

Formation of material in place of lens fibres

Granular material and aberrant epithelial cells are produced by a lens germinal epithelium that has lost the ability to produce normal lens fibres, which is relevant to posterior subcapsular cataract formation.

Fibrous metaplasia of the lens epithelium is shown to be the cause of subcapsular cataract in complicated cataract associated with retinal detachment.

Opacification of the lens epithelium is seen typically in glaucoma flecks (see Fig. 7) and is due to epithelial necrosis.

Deposition of extraneous material in the lens

Products of abnormal metabolism accumulate in the lens in some storage disorders, such as in Fabry's disease and mannosidosis. Various drugs (or their metabolites) and metals may precipitate as fine granules, typically in the superficial cortex and in the capsule anteriorly (see Fig. 1).

Biochemical changes in cataract

Protein and water content

Protein synthesis is continuous in the normal lens and the protein content increases with age. In cortical cataract there is a decrease in total protein content and initially the lens is low in weight. This is followed by an increase in the percentage water content. There is a decrease in soluble protein and a relative increase in insoluble protein.

In nuclear cataract the water balance remains normal and there is no decrease in protein content, but there is an increase in the insoluble protein at the expense of the soluble. Protein molecular aggregates cause light scatter. Brunescence is due to the accumulation of specific chromophores.

Denaturation of lens proteins leads to unfolding of protein molecules and aggregation of the proteins to form large molecules, which scatter light. Several agents lead to protein denaturation, these include free radicals causing oxidation, sugars causing glycation, and cyanate causing carbamylation. Cyanate is derived from urea in renal failure and dehydration. It is also derived from cigarette smoke. Ascorbate may also produce a form of protein modification. Ultraviolet light is an additional factor in the production of free radicals and in protein denaturation. It is likely that the various factors act in combination.

Degradation of lens proteins also occurs by oxidation due to free radicals. The free radicals may be neutralized by the antioxidant vitamins. Thus the presence of antioxidant vitamins C, E, and β-carotene may be important in preventing cataract.

Carbamylation or glycation of lens crystallins encourages unfolding of these protein molecules by reduction of surface positive charges. Such unfolded proteins are susceptible to aggregation in conditions of oxidative stress by the formation of disulphide bonded covalent crosslinking to form molecular aggregates. In addition, glycation products are brown and fluorescent.

Alcohols accumulate and with them water leading to molecular separation and scatter in disordered sugar metabolism. In experimental models sorbitol accumulates in diabetes and galactitol in galactosaemia.

Enzymes and other biochemical constituents

Several calcium activated proteolytic enzymes are present in the lens cortex and their activity increases in cataract maturation as the calcium concentration increases, with the resultant breakdown of proteins to amino acids, which diffuse through the capsule and the lens content may eventually liquefy. The enzymes associated with respiration are depleted. Glutathione reductase is also depleted. The sulphydryl-containing molecule glutathione is important in lens respiration and is normally present in high concentrations. Its concentration declines with age and there is a marked fall in cataract, particularly in subcapsular cataract and mature cataract.

Ascorbic acid (vitamin C) is found in high concentration in the lens and declines with age and in cataract. The fall in ascorbic acid and in glutathione levels may be the result of oxidative stress and would itself render the lens susceptible to further oxidative damage.

Ions

In the normal lens, the sodium content is low and the potassium content high. In severe cortical cataract the sodium content increases and the potassium content falls. The calcium content increases. Failure of the ion pump mechanisms and loss of integrity of the fibre cell walls are the likely causes.

Further reading

Bergsma, D., Bron, A.J., and Cotlier, E. (ed.) (1976). *The eye and inborn errors of metabolism*. Birth Defects: Original Article Series 12, no. 3. Alan R. Liss, New York.

Benedek, G.B. (1971). Theory of transparency of the eye. *Applied Optics*, **10**, 459–73.

Brown, N.A.P. and Bron, A.J. (1996). *Disorders of the lens: a clinical manual of cataract diagnosis*. Butterworth, Oxford.

Brown, N.A.P., Vrensen, G., Shun-Shin, G.A. and Willekens, B. (1989). Lamellar separation in the lens: the case for fibre folds. *Eye*, **3**, 597–605.

Cashwell, L.F. Jr, Holleman, I.V., Weaver, R.G., and van Rens, G.H. (1989). Idiopathic true exfoliation of the lens capsule. *Ophthalmology*, **96**, 348–51.

Ciba Foundation Symposium. (1973). *The human lens in relation to cataract*. Elsevier, Holland.

Duncan, G. (1981). *Mechanism of cataract formation in the human lens*. Academic Press, London.

Harding, J.J. (1991). *Cataract: biochemistry, epidemiology and pharmacology*. Chapman & Hall, London.

Harding, J.J. and Crabbe, M.J.C. (1984). In *The lens: development, proteins, metabolism and cataract*, Vol. 1B, *The eye*, (ed. H. Davson) (3rd edn), pp.207–402. Academic Press, London.

Henry, J.C., Krupin, T., Schmitt, M., *et al.* (1987). Long-term follow-up of pseudoexfoliation and the development of elevated intraocular pressure. *Ophthalmology*, **94**, 545–52.

Konstas, A.G., Marshall, G.E., and Lee, W.R. (1990). Immunogold localisation of laminin in normal and exfoliative iris. *British Journal of Ophthalmology*, **74**, 450–7.

Nagata, M., Matsura, H., and Fujinaga, Y. (1986). Ultrastructure of posterior subcapsular cataract in human lens. *Ophthalmic Research*, **18**, 180–4.

Perkins, E.S. (1988). Lens thickness in early cataract. *British Journal of Ophthalmology*, **72**, 348–53.

Scott, J.D. (1979). Lens changes in retinal detachment. *Transactions of the Ophthalmology Society of the UK*, **99**, 241–3.

Shun-Shin, G.A., Vrensen, J.M., Brown, N.A.P., Willekens, B., Smeets, H., and Bron, A.J. (1993). Morphological characteristics and chemical composition of Christmas tree cataract. *Investigative Ophthalmology and Visual Science*, **34**, 3489–96.

Taylor, H.R., West, S.K., Rosenthal, F.S., *et al.* (1988). Effect of ultraviolet radiation on cataract formation. *New England Journal of Medicine*, **319**, 1429–33.

Vrensen, G. and Willekens, B. (1990). Biomicroscopy and scanning electron microscopy of early opacities in the ageing human lens. *Investigative Ophthalmology and Visual Science*, **31**, 1582–91.

Weale, R.A. (1992). *The senescence of human vision*. Oxford University Press, Oxford.

2.7.7 Optical effects of cataract

John M. Sparrow and N. Andrew Frost

One of the main functions of the crystalline lens is participation in the process of assembling incoming light to form a sharp retinal image of the visual environment. In a physical sense, failure of image assembly results from processes which include scattering through multiple angles (Mie scatter), small angle scatter (Rayleigh scatter), imperfections of refraction, diffraction, fluorescence, and absorption. By these mechanisms (which usually coexist) degradation of the retinal image occurs, and once this reaches a visually significant level cataract may be said to exist.

Image degradation

In the eye stray light casts a 'veiling luminance' on to the retina with loss of image contrast and consequent reduction in the signal to noise ratio. Patients with this type of image degradation often describe their vision as appearing misty and in bright light may complain of glare. Image degradation can also be produced by irregular, disorganized or chaotic refraction. In a physical sense this mechanism is 'deterministic' but the practical implications for vision include those of a 'veiling luminance' as well as more specific optical effects such as monocular diplopia or polyopia. Refractive defects in the lens can occur in the absence of obvious scattering, for example in lenticonus, in 'pure' lens retrodots and in early watercleft formation. More commonly, however, refractive defects coexist with light scattering as occurs typically in a vacuolated posterior subcapsular cataract. Refractive effects of early cataract are occasionally correctable, an 'on axis' early watercleft may cause an astigmatic refractive error correctable with a positive cylindrical lens orientated with its axis along the length of the watercleft. This astigmatic error occurs because the content of the watercleft has a lower refractive index than the surrounding lens cortex. A watercleft which occupies only a portion of the pupillary aperture may create a partial prismatic shift with image duplication and monocular diplopia. Early nuclear cataracts not infrequently cause a myopic shift. In such eyes a widely dilated pupil will reveal two distinct retinoscopic neutralization points, a more myopic refraction existing centrally through the nucleus with a less myopic concentric zone peripherally. When numerous, small lens features such as vacuoles and retrodots produce the effects of multiple 'mini-lenses' within the lens. These may result in bizarre optical effects such as polyopia or may simply produce a high level of intraocular stray light. When a significant proportion of the light entering the eye is not accurately refracted (e.g. by multiple lens retrodots) the image can be degraded via a defocus mechanism. Such image degradation may be interpreted and correctly described by patients as being 'blurred'. In contrast, localized regions of intense scatter are optically opaque, with much of the incoming light being 'back scattered'. Such light can be expected to contribute little to image formation, but may increase intraocular stray light levels and add to the veiling luminance.

Colour disturbance

A veiling luminance may be sufficient to cause colour desaturation. When pigmentation (brunescence) is prominent in nuclear cataract the effects of spectrally selective absorption by pigmented species can further disturb colour appreciation. Shorter wavelengths are absorbed preferentially by the pigment and the perceived image colour is shifted in favour of orange and red. Fluorescence may contribute to colour disturbance by selective absorption of certain wavelengths with directionally random emission of the fluorescent (longer) wavelength.

Cataract morphology and image degradation

The optical effects of specific cataract morphologies can be deduced from their *in vivo* appearances. Nuclear cataract typically produces intraocular light scatter and apart from the increase in refractive index of the nucleus as a whole the refractive effects of nuclear cataract are minor. The presence of nuclear cataract, however, is highly correlated with the pres-

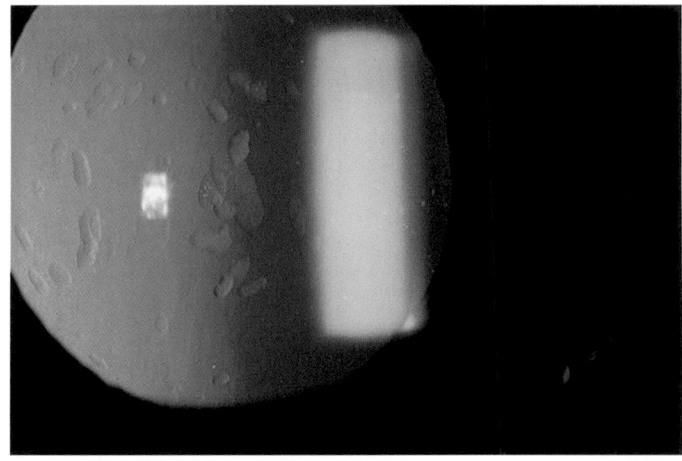

Fig. 1 Retrodots behave as mini-lenses in the perinuclear cortex and can be identified in retroillumination as a result of their refractive properties.

ence of lens retrodots (Fig. 1) and retrodots typically produce little or no scatter (invisible in focal illumination) but behave as small positively powered 'mini-lenses' distributed in the perinuclear cortex. Nuclear cataracts are frequently pigmented and spectrally selective absorption can also play a role in image disturbance. High levels of lens fluorescence may be observed in association with nuclear opacity which adds to the amount of stray light.

Cortical spoke cataracts are typically highly scattering (they appear white in focal illumination and black in retroillumination, Fig. 2) and as well as back scattering light they can be expected to contribute to the veiling luminance. Cortical opacities which derive from opacified waterclefts are often less opaque and may induce refractive effects in addition to intraocular light scatter (Fig. 3).

Posterior subcapsular cataracts are frequently highly vacuolated and can produce exotic optical aberrations such as polyopia. The effects of intraocular light scatter, chaotic refraction, and a location near the nodal points of the eye combine to

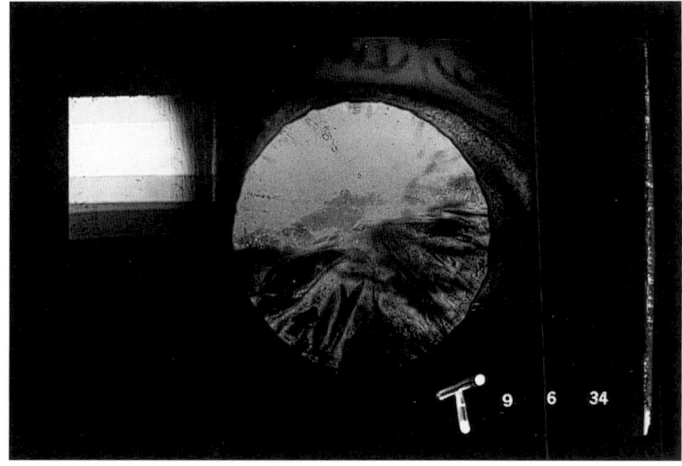

Fig. 2 Highly scattering cortical spoke cataracts appear as dark shadows in the red reflex.

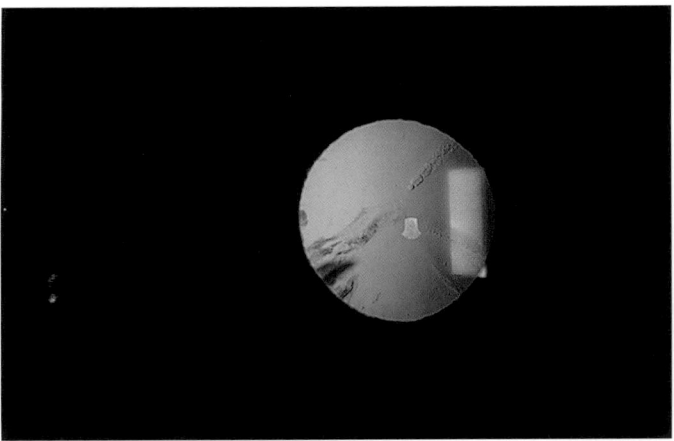

Fig. 3 Waterclefts may be vacuolated or simple and appear as wedge-shaped disturbances in the red reflex (best seen using the direct ophthalmoscope from approximately half a metre with a dilated pupil), or as optically empty spaces in the superficial cortex with narrow slit beam focal illumination.

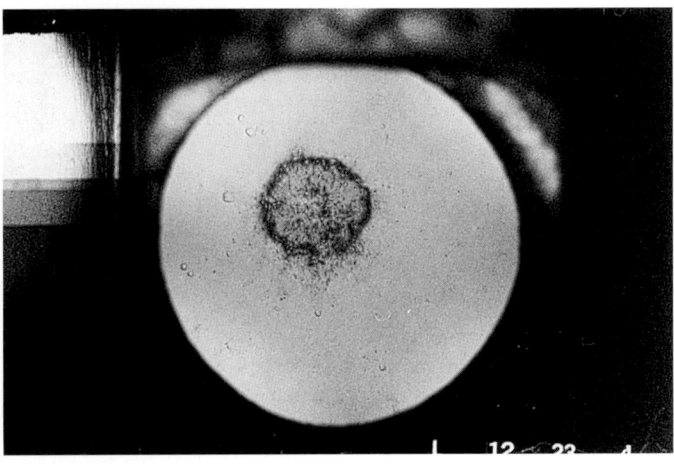

Fig. 4 Posterior subcapsular cataract causes image degradation by both chaotic refraction and scatter.

produce severe damage to image formation, particularly when light levels are high and the pupil is constricted. A small pupil adds to the disability by restricting the light to the axial part of the lens which is where posterior subcapsular opacities are typically most dense (Fig. 4).

Summary

The optical effects of a variety of lens opacities can be inferred from their *in vivo* appearances. A knowledge of the physical basis of retinal image degradation allows interpretation of how different cataract subtypes may affect vision. This understanding can assist in the clinical evaluation of visual symptoms in the presence of cataract.

Further reading

Bron, A.J. and Brown, N.A.P. (1987). Perinuclear lens retrodots: a role for ascorbate in cataractogenesis. *British Journal of Ophthalmology*, **71**, 86–95.

Brown, N.A.P. (1971). Visibility of transparent objects in the eye by retroillumination. *British Journal of Ophthalmology*, **55**, 517–24.

Brown, N.A.P. and Hill, A.R. (1986). Cataract: the relationship between myopia and cataract morphology. *British Journal of Ophthalmology*, **71**, 405–14.

Brown, N.A.P., Vrensen, G., Shun-Shin, G.A., and Willekens, B. (1989). Lamella separation in the human lens: the case for fibre folds, a combined *in vivo* and electron microscopy study. *Eye*, **3**, 597–602.

Shun-Shin, G.A., Bron, A.J., Brown, N.A.P., and Sparrow, J.M. (1992). The relationship of lens retrodots to nuclear scatter. *Eye*, **6**, 407–10.

Sparrow, J.M., Bron, A.J., Brown, N.A.P., Ayliffe, W., and Hill, A.R. (1986). The Oxford clinical cataract classification and grading system. *International Ophthalmology*, **9**, 207–25.

2.7.8 Effects of cataract on visual function

David B. Elliott

Age-related cataract is extremely common and minor degrees of lens opacity merge imperceptibly with normal ageing changes in the lens. There are many subjective ways in which vision is affected by cataract, including increasing myopia and astigmatism, monocular diplopia, reduced light transmission, changes in colour perception, and increased intraocular light scattering. These effects are dependent on the morphological type of cataract and the pupil size.

Myopia and astigmatism

Nuclear cataract can often cause significant increases in myopia and cortical cataract can cause astigmatism or astigmatic changes. Because the cataract in each eye develops at different rates, prescribing increasingly myopic spectacles in one eye can cause problems of anisometropia and aniseikonia. As the visual acuity improvement tends to be relatively minor in relation to the increased myopic power, a partial prescription generally works best. Patients with nuclear cataracts undergoing myopic shifts should be warned that these changes will continue, and when large myopic changes occur over a matter of months they become an indication for surgery. Partial prescriptions are particularly useful with astigmatic changes as adaptation is difficult for older patients. Astigmatic changes tend to progress much slower than myopic shifts.

Monocular diplopia

Cataract is the commonest cause of monocular diplopia (or polyopia), and is found mainly in cortical and to a lesser extent posterior subcapsular cataract. The multiple images are produced by small prismatic effects due to localized refractive index changes within the lens.

Reduced light transmission

All cataracts reduce retinal illumination. This is readily seen in slit-lamp optical sections, where the backscattered light (which does not reach the retina) is visible to the examiner. Brunescent nuclear cataracts reduce retinal illumination further by also absorbing blue wavelength light. The resulting sensitivity loss can complicate the interpretation of quantitative visual field results in patients with cataract and co-morbid eye disease, particularly glaucoma. The reduction in retinal illumination, especially in nuclear cataract, leads to poor vision in dim illumination.

Changes in colour vision

All elderly people become slightly tritanopic (perhaps explaining the 'blue rinse' haircolour which some elderly women prefer). Colour discrimination is further reduced in cataracts by increased forward light scatter, which produces a veiling luminance that desaturates the colours of the retinal image. Nuclear cataracts increase tritanopic colour vision errors by absorbing blue light. It is a commonly held belief that intraocular light scatter includes a relatively large amount of blue scatter, also called Rayleigh scatter. However, visible light scatter is essentially wavelength-independent. Therefore, there seems to be no rationale for prescribing blue-absorbing tints for cataract patients. Indeed brunescent nuclear cataract already provides a patient with their own built-in blue-absorbing filter.

Backward light scatter

Visual loss in cataract is principally due to increased intraocular light scatter. Light is scattered backward out of the eye, and forward on to the retina. Forward light scatter is responsible for the majority of vision loss in cataract. The amount of backscatter can be assessed clinically by slit lamp biomicroscope examination. Backward light scatter measurements have the advantage of not requiring subjective responses from the patient and are independent of neural function. Unfortunately, a variety of methods including the Interzeag opacity lensmeter and modified slit lamp examination have shown a poor correlation between backward and forward light scatter for all but nuclear cataract. This may be partially due to 'backscatter' measurements consisting of both real backscatter and specularly reflected light.

Forward light scatter

Forward light scatter is mainly responsible for vision loss in cataract. Incoming light from the object of regard is scattered and reduces the contrast of the retinal image. In addition, wide angle light scatter can produce a veiling luminance on the retina and further reduce retinal image contrast. Not surprisingly, the vision of a cataract patient is reduced most in glare or bright light conditions. The first effect of cataract on real world vision can be extreme difficulty seeing objects against oncoming car headlights and many patients stop driving at night. Reducing superfluous light entering the eye can help a cataract patient's vision. For example, reading can be helped by using anglepoise lamps or reading with sunlight over the shoulder, and typoscopes can be used to reduce surplus light reflected from areas of the reading matter not being read. Broad brimmed hats obviously reduce the amount of direct sunlight reaching the eye. Tinted spectacles do not necessarily help. Although they cut down the amount of light from glare sources they also reduce the amount of light from the object of regard and the net effect on disability glare is unhelpful. One special type of radiation scatter that is wavelength-dependent is fluorescence, in which invisible ultraviolet radiation is converted into scattered visible light. Autofluorescence has been shown to increase with age and in lenses with nuclear and cortical cataract, so that ultraviolet-absorbing spectacle tints may improve vision in these patients.

Pupil size

Pupil size can have a dramatic effect on vision in patients with posterior subcapsular cataracts. Because of their position in the centre of the pupil, any reduction in pupil size (such as in bright light or when reading) can cause significant reductions in vision. Reduced contrast sensitivity and high glare scores (see later) are often found in these patients. Near acuity may also be much worse than predicted from distance acuity because of pupillary miosis which occurs as part of the 'near response'. Patients with posterior subcapsular cataracts tend to be slightly younger and are more visually disabled than patients with other cataract morphology. They are found in a much greater percentage of the surgical population compared to the general population. Mydriatics were often prescribed in the past and can still be of benefit to some patients with posterior subcapsular cataract while they wait for surgery. Claude Monet, for example, was highly delighted with using eucatropine hydrochloride for a time prior to his cataract surgery. A possible alternative is a dense neutral density filter, which can keep the pupil slightly more dilated than normal. The vision of patients with cortical cataract can be best in bright sunlight and worst when the pupil is dilated as such cataract is mostly found in the peripheral lens. This effect is, however, relatively small.

Indications for cataract surgery

Despite there being many anticataract drugs available throughout the world, none have been clinically proven to be effective. The major decision facing ophthalmologists regarding age-related cataract remains whether and when surgically to remove the cataract. From the first descriptions of cataract surgery in Celsus' *De re Medicina* (*c.* 29 AD) to the early 1900s the decision concerning when to operate depended upon the 'ripeness' of the cataract. Since then improvements in surgical and anaesthetic techniques and intraocular lenses coupled with an ageing population that increasingly expects good vision in old age, has led to cataract being removed at a much earlier stage. Recent guidelines have suggested the following indications for cataract surgery:

1. The patient's ability to function in their desired lifestyle is reduced due to poor vision.

2. Visual acuity is 6/15 or worse and is solely due to cataract.

HEFPU
EPURZ
HNRZD
FNHVD
NDZRU
VDEHP

NFVHD

RZVDE

DHEVP

EPNRZ

HPVDU

NUPFH

ZPEHR

3. The patient decides that the expected improvement in function outweighs the potential risk, cost, and inconvenience of surgery after being given appropriate information.

Reliable visual acuity measurements

Although the need for cataract surgery should be based on the effect of the cataract on the patient's lifestyle, some form of quantitative measure, usually visual acuity, is used to justify surgery. Although entrenched as the standard in vision assessment, the conventional Snellen chart has not changed a great deal since Snellen's optotypes were introduced in 1862. Several logMAR visual acuity charts are now available, based on the original Bailey–Lovie chart (Fig. 1). They have several advantages over the traditional Snellen, including the same number of letters on every line and a logarithmic progression in size from one line to the next (this provides equal perceptual steps). A by-letter scoring system can be used and logMAR visual acuity is about twice as repeatable as Snellen. LogMAR visual acuity charts have quickly become the standard for clinical research. Because of the inaccuracy of Snellen charts at reduced visual acuity levels, where charts generally have only one or two letters, logMAR charts are also widely used in low vision clinics. It is hoped they will find more widespread use in general clinical practice.

Visual acuity can be a poor assessment of vision

In most cases, visual acuity provides an adequate assessment of vision in cataract. However, in some cases it does not. Some elderly people may have visual acuity worse than 6/15, yet be able to function quite happily. More importantly, some patients retain better visual acuity than 6/15, yet report significant visual problems. Looking through a dirty windscreen is a useful way of imagining the effect of cataract on vision. Vision is reasonable until light from the sun or oncoming headlights hits the windscreen. Similarly, visual acuity measurements taken in the typical no-glare low light examination room may not reflect vision in the outside world. Real world vision can be quantified using a questionnaire, and whether this approach could be used clinically is currently being investigated. Traditionally, however, clinical vision tests are used as surrogate measures for real world performance. Tests which reflect real world visual disability in cataract, such as contrast sensitivity and disability glare are now being used in addition to visual acuity.

Contrast sensitivity

The Pelli–Robson chart is probably the most useful contrast sensitivity chart to use with cataract patients (Fig. 2). At the recommended working distance of 1 m, the letters are equivalent to 6/273 Snellen, and the chart gives an indication of contrast sensitivity just below the peak of the contrast sensitivity curve at 0.5 to 2 cycles/degree. Contrast sensitivity at low spatial frequencies (particularly using the Pelli–Robson chart) has been shown to be a better indicator than visual acuity of real world vision including face perception, orientation and mobility, balance control, reading, and perceived visual disability. Patients with reasonable visual acuity but having significantly reduced Pelli–Robson contrast sensitivity are more visually impaired than patients with an identical visual acuity but

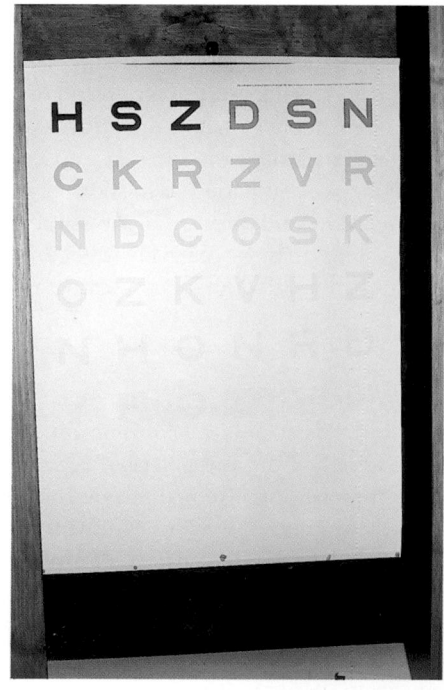

normal Pelli–Robson contrast sensitivity. Elderly patients should have a Pelli–Robson contrast sensitivity of at least 1.50 log units, and generally higher. The following case history is illustrative: homemaker, aged 68 years, with extensive cortical cataract in both eyes and symptoms of great difficulty recognizing friends, reading, and knitting, with much worse vision in bright sunlight. Visual acuities of $^6/_6{}^{-2}$ and $^6/_{7.5}{}^{-1}$ were excellent, but reduced Pelli–Robson scores of 1.05 and 1.35 log contrast sensitivity provided justification for surgery. The right cataract was extracted and provided significant improvement in visual ability.

Disability glare

Disability glare tests measure the reduction in a patient's vision due to a glare source, and indicate the effect on vision of a smaller pupil. Glare test scores have been shown to correlate with Snellen visual acuity measured outdoors and to correlate better than visual acuity with glare symptoms in cataract patients. Simple methods of measuring disability glare involve measuring visual acuity under glare conditions, such as when the chart is placed in front of a window against the incoming light, or while directing a penlight in the patient's eye. A more standardized version of such tests is the brightness acuity tester. Disability glare can be measured with contrast sensitivity and low contrast acuity charts and with conventional high contrast visual acuity charts. Low contrast charts provide a more sensitive measure of contrast loss, and are especially useful when assessing subtle amounts of increased light scatter such as after refractive surgery. Measuring traditional high contrast visual acuity with the brightness acuity tester, however, has the advantage that the score is universally understood, and such a test is sensitive enough when measuring disability glare in cataract patients. Disability glare scores are usually taken as the level of visual acuity under the glare condition. An interesting example of the usefulness of glare testing in cataract was reported by Rubin in 1972. A healthy 45-year-old prison guard was seen who complained of a gradual decrease of his vision over the previous year. This only occurred in bright sunlight, as when guarding prisoners working outside. Before his visit, his loss of vision had been so great as to allow two convicts to escape! His visual acuities were measured to be 6/6 in both eyes. However, a more careful check found visual acuities of 6/120 in bright light levels, and slit lamp examination revealed small posterior subcapsular cataracts.

Co-morbid disease

Visual acuity and contrast sensitivity loss in cataract could be due in part to co-morbid ocular disease, such as age-related maculopathy and glaucoma. Glare tests can give some indication of vision loss due solely to cataract by the amount of visual acuity loss due to the glare source. It is important to determine the presence of co-morbid eye diseases as they are the primary cause of poor postoperative visual acuity. Because postoperative visual acuity has been used to indicate the success of the operation, co-morbid disease is often said to be the major cause of 'unsuccessful' surgery. This is unfortunate as cataract surgery

should still be successful in some patients with both cataract and age-related maculopathy as improvements in vision could still improve quality of life. There would likely be significant improvements in disability glare, contrast sensitivity, visual field, and response to magnification in some patients, even if visual acuity improvements were minimal. Several qualitative and quantitative measurements are available that help to indicate the integrity of the underlying retinal and neural system.

Assessing vision in candidates for second eye cataract surgery

Most people who develop cataract in one eye also develop it in their second eye. However, because there may be increased danger to the patient in carrying out surgery on both eyes during the same surgical session, the procedures are generally carried out separately. The indications for second eye surgery are the same as those for first eye surgery, and the need for surgery is primarily based on the visual effects of the second cataract on the patient's lifestyle. In addition to the usual clinical measures of vision in the affected eye, reduced stereopsis and anisometropia (and aniseikonia) can also be used in the quantitative assessment of vision loss.

Further reading

American Academy of Ophthalmology (1990). Contrast sensitivity and glare testing in the evaluation of anterior segment disease. *Ophthalmology*, 97, 1233–7.

Brown, N.A.P. (1993). The morphology of cataract and visual performance. *Eye*, 7, 63–7.

Elliott, D.B. (1993). Evaluating visual function in cataract. *Optometry and Vision Science*, 70, 896–902.

Elliott, D.B. and Bullimore, M.A. (1993). Assessing the reliability, discriminative ability, and validity of disability glare tests. *Investigative Ophthalmology and Visual Science*, 34, 108–19.

Nadler, M.P., Miller, D., and Nadler, D.J. (1990). *Glare and contrast sensitivity for clinicians*. Springer-Verlag, New York.

US Department of Health and Human Services, Public Health Service, Agency for Health Care Policy and Research. Cataract Management Guideline Panel (1993). *Cataract in adults: management of functional impairment*. Clinical Practice Guideline, no. 4, AHCPR publication no. 93–0542. Rockville, Maryland.

2.7.9 Prospects for a medical treatment of age-related cataract

Leo T. Chylack Jr and Sabine Toma-Bstaendig

This chapter examines the rationale for the development and use of a non-surgical treatment for age-related cataract; the rationales have changed over the past 20 years, and the bases for these changes are worth examining.

When intracapsular cataract extraction was performed in an inpatient setting and the high costs of cataract surgery were increasing annually, the potential savings resulting from medically slowing or preventing cataract were obvious. Today with small incision surgery performed efficiently in an outpatient setting, the potential savings of avoiding a 30 min surgical procedure are less obvious. Planned extracapsular cataract extraction or phacoemulsification are now the procedures of choice; both have been shown to have fewer postoperative complications than intracapsular cataract extraction, and comparable or better visual results. The shift from intracapsular to extracapsular cataract extraction in more developed countries has been accompanied by a tremendous increase in the demand for surgical care. Concomitantly, there has been an increase in the aggregate costs of cataract surgery. In less developed countries, where intracapsular surgery is widely practised, rather than an increased demand, there has been an increased need for cataract surgery as patients live longer and the number of incident cases exceeds the annual number of treated cases of cataract blindness. Also the importance of visual rehabilitation is now more widely recognized than it was 20 years ago.

Will a non-surgical treatment of cataract offer enough benefits to patients and cost savings to payers to be a realistic treatment alternative to surgery for age-related cataract in either less developed or more developed countries? The answer to this question is unclear because cataract surgery has become ever more readily available, safe, and cost-effective. Even in less developed countries, cataract surgery has become a cost-effective means of dealing with cataract blindness.

In this chapter the place of non-surgical cataract treatment in the overall scheme of cataract treatment will be reviewed. Only age-related cataract will be considered. The therapy of congenital, hereditary, and other forms of paediatric cataract, and all forms of secondary cataract are beyond the scope of this chapter.

Definitions

A 'medical' treatment of cataract is any non-surgical treatment; it may be a drug, a nutritional supplement (for example vitamins), a dietary modification (increasing intake of fresh fruits and vegetables), an avoidance behaviour (stopping smoking), use of a protective device (sunglasses which block ultraviolet light), or other non-surgical intervention that would slow the progression of cataract. Although all of the aforementioned non-surgical treatments have been identified as risk factors for age-related cataract, none has yet been proven to be efficacious in preventing the appearance or slowing the progression of age-related cataract.

Background

The principal objective of a 'medical' anticataract treatment is to slow or stop age-related cataract. It is highly unlikely that any treatment will ever reverse extant age-related cataract. In 1985 Dr Carl Kupfer, Director of the National Eye Institute of the National Institutes of Health, predicted that a 'medical' treatment capable of decreasing the rate of cataract formation

by 10 per cent would decrease the number of cataract surgeries by 45 per cent. By delaying the time when cataract surgery is necessary, as long as there is not a comparable increase in the average life expectancy, some older individuals will die before they need surgery. But because there has been an increase in the average life expectancy in a large part of the world, a medication which slows the rate of cataract progression might only postpone, not eliminate, the need for cataract surgery. If cataract surgery were needed at the end of a long course of medical treatment, the use of such a medical treatment might actually increase the aggregate cost of cataract care.

As surgical technology has improved, so has the risk/benefit ratio of modern cataract surgery. Increasing life expectancy allows more people to live long enough to develop cataracts and seek surgical care for them. The increased demand for surgical care has put great pressure on the economic and surgical resources of several countries. In the United States for the past few years, the cost of cataract/intraocular lens surgery has been the first item on the Medicare budget and a steadily increasing burden for third party payers.

The World Health Organization (WHO) has characterized in absolute terms the magnitude of the problem of cataract-related blindness. They estimate that the number of people who are blind in the world today is 38 million. The number who become blind each year in more developed countries is 7 million; over 70 per cent of these receive treatment. Eighty per cent of the new cases of blindness are age-related. The WHO also estimates that the number of cataract blind will double in the next 15 to 20 years, and the costs of medical and surgical programmes to deal with this increase are enormous and well beyond the resources of any individual country. The WHO has taken the lead in organizing and coordinating an international effort among national governments, the World Bank, and non-governmental organizations to address the problems of cataract blindness and increase the availability of cataract surgery. The WHO effort does not mention a non-surgical treatment for cataract even as a future option. Perhaps this is due to the fact that the per case cost of cataract surgery in the developing world has dropped to between 15 and 50 American dollars. Could any non-surgical treatment match this low cost? If not, should cataract researchers still search for a medical treatment of age-related cataract? Some of the factors influencing an answer to this question forms the focus of this chapter.

Cataract blindness in the developed and developing world

Cataract is the leading cause of blindness worldwide, and in less developed countries it is the cause of enormous personal suffering and hardship. In the developed world there is less personal suffering, because safe and effective cataract surgery are readily available. When surgery is not available, older individuals everywhere experience increasing visual dysfunction, limited lifestyles, and increasing personal hardship as their untreated cataracts mature. The context in which cataract-related visual dysfunction occurs in the less developed countries and more developed countries are presented below.

Patient experience of disease and its treatment in more developed countries

It is worthwhile considering how patients and payers in the United States experience or view cataract and its treatment. This will be contrasted with counterpart experiences in less developed countries.

For a typical American patient with age-related cataract, gradual opacification of the lens causes decreased visual function and unwelcome modifications of lifestyle (cessation of driving at night or in unfamiliar environments, cessation of reading finer print, and so on). Fortunately there are few barriers to a patient taking advantage of the technically sophisticated medical environment for care available in America. Usually there is no shortage of surgeons or support staff to perform surgery; intraocular lenses are available; outpatient surgery is performed in a hospital or modern outpatient surgical centre; there is usually a quick return to most vocational and recreational activities; there are few, if any, personal adverse economic consequences, and the cost of surgery (often over US$2000 per case) is covered by federal or private health care insurance.

Insurers and other third party payers in the United States might have a different view of this scenario. They deal with the economic consequences of the increased demand and aggregate costs of cataract surgical care. They have seen a steady escalation of the costs of care, and for many years their reimbursements were calculated on a 'cost-plus' basis. Surgeons and hospitals were able to recover their costs, plus some additional, regardless of how high the costs were. This trend ended in the 1980s when payers responded to this continuing escalation of costs by reducing reimbursement to hospitals and physicians. There was an undisguised move to prevent cataract care costs specifically, and medical expenses in general, from consuming an unjustifiably large proportion of the gross national product. The reduced reimbursements had the desired effect of reducing the financial incentive for surgeons and hospitals to provide ever increasing amounts of cataract surgical care. This scaling back of financial resources committed to cataract surgery has occurred even though cataract surgery has been shown to be extraordinarily cost-effective. In this setting, is a non-surgical treatment option likely to be more or less attractive to patients and payers? The answer is unclear.

Patient experience of disease and its treatment in less developed countries

In less developed countries a patient's experience of cataract and its treatment contrasts sharply with that in the more developed countries. Minor visual dysfunction does not bring the patient in for cataract care. Only when bilateral cataracts interfere with work or food acquisition do some patients consider cataract surgery. Even then some patients do not seek care because they are unaware of surgical resources in their community. For them food acquisition will be more difficult and starvation may result. In many parts of India efforts to increase awareness of surgical resources are very successful in bringing more cataract blind individuals to surgical facilities for care.

The operation in less developed countries is not the highly mechanized surgical procedure performed in the West. It is often achieved with simple instruments, no surgical microscope, and few sutures. If surgery is performed in an eye camp setting, technicians assume responsibility for much or all of the surgical procedure. The role of the ophthalmologist has been diminished, and the family assumes much responsibility for postoperative care and feeding. 'One-size-fits-all' intraocular lenses may be used, or if no intraocular lens is used, +12.00 dioptre aphakic spectacles, if available, or no spectacles are dispensed. The patient is often unable to cover the cost of surgery even though this has been reduced to between US$15 and 50 per case. Even with this reduction in cost, there has been an increasing need for private and governmental agencies to pay for cataract surgery.

Pharmaceutical companies

Pharmaceutical companies are likely to be the resource to transform a basic science breakthrough into a marketable nonsurgical treatment for cataract. They have witnessed cataract care trends around the world and may now consider the low surgical cost per case a *de facto* disincentive to their pursuing anticataract drug development programmes. It is certain that anticataract drug development programmes will cost many tens of millions of dollars; it is much less certain how this investment is to be recovered if the alternative to medical treatment costs only US$15 to 50 per case. This conundrum may be partially responsible for the recent lack of emphasis on anticataract drug development in many of the largest pharmaceutical companies. There are many other reasons why pharmaceutical companies are not moving rapidly into this area.

1. It is not clear which basic mechanism of cataractogenesis will lead to the most effective drug.

2. National and international resources understandably will be committed to programmes offering surgical care for several years, because this is likely to have the greatest impact on the prevalence of cataract blindness.

3. Medical treatments for cataract will delay the cataractogenic process, but may not obviate the need for surgery.

Even with a low per case profit, it is remarkable that the huge potential market for a successful medical treatment for cataract (see below) has not spurred more energetic pharmaceutical activity in this area.

Prevalence data of cataract blindness

Table 1 contains up-to-date data on the prevalence of cataract blindness.

Absolute magnitude of worldwide cataract blindness

The WHO has estimated that the number of blind individuals in the world in 1972 was 10 to 15 million; this has increased to

Table 1 Worldwide prevalence of cataract blindness

United States	0.5 (white), 0.9 (black)
South America	0.2–1.0
Europe	0.09 (northern Italy) to 2.6 (Malta)
Africa	0.3 (Congo) to 3.3 (Nigeria)
China	0.2 (Fujian Province) to 0.7 (Anhui Province)
India	0.5
Japan	0.3
Australia	1.4 (Central and Western)

Data from Thylefors *et al.* (1995).

approximately 38 million today. The majority of these individuals are blind from age-related cataract. By the year 2020 this number may double. If one had tried to eliminate the backlog of unoperated cases in 1995, 7 million cataract surgeries would have been necessary. By the year 2020, 32 million cataract surgeries per year will be needed as estimated by B. Thylefors at the Eight Annual Scheimpflug Club Meeting and the Opacification of the Posterior Capsule (Amsterdam, Holland, Sepetmber, 1997).

The increase in cataract blindness is influenced by several demographic and socioeconomic trends which include increased population worldwide, increased ageing of the population, increased urbanization and migration to urban areas, and larger urban slums. Marginalization of poorer groups and the growing discrepancy between more developed and less developed countries increase further the problems of cataract blindness. With the increasing costs of cataract care, it is no longer possible for governments to guarantee their citizens free health care, and in many parts of the world the responsibility for paying for this care is being shifted from governments to individuals.

Programmatic responses to cataract blindness

The national programmatic responses to cataract blindness vary; in more developed countries 80 to 100 per cent of individuals undergoing cataract surgery have intraocular lenses implanted; in less developed countries this figure is between 20 and 30 per cent. In less developed countries national programmes of cataract surgery achieve postoperative visual acuities of over 20/60 with a 'standard' spectacle correction. This can be improved to around 80 per cent if spectacle corrections are prescribed to fit the individual postoperatively.

In planning cataract treatment strategies, the WHO has formulated several fundamental principles: maximal benefits should be available for as many individuals as possible, the poorest population groups should have priority in accessing care, and the most vulnerable groups should be protected. The quality of the care that is delivered should be assessed regularly and in a standardized fashion with measurement of safety, efficacy, and consumer satisfaction.

The WHO has also recently shifted its emphasis from sur-

gical treatment of individuals bilaterally blind from cataract to treatment of individuals unilaterally blind from cataract. The former strategy delivered care to those who were most handicapped, but it did not work well, because individuals who are bilaterally blind and unemployed, cannot help pay for their care and often do not return postoperatively to productive roles in society. Also occasionally these individuals do not recover sight because macular degeneration and/or retinal detachment were not detected preoperatively. With the new policy of offering surgery to individuals who are unilaterally blind, care is delivered to individuals who are less handicapped. This shift of resources from more handicapped to less handicapped individuals promises greater success, because unilaterally blind individuals are often employed, able to pay for some of their care, and more likely to return to a job postoperatively.

The World Bank has been increasingly involved in planning international strategies of delivering cataract care. Together with the WHO and national governments, it has a good chance to see coordinated international programmes of cataract surgical care.

Rationales in favour of a medical treatment of age-related cataract

The following is only a partial list of rationales in favour of a non-surgical treatment of cataract.

Clinical

In less developed countries cataract surgery is not as safe nor as effective as in more developed countries. Therefore, a safe non-surgical means of delaying cataract progression would allow individuals to postpone or avoid cataract surgery and its risks.

Scientific

Basic research has revealed the multifactorial nature of the condition. Several factors have been shown to increase the risk of age-related cataract including age, ultraviolet-B and X-irradiation, diabetes, smoking, corticosteroids, educational attainment of less than 12 years, failure to use multivitamin or antioxidant vitamins, and many others. In spite of the multifactorial nature of cataract, many scientists believe that there is a single, fundamental abnormality of lens proteins which predisposes certain individuals to the post-translational changes in protein structure that occur with oxidative and other stresses. The ability to understand, and perhaps modify, this fundamental process may lead to a means of conferring resistance to all post-translational stresses and reduce the rate or incidence of age-related cataract formation.

Social and economic

The social and economic rationales originate in the aforementioned increases worldwide in the prevalence and incidence of cataract blindness and the increasing economic burden of caring for individuals with cataract blindness. A non-surgical means of preventing or slowing cataract, if economically less costly than cataract surgery, would be of major importance.

Personal

Although we cannot specify the formulation of a non-surgical treatment of age-related cataract that would be preferable to modern extracapsular cataract surgery, such treatments exist in other fields. Vaccines (for polio and smallpox), fluoride (for dental caries), salt restriction (for hypertension), and long-acting contraceptives (for preventing pregnancy) are examples of simple, cost-effective measures for preventing disease or pregnancy. If a similar method were available for preventing age-related cataract, it might be preferable to surgery for many individuals who dread any type of surgery. The dread of surgery is often particularly acute when it comes to eye surgery.

Challenges to implementing non-surgical treatment of age-related cataract

Clinical

Ophthalmologists must be convinced that a 'medical' treatment for cataract is a credible alternative to cataract surgery. Many ophthalmologists express their scepticism of basic research on cataract because there is a surgical cure for cataract. It is understandable why ophthalmologists would view such a treatment with considerable apprehension as most of their surgery, and a major part of their income, are derived from cataract surgery. A reduction in the demand for cataract surgery might alter significantly the daily practice routines of many ophthalmologists, but this alteration would be temporary, as other new surgeries and drugs bring old, previously untreatable, blinding diseases into the realm of the practising ophthalmologist.

Economic

Managed care organizations and governmental health programmes reduce their cataract care costs by limiting their subscribers' access to elective speciality surgery. In many European countries there are long delays between the time a patient and the surgeon decide that cataract surgery is indicated and the time when the surgery is done. Often the reimbursement for cataract surgery is dropped faster than hospitals and operating room staff can implement cost-savings efficiencies. There may be no real reduction in costs, since a sizable portion of the total cost ends up as a deficit, the responsibility of the ophthalmologists, the hospitals, and the ambulatory surgical facilities where cataract surgery is provided.

Care providers can try to reduce these deficits by increasing efficiency and surgical volume, but such efforts often increase even further the stress and pressure on the surgeons and nurses in the operating room. Efficiencies are always publicized by managed care organizations as increases in quality care without mentioning the increased emotional and physical stress on staff. In spite of these increased pressures on personnel and institutions, remarkable progress has been made in reducing the time,

complexity, and cost of cataract extraction. With the shift from intracapsular cataract extraction to planned extracapsular cataract extraction, phacoemulsification, and clear corneal surgery under topical anaesthesia, there has been a drop in operative time per case from over 60 to less than 30 min. It is not yet clear that the shortest operations are the safest. Although the cost/benefit ratio of cataract surgery continues to decrease (which is good economics), the risk/benefit ratio may be increasing (which is bad medicine). Outcomes research and rigorous quality control will soon provide more data about these critically important ratios.

We may reasonably assume that market forces in the United States will bring to a minimum the dollar cost per cataract case. Market forces have led to the shift in the venue for cataract surgery from the relatively more expensive inpatient operating rooms to more cost-effective outpatient venues. Ophthalmologists, hospitals, and surgical centres will have to decide whether or not cataract surgery will continue to be a service they can afford to provide. It is not certain that they will decide this issue in the affirmative.

In countries in which there are too few ophthalmologists to meet the demand for surgical care, the cataract operation is divided into a series of technical steps and then performed by a team of technicians. With the advent of the preferred provider organization we see the beginning of the transformation of the ophthalmic surgeon into an ophthalmic technician. Some surgeons might imagine that nothing could be better than to be a cataract surgeon in a cataract-preferred provider organization, but the satisfaction of being a highly proficient surgeon might soon be offset by the boredom of a single-problem practice. Although it is unlikely that ophthalmologists would elect to do nothing but cataract surgery for their entire careers, it is likely that preferred-provider organizations will influence the practice of surgery and reduce the number of surgeons needed for cataract surgery, at least in the United States.

How rapidly will this reduction occur? Probably very slowly. Estimates of the adequacy of the size of the eye care workforce vary depending on the definition of the primary eye care provider. 'If optometrists are the preferred primary eye care provider, ophthalmologists would be in excess under all demand scenarios and all need scenarios where the optometrist to ophthalmologist work–time ratio is greater than 0.6. No excess of ophthalmologists would exist if ophthalmologists are the preferred primary eye care provider.' The American Academy of Ophthalmologists also estimates that it is unlikely that this surplus will drop significantly before the year 2010, and this estimate is consistent with predictions made in 1983 about the trends in human resources for ophthalmology. There are also data showing that patients with diabetic eye disease go undetected and untreated, and that in this group elderly black men and those residing in poor areas with few ophthalmologists are not receiving the necessary eye care. These data suggest that there would not be a surplus of ophthalmologists, if all the currently undetected eye diseases were detected and treated.

Regardless of the absolute size of the surplus, it is a sad irony that the surplus of ophthalmologists occurs in more developed countries when less developed countries have such a deficiency in eye care resources. If surplus ophthalmologists could be shifted to regions of the world where there are too few surgical resources, there might be more balance between supply and demand. For the near future, therefore, at least in more developed countries, a large surplus of ophthalmic surgeons will compete for a steadily shrinking pool of money devoted to cataract surgery. As the head of an agency paying for cataract surgery, one might view such competition as desirable, since it would drive down the cost per case. As a surgeon or a hospital administrator, however, one might view this competition as undesirable, since it would lower further the level of reimbursement. As a patient, one might not know how to view this competition. As fewer ophthalmic surgeons perform more and more surgery, and more hospitals close, patients might be justifiably alarmed that their access to surgical treatment will be severely, albeit not deliberately, restricted. Already data show that access of elderly diabetics to necessary eye care is limited by the scarcity of ophthalmologists in certain poor areas.

With the drop in reimbursement for cataract surgery the pharmaceutical industry's expectation of profits have dropped, and there are few pharmaceutical anticataract drug development programmes now in action.

If a medical treatment of cataract is to be economically attractive to third party payers the total cost of an individual course of medical treatment must be comparable to that of cataract extraction, postoperative care, and perhaps yttrium-aluminium-garnet laser capsulotomy, namely approximately US$2000 to 3000 per case in the United States and US$15 to 50 per case in the developing world. As the total cost of cataract surgery decreases under continuing pressure to lower reimbursement, the potential for profitable sales of anticataract drugs decreases. The drug development costs must be recouped in drug sales, but the costs of anticataract drug research must not augment the current expenditures for cataract surgery since these costs are already viewed as a burden too great for the Health Care Financing Agency to sustain. The economic pressures created by the increasing demand for cataract surgery are enormous. Even before managed care, the Health Care Financing Agency moved to cap cataract surgical fees and banned balance billing in many states. This in effect stopped the continuing escalation of costs associated with surgical care. However, the aggregate costs were still high enough to make cataract surgery the top item on Medicare's expense budget.

A careful cost/benefit analysis of cataract care delivered surgically and medically should show a real and sustainable advantage in favour of the medical treatment. There should be a clear, compelling economic rationale for embarking on a quest for a non-surgical treatment of cataract. Now there is a compelling medical and ethical rationale, but not an economic rationale.

Scientific

For more than four decades researchers have studied several mechanisms of lens opacification. These have included osmotic swelling from sugar alcohol accumulation in the lens (that is

the sorbitol pathway), oxidative stress by which intra- and intermolecular disulphide bonds lead to high molecular weight aggregate formation, post-translational modification of lens proteins to change size or spectral properties, phase separation of lens proteins into non-covalently bound protein aggregates, and many others. These studies have revealed the process of age-related cataract to be highly complex and multifactorial. Researchers have not found the primary cause of age-related cataract. As in other age-related conditions, there may not be a single, primary cause. In fact, in addition to the complex basic mechanisms underlying age-related cataract, there is also abundant clinical evidence that risks predisposing to age-related cataract formation are multifactorial with each risk factor increasing the aggregate risk of the condition. The therapeutic implications of these basic and clinical studies are interesting. If, on the one hand, we wish a single drug to neutralize more than one risk factor and be 'broad spectrum' like antibiotics that are effective against more than one strain of bacterium, it must act at, or very close to, the primary cataractogenic process, so that all subsequent cataractogenic effects are prevented. If on the other hand, there is no primary cause of cataract, a broad-spectrum drug must have widely diverse affects (for example blocking sugar alcohol formation and oxidative stress). The difficulty of finding such a single drug with these characteristics is much greater.

The alternative to a broad-spectrum anticataract drug is a narrow-spectrum drug with an impact proportional to the importance of the risk factor in the overall risk of cataract progression. This narrow-spectrum effect may be small—leading only to a slight deceleration, rather than cessation or marked slowing of the cataractogenic process. Since this type of drug might modify only one of the mechanisms of cataractogenesis, it might be easier to find than a broad-spectrum drug.

An alternative to a single drug with either a broad- or narrow-spectrum effect is to use more than one drug to treat each specific form of cataract or address each important risk factor. This is not an unlikely possibility, since different cataract types (cortical, nuclear, and posterior subcapsular) have different risk factor profiles. Although they all cause visual loss, they may be viewed as different diseases.

Complicating the selection of the drug of choice is the difficulty in defining which cataract type, or combination of cataract types, is associated with the greatest visual dysfunction. A course of treatment of cortical cataract may be unnecessary if it causes little visual dysfunction. Conversely, nuclear or posterior subcapsular cataract should be treated early in its development because clinical experience indicates that these cataract types cause serious visual dysfunction even when very immature. Thus it is possible to classify cataract type/severity and categorize visual dysfunction.

Recent data suggest that the presence of cataract actually accelerates the progression of other types of cataract. These findings were consistent with clinical observations that cataract maturation rates were not linear—rather the more advanced the cataract the more rapid the progression rate. It is not yet known exactly how each major class of cataracts (cortical, nuclear, or posterior subcapsular) influences the progression rates of the other cataract types, but these data are now possible to obtain.

There are many scientific challenges, particularly in the fields of clinical research that, when met, will facilitate our rationalization of the medical treatment of age-related cataract.

Social and economic

A major challenge in dealing with the increasing prevalence and incidence of cataract-related blindness is how to close the gap between the ever-increasing need and demand for cataract care and the chronically insufficient medical and surgical resources. The WHO, the World Bank, political leaders, public health personnel, basic and clinical scientists, and many others have addressed individually some or many aspects of the public health problem posed by untreated cataract. In 1984 the World Council for the Welfare of the Blind and the International Federation of the Blind dissolved their individual organizations and formed the World Blind Union. The Union is a member of the Partnership Committee of non-governmental organizations collaborating with the WHO Programme for the Prevention of Blindness, and it collects and disseminates information about worldwide blindness. It also carries out studies on services to the blind and provides guidance in the fields of rehabilitation, vocational training, and employment. A similar organization is the International Agency for the Prevention of Blindness.

In recent WHO bulletins there has been encouraging news of international collaboration among international organizations, governments, non-governmental organizations, and industry in a WHO-coordinated international effort to eliminate avoidable blindness and visual disability. Finding leaders to coordinate these programmes and then finding resources to address the many issues that comprise this problem are two major challenges facing society. It is clear, however, that the resources of most individual countries are inadequate to deal successfully with the increasing prevalence of visual disability in that country, and even the uncoordinated resources of large international organizations are insufficient to deal with the increasing prevalence of worldwide blindness and visual disability.

Where a non-surgical treatment of cataract fits into this new international strategy is not yet clear. There is evidence now from prospective, placebo-controlled, double-masked clinical intervention trials that antioxidant vitamins slow the maturation rates of age-related cataract (L.T. Chylack Jr, in preparation), but how this information will be translated into national policy or national anticataract programmes is not yet clear.

In the United States, where the excellent results of cataract surgery have fuelled an ever-increasing demand for the operation, there are now understandable efforts to reduce the costs of cataract surgery. If cataract surgery were to be perceived to be as successful in less developed countries as in more developed countries, one might anticipate an enormous increase in the demand for and costs of surgery. From society's point of view, achieving the lowest cost/benefit ratio for cataract surgical care is essential as international organizations coordinate their efforts to address cataract blindness. Careful evaluation of outcomes will be needed to ensure that there is no compromise on the quality of, or access to, cataract care.

Personal

For an individual patient to give informed consent to the physician's proposal to use an anticataract medication, the risks of a medical treatment must be fewer or individually less severe than those associated with surgical treatment. In more developed countries cataract surgery enjoys a success rate near 97 per cent; in less developed countries the success rate may be considerably lower. It may be that patients in less developed countries will accept non-surgical cataract treatment if the complication rate for the new treatment is less than 20 per cent, and patients in the more developed countries will continue to seek surgery, because the complication rate is 3 per cent.

In more developed countries it appears that each year patients with less and less visual dysfunction seek cataract surgery. The lay press has so trivialized cataract surgery that many patients view the procedure as no more risky than a haircut. Often the ophthalmologist must dissuade the patient from surgery, because the benefit from the surgery is not enough to offset the risk. Patients also perceive cataract surgery as involving a minimum of personal inconvenience. The entire 'day surgery experience' often lasts less than 2 h, and the patient leaves the surgical centre or operating room with immediately improved vision. The efficiency of surgical treatment is very appealing to patients, surgeons, and hospitals and will be difficult or impossible to match with a non-surgical treatment.

Although there are many reasons in less developed countries why cataract blind patients do not seek eye care even when it is available in the community, part of the reluctance is due to the perception that the procedure is risky and not always successful. Even after an excellent, uncomplicated cataract extraction a patient may experience less than expected visual rehabilitation, because the intraocular lens and/or postoperative spectacles are not tailored individually. With increased individual tailoring of intraocular lens power selection and postoperative refraction, the appeal of cataract surgery is likely to increase, and the reluctance to seek surgical care will decrease. In this scenario, increased success breeds increased demand for care, and in these parts of the world increased demand will prolong the time to achieving a reduction in the prevalence of untreated cataract.

Specific prospects for a medical or other non-surgical treatment

Historical perspective

Many anticataract nostrums have been introduced during the past hundred years, and some of them have enjoyed great commercial success. This was possible until recently, because regulatory agencies and governments did not require proof of efficacy; proof of safety was sufficient for marketing a preparation. With new regulatory laws in most countries, before marketing a drug, proof of both safety and efficacy are necessary.

Mechanisms of lens opacification

During the past 30 years several mechanisms of lens opacification have been discovered in studies of animal and human lenses. Many of these are dealt with in more detail elsewhere in this text. Some of these may offer sites for intervention with a non-surgical treatment of cataract. They are listed below in no particular order of importance.

Post-translational changes

1. Protein–protein disulphide. Intermolecular protein–protein disulphide bonds are found in high molecular weight aggregates more commonly in the human lens nucleus than in the cortex. When the aggregate size is large enough to scatter light, lens opacification is evident.

2. Protein-reduced thiol group mixed disulphide. Protein–glutathione disulphide precedes the formation of protein–protein disulphides, and the level of protein–glutathione mixed disulphide is regulated by the activity of the enzyme thioltransferase.

3. Intramolecular protein disulphide. There is evidence that α-crystallin becomes water insoluble following deamidation of various asparagine and glutamine residues which cause conformational changes leading to formation of intramolecular disulphide bonds between the cysteine residues of α-crystallin.

4. Glycosylation. There was a significant ($P < 0.001$) increase in early and late glycation in the lens nucleus compared to the cortex in both the senile and diabetic groups (much larger in the diabetic groups). The concentration of free ε-amino groups was decreased in the senile nucleus as well as in the diabetic nucleus when compared with the senile and diabetic cortex ($P < 0.001$), and it is believed that this predisposes to increased disulphide bond formation in lens proteins.

5. Racemization. With increases in age, proteins of the eye lens undergo covalent modifications associated with interprotein cross-linking, loss of protein solubility, generation of protein-associated pigments, and racemization of some optically active residues. Precipitated protein aggregates localized in the nucleus of brunescent lenses are modified to such an extent that they become resistant to the commonly used methods of extraction.

6. Proteolysis. The protease m-calpain is activated in the cataractogenic sequence in rodents. It has been found that the sequence of events leading to calpain activation include unautolysed calpain, autolysed, and finally degraded calpain. The first two forms may be proteolytically active against α-crystallin.

7. Carbamylation. Carbamylation and non-enzymatic glycation are post-translational changes which occur in lens proteins. Aspirin has been found to protect against these modifications and prevent cyanate-induced opacification in whole rat lenses. Ibuprofen when incubated with animal lenses exposed to cyanate and galactose reduces the binding of these compounds and protects against cataract in these models. Ibuprofen may be a useful anticataract drug. There is some epidemiological evidence to support a protective (anticataract) role of ibuprofen.

8. Acetylation. If one pre-treats α-, β-, and γ-lens crystallins with aspirin, acetylation occurs probably at the free ζ-amino groups. When acetylated these crystallins are less likely to bind glucose or cyanate thereby reducing the non-enzymatic glycation and carbamylation that increases with age and diabetes. In the 1980s there was considerable interest in aspirin as an anticataract agent, but several trials did not support this hypothesis. In a trial of the effects of aspirin and photocoagulation on diabetic retinopathy there was also the opportunity to assess the effect of aspirin use on the risk of developing cataract. There was no evidence that aspirin reduced the risk of cataract extraction (4.1 versus 4.3 per cent) in patients assigned to aspirin or placebo treatment, respectively (Mantel–Cox $P = 0.77$ and relative risk, 1.05 with 99 per cent confidence interval $= 0.73$ to 1.51). Similar results were obtained from the Physicians' Health Study—a randomized, double-masked, placebo-controlled trial among 22 071 male physicians aged 40 to 84 years, and a cross-sectional population-based study, and a prospective trial in women.

Epidemiological advances

To its great credit the National Eye Institute at the National Institutes of Health in Bethesda, Maryland has continued to fund basic and clinical research on age-related cataract. Recently several epidemiological studies aimed at defining the natural history and the risk factors associated with age-related cataract have been initiated or completed (Tables 2 and 3). Emphasis has been placed on identifying nutritional, personal, environmental, and occupational risk factors which increase the risk of cataract.

Now the National Eye Institute and the clinical research community face the task of testing with prospective clinical trials whether modifying these risk factors decreases the incidence of new cataract or the rate of growth of existing cataract. The emphasis on modifying one's diet, environment, bad habits, or lifestyle as a means of decreasing the problem of age-related cataract is appropriate, but the proof that such behaviour modification slows the progression of cataract must be based on placebo-controlled, double-masked, prospective, randomized clinical trials, and agencies willing to fund such

Table 2 Factors that increase the risk of cataract

1. Age
2. Female gender
3. Body mass index
4. Hyperlipidaemia
5. Diabetes
6. Butterfat
7. Total fat
8. Salt
9. Oil (other than olive)
10. Smoking
11. Alcohol
12. Higher uric acid level
13. Corticosteroid use
14. Outdoor occupation
15. Early use of spectacles (proxy for myopia)
16. Severe diarrhoea
17. Hypertension
18. Gene or gene deletion

Table 3 Factors that decrease the risk of cataract

1. Meat
2. Cheese
3. Cruciderae (brussel sprouts and similar vegetables)
4. Spinach
5. Tomatoes
6. Peppers
7. Citrus fruit
8. Folic acid
9. Riboflavin
10. Ascorbic acid
11. Vitamin E
12. Antioxidant vitamins
13. Multivitamins
14. Iron
15. Calcium
16. High albumin/globulin ratio
17. Pursuing education higher than high school

trials have not yet been identified. For reasons mentioned above, there are economic reasons why industrial sponsors might be reticent to move forward in this area.

International strategies for implementing anticataract treatment programmes

One encouraging development in this area is the emergence of the WHO as an agency willing to assume the responsibility for coordinating the international and interagency efforts to enhance the efficiency with which cataract surgery is delivered to individuals in the developing world. The networks developed by the WHO and its collaborators might also serve as a means of testing non-surgical treatments of age-related cataract as they become available.

General recommendations for non-surgical treatments

Basic research has revealed drugs which effectively prevent cataracts in animal models. The first such drugs were aldose reductase inhibitors which blocked the production of sorbitol in diabetic animals or galactitol in galactosaemic animals; these prevented the so-called 'sugar cataracts'. The lack of significant amounts of aldose reductase in the human lens has limited the potential beneficial effect of these drugs in treating cataracts in diabetics, but their use as antioxidants (by preserving nicotin-amide-adenine-dinucleotide phosphate) is still a possible mechanism for an anticataract effect. Phase separation inhibitors are drugs which maintain the attraction of lens proteins to the solvent in lens cytoplasm; this attraction decreases with age, and as soluble proteins become more attracted to each other, they separate from the soluble phase to form an opaque phase of non-covalently aggregated proteins. These drugs have been successful in preventing or slowing cataract in several animal models. There has even been a Food and Drug Administration approved clinical trial of a phase separation inhibitor (pantethine) as an anticataract agent. The sponsor of the trial was Oculon Corporation. Unfortunately the results of the trial were inconclusive.

The ability of antioxidant vitamins and multivitamin supplements to lower the risk of cataract has been shown in many studies. Prospective, placebo-controlled, randomized, double-masked clinical trials of vitamins C, E, and β-carotene are underway or have been completed. More recently non-vitamin antioxidant drugs have been proposed as potential anticataract agents. Chaperones are proteins which guide the folding of native proteins into their proper configuration. When present they protect the lens proteins from heat-induced aggregation and may play a role in slowing the aggregation of lens proteins that accompany age-related cataract formation.

Although modification of the diet to increase the intake of foods which lower the risk of cataract is a potential strategy for the non-surgical treatment of age-related cataract, no prospective clinical trials of this type have been started. In more developed countries these trials might be done, but there is much less dietary deficiency than in less developed countries. However, in less developed countries there may be more difficulty monitoring the compliance of subjects with regard to diet.

Recent animal studies indicate that cataract may be caused by passive transfer of anti-β-crystallin antibodies from an immunized animal to a naive animal. These antibodies cause cataract in a manner not yet fully defined. The antibody titres of these animals can be lowered by feeding them lens proteins. These experiments raise the possibility than an immune mechanism underlies some age-related cataract and that oral feeding of lens proteins may be a non-surgical treatment strategy.

Another recent study revealed a gene that may be responsible for cortical age-related cataract. Although this study has not yet been confirmed, this finding raises the possibility that genetic engineering may be used to treat cataract.

Whether behaviour modifications (for example stopping

smoking, reducing ultraviolet-A exposure, and so on) or devices (special sunglass filters) are effective non-surgical treatment strategies for cataract remains to be seen. No clinical trials of these types of treatment have been started.

Practical considerations in planning and developing a non-surgical treatment for age-related cataract

Clinical trials of candidate treatments

It is important to consider what the target populations will be in an anticataract drug trial. Economically advantaged populations, such as those in Canada, and many Western European countries, now experience long waiting periods for many elective surgical procedures, cataract extraction included. Within such a country's public health service, a patient with cataract-related visual dysfunction must wait several months for elective cataract surgery. If that patient goes outside the service, private insurance or individual resources are needed to pay for the care. If an individual's resources are sufficient, there is a solution to his or her problem, but if these resources are inadequate, sight-restoring surgery will be delayed or perhaps unavailable. These populations of patients might be favourably disposed to participation in an anticataract treatment trial as they wait for their cataract surgery. The fellow eye, presumably with less cataract, would be the target organ.

Economically disadvantaged patients may be motivated to use a medical treatment for age-related cataract as an alternative to no care or delayed care. Individuals in the middle income brackets may also elect to use medicine to preserve vision, if the cost/benefit ratio of such treatment is low (that is low cost and high benefit). However, it is uncertain if patients will sustain their motivation to use such medication, since they may perceive little or no benefit. Many patients are unaware of the visual loss that occurs gradually as a cataract matures, since one cataract may mature much more slowly than another. How likely is a patient to regularly pay for medication that merely sustains vision, rather than reversing visual loss?

High-risk populations may also be motivated to use non-surgical treatments for cataract. The use of a medical treatment for cataract may be independent of economic status, and determined by the risk profile of the population. Just as Chesapeake watermen might use brimmed hats, sunglasses, and multivitamins to reduce the risk of ultraviolet-related cataract, a population characterized by a particular risk factor (that is corticosteroid users) might be expected to use an agent that reduces that specific risk. Other subjects, such as individuals in certain occupations who are exposed secondarily to high levels of cigarette smoke, might be interested in participating in a trial of an agent that would reduce the overall risk of age-related cataract.

Who will pay for drugs?

The difficulty in predicting who will use and who will pay for drugs to prevent cataract may explain at least in part why few pharmaceutical companies are trying to develop anticataract drugs. In the mid-1970s Dr Carl Kupfer, Director of the National Eye Institute, expressed his concern (unpublished) that drugs with anticataract potential might be produced by the pharmaceutical industry before clinical methods were available to test their efficacy. Nearly 20 years later the methods for measuring cataract growth rates are available throughout the world, and few drugs have been forthcoming. Formerly, medical treatment of cataract was viewed as a less expensive alternative than surgery, but it is no longer obvious that this is true today.

Trial design and endpoint selection

It is essential to select one primary endpoint as a measure of efficacy of anticataract effect. Secondary endpoints may be used as well, but the results of a trial are usually based on a key endpoint designated before the trial begins. There is no shortage of potential endpoints to serve as measures of cataract severity. They are listed below. The challenge is to select one, and only one, that will possess sufficient sensitivity to avoid a lengthy and costly trial. The advantage of high sensitivity might be offset by the disadvantage of limited power to predict subsequent deterioration in visual function. The predictive power of individual measures of cataract risk is unknown, but it is now possible to begin gathering these data.

The technical complexity of film-derived measures of lens opacification (for example 'pixel density' for nuclear cataract, and 'area pixels opaque' for cortical and subcapsular cataract) has frustrated some attempts to use changes in these endpoints to predict subsequent cataract formation. The improved simplicity of digital counterparts of these measures undoubtedly will simplify the definition of the predictive power of these endpoints. Not only are sensitive methods to predict subsequent cataract formation needed, but methods to predict changes in visual function are also necessary.

Although Snellen, and more recently logMAR, measures of high contrast visual acuity continue to be used as an index of cataract severity in clinical practice (for example the need to have decreased visual acuity to 20/50 or less in order to qualify for cataract surgery in many Health Maintenance Organization plans), there is less reliance on this index in clinical cataract research.

Visual function, contrast sensitivity function, glare disability, the National Eye Institute Visual Function Questionnaire score, and other questionnaire scores have all been used as measures of cataract severity. The questionnaire scores are recommended as valid, sensitive measures of significant cataract-related visual dysfunction. The potential impact of a drug with a significant effect on a questionnaire score might be more easily understood by patients considering alternatives to cataract surgery, but a trial demonstrating such an effect might be lengthy and costly.

Ordinal, subjective, cataract classification scores, such as lens opacity classification system version II scores, are less sensitive to significant changes in cataract severity than are objective measures of cataract, so these types of cataract classification systems will probably not be used in clinical trials. If they were, the trial cost and length would be too high.

Continuous, subjective, cataract classification scores, such as lens opacity classification system version III scores, have been shown to be valid measures of cataract change. Lens opacity classification system version III can detect a change in cataract classification in a 1-year period. It is probably less sensitive than some of the objective measures of cataract, but it may be easier to interpret a significant change in lens opacity classification system version III to a patient than a significant change in a more sensitive objective measure.

Continuous objective measures of cataract include measures of pixel density for nuclear cataract, and areas of pixel opacification for cortical and posterior subcapsular cataract opacification. The density or areal measures are derived from digital images of the lens.

Continuous objective measures of light scattering, from a photometer or a quasi-elastic measure of light scattering device, are probably the most sensitive detectors of increased light scattering in the lens. The ability of such changes in light scattering to predict subsequent clinical cataract formation has not yet been demonstrated.

Statistical and clinical significance levels

The focus needs to be on clinical rather than statistical significance. While the ability to base a prediction of eventual visual dysfunction on one of the highly sensitive measures of cataract is lacking, there will be some difficulty defining the clinical significance of a clinical trial result. Statistical significance involves a decision is a to whether one chooses a P-value of 0.01 or 0.05 to define the critical level of statistical significance. This is more a practical decision than a scientific one. With no limits on time and cost, the 0.01 level would be chosen, but striving to achieve this may require impossibly long patient compliance and larger budgets than most sponsors can afford.

Drug (or non-drug) manufacture

Manufacture of anticataract drugs will be by pharmaceutical companies. It is highly unlikely that governments or charitable agencies will become involved in this area. In order to offset the costs of anticataract drug development, manufacture, and distribution, companies will need patent protection, guaranteed markets, and sufficient profits to sustain such an effort. The difficulty in predicting patient compliance with such a drug is preventing vigorous pharmaceutical involvement in this area. For example, if a drug was effective in slowing, but not preventing a cataract, would the use of an anticataract drug simply delay the time of cataract surgery thereby increasing the total cost of cataract care? For long-lived patients this would be true; for those who died not needing cataract surgery, the total cost of cataract care might be less.

Postmarketing monitoring

Following the introduction of an anticataract drug, ophthalmologists and optometrists will have to monitor patients for therapeutic and possible adverse effects. Monitoring for therapeutic efficacy might prove to be a challenge for eye care specialists not trained in cataract measurement methods. It should prove less of a problem to detect adverse effects.

Role of public and private health programmes

As in vaccination and vitamin A supplementation programmes, governmental health programmes might have to assume responsibility for directing such programmes, since there would be little if any profit potential to attract industry to assume this important role. However, if drugs are developed and applied, the role of public health programmes might be more in the area of support, and in the assessment of outcomes, than in the area of distribution.

Role of international organizations

Organizations such as the WHO and the World Bank may have to play a more active role in organizing and coordinating national efforts in these areas, simply because in many countries international, not national, resources are needed to address these problems.

Summary and conclusion

A non-surgical treatment for age-related cataract is not only a reasonable alternative to surgery, it also may be a matter of necessity in the United States as the availability of cataract surgeons and funds to pay for cataract surgery are further decreased. It is already a matter of necessity in the developing world, since it is unlikely that surgical resources there will ever be sufficient to meet the ever-increasing need for surgical care.

Further reading

Alberti, G., Oguni, M., Podfor, M., et al. (1996). Glutathione-S-transferase-M1 genotype and age-related cataracts. Lack of association in an Italian population. Investigative Ophthalmology and Visual Science, 37, 1167–73.

Azuma, M., Fukiage, C., David, L.L., and Shearer, T.R. (1997). Activation of calpain in lens: a review and proposed mechanism. Experimental Eye Research, 64, 529–38.

Benedek, G.B. (1997). Cataract as a protein condensation disease. The Proctor Lecture. Investigative Ophthalmology and Visual Science, 38, 1911–21.

Black, R.L., Oglesby, R.B., von Sallman, L., et al. (1960). The occurrence of posterior subcapsular cataracts in patients with rheumatoid arthritis treated with corticosteroids. Arthritis and Rheumatology, 3, 432–3.

Chatterjee, A., Milton, R.C., and Thyle, S. (1982). Prevalence and aetiology of cataract in Punjab. British Journal of Ophthalmology, 66, 35–42.

Chew, E.Y., Williams, G.A., Burton, T.C., Barton, F.B., Remaley, N.A., and Ferris, F.L. (1992). Aspirin effects on the development of cataracts in patients with diabetes mellitus. Early treatment diabetic retinopathy study report 16. Archives of Ophthalmology, 110, 339–42.

Chiang, Y.P., Bassi, L.B., and Javitt, J.C. (1992). Federal budgetary costs of blindness. Milbank Quarterly, 70, 319–40.

Christen, W.G., Glynn, R.J., and Hennekens, C.H. (1996). Antioxidants and age-related eye disease. Current and future perspectives. Annals of Epidemiology, 6, 60–6.

Chylack, L.T. Jr and Friend, J. (1990). Intermediary metabolism of the lens. A historical perspective, 1928–1989. Experimental Eye Research, 50, 575–82.

Chylack, L.T. Jr, Wolfe, J.K., Singer, D.M., et al. and the LSC Study Group (1993). The lens opacities classification system, version III (LOCS III). Archives of Ophthalmology, 111, 831–6.

Chylack, L.T. Jr, Wolfe, J.K., Friend, J., et al. (1995). Validation of methods for the assessment of cataract progression in the Roche European-American Anticataract Trial (REACT). *Ophthalmic Epidemiology*, **2**, 59–75.

Duhaiman, A.S. (1995). Glycation of human lens proteins from diabetic and (nondiabetic) senile cataract patients. *Glycoconjugate Journal*, **12**, 618–21.

Ederer, F., Hiller, R., and Taylor, H.R. (1981). Senile lens changes and diabetes in two population studies. *American Journal of Ophthalmology*, **91**, 381–95.

Ferris, F.L. (Principal Investigator). *Age-related Eye Disease Study*. National Eye Institute, National Institutes of Health, Bethesda, MD.

Glynn, R.J., Christen, W.G., Manson, J.E., Bernheimer, J., and Hennekens, C.H. (1995). Body mass index. An independent predictor of cataract. *Archives of Ophthalmology*, **113**, 1131–7.

Hankinson, S.E., Stampfer, M.J., Seddon, J.M., *et al.* (1992). Nutrient intake and cataract extraction in women: a prospective study. *British Medical Journal*, **305**, 335–9.

Hankinson, S.E., Seddon, J.M., Colditz, G.A., *et al.* (1993). A prospective study of aspirin use and cataract extraction in women. *Archives of Ophthalmology*, **111**, 503–8.

Harding, J.J. and Rixon, K.C. (1980). Carbamylation of lens proteins. A possible factor in cataractogenesis in some tropical countries. *Experimental Eye Research*, **31**, 567–71.

Harding, J.J. and van Heyningen, R. (1988). Drugs, including alcohol, that act as risk factors for cataract, and possible protection against cataract by aspirin-like analgesics and cyclopenthiazide. *British Journal of Ophthalmology*, **72**, 809–14.

Heiba, I.M., Elston, R.C., Klein, B.E., and Klein, R. (1995). Evidence for a major gene for cortical cataract. *Investigative Ophthalmology and Visual Science*, **36**, 227–35.

Hiller, R., Sperduto, R.D., and Ederer, F. (1983). Epidemiologic associations with cataract in the 1971–1972 National Health and Nutrition Examination Survey. *American Journal of Epidemiology*, **118**, 239–49.

Hirvela, H., Luukinen, H., and Laatikainen, L. (1995). Prevalence and risk factors of lens opacities in the elderly in Finland. A population-based study. *Ophthalmology*, **102**, 108–17.

Hodge, W.G., Whitcher, J.P., and Satariano, W. (1995). Risk factors for age-related cataract. *Epidemiology Review*, **17**, 336–46.

Horwitz, J. (1992). Alpha-crystallin can function as a molecular chaperone. *Proceedings of the National Academy of Science USA*, 89, 10 449–53.

Hu, T.S., Zhen, Q., Sperduto, R.D., Zhao, J.L., Milton, R.C., and Nakajima, A. (1989). Age-related cataract in the Tibet Eye Study. *Archives of Ophthalmology*, **107**, 666–9.

Jacques, P.F., Chylack, L.T. Jr, McGandy, R.B., and Hartz, S.C. (1988). Antioxidant status in persons with and without senile cataract. *Archives of Ophthalmology*, **106**, 337–40.

Javitt, J.C. (1993). The cost-effectiveness of restoring sight. *Archives of Ophthalmology*, **111**, 1615.

Javitt, J.C. (1994). Measuring the benefit and value of services. *Archives of Ophthalmology*, **112**, 32.

Jedziniak, J.A., Chylack, L.T. Jr, Cheng, H.M., Gillis, M.K., Kalustian, A.A., and Tung, W.H. (1981). The sorbitol pathway in the human lens: aldose reductase and polyol dehydrogenase. *Investigative Ophthalmology and Visual Science*, **20**, 314–26.

Kador, P.F. (1983). Overview of the current attempts toward the medical treatment of cataract. *Ophthalmology*, **90**, 352–64.

Kahn, H.A., Leibowitz, H.M., Ganley, J.P., *et al.* (1977). The Framingham Eye Study. I. Outline and major prevalence findings. *American Journal of Epidemiology*, **106**, 17–32.

Klein, B.E. and Klein, R. (1982). Cataracts and macular degeneration in older Americans. *Archives of Ophthalmology*, **100**, 571–3.

Klein, B.E., Klein, R., Jensen, S.C., and Linton, K.L. (1995). Hypertension and lens opacities fro the Beaver Dam Eye Study. *American Journal of Epidemiology*, **19**, 640–6.

Kupfer, C. (1985). Bowman Lecture. The conquest of cataract: a global challenge. *Transactions of the Ophthalmology Society UK*, **104**, 1–10.

Lee, P.P., Jackson, C.A., and Relles, D.A. (1995). Estimating eye care workforce supply and requirements. *Ophthalmology*, **102**, 1964–71.

Leske, M.C., Chylack, L.T. Jr, and Wu, S.-Y. (1991). The lens opacities case-control study. Risk factors for cataract. *Archives of Ophthalmology*, **109**, 244–51.

Leske, M.C., Wu, S.-Y., Hyman, L., *et al.*, and the Lens Opacities Case–Control Study Group (1995). Biochemical factors in the Lens Opacities Case–Control Study. *Archives of Ophthalmology*, **113**, 1113–19.

Leske, M.C., Chylack, L.T. Jr, Wu, S.-Y., *et al.* (1996). Incidence and progression of nuclear opacities in the longitudinal study of cataract. *Ophthalmology*, **103**, 705–12.

Leske, M.C., Chylack, L.T. Jr, Qimei, H., *et al.* and the LSC Group (1997). Incidence and progression of cortical and posterior subcapsular opacities. *Ophthalmology*, **104**, 1987–93.

Li, J.Y., Li, B., Blot, W.J., and Taylor, P.R. (1993). Preliminary report on the results of nutrition prevention trials of cancer and other common diseases among residents in Linxian, China. *Chung Hua Chung Liu Tsa Chih*, **15**, 165–81.

Lund, A.L., Smith, J.B., and Smith, D.L. (1996). Modification of the water-insoluble human lens alpha-crystallins. *Experimental Eye Research*, **63**, 661–72.

Luthra, M., Ranganathan, D., Ranganathan, S., and Balasubramanian, D. (1994). Racemizatrion of tyrosine in the insoluble protein fraction of brunescent aging human lenses. *Journal of Biological Chemistry*, **269**, 22 678–82.

Mangione, C.M., Orav, E.J., Lawrence, M.G., Phillips, R.S., Seddon, J.M., and Goldman L. (1995) Prediction of visual function after cataract surgery. A prospectively validated model. *Archives of Ophthalmology*, **113**, 1305–11.

Minassian, D.C., Mehra, V., and Jones, B.R. (1984). Dehydrational crises from severe diarrhea or heat stroke and risk of cataract. *Lancet*, **1**, 751–3.

Muñoz, B., Tajchman, U., Bochow, T., and West, S. (1993). Alcohol use and risk of posterior subcapsular opacities. *Archives of Ophthalmology*, **111**, 110–12.

Naeser, K., Hansen, T.E., and Nielsen, N.E. (1990). Visual outcome and complications following extracapsular cataract extraction. A prospective, controlled follow-up study. *Acta Ophthalmologica (Copenhagen)*, **68**, 733–8.

Pelli, D.G., Robson, J.G., and Wilkins, A.J. (1988). The design of a new letter chart for measuring contrast sensitivity. *Clinics of Vision Science*, **2**, 187–99.

Rao, G.N., Lardis, M.P., and Cotlier, E. (1985). Acetylation of lens crystallins: a possible mechanism by which aspirin could prevent cataract formation. *Biochemistry and Biophysics Research Communications*, **128**, 1125–32.

Roberts, K.A. and Harding, J.J. (1990). Ibuprofen, a putative anticataract drug, protects the lens against cyanate and galactose. *Experimental Eye Research*, **50**, 157–64.

Robertson, J.M., Donner, A.P., and Trevethick, J.R. (1990). Vitamin E intake and risk of cataracts in humans. *Annals of New York Academy of Science*, **503**, 372–82.

Rouhiainen, P., Rouhiainen, H., and Salonen, J.T. (1996). Association between low plasma vitamin E concentration and progression of early cortical lens opacities. *American Journal of Epidemiology*, **144**, 496–500.

Schmitt, C. and Hockwin, O. (1990). The mechanisms of cataract formation. *Journal of Inherited Metabolic Disease*, **13**, 501–8.

Seddon, J.M., Christen, W.G., Manson, J.E., Buring, J.E., Sperduto, R.D., and Hennekens, C.H. (1991). Low-dose aspirin and risks of cataract in a randomized trial of US physicians. *Archives of Ophthalmology*, **109**, 252–5.

Sekine, Y., Hommura, S., and Harada, S. (1995). Frequency of glutathione-*S*-transferase-1 gene deletion and its possible correlation with cataract formation. *Experimental Eye Research*, **60**, 159–63.

Singh, D.P., Guru, S.C., Kikuchi, T., Abe, T., and Shinohara, T. (1995). Autoantibodies against β-crystallins induces lens epithelial cell damage and cataract formation in mice. *Journal of Immunology*, **155**, 993–9.

Spaeth, G.I. and von Sallman, L. (1966). Corticosteroids and cataracts. *International Ophthalmology Clinics*, **6**, 915–28.

Spector, A. (1995). Oxidative stress induced cataract: mechanism of action. *FASEB J*, **9**, 1173–82.

Spector, A., Ma, W., Wang, R.-R., and Kleiman, N. (1997) Microperoxidases catalytically degrade reactive oxygen species and may be anti-cataract agents. *Experimental Eye Research*, **65**, 457–70.

Steinberg, E.P., Javitt, J.C., Sharkey, P.D., *et al.* (1993). The content and cost of cataract surgery. *Archives of Ophthalmology*, **111**, 1041–9.

Sueno, T., Inoue, E., Singh, D.P., Awata, T., Chylack, L.T. Jr, and Shinohara, T. (1997). Oral administration of lens homogenate suppresses antibody production in mice injected with β-crystallin emulsified in CFA. *Experimental Eye Research*, **64**, 379–85.

Takemoto, L.J. (1997). Disulfide bond formation of cysteine-37 and cysteine-66 of beta B2 crystallin during cataractogenesis of the human lens. *Experimental Eye Research*, **64**, 609–14.

Tavani, A., Negri, E., and LaVecchia, C. (1995). Selected diseases and risk of cataract. A case–control study from northern Italy. *Annals of Epidemiology*, **5**, 234–8.

Tavani, A., Negri, E., and LaVecchia, C. (1996). Food and nutrient intake and risk of cataract. *Annals of Epidemiology*, **6**, 41–6.

Thylefors, B., Negrel, A.D., Pararajasegaram, R., and Dadzie, K.Y. (1995). Available data on blindness (update 1994). *Ophthalmological Epidemiology*, **2**, 5–39.

Trobe, J.D. and Kilpatrick, K.E. (1983). Ophthalmology manpower: shortfall or windfall? *Survey of Ophthalmology*, **27**, 271–5.

Urbak, S.F. and Naeser, K. (1993). Retinal detachment following intracapsular and extracapsular cataract erxtraction. A comparative, retrospective follow-up study. *Acta Ophthalmologica (Copenhagen)*, **71**, 782–6.

Wang, F. and Javitt, J.C. (1996). Eye care for elderly Americans with diabetes mellitus. Failure to meet current guidelines. *Ophthalmology*, **103**, 1744–50.

Wang, G.M., Raghavachari, N., and Lou, M.F. (1997). Relationship of protein–glutathione mixed disulfide and thioltransferase in H_2O_2-induced cataract in cultured pig lens. *Experimental Eye Research*, **64**, 693–700.

West, S.K. and Valmadrid, C.T. (1995). Epidemiology of risk factors for age-related cataract. *Survey of Ophthalmology*, **39**, 323–34.

West, S.K., Muñoz, B.E., Newland, H.S., Emmett, E.A., and Taylor, H.R. (1987). Lack of evidence for aspirin use and prevention of cataracts. *Archives of Ophthalmology*, **105**, 1229–31.

Wolfe, J.K., Friend, J., Singer, D.M., and Chylack, L.T. Jr (1994). Assessment of the ability of methods of measuring cataract to detect clinically significant change. *Ophthalmic Research*, **26**, 55–60.

World Bank (1995). *The essential package of health services in developing countries. The minimum package of health services: criteria, methods and data.* The World Bank, February 14.

World Health Organization (1997a). *Blindness and visual disability—Part V of VII: Seeing ahead—projections into the next century.* WHO Fact sheet no. 146, February.

World Health Organization (1997b). *WHO sounds the alarm: visual disability to double by 2020.* Press Release WHO, no. 15, 21 February.

2.8 Uvea

2.8.1 Anatomy and physiology of the uveal tract

Jane M. Olver and A. Sharma

The uveal tract is the middle layer of the three eye-coats, with the outer sclera and inner retina. It is a continuous, highly vascular, pigmented layer consisting of the iris, ciliary body, and choroid. Each part of the uvea has defined specialist functions (Table 1). In order to understand the functions of the uvea, it is important to understand the anatomy.

The eviscerated eye, with the uvea surrounding the retina, lens, and vitreous, has the appearance of a grape, hence the term uvea (*uva* is Latin for grape).

Iris

Anatomy

Macroscopic anatomy

The iris forms the anterior part of the uveal tract. It is a thin disc forming a diaphragm approximately 12 mm diameter in front of the lens and ciliary body, separating the aqueous in the anterior chamber from that in the smaller posterior chamber. It extends from its root at the anterior chamber angle where it is attached loosely to the ciliary spur, to the edge of the pupil, its central opening. The pupil lies just inferonasal to its centre. The iris is thinnest at its root. Its posterior surface is supported in part by contact with the anterior lens capsule.

There are two zones visible on its anterior surface, separated by a wavy circumferential ridge, the collarette: (a) the central pupillary zone (1.5 mm wide) with a flattish surface, and (b) the wider peripheral ciliary zone with radial interlacing ridges.

Microscopic anatomy

There are two main layers: (a) the anterior stroma (mesodermal origin), consisting of the anterior border layer and the deep stroma; and (b) the pigmented epithelium (neuroectoderm origin) consisting of bilayered cuboidal epithelium cells with adjacent apices (Fig. 1).

The anterior border layer consists of loose collagen, fibroblasts, and melanocytes. It has an incomplete surface layer of flattened connective tissue, which is absent in Fuchs' crypts. It may contain aggregates of pigmented melanocytes, recognized on the slit lamp as naevi. The anterior border layer is partially atrophic in the pupillary zone.

The stroma forms the bulk of the iris tissue and is found in both the pupillary and ciliary zones. It consists of loose connective tissue around radial blood vessels and nerves, with pigmented and non-pigmented cells. The capillaries are non-fenestrated and their endothelium has tight junctions (zonulae occludens).

Table 1 Functions of the uvea

Iris	*Aquecus*	*Pupils*
	Blood–aqueous barrier	Regulates light entry
	Aqueous humour circulation	Alters depth focus near
	Aqueous drainage (uveoscleral outflow)	Minimizes optical aberrations
	Maintains eye shape	
Ciliary body	*Aqueous*	*Lens*
	Blood–aqueous barrier	Zonule formation
	Aqueous humour formation	Accommodation
	Aqueous drainage (uveoscleral outflow)	
Choroid	*High blood flow and large surface area*	
	Nutrition outer retina	Heat dissipation
	Removal metabolic products	Absorption light
	Immune cells	Visible pigmentation
	Maintains intraocular pressure	

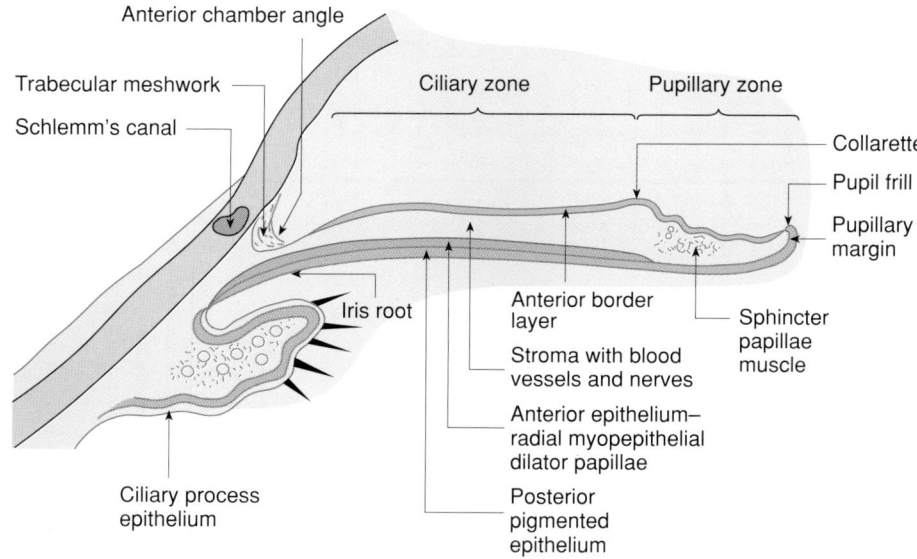

Fig. 1 Microscopic anatomy of the iris. The posterior pigmented epithelium is bathed by posterior chamber aqueous and is partly in contact with the anterior lens capsule. Note that there is a switch in location of the pigmented epithelium from iris to ciliary body.

The sphincter pupillae muscle (neuroectoderm origin) is a 1 mm wide annulus of true smooth muscle located in the posterior stroma in the pupillary zone.

The pigmented epithelium has an anterior and a posterior layer. The anterior layer of cells contain radial myoepithelial extensions which form the dilator pupillae. The dilator cells extend from the iris root to the sphincter muscle, with the myofilaments attaching to the posterior iris stroma. The myoepithelial cells are regarded as incompletely differentiated smooth muscle cells. This layer is only lightly pigmented. It is continuous with the outer layer of pigmented epithelium of the ciliary processes.

The posterior pigmented epithelium consists of cuboidal cells densely packed with melanin. This layer extends to the pupillary ruff. Their apices face the anterior epithelial layer and their basement membrane lies on the lenticular surface. The basement membrane is in continuation posteriorly with that of the ciliary body. This layer is continuous posteriorly with the inner non-pigmented epithelium of the ciliary processes, that is there is a big switch in the location of pigmentation between the iris and ciliary processes.

Iris colour

The iris colour is from melanin in the anterior border layer. The pigmented epithelium provides only some bluish colour. Neonates have light blue irides because the unpigmented iris preferentially absorbs longer wavelength light.

Blood supply

The blood supply of the iris is centripetal by radial iris arterioles from the partially overlapping segments of the major arterial circle at the root of the iris. The iris arterioles have a cork-screw configuration to allow for rapid changes in pupil size. The major arterial circle is supplied from the two long posterior ciliary arteries and more numerous anterior ciliary arteries. There is a sectoral blood supply, based upon the long posterior ciliary arteries horizontally and the vertical ciliary arteries superiorly and inferiorly, with potential deep and superficial anastomoses between the four sectors (Fig. 2). The radial iris arterioles anastomose at the collarette to form the minor arterial circle.

Nerve supply

The autonomic nervous system supplies the iris which is richly innervated by a short ciliary nerve (cranial nerve III) and by two long ciliary nerves (cranial nerve V1).

The sphincter pupillae muscle is under parasympathetic control from cholinergic fibres from the Edinger-Westphal nucleus of the oculomotor nerve, which synapse in the ciliary ganglion and are distributed in the short posterior ciliary nerves. The dilator pupillae is under sympathetic control along the long posterior ciliary nerves. There is an adrenergic (sympathetic) supply to the iris arterioles via the short posterior ciliary nerves.

Physiology

Aqueous functions

Blood–aqueous barrier

The tight junctions between iris capillary endothelial cells form a barrier to free diffusion of molecules, including water and ions. Lipid soluble substances such as oxygen and carbon dioxide can pass through easily. Metabolic substrates have to be transported by active carriers across these cells. Under normal conditions, iris fluorescein angiography demonstrates little leakage of fluorescein even though fluorescein is highly water soluble.

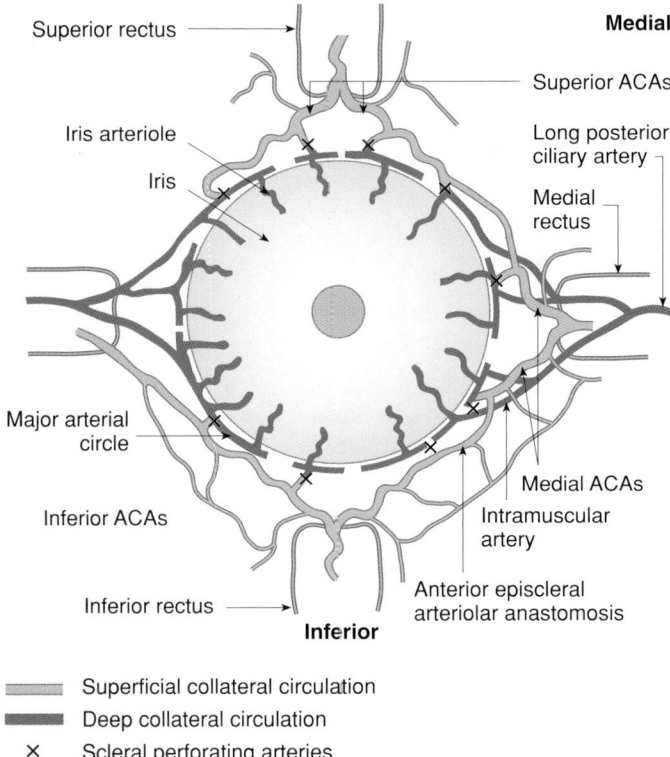

Superior rectus

Iris arteriole

Iris

Medial

Superior ACAs

Long posterior
ciliary artery

Medial
rectus

Major arterial
circle

Inferior ACAs

Medial ACAs

Intramuscular
artery

Inferior rectus

Anterior episcleral
arteriolar anastomosis

Inferior

━━━ Superficial collateral circulation
━━━ Deep collateral circulation
  ×   Scleral perforating arteries

Fig. 2 The blood supply of the anterior segment of the human eye is from anterior ciliary arteries (superficial) and long posterior ciliary arteries (deep). The superficial and deep collateral circulations are linked by several scleral perforating arteries.

Trauma and inflammation causes the blood–aqueous barrier to break down, with resultant cells and protein leaking into the aqueous. This may be seen clinically as aqueous flare and cells using the slit lamp. Ocular fluorophotometry can be used to measure even small permeability increases of the blood–aqueous barrier.

Aqueous humour circulation
The aqueous is formed by the ciliary processes and circulates from the posterior chamber through the pupil into the anterior chamber. The heat of the iris and the cooler corneal posterior surface causes aqueous convection currents in the anterior chamber.

Aqueous drainage (uveoscleral outflow)
The major aqueous outflow is through the trabecular meshwork into Schlemm's canal and the episcleral vessels. Minor aqueous outflow (10–20 per cent) occurs at the root of the iris, through the ciliary body to the suprachoroidal space, the uveoscleral route.

Pupil functions

Regulation light entry
The pupil is small in the newborn, largest in young children, and gradually diminishing again into older age. Physiological anisocoria of 0.4 to 1.0 mm in dim light occurs in almost

20 per cent of the adult population, but is only noticeable in 4 per cent. With pharmacological agents the pupil size can range from 1 to 9 mm in an adult: normally it has a range of 2 to 4 mm which regulates the amount of light entering the eye.

Light causes miosis of the pupil with a similar constriction occurring in both pupils (direct and consensual light response). The afferent part of the light reflex is via retinal ganglion cells, optic nerve, optic chiasm, optic tract to the pretectal nucleus relaying in the Edinger–Westphal nucleus. Parasympathetic efferent fibres pass to the third nerve nucleus and leave the brainstem in the third cranial nerve, synapse in the ciliary ganglion, and run in the short posterior ciliary nerves which supply the sphincter pupillae muscle.

The amount of miosis depends on factors including retinal adaptation, intensity of light, emotional status, and age of the subject. Miosis also occurs as part of the near reflex.

Depth of focus and optical aberrations
Miosis increases the depth of focus, and reduces spherical and chromatic aberrations. Conversely, a dilated pupil increases spherical and chromatic aberrations. An example is that of night-induced myopia which many myopic subjects find makes night driving uncomfortable.

Ciliary body

Anatomy

Macroscopic anatomy
The ciliary body is an annular structure extending from the ora serrata posteriorly, to the scleral spur anteriorly, over approximately 5 to 6 mm. The scleral surface of the ciliary body is the suprachoroid (lamina fusca) and its inner surface is adjacent to the anterior vitreous cavity, the posterior chamber, and lens equator. It is triangular on section, with the apex posterior and base anterior. It is divided into two zones, the posterior pars plana (orbiculus ciliaris) 4 mm wide and the anterior pars plicata (corona ciliaris) 2 mm wide. The posterior margin is scalloped to correspond with the anterior margin of the sensory retina. The pars plicata is functionally the most important zone since its 60 to 80 radiating ridges (ciliary processes) form the aqueous humour. Each ciliary process is 0.5 to 0.8 mm high and 0.5 mm wide, with minor ciliary processes found between the larger ones. The zonule fibres which support the lens arise from the ciliary process crypts and pars plana ciliary epithelium.

Microscopic anatomy
The ciliary body is divided microscopically into three parts (a) stroma, (b) epithelium, and (c) muscle. The stroma (mesenchyme origin) is a loose net of connective tissue in which the ciliary muscle intermingles. It contains blood vessels with fenestrated capillary endothelium and cells including melanocytes, fibroblasts and mast cells, macrophages and lymphocytes.

The ciliary epithelium (neuroectoderm origin) consists of

two layers of cuboidal epithelium lying apex to apex over the entire inner aspect of the ciliary body. The inner non-pigmented epithelium is continuous with the retinal nerve layer posteriorly and the posterior pigmented iris epithelium anteriorly. The basement membrane of the inner layer is continuous with the internal limiting membrane of the retina.

The non-pigmented epithelium cells contain many organelles for secretory function; Golgi apparatus, rough endoplasmic reticulum, and mitochondria. There are tight junctions between the apices of the non-pigmented epithelium but not between the non-pigmented epithelium and outer layer of pigmented epithelium. The zonule fibres arise from non-pigmented epithelium cells lying in the crypts between the ciliary processes and from the ciliary epithelium extending back to the ora serrata.

The pigmented epithelium is continuous with the retinal pigment epithelium posteriorly and its basement membrane continuous with that of the retinal pigment epithelium. The cells contain numerous organelles indicating some metabolic activity, and many melanosomes. There are no tight junctions between pigmented epithelium cells in the outer layer, only gap junctions.

Each ciliary process contains a central vascular core of fenestrated capillaries surrounded by the two layers of ciliary epithelium (Fig. 3).

The ciliary muscle consists of three groups of interwoven smooth muscle—longitudinal, circular, and oblique—and forms the bulk of the uveal portion of the ciliary body adjacent to the sclera. The outer longitudinal fibres (Brucke's muscle)

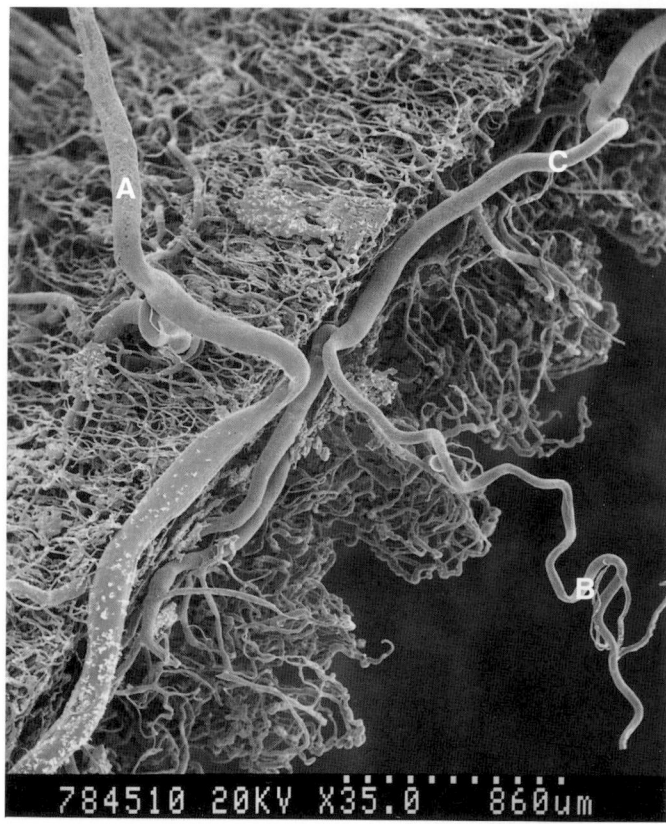

Fig. 4 Scanning electron photomicrograph of part of a corrosion cast of the human anterior uvea. It shows a scleral perforating artery (A), part of the incomplete major arterial circle (MAC) at the root of the iris, and a corkscrew-shaped iris arteriole (B). The vascular cores of the ciliary processes are seen in the background supplied by branches from the major arterial circle (C). The ciliary muscle vasculature is upper left.

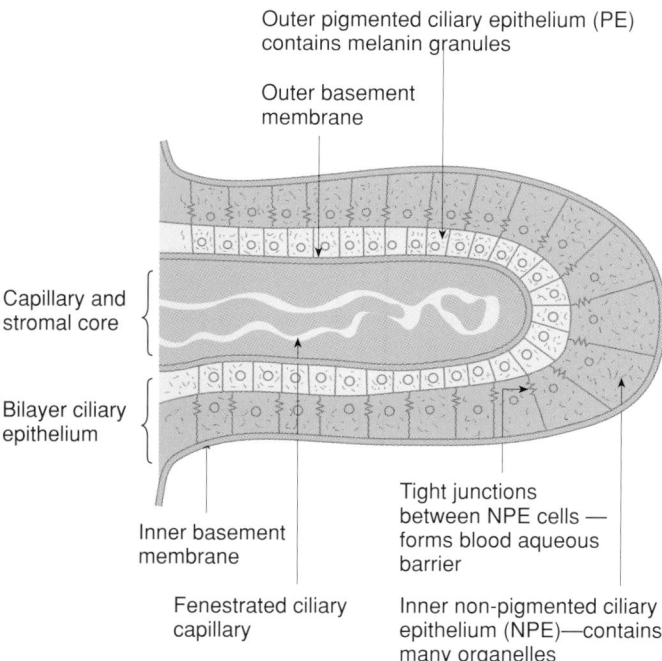

Outer pigmented ciliary epithelium (PE) contains melanin granules

Outer basement membrane

Capillary and stromal core

Bilayer ciliary epithelium

Inner basement membrane

Fenestrated ciliary capillary

Tight junctions between NPE cells — forms blood aqueous barrier

Inner non-pigmented ciliary epithelium (NPE)—contains many organelles

Fig. 3 Microscopic anatomy of a ciliary process. Each of the 60 to 80 ciliary processes consist of a vascular core covered by two layers of highly specialized epithelium.

run parallel to the sclera, extending from the choroidal stroma at the ora serrata to the scleral spur. Contraction pulls the anterior choroid and ciliary body forwards. The inner circular muscle (Müller's muscle) are parallel to the lens equator; contraction pulls the ciliary body centripetally which relaxes the zonules and allows the lens to accommodate. The middle oblique fibres run radially from the scleral spur and their contraction may facilitate aqueous outflow.

Blood supply

The long posterior ciliary and anterior ciliary arteries form the intermuscular arteries (within the ciliary muscle) and major arterial circle, branches of which supply the ciliary body (Fig. 4).

Venous drainage

Venous drainage of the ciliary muscle is in part to the episcleral veins whilst the ciliary processes drain solely to the vortex veins.

Nerve supply

Parasympathetic nerve supply from the Edinger–Westphal nucleus is via the third cranial nerve, synapsing in the ciliary ganglion and travelling to the eye in the short ciliary nerves.

Sympathetic nerves synapse in the superior cervical ganglion, fibres travel mainly via the nasociliary nerve (cranial nerve Va), pass through the ciliary ganglion without synapse, then reach the ciliary body via the short ciliary nerves.

Physiology

Aqueous functions

Blood–aqueous barrier

The blood–aqueous barrier in the ciliary body is formed by the tight junctions between adjacent inner non-pigmented epithelial cells. These junctions are lipid soluble, allow O_2, and carbon dioxide, to pass through easily whilst sodium ions, larger molecules, and proteins cannot. These tight junctions are leaky as they will allow low molecular weight ions and solutes to pass through; the pore size for the blood–aqueous barrier is 104 nm.

There are no tight junctions between the bilayered epithelial cells or between adjacent outer pigmented epithelium cells and since the ciliary process capillaries are fenestrated (300–1000 nm) they do not contribute to the blood–aqueous barrier.

Aqueous humour formation

Aqueous is formed by the non-pigmented epithelium of the ciliary processes at a rate of approximately 2.5 µl/min. It is formed by cells on the anterior crests of the processes (non-pigmented epithelium cells lying in the crypts between processes are concerned with zonule fibres). Three mechanism combine to produce aqueous (a) active secretion (70 per cent), (b) passive diffusional exchange, and (c) ultrafiltration.

Active secretion of aqueous depends on two enzyme-mediated processes in the non-pigmented epithelium. N^+/K^+ adenosine triphosphatase pump, in lateral cellular interdigitations, creates an Na^+ concentration gradient that produces an osmotic flow of water. (This system can be poisoned by ouabain.)

Carbonic anhydrase (inhibited by acetazolomide) creates electrochemical neutrality by H^+ and HCO_3^- production which further augments the osmotic gradient and aqueous flow. Adenylate cyclase (stimulated by adrenergic agents) inhibits aqueous formation by raising cyclic adenosine monophosphate level. β-Blockers reduce cyclic adenosine monophosphate mediated NA^+/K^+ adenosine triphosphatase function in non-pigmented epithelium and thereby diminishes aqueous production.

Ultrafiltration of plasma into the aqueous is a less important mechanism in which the capillary hydrostatic pressure exceeds the oncotic pressure.

The aqueous humour is optically clear and colourless. It is important for ocular metabolism. It nourishes the lens and posterior cornea with O_2 and amino acids, and removes waste products of metabolism such as lactate and carbon dioxide. It maintains the intraocular pressure and shape of the eye.

Aqueous drainage

The uveoscleral outflow is a minor but important route, Intraocular pressure can be reduced by prostaglandin $F_{2\alpha}$ analogues which increase uveoscleral outflow. Cholinomimetic drugs (pilocarpine) contract the longitudinal ciliary muscle which pulls the ciliary spur centripetal and posteriorly, opening the trabecular meshwork to increase aqueous trabecular outflow.

Lens zonule fibres These arise from the non-pigmented epithelium cell basement membrane forming the zonule of Zinn around 360°. They attach to the lens equator.

Accommodation When the ciliary muscle contracts the zonule fibres relax and the lens becomes more spherical, increasing its refractive power.

Choroid

Anatomy

Macroscopic anatomy

The choroid is a thin, brown, continuous membrane composed of blood vessels, melanocytes, and connective tissue. It forms the posterior part of the uveal tract and extends from the optic disc to the ora serrata. It is derived from mesoderm and neuroectoderm. There exists a potential space between the choroid and inner sclera, the suprachoroid, which may become separated in the diseased eye. The choroid at the posterior pole is thicker (0.22–0.3 mm) than in the periphery (0.1–0.15 mm).

The choroidal appearance has racial variations, being darker in pigmented races and, in the pale-skinned or albinos the choroidal, ciliary, and vortex vessels are easily seen.

Microscopic anatomy

The choroid has four layers:

1. Suprachoroid
2. Stroma with vessels—large vessels in Haller's and intermediate sized vessels in Sattler's layers
3. Choriocapillaris
4. Bruch's membrane.

Suprachoroid

The suprachoroid is the transition zone (30 µm) between the large vessel layer of the choroidal stroma and the inner layer of pigmented sclera and is traversed by numerous lamellae of melanocytes, fibroblasts, and nerve fibres. No endothelial cells or lymphatics are present in the suprachoroid. The deep brown colour of the choroid derives from the many melanocytes found in the suprachoroidal lamellae, as well as around blood vessels and in the outer choroidal stroma (where they are most dense and form an almost continuous layer). Melanocyte density is greatest near the optic nerve head.

Stroma

The stroma consists of an outer large vessel layer (Haller's) consisting of many large veins, arteries, melanocytes, and ciliary nerves. The arteries in Haller's layer have an internal elastic lamina and smooth muscle media. The medium vessel layer (Sattler's) contains many interlinked and intertwined vessels

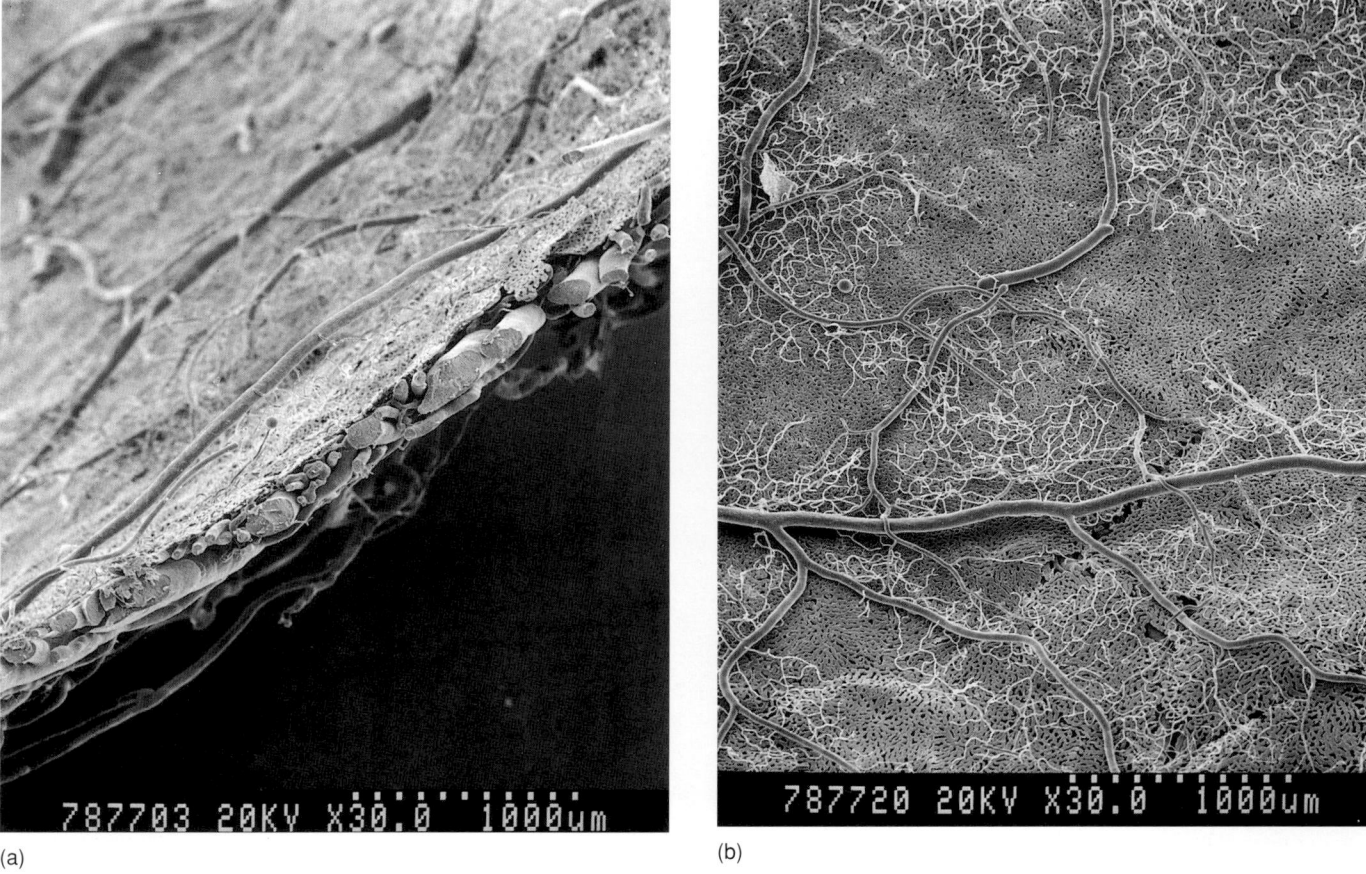

(a)

(b)

Fig. 5 (a) Scanning electron photomicrograph of a corrosion cast of human choroid cut to show a cross-section of the choroidal layers, with inner thin choriocapillaris and outer larger choroidal vessels. Remnants of the retinal vasculature are visible on the surface of the choriocapillaries; since these are corrosion casts there is no intervening tissue. (b) Retinal aspect of the choriocapillaris at the posterior pole with a retinal arteriole and residual retinal capillaries in front.

that lack fenestrations. There are interarteriolar and intervenous anastomoses in Sattler's layer, particularly at the posterior pole—choroidal arterioles supply the choriocapillaris, but are not truly endarterial because of these anastomoses.

Choriocapillaris

The choriocapillaris is a single layer of wide diameter capillaries internal to the arterioles and venules of Sattler's layer and external to Bruch's membrane. Anteriorly the choriocapillaries terminate at the ora serrata and posteriorly, end in a well-defined margin around the optic nerve head. Connective tissue lies between the choriocapillaries. The choriocapillaries are thin walled and have endothelial nuclei on their sclerad surface and many fenestrations on the retinal aspect, with only occasional pericytes present. They are flattened anteroposteriorly with an elliptical cross-section, providing a large surface area for unim-

peded metabolic exchange across Bruch's membrane (Fig. 5). The choriocapillaries at the posterior pole appear anatomically continuous when viewed from their retinal aspect, but form functional small lobules supplied by arterioles entering at right angles to the plane of the choriocapillaris and draining by several surrounding venules. Towards the equator choriocapillary lobules become anatomically more evident and spindle shaped whilst at the periphery they form obvious fan-shaped lobules, with the arterioles and venules almost parallel in the same plane as the choriocapillaries, with wider choriocapillaries with wider intercapillary tissue (Table 2). The arteriole to venule ratio changes from the posterior pole (1 to 5–7) to the periphery (1 to 1–2).

Electron microscopy has failed to show the existence of precapillary muscular sphincters, unlike capillary beds elsewhere in the body.

Table 2 Choriocapillary normal regional variation

	Lobule size (μm)	Capillary lumen diameter (μm)	Intercapillary distance (μm)
Posterior pole	200–300	16–20	5–20
Equator	300–400	20–50	20–200
Periphery	500–1000	20+	20–300

Bruch's membrane

Bruch's membrane is a thin, acellular, well-delineated zone lying between the retina and choroid. It is thickest near the disc (2–4 μm) and is an integral part of the choroid anatomically. It contains no nerve fibres. Its innermost layer is part of the retinal pigment epithelium.

Bruch's membrane has five layers on electron microscopy:

1. basement membrane of retinal pigment epithelium

2. inner collagenous zone

3. middle elastic fibre zone

4. outer collagenous zone

5. basement membrane of the choriocapillaris.

Blood supply

The blood supply of the choroid arises from posterior ciliary branches of the ophthalmic artery and is separate from the retinal circulation. Short posterior ciliary arteries are grouped in temporal and medial bundles either side of the optic nerve. Within each short posterior ciliary artery bundle there are numerous distal (away from the optic nerve) short posterior ciliary arteries which supply the choroid, and a single paraoptic (close to the optic nerve) short posterior ciliary artery which branches to form the circle of Haller or Zinn (also known as the perioptic nerve arteriolar anastomoses) (Figs 6, 7). Branches from the circle of Haller supply the peripapillary choroid and laminar/retrolaminar optic nerve.

The long posterior ciliary arteries lie within each short posterior ciliary artery bundle, then leave to pierce the sclera anterior to the short posterior ciliary arteries, travelling via the suprachoroidal space towards the ciliary body. Immediately posterior to the ciliary body they form superior and inferior branches which become intramuscular arteries, so named because they cross through the ciliary muscle to the iris root. Intermuscular arteries and perforating scleral branches of anterior ciliary arteries form the major arterial circle which supplies the iris and ciliary body. Several recurrent choroidal arteries from the anterior segment supply the anterior choroid. Intercapillary and interarteriolar anastomoses are noted between the anterior and posterior supply to the choroid.

Venous drainage

The venous drainage of the entire choroid and most of the anterior uvea is by way of the vortex veins. The vortex veins subsequently drain into the superior and inferior orbital veins which exit the orbit through the superior and inferior orbital fissures.

Nerve supply

About 20 short posterior ciliary nerves innervate the choroid. They arise from the ciliary ganglion and pierce the posterior sclera 3 to 4 mm from the optic nerve to enter the suprachoroidal space, where they lose their myelination. Extensive plexuses exist in the suprachoroid and choroid which ramify in all three dimensions. Axons terminate in the subcapillary layer and not in the choriocapillaris. They provide sensory, motor, and sympathetic fibres. The two long posterior ciliary nerves innervate the anterior part of the choroid, but are largely providing the sympathetic supply to the dilator pupillae.

Physiology

Choroidal circulation

The ocular blood flow is divided as follows:

- choroid: 85 per cent

- retina: 2 to 4 per cent

- ciliary body: 10 to 28 per cent

- iris: 1 to 5 per cent.

Choroidal vessels are similar to renal glomerular capillaries in that they have a very high flow rate, one of the highest in relation to tissue mass. Blood flow through the choroid is under autonomic control, via sympathetic fibres of the short posterior ciliary nerves. The simple relationship:

perfusion pressure = arterial pressure – venous pressure

has to be modified by a third variable, intraocular pressure. Raised intraocular pressure will drop the perfusion pressure by increasing venous pressure. A low blood pressure will reduce perfusion by decreasing arterial pressure. Retinal blood flow demonstrates almost no change with intraocular pressure and perfusion pressure changes because of local autoregulation. Autoregulation controls blood flow in the body's organs but, choroidal vessels show no autoregulation and are strongly influenced by sympathetic stimulation. Autoregulation is mediated by vasoactive substances such as carbon dioxide and adenosine diphosphate. In the eye choroidal venous saturation is relatively high (90 per cent of arterial $P\text{O}_2$) reflecting the high choroidal blood flow—only 5 to 10 per cent of oxygen is extracted during passage through the eye. Reduced blood flow increases O_2 extraction with little change in venous $P\text{CO}_2$ because of the relatively low metabolic rate of the uvea. This explains the lack of autoregulation in the choroidal circulation.

Nutrition of the outer retina

The choroidal circulation provides O_2 and nutrients to the outer retina. The wide diameter flattened choriocapillaries provide a large surface area for metabolic exchange with the retinal pigment epithelium. The retinal surface of the choroidal capillaries is further adapted anatomically for unimpeded metabolic exchange by location of endothelial nuclei on the sclerad surface. The breadth of the choriocapillaries allows between three and seven red blood cells to pass without being deformed. The choroidal circulation is a very 'leaky' system and transport systems are not required for essential substances. This leakiness is well demonstrated by the high permeability to fluorescein on angiography. Indocyanine green, being highly protein bound, remains intravascular and highlights the choroidal circulations well.

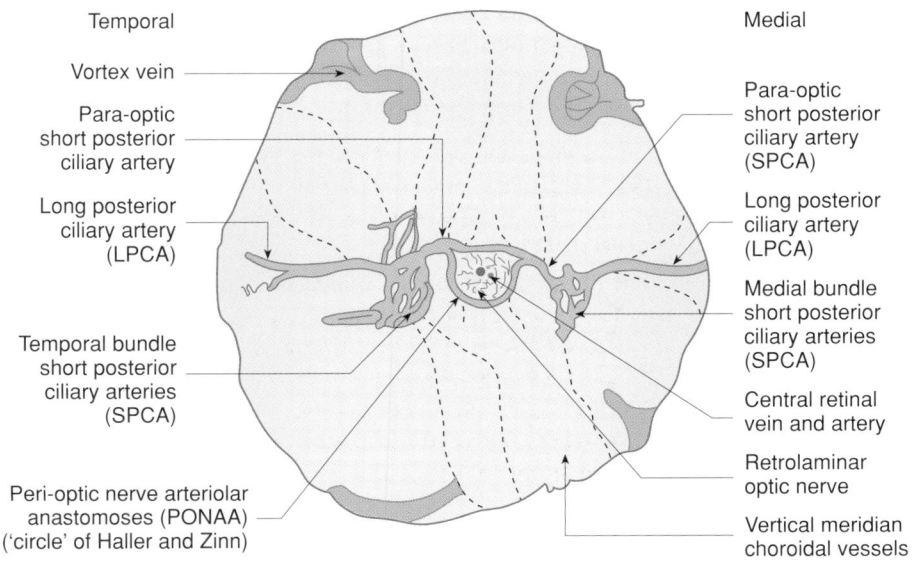

Temporal

Vortex vein

Para-optic
short posterior
ciliary artery

Long posterior
ciliary artery
(LPCA)

Temporal bundle
short posterior
ciliary arteries
(SPCA)

Peri-optic nerve arteriolar
anastomoses (PONAA)
('circle' of Haller and Zinn)

Medial

Para-optic
short posterior
ciliary artery
(SPCA)

Long posterior
ciliary artery
(LPCA)

Medial bundle
short posterior
ciliary arteries
(SPCA)

Central retinal
vein and artery

Retrolaminar
optic nerve

Vertical meridian
choroidal vessels

(a)

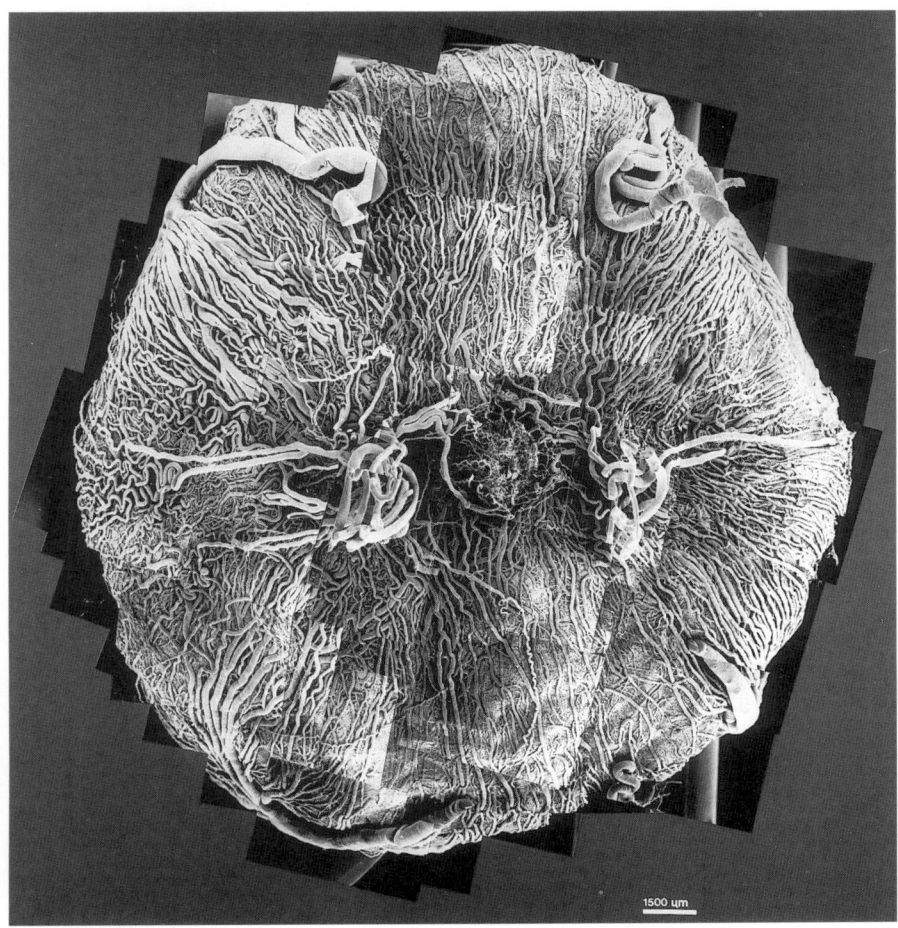

(b)

1500 µm

Fig. 6 (a) Diagrammatic representation of the short posterior ciliary artery supply of the posterior choroid and retrolaminar optic nerve. (b) Scanning electron photomicrograph (montage) of the scleral aspect of the posterior segment from a microvascular corrosion cast of a left human eye. The temporal and medial short posterior ciliary arteries supply the choroid and retrolaminar optic nerve.

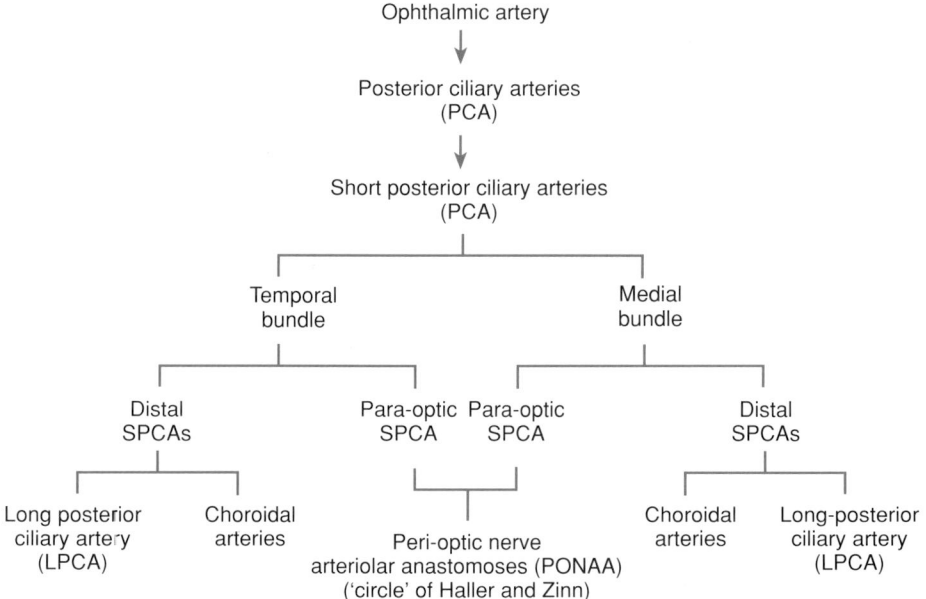

Fig. 7 Scheme to demonstrate the blood flow from the ophthalmic artery into the choroidal vascular system via the short posterior ciliary arteries (SPCAs).

Other functions

The choroidal circulation helps maintain intraocular pressure and heat dissipation. The pigmentation absorbs light.

There is no intraocular lymphatic system. The choroid is regarded as important immunologically as it contains many immune cells such as mast cells, macrophages, and dendritic cells.

Further reading

Auker, C.R., Parver, L.M., Doyle, T., and Carpenter, D.O. (1982). Choroidal blood flow. I. Ocular tissue temperature as a measure of flow. *Archives of Ophthalmology*, **100**, 1323–6.

Bill, A. (1975). Blood circulation and fluid dynamics in the eye. *Physiology Review*, **55**, 383.

Hayreh, S.S. (1975). Segmental nature of the choroidal vasculature. *British Journal of Ophthalmology*, **59**, 631.

Maepea, O. (1992). Pressures in the anterior ciliary arteries, choroidal veins and choriocapillaris. *Experimental Eye Research*, **54**, 731–6.

Olver, J.M. (1990). Functional anatomy of the choroidal circulation: methyl methacrylate casting of human choroid. *Eye*, **4**, 262–72.

Olver, J.M. and Lee, J.P. (1992). Recovey of anterior segment circulation after strabismus surgery in adult patients. *Ophthalmology*, **99**, 305–15.

Olver, J.M., Spalton, D.J., and McCartney, A.C.E. (1994). Quantitative morphology of human retrolaminar optic nerve vasculature. *Investigative Ophthalmology and Visual Science*, **35**, 3858–66.

Parver, L.M., Auker, C.R., Carpenter, D.O., and Doyle, T. (1982). Choroidal blood flow. II. Reflexive control in the monkey. *Archives of Ophthamology*, **100**, 1327–30.

Williamson, T.H. and Harris, A. (1994). Ocular blood flow measurements. *British Journal of Ophthalmology*, **78**, 939–45.

2.8.2 Classification and epidemiology of uveitis

C.S. Ng and A. Ralph Rosenthal

Definitions and classification

Intraocular inflammatory diseases involving the uveal tract directly or indirectly (secondary to inflammation of adjacent tissues) are collectively known as uveitis in the clinical setting. The term uveitis therefore covers a substantial number of pathological entities varying in aetiology and natural history, which require significantly different approaches to investigations and management. It is therefore important that there is a suitable system of classification for this group of diseases in order that clinicians may have a uniform framework for describing a given condition. Various methods of categorising the subtypes of uveitis have been proposed, and these include anatomical, clinical, pathological, and aetiological classifications. As the causes for a substantial number of cases of uveitis are unknown, the nosology of uveitis has depended largely on the description of the clinical manifestations and natural history of the disease process. The first three ways of classifying the uveitides was devised entirely on clinical features. Advances in laboratory techniques, an improved understanding of the pathophysiological basis of many more uveitic entities, as well as the recognition of and new definitions for previously uncategorized diseases have allowed a classification system based on

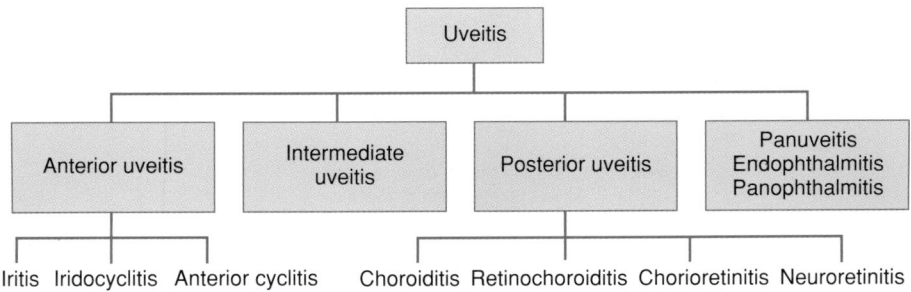

Fig. 1 Anatomical classification of intraocular inflammation diseases.

aetiology which is more practical in terms of patient management.

Anatomical classification

Uveitis may be classified according to the site of the inflammatory activity (Fig. 1). Anterior uveitis affects the iris and ciliary body: if the former is predominantly involved, the term iritis is used, if the pars plicata is principally affected, the condition is then classed as an anterior cyclitis, whereas when they are equally involved, the term iridocyclitis is applied.

Intermediate uveitis predominantly involves the pars plana and the extreme periphery of the retina and was previously known as pars planitis, chronic cyclitis, posterior cyclitis, hyalitis, and basal retinochoroiditis.

Inflammation involving tissues posterior to the posterior border of the vitreous base is known as posterior uveitis and may be focal, multifocal (involving more than one site), depending on the number of sites involved, or diffuse (when large, confluent areas are involved). Based on the site of primary involvement, posterior uveitis can be further subdivided into choroiditis, retinochoroiditis, chorioretinitis, or neuroretinitis.

If the entire uveal tract is involved, the term panuveitis is used, while endophthalmitis refers to the inflammation of intraocular tissues not extending beyond the bounds of the sclera, and panopthalmitis refers to the inflammation of ocular tissues, including structures beyond the scleral wall.

This method of classifying uveitides allows the clinician to describe the main site of the inflammatory response.

Clinical classification

Uveitis may also be described with respect to the clinical characteristics of the disease process. The character of each episode is individually considered. The onset of the disease can be insidious or sudden, the pattern of the disease can be described as single or recurrent, the duration may be short (less than 3 months) or long, and the severity of the inflammatory activity can be classed as mild or severe. In this type of classification, the clinical signs and symptoms provide a framework which allows certain ocular inflammatory syndromes to be defined.

Pathological classification

Uveitis can be classified into granulomatous or nongranulomatous types. Granulomatous uveitis generally has a propensity to present with 'mutton fat' keratic precipitates which are large and greasy in appearance and are composed of macrophages. It is often of insidious onset and runs a chronic course. Aggregates of inflammatory cells such as Koeppe nodules on the pupillary margin of the iris or Busacca spots on the iris surface may also be present. Eyes with non-granulomatous uveitis by contrast develop small keratic precipitates consisting of neutrophils and lymphocytes, have a more acute onset with a short course, and do not usually form iris nodules. Some cases exhibiting clinical characteristics of granulomatous uveitis do not necessarily show histopathological properties of granulomatous inflammation and features of both may be present at the same time. Changes from one to the other may also occur during the course of the disease. Nevertheless, this classification, taken together with the other clinical features in a particular case should help indicate a set of working differential diagnoses.

Aetiological classification

Historically, uveitis has been classified as exogenous if caused by trauma or from infection introduced into the eye from an external source, and endogenous if the inflammation originated from within the patient. Patients can be more usefully categorized according to whether they have uveitis:

- of infectious origin

- related to specific ocular disease

- related to specific systemic disease

- with well-established disease patterns but of unknown pathophysiological origin

- which is idiopathic, non-specific, and does not fall into any of the above categories.

Examples of each are given in Table 1. This classification system takes into account the current understanding of the pathological origins and clinical associations of uveitic entities and is helpful to the clinician in the practical aspects of clinical

Table 1 Aetiological classification of uveitis

Uveitis of infectious origin
Parasitic infestations (e.g. toxoplasmosis, toxocariasis, onchocerciasis)
Viral infections (e.g. HSV, HZV–HVV, EBV, CMV, HTLV-1)
Bacterial infections (e.g. tuberculosis, borreliosis, leprosy, syphilis, pyogenic organisms)
Fungal infections (e.g. *Candida*, *Histoplasma capsulatum*, coccidioidomycosis)

Uveitis related to specific ocular disease
Intraocular lens induced uveitis
Phacoanaphylactic endophthalmitis
Postsurgical/traumatic uveitis

Uveitis related to specific systemic disease
Behçet's disease
Connective tissue diseases (e.g. SLE, juvenile chronic arthritis, Wegener's granulomatosis, PAN, HLA B27-related uveitis including ankylosing
  spondylitis, Reiter's syndrome, psoriasis)
Inflammatory bowel diseases
Multiple sclerosis
Sarcoidosis
Vogt–Koyanagi–Harada syndrome

Specific uveitis entities of unknown origin
Acute multifocal placoid pigment epitheliopathy
Birdshot choroidopathy
Eales' disease
Fuchs' heterochromic uveitis
Intermediate uveitis
Punctate inner choroidopathy
Serpiginous choroidopathy

Non-specific uveitis entities of unknown origin (idiopathic)

CMV, cytomegalovirus; EBV, Epstein–Barr virus; HLA, human leucocyte antigen; HSV, herpes simplex virus; HTLV-1, human T-cell leukaemia virus; HZV–HVV, herpes zoster and/or varicella virus; PAN, polyarteritis nodosa; SLE, systemic lupus erythematosus.

management of the patient in terms of investigations and therapy.

Epidemiological aspects of uveitis

The prevalence of uveitis is estimated to be 38/100 000 in predominantly Caucasian communities in developed countries, with about 17/100 000 new cases annually. The incidence and prevalence of each individual type of uveitis varies between different populations and Table 2 presents a comparison of the frequencies of specific uveitis diagnoses encountered in a selection of studies. Statistical data on patients suffering from uveitis collected from tertiary referral centres that are under the charge of ophthalmologists with a special interest in particular forms of uveitides can lead to a bias in patient selection. Cases which are less difficult to manage such as acute anterior uveitis are less likely to be seen at these centres and can consequently lead to an apparent decrease in the observed occurrence of these diseases and an apparent increase in the other possibly less common conditions. In addition, the diagnostic criteria used for the individual disease entities are not specified in detail in all such studies and may be different between each centre. These problems need to be taken into account in the interpretation of such comparisons but they nevertheless serve to illustrate some of the differences in the distribution of aetiology

of uveitis in various patient groups. These differences depend broadly upon demographic, environmental, and genetic influences as discussed below.

Demographic considerations

Age and sex

Uveitis is a relatively uncommon condition in childhood (below the age of 16). The incidence of uveitis then increases with age, rising to its highest amongst individuals in their third or fourth decade, followed by a decline, such that primary uveitis first appearing in patients over the age of 65 again becomes uncommon. In older people the presence of other diseases masquerading as uveitis should be considered. While many conditions have been noted to occur at any age, the age of an individual has striking effects on the onset of many types of uveitic entities. An extreme example of this is the paucity of patients suffering from birdshot choroidopathy below the age of 15 years, and the decidedly low incidence of *Toxoplasma* retinitis in individuals over 65 year old. It is therefore useful to consider the occurrence of uveitis within broad age bands as a framework for the differential diagnosis in each age group (Table 3). Diseases such as chronic uveitis associated with juvenile chronic arthritis, postviral neuroretinitis, and toxocariasis typically occur in young children, while in slightly older

Table 2 Studies reporting the frequency of uveitis diagnoses

	Leicester, UK (Thean) n = 712 (%)	Los Angeles, USA (Henderly) n = 600 (%)	Lausanne, Switzerland (Tran) n = 435 (%)	Tokyo, Japan (Yokoi) n = 693 (%)	Amsterdam, the Netherlands (Rothova) n = 865 (%)
Toxoplasmosis	5	7	9	2	10
Herpes simplex uveitis	5	2	5	<1	5
Herpes zoster uveitis	2	1	9	<1	(Classed with above)
Other infective uveitides	4	11	1	11	<0.5
HLA B27 related uveitis	15	3	15	4	12
Sarcoidosis	5	4	7	13	9
Behçet's disease	2	2	1	12	<0.5
Vogt–Koyanagi–Harada disease	1	3	1	9	<0.5
Other uveitides associated with systemic diseases	7	8	2	4	15
Fuchs' heterochromic uveitis	13	2	6	1	6
Intermediate uveitis	8	15	7	3	6
Other classified uveitides	4	10	4	6	6
Idiopathic uveitis	27	33	28	32	27

HLA, human leucocyte antigen

Table 3 Common ages of initial onset of some uveitides

Age (years)	Anterior uveitis	Intermediate uveitis	Posterior uveitis	Panuveitis
<5	Juvenile chronic uveitis		Toxocariasis Postviral neurotetinitis	
5–15	Juvenile chronic uveitis	Intermediate uveitis	Toxocariasis Postviral neuroretinitis	
16–25	Anterior uveitis (HLA B27 +ve/-ve)	Intermediate uveitis	Toxocariasis POHS	Sarcoidosis
25–45	Anterior uveitis (HLA B27 +ve/-ve Fuchs' uveitis	Intermediate uveitis	AMPEE Eales' disease HIV-related uveitidis MEWDS PIC POHS Toxoplasmosis	Behçet's disease Multifocal choroiditis Sarcoidosis VKH disease
45–65			Acute retinal necrosis Birdshot choroidopathy Serpiginous choroidopathy	Behçet's disease Sarcoidosis
>65			Serpiginous choroidopathy	

AMPEE, acute multifocal placoid pigment epitheliopathy; HIV, human immunodeficiency virus; HLA, human leucocyte antigen; MEWDS, multiple evanescent white dot syndrome; PIC, punctate inner choroidopathy; POHS, presumed ocular histoplasmosis syndrome; VKH, Vogt–Koyanagi–Harada syndrome.

children and young adults, intermediate uveitis, Fuchs' heterochromic iridocyclitis, and human leucocyte antigen B27 related acute anterior uveitis are often seen. Conditions like acute multifocal placoid pigment epitheliopathy, multiple evanescent white dot syndrome, punctate inner choroidopathy, Vogt–Koyanagi–Harada syndrome, and Behçet's disease often first appear in slightly older individuals (between 25 and 45 years old), whereas uveitides like serpiginous choroidopathy and birdshot choroidopathy are usually diagnosed in individuals over the age of 45 years. For those patients over the age of 65 diagnosed as having uveitis, the relative frequencies of acute anterior, chronic anterior, intermediate, and posterior uveitides do not appear to be different from those in younger patients.

In terms of gender, the occurrence of uveitis appears broadly to divide equally. A few conditions such as uveitis associated with juvenile chronic arthritis, birdshot choroidopathy, multiple evanescent white dot syndrome, and punctate inner choroidopathy have a predilection for female patients whereas Behçet's disease and human leucocyte antigen B27 related uveitis (including patients with Reiter's syndrome and ankylosing spondylitis) are more often encountered in male patients. Sympathetic ophthalmitis also occurs more often in males, but this is attributed to the higher frequency of ocular injuries.

Race

Table 4 summarizes the principal racial influences in uveitic entities. These racial differences in the occurrence of uveitis are of clinical interest in terms of providing indications of the formulation of differential diagnoses. The ethnic groups are, however, different in terms of their genetic make-up and the environment in which they live, both of which can have profound effects in the development of disease. Having taken these into account, there remain some conditions where race appear to be a significant risk factor. Vogt–Koyanagi–Harada syndrome, for example, is much more common in the more darkly pigmented races such as oriental people (including Japanese, Asian Indians, and American Indians) and Hispanics. 'Caucasians' who suffer from this condition often report at least having a remote ancestor belonging to one of the above races.

Genetic factors—human leucocyte antigens

Whilst uveitis entities are as a rule not directly inherited in the mendelian fashion, the genetic make-up of the individual may carry a predisposition to uveitis. This is illustrated in the link between human leucocyte antigens and the predisposition to various forms of uveitides, notably acute anterior uveitis and birdshot choroidopathy (Table 5). The prevalence of a particular human leucocyte antigen allele in different races

Table 4 Racial predilection in the occurrence of uveitis

Disease	Race
Afro-Caribbean	Sarcoidosis
American Indian	Vogt–Koyanagi–Harada disease
Caucasian	HLA B27 related uveitis Birdshot choroidopathy
Mediterranean	Behçet's disease
Oriental	Behçet's disease Sarcoidosis Vogt–Koyanagi–Harada disease

HLA, human leucocyte antigen.

varies considerably, and therefore, in epidemiological terms, the establishment of the relative risk for a disease linked to a particular human leucocyte antigen status requires the examination of an appropriate number of individuals who are free of the disease:

$$\text{relative risk} = \text{number of antigen-positive patients} \times \text{number of antigen-negative controls} / \text{number of antigen-negative patients} \times \text{number of antigen-positive controls}$$

In order for such calculations to be valid, the control population need to be derived from a gene pool that is not significantly different to that of the reference population. The study of the human leucocyte antigen and its clinical applications is a rapidly expanding field and further associations between human leucocyte antigen status and disease entities are likely to be uncovered.

Human leucocyte antigens are protein molecules found on the surfaces of nucleated cells. They appear to play a major role in the immune response as recognition antigens for immunocompetent cells during allograft rejection and also in cytotoxic reactions against infected cells. The pathophysiology of these associations has not been completely elucidated, but clinical evidence in studies of human leucocyte antigen B27 related acute anterior uveitis supports an immunopathogenetic mechanism involving the autosensitisation of cytotoxic lymphocytes in susceptible patients by an infectious agent(s) ultimately leading to an autoimmune response against ocular tissues. The infectious organisms implicated include *Chlamydia* trachomatis, and Gram-negative bacteria. The pathophysiological mechanism for the other human leucocyte antigen-related uveitides may be similar.

The association between diseases and human leucocyte antigen varies significantly between populations of different ethnicity. For example, human leucocyte antigen B7 is more commonly associated with ankylosing spondylitis in Afro-Caribbean patients than human leucocyte antigen B27, and the relative risk of the development of Behçet's disease varies between patients of different races (see Table 5). The distribution of human leucocyte antigen A29, which is known to be very strongly linked to birdshot choroidopathy does not appear to correlate exactly with the variation in the geographical distribution of the disease in Europe, which further suggests that other factors are necessary to trigger the development of this condition. In addition, individuals with human leucocyte antigen B27 and a family history of acute anterior uveitis have a 13-fold increase in their risk of also developing acute anterior uveitis when compared with those individuals with the antigen but a negative family history. The presence of a particular human leucocyte antigen in an individual, therefore, does not on its own lead to the development of disease; other factors such as racial and environmental influences also play significant roles.

Environmental factors

Geographical influences

Racial and genetic factors discussed above need to be examined in the context of the geographical distribution of disease as

Table 5 Association of human leucocyte antigens with uveitis entities

Disease	Antigen (HLA)	Race	Relative risk
Acute anterior uveitis	B27	Causcasian	13
	B8	Afro-Caribbean	5
Ankylosing spondylitis	B27	Caucasian	100
Behçet's disease	B51	Oriental	10
	B51	Caucasian	2
	B51	Middle Eastern	14
Birdshot choroidopathy	A29	Caucasian	49
Presumed ocular histoplasmosis	DR2	Caucasian	10
	B7	Caucasian	5
Psoriasis	B27	Caucasian	13
Reiter's syndrome	B27	Caucasian	26
Rheumatoid arthritis	DR4	Caucasian	11
Serpiginous choroidopathy	B7	Caucasian	2
Sympathetic ophthalmitis	A11	Mixed	3.9
Vogt–Koyanagi–Harada disease	DR4	Oriental	16
	Dw53	Oriental	34

well. Some striking differences in the distribution of certain uveitic entities have been noted, which serves to illustrate the environmental impact on the development of particular diseases. A selection of these conditions are considered below.

Onchocerciasis
Onchocerciasis (river blindness), due to the infestation by the microfilaria *Onchocerca volvulus* is found where the *Simulium* blackfly vector is commonly found to breed in rivers. This includes countries in Central and West Africa, and Latin America. Blindness due to onchocercal panuveitis is the second most common cause of blindness in some West African countries after cataracts. The use of larvicides in rivers to reduce the numbers of the *Simulium* flies and the mass distribution of the filaricidal drug ivermectin in endemic onchocercal communities since 1989 has led to a decline in the incidence of this condition.

Presumed ocular histoplasmosis syndrome
Histoplasma capsulatum is a fungus found throughout the world in river valleys including the Ohio–Mississippi valley in the Midwest of the United States. This condition is however, almost exclusively found in the United States, especially in the Midwest, where there is a high incidence of individuals with a positive histoplasmin skin test. Factors including (a) the presence of a number of patients meeting the diagnostic criteria for this ocular condition who do not appear to react to the histoplasmin skin test; (b) the development in some patients of the disease many years after leaving the endemic area; (c) the rarity of this disease in other areas of the world where this fungus is found; (d) its uncommon occurrence in non-Caucasians, all suggest that other factors may be important in the pathogenesis

of presumed ocular histoplasmosis syndrome, including the presence of human leucocyte antigens B7 and Dr2.

Other environmental considerations

Diet and toxoplasmosis
Toxoplasma gondii is a ubiquitous obligatory intracellular parasite. Human infection may be congenital if a woman develops a parasitaemia during pregnancy, or acquired via the ingestion of the parasite through eating undercooked meat. Ocular toxoplasmosis is the commonest cause of uveitis in Brazil, accounting for over a half of uveitis cases, with a prevalence of 18 per cent in some rural areas. This is attributed to the practice in these communities of ingesting raw pork which may be contaminated with *Toxoplasma* cysts. A study comparing immigrant groups from West Africa and subjects born in England revealed that the incidence of this condition was a 100-fold higher in the former (77/100 000/year) compared with the latter (0.8/100 000/year). This may be attributed to different dietary practices in these communities.

Living standards
While infective conditions such as tuberculosis and leprosy have been common in the past, improvements in living standards, and to a lesser extent the advent of antimicrobial therapy, have contributed to the decline in their prevalence in Western countries. They unfortunately remain important causes of disease in more deprived areas of the world.

Lifestyle
The lifestyle of a individual has a significant effects on the risks of developing human immunodeficiency virus (HIV)-related diseases including acquired immune deficiency syndrome (AIDS) with the attendant opportunistic uveitides. High-risk

groups include homosexual/bisexual men and their sexual contacts, and intravenous drug abusers. Recipients of blood products are also at risk. Fungal intraocular infections such as *Candida* endopthalmitis are also more common amongst intravenous drug abusers as well as patients requiring indwelling urinary catheters. In addition syphilis should be considered in uveitis in sexually promiscuous individuals.

Animal vectors

Toxocariasis is transmitted through the ingestion of the ova of the larva *Toxocara canis* (in dogs) and *T. catis* (in cats). The prevalence of seropositivity in humans in the West is in the order of 10 per cent, but most cases are subclinical. Regular worming of pets helps reduce infestations in pet animals. Young children are particularly at risk. Borreliosis (Lyme disease) can be transmitted through ticks infesting deer, birds, and field mice and may manifest as uveitis, often occurring in the summer months in association with outdoor activity. This condition is endemic in southern New England and the mid-Atlantic states of the United States.

Immunosuppression

Patients who are immunocompromised such as patients receiving cytotoxic chemotherapy for cancer, immunosuppressive therapy for autoimmune diseases, following organ transplantation, or with AIDS, are at risk of developing infective uveitides such as cytomegalovirus retinitis or ocular candidiasis.

Uveitis and systemic diseases

Underlying systemic diseases are diagnosed in between a fifth and a half of patients with uveitis. The ophthalmologist may encounter (a) patients with uveitis related to systemic diseases when patients present directly with ocular symptoms as the initial manifestation of the disease; (b) patients with known systemic disease who present with ocular manifestations of their systemic condition; or (c) patients referred by other medical practitioners for screening for ocular involvement in the absence of eye symptoms (e.g. in the case of juvenile chronic arthritis). The most common systemic condition associated with uveitis in Western populations is acute anterior uveitis related to human leucocyte antigen B27 (including ankylosing spondylitis, Reiter's disease, and psoriasis). There are many other systemic diseases associated with uveitis, examples of which are listed in Table 1. Evaluation and planning of investigations for uveitis patients are guided by the clinical picture, and blanket investigation of such patients should be avoided.

Changing patterns in uveitis

Diagnostic entities in uveitis have changed over time as a result of the following:

1. Recent advances in laboratory sciences have led to the discovery of aetiological agents for uveitic entities of previously unknown pathogenesis (for example in the definition of human T-cell leukaemia virus type 1 related uveitis through the development of the use of polymerase chain reaction in the detection of DNA from infective agents in ocular fluids), and the association of some uveitides with particular human leucocyte antigens.

2. The discovery and/or better definition of new uveitic conditions (e.g. acute multifocal placoid pigment epitheliopathy and punctate inner choroidopathy).

3. The increased occurrence of some previously uncommon diseases (e.g. cytomegalovirus retinitis in immunocompromised patients).

4. The emergence of new uveitic diagnoses (e.g. hypopyon uveitis due to therapy with rifabutin in patients with AIDS).

5. The decrease in occurrence of some conditions more commonly encountered previously (e.g. syphilitic and tuberculous uveitis).

Despite recent advances there remains a group of patients for whom no specific diagnosis can be made. It is imperative that effort be directed to improvement in diagnostic techniques which can lead to a decrease in the number of uncategorized uveitides encountered in ophthalmic practice. This will lead in turn to a better understanding of the pathogenesis and management of intraocular inflammatory diseases.

Further reading

Baarsma, G.S. (1992). The epidemiology and genetics of endogenous uveitis: a review. *Current Eye Research*, **11**, 1–9.

Barton, K., Pavesio, C.E., Towler, H.M.A., and Lightman, S. (1994). Uveitis presenting *de novo* in the elderly. *Eye*, **8**, 288–91.

Bloch-Michel, E. and Nussenblatt, R.B. (1987). International Uveitis Study Group recommendations for the evaluation of intraocular inflammatory disease. *American Journal of Ophthalmology*, **103**, 234–5.

Darrell, R.W., Wagener, H.P., and Kurland, L.T. (1962). Epidemiology of uveitis: incidence and prevalence in a small urban community. *Archives of Ophthalmology*, **68**, 100–12.

de Boer, J.H., Luyendijk, L., Rothova, A., and Kilstra,A. (1995). Analysis of ocular fluids for local antibody production in uveitis. *British Journal of Ophthalmology*, **79**, 610–16.

Forrester, J.V. (1992). Uveitis. In *Recent Advances in Ophthalmology*, Vol. 8, (ed. S.I. Davidson and B. Jay), pp. 107–27. Churchill Livingstone, Edinburgh.

Gilbert, R.E., Stanford, M.R., Jackson, H., *et al.* (1995). Incidence of acute symptomatic *Toxoplasma* retinochoroiditis in south London according to country of birth. *British Medical Journal*, **310**, 3134–40.

Goto, K., Saeki, K., Kurita, M., and Ohno, S. (1995). HTLV-1 associated uveitis in central Japan. *British Journal of Ophthalmology*, **79**, 1018–20.

Henderly, D.E., Genstler, A.J., Smith, R.E., and Roa, N.A. (1987). Changing patterns of uveitis. *American Journal of Ophthalmology*, **103**, 131–6.

Holland, G.N. and the Executive Committee of the American Uveitis Society (1994). Standard diagnostic criteria for the acute retinal necrosis syndrome. *American Journal of Ophthalmology*, **117**, 663–7.

Moorthy, R.S., Inomata, H., and Roa, N.A. (1995). Vogt–Koyanagi–Harada syndrome. *Survey of Ophthalmology*, **39**, 265–92.

Nussenblatt, R.B. and Palestine, A.G. (1989). *Uveitis: fundamentals and clinical practice*. Year Book Medical, Chicago.

Ronday, M.J.H., Stilma, J.S., Barbe, R.F., and Rothova, A. (1994). Blindness from uveitis in a hospital population in Sierra Leone. *British Journal of Ophthalmology*, **78**, 690–3.

Rosenbaum, J.T. (1989). Uveitis: an internist's view. *Archives of Internal Medicine*, **149**, 1173–6.

Rothova, A. (1993). Ocular invovement in toxoplasmosis. *British Journal of Ophthalmology*, **77**, 371–7.

Rothova, A., Buitenhuis, H.J., Meenken, C., *et al.* (1992). Uveitis and systemic disease. *British Journal of Ophthalmology*, **76**, 137–41.

Smith, R.E. and Nozik, R.A. (1989). *Uveitis: a clinical approoch to diagnosis and management*, (2nd edn). Williams & Wilkins, Baltimore.

Thean, L.H., Thompson, J., and Rosenthal, A.R. (1996). A uveitis register at the Leicester Royal Infirmary. *Ophthalmic Epidemiology*, **3**, 151–8.

Tran, V.T., Auer, C., Guex-Crosier, *et al.* (1995). Epidemiological characteristics of uveitis in Switzerland. *International Ophthalmology*, **18**, 293–8.

Wakefield, D., Montanaro, A, and McCluskey, P.M.C. (1991). Acute anterior uveitis and HLA-B27. *Survey of Ophthalmology*, **36**, 223–32.

Yokoi, H., Goto, H., Sakai, J.-I., *et al.* (1995). Incidence of uveitis at Tokyo Medical College Hospital. *Nippon Ganka Gakkai Zasshi*, **99**, 710–14.

2.8.3 Immunological aspects of uveitis

Harminder S. Dua

Over the last decade, our knowledge and understanding of the management, diagnosis, and underlying pathogenetic mechanisms of uveitis have developed at a rapid pace. Uveitis is now firmly established as an ophthalmic subspeciality. Much of this development has stemmed from our improved understanding of molecular, experimental, and clinical aspects of the immune system and, though not yet fully refined, our ability to manipulate it to the patient's advantage is improving.

Fundamental to the understanding of immune mechanisms in uveitis is a broad understanding of various facets of the immune system and more specifically, its unique interactions with the eyes given their 'immunologically privileged' status.

Antigen

By definition, any substance that can specifically bind to an antibody is an antigen. Substances that initiate an immune response, the generation of an antibody for instance, are called immunogens. Whereas almost all biological molecules are potential antigens, only macromolecules (of phospholipids, carbohydrates, and proteins) can act as immunogens. Furthermore, only certain segments or peptides of an antigen/immunogen can bind to antibody or to an immune cell. These segments are called epitopes or determinants. A given protein molecule can have several peptides some of which are antigenic and some immunogenic.

The vast majority of clinical uveitides, both anterior and posterior, have an (auto)immune aspect in their initiation, perpetuation or recrudescence. Although an antecedent viral, bacterial or parasitic infection is evident in some forms of uveitis, most of them are labelled idiopathic or autoimmune. Several ocular proteins are sequestered during embryogenesis and are there-fore potential autoantigens. The lens crystallins and retinal proteins—namely S antigen, interphotoreceptor retinoid binding protein, rhodopsin, phosducin, and recoverin—are significant in this regard and have been incriminated in the aetiology and pathogenesis of uveitis. Melanin granules from the uveal tissue are also immunogenic. Retinal S antigen has been quite extensively studied and several antigenic and immunogenic epitopes have been identified. Interestingly not all immunogenic epitopes initiate disease. In the experimental autoimmune uveitis model it has been observed that the disease initiating (pathogenic) epitopes are located towards the C-terminal portion of the molecule. Since most epitopes are approximately 15 amino acids long or less, it is quite conceivable that several naturally occurring proteins have epitopes that are similar or near identical to immunogenic/pathogenic epitopes of autologous proteins. This is referred to as molecular mimicry. Molecular mimicry between certain viral and yeast protein epitopes and retinal S antigen has been observed. This provides a basis for the concept that microbial infections can trigger an immune response which, through molecular mimicry, can evolve into an 'auto' immune uveitis.

Antibody

Antibodies are immunoglobulin (glycoprotein) molecules in the blood that are responsible for the specific recognition and elimination of antigens. Each antibody molecule has a variable region, that varies from antibody to antibody, and a constant region. The antigen binding site (idiotype) of an antibody is located in its variable region and it is this site that gives an antibody its unique antigen specificity. There over 10^9 different antibody molecules in every individual, each with its specific antigen binding site. This enormous repertoire is genetically determined by a process of DNA recombination in genes coding for the variable region of antibodies. Antibodies exist in a bound form on the membrane of B cells where they act as antigen recognition receptors for the cell, and in a secreted form in the serum. When antigen binds to membrane-bound antibody it initiates an expansion of that particular clone of B cells, with the progeny cells producing secreted antibody. Secreted antibody in turn binds to antigen (immune complex) and triggers several effector functions such as neutralisation (of drugs, microbes, or toxins), activation of complement (immunoglobulin G or M), opsonisation of antigen (microbe) for enhanced phagocytosis (immunoglobulin G), antibody-dependent cell-mediated cytotoxicity (immunoglobulin G, E, and A), immediate hypersensitivity reactions (immunoglobulin E) and mucosal immunity (immunoglobulin A). The cognitive phase of this response is very specific but the effector phase is not specific for the eliciting antigen. It is these effector responses that, in some instances, lead to inflammation in the tissue where they occur and produce clinical signs and symptoms. Of these, immune-complex mediated reactions (type III, arthus reaction) are probably involved in many types of uveitis such as reactive iridocyclitis, reactivation of *Toxoplasma* chorioretinitis, lens-induced uveitis, Behçet's disease, and importantly, idiopathic and other forms of retinal vasculitis that may be associated with collagen vascular disease like systemic lupus erythematosus.

Antibodies being protein molecules, can themselves elicit an antibody response, particularly against their variable regions or idiotype. Such anti-idiotypic antibodies are believed to act as feedback molecules to regulate the immune response. Interestingly, in the experimental situation, anti-idiotypic antibodies generated against certain anti-retinal S-antigen antibodies have been shown to offer protection against S-antigen induced uveitis.

Cells and cytokines

The cellular arm of the immune response involves T lymphocytes, predominantly T-helper cells (CD4$^+$ Th) and suppressor/cytotoxic cells (CD8$^+$). The sequence of events leading to activation of cell-mediated immune responses include: (a) antigen capture by antigen-presenting cells such as macrophages. In the eye, lymphoid cells and resident non-lymphoid cells like the retinal pigment epithelium, ciliary epithelium, and perhaps Müller cells can also present antigen. (b) Antigen processing, whereby captured antigen is lysed by intracellular enzymes. Peptide fragments generated by enzymatic action are linked to major histocompatibility complex molecules and expressed on the surface of the cell where they are (c) presented to T cells. T-cell receptors recognize antigen in association with major histocompatibility complex class I (CD8$^+$) and II (CD4$^+$), and are as specific for antigen as are the antigen binding sites of antibodies. T-cell receptors of the vast majority of peripheral blood T-cells have an α-chain and a β-chain. These polypeptide chains are analogous to antibody molecules and have variable and constant regions. The variable regions are divided into several subtypes. It has been shown that in human endogenous posterior uveitis the levels of variable β1 bearing T cells are elevated. This may indicate that a specific subtype of T lymphocyte is involved in endogenous posterior uveitis and is significant because it may allow specific targeting of this subtype in future strategies for the management of uveitis. T-cell receptors are closely linked to another cell surface molecule, CD3, that is expressed on all thymus-derived T cells. When T-cell receptor/CD3 interaction with major histocompatibility complex coupled antigen occurs, it is the CD3 molecule that transduces the activating signals to the cytoplasm of the T cell. Activated T cells produce cytokines and also undergo clonal expansion.

Cytokines are soluble factors which (a) function in cell–cell communication and interactions; (b) initiate and support cell proliferation, migration, and differentiation; (c) possess chemotactic, cytotoxic, and antiviral activity; and (d) initiate local inflammation in target tissues and systemic responses such as fever. One subset of T cells (Th1) produce cytokines that initiate cell-mediated immunity and delayed-type hypersensitivity responses; another subset (Th2) produces cytokines (IL4) that in turn activate B cells and initiate the humoral immune response. The cytokines, interleukin 1, 2, 6, and 8, tumour necrosis factor, and interferon-γ are known to be associated with posterior and anterior (particularly interleukin 6 and interferon-γ) uveitis. Another group of inflammatory mediators, prostaglandins are implicated in anterior uveitis. Ocular responses elicited by prostaglandins in experimental models are similar to those seen in anterior uveitis and levels of prostaglandin 1 and 2 in the aqueous correlate to intensity of inflammation.

Immunological suppression

Although both humoral and cell-mediated immune responses occur in the eye and are implicated in almost all types of anterior and posterior uveitis, the natural response of ocular tissue is that of immunosuppression, that is limiting the immune responses such that elimination of the offending 'antigen' can occur avoiding the devastating consequences of inflammation that follow a full-blown immunological response. The aqueous humour contains factors and cytokines that downregulate antigen-driven T-cell responses. Tissue growth factor-β is important in this regard. Anterior chamber-associated immune deviation is a unique phenomenon that permits immunological suppression to occur within the eye. Antigens accessing the anterior chamber interact with the immune system via the aqueous veins and blood stream rather than the usual pathway of lymphatics and lymph nodes. This allows for a different kind of immune response wherein delayed-type hypersensitivity responses are suppressed but humoral and normal cytotoxic responses are preserved. Transforming growth factor-β is believed to play an important role in anterior chamber-associated immune deviation.

Human leucocyte antigen and uveitis

The major histocompatibility complex is also known as the human leukocyte antigen complex and is encoded by genes located on chromosome 6. These genes control the production and expression of three classes of antigens, I, II, and III. Class I is represented by three gene loci, A, B, and C. They are present on all nucleated cells and are targets of cytolytic cells in virus infections and allograft rejection. Class II molecules are coded by the human leucocyte antigen D/DR locus. They are expressed on cell surfaces and, as explained above, in association with antigen, are recognized by T cells during the initiation of an immune response. The class III locus encodes components of the complement system.

The association of human leucocyte antigen molecules to different forms of uveitis is well documented but the exact aetiopathogenetic significance of this association remains unclear. Human leucocyte antigen molecules or antigens do not themselves cause uveitis. It is likely that certain exogenous or endogenous antigens associate more readily with specific human leucocyte antigen molecules thereby facilitating the initiation of an immune response. Molecular mimicry between certain bacterial antigens and human leucocyte antigen class I molecules has been described and may be a relevant factor in the association of human leucocyte antigen and uveitis. Bacterial enterocolitis with *Yersinia* and *Klebsiella* in combination with human leucocyte antigen B27 has a strong link with ankylosing spondylitis, Reiter's disease, and anterior uveitis. Antigenic similarity between human leucocyte antigen B27 and a nitrogenase enzyme derived from *Klebsiella* pneumonia has been reported.

The significant human leucocyte antigen associations are:

- anterior uveitis with human leucocyte antigen B27

- Behçet's syndrome with human leucocyte antigen B5 and B51

- birdshot choroidopathy with human leucocyte antigen A29.

A B-cell specific antigen MT3 has a strong association with Vogt–Koyanagi–Harada syndrome. This syndrome also has an association with human leucocyte antigen DR4 and DQ3 in North Americans and with human leucocyte antigen DR53 in Japanese patients. Several of these associations have multisystem involvement of which uveitis is one part.

To summarize, an exogenous or autologous antigen, either ocular or extraocular, may interact with the immune system and trigger the humoral and/or cell-mediated arms of the immune response. This results in activated cells producing antibodies or cytokines and an expansion of the particular clone of cells, specific for the particular antigen, most probably at an extraocular site (spleen or regional lymph node) but may occur within the eye. The function of these cells, antibodies, and cytokines is to contain the invading antigen (organism) and neutralize or destroy it. Activated cells from extraocular sites travel to the eye via the blood stream. Various homing mechanisms are involved in this process. Expression of intercellular adhesion molecules on lymphocytes and on the vascular endothelium (addressins) allows lymphocytes to adhere to the vascular endothelium. This facilitates the migration of lymphocytes through the vascular endothelium and access to intraocular antigens. In lymph nodes, where a constant traffic of lymphocytes to and from the vascular compartment occurs, the vascular endothelium is modified (high endothelial venules) to facilitate this transgression. It has been shown that the retinal vascular endothelium can assume characteristics of high endothelial venules in autoantigen-mediated experimental uveitis. This may be one of the mechanisms in intraocular homing. Once inside the eye, activated cells will target the sensitizing antigen or its mimotopes and initiate inflammation (uveoretinitis). The various clinical types of uveitis represent different aspects of this inflammatory response: intra- and perivascular infiltration of cells (retinal vasculitis), vitreous cellular infiltration, dispersed or in aggregates (vitreous cells and snowballs), focal or diffuse chorioretinal infiltrates (choroidal nodules or patches of chorioretinitis), and retinal or optic disc oedema (cystoid macular oedema or papilloedema).

It is not surprising therefore that immunosuppression is the mainstay in the management of uveitis. Non-specific immunosuppression is achieved with steroids, cyclophosphamide, and azathioprine, and T-helper cell targeted immunosuppression with cyclosporin, rapamicin, or FK506. Newer, more specific immune intervention in uveitis is being explored using anti-bodies against receptors expressed by specific subsets of activated lymphocytes.

Further reading
Abbas, A.K., Lichtman, A.H., and Pober, J.S. (1991). *Cellular and molecular immunology*. Saunders, Philadelphia.
Nozik, R.A. and Michelson, J.B. (guest ed.) (1993). *Ophthalmology Clinics of North America, Uveitis*. Saunders, Philadelphia.
Tabbara, K.F. and Nussenblatt R.B. (1994). *Posterior uveitis, diagnosis and management*. Butterworth-Heinemann, Boston.
Dua, H.S. and Donoso, L.A. (1993). Function in the immune system of antigenic peptides from S-antigen (Arrestin). *Methods: A Companion to Methods in Enzymology*, 5, 242–51.

2.8.4 Clinical features of uveitis

Carlos E. Pavésio

Knowledge of the symptoms and signs of the different presentations of uveitis is essential for the establishment of a complete list of differential diagnoses which will help to reach a final diagnosis. The classification system in uveitis, as discussed in Chapter 2.8.2, is usually artificial, but helps to define a group of findings and the diseases most likely to be associated with them. This chapter discusses the clinical manifestations of uveitis according to the anatomical classification, which is the most commonly used.

Acute anterior uveitis

Anterior uveitis includes both iritis and iridocyclitis, and is probably the most common form of uveitis accounting for approximately three-quarters of all cases. It may also be the most difficult for which to obtain a correct aetiological diagnosis. The clinical presentation of anterior uveitis (iritis or iridocyclitis) depends on its acute or chronic behaviour.

Acute anterior uveitis is characterized by rapid onset of pain, redness, and photophobia. Signs include ciliary injection, pupillary miosis, and small keratic precipitates. Keratic precipitates are small aggregates of inflammatory cells that accumulate on the endothelial surface of the cornea, and, when fresh, indicate an active inflammatory process. A more detailed discussion on keratic precipitates will come under chronic anterior uveitis, since this is where it is most frequently found .

There is marked inflammatory activity at the anterior chamber with variable flare (protein) and cells. Flare represents a breakdown of the blood–ocular barrier. There are different ways of grading flare, but the way it interferes with visualization of iris details, as proposed by Hogan *et al.* in 1959, is probably the easiest to remember:

0 absent
1 very slight
2 moderate (iris and lens clear)
3 marked (iris and lens hazy)
4 intense (fibrin, plastic aqueous)

Cells in the anterior chamber are more indicative of active inflammation and they can be counted using a 1×1 mm slit lamp on higher magnification. The system proposed by Hogan et al. (Hogan et al. 1959) allows a grading from 0 to 4+:

0	0 cells
Rare cells	1–2
Occasional	3–7
1+	7–10
1–2+	10–15
2+	15–20
3+	20–50
4+	>50

This grading is very useful for assessing response to therapy and also for the planning of cataract extraction in these patients, since persistence of more than a rare cell indicates higher risk of complications and a poorer prognosis. Hypopyon is a collection of inflammatory cells (leucocytes), and also fibrin, that settles in the lower angle of the anterior chamber. It is a sign of intense inflammation and, in some cases, it may be very short lived (Fig. 1).

Intraocular pressure is usually low at the beginning of the attack, which is due to inflammation of the ciliary body, but later it may become elevated, which occurs secondary to blockage of the outflow channels. Blurring of vision is another feature, and in some cases is due to cystoid macular oedema which may be seen in the severe cases of acute anterior uveitis.

Most of the time the condition presents unilaterally, but carries the risk of recurrence in the same or the fellow eye. Bilateral simultaneous presentation should raise the suspicion for a systemic association and should be investigated as such.

The most commonly associated conditions with acute anterior uveitis are the HLA B27 syndromes, but the differential diagnoses also include trauma, infectious diseases such as tuberculosis, syphilis, herpes viruses, and idiopathic anterior uveitis.

Patients who are HLA B27 positive may have ocular disease alone or in association with systemic inflammatory diseases such as ankylosing spondylitis, Reiter's syndrome, psoriatic arthritis, and inflammatory bowel disease. The incidence of anterior uveitis in HLA B27 positive patients without systemic disease ranges from 43 to 58 per cent, and both eyes are affected in 80 per cent of the cases, but very rarely simultaneously. Ankylosing spondylitis is a condition seen two to three times more frequently in men and has as its most common initial symptom low back pain (70 per cent). Ocular involvement occurs in 25 per cent of the patients, and may be the initial presentation of the disease. The association with an HLA B27 positive test is 90 per cent (normal Caucasian population has a positive HLA-B27 in 8–10 per cent).

Anterior uveitis occurs in 3 to 12 per cent of patients with Reiter's syndrome, and the first attack tends to be more severe than the recurrences. The diagnosis is clinical and based on the association with systemic findings (non-gonococcal urethritis, keratoderma blennorrhagicum, balanitis, sacroiliitis). Association with HLA B27 occurs in 85 to 90 per cent of cases.

Iridocyclitis may occur in patients with psoriasis, but mainly those with psoriatic arthritis.

The association of acute anterior uveitis and inflammatory bowel disease occurs mainly with granulomatous enterocolitis or Crohn's disease, with rare cases associated with ulcerative colitis. The uveitis in Crohn's disease is usually exacerbated during intestinal disease activity, and in patients with arthritis the incidence of iritis increases from 2 to 30 per cent.

Apart from the HLA B27 uveitis, hypopyon can be found characteristically in Behçet's disease, and an infectious origin should be suspected in cases of recent intraocular surgery or perforating injuries. The development of posterior synechiae is a complication of this type of uveitis, especially in those cases with intense flare. In uveitis the pupil is usually miotic, which increases the contact surface with the lens thus facilitating the development of synechiae. In advanced cases an iris bombé picture can occur which will then lead to elevated intraocular pressure. Usually in inflammatory conditions affecting the ciliary body, there is a reduction in the secretion of the aqueous humour, and in consequence a reduction in intraocular pressure. A few uveitic entities are associated with raised intraocular pressure, even in the absence of posterior synechiae. This is known as hypertensive uveitis, and can be seen in toxoplasmic retinitis, herpetic keratouveitis, sarcoidosis, and masquerade syndrome. Chronic glaucoma occurs either as a consequence of synechiae or damage to the trabecular meshwork associated with persistent inflammation. In Fuchs' heterochromic cyclitis, a condition many times associated with open angle glaucoma, fine blood vessels can be seen crossing the angle by gonioscopy. This is the anatomical basis for the well-known bleeding seen during paracentesis or intraocular surgery in these patients (Amsler sign).

Cells can be seen in the anterior vitreous in cases of iridocyclitis, and the number of cells will depend on the intensity

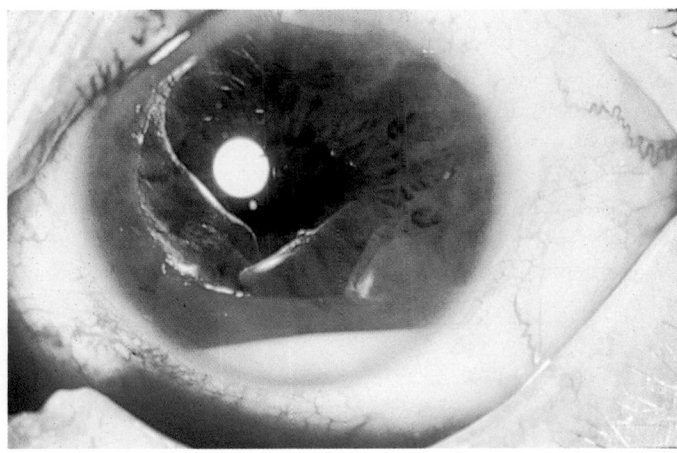

Fig. 1 Hypopyon in a patient with a severe attack of acute anterior uveitis.

of the inflammatory reaction. Most anterior uveitis associated conditions will not lead to significant posterior segment disease (which can occur in Behçet's syndrome, Crohn's disease, and Reiter's syndrome), but it is not uncommon to find cystoid macular oedema in severe cases. The treatment of the anterior uveitis is usually enough to reverse the oedema.

Chronic anterior uveitis

Chronic anterior uveitis may present either as a very quiet eye, such as in juvenile chronic arthritis, Fuchs' cyclitis, or in masquerade syndromes, or with inflammatory signs, such as in granulomatous uveitis. In the latter, there is ocular discomfort and variable photophobia. Keratic precipitates are more typical of this form of presentation and can be small, non-granulomatous, medium, as classically described in Fuchs' cyclitis, or large, usually granulomatous in nature. Keratic precipitates tend to concentrate in a triangular pattern in the inferior central portion of the cornea (Arlt's triangle), which is due to the influence of gravity and the normal convection pattern of the aqueous humour (Fig. 2). Diffuse scattering of the keratic precipitates over the endothelium is very typical of Fuchs' cyclitis (Fig. 3), and may also be found concentrated in other areas, usually associated with a corneal lesion, in cases of herpes simplex keratitis. Keratic precipitates tend to disappear without leaving any signs, apart from the granulomatous type that can leave ghost images ('fingerprints'), due to the damage they cause to the endothelial cells. Large numbers of granulomatous keratic precipitates can lead to corneal oedema. Pigmentation of the keratic precipitates, or keratic precipitates in the absence of anterior chamber reaction, is an indication of previous uveitis.

Iris nodules are also more typical of the chronic uveitis, and they can occur at the pupillary margin (Koeppe's nodules) or at the iris stroma (Busacca's nodules). Koeppe's nodules are not specific, but are an important clue to the activity of the uveitis (Fig. 4). Posterior synechiae occur more frequently at sites where these nodules are found. Busacca's nodules repres-

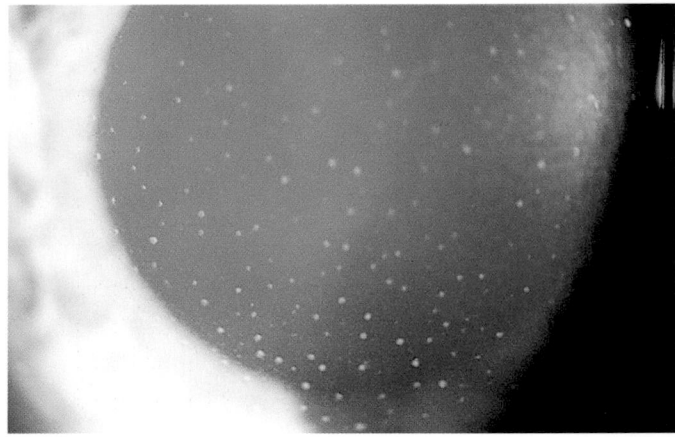
Fig. 3 Small keratic precipitates evenly distributed on the corneal endothelium as typically seen in Fuch's cyclitis.

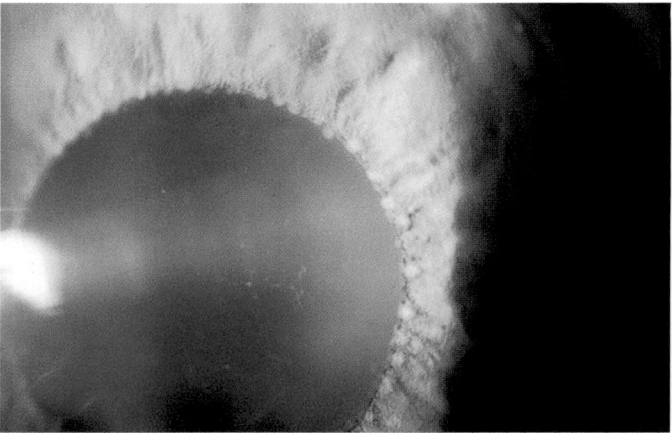
Fig. 4 Inflammatory nodules at the pupillary margin (Koeppe's nodules).

ent a sign of a granulomatous process and present in variable sizes. The nodules are usually white, although large pink nodules can be found in conditions such as sarcoidosis (iris granulomas). Peripheral anterior synechiae can develop in chronic anterior uveitis and can lead to glaucoma due to involvement of the angle.

The texture of the iris may be altered by infiltration of inflammatory or neoplastic cells, with the presence of diffuse or localized thickening of the iris. Especially in sarcoidosis, the iris may show complete loss of its crypts and ridges, acquiring what has been described as a 'succulent' quality. In other conditions, the iris stroma will be atrophic, which can easily be seen by retroillumination. In Fuchs' cyclitis this is usually seen along the pupillary border, while it will be sectorial in association with herpes zoster uveitis and multifocal in cases associated with herpes simplex uveitis.

Cataract can develop either as a consequence of intense or recurrent uveitis, or as a consequence of the prolonged use of topical steroids, sometimes required to control the inflammation, and it is typically a posterior subcapsular type (Fig. 5). Band keratopathy can develop in cases of chronic anterior

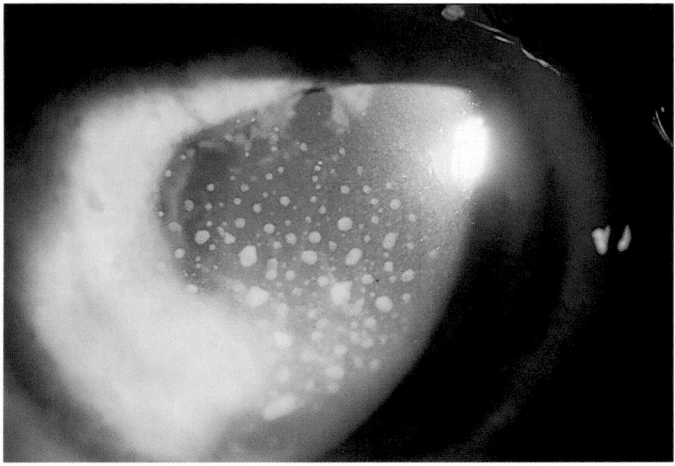
Fig. 2 Large and small keratic precipitates concentrated mainly inferiorly; also note the presence of posterior synechiae.

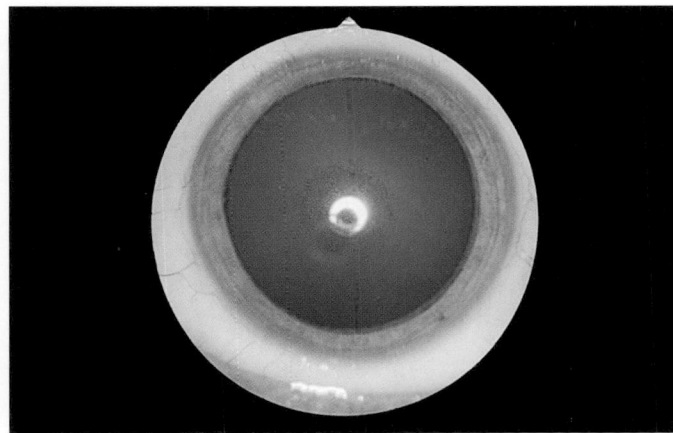

Fig. 5 Posterior subcapsular cataract associate with uveitis and chronic use of topical steroids.

segment inflammation, especially in cases of juvenile chronic arthritis and sarcoidosis, and represents the accumulation of calcium hydroxyapatite in Bowman's membrane. It is localized in the interpalpebral cornea, which is probably related to local pH, and starts 1 mm inside the cornea (not continuous with the limbus).

From the chronic anterior uveitis group, juvenile chronic arthritis deserves especial consideration since it is usually asymptomatic ('white' eye) and these young patients tend to be seen only when severe complications have already developed leading to severe loss of vision. Approximately 20 per cent of juvenile chronic arthritis patients develop anterior uveitis which is usually bilateral. From the three subgroups that have been identified (Still's disease, polyarticular juvenile chronic arthritis, and pauciarticular juvenile chronic arthritis) the latter is closely associated with iridocyclitis, and it can be divided into early onset (before 8 years) and late onset. It is in the early onset subgroup, which occurs more frequently in females, that the highest association with chronic iridocyclitis is found. The first symptom is usually reduced vision or a white pupil due to cataract. The disease tends to be progressive, often resulting in severe visual loss or blindness. In most cases, the interval between the onset of juvenile chronic arthritis and the diagnosis of uveitis occurs between 2 and 7 years, with the risk of uveitis decreasing when the patient is older than 7 years. Since the risk of developing uveitis is different for the different groups, a schedule of ophthalmological examinations for at least 7 years has been proposed by Kanski: patients with systemic onset (Still's disease) should be examined annually; the polyarticular onset should be seen every 6 months; the pauciarticular every 3 months; and those with a positive antinuclear antibody every 2 months. The antinuclear antibody is positive in approximately 80 per cent of the cases presenting with ocular involvement.

Intermediate uveitis

Intermediate uveitis is a term proposed to describe a condition that primarily involves the vitreous and peripheral retina. Several conditions have been reported to produce this type of picture, the most frequent being pars planitis. The picture is usually bilateral, but frequently asymmetrical, with one symptomatic eye and the other already showing signs of the disease. Other conditions include multiple sclerosis, sarcoidosis, toxocariasis, peripheral toxoplasmosis, Fuchs' cyclitis, and infectious causes such as tuberculosis, syphilis, and Lyme disease.

The clinical presentation is usually with a history of floaters, with or without hazy vision, in the absence of pain, redness, and photophobia. Rarely it may begin as a typical attack of acute anterior uveitis, with the possibility of formation of posterior synechiae; following this, it tends to behave more typically, with minimal anterior chamber reaction. The most important diagnostic findings are in the vitreous cavity, with the typical snowball opacities mainly inferiorly and at the peripheral retina where retinal periphlebitis is common. The vitreous opacities are described as floaters, and they may vary from only a few to numerous. They may cause important visual disturbance when in large numbers (Fig. 6).

Snowbanking is an organized fibrous or fibrovascular tissue seen at the pars plana/ora serrata region, and represents a hallmark for pars planitis. Its presence for the diagnosis of this condition is questionable and some believe that it only represents a sign of chronicity and severity. It is most frequently found inferiorly, but may be seen in all quadrants. New vessels at the snowbanking are a sign of aggressive inflammation and may be associated with vitreous haemorrhage. As mentioned above, sheathing of vessels in the retinal periphery (Fig. 7) is a common finding, and both these vessels, as well as posterior vessels, may show leakage during a fluorescein angiography. Peripapillary retinal oedema and cystoid macular oedema may occur with the latter being usually responsible for the poor vision in these patients, and it represents the main reason for initiating therapy. Vision can also be affected by dragging of the macula towards the area of organized exudation in the retinal periphery. Posterior subcapsular cataract can also develop and is another reason for reduced vision.

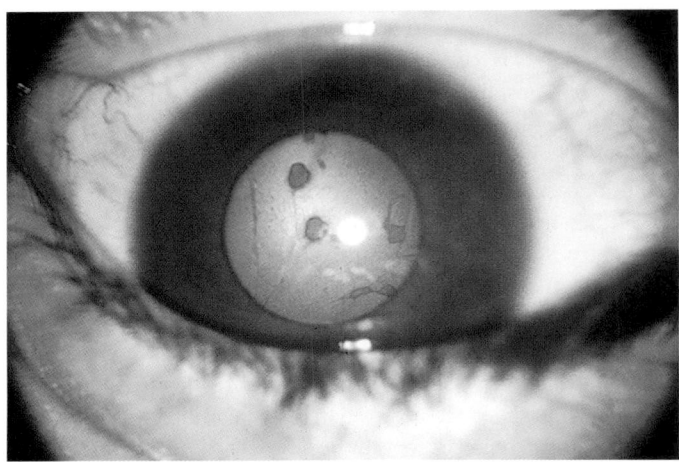

Fig. 6 Vitreous condensations (floaters) in a patient with intermediate uveitis.

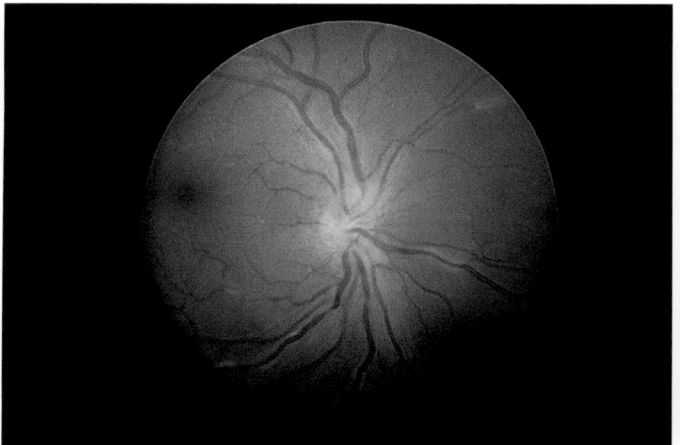

Fig. 7 Vascular sheathing in a patient with systemic sarcoidosis.

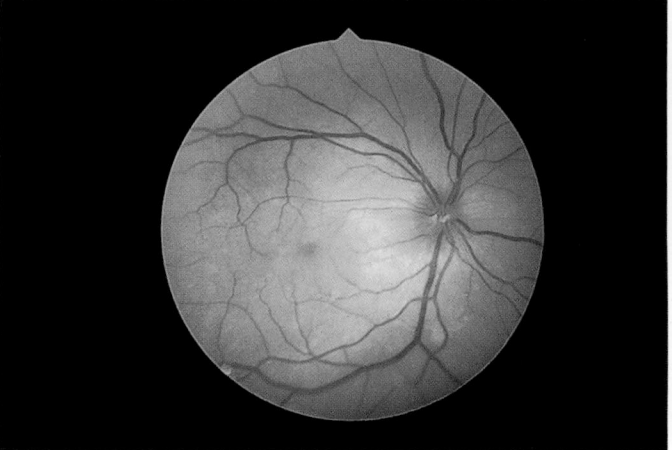

Fig. 8 Optic disc is hyperaemic but not swollen with the presence of choroidal hypochromic lesions temporal to the disc (Vogt–Koyanagi–Harada syndrome).

Multiple sclerosis is a demyelinating disease of the central nervous system, of probable autoimmune origin, and has as its main ocular manifestation optic neuritis. The duration of the multiple sclerosis does not correlate with the incidence of uveitis, which may actually antedate the neurological involvement by many years. Chronic intermediate uveitis has been reported in 27 per cent of patients with multiple sclerosis.

Posterior uveitis

Posterior uveitis is the general descriptive term for retinitis, retinochoroiditis, choroiditis, and chorioretinitis. Inflammatory changes may be limited or may start as retinitis or choroiditis, but in most cases there will be involvement of both. Clinical manifestation of choroidal lesions will depend on their location, size, and severity. While peripheral lesions may remain relatively asymptomatic, a lesion in the posterior pole is more likely to induce visual symptoms. Lesions of the choroid will usually appear as individual round yellow nodules, but may also be more confluent and placoid in appearance. These lesions may affect the function of the retinal pigment epithelium, with consequent disturbance of photoreceptors function, and in more severe cases, may lead to accumulation of fluid in the subretinal space (exudative retinal detachment).

The vitreous remains free of inflammatory cells if the disease process remains limited to the choroid, but will be involved when the retina or retinal vessels become affected. Vitreous haze seems to be a good indicator of inflammatory activity and a grading scale, based on the view of the optic disc and posterior retina, with the use of an indirect ophthalmoscope and a 20-dioptre lens has been developed by Nussenblatt *et al.* (Nussenblatt *et al.* 1985).

Some cases present as multifocal choroiditis and leave areas of atrophy, some of which may have a characteristic punched out appearance. In some conditions such as sympathetic ophthalmia, Vogt–Koyanagi–Harada (Fig. 8), and sarcoidosis, cellular infiltrates may occur at the level of the retinal pigment epithelium, which are known as Dalen–Fuchs nodules.

Retinitis may present with blurring of vision when there is involvement of the macula or secondary cystoid macular oedema. Peripheral lesions may be less noticeable but may still produce cells in the vitreous which will be seen as floaters. In the absence of vitreous haze, cystoid macular oedema can be easily seen with a contact lens, which will also allow determination of macular thickening. Macular oedema may be obscured by vitreous haze, and in these cases, an indirect illumination, with the light slightly to one side of the fovea, will reveal the cystic changes. Objective documentation of cystoid macular oedema can be obtained with fluorescein angiography (Fig. 9).

Scotomas will correspond to the location of the retinal lesion. Acute retinal lesions will appear as clouded areas with indistinct borders and overlying vitreous cells. Sheathing of retinal vessels may also be seen in the vicinity of the active retinitis and does not represent primary vasculitis. As the lesion resolves the borders become more demarcated and, at the time of complete resolution, will leave behind a central area of necrosis, which can be limited to the retina, such as seen in cytomegalovirus retinitis, or affecting deeper layers (choriocapillary and choroid)

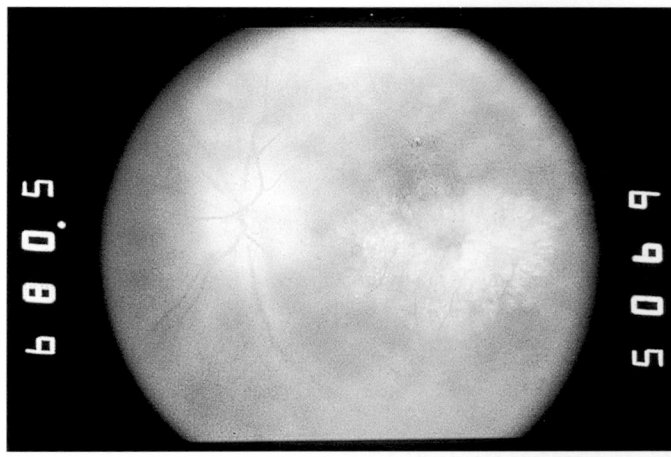

Fig. 9 Late phase of fluorescein angiogram showing posterior pole leakage and marked cystoid macular oedema.

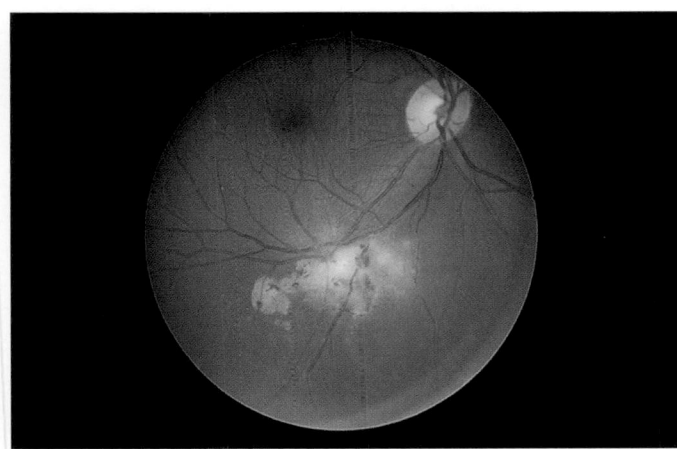

Fig. 10 Retinal scar with the presence of an active retinitis next to it (satellite lesion), typical of toxoplasmic retinochoroiditis.

such as in toxoplasmosis (Fig. 10). In severe cases of inflammation the posterior vitreous may detach and clumps of cells can precipitate on the posterior vitreous face.

In acute vascular occlusions, ischaemic retinal oedema will be seen, but in cases of old vascular loss, the retina will look atrophic, usually with pigmentary changes (retinal pigment epithelium stippling). Cotton-wool spots and haemorrhages may also be present in retinal vasculitis, which are secondary to ischaemia, and associated with involvement of the microvascular system or larger vessels, respectively. Another form of vascular complication in uveitis is the development of choroidal neovascular membranes which should be suspected in the presence of grey–white elevations of the retina, subretinal haemorrhages, and hard exudates. They are associated with lesions affecting the integrity of Bruch's membrane, and may induce severe loss of vision in cases of macular involvement.

Optic nerve involvement may occur directly as in cases of some viral infections (acute retinal necrosis), sarcoidosis, or Vogt–Koyanagi–Harada syndrome, but most frequently occurs secondarily to the primary inflammatory focus, such as in toxoplasmosis or cases of intermediate uveitis. The optic nerve may look hyperaemic, with little or no swelling as is typical of Vogt–Koyanagi–Harada, but may also look grossly swollen which may be due to oedema or optic nerve cellular infiltration. In primary involvement, vision is severely affected and a relative afferent pupillary defect is obvious.

Further reading

Aaberg, T.M. (1987). The enigma of pars planitis. *American Journal of Ophthalmology*, **103**, 828–30.

Bloch-Michel, E. and Nussenblatt, R.B. (1987). International Uveitis Study Group recommendations for the evaluation of intraocular inflammatory disease. *American Journal of Ophthalmology*, **103**, 234–5.

Dreyer, R.F. and Gass, J.D.M. (1984). Multifocal choroiditis and panuveitis. *Archives of Ophthalmology*, **102**, 1776–84.

Gass, J.D.M. and Olson, C.L. (1976). Sarcoidosis with optic nerve and retinal involvement. *Archives of Ophthalmology*, **94**, 945–50.

Henderly, D.E., Haymond, R.S., Rao, N.S., *et al.* (1987). The significance of the pars plana exudate in pars planitis. *American Journal of Ophthalmology*, **103**, 669–71.

Hogan, M.J., Kimura, S.J., and Thygeson, P. (1959). Signs and symptoms of uveitis: I. Anterior uveitis. *American Journal of Ophthalmology*, **47**, 155–70.

Jabs, D.A. and Johns, C.J. (1986). Ocular involvement in chronic sarcoidosis *American Journal of Ophthalmology*, **102**, 297–301.

Kanski, J.J. (1977). Anterior uveitis in juvenile rheumatoid arthritis. *Archives of Ophthalmology*, **95**, 1794–7.

Kanski, J.J. (1989). Screening for uveitis in juvenile chronic arthritis. *British Journal of Ophthalmology*, **73**, 225–8.

Jones, N.P. (1993). Fuchs' heterochromic uveitis: an update. *Survey of Ophthalmology*, **37**, 253–72.

Marak, G.E. Jr (1979). Recent advances in sympathetic ophthalmia. *Survey of Ophthalmology*, **24**, 141–56.

Michaelson, J.B. and Chisari, F.V. (1982). Behçet's disease. *Survey of Ophthalmology*, **26**, 190–203.

Nussenblatt, R.B., Palestine, A.G., Chan, C.C., *et al.* (1985). Standardisation of vitreal inflammatory activity in intermediate and posterior uveitis. *Ophthalmology*, **92**, 467–71.

Nussenblatt, R.B., Whitcup, S.M., and Palestine, A.G. (1996). *Uveitis: fundamentals and clinical practice*, (2nd edn). Mosby, St Louis.

Pavésio, C.E. and Lightman, S.L. (1996). *Toxoplasma gondii* and ocular toxoplasmosis: pathogenesis. *British Journal of Ophthalmology*, **80**, 1099–107.

Pavésio, C.E. and Nozik, R.A. (1990). Anterior and intermediate uveitis. *International Ophthalmology Clinics*, **30**, 244–51.

Rosenberg, A.M. (1987). Uveitis associated with juvenile rheumatoid arthritis. *Seminars on Arthritis and Rheumatology*, **16**, 158–73.

Rothova, A., Veenedaal, W.G., Linseen, A. *et al.* (1987). Clinical features of acute anterior uveitis. *American Journal of Ophthalmology*, **103**, 137–45.

Schlaegel, T.F. Jr (1973). Differential diagnosis of uveitis. *Ophthalmology Digest*, **35**, 34.

Shields, J.A. (1984). Ocular toxocariasis: a review. *Survey of Ophthalmology*, **28**, 361–81.

Smith, R.E. and Nozik, R.A. (1989). *Uveitis: a clinical approach to diagnosis and management*, (2nd edn). Williams & Wilkins, Baltimore.

Spalton, D.J. and Sanders, M.D. (1981). Fundus changes in histologically confirmed sarcoidosis. *British Journal of Ophthalmology*, **65**, 348–58.

Stillermen, M.L. (1951). Ocular manifestations of diffuse collagen disease. *Archives of Ophthalmology*, **45**, 239–50.

Sugiura, S. (1978). Vogt–Koyanagi–Harada disease. *Japan Journal of Ophthalmology*, **22**, 9–35.

Wakefield, D., Montanaro, A., and McCluskey, P. (1991). Acute anterior uveitis and HLA-B27. *Survey of Ophthalmology*, **36**, 223–32.

2.8.5 Uveitis associated with infections

A. Tufail and Gary N. Holland

Infectious diseases account for a higher percentage of uveitis cases at the extremes of ages and in immunosuppressed hosts. Uveitis caused by infectious disease is often only one manifestation of a systemic illness. Clinicians should always consider the possibility of an infectious cause before treating a case of 'idiopathic' uveitis with anti-inflammatory or immunosuppressive drugs. In many cases an infectious disease can be identified at an early stage with a careful history, review of systems, and thorough ophthalmological examination. An infectious disease

Table 1 Usual sites of primary intraocular disease causes by infectious agents

	Keratouveitis	Iridocyclitis	Intermediate uveitis	Retinitis	Reinochoroiditis/ chorioretinitis	Choroiditis	Retinal vasculitis	Neuroretinitis	Panuveitis	Endophthalmitis
Bacteria										
Syphilis	Yes	Yes	Yes	Yes	Yes	Yes	Yes	Yes	Yes	
TB	Yes	Yes		Rare	Yes	Yes	Yes		Yes	Yes
Non-TB mycobacteria disease						Yes (multifocal)				
Lyme disease	Yes	Yes	Yes			Yes	Yes	Optic neuritis	Yes	
Relapsing fever		Yes	Yes					Optic neuritis		
Leptospirosis		Yes		Yes (rare)						
Leprosy	Yes	Yes							Rare	
Whipple's disease		Yes	Yes	Yes		Yes	Yes			
Catscratch disease				Yes				Yes		
Poststreptococcal disease		Yes								
Endogenous bacterial infection		Yes			Yes					Yes
Brucellosis		Yes	Yes		Yes		Rare		Rare	Rare
Viruses										
HSV disease	Yes	Yes		Yes, ARN	Yes			Optic nueritis		
HIV disease		?Yes	?Yes					?Optic neuritis		
CMV retinitis				Yes			Yes			
HTLV-1 disease		Yes	Yes				Yes			
EBV disease		Yes				?Yes				
Measles		Yes		Yes				Yes		
Mumps		Yes		Yes						
Rubella		Yes			Yes					
Rift valley fever				Yes			Yes			
VZV disease	Yes	Yes		Yes, ARN				Optic neuritis		
Protozoa										
Toxoplasmosis				Yes	Yes				Yes	
Pneumocystosis						Yes (multifocal)				
Helminths										
Toxocariasis					Yes					Yes
Cysticercosis				Yes						
Onchocerciasis	Yes	Yes			Yes			Optic neuritis		
Trypanosomiasis	Yes	Yes		Yes				Optic neuritis		
Ophthalmomyiasis		Yes			Yes				Yes	Yes
Giardiasis		Yes			Yes					
Fungal										
POHS						Yes				
Infectious histoplasmosis		Yes		Yes					Yes	Yes
Cryptococcosis						Yes (multifocal)				
Coccidioidomycosis						Yes (multifocal)				
Candidiasis				Yes	Yes	Yes				Yes

ARN, acute retinal necrosis; CMV, cytomegalovirus; EBV, Epstein–Barr virus; HSV, herpes simplex virus; HTLV, human T-lymphotrophic virus; VZV, varicella-zoster virus; POHS, presumed ocular histoplasmosis syndrome; TB, tuberculosis.

should be suspected if the inflammation does not resolve or improve greatly with aggressive corticosteroid therapy; suspicious signs would include persistent keratic precipitates or fibrin in the anterior chamber, chemosis, and hypopyon.

Specific infectious agents usually affect a particular group of ocular structures. Primary sites of intraocular infectious diseases are summarized in Table 1.

This chapter will concentrate on the more common causes of infectious uveitis. Postsurgical infectious uveitis, various forms of endophthalmitis, and infectious uveitis associated with immunosuppression are discussed elsewhere.

Bacterial infections

Syphilis

Syphilis is a systemic disease with diverse ocular manifestations caused by the spirochaete *Treponema pallidum*. The prevalence of early acquired syphilis has increased over the last two decades due to altered sexual practices, drug abuse, and acquired immune deficiency syndrome (AIDS). There are now approximately 50 cases per 100 000 population in Western countries.

Syphilis is usually transmitted sexually and therefore the chancre lesion, which occurs during primary syphilis, is commonly situated in the genital area. A chancre is a painless, hard nodule caused by mononuclear cell infiltration at the site of spirochaete entry. It typically heals in 3 to 6 weeks. The organism is then disseminated via blood vessels and lymphatics, causing a more diffuse mononuclear reaction that results in secondary syphilis. The secondary stage occurs in most untreated patients about 6 weeks after the primary stage, and is commonly associated with a maculopapular rash and with large papules, called condyloma lata, in the intertriginous regions. The ocular and systemic features of acquired syphilis are summarized in Table 2.

Table 2 Syphilis

Stage	Time from infection	Serological testing	General systemic complications	Ocular complications	Neurological complications
Primary syphilis	2–6 weeks	VDRL and FTA (about 75% positive after 1 month)	Genital chancre, occasionally extragenital	Rarely lid or conjunctival chancre	
Secondary syphilis	6 weeks to 6 months	Postprimary syphilis VDRL and FTA almost always both positive (rare exceptions*)	Maculopapular rash, fever/malaise/lymph-adenopathy, condyloma lata, alopecia	Anterior uveitis, iris roseola, papillary conjunctivitis, conjunctival erosion and nodule, margins, corneal infiltrates epi/scleritis, chorioretinitis and retinal vasculitis, neuroretinitis, optic neuritis papilloedema, periostitis	Acute meningitis, optic neuritis, cranial nerve palsy, stroke due to meningovascular syphilis, rare at this stage except if immunosuppressed
Relapsing secondary syphilis	Occurs in about 25% of patients in latency			As above	
Latent syphilis	About 1 year	FTA mostly positive, VDRL often (about 25%) negative, if present low titre	Signs of inactive disease	Signs of inactive disease	
Tertiary syphilis	2 years to decades† (parenchymatous syphilis tends to occur after about 10–15 years)	FTA mostly positive, VDRL often (about 25%) negative, low titre if present, CSF VDRL often positive in neurosyphilis	Gummatous disease (granulomatous endarteritis) affecting skin, lungs, bones, liver and CNS. Obliterative endarteritis causing cardiovascular problems (aortic aneurysm, aortic valve regurgitation)	Anterior uveitis, stromal keratitis (often unilateral), scleritis, chorioretinitis (focal or multifocal), retinal vasculitis leading to occlusion, granulomas affecting conjunctiva, lid, orbit, iris and optic nerve, neuro-ophthalmic manifestations	Meningovascular (periarteritis leading to stroke syndromes: can cause field defects and Horner's syndrome) parenchymatous (postinflammatory neuronal degeneration) leading to a number of disorders: (i) general paresis (personality change, Argyll Robertson pupil, fits, dementia, paresis), (ii) tabes dorsalis, (iii) isolated optic atrophy

*If secondary syphilis is strongly suspected on clinical grounds a diluted blood sample should be retested, as occasionally excess antigen may give a false-negative result (prozone reaction).
†In HIV-positive patients, the stages may progress more rapidly.
CNS, central nervous system; CSF, cerebrospinal fluid; FTA, fluorescent treponemal antibody test; VDRL, Venereal Disease Research Laboratory.

Granulomatous or non-granulomatous anterior uveitis of varying severity is the most common eye manifestation of the secondary stage, and is present in up to 5 per cent of cases. Anterior uveitis is often unilateral initially and may be of sudden onset. It may be accompanied by the presence of engorged iris vascular fronds called roseola. Posterior uveitis may be focal or diffuse and may take the form of a choroiditis or a chorioretinitis. Plaque-like areas of chorioretinitis may be associated with vitreous inflammatory reaction and serous retinal detachment. Chorioretinitis gives a 'leopard-spot' appearance to the early phases of the fluorescein angiogram, and late staining. The chorioretinitis may resolve, leaving a pigmentary retinopathy with hypopigmented chorioretinal scars. Complica-

tions of posterior uveitis include uveal effusion, exudative retinal detachment, and optic disc oedema.

It is not clear why second-stage disease is able to progress to an asymptomatic latent phase despite the presence of an intact immune response including circulating antibodies. Relapses of disorders associated with secondary syphilis may occur during the early latent phase.

About a quarter of untreated patients eventually develop tertiary syphilis. Anterior uveitis, which may be associated with uniocular interstitial keratitis or punctate stromal keratitis, is the most common ocular manifestation of tertiary syphilis, affecting up to 5 per cent of patients at this stage. Uveal inflammation may produce iris nodules, masses in the

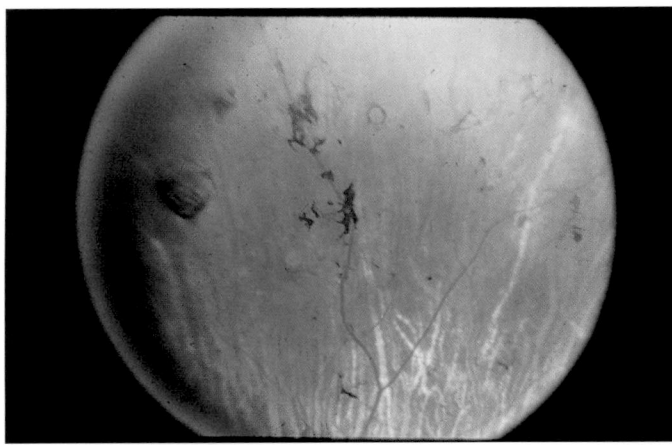

Fig. 1 Mottled fundus pigmentation in a patient with a history of syphilitic retinitis. (By courtesy of Allan E. Kreiger.)

iridocorneal angle, focal or multifocal chorioretinitis, and retinal vasculitis. The clinical presentation of syphilitic uveitis may be more severe in human immunodeficiency virus (HIV) positive individuals as described elsewhere in this text. Obliterative endarteritis occurs in this stage, which may produce granulomatous lesions, termed gummas, that can affect the eyelids, anterior segment structures, orbit, optic nerve, and uvea.

Congenital syphilis may be divided into an early stage, occurring before 2 years of age, and late stages that approximate the secondary and tertiary stages of acquired disease (see Table 2). Chorioretinitis and anterior uveitis are the most common complications of early, congenital syphilis and may appear as early as 6 months of age. Sequelae of uveitis include glaucoma, cataract, and postinflammatory pigmentary changes of the posterior pole. Untreated late congenital syphilis differs from acquired disease by the occurrence of bilateral (80 per cent of cases) interstitial keratitis, which is rare in acquired disease and is usually unilateral if present. Periostitis may result in an array of bone and dental abnormalities, such as peg-shaped incisors (Hutchinson's teeth), abnormal molars, 'sabre tibia', and saddle-nose deformities.

Diagnosis of ocular syphilis is based on a combination of serological tests and clinical findings, because isolation of the organism is usually not possible in late syphilis or isolated ocular disease. If tissue specimens are available, then dark-field microscopy, silver staining, or fluorescence microscopy may be useful for detecting the organism. Serological tests can be divided into direct specific tests for immunoglobulins against *T. pallidum* (indirect fluorescent treponemal antibody absorbed test (FTA-Abs), and microhaemagglutination *T. pallidum* test (MHA-TP)) and indirect tests for non-specific antibodies against altered host lipids (Venereal Disease Research Laboratory test (VDRL) and the rapid plasmin reagin test (RPR)). Both types of test should be performed in the setting of suspected syphilitic uveitis, as this disease usually occurs in the setting of late syphilis when the sensitivity of the indirect tests are only about 70 per cent. The

indirect tests reflect disease activity and the direct tests are used to detect previous or current syphilis infection. Both tests are prone to false positives and negatives due to other disease states, and their rates of positivity vary according to disease stage (see Table 2). Evaluation of cerebrospinal fluid for an inflammatory cellular reaction, elevated protein, and reactivity on VDRL testing should be performed when active ocular disease or neurosyphilis is suspected or in the setting of HIV infection.

The treatment of choice for syphilis is systemic penicillin. The exact formulation of penicillin and the length of treatment depends on the stage and manifestation of syphilis. For neurosyphilis, ocular disease, and HIV-positive hosts, more prolonged treatment at higher doses may be necessary, and the addition of probenecid may be beneficial in boosting drug levels in these cases. Patients with interstitial keratitis and anterior uveitis should also receive topical corticosteroids and mydriatics. The use of systemic corticosteroids in conjunction with antibiotics should not be used routinely, but may have a role in severe sight-threatening inflammatory ocular disease such as posterior uveitis and scleritis. Response to treatment is reflected by improvement in clinical signs and decline in VDRL titres. After initiating penicillin therapy, uveitis rarely may become worse as part of the Jarisch-Herxheimer reaction, a hypersensitivity response to released antigen.

Lyme disease

Lyme disease is a tick-borne infection caused by the spirochaete *Borrelia burgdorferi*. Although the disease was described at the beginning of the twentieth century, its name is derived from an outbreak of the disease in Lyme, Connecticut, in the United States during the 1970s. The primary reservoirs for this spirochaete are small rodents, although other animals, such as deer and racoons, can provide mating grounds and blood meals for the ticks. *Ioxedes* ticks (of various species) acquire and spread the spirochaete while taking a blood meal, which it does once in each of the three stages in its lifecycle. The peak seasonal incidence in the northern hemisphere occurs in the spring and early summer, corresponding to when the second-stage organism, the nymph, takes its blood meal. Disease features can be grouped into early and late manifestations. In the early stage, a pathognomonic rash called erythema migrans is noted in about 60 per cent of patients. The rash starts days to weeks after a tick bite that is usually painless; it begins as a macule, then typically expands into a circular or annular lesion greater than 5 cm in diameter. In about 50 per cent of patients multiple, smaller annular lesions may occur after several days at sites distal to the original tick bite. Fever, headache, arthralgia, and conjunctivitis may occur at this stage, but these features all resolve typically in 2 to 4 weeks. The late stage can involve the nervous system in about 15 per cent of cases (causing meningitis, Bell's palsy and other cranial neuropathies, encephalitis, and encephalomyelitis), the heart in about 10 per cent of cases (causing myocarditis and heart block), the musculoskeletal system in about 60 per cent of cases (typically a pauciarticular large joint arthropathy), and occasionally the eye. Anterior uveitis that may include iris nodules and posterior synechiae can develop at this stage. Vitreous inflammatory reactions, snowbanks, panuveitis, choroiditis, and exudative retinal detachments may also occur. Other ocular findings include stromal keratitis, optic neuritis, papilloedema (secondary to meningitis), and optic atrophy.

A diagnosis of Lyme disease is made when the erythema migrans rash is documented or serological tests are positive in the appropriate clinical setting. One should be wary of making the diagnosis outside an endemic area; serological tests are unreliable, having a high false-positive rate of up to 5 per cent, which gives a very low positive predictive value in non-endemic areas. *Borrelia burgdoferi* is difficult to culture and it is also difficult to demonstrate a four-fold increase in anti-*B. burgdoferi* immunoglobulin M antibodies. A two-test approach, looking for antibodies to *B. burgdoferi*, is most reliable, using a sensitive enzyme immunoassay or immunofluorescence assay followed by a Western immunoblot, if the initial test is positive. Other diseases such as syphilis, multiple sclerosis, sarcoidosis, juvenile chronic arthritis, and other inflammatory diseases should be ruled out. Serological tests for Lyme disease titres may be positive in up to 60 per cent of patients with syphilis, and conversely, the fluorescent treponemal antibody absorbed test may be positive in about 20 per cent of patients with Lyme disease. Autoimmune disorders and infectious mononucleosis may also give rise to false-positive serological tests.

Current recommendations for treatment include the use of amoxycillin or doxycycline for early infections (although the latter should be avoided in children or pregnant women) and intravenous ceftriaxone for late infections or cardiac and central nervous system complications. Iridocyclitis responds to topical corticosteroid and cycloplegic treatment.

Leptospirosis

Leptospirosis is caused by the spirochaete *Leptospira interrogans*. The usual hosts for the spirochaete include rats and domestic animals. Humans acquire disease most commonly by contact with water infected by animal urine. Occupations at greatest risk of encountering leptospirosis are farmers, and sewer and abattoir workers.

After an incubation period of up to a month a primary leptospiraemic phase occurs, characterized by headache, fever, and conjunctival suffusion. The secondary, immune phase of disease commences between day 6 and 12 of the illness. The immune phase has variable manifestations including fever, meningism, cranial nerve palsies, optic neuritis, and renal and liver dysfunction. Up to 44 per cent of patients may develop uveitis that usually takes the form of a bilateral panuveitis, although retinal periphlebitis and isolated anterior uveitis or vitreous humour inflammation may also occur. Occasionally the posterior segment can be involved with the appearance of retinal haemorrhages and exudates. Diagnosis is made serologically or by isolation of the spirochaete. Treatment for mild disease is with oral ampicillin or doxycyline, and with intravenous penicillin reserved for severe disease.

Tuberculosis

Tuberculosis is a disease caused by the acid-fast bacillus *Mycobacterium tuberculosis*. It is increasing in prevalence in some Western countries due to a combination of factors, including HIV infection, immigration from endemic areas, homelessness, and intravenous drug use. Tuberculosis usually affects the lungs, but may also affect extrapulmonary sites in up to 15 per cent of all cases and in an even larger proportion of immunosuppressed patients. In developed countries primary infection only causes clinical disease in about 5 to 10 per cent of cases. Ocular manifestations occur in only about 1 per cent of those affected. In asymptomatic patients disease is controlled by cell-mediated immunity. Postprimary tuberculosis is triggered by altered immune function and usually occurs within a few years of the primary infection. Clinical signs result from local lung disease, miliary tuberculosis, or infection of individual organs.

Tuberculosis may cause a variety of ocular inflammatory disorders, which, although uncommon in developed countries, have been estimated to cause up to a third of childhood uveitides in India. Anterior uveitis is usually chronic and granulomatous in type, and is often complicated by posterior synechiae and glaucoma. Tuberculosis is not expected to result in non-specific anterior chamber cellular reactions as the sole manifestation of disease; there will commonly be a focus of infection, such as an iris mass. Iris nodules may be due to either granulomatous inflammation, mycobacterial infection in miliary disease (that takes the form of greyish masses), or a tuberculoma (that typically presents as a single large lesion). The posterior segment is most commonly affected either a single large or, more commonly, by multiple grey or yellow choroidal tuberculomas that may be associated with a local serous retinal detachment. Vitreous inflammatory reaction is usually mild. A retinal vasculitis may occur in association with or independent of choroiditis, but retinal vasculitis is not believed to be a manifestation of vessel wall infection. A severe endophthalmitis may occasionally occur. Other ocular abnormalities include phlyctenular conjunctivitis, interstitial keratitis, orbital periostitis, and neuro-ophthalmic abnormalities.

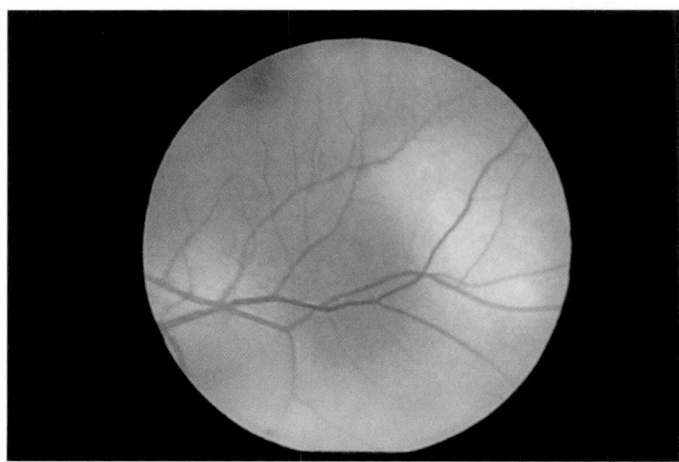

Fig. 2 Choroidal tuberculoma. (By courtesy of Careen Y. Lowder. Reprinted with permission from Helm and Holland 1993.)

The diagnosis of ocular tuberculosis is often difficult to make, and is based on clinical findings, chest X-ray, skin testing, and, if necessary, sputum or other body fluid culture and histology. Chest radiographic abnormalities are common in immunocompetent individuals, although they may be less common in the immunosuppressed or in those presenting with extrapulmonary disease. Skin testing involves development of a hypersensitivity response to a subcutaneous injection of purified protein derivative. A false-positive reaction occurs in patients who have received bacille Calmette–Guérin vaccination and false negatives can occur in those with sarcoidosis, the elderly, immunosuppressed individuals, and those with viral illnesses. Strongly reactive skin tests should not be attributed to prior bacille Calmette–Guérin immunization. Acid-fast bacilli are detected in tissue smears by fluorescence testing or by Ziehl-Neelsen staining. Experimental polymerase chain reaction techniques on vitreous humour samples are under evaluation. Diagnosis may be made by finding the classic lesion of caseating granuloma with epithelioid and Langerhans' giant cells and the presence of acid-fast bacilli on staining of tissue sections. Isoniazid therapeutic testing to diagnose tuberculosis is controversial and probably unreliable. Consideration should be given to the possibility of coinfection with HIV.

Treatment of tuberculosis requires multidrug therapy because of the high rate of resistant organisms and/or the development of resistance during treatment. Treatment initially consists of a three or four drug regimens, depending on knowledge of local resistance. The drugs generally used are rifampicin and isoniazid for a minimum of 6 months and pyrazinamide for at least the first 2 months with the possible addition of either ethambutol or streptomycin. It should be noted that rifampicin is hepatotoxic and causes a red discoloration of body fluids including tears that can stain contact lenses. Isoniazid is also hepatotoxic and may cause optic neuropathy. Ethambutol may cause retrobulbar optic neuritis. Multiple drug resistant strains are emerging and are common in patients with AIDS. Patients should have regular monitoring to check for compliance and drug toxicity. The treatment of resistant strains and of non-tuberculous mycobacterial infection are covered elsewhere in this text.

Leprosy

Leprosy, or Hansen's disease, is caused by the acid-fast bacillus *Mycobacterium leprae*. Leprosy is endemic in many parts of Central and South America, Africa, and Asia. Leprosy is only mildly contagious and is transmitted via the upper respiratory tract or skin lesions. Ocular complications are very common because the bacillus prefers cool, nerve- and pigment-rich environments. Infection causes an inflammatory response that results in atrophy, deformity, and loss of function of many tissues. Leprosy results in blindness in up to 10 per cent of those with eye disease. The disease manifestations and type of ocular complications depend on the host's immune response. The extremes of the disease spectrum are the tuberculoid type, with limited infection and marked cell-mediated immune reaction, and the lepromatous type, with extensive infection and poor cell-mediated immunity. Leprosy can also be divided by skin smear tests into a paucibacillary type, corresponding to the tuberculoid type of disease, and a multibacillary type, corresponding to the lepromatous end of the spectrum. Between these extremes lie 'borderline' cases.

Anterior uveitis is a common complication of multibacillary disease. It usually has few cells and little flare, and takes a chronic, insidious course that tends to result in iris atrophy and small pupil due to concomitant sympathetic neuropathy. The small pupil combined with cataract results in profound vision loss. Microlepromas, appearing as small white pearls, are sometimes found on the iris early in the disease. A more acute, granulomatous iridocyclitis that results in synechiae and secondary glaucoma may also occur, often in association with erythema nodosum. Other ocular manifestations include madarosis, entropion and ectropion, trichiasis, dry eyes, lagophthalmos, and anaesthetic cornea that leads to exposure keratitis and scarring (fifth and seventh cranial nerve palsies are common), episcleritis, scleritis, enlarged corneal nerves, interstitial keratitis, corneal lepromas, hypotony or glaucoma, cataracts, and dacroadenitis.

A clinical diagnosis of leprosy can be made if two of the following three disorders are found: characteristic skin lesions, sensory loss associated with peripheral nerve or skin lesions, and enlarged peripheral nerves. The presence of iris pearls are also highly suggestive of leprosy. Skin biopsies and the lepromin test are reserved for differentiating multibacillary and paucibacillary forms, which will determine the appropriate treatment regimen. Patients with paucibacillary disease require dapsone and rifampicin for a minimum of 6 months, whereas multibacillary disease requires clofazimine in addition. Chronic iridocyclitis requires topical corticosteroid and mydriatic in addition to systemic antimicrobial treatment. Patients with acute iridocyclitis may also require treatment with clofazimine or thalidomide because of the accompanying erythema nodosum leprosum.

Whipple's disease

Whipple's disease is a rare systemic disorder caused by the Gram-positive bacillus *Tropheryma whippelii*. Infection most often affects the gastrointestinal system resulting in malabsorption, weight loss, abdominal tenderness, and regional lymphadenopathy. Low grade fever, arthralgia, endocarditis, and skin hyperpigmentation may also occur. Central nervous system involvement may result in dementia, myoclonus, papilloedema, and ocular motility disorders, including the specific motility disorder of oculomasticator myorhythmia. Other ocular manifestations include iridocyclitis, vitreous inflammatory reaction, retinitis, and retinal vasculitis. Experimental polymerase chain reaction techniques have been used to confirm the diagnosis of *T. whippelii* infection on tissue and vitreous humour samples, as culture of the bacillus is not possible. Diagnosis can also be made by showing periodic acid–Schiff-positive staining of bacteroid structures in macrophages in biopsy specimens. Treatment is initially with parenteral penicillin and streptomycin followed by oral trimethoprim/sulphamethoxazole combination.

Cat-scratch disease

Cat-scratch disease is caused by the Gram-negative bacillus *Bartonella* (formally *Rochalimaea*) *henselae*. Cats, the principal host, transmit infection to humans by bites, scratches, or possibly via fleas. Human infection can result in a localized skin reaction at the site of inoculation and a regional lymphadenitis. Cat-scratch disease is most common in people less than 20 years old, and the prevalence decreases with age. The ocular disease can take two forms: Parinaud's oculoglandular syndrome, caused by direct inoculation near the eye; and a spectrum of intraocular disorders, including optic neuritis, neuroretinitis, retinitis, and vitreous inflammatory reaction, caused by disseminated infection. Disease may take a form similar to Leber's idiopathic stellate neuroretinitis, which causes variable vision loss, and possibly an afferent pupillary defect. In such cases fundoscopy reveals a swollen optic disc and macular star, which usually resolve within 2 to 12 months leaving good final vision. The diagnosis can be confirmed by the indirect fluorescence antibody test for *Bartonella henselae* specific antigen. A variety of antibiotics, including doxycycline and ciprofloxacin, have been used successfully for treatment of the uveitis. Concomitant use of oral corticosteroids has been advocated by some authorities.

Brucellosis

Several species of the Gram-negative bacillus *Brucella* have been implicated in human disease. Brucellosis is a zoonotic infection, with different species having different specific hosts. Cattle, sheep, pigs, and goats are the primary hosts for the species causing human disease. Brucellosis occurs worldwide and is transmitted to humans via unpasturized dairy products or by contact with infected meat.

The disease has two stages: acute and chronic. The acute stage is associated with non-specific symptoms, such as fever, fatigue, abdominal pain, and night sweats, and the chronic stage with arthropathy and neurological involvement. The eye may become involved in both stages, with uveitis being the most common manifestation. Uveitis may range from a mild granulomatous or non-granulomatous anterior uveitis to vitreous inflammatory inflammation, chorioretinitis, and panuveitis. Retinal vasculitis, optic neuritis, and scleritis may also occur. Rarely an endogenous endophthalmitis may occur early in the disease course.

The diagnosis can be made either serologically or by isolation of the organism from blood or ocular fluid samples. Treatment is with a combination of doxycycline and either streptomycin or rifampicin.

Viral infections

Herpes simplex virus associated diseases

Herpes simplex virus, both types 1 and 2, may cause an anterior uveitis that is usually associated with corneal disease. Herpes simplex virus 1 is transmitted by close contact with infected skin or secretions. Herpes simplex virus 2 is spread to the eye from genital tissues, either directly or via the hands. Transmission of herpes simplex virus 2 can occur by these mechanisms at the time of birth in the case of neonatal infections, but both type 1 and 2 may also cause congenital infection *in utero*.

Primary herpes simplex virus infection is usually asymptomatic. Following a primary cutaneous infection in the trigeminal area, herpes simplex virus spreads via retrograde axonal transport and remains latent in the trigeminal or ciliary ganglia. Reactivation results in active virus production and anterograde movement along nerves to the skin or eye.

Herpetic iridocyclitis is usually a manifestation of recurrent disease. It is often granulomatous, and may be accompanied by keratic precipitates, posterior synechiae, and patchy transillumination defects of the iris. The diagnosis is usually made clinically, on the basis of its unilateral presentation, associated iris atrophy, and frequently on accompanying corneal scarring, a sign of previous herpetic keratitis. Usually there will not be a dendritic lesion that can be cultured to confirm disease. Glaucoma is a common complication, either due to trabeculitis, or blockage of outflow by inflammatory cells or debris.

A full thickness, often bilateral, retinitis may rarely occur in patients with disseminated herpes simplex virus infection, and usually in association with encephalitis. This form of retinitis is characterized by retinal oedema, vasculitis with occlusion, and scant haemorrhage. It is often complicated by rhegmatogenous or exudative retinal detachment. The retinitis may also take the form of acute retinal necrosis and may be more severe in the immunosuppressed hosts.

Disseminated infection acquired *in utero* may result in keratitis, iridocyclitis, cataract, optic atrophy, and retinitis. The retinitis usually appears as extensive areas of retinal whitening as described above for patients with encephalitis.

Dendritic ulcer with accompanying iridocyclitis is initially treated with topical antiviral medication (acyclovir or trifluridine). Iridocyclitis is treated with topical corticosteroids and cycloplegia. If corticosteroid is being used frequently, concurrent administration of topical antiviral should be considered to prevent severe epithelial disease if virus shedding recurs. A benefit of systemic antiviral therapy has been suggested in the treatment of keratouveitis. Topical antiviral agents, such as trifluridine or acyclovir, must be given concurrently with topical corticosteroids to treat active epithelial viral infection if it should occur during treatment of the anterior uveitis. Disciform keratitis should be treated with a topical antiviral agent and the minimal dose of topical corticosteroid required to control oedema and inflammation. Topical corticosteroid therapy must be tapered slowly either by reducing frequency of dosing (not more than a 50 per cent reduction at one time) or potency of the corticosteroid preparation to prevent flare-ups of keratitis and uveitis, which are common. Associated elevations of intraocular pressure should be treated as necessary. Retinitis requires systemic acyclovir or other systemic antiviral treatment.

Varicella zoster virus associated disease

Varicella zoster virus usually causes ocular disease during recurrences although the primary infection (chickenpox or

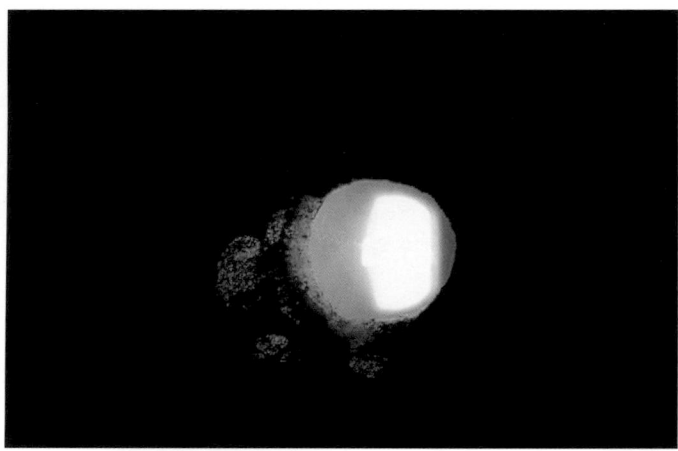

Fig. 3 Retroillumination of the iris in a patient with a history of herpes zoster ophthalmicus. Sectoral iris atrophy is characteristic of varicella zoster virus associated iridocyclitis. (By courtesy of Thomas H. Pettit.)

varicella) can occasionally cause ocular disease. Varicella is a common infection in children and is spread by skin contact or the respiratory route. Disseminated infection causes skin and mucous membrane vesicular lesions. Mild anterior uveitis may complicate this stage of disease, and occasionally patients will develop necrotizing retinitis. The most common complication of varicella is a superficial keratitis, but a disciform or stromal keratitis can also occur.

Following the primary infection varicella zoster virus migrates to the sensory ganglion where it remains latent. Reactivation of the virus, which tends to occur in elderly or immunosuppressed hosts, commonly involves the ophthalmic branch of the trigeminal nerve, resulting in herpes zoster ophthalmicus. Common ocular manifestations include conjunctivitis, keratitis, uveitis, episcleritis, and scleritis, but retinitis, cranial nerve palsies, orbital apex syndrome, and optic neuritis may also occur. Rarely cerebral vasculitis may complicate the course. Iridocyclitis develops in up to 50 per cent of patients with eye disease. It shares many features in common with herpes simplex virus iridocyclitis: iris atrophy, prolonged inflammation with frequent recurrences, granulomatous changes, including mutton-fat keratic percipitates, and a high rate of posterior synechiae and secondary glaucoma. The iris atrophy is often segmental or sectorial, in contrast to diffuse patchy atrophy associated with diffuse herpes simplex virus disease. The atrophy is believed to be a result of local iris vessel occlusion. Intraocular pressure rise, which occurs in up to 40 per cent of patients, can result from a trabeculitis, obstruction of the anterior chamber angle with inflammatory cells or by pupillary seclusion. In the posterior segment inflammatory vascular sheathing or a necrotizing retinitis may develop (see section on acute retinal necrosis and progressive outer retinal necrosis syndrome).

Treatment of herpes zoster ophthalmicus in the immunocompetent patient is with oral acyclovir, valaciclovir, or famciclovir given early in the disease course to reduce the severity and rate of late ocular inflammatory complications. If anterior uveitis occurs, it is treated with topical corticosteroid and cycloplegics. Topical antivirals play no role in the therapy of anterior uveitis.

Measles

Measles is a highly contagious disease caused by a paramyxovirus. Congenital infection may cause cataracts and retinitis. Acquired infection is characterized by fever, maculopapular rash, mucosal Koplik's spots, cough, and conjunctivitis. An acquired retinitis with macular and optic disc oedema, and neuroretinitis can occur rarely. In developing countries, measles is a major cause of blindness through delayed complications that include corneal scarring and rarely an optic neuritis and chorioretinitis. Herpes simplex virus coinfection and vitamin A deficiency may contribute to some of these complications in developing countries.

Subacute sclerosing panencephalitis

Subacute sclerosing panencephalitis is a rare, progressive disease, believed to be a late complication of infection with a measles-type virus that differs from the normal wild type. It usually occurs 6 to 7 years following the initial episode of measles, and often presents with behavioural changes and decreasing school performance followed by seizures. About 50 per cent of those affected have ocular signs, which include focal pigmentary changes at the fovea, white areas of retinitis that may be associated with haemorrhage, papilloedema, and optic atrophy. Ocular motility disorders and cortical blindness may also occur. The prognosis is poor with death occurring within 3 years. There is no treatment for the retinitis, although isoprinisone delays the rate of neurological deterioration.

Mumps

Mumps is caused by a paramyxovirus infection that predominantly affects young children. It causes fever, headache, and malaise, and is followed by parotitis and occasional orchitis and dacroadenitis. Anterior uveitis may occur, and can last for up to a month. Uveitis is treated with topical corticosteroids and cycloplegics. There are usually no long-term sequelae of the inflammation. Rarely an episcleritis, scleritis, and optic neuritis can occur.

Rubella

Rubella is caused by a togavirus infection. Congenital disease results in a syndrome consisting of ocular, as well as cardiac and central nervous system problems. Retinopathy affects about 20 per cent of patients; it causes pigmentary mottling, and has variable retinal distribution. A chronic nongranulomatous anterior uveitis may also develop in the neonatal period. Other ocular problems include microphthalmos, corneal haze, atrophic iris, glaucoma, and cataract. Because virus persists in the lens, care should be taken during cataract surgery to minimize dissemination of virus from lens material, which can cause severe inflammation. Intensive topical corticosteroid therapy is usually required in the postoperative period to control the inflammation. Diagnosis of the congenital rubella syndrome is made on clinical appearance, virus isolation from the oropharynx, and the presence of immunoglobulin M antibodies.

Ocular manifestations of acquired rubella infection are conjunctivitis, superficial keratitis, iritis, and rarely a retinitis that may be associated with exudative retinal detachment.

Epstein–Barr virus associated disease

Epstein–Barr virus is a member of the herpeviridae group. It is endemic in most parts of the world, and is a cause of infectious mononucleosis. Infection with Epstein–Barr virus has been implicated as an infrequent cause of conjunctivitis, numular keratitis, Parinaud's oculoglandular syndrome, Sjögren's syndrome, optic neuritis, cranial nerve palsies, ophthalmoplegia, scleritis, retinitis, choroiditis, and anterior uveitis. Evidence supporting the association between these disorders and Epstein–Barr virus has been limited, however, with published reports of the association failing to rule out other possible causes. Intraocular disease may present as an anterior uveitis or rarely as a panuveitis. Diagnosis is made on the appropriate haematological finding and serological tests for heterophile antibodies. The anterior uveitis responds to topical corticosteroid therapy and resolves without sequelae. Panuveitis and choroiditis although often self-limited have been reported to improve with acyclovir and corticosteroid therapy.

Human T-lymphotrophic virus type 1 associated disease

Human T-lymphotrophic virus type 1 is a single-stranded RNA retrovirus that can cause adult T-cell leukaemia, tropical spastic paraparesis (a myelopathy), and uveitis. Carriers of human T-lymphotrophic virus type 1 are common in Japan and central and western equatorial Africa but are rare in Europe apart from migrant communities. The infection may be transmitted from mother to child (in utero or via breast milk), sexually, and via blood transfusions.

Ocular manifestations occur either as a complication of leukaemia, or as an isolated uveitis in otherwise asymptomatic patients. Leukaemia may cause retinal vasculitis, vitreous inflammatory reaction, cotton-wool spots, or be associated with opportunistic infections, such as cytomegalovirus retinitis. Human T-lymphotrophic virus type 1 has been implicated by seroepidemiological studies to be commonly associated with 'idiopathic' uveitis in endemic areas of Japan. Uveitis may take either a granulomatous or non-granulomatous form and may be either unilateral or bilateral. Intermediate uveitis with lacy, membranous opacities and iritis are the most common reported presentations, although retinal vasculitis and retinal haemorrhages may occur. Up to 15 per cent of patients may develop a transient grey–white deposit on the retinal vessels. Diagnosis of human T-lymphotrophic virus type 1 uveitis is based on the presence of type 1 antibodies in the absence of human T-lymphotrophic virus type 1 related leukaemia and other defined causes of uveitis. Treatment with topical corticosteroids and cycloplegia is usually adequate to cause resolution of uveitis

in 4 to 6 weeks, although periocular or systemic corticosteroids are occasionally required. Relapses of uveitis occur in 50 per cent of patients.

Viral retinitis syndromes

Acute retinal necrosis syndrome

Acute retinal necrosis syndrome is a specific pattern of necrotizing retinitis and associated intraocular inflammatory reactions, known to be caused by either the varicella-zoster virus or herpes simplex virus. It tends to affect patients between 20 and 60 years old, but may affect any age group and has no clear racial predilection. Acute retinal necrosis syndrome may occur both in immunocompetent and immunosuppressed patients.

Patients typically present with complaints of hazy vision or floaters accompanied by moderate ocular discomfort that may be made worse by ocular movement. Anterior uveitis may be present, which does not respond to topical corticosteroid therapy. The patient may give a history or suffering from recent cutaneous herpes simplex virus or varicella-zoster virus infection.

Diagnosis is based solely on clinical appearance and course of infection. Characteristic findings on examination are an occlusive arteriolar vasculopathy, a full thickness retinal necrosis in the periphery that spreads circumferentially, and a prominent inflammatory reaction in the vitreous humour and anterior chamber. The areas of necrosis usually have very discrete margins and may develop as wedge-shaped areas pointing posteriorly. They are generally peripheral to the major vascular arcades; macular involvement occurs late or not at all. An optic neuropathy with disc swelling may be present, which causes vision loss out of proportion to retinal findings. Bilateral involvement occurs in about one-third of patients. Both eyes may be involved simultaneously or second eye involvement can occur weeks or even years later.

Retinal detachment is currently the main cause of severe

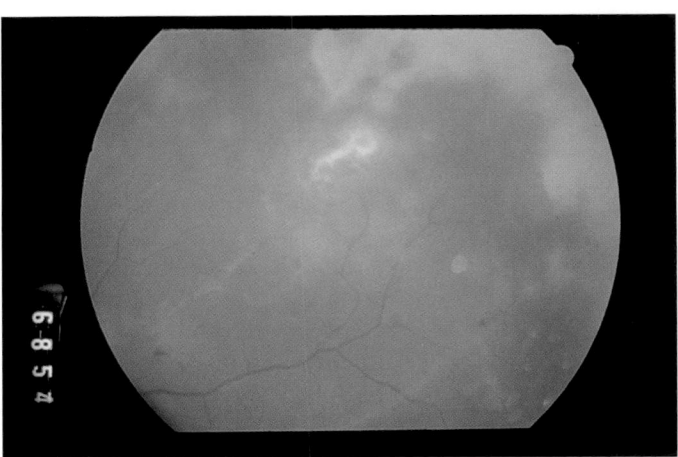

Fig. 4 The fundus of an immunocompetent patient with acute retinal necrosis syndrome. There is a sharp demarcation at the posterior border of an area of retinal necrosis. There is also retinal vasculopathy.

vision loss, and occurs in up to 75 per cent of cases. Multiple full thickness retinal holes that can occur in a posterior location frequently develop during the recovery phase of the disease. Vitreous fibrosis leads to tractional retinal detachments that are complicated by proliferative vitreoretinopathy. Neovascularization of the optic disc or retina is an occasional complication.

Treatment of acute retinal necrosis syndrome in the immunocompetent patient involves antiviral therapy, usually intravenous acyclovir, which is given for 10 to 14 days, followed by oral acyclovir or valaciclovir for 3 to 4 months or longer. Evidence suggests that acyclovir therapy reduces the rate of eventual bilateral disease. The benefits of concomitant corticosteroid and anticoagulant therapy is uncertain, but are used by many clinicians.

Retinal detachment repair is complex because of the presence of multiple posterior breaks and the high rate of proliferative vitreoretinopathy, but vitrectomy with silicone oil tamponade can often achieve anatomical reattachment. Prophylactic photocoagulation to prevent retinal detachment is sometimes used for patients with small discrete lesions, but its benefit has not yet been confirmed for most patients.

Management of acute retinal necrosis in the immunosuppressed is described elsewhere.

Progressive outer retinal necrosis syndrome
See Section 2.9.

Parasitic infections

Protozoa

Toxoplasmosis
Toxoplasma gondii, an intracellular protozoan parasite, is the most common cause of posterior uveitis in many Western countries. Cats are the definitive hosts for *T. gondii*, but infection can be found in other animals, including cattle, sheep, and pigs. Human beings are infected mainly by the ingestion of tissue cysts in undercooked meat or ingestion of oocytes from cat faeces that contaminate the soil and environment. The organisms can invade the intestinal wall after ingestion, go through an asexual reproductive cycle, and then disseminate to other organs in the form of tachyzoites. If the primary infection occurs during pregnancy, then tachyzoites can pass through the placenta and infect the developing fetus. Transmission to the fetus occurs in about 40 per cent of cases, with the most severe congenital disease resulting from infection in the first trimester of pregnancy.

Toxoplasma gondii can cause both congenital and acquired disease. The most common manifestation of congenital disease is retinochoroiditis, which occurs in 70 to 90 per cent of cases. A minority of infants suffer a disseminated infection characterized by jaundice, fever, pneumonitis, and hepatosplenomegaly. Infection of the central nervous system may result in intracranial calcification, hydrocephalus, and mental retardation. The retina is the only site of infection in ocular toxoplasmosis, but there will be secondary inflammation of the choroid, vitreous humour, and anterior segment. A discrete, yellow–white

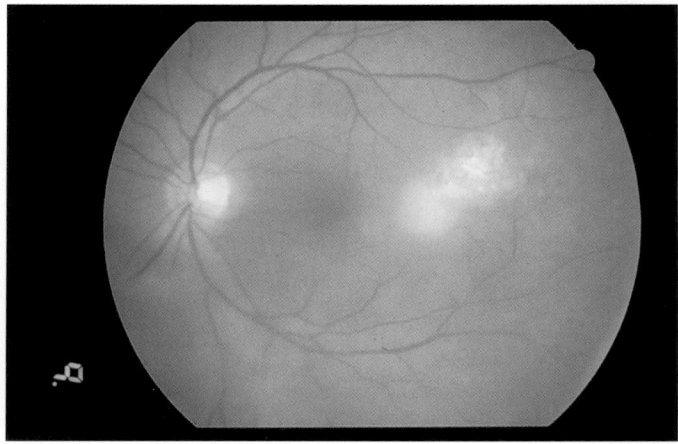

Fig. 5 A focus of recurrent toxoplasmic retinochoroiditis adjacent to an atrophic retinochoroidal scar. The associated inflammatory response results in a 'headlight-in-the-fog' appearance. (Reprinted from Pepose *et al.* 1996, with permission.)

scar with a hyperpigmented border is left after an episode of active infection. Live organisms may persist for many years after birth in the form of tissue cysts within clinically quiescent lesions. Reactivation of these organisms results in recurrent inflammation, appearing as a dense, yellow–white infiltrate with surrounding retinal oedema, and a marked overlying vitreous reaction at the border of an old hyperpigmented scar. Active ocular toxoplasmosis may occasionally result in a vasculitis, vascular occlusion, or papillitis (termed Jensen's juxtapapillary retinitis). Atypical presentations include a punctate inner retinitis characterized by multifocal grey lesions and some vitreous humour cells, and punctate outer retinitis with multifocal white lesions but no vitreous reaction. Complications of ocular toxoplasmosis include secondary glaucoma, cataract, choroidal neovascularization, and retinal detachment.

Diagnosis of ocular toxoplasmosis is usually made on clinical appearance alone. In atypical cases serological tests may be helpful in diagnosis. There are a large number of serological tests available but all suffer from the fact that there is a high prevalence of antibodies in the general population of many communities, making the presence of immunoglobulin G antibody unreliable for confirming disease causation. Immunoglobulin M antibody can also persist for up to 2 years after acute infection.

In immunocompetent patients, only lesions that are threatening the optic nerve or macula, or are causing a two or more line reduction in visual acuity due to severe vitreous inflammatory response, are treated by most clinicians. Standard therapy utilizes a combination of pyrimethamine, sulphadiazine, and oral corticosteroid given for 4 to 6 weeks depending on clinical response. Folinic acid is given to prevent suppression of the bone marrow by pyrimethamine. Fluid intake should be encouraged to prevent drug-related side-effects and blood count should be monitored if the patient is receiving pyrimethamine. Corticosteroids should never be used without concurrent antimicrobials, and it may be prudent to initiate use of corticosteroids 24 h after starting antimicrobials. Periocular corticosteroid injections should be avoided as there are reports of disease becoming uncontrolled following such therapy. In patients allergic to or intolerant of pyrimethamine or sulphadiazine, clindamycin is an alternative agent. Currently available antimicrobial agents do not eliminate tissue cysts from the eye, and therefore, treatment does not prevent recurrences.

Helminths

Toxocariasis

Toxocariasis is usually caused by the nematode *Toxocara canis*. Children between 3 and 13 years of age are the main group in which ocular disease occurs. The systemic form of the disease, visceral larval migrans, in which ocular involvement is uncommon, usually occurs before 6 years of age. The local form, ocular toxocariasis, most commonly affects older children (mean 8 to 9 years old).

The primary host for *T. canis* is the dog. Dogs ingest ova which migrate through the intestine and become disseminated to various organs, including the heart, liver, lung, brain, and eye, and become encysted there. During pregnancy in dogs the encysted form reactivates, migrates, and crosses the placenta infecting the puppy. Up to 80 per cent of puppies are infected. Ova can be excreted by puppies and dogs into the soil allowing for infection to be transmitted to other dogs or humans by soil ingestion. In the human who ingests the ova the cycle is incomplete, stopping at the encysted form after dissemination to the organs. Humans cannot excrete ova, nor will reactivation and migration occur during pregnancy. A history of pica and exposure to puppies are risk factors for acquiring ocular toxocariasis in children.

Fever, hepatomegaly, pneumonitis, and encephalitis due to disseminated larvae are the complications of visceral larval migrans. Ocular larva migrans patients may present with secondary strabismus, leucocoria, hypopyon uveitis, or decreased vision picked up on a routine screening examination. Ocular disease is without systemic features in the majority of cases.

In the eye the parasites may encyst or die exciting a predominately eosinophilic granulomatous response. Toxocariasis can affect the eye in three patterns. A chronic endophthalmitis may occur, which may be severe enough to cause a hypopyon. The inflammation results in secondary cicatrization with synechiae, and with cyclitic and vitreous membrane formation. A peripheral granuloma may occur causing local traction resulting in retinal folds, macula drag, and retinal detachment. The third form of presentation is a posterior pole granuloma which may result in traction band formation. Granulomas appear grey–white raised masses with a variable amounts of vitritis which may have a darker area indicating the larval position.

There are some important differential diagnoses that need to be considered that include retinoblastoma, Coats' disease, familial exudative vitreoretinopathy, and persistent hyperplastic primary vitreous. Ultrasound and/or computed tomography (CT) investigations will help in the differentiation of retinoblastoma and persistent hyperplastic primary vitreous. Cholesterol deposits are often seen in Coats' disease but not in toxocariasis. The enzyme-linked immunoadsorbent assay test for larval antigen in ocular fluid and the presence of eosinophilia in ocular fluid samples may be used to aid diagnosis in difficult cases. Enzyme-linked immunoadsorbent assay testing of serum is less reliable than ocular testing but is less invasive.

Anterior segment inflammation is treated with topical corticosteroids and cycloplegia. Significant posterior segment inflammation is treated with periocular corticosteroids; systemic corticosteroids are reserved for severe disease. Antihelminthic drugs are not used in isolated ocular disease but are reserved for the treatment of selected cases of visceral larval migrans, as larval death may worsen the inflammatory reaction. Retinal detachments usually require vitrectomy techniques due to the tractional element and the presence of membranes.

Onchocerciasis

See Chapter 1.2.1.

Fungal infections

Candidiasis

See Chapter 1.2.1.

Histoplasmosis

The dimorphic soil fungus *Histoplasma capsulatum* is endemic in many parts of the world including Italy, Turkey, Australia, central and south-eastern America, and Asia, but not in the United Kingdom. It can cause ocular disease directly by productive infection and has also been implicated as a cause of the presumed ocular histoplasmosis syndrome through immune-mediated mechanisms.

Infectious histoplasmosis is usually a subclinical or mild flu-like illness with the rare severe disseminated disease usually confined to infants and the immunosuppressed. Ocular involvement includes uveitis, retinitis, vitritis, panuveitis, and endophthalmitis. The retinal lesions are multiple, usually less than one-quarter disc diameter in size, and yellow–white in colour. Diagnosis can be confirmed by culture of ocular fluid and blood. Treatment is with amphotericin B, or alternatively, ketoconazole in those without central nervous system infection or immunosuppression.

The prevalence of presumed ocular histoplasmosis syndrome is much greater than that of infectious histoplasmosis. Epidemiological studies and animal models have implicated *H. capsulatum* as a cause of presumed ocular histoplasmosis syndrome although the syndrome occurs in non-endemic regions. There are no undisputed histopathological studies that have recovered *H. capsulatum* from eyes with presumed ocular histoplasmosis syndrome. The syndrome is most common in the 30 to 40 year age group and the presence of disciform macular lesions are associated with HLA B7.

Features of presumed ocular histoplasmosis syndrome include multiple, round yellow lesions up to one-half disc diameter in size which, in their atrophic stage, appear 'punched-out'. A pigmented crescent around the optic disc inside a depigmented area signifying peripapillary choroiditis is frequently seen. Mottled circumlinear chorioretinal scars may

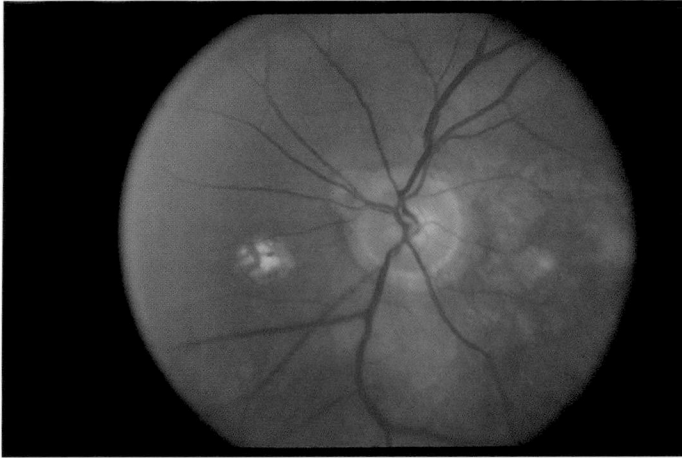

Fig. 6 The left fundus of a patient with presumed ocular histoplasmosis syndrome. A prominent 'histo spot' is present nasal to the optic disc. There is peripapillary atrophy and scarring in the macula.

occasionally be seen in the periphery. There is little or no vitritis in the presumed ocular histoplasmosis syndrome and the presence of cells should alert the examiner to other diagnoses. The development of choroidal neovascular membranes is the most significant complication. If a membrane, is suspected then fluorescein angiography should be used to delineate the lesion. Patients with symptomatic membranes at 1 to 2500 μm from the centre of the foveal avascular zone have been shown to have a better visual outcome if treated with either argon or krypton laser. The role of corticosteroids is unclear. Oral corticosteroids have been used in cases of acute macular neovascular membranes. Surgical removal of subfoveal neovascular membranes may be of benefit, but this technique requires long-term follow-up studies before its true efficacy can be assessed.

Conclusion

Most of the tissue destruction in necrotizing infectious disease is believed to be due to the proliferation of organisms and not to the associated inflammatory response. Some infectious diseases such as the presumed ocular histoplasmosis syndrome do cause destructive immunologically mediated disorders in the eye, however, and these problems can persist after control of the infection. Inflammatory reactions can also lead to complications such as secondary glaucoma, cataract formation, macula oedema, and vitreous haze.

In the treatment of ocular infectious diseases, corticosteroids may play an important role in therapy by suppressing secondary inflammation caused by antigen release, but in general, these agents should not be used without concurrent administration with antimicrobials.

Further reading

Breeveld, J., Rothova, A., and Kuiper, H. (1992). Intermediate uveitis and lyme borreliosis. *British Journal of Ophthalmology*, **76**, 181–2.

Dadzie, K.Y., Bird, A.C., Awadzi, K., *et al.* (1987). Ocular findings in a double-blind study of invermectin versus placebo in the treatment of onchocerciasis. *British Journal of Ophthalmology*, **72**, 78–85.

Engstrom, R.E. Jr, Holland, G.N., Nussenblatt, R.B., and Jabs, D.A. (1991). Current practices in the management of ocular toxoplasmosis. *American Journal of Ophthalmology*, **111**, 601–10.

Helm, C.J. and Holland, G.N. (1993). Ocular tuberculosis. *Survey of Ophthalmology*, **38**, 229–56.

Holland, G.N. and the Executive Committee of the American Uveitis Society (1994). Standard diagnostic criteria for the acute retinal necrosis syndrome. *American Journal of Ophthalmology*, **117**, 663–6.

Karma, A., Seppala, I., Mikkila, H., *et al.* (1994). Diagnosis and clinical characteristics of ocular lyme borreliosis. *American Journal of Ophthalmology*, **108**, 651–7.

Mendelsohn, A.D. and Jampol, L.M. (1985). Syphilitic retinitis: a cause of necrotizing retinitis. *Retina*, **4**, 221–43.

Mets, B., Hlfels, E., Boyer, E.M., *et al.* (1996). Eye manifestations of congenital toxoplasmosis. *American Journal of Ophthalmology*, **122**, 309–24.

Mochizuki, M., *et al.* (1994). Human T lymphotropic virus type 1 uveitis. *British Journal of Ophthalmology*, **78**, 149–54.

Murdoch, D. (1980). Leptospiral uveitis. *Transactions of the Ophthalmology Society*, **32**, 73–5.

Newland, H.S., White, A.T., Greene, B.M., *et al.* (1991). Ocular manifestations of onchocerciasis in a rain forest area of West Africa. *British Journal of Ophthalmology*, **75**, 163–9.

O'Connor, G.R. (1976). Recurrent herpes simplex uveitis in humans. *Survey of Ophthalmology*, **21**, 165–70.

Pepose, J., Holland, G.N., Wilhelmus, K. (1996). *Ocular infection and immunity*. Mosby Year Book, St Louis. [This covers all of the infectious causes of uveitis in detail.]

Rathinam, S.R., Rathnam, S., Selvaraj, S., Dean, D., Nozik, R.A., and Namperumalsamy, P. (1997). Uveitis associated with an epidemic outbreak of leptospirosis. *American Journal of Ophthalmology*, **124**, 71–9.

Rothova, A., Meenken, C., Buitenhuis, H.J., *et al.* (1993). Therapy for ocular toxoplasmosis. *American Journal of Ophthalmology*, **115**, 517–23.

Shields, J.A. (1984). Ocular toxocariasis: a review. *Survey of Ophthalmology*, **28**, 361–81.

Tabbara, K.F. and al Kassimi, H. (1990). Ocular brucellosis. *British Journal of Ophthalmology*, **74**, 249–50.

Womack, L.W. and Leisegang, T.J. (1983). Complications of herpes zoster ophthalmicus. *Archives of Ophthalmology*, **101**, 42–5.

2.8.6 Uveitis confined to the eye

P. I. Murray

Acute anterior uveitis

Definition and aetiology of disease

Acute anterior uveitis (also known as acute iritis, acute iridocyclitis) is defined as inflammation in the anterior chamber of the eye which requires therapy for less than 3 months. Approximately 50 per cent of cases are HLA-B27-positive as compared to 8 per cent of the normal population. Mucosal infection of the gastrointestinal and urogenital tract with Gram-negative bacteria and *Chlamydia trachomatis* potentially triggers

HLA B27 associated reactive arthritis. Therefore, studies have concentrated on the role of these infections in B27-positive acute anterior uveitis and most reports of associations between acute anterior uveitis and micro-organisms concerned possible induction of acute anterior uveitis by *Yersinia*. Nevertheless, to date the mechanisms that are involved in the pathogenesis of B27-related acute anterior uveitis have not been indentified. The B27-negative acute anterior uveitis may be associated with herpesvirus, the Posner–Schlossman syndrome, and sarcoidosis but the majority are idiopathic in nature.

Basic epidemiology

Most patients are aged 20 to 50 years and the disease is often unilateral and recurrent. The B27-related acute anterior uveitis peaks at 30 years, is commoner in males, is associated with low back pain, and there is a higher incidence of B27-positive first-degree relatives suffering with acute anterior uveitis. The commonest disease associations are with ankylosing spondylitis (30–40 per cent of these patients will develop acute anterior uveitis) then Reiter's disease, and occasionally psoriatic arthritis and inflammatory bowel disease. The B27-negative patients show a biphasic peak at 30 and 60 years.

Clinical features including special investigations

The usual symptoms are of a red, painful, photophobic eye and unless complications occur most patients maintain good vision. Recurrences are frequent (particularly in the B27-positive group) with gaps between attacks of months to many years. The B27-positive acute anterior uveitis is usually recurrent, unilateral but alternating, often severe anterior chamber inflammation with extensive posterior synechiae, hypopyon, and fibrin. The latter is almost pathognomonic although it can occur in acute anterior uveitis associated with type II diabetes mellitus. Occasionally the B27-positive patient presents with a white eye and very mild acute anterior uveitis but reduced vision resulting from cystoid macular oedema. The B27-negative acute anterior uveitis may be bilateral, less severe, often with mutton fat keratic precipitates. The presence of pigment on the anterior lens capsule (from posterior synechiae formation) is a sign of a previous attack of acute anterior uveitis. It is important to recognize herpetic disease which is unilateral, often has increased intraocular pressure, keratic precipitates may be central, and there is segmental iris atrophy.

Complications

One of the main complications is missed pathology of the posterior segment and examination must include dilation of both pupils. Missed pathology includes posterior uveitis, retinitis, posterior scleritis, and retinal detachment. Other complications are posterior synechiae, failure of topical therapy, secondary glaucoma, and cataract. After multiple attacks there are a small number of B27-positive patients whose anterior uveitis becomes chronic requiring continuous topical steroid therapy.

Investigations

There is much debate as to whether investigations are necessary and if so what tests should be ordered. In a number of centres an uncomplicated first attack is not investigated but recurrent attacks are. Baseline tests as mentioned under chronic anterior uveitis (see below) can be performed and other investigations, such as X-rays of the sacroiliac joints tailored to the index of clinical suspicion. Routine tissue typing for HLA B27 is not normally undertaken but may be of use in certain patients. In cases of fibrinous uveitis, particularly in the middle aged and elderly subject, urinalysis is mandatory to detect glycosuria and possible diabetes mellitus.

Principles of treatment

Medical

Prompt treatment is vital if complications such as posterior synechiae are to be avoided. There is usually only one chance to prevent posterior synechiae and this is when the patient presents to the accident and emergency department. At that stage intensive pupillary dilation is essential and every attempt should be made to ensure that the pupil is fully dilated (even with the use of old-fashioned remedies, such as hot spoon bathing) before the patient leaves the department. In those patients where the pupil cannot be dilated a subconjunctival injection of Mydricaine no. II can be given and this is often combined with betamethasone. In severe attacks the pupil should be dilated with atropine 1 per cent but in milder attacks cyclopentolate 1 per cent can be used. The choice of topical steroid usually depends on the degree of anterior chamber activity. Mild attacks may warrant prednisolone 0.5 per cent but severe attacks may need dexamethasone 0.1 per cent or prednisolone forte 1 per cent. Frequency of use also depends on the degree of activity; they can be given 1 to 2 hourly and tapered over a number of weeks. Most patients attain a great improvement in their symptoms in the first 1 to 2 weeks and treatment is usually stopped after approximately 6 weeks. One of the best signs of the degree of severity is fibrin formation as this indicates massive blood–aqueous barrier breakdown. Occasionally, even intensive topical therapy fails to resolve the inflammation and in a very small number of cases (usually B27-positive with hypopyon and fibrin) a short course of systemic steroids is needed. Only a moderate dose is required, such as prednisolone 40 mg and this usually results in a rapid improvement; the steroids can be tapered quite quickly over the next few weeks. In those B27-positive patients with cystoid macular oedema, a periocular injection of depot steroid, such as methylprednisolone 40 mg or triamcinolone 40 mg is usually highly effective. When acute anterior uveitis occurs in a patient who has previously undergone penetrating keratoplasty this should be treated as graft rejection until proved otherwise.

Fuchs' heterochromic cyclitis

Definition and aetiology of disease

Fuchs' heterochromic cyclitis is a painless, low grade, chronic uveitis of unknown aetiology comprising about 5 per cent of

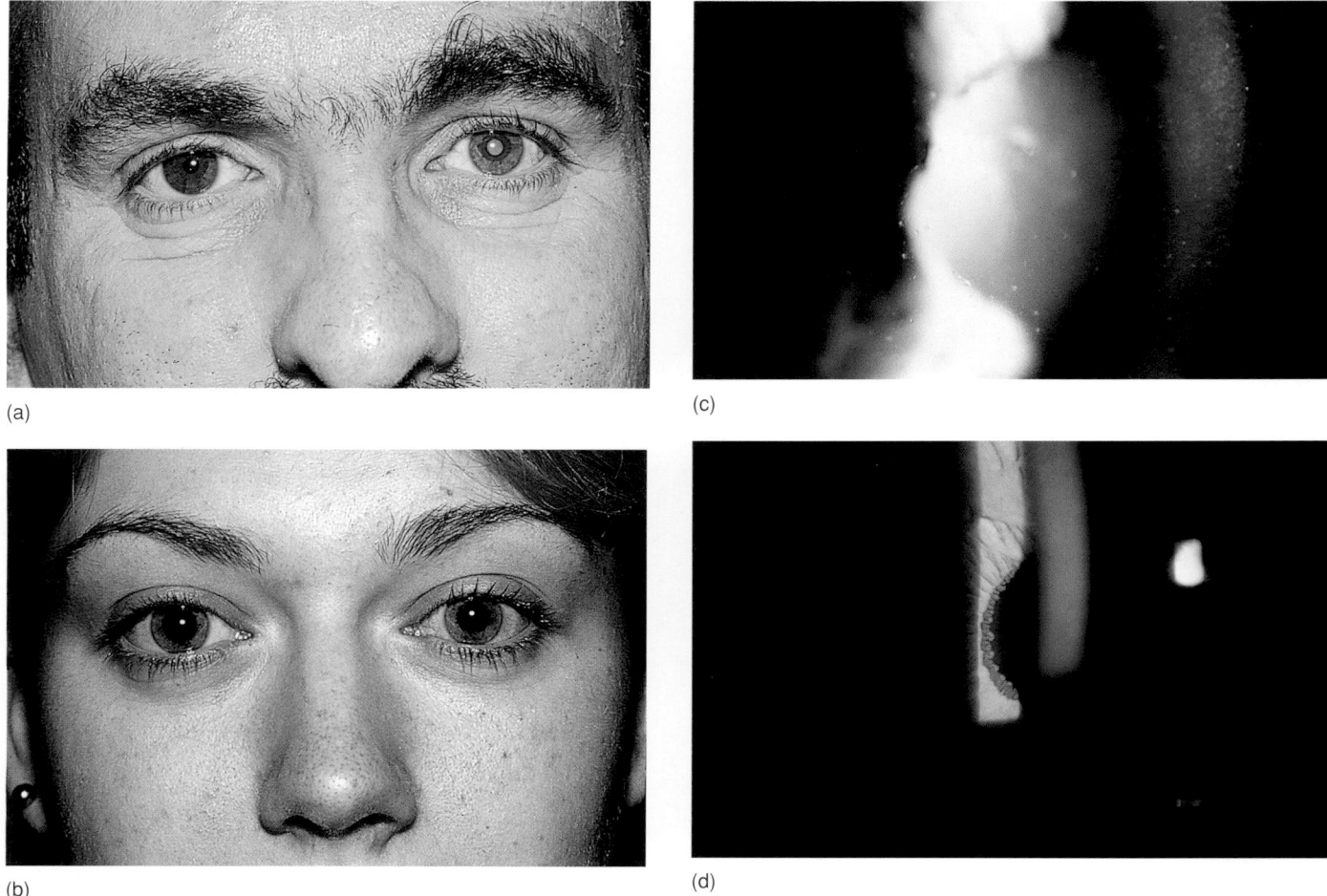

Fig. 1 (a) Left Fuchs' heterochromic cyclitis in a brown-coloured iris. (b) Left Fuchs' heterochromic cyclitis in a blue-coloured iris. (c) Characteristic keratic precipitates. (d) Iris pupillary (Koeppe) nodules.

all uveitis entities. The first comprehensive clinical description was made by Ernst Fuchs in 1906, and since then the condition has remained one of the most puzzling of all the uveitis syndromes. As yet no single cause has been identified (Fig. 1).

Basic epidemiology

Most patients present between 20 and 50 years although a number are older children. There is an equal sex distribution. The condition is almost invariably unilateral (> 90 per cent) and signs of bilateral inflammation should promote the search for an alternative diagnosis, such as intermediate uveitis.

Clinical features including special investigations

Patients usually present with floaters as a result of vitreous opacification or reduced vision due to cataract. The diagnosis may not be immediately obvious at initial presentation and other features may develop over many years. The characteristic physical signs are of a white eye with stellate, filamentary keratic precipitates scattered all over the corneal endothelium, with

pigmented keratic precipitates rarely seen. The keratic precipitates may be absent if the patient is being treated with topical steroids making the diagnosis more difficult. Iris heterochromia may range from subtle changes around the pupillary zone to widespread iris atrophy. Usually the colour of the affected iris becomes lighter and colour changes are more easily seen in daylight rather than at the slit lamp. The iris assumes a smooth, pale surface with blunting of crypts, a dull stroma, and loss of crispness of iris architecture. Iris nodules on the pupil margin (Koeppe) or the pupillary zone (Busacca) are found in up to one-third of patients and the presence of these nodules should alert one to this condition. There is mild anterior chamber activity and an absence of posterior synechiae. Posterior subcapsular cataract develops in at least 80 per cent of eyes. Vitreous opacification, in the form of veils and cells, is found in most patients and sometimes may be so severe as to limit the fundal view. This finding should not divert the ophthalmologist from the diagnosis. Small, punched out, pigmented, peripheral chorioretinal scars are seen in about 7 per cent of eyes. Secondary glaucoma can occur in up to 25 per cent of patients and fine, radial new vessels may be seen in the angle on gonioscopy.

It is more common for patients to present with raised intraocular pressure than to develop it at subsequent follow-up.

Principles of treatment

Medical

Usually nil as the inflammation is mild and topical steroids appear to have little effect. In a small percentage of patients large numbers of keratic precipitates may reduce vision by obstructing the visual axis and a short course of topical steroids can be prescribed. Secondary glaucoma may be refractory to topical therapy and surgery is often required.

Surgical

Of all the types of uveitis, patients with Fuchs' heterochromic cyclitis fare the best from cataract extraction and 90 per cent should achieve a return of vision to at least the 6/9 level. Either phacoemulsification or extracapsular extraction is performed and posterior chamber intraocular lenses can be safely implanted. A flare-up of inflammatory activity may be seen in patients in the immediate postoperative period and under these conditions posterior synechiae can form. It is not necessary to cover the patient with systemic steroids during the operative period. A filiform haemorrhage (Amsler's sign) from the angle, starting opposite to the site of entry into the eye, is a characteristic finding. Trabeculectomy (with or without an antimetabolite, such as 5-fluorouracil or mitomycin C) appears to be successful in controlling the glaucoma.

Other related information

The aetiology of Fuchs' heterochromic cyclitis has remained an enigma since the condition was first described. A number of theories have been put forward and these include the following.

Sympathetic nervous system

As iris hypochromia can result from a lesion of the sympathetic nervous system, a neurogenic cause for Fuchs' heterochromic cyclitis has been postulated. Cases of Fuchs' heterochromic cyclitis exist in association with conditions due to a sympathetic defect, such as Horner's syndrome, status dysraphicus (unilateral syndrome of dysmorphism and asymmetry), and Parry–Romberg syndrome (progressive facial hemiatrophy). Despite this, evidence for Fuchs' heterochromic cyclitis resulting from a sympathetic defect remains weak.

Hereditary

A genetic basis for Fuchs' heterochromic cyclitis remains unlikely despite reports of more than one family member having the disease, including sets of monozygotic twins. HLA studies have not been shown to be helpful.

Infective

Some authors believe that an association exists between Fuchs' heterochromic cyclitis and ocular toxoplasmosis. The presence of 'Toxoplasma-like' scars in the fundi of Fuchs' heterochromic cyclitis patients and reports of a few cases of active Toxoplasma retinochoroiditis in association with Fuchs' heterochromic cyclitis have led to this theory. Nevertheless, this association cannot be substantiated by laboratory tests for toxoplasmosis. The search for other infective agents such as viruses has not been fruitful with the failure to detect herpesviral DNA in aqueous humour samples from Fuchs' heterochromic cyclitis patients.

Vascular

The basis for this theory has come from the presence of vascular abnormalities in the form of new vessels in the angle, and leakage from iris vessels with areas of ischaemia associated with neovascularization as seen on iris fluorescein angiography. An immune complex vasculitis has been suspected but there is no good evidence to support this.

Immunological

This is the most interesting theory as large numbers of immunological aberrations have been identified in the serum and aqueous humour of Fuchs' heterochromic cyclitis patients. These include intraocular immunoglobulin G production with oligoclonal immunoglobulin G bands and raised levels of circulating soluble interleukin-2 receptors (a T-cell activation marker). The finding of antiendothelial cell antibodies and various adhesion molecules in the circulation add further support to this theory. Despite these abnormalities patients are free of the systemic manifestations of immune-mediated disease.

Recent reviews have suggested that far from being a specific clinical entity, Fuchs' heterochromic cyclitis may be a secondary response to a variety of different aetiological agents, with the triggering stimulus being possibly immunological, infectious, or a combination of both.

Chronic anterior uveitis

Definition and aetiology of disease

Chronic anterior uveitis is defined as inflammation in the anterior chamber of the eye which requires therapy for more than 3 months. Although chronic anterior uveitis may be part of a systemic disease process, such as sarcoidosis, the majority of cases are idiopathic. A small proportion of patients who are HLA-B27-positive with recurrent acute anterior uveitis may go on to pursue a chronic course. Juvenile chronic arthritis associated uveitis has been excluded as it is covered elsewhere.

Basic epidemiology

Most patients are aged between 20 and 50 years and it is unusual for the inflammation to persist over the age of 60 years.

Clinical features including special investigations

Symptoms may vary from eye(s) being painful, red, and photophobic to being white and painless. A variety of keratic precipitates may be seen from fine to 'mutton fat', there is anterior chamber flare (usually persistent due to chronic breakdown of the blood–aqueous barrier) and cells. Iris nodules may be present but are usually non-specific as they can occur in many types of uveitis. Posterior synechiae can range from absent to extensive. The main complications are secondary glaucoma and posterior subcapsular cataract formation. If the intraocular pressure is elevated it is vital that gonioscopy is undertaken. This will help to differentiate between occlusion of the angle due to the formation of peripheral anterior synechiae and an open angle thereby raising the possibility of a trabeculitis or a steroid-induced rise in pressure. Pupil block with iris bombé can occur with 360° posterior synechiae. All patients with raised intraocular pressures should have their visual fields plotted on a regular basis. Detailed examination of the posterior segment is vital to exclude a diagnosis of panuveitis, retinal vasculitis, or intermediate uveitis. Many patients retain good visual acuities unless cataract or glaucoma develops. Unilateral disease which flares up soon after topical steroids are stopped should alert the ophthalmologist to the possibility of herpesviral infection, such as herpes simplex or varicella zoster. Often there is reduced corneal sensation and sector iris atrophy but not all patients will give a history of the typical skin rash of herpes zoster ophthalmicus. In patients with an associated scleritis a systemic vasculitis will need to be excluded. Rarely, anterior segment ischaemia due to the ocular ischaemic syndrome can result in a chronic anterior uveitis although a panuveitis is more likely. Ocular ischaemia may be associated with iris neovascularization, secondary glaucoma, and cataract. A history of vascular disease elsewhere, such as vertebrobasilar insufficiency may be elicited and a carotid bruit may be audible.

Investigations

As the cause of the uveitis is closely linked to other notable issues, such as the natural course of the disease and the most appropriate therapy, pathogenesis is of prime importance. Thus, performing various investigations may be of value in determining the cause of the intraocular inflammation. In view of the puzzling nature of uveitis and that it may form part of a systemic disease process, many patients are frequently over-investigated by being subjected to a vast battery of unnecessary tests. It is important to discriminate between the sensitivity and specificity of a particular test. Ordering large numbers of investigations in the hope that one may turn out to be positive should be actively discouraged. It is often the history and examination findings that are far more informative than the investigation results and a detailed ocular and general history is essential. In the clinical setting, one should perform the minimum number of investigations that will give the maximum information regarding the management of the patient. There are a number of tests that would be common to all uveitis patients, and additional tests that might be relevant depending on the history and examination findings. Baseline investigations that could be ordered include: chest radiograph, full blood count, plasma viscosity or erythrocyte sedimentation rate, syphilis serology, and urinalysis. Specific investigations, such as serum angiotensin-converting enzyme and a purified protein derivative test can be performed if clinically indicated. In some patients whose uveitis is of unknown aetiology, repeating investigations years later may increase the yield of positive results. Those patients in whom an underlying systemic disease is suspected may require more detailed and invasive investigations.

Principles of treatment

Medical

Topical treatment is usually all that is required. The weakest preparation of topical steroid should be prescribed that will keep the inflammation under control. In very mild cases it is disputable whether long-term treatment with topical steroids is justified. Some patients, particularly those who are prone to posterior synechiae formation, should have their pupil dilated or just have dilating drops at night to keep the pupil mobile. Periocular and systemic steroids are not usually required unless macular oedema develops. Secondary glaucoma can be treated with a topical β-blocker but if this is not adequate to control the intraocular pressure then a carbonic anhydrase inhibitor (either oral or topical), or topical α_2-agonist can be added. Where a trabeculitis is suspected, even if the anterior chamber is quiet, topical steroids should be increased in strength and frequency in the first instance. For a steroid-induced rise in pressure it may be necessary to reduce the strength of the steroid preparation, such as clobetasone 0.1 per cent. Fluoromethalone 0.1 per cent drops are of little value for controlling the uveitis as it has almost no penetration into the anterior chamber. Patients with herpetic uveitis may need to be maintained on a weak topical steroid even on an alternate day basis for many months or even years as discontinuation could result in a flare-up. The uveitis due to ocular ischaemia usually responds poorly to steroid therapy.

Surgical

For patients with cataract, phacoemulsification or extracapsular extraction can be performed and a posterior chamber intraocular lens is usually implanted. Where many posterior synechiae are present, iris hooks and a high viscosity viscoelastic may be helpful. Although there are no good controlled clinical trials, some authors advocate that the implant should be heparin surface modified. To date, the best material for a foldable implant is not known. Extreme vigilance is required to control pre- and postoperative inflammation if a successful visual outcome is to be achieved. It is imperative to have a quiet anterior chamber (< 1+ cells) for a minimum of 3 months prior to surgery and all efforts should be made to achieve this. Many authors prescribe high-dose systemic corticosteroid prior to surgery, slowly tailing it off in the postoperative period. The rationale for this is to minimize the inflammatory reaction following surgical trauma on an already inflamed eye and it may also prevent the development of cystoid macular oedema. Cataract extraction in the ocular ischaemic syndrome may be fraught as neovascularization of iris and retina may occur in the early postoperative period leading to neovascular glaucoma and subsequent blindness if aggressive therapy is not instigated.

Trabeculectomy (with or without an antimetabolite, such as 5-fluorouracil or mitomycin C) will be necessary if the intraocular pressure is uncontrollable on maximum medical therapy and the results of surgery are encouraging.

Intermediate uveitis

Definition and aetiology of disease

Intermediate uveitis is an anatomical classification of uveitis proposed by the International Uveitis Study Group. It comprises intraocular inflammation predominantly involving the vitreous and peripheral retina, although anterior segment inflammation also occurs. The aetiology is unknown although some evidence exists for an autoimmune cause and a number of younger patients give a history of atopy. Like other forms of uveitis it may be associated with an underlying systemic disease process, such as sarcoidosis or demyelination. A similar clinical picture has been reported in association with Lyme disease. The differential diagnosis includes intraocular inflammation associated with toxocariasis, inflammatory bowel disease, intraocular B-cell lymphoma, and human T-cell leukaemia virus type 1 (HTLV-1).

Basic epidemiology

Intermediate uveitis forms about 10 to 15 per cent of all uveitis cases and the largest subset is the condition previously described as pars planitis. It is bilateral in 80 per cent but the disease is often asymmetrical. Most cases present from late teens to early forties, but there is a bimodal peak, the latter in the elderly. About 10 per cent of cases occur in young children and it forms up to 25 per cent of all childhood uveitis. There is no sex or race predilection and in some patients there is an association with HLA DR2.

Clinical features including special investigations

Most patients present with floaters due to vitreous opacities, or reduced vision due to vitreous opacities with or without cystoid macular oedema. Although symptoms are usually unilateral, examination often reveals signs in the asymptomatic eye. Usually the eyes are white with minimal anterior segment activity, but redness, pain, and photophobia can occur. Rarely, vitreous haemorrhage is a presenting feature. The main findings are of vitreous cells and opacities, the latter described as snowballs. These are aggregates of multinucleated giant cells and epithelioid cells. A white exudate, or snowbank, is characteristically found at the ora serrata and is easiest seen inferiorly although it can extend over 360° and involve peripheral retina and pars plana. Snowbanks are best visualized using the binocular indirect ophthalmoscope with scleral indentation. Histopathology of the exudate reveals fibroglial cells including fibrous astrocytes and some inflammatory cells, mainly lymphocytes. Peripheral retinal periphlebitis may also be a feature of this condition.

The course of the disease can be variable, from a self-limiting process to an unrelenting disease with multiple exacerbations.

About two-thirds of eyes will maintain 6/12 vision or better on no treatment or just topical steroids. The other third may have a moderate or severe form of inflammation. Posterior subcapsular cataract formation is a frequent finding, particularly in patients on long-term systemic steroid therapy. Secondary glaucoma also occurs. The most serious sight-threatening complication is cystoid macular oedema. Vitreous haemorrhage is unusual but may result from retinal neovascularization at the vitreous base, peripheral retina, or at the optic disc. Vitreous inflammation and traction can lead to a retinal tear and subsequent detachment.

Investigations

Taking a detailed ocular and general history is essential. Routine uveitis investigations are usually performed as it is important to rule out coexisting systemic disease, such as sarcoidosis or demyelination. Fundus fluorescein angiography may be of value in those patients with macular oedema and retinal neovascularization.

Principles of treatment

In patients with visual acuities better than 6/12 due to vitreous haze, observation rather than therapy may be all that is required. Topical steroids are prescribed for anterior segment activity and dilation of the pupil may be necessary. Periocular injections of a depot steroid preparation, such as methylprednisolone or triamcinolone are a valuable addition to the standard therapeutic options and can be given for unilateral cystoid macular oedema or visually disabling vitreous opacities. Unfortunately, the efficacy of this treatment is unpredictable and the injection should be repeated if the first injection is ineffective. A rise in intraocular pressure following injection has been reported. In children, injections require a general anaesthetic.

In patients with vision-threatening disease who have not responded to periocular steroids, oral steroids are prescribed. It is important to start the patient on a large dose, such as prednisolone 60 mg/day for 2 weeks as a failure to respond could be due to an inadequate steroid dose rather than steroid-resistant disease. Patients should be warned of the major side-effects that they could encounter and advised not to stop the steroids suddenly. A minimum monitoring of the steroids should involve regular urinalysis, blood pressure measurement, and checking of weight. The oral steroids are slowly tapered and can be given as alternate day therapy to minimize sytemic side-effects. If the patient responds to the treatment then an attempt should be made to try to stop the steroids; however, a number of patients will flare-up below a certain level and those patients will require a maintenance dose to keep the disease in remission. In patients whose disease progresses unrelentingly or have intolerable steroid side-effects then immunosuppressives, such as cyclosporin or azathioprine are added. Other therapeutic options include cryotherapy and vitrectomy. Cryotherapy appears most beneficial in the treatment of peripheral snowbanking associated with neovascularization and a double freeze–thaw technique is applied to the vitreous base under local or general anaesthesia depending on the age of the patient. Pars plana vitrectomy (or a combined vitreolensectomy) is often reserved for patients with a dense vitritis who have failed to respond to steroids and immunosuppressives or eyes with a persistent vitreous haemorrhage. In patients with retinal neovascularization, laser photocoagulation and/or oral steroids are required depending on the degree of retinal ischaemia as seen on fluorescein angiography. For cataract surgery the same principles as outlined on chronic anterior uveitis (see above) should be applied and a posterior chamber intraocular lens is usually implanted. Glaucoma surgery may require the use of an anti-metabolite.

Multifocal choroiditis

Definition and aetiology of disease

White dots in the fundus can be observed in a number of diverse uveitis entities. These include a collection of overlapping clinically similar conditions that can be grouped together known as multifocal choroiditis and a variant of this, punctate inner choroidopathy. The aetiology is unknown although Epstein–Barr virus has been suspected (Fig. 2).

Basic epidemiology

The vast majority of patients are young adults. Approximately 90 per cent are female, the majority being moderate myopes. It is bilateral in up to 80 per cent.

Clinical features including special investigations

Presenting symptoms include blurred vision, metamorphopsia, and central vision loss. Patients with multifocal choroiditis are more likely to have signs of intraocular inflammation, whereas patients with punctate inner choroidopathy often complain of multiple scotomas. The most striking feature is of few to multiple round, grey/yellow lesions 50 to 200 μm in size at the level of the retinal pigment epithelium/inner choroid. They occur at the posterior pole and in the periphery mainly posterior to the equator and eventually progress to atrophic pigmented scars. Vitreous cells and occasionally anterior segment activity may be seen as well as mild disc oedema and subretinal fibrosis. The condition can be recurrent and findings may mimic those seen in the presumed ocular histoplasmosis syndrome. The major complication is macular disease and up to 50 per cent will develop a subfoveal neovascular membrane or cystoid macular oedema.

Principles of treatment

Up to 50 per cent of patients with cystoid macular oedema improve with periocular or systemic steroids but it is not possible to predict which patients will respond. The visual prognosis is good if a subfoveal neovascular membrane does not occur. In patients with a membrane the therapeutic options include laser photocoagulation and submacular surgery. Des-

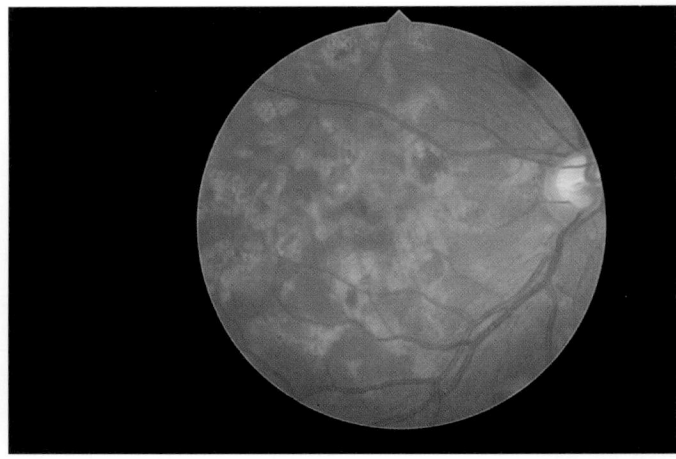

(a)

(b)

Fig. 2 (a) Multifocal choroiditis. (b) Punctate inner choroidopathy with subretinal fibrosis.

pite subretinal neovascularization the final visual acuity may be as good as 6/18 (20/60).

Vogt–Koyanagi–Harada syndrome

Definition and aetiology of disease

This is a severe bilateral panuveitis associated with multifocal serous retinal detachments, signs of meningeal irritation, with or without auditory disturbances. Current thinking favours an autoimmune response against melanocytes (Fig. 3).

Basic epidemiology

Occurs more frequently in darkly pigmented races, such as Orientals (common in Japan), Asians (Indo-Pakistani origin), Hispanics, American-Indians, and is unusual in Caucasians. The age range is from the second to fifth decade although it can occur in children. It is commoner in females and there is an association with HLA DR4.

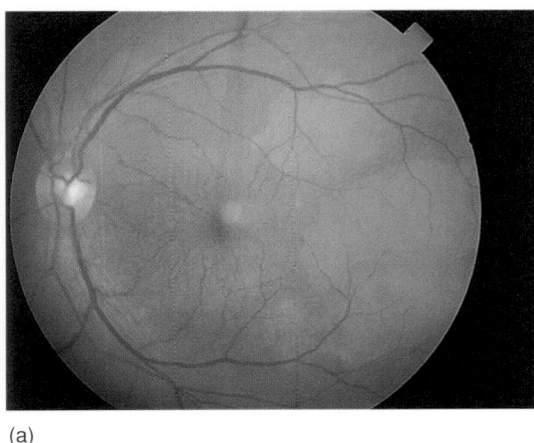

(a)

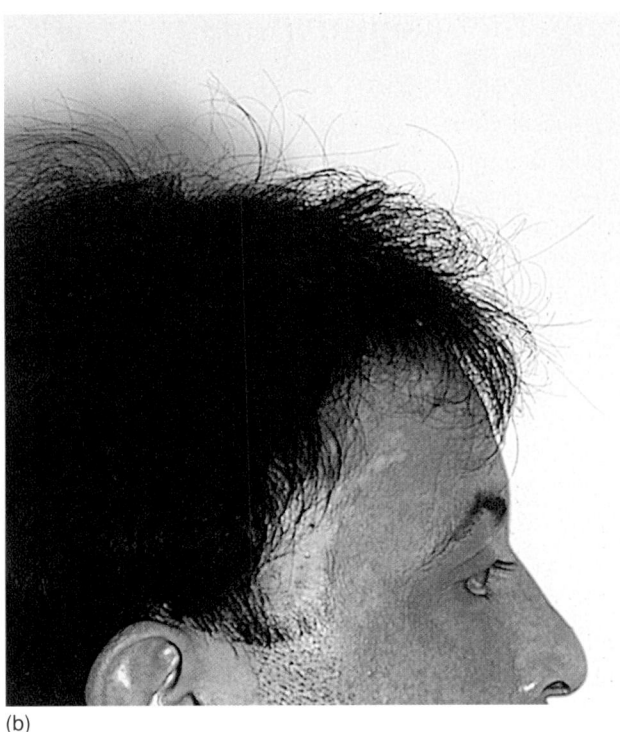

(b)

Fig. 3 (a) Multiple serous retinal detachments characteristic of Vogt–Koyanagi–Harada syndrome. (b) Facial vitiligo occurring 1 year after the onset of uveitis.

Clinical features including special investigations

There is an initial prodromal stage with fever, nausea, and neurological signs and symptoms including meningism, headache, tinnitus, and hearing loss, which lasts only a few days. Lumbar puncture reveals a cerebrospinal fluid lymphocytic pleocytosis. The acute uveitic phase develops which may last several weeks. Symptoms are of blurred vision or profound visual loss. The majority of patients present with bilateral panuveitis often with mutton fat keratic precipitates, optic disc swelling, and serous retinal detachments or there may be a delay of a few days before the second eye is involved. Breakdown of the retinal pigment epithelial barrier to the subretinal space leads to areas of subretinal fluid accumulation and subsequently multifocal serous detachments. Occasionally the anterior chamber is shallowed. The convalescent or chronic phase follows with cutaneous and uveal depigmentation developing months or years after the acute phase. Depigmentation of the choroid leads to the sunset glow/blond fundus and patchy vitiligo occurs in up to two-thirds of patients. Poliosis of lashes/eyebrows and alopecia are also a feature. Multiple, small, yellow/cream coloured Dalen–Fuchs nodules are found and the fundal appearance can resemble that seen in sympathetic ophthalmitis. Relapses of uveitis can occur in the chronic recurrent phase and complications include cataract, secondary glaucoma, subretinal fibrosis, subretinal neovascular membranes, and pigment clumping/retinal pigment epithelial stippling at the macula.

Investigations

The diagnosis is usually made clinically but fluorescein angiography is particularly helpful in evaluating the extent of the disease and the presence of subretinal neovascular membranes. B-scan ultrasound will show low to medium reflective choroidal thickening. A lumbar puncture may be a useful adjunctive test in atypical cases as the cerebrospinal fluid pleocytosis may last up to 8 weeks.

Principles of treatment

Early aggressive treatment is essential and 60 per cent of patients may get return of vision to about the 6/9 level as the intraocular inflammation improves with resolution of the disc swelling and reattachment of the non-rhegmatogenous detachments. Initial therapy is with high dose systemic steroids, such as prednisolone 100 mg/day. In some cases pulsed intravenous methylprednisolone may be required to arrest the disease process. Tapering the steroids too quickly may result in a recurrence and patients may need to remain on oral steroids for at least a year. If systemic steroids are ineffective or the side-effects become intolerable then an immunosuppressive agent, such as cyclosporin A can be added. The prognosis is worse if the disease recurs in the first 2 years after presentation. The principles of cataract surgery are similar to those described for chronic anterior uveitis (see above). Systemic steroid cover is given over the operative period and an intraocular lens is usually implanted. Surgery may be complicated as there is often extensive posterior synechiae. Postoperatively, giant cells accumulate on the optic of the implant and there may be 'pupil capture' of the optic by the iris. The secondary glaucoma can be difficult to manage medically and if a trabeculectomy is required it will probably require augmentation with 5-fluorouracil or mitomycin C. Patients with subretinal neovascular membranes may need laser photocoagulation.

Sympathetic ophthalmia

Definition and aetiology of disease

Sympathetic ophthalmia is a bilateral granulomatous panuveitis that occurs after a penetrating injury either produced by accidental trauma or surgery. Trauma to one eye (the exciting eye) will result not only in an inflammatory response in that eye but also the contralateral eye (the sympathizing eye) and potentially devastating visual consequences. The interval between ocular injury and the onset of sympathetic ophthalmia is highly variable ranging from 5 days to as long as 66 years. In general 65 per cent of cases occur between 2 weeks to 2 months after injury, 70 per cent of cases before 3 months, and 90 per cent occur within 1 year. Clinical and immunological features indicate that T-lymphocyte-mediated delayed hypersensitivity plays an important role in the pathogenesis of this disease.

Basic epidemiology

Sympathetic ophthalmia is rare with a prevalence of 0.1 to 0.2 per cent following penetrating ocular trauma. In a 5-year histopathological review Gass diagnosed sympathetic ophthalmia in 53 eyes (two out of 1000 eyes examined), of which 55 per cent were post-traumatic. The same study reported an incidence of 0.01 per cent of sympathetic ophthalmia after vitrectomy alone but a rate of 0.06 per cent when vitrectomy was associated with other penetrating wounds. Sympathetic ophthalmia can follow not only any intraocular procedure such as cataract extraction or glaucoma surgery, but also retinal detachment repair particularly after multiple procedures and even laser photocoagulation. Although some authors have reported a number of HLA associations with sympathetic ophthalmia, small numbers of patients have precluded any firm conclusions. There is no racial predilection for the disease.

Clinical features including special investigations

The onset of sympathetic ophthalmia is usually insidious. Presenting symptoms include slight pain, photophobia, and reduced vision in both the exciting and sympathizing eye. Usually, the exciting eye is chronically inflamed, painful, and sometimes phthisical. The classic anterior chamber findings include mutton fat keratic precipitates, but occasionally there is a non-granulomatous milder type of inflammation. Features are of a bilateral panuveitis with a moderate to severe vitritis, choroidal thickening and infiltration, and optic disc swelling. A typical feature is the presence of Dalen–Fuchs nodules. These are small yellowish-white granulomas seen in relation to the retinal pigment epithelium and most commonly located in the periphery of the fundus. Although they are a characteristic feature they are not pathognomonic for sympathetic ophthalmia as they can occur in granulomatous inflammation due to any cause, particularly Vogt–Koyanagi–Harada syndrome.

Complications

These include cataract, secondary glaucoma, macular oedema, optic atrophy, iris rubeosis, exudative retinal detachment, and chorioretinal scarring.

Histopathology

Characteristically there is granulomatous inflammation primarily involving the choroid with diffuse thickening and lymphocytic infiltration interrupted at multiple sites with collections of epithelioid cells and a few multinucleated giant cells both containing pigment. There is absence of apparent choroidal necrosis, sparing of choriocapillaris from inflammatory cell infiltration, and preservation of retinal pigment epithelium and retina except at the sites of Dalen–Fuchs nodules and other foci where retinal pigment epithelium junctions are disrupted. Choroidal infiltrates are composed predominantly of T lymphocytes (CD3$^+$) with a predominance of helper T lymphocytes (CD4$^+$) in early stages of the disease compared with a relatively larger number of cytotoxic T lymphocytes (CD8$^+$) in the later stages. Expression of adhesion molecules and major histocompatibility complex (MHC) class II molecules are observed on infiltrating and ocular resident cells. All these findings suggest a T-lymphocyte-mediated mechanism in the induction and/or perpetuation of the uveal inflammation, possibly directed to uveal melanocytes or other antigens in the uveal tract. The histopathological features are almost identical to that seen in Vogt–Koyanagi–Harada syndrome.

Investigations

There are no specific tests for diagnosing sympathetic ophthalmia. Clinical findings and a high index of suspicion are important if prompt and appropriate therapy is to be instigated.

Principles of treatment

Surgical

The only way to prevent sympathetic ophthalmia is enucleation of the exciting eye prior to inflammation developing in the sympathizing eye. As sympathetic ophthalmia is unlikely to occur less than 10 days following injury one has a small window of opportunity in which to decide about enucleation. Unfortunately, it is not possible to predict from the type of injury which eyes will go on to develop sympathetic ophthalmia. Enucleation is not a difficult decision to make if the traumatized eye is blind and painful. With advances in microsurgical techniques and increasing surgical success in repairing wounds, eyes that would have been excised in the past have now been saved possibly even regaining navigational vision so the decision to enucleate in these circumstances is very difficult. There is some controversy regarding the indication for enucleating the exciting eye once sympathetic ophthalmia has developed. Some authors suggest that enucleation within 2 weeks of symptoms developing in the sympathizing eye leads to milder inflammation and a more favourable prognosis.

Medical

The mainstay of therapy is systemic and topical steroids. High-dose oral steroids should be given at the onset of the disease and slowly tapered once the inflammation comes under control. Failure to respond, unacceptable steroid side-effects, or difficulty in reducing the steroids to an acceptable maintenance dose requires the addition of another immunosuppressive agent, usually cyclosporin A. With aggressive therapy approximately 60 per cent of patients can achieve a good visual outcome (6/18 or better) in the sympathizing eye.

Birdshot retinochoroidopathy

Definition and aetiology of disease

A bilateral posterior uveitis of unknown aetiology characterized by multiple, cream-coloured lesions mainly in the posterior pole and surrounding area. A strong genetic predisposition is suggested as approximately 90 per cent of patients are HLA-A29-positive (Fig. 4).

Basic epidemiology

Patients are invariably Caucasian with a slight female preponderance. Ages range from 23 to 79 years with a mean of 53 years.

Clinical features including special investigations

Patients present with blurred/reduced vision and floaters. Questioning may reveal difficulties with night and colour vision. The most striking feature is multiple, small, oval, cream-coloured lesions at the level of the retinal pigment epithelium and inner choroid. They are scattered mainly around the optic disc radiating towards the equator, the largest being up to three-quarters of a disc diameter. The lesions are associated with the large choroidal vessels and are more common nasally inferior to the optic disc. Eventually the lesions become atrophic, occasionally confluent, and remain non-pigmented. There is an associated vitritis, retinal vasculitis, and narrowing of the retinal arterioles. Cystoid macular oedema is a frequent cause of poor vision. With disease progression subretinal neo-

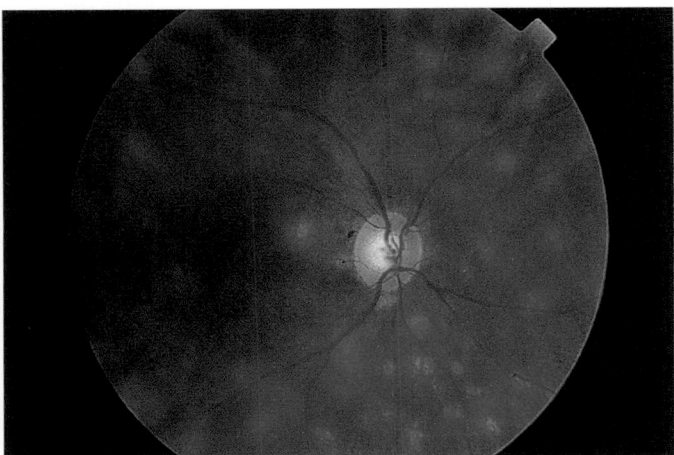

Fig. 4 Classical lesions of birdshot retinochoroidopathy.

vascular membranes, preretinal membranes, and optic atrophy can develop. The condition is usually bilateral but may be asymmetrical. Investigations reveal an abnormal electroretinogram with reduced amplitude and latency of the b wave, and a subnormal light/dark ratio of the electro-oculogram. There is also abnormal dark adaptation and reduced colour vision. HLA testing can be carried out and if the patient is HLA-A29-negative then sarcoidosis should be suspected as a similar clinical picture can occur.

Principles of treatment

Treatment of the cystoid macular oedema is with periocular and/or oral steroids. Failure to respond usually requires the addition of an immunosuppressive agent, such as cyclosporin A. Although good results are seen in some patients it is not yet known if it influences the final visual outcome. Laser photocoagulation may be required for subretinal neovascular membranes.

Serpiginous choroidopathy

Definition and aetiology of disease

This is a rare, usually recurrent, invariably bilateral disease of unknown aetiology primarily affecting the inner choroid and retinal pigment epithelium and secondarily the retina. Debate exists as to whether this condition is a true inflammation or an abiotrophic process. There is no association with a systemic disorder. The condition is also known as geographic choroidopathy (Fig. 5).

Basic epidemiology

It is seen more commonly in the middle-aged although it can occur in younger patients. There is an equal sex distribution.

Clinical features including special investigations

The condition may be asymptomatic until the macula is involved then patients complain of blurred vision or describe a central or paracentral scotoma with metamorphopsia. Although symptoms may be unilateral, examination may reveal bilateral signs and the appearance of one eye may not resemble that of the other. Chorioretinal disease manifests as greyish-white or yellowish acute lesions involving the choriocapillaris and retinal pigment epithelium. They usually start at the optic disc and fan out in a centrifugal (serpentine) fashion, spreading out towards the equator and involving the macular region. Often they are confluent but 'skip' lesions can occur. Occasionally lesions start at the macula and spread towards the disc. A mild vitritis is seen in up to one-third of patients. After several weeks or months the natural history of these lesions is to become atrophic. Fibrous scar tissue forms with loss of the choriocapillaris and clumps of retinal pigment epithelial hyperplasia. Foveal and parafoveal lesions can severely damage central vision. Recurrences are usual and can happen several years after the initial attack with active lesions frequently occurring

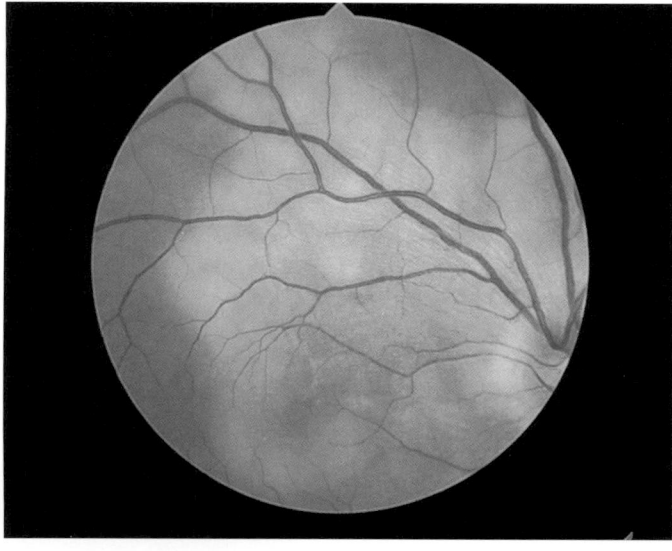

(a)

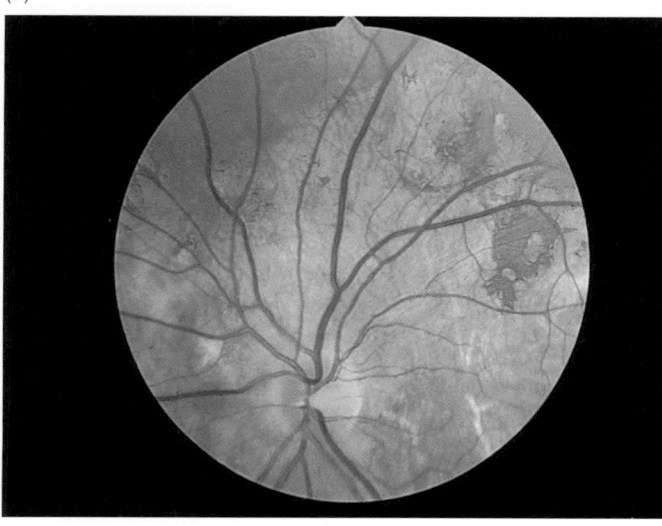

(b)

Fig. 5 Serpiginous choroidopathy. (a) Acute lesions in right eye. (b) Chronic lesions in left eye.

at the edge of older ones. Diagnosis is made on clinical grounds but fluorescein angiography shows early hypofluorescence of acute lesions then late staining with hyperfluorescence at the edges of the lesion which then spreads inwards. Older lesions may also hypofluoresce due to loss of the choriocapillaris but late hyperfluorescence and staining occurs in areas of fibrous scar tissue and retinal pigment epithelial clumping. Associated findings include retinal periphlebitis, branch retinal vein occlusion, retinal pigment epithelial detachment, and serous retinal detachment. It is important not to miss a macular subretinal neovascular membrane which occurs in up to 25 per cent of patients as the symptoms could easily be mistaken for a new acute lesion. The differential diagnosis includes acute posterior multifocal placoid pigment epitheliopathy where the acute lesions have the same features on fluorescein angiography but these lesions resolve in a few weeks and recurrences are uncommon.

Principles of treatment

In the acute phase, systemic steroids with or without immuno-suppressives are often prescribed but these are not always effective, raising the possibility that the condition may not be a true inflammation. As yet, there are no good clinical trials on the benefits of treatment. Occasionally, acute macular lesions may heal without treatment with an apparent sparing of the fovea and an improvement in central vision several months later. For subretinal neovascular membranes, which usually arise from an older lesion, laser photocoagulation may be appropriate.

Further reading

Aaberg, T.M. (1987). The enigma of pars planitis. *American Journal of Ophthalmology*, **103**, 828–30.

Beckingsale, A.B., Davies, J., Gibson, J.M., *et al.* (1984). Acute anterior uveitis, ankylosing spondylitis, back pain and HLA B27. *British Journal of Ophthalmology*, **68**, 741–45.

Beniz, J., Forster, D.J., Lean, J.S., *et al.* (1991). Variations in clinical features of the Vogt–Koyanagi–Harada syndrome. *Retina*, **11**, 275–80.

Brewerton, D.A., Caffrey, M., Nicholls, A., *et al.* (1973). Acute anterior uveitis and HLA B27. *Lancet*, ii, 994–6.

Brockhurst, R.J., Schepens, C.L., and Okamura, I.D. (1960). Uveitis II. Peripheral uveitis: clinical description, complications and differential diagnosis. *American Journal of Ophthalmology*, **49**, 1257–66.

Brown, J., Folk, J.C., Reddy, C.V., *et al.* (1996). Visual prognosis of multifocal choroiditis, punctate inner choroidopathy, and the diffuse subretinal fibrosis syndrome. *Ophthalmology*, **103**, 1100–5.

Chan, C.-C., Roberge, F.G., Whitcup, S.M., *et al.* (1995). Thirty-two cases of sympathetic ophthalmia: a retrospective study at the National Eye Institute, Bethesda, MD, from 1982 to 1992. *Archives of Ophthalmology*, **113**, 597–600.

Chisholm, I.H., Gass, J.D.M., and Hutton, W.L. (1976). The late stage of serpiginous (geographic) choroiditis. *American Journal of Ophthalmology*, **82**, 343–51.

Devenyi, R.G., Mieler, W.F., Lambrou, F.H., *et al.* (1988). Cryopexy of the vitreous base in the management of peripheral uveitis. *American Journal of Ophthalmology*, **106**, 135–8.

Dreyer, R.F. and Gass, J.D.M. (1984). Multifocal choroiditis and panuveitis: a syndrome that mimics ocular histoplasmosis. *Archives of Ophthalmology*, **102**, 1776–84.

Dugel, P.U., Rao, N.A., Ozler, S., *et al.* (1992). Pars plana vitrectomy for intraocular inflammation-related cystoid macular edema unresponsive to corticosteroids. A preliminary study. *Ophthalmology*, **99**, 1535–41.

Ebringer, R., Cawdell, D., and Ebringer A. (1979). Association of *Klebsiella pneumoniae* with acute anterior uveitis in ankylosing spondylitis. *British Medical Journal*, **1**, 383.

Foster, R.E., Lowder, C.Y., Meisler, D.M., *et al.* (1992). Extracapsular cataract extraction and posterior chamber intraocular lens implantation in uveitis patients. *Ophthalmology*, **99**, 1234–41.

Gass, J.D.M. (1982). Sympathetic ophthalmia following vitrectomy. *American Journal of Ophthalmology*, **93**, 552–8.

Hakin, K.N., Pearson, R.V., and Lightman, S.L. (1992). Sympathetic ophthalmia: visual results with modern immunosuppressive therapy. *Eye*, **2**, 453–5.

Hamilton, A.M. and Bird, A.C. (1974). Geographical choroidopathy. *British Journal of Ophthalmology*, **58**, 784–97.

Helm, C.J. and Holland, G.N. (1995). The effects of posterior subtenon injection of triamcinolone acetonide in patients with intermediate uveitis. *American Journal of Ophthalmology*, **120**, 55–64.

Henderly, D.E., Haymond, R.S., Rao, N.S., *et al.* (1987). The significance of the pars plana exudate in pars planitis. *American Journal of Ophthalmology*, **103**, 669–71.

Jampol, L.M., Orth D.D, Daily, M.J., *et al.* (1979). Subretinal neovascularization with geographic (serpiginous) choroiditis. *American Journal of Ophthalmology*, **88**, 683–9.

Jones, N.P. (1993). Fuchs' heterochromic uveitis: an update. *Survey of Ophthalmology*, 37, 253–72.

Kuppner, M.C., Liversidge, J., McKillop-Smith, S., *et al.* (1993). Adhesion molecule expression in acute and fibrotic sympathetic ophthalmia. *Current Eye Research*, 12, 923–34.

La Hey, E., de Jong, P.T.V.M., and Kijlstra, A. (1994). Fuchs' heterochromic cyclitis: review of the literature on the pathogenetic mechanisms. *British Journal of Ophthalmology*, 78, 307–12.

Laatikainen, L. and ErkkilŠ, H. (1974). Serpiginous choroiditis. *British Journal of Ophthalmology*, 58, 777–83.

Liversidge, J., Dick, A., Cheng, Y.F., *et al.* (1993). Retinal antigen-specific lymphocytes, TCR gamma delta T cells and CD5+ B cells cultured from the vitreous in acute sympathetic ophthalmitis. *Autoimmunity*, 15, 257–66.

Lubin, J.R., Albert, D.M., and Weinstein, M. (1980). Sixty-five years of sympathetic ophthalmia: a clinicopathologic review of 105 cases (1913–1978). *Ophthalmology*, 87, 109–21.

Malinowski, S.M., Pulido, J.S., Goeken, N.E., *et al.* (1993). The association of HLA-B8, B51, DR2, and multiple sclerosis in pars planitis. *Ophthalmology*, 100, 1199–205.

Malinowski, S.M., Pulido, J.S., and Folk, J.C. (1993). Long-term visual outcome and complications associated with pars planitis. *Ophthalmology*, 100, 818–25.

Miller, W.F., Will, B.R., Lewis, H., *et al* (1988). Vitrectomy in the management of peripheral uveitis. *Ophthalmology*, 95, 859–64.

Moorthy, R.S., Inomata, H., and Rao, N.A. (1995). Vogt–Koyanagi–Harada syndrome. *Survey of Ophthalmology*, 39, 265–92.

Morgan, C.M. and Schatz, H. (1986). Recurrent multifocal choroiditis. *Ophthalmology*, 99, 1138–47.

Murray, P.I. (1995). Fuchs' heterochromic cyclitis: an immunological disease or an immunological response? *International Ophthalmology*, 18, 313–14.

Murray, P.I., Hoekzema, R., Luyendijk, L., *et al.* (1990). Analysis of aqueous humor immunoglobulin G in uveitis by enzyme linked immunosorbent assay, isoelectric focusing and immunoblotting. *Investigative Ophthalmology and Visual Science*, 3, 2129–35.

Murray, P.I., Pall, A., Rene, C., *et al.* (1994). Markers of endothelial dysfunction in Fuchs' heterochromic cyclitis. *Regional Immunology*, 6, 35–7.

Nussenblatt, R.B., Mittal, K.K., Ryan, S., *et al.* (1982). Birdshot retinochoroidopathy associated with HLA A29 antigen and immune responsiveness to retinal S-antigen. *American Journal of Ophthalmology*, 94, 147–58.

O'Neill, D., Murray, P.I., Patel, B.C., *et al.* (1995). Extracapsular cataract surgery with and without intraocular lens implantation in Fuchs heterochromic cyclitis. *Ophthalmology*, 102, 1362–8.

Power, W.J. and Foster, C.S. (1995). Update on sympathetic ophthalmia. *International Ophthalmology Clinics*, 35, 127–37.

Priem, H.A. and Oosterhuis, J.A. (1988). Birdshot chorioretinopathy: clinical characteristics and evolution. *British Journal of Ophthalmology*, 72, 646–59.

Rao, N.A. (1997). Mechanisms of inflammatory response in sympathetic ophthalmia and Vogt–Koyanagi–Harada syndrome. *Eye*, 11, 213–16.

Riordan-Eva, P. and Lightman, S. (1994). Orbital floor steroid injections in the treatment of uveitis. *Eye*, 8, 66–9.

Rothova, A., van Veenendaal, W.G., Linssen, A., *et al.* (1987). Clinical features of acute anterior uveitis. *American Journal of Ophthalmology*, 103, 137–45.

Rubsamen, P.E. and Gass, J.D.M. (1991). Vogt–Koyanagi–Harada syndrome: clinical course, therapy and long-term visual outcome. *Archives of Ophthalmology*, 109, 682–7.

Ryan, S.J. and Maumenee, A.E. (1980). Birdshot retinochoroidopathy. *American Journal of Ophthalmology*, 89, 31–45.

Sprenkels, S.H., Van Kregten, E., and Feltkamp, T.E. (1996). IgA antibodies against *Klebsiella* and other Gram-negative bacteria in ankylosing spondylitis and acute anterior uveitis. *Clinical Rheumatology*, 15 (suppl 1), 48–51.

Stavrou, P. and Murray, P.I. (1994). Heparin surface modified intraocular lenses in uveitis. *Ocular Immunology and Inflammation*, 2, 161–8.

Stavrou, P., Misson, G.P., Rowson, N.J., *et al.* (1995). Trabeculectomy in uveitis: are antimetabolites necessary at the first procedure? *Ocular Immunology and Inflammation*, 3, 209–16.

Watzke, R.C., Packer, A.J., Folk, J.C., *et al.* (1984). Punctate inner choroidopathy. *American Journal of Ophthalmology*, 98, 572–84.

Weiss, H., Annesley, W.H. Jr, Shields, J.A., *et al.* (1979). The clinical course

of serpiginous choroidopathy. *American Journal of Ophthalmology*, 87, 133–42.

Welch, R.B., Maumenee, A.E., and Wahlen, H.E. (1960). Peripheral posterior segment inflammation, vitreous opacities, and edema of the posterior pole. *Archives of Ophthalmology*, 64, 540–9.

2.8.7 Uveitis associated with systemic disease

Elizabeth M. Graham and Miles R. Stanford

Retinal vasculitis is an associated feature of a number of systemic diseases. In this chapter the clinical and ocular features of each disease are given; the retinal signs often overlap but some of them are more prevalent in some diseases than others. It is worth identifying the retinal vessels that are predominantly involved, whether arteries, veins, or capillaries, as this helps define the differential diagnosis (Table 1). In the majority of patients the underlying disorder may be detected from the clinical history and the examination (Table 2). Multiple sclerosis and sarcoidosis are exceptions; in the former intraocular inflammation may precede the diagnosis by some years, in the latter the diagnosis may be notoriously difficult to prove despite all modern investigations. The systemic vasculitides do not, as a rule, present with retinal vasculitis, their main retinal features being arterial obstruction in the absence of intraocular inflammation. The exceptions to this are the rare cases of systemic lupus erythematosus with antiphospholipid antibody where retinal venous obstruction and mild vitritis may also occur.

Behçet's disease

The clinical diagnosis of Behçet's disease is based on the combination of orogenital ulceration, uveitis, and dermatological disease which may be complicated by arthritis and neurological involvement. It is rarely life-threatening and the major cause of morbidity in this disease is blindness. It is common in patients from countries surrounding the Mediterranean basin, the Middle East, and in Japan but cases from other populations are not unusual. The genetic marker for this condition is the human leucocyte antigen (HLA) B51 haplotype which is increased in prevalence in all populations studied. The underlying aetiology and pathogenesis are not clearly understood but an infective agent acting in patients with the appropriate genetic make-up is likely. It is predominantly a disease of young people, tending to burn out in middle age and both sexes are equally affected.

Ocular features

The commonest ocular presentation of Behçet's disease is recurrent anterior uveitis with hypopyon formation. This may

Table 1 Ophthalmological features of patients with retinal vasculitis associated with systemic diseases

Feature	Behçet's syndrome (%)	Sarcoidosis (%)	Uveomeningitic syndrome (%)	HLA B27 arthritis (%)
Anterior uveitis	50	40	36	100
Macula oedema	67	35	73	90
Peripheral vascular sheathing	36	18	45	0
Periphlebitis	23	65	27	0
Retinal vein occlusion	50	12	18	0
Neovascularization	15	18	25	0
Retinal infiltrates	33	0	0	0
Pigment epithelial disease	21	29	9	0

HLA, human leucocyte antigen.

Table 2 Physical signs found in different systemic diseases associated with posterior uveitis

Disease	Mouth ulcers	Chest signs	Joint involvement	Skin involvement	CNS involvement
Behçet's syndrome	++	−	+	+	+
Sarcoidosis	−	++	+	+	+
Multiple sclerosis	−	−	−	−	++
Inflammatory bowel disease	+	−	+	−	−
Seronegative arthropathy	−	−	++	−	−

CNS, central nervous system.

be unilateral initially but eventually both eyes are affected. Interestingly, in the majority of patients, the hypopyons may resolve spontaneously without specific treatment and are a marker of exacerbation of systemic disease. The main cause of visual morbidity in this condition is retinal vasculitis. Retinal infiltrates (Fig. 1) are characteristic and are not seen in any other idiopathic posterior uveitis. These tend to be larger and more fluffy than cotton-wool spots, often occurring in the retinal periphery where cotton-wool spots do not occur. Recurrent ischaemic retinal branch vein occlusions are common (Fig. 2) and lead to progressive retinal and optic atrophy with extensive sheathing of retinal vessels. Visual loss may also occur secondary to macular oedema and diffuse microvascular leakage on fluorescein angiography is common. Occasionally these patients also show macular ischaemia. Choroidal disease does not occur. Secondary complications including neovascularization, rubeotic glaucoma and phthisis are rare but may lead to enucleation. Pathological specimens of the eye show a central perivasculitis with surrounding tissue destruction.

Ocular disease is usually associated with other signs of Behçet's disease but the characteristic retinal signs may be seen without other evidence of systemic disease or only oral ulceration. The visual prognosis, despite modern immunosuppres-

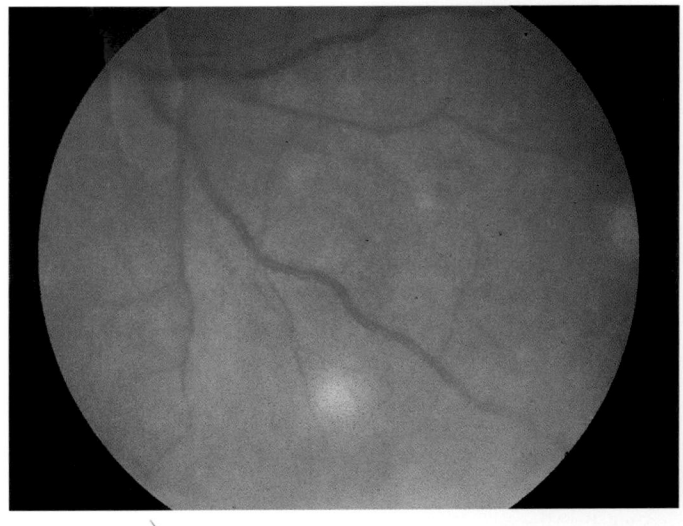

Fig. 1 Colour fundus photograph of the retinal periphery in a young man with Behçet's disease showing an intraretinal infiltrate.

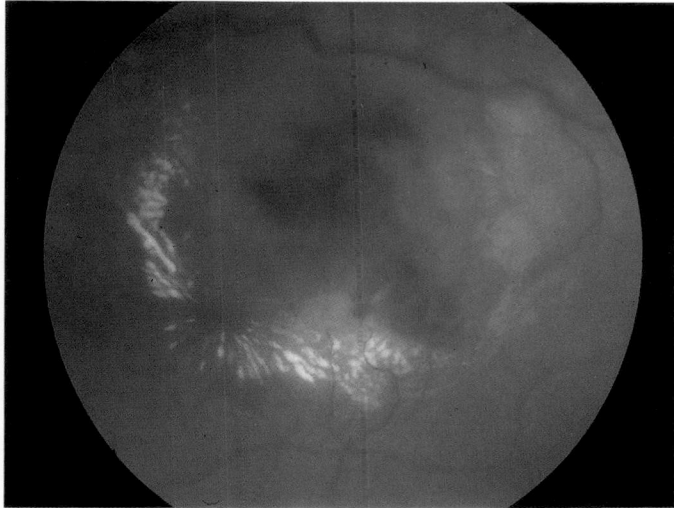

(a)

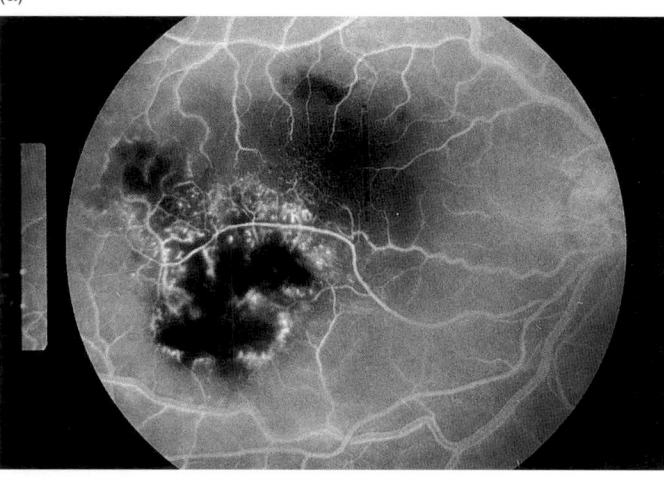

(b)

Fig. 2 (a) Fundus photograph of a patient with Behçet's disease showing a haemorrhagic macula branch retinal vein occlusion; (b) mid-phase fluorescein angiogram in the same patient demonstrating capillary closure within the venous occlusion.

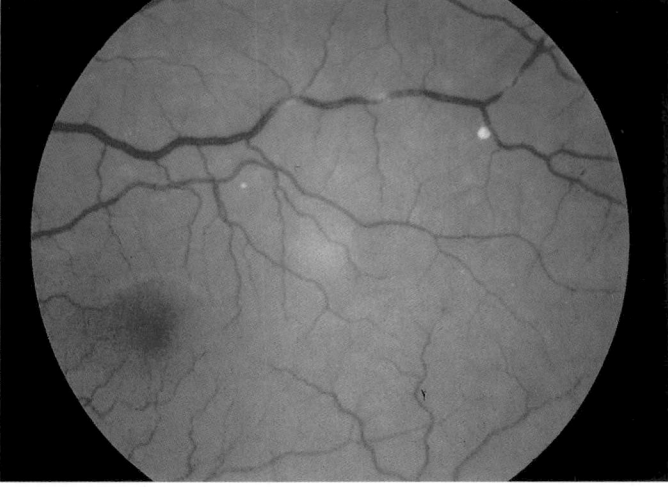

Fig. 3 Fundus photograph of a patient with ocular sarcoidosis. There are three discrete areas of periphlebitis along the retinal vein at the top.

sives, is poor with 75 per cent of patients being blind in one eye within 5 years of onset.

Sarcoidosis

Sarcoidosis is a chronic granulomatous condition of unknown aetiology which can affect any organ system in the body. Ocular involvement is found in 25 per cent of patients with sarcoidosis at some time. Ocular involvement has been reported in up to 50 per cent of patients with chest disease and of patients presenting with uveitis about 7 per cent will have underlying sarcoidosis which rises to 20 per cent in those with a panuveitis. The most common ocular manifestation of sarcoidosis is anterior uveitis which occurs in 60 per cent of patients. Sarcoidosis has two clinical forms: (a) an acute form associated with erythema nodosum, hilar lymphadenopathy, and acute anterior uveitis which resolves spontaneously; or (b) a chronic form associated with chronic uveitis, arthritis, skin lesions, and cent-

ral nervous system involvement which may wax and wane over 50 years.

Anterior uveitis in sarcoidosis is characterized by a chronic relapsing and remitting uveitis, often with mutton fat keratitic precipitates and is associated with iris granulomas and posterior synechiae. Hypopyons are never seen. The anterior chamber reaction is variable ranging from a low grade uveitis with a few keratitic precipitates to a marked plastic reaction with multiple keratic precipitates which may cover the corneal endothelium. In a few patients the disease may be restricted to one eye and quickly remit but in the majority it is bilateral and chronic. Intraocular pressure may or may not be raised and gonioscopy often reveals mutton fat keratitic precipitates on the trabecula meshwork.

Posterior segment disease in sarcoidosis provides a wide variety of signs. In the vitreous cellular infiltrates, opacities and haemorrhage from retinal new vessels may occur. Periphlebitis (Fig. 3) is the most common and diagnostic retinal feature and occurs in about 10 per cent of patients with ophthalmic sarcoid. It tends to involve small retinal venules in the equatorial retina and generally affects a smaller section of vessel and is whiter than the perivenous sheathing seen in patients with multiple sclerosis. On fluorescein angiography there is intense focal leakage at the areas of periphlebitis and this clinical feature very rarely occurs in any other form of intraocular inflammation. Mild peripheral venous occlusion (and, rarely, major branch vein occlusions) with capillary closure may occur and occasionally the perivenous infiltration becomes so extensive as to resemble candle-wax drippings. This latter feature is not common and not pathognomonic. As with other forms of inflammatory retinal disease cystoid macular oedema occurs in sarcoidosis and is a major cause of visual loss in the condition. Occasionally, subtle macular ischaemia characterized by perifoveal capillary dropout with enlargement and irregularity of the avascular zone is seen.

Retinal neovascularization, either at the disc or in the periphery, may occur in 15 per cent of patients with posterior seg-

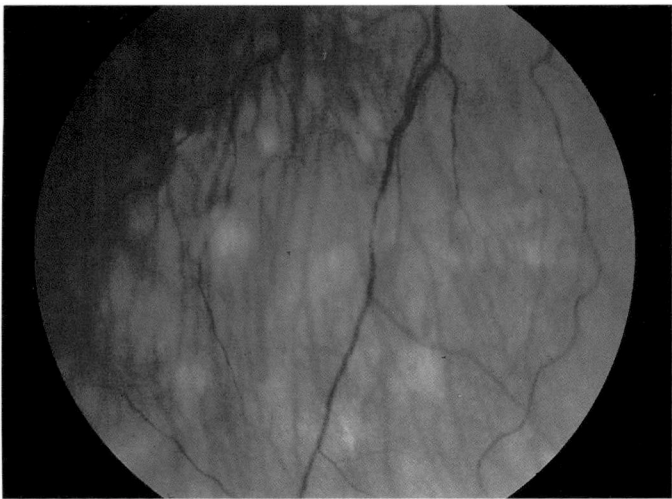

Fig. 4 Fundus photograph of a patient with ocular sarcoidosis showing peripheral choroidal/retinal pigment epithelial scars which are presumed to result from previous choroidal granulomas.

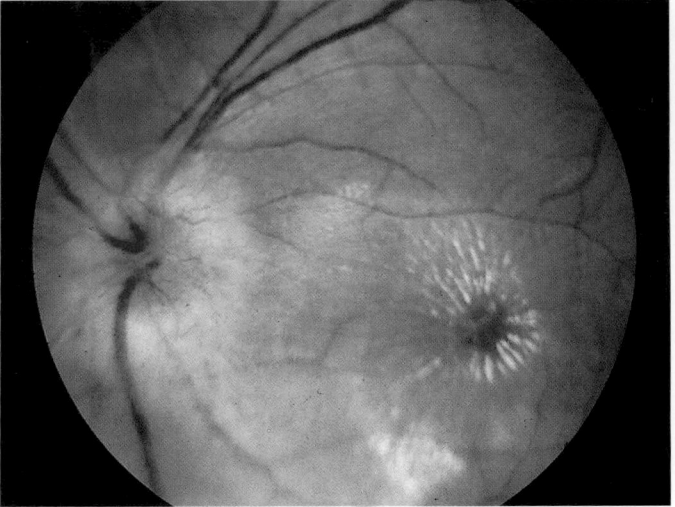

Fig. 5 Fundus photograph of the posterior pole in a patient with sarcoidosis and optic neuropathy. The optic disc is pink and swollen and there is a well-defined macula star.

ment disease. If neovascularization at the disc does occur in the presence of intraocular inflammation, sarcoidosis is by far the most likely diagnosis. Whilst, in some patients, it is associated with peripheral capillary closure and behaves in much the same way as other ischaemic retinopathies, in some it is caused by inflammation alone; these new vessels may regress spontaneously or on steroid treatment. Vitreous haemorrhage and traction retinal detachment are much more uncommon than in the ischaemic retinopathies.

Acutely, choroidal nodules may be seen in 6 per cent of patients and are usually bilateral. More commonly areas of retinal pigment epithelium atrophy (Fig. 4), particularly in the inferior equatorial region may be found and are thought to arise from resolved choroidal granulomas. Occasionally sarcoidosis may be a cause of multifocal choroiditis and rarely can give a picture reminiscent of serpiginous choroiditis.

Optic nerve involvement (Fig. 5) occurs in under 10 per cent of cases of ophthalmic sarcoid. Swelling of the disc may be due to posterior uveitis, direct infiltration of the nerve head, or raised intracranial pressure secondary to chronic meningitis or the mass effect of a large central nervous system granuloma.

The long-term visual outcome of patients with sarcoidosis is varied. Some patients may have a few attacks of isolated anterior uveitis with no subsequent sequelae whilst others have long-term intraocular inflammation requiring chronic immunosuppression to prevent permanent visual loss. A proportion of patients will develop glaucoma or cataract as part of their disease and up to 15 per cent may subsequently develop symptoms and signs attributable to neurosarcoidosis.

Multiple sclerosis

Retinal vasculitis may precede or complicate multiple sclerosis and may be either asymptomatic or symptomatic. Initial reports of peripheral venous sheathing have appeared in the literature in the past but it is now becoming apparent that the true pre-

valence of intraocular inflammation is high. Asymptomatic uveoretinal inflammation may be seen ophthalmoscopically in 1–5 per cent of unselected outpatients with multiple sclerosis, 20 per cent of unselected inpatients, and in up to 40 per cent of patients with the progressive form of the disease. In 12 per cent of patients with isolated optic neuritis asymptomatic intraocular inflammation may be detected and fluorescein angiography will reveal abnormal vascular leakage in a further 12 per cent. Symptomatic uveoretinitis is rarer but increasingly recognized. The occurrence of retinal vasculitis in a tissue that lacks myelin has pathogenetic significance in that it supports a primary vasculitic rather than a myelinodestructive process in causing disease. Postmortem findings of segmental perivenous lymphocytic retinal infiltration have shown these changes to be comparable to those found within the central nervous system.

Symptomatic uveoretinitis is commoner in females with multiple sclerosis and these patients have a higher prevalence of the established HLA association A3, B7, DR2, and DR3. Female patients presenting with isolated (idiopathic) retinal vasculitis and the HLA B7 haplotype have a 30-fold higher chance of developing multiple sclerosis in subsequent years than patients with this disease but without this haplotype.

The ocular findings in patients with multiple sclerosis are not distinctive. Both granulomatous and non-granulomatous anterior uveitis have been reported but this rarely gives rise to a painful, photophobic red eye. In the posterior segment perivenous sheathing is the commonest sign and this may be distinguished from the periphlebitis seen in sarcoidosis although the distinction is probably arbitrary. Ophthalmoscopically perivenous sheathing is characterized by a greyish reflex over the retinal veins, often with some mild sclerotic change. Conversely, periphlebitis is characterized by a localized white cuffing of retinal veins often at areas of vascular bifurcation. Available pathological studies of retinal venous sheathing in multiple sclerosis and periphlebitis in sarcoidosis reveal an essentially common microscopic picture and it is likely therefore that venous sheathing represents a more advanced stage of venular inflammation than periphlebitis. This is supported by the finding of universal fluorescein leakage with periphlebitis whilst this may or may not be present with venous sheathing. In addition to these vascular signs patients may present with intermediate uveitis and others with frank macular oedema with its attendant visual loss. Capillary closure is extremely uncommon although neovascularization at the disc has been reported. Retinal pigment epithelial inflammation or choroiditis is practically unknown in multiple sclerosis and the absence of this is a more important diagnostic sign of multiple sclerosis than the presence of anterior uveitis or retinal vascular involvement. Patients with choroiditis and a uveomeningitic syndrome must be evaluated for other disease, the most common being neurosarcoidosis.

There do not appear to be any unusual features of the neurological involvement in patients with multiple sclerosis and ocular inflammation. Thus, the age of onset, pattern of neurological involvement, and degree of disability do not differ from other patients with multiple sclerosis without uveitis. Overall, the retinal inflammation seen in multiple sclerosis is relatively benign; if treatment is required inflammation responds readily to corticosteroids and second-line immunosuppression is rarely required.

Inflammatory bowel disease

The incidence of intraocular inflammation in inflammatory bowel disease (whether granulomatous or ulcerative) has varied from 0.5 to 11.8 per cent. The commonest form of ocular involvement is a recurrent anterior uveitis similar to that seen in HLA B27-positive patients but posterior segment inflammation also occurs, albeit more rarely.

Crohn's disease

This form of inflammatory bowel disease is characterized by a chronic, segmental, granulomatous inflammation of the bowel wall that is usually transmural. The small bowel is mainly affected but perirectal complications are common. Extraintestinal complications include disorders of the skin, mucous membranes, lungs, kidneys, muscles, and eyes. Sacroiliitis, ankylosing spondylitis, and liver changes also occur but tend to be independent of the main disease.

Retinal vasculitis is a rare complication of Crohn's disease, but some cases with occlusive arteritis and phlebitis have been reported. Fluorescein angiography shows leakage from vessel walls and the optic disc, and visual loss may occur from macular oedema. High dose immunosuppression is often required to control the acute disease.

Ulcerative colitis

The incidence of any form of ocular inflammation (scleritis, uveitis, etc.) in ulcerative colitis is up to 11 per cent. However, when only uveitis is present, this falls to 1 per cent making it a rare complication of the disorder. Classically patients present with a systemic upset and chronic bloody diarrhoea, and the diagnosis is made on colonic biopsy. Ocular and colonic disease occur together, but rarely the ocular disease precedes bowel symptoms by some years. Interestingly, where uveitis is present as an extracolonic manifestation other complications are present at a higher than expected rate. Thus, 50 per cent of patients also have sacroiliitis compared with 4 per cent who do not have uveitis, and 85 per cent have peripheral arthritis compared with 17 per cent without associated uveitis.

The uveitis, like the bowel disease, tends to be chronic and relapsing in young adults. Topical and systemic treatment are often required to control intraocular inflammation.

Whipple's disease

Patients with this rare malabsorption state usually present with malaise, weight loss, diarrhoea, and arthritis. Extraintestinal disease includes pulmonary, skin, cardiac, and neurological involvement but some of these complications are due to secondary nutritional deficiencies consequent on the malabsorption. Patients may develop a mild granulomatous panuveitis with retinal involvement affecting the capillaries with haemorrhage, exudate, and capillary closure.

Ankylosing spondylitis and the seronegative arthropathies

Acute anterior uveitis is the most important ocular complication of these diseases and affects 25 per cent of patients with ankylosing spondylitis and 5 to 10 per cent of patients with other causes of seronegative arthropathy. The majority (60–90 per cent) of these patients with acute anterior uveitis and seronegative arthropathy are HLA B27-positive. The attacks of uveitis are usually unilateral but both eyes are affected during the course of the disease, usually alternately and rarely simultaneously. The pattern of uveitis is identical regardless of the aetiology of the seronegative arthropathy. The patients complain of severe pain and drop in visual acuity during attacks which are characterized by a fibrinous exudate in the anterior chamber and the absence of mutton fat keratic precipitates. In half the patients posterior synechiae develop and cataract in 15 per cent but blindness is rare. Posterior segment complications are also unusual: a few patients (5 per cent) develop severe exudative disease with cystoid macular oedema, disc oedema, and serous retinal detachment. Retinal vascular occlusions do not occur. These posterior segment complications may only respond to very high doses of corticosteroids. The severity of the uveitis does not correlate with the severity of the ankylosing spondylitis or other joint disease: in fact there is a suggestion that progression of joint disease is slower in patients under regular observation for uveitis.

Systemic vasculitides

As a general rule uveitis is not a feature of the systemic vasculitides (systemic lupus erythematosus, polyarteritis nodosa, Churg–Strauss syndrome). However, if the patient has a very severe scleritis, particularly posterior scleritis, an 'overflow' intraocular inflammation may develop with cells in the vitreous, and disc oedema.

Wegener's granulomatosis, particularly the non-sarcoidal variant, may produce identical ocular complications to sarcoidosis with a granulomatous anterior uveitis and a posterior uveitis characterized by retinal periphlebitis and retinal pigment epithelial and choroidal changes.

Primary Sjögren's syndrome

Primary Sjögren's syndrome is an autoimmune disorder characterized by dry eyes and dry mouth but complicated by vasculitis which may produce arthritis, peripheral and central nervous system disease, as well as myositis, pneumonitis, and renal disease. Very high levels of extractable nuclear antibodies and rheumatoid factor are pathognomonic of this disease. Rarely, these patients present with panuveitis and retinal periphlebitis but these features should alert the doctor to an alternative diagnosis such as sarcoidosis.

Scleroderma en coup de sabre

This rare, disfiguring dermatological disease may be complicated by uveitis on the affected side presumably as a result of ischaemia. Heterochromia and retinal vein occlusions may develop.

Ocular lymphoma

Ocular lymphoma has long been known to masquerade as a chronic uveitis particularly in elderly patients. Originally known as reticulum cell sarcoma of the eye, modern immunophenotyping techniques have now clearly established that the tumour is derived from lymphocytes, almost exclusively of B-cell lineage. Eye involvement is usually seen in primary disease of the eye and brain rather than as part of systemic lymphoma, although the latter is recognized in immunocompromised patients. Twenty per cent of patients with primary central nervous system lymphoma have ocular disease and 60 to 89 per cent of patients who present with isolated ocular disease progress to central nervous system involvement depending on the length of follow-up. Ocular lymphoma may be becoming more common, probably due to heightened recognition of the disease, although true figures are not available.

The clinical features of ocular lymphoma are summarized in Table 3. Patients usually present with floaters and blurred vision and rarely with pain. Colour vision is often unexpectedly reduced and patients may have constricted visual fields. Patients are usually elderly (more than 60 years of age); in younger age groups predisposing conditions such as long-term immunosuppression, acquired immune deficiency syndrome, or ataxia telangiectasia must be considered. Anterior segment involvement is usually mild and posterior segment signs include large cells in the vitreous of both eyes in association with subretinal infiltrates (Fig. 6) and pigment epithelial lesions (Fig. 7) which often progress to attenuation of retinal vessels and optic atrophy. The differential diagnosis of chronic panuveitis in such elderly patients includes ocular ischaemia,

Table 3 Clinical features of patients with ocular lymphoma

Age more than 55 years at presentation

Bilateral disease

Constricted visual field with reduced or absent colour vision

Fine pigmented keratic precipitates, large vitreous cells, and subretinal infiltrates

Pigment epithelial abnormality without associated macular oedema on fluorescein angiography

Poor response to treatment with systemic corticosteroids

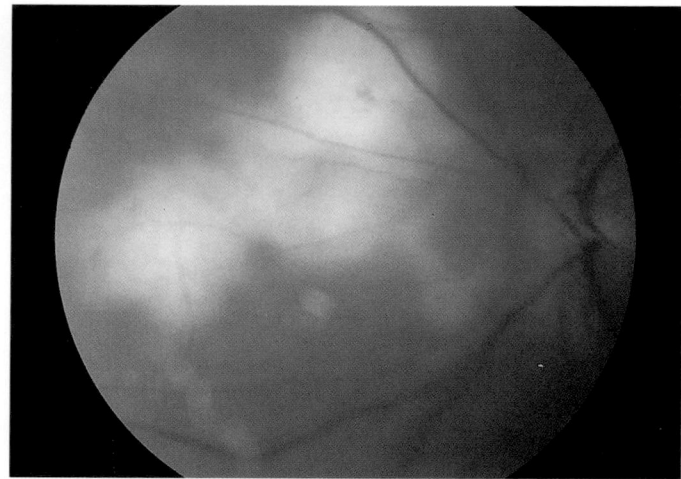

Fig. 6 Fundus photograph of a patient with ocular lymphoma. There are widespread white–yellow subretinal infiltrates.

sarcoidosis, and viral retinitis. Fluorescein angiography may reveal the presence of extensive pigment epithelial disease with attenuation of retinal vessels. Marked leakage from retinal vessels, the optic disc, or macular oedema is rare and helps to differentiate this condition from other causes of inflammatory uveitis in this age group. Pathological studies show tumour cells present between the pigment epithelium and Bruch's membrane, often infiltrating the optic nerve head at the level of the lamina cribrosa. Perivascular cuffing is frequently seen in the retinal blood vessels but tumour cells rarely infiltrate the vessel wall. Involvement of the choroid is unusual but the iris, ciliary body, and vitreous may be heavily infiltrated. Another classical clinical feature is the initial response of this tumour to systemic corticosteroids with reduction of the vitreous infiltrate, presumably due to a reduction in the accompanying inflammation, with a subsequent loss of control as the tumour cells become more proliferative. The diagnosis may be made on the characteristic clinical symptoms and signs, and should be confirmed by vitreous biopsy with immunostaining of the cellular infiltrate. In addition these patients must undergo evaluation for concomitant central nervous system and systemic disease and should have bone marrow examination, magnetic resonance imaging scans, plasma protein and immunoglobulin estimation,

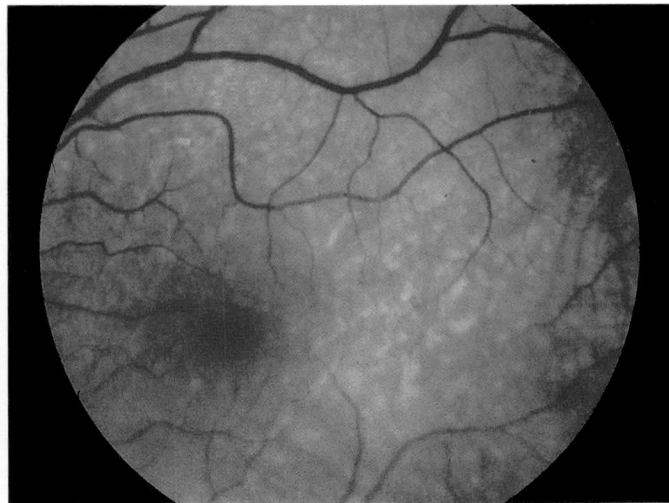

(a)

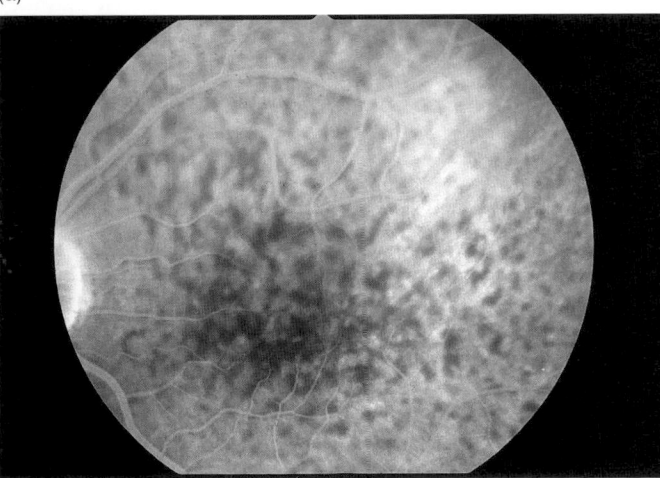

(b)

Fig. 7 (a) Fundus photograph and (b) fluorescein angiogram of a patient with ocular lymphoma showing characteristic pigment epithelial changes.

and cytological evaluation of cerebrospinal fluid following cytospin.

The treatment of choice is localized radiotherapy but given the high risk of developing central nervous system disease these patients should be kept under close review from the neurological point of view. The prognosis for vision in this condition is good although the majority of patients will eventually succumb to central nervous system disease in time.

Malignant disease

Uveitis and retinal vasculitis can be the presenting features of malignant disease. Choroidal melanoma is associated with ipsilateral ocular inflammation in 10 per cent of cases, particularly those tumours with necrosis and mixed or epithelioid tumours. Metastatic melanoma may deposit in the eye but in this circumstance the cells in the anterior segment and vitreous are pigmented. The choroid is a common site for bloodborne metastases, particularly from breast and lung but these metastases

are rarely associated with intraocular inflammation. Leukaemia and lymphoma can both involve the retina and the iris and masquerade as uveitis. Similarly, retinoblastoma is a rare cause of uveitis in children when the cells of the aqueous may be either tumour cells or inflammatory cells. Both the paraneoplastic conditions, carcinoma-associated retinopathy and melanoma-associated retinopathy, have been reported with intraocular inflammation with cells in the vitreous and bilateral retinal vasculitis with either sheathing of the retinal veins or attenuation of the vessels. These patients present with problems of retinal dysfunction such as troublesome photopsia or nightblindness and their ocular symptoms may antedate the discovery of their tumours.

Vogt–Koyanagi–Harada syndrome

Vogt–Koyanagi–Harada syndrome is a severe bilateral panuveitis associated with serous retinal detachment and retinal pigment epithelial changes accompanied by poliosis, vitiligo, alopecia, and central nervous system and auditory signs. It is unusual for all the signs to be present together; the most common manifestation is bilateral panuveitis with serous detachments and meningism. It is commoner in pigmented races and is seen more frequently in women. Most patients are young and present between the ages of 20 and 50. The aetiology and pathogenesis of this disorder are not understood but, given the predilection for immunological damage to melanocytes of the skin, choroid, meninges, and inner ear, autoimmune disease against components of melanocytes has been suggested. A high prevalence of HLA DR4, particularly in Japanese patients, has been noted.

The disease divides itself into a number of phases. During the prodromal phase patients may experience meningitic signs of headache, nausea, vertigo, neck stiffness, and photophobia. Soon after this, blurring of vision becomes evident and this is usually bilateral. Thickening of both the retina and choroid is initially focal but then becomes diffuse with signs of exudative retinal detachments. Granulomatous anterior uveitis may then supervene and, in rare cases, patients may experience acute angle closure glaucoma. Some weeks after the inflammatory phase the disease enters a convalescent stage when depigmentation of the choroid—'sunset-glow' fundus—and the perilimbal area both occur. Areas of pigment epithelial clumping and multiple discrete small areas of chorioretinal atrophy occur. In some patients the disease enters a chronic, recurrent phase characterized by repeated attacks of granulomatous anterior uveitis which can be quite steroid-resistant. The ocular complications of the disease include cataract, glaucoma, and subretinal neovascular membranes.

Whilst Vogt–Koyanagi–Harada syndrome is predominantly a clinical diagnosis, both fluorescein angiography and cerebrospinal fluid examination are useful in confirming the disease. In the acute phase of disease, fluorescein angiography may reveal hyperfluorescent dots at the level of the retinal pigment epithelium with subsequent pooling of dye which delineates the overlying retinal detachment. Inflammatory disc leakage and occasional retinal venous staining may also occur. Cerebrospinal fluid examination shows an increased white count, especially lymphocytes, that lasts for about 8 weeks after the initial acute inflammatory episode.

In general, patients with Vogt–Koyanagi–Harada syndrome who are adequately treated have a reasonable visual prognosis and two-thirds of patients should retain 6/12 vision or better in the long term.

Uveitis in children

Uveitis in children is approximately four times less common than in people over 16 years of age. The essentials of diagnosis and management of uveitis in children is the same as in adults. With the exception of uveitis associated with juvenile chronic arthritis, all the disease entities seen in adults may occur in children, albeit often with reduced frequency, as the incidence of systemic inflammatory disease such as Behçet's or sarcoidosis is much less in children and accounts for less than 10 per cent of all cases of uveitis in childhood.

Juvenile chronic arthritis

Smiley identified 30 years ago the characteristics of the chronic anterior uveitis which affects 30 per cent of children with juvenile chronic arthritis. The classic features of the eye disease are painless uveitis occurring in white eyes, often with granulomatous keratic precipitates and posterior synechiae in the acute phase and complicated by glaucoma, cataracts, and band keratopathy (Fig. 8). Posterior segment disease with vitritis and cystoid macular oedema is rarely seen but a few aphakic children may develop retinal detachments. The insidious nature of the disease results in delayed referral to the ophthalmologist and in 10 to 30 per cent of patients the potentially blinding complications of glaucoma and cataract may develop. Cataract should not be a cause for blindness but the glaucoma in this condition remains a difficult therapeutic problem and accounts for the majority of the 8 per cent of children who go blind from the uveitis associated with juvenile chronic arthritis.

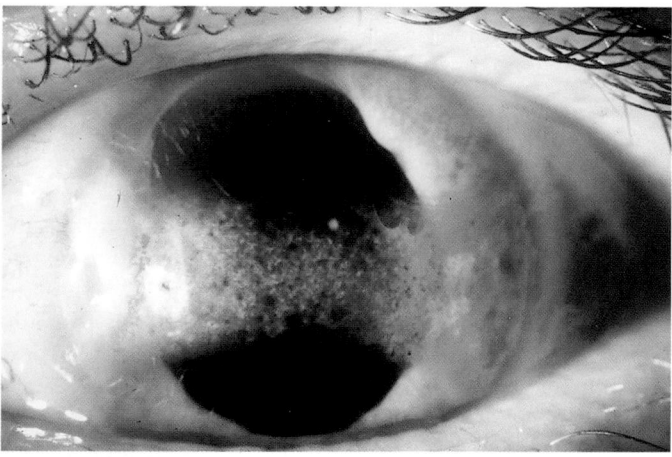

Fig. 8 Anterior segment photograph of a child with established juvenile chronic arthritis. There is a marked band-shaped keratopathy and a surgically enlarged pupil secondary to cataract surgery.

Table 4 Recommended ophthalmic screening programme for patients with juvenile chronic arthritis (i.e. patients with normal eyes at first visit to ophthalmologist); all patients except those with juvenile ankylosing spondylitis and systemic onset

3 monthly	1st year
4 monthly	2nd year
6 monthly	3, 4, 5 years
Annually	Thereafter

As the condition is a potentially blinding disorder and it occurs in a well-recognized disease the validity of screening for eye disease is a perpetual question. The children most likely to develop uveitis are girls with pauciarticular disease with early age of onset (less than 3 years) of arthritis and positive antinuclear antibodies. However, with the exception of systemic onset disease any other child with any of the other categories of juvenile chronic arthritis (polyarticular, extended pauciarticular) may develop uveitis and its blinding complications. A low risk of disease development is not necessarily associated with good visual outcome. Early onset of uveitis, the presence of posterior synechiae at the initial examination, disease persistence for more than 12 months, and the male sex are factors associated with poor visual outcome.

A vital point in managing these children is to give priority to early ocular examination. These children do not complain about their eyes as they are neither red nor painful. Therefore, patients with 'normal eyes' should be seen as suggested in Table 4. Treatment is essentially with local steroids (dexamethasone or Pred Forte) and mydriatrics (cyclopentolate). Glaucoma is very rarely a feature of active uveitis but occurs in quiescent disease. Topical treatment regimes and oral acetazolamide must be exhausted before surgical treatment is attempted as even with the best microsurgical expertise these eyes fare badly after surgery. Systemic immunosuppressives are rarely required to control ocular inflammation although occasional high dose corticosteroids are needed to reduce posterior pole oedema and serous elevation of the retina. The impact of other drugs such as chloroquine or methotrexate on activity and severity of uveitis has not been clarified although many children take these drugs to control their joint disease.

Other rheumatological diseases in childhood

Rare conditions which may mimic juvenile chronic arthritis, as they are characterized by both arthritis and granulomatous uveitis, are infantile onset multisystem inflammatory disease, which is a familial arthropathy with rash, uveitis, and mental retardation and Farber's lipogranulomatosis when the unfortunate children rarely reach more than 2 years of age and succumb to pulmonary disease.

Spondyloarthropathies

Ten per cent of patients with ankylosing spondylitis develop the first symptoms of disease before the age 16 (juvenile spondylitis). These patients are usually adolescent boys with lower limb arthritis. With long follow-up of these children 27 per cent suffer episodes of acute anterior uveitis characterized by pain, redness, and florid anterior chamber inflammation.

Psoriasis

Children with psoriasis complicated by arthritis may suffer uveitis. The inflammation of these eyes is clinically indistinguishable from the uveitis seen with juvenile chronic arthritis.

Multisystem systemic illnesses in childhood

Behçet's disease and sarcoidosis are rarely seen before adolescence but are indistinguishable from the adult disease. The systemic vasculitides, systemic lupus erythematosus, and polyarteritis nodosa rarely present with uveitis or retinal vasculitis. Children with Kawasaki's disease commonly have bilateral uveitis in addition to a non-suppurative bulbar conjunctivitis.

Tubulointerstitial nephritis and uveitis syndrome

Acute tubulointerstitial nephritis and uveitis syndrome is a condition primarily of young people. Patients develop a bilateral uveitis characterized by keratic precipitates and posterior synechiae; these respond well to local therapy. The uveitis may antedate or coincide with the onset of nephritis.

Further reading

Atmaca, L.S. (1989). Fundus changes associated with Behçet's disease. *Graefes Archives of Ophthalmology*, 227, 340–4.

Duber, J.S., Brown, G.C., and Brooks, L. (1987). Retinal vasculitis in Crohn's disease. *American Journal of Ophthalmology*, 103, 664–8.

Giles, C.L. (1989). Uveitis in childhood—parts I–III. *Annals of Ophthalmology*, 21, 13–28.

Graham, E. (1987). Intraocular treatment of T and B cell lymphomas. *Eye*, 1, 691–8.

Graham, E.M., Stanford, M.R., Sanders, M.D., Kasp, E., and Dumonde, D.C. (1989). A point prevalence study of 150 patients with idiopathic retinal vasculitis. I. Diagnostic value of ophthalmological features. *British Journal of Ophthalmology*, 73, 714–21.

Hoover, D.L., Khan, J.A., and Giangiacomo, J. (1986). Paediatric ocular sarcoidosis. *Survey of Ophthalmology*, 30, 215–28.

Kanski, J.J. and Shun Shun, A. (1984). Systemic uveitis syndromes in childhood: an analysis of 340 cases. *Ophthalmology*, 91, 1247–52.

Kerrison, J.B., Flynn, T., and Green, W.R. (1994). Retinal pathologic changes in multiple sclerosis. *Retina*, 14, 445–51.

Leak, A.M. and Wenberg, D.A. (1989). Autoimmune rheumatic disorders in childhood—a comparison with adult onset disease. *Quarterly Journal of Medicine*, 73, 270, 875–93.

Lightman, S., McDonald, W.I., Bird, A.C., *et al.* (1987). Retinal venous sheathing in optic neuritis. *Brain*, 110, 405–14.

Malinowski, S.M., Pulido, J.S., and Folk, J.C. (1993). Long-term visual outcome and complications associated with pars planitis. *Ophthalmology*, 100, 818–24.

Michelson, J.B. and Chisari, F.V. (1982) Behçet's disease. *Survey of Ophthalmology*, 26, 190–203.

Michelson, J.B. and Friedlander, M.H. (1990) Behçet's disease. *International Ophthalmology Clinics*, 30, 271–8.

Moorthy, R.S., Inomata, H., and Rao, N.A. (1995). Vogt–Koyanagi–Harada syndrome. *Survey of Ophthalmology*, 39, 265–91.

Nussenblatt, R.B. and Palestine, A.G. (ed.) (1989). *Uveitis. Fundamentals and clinical practice*. Year Book Medical, Chicago.

Pepose, J., Holland, G.N., and Wilhelmus, K.R. (ed.) (1996). *Ocular infection and immunity*. Mosby Year Book, St Louis.

Perkins, E.S. (1966). Pattern of uveitis in childhood. *British Journal of Ophthalmology*, 50, 169–85.

Rodriguez, A., Akova, Y.A., Pedroya-Seres, M., and Foster, C.S. (1994). Posterior segment ocular manifestations in patients with HLA-B27-associated uveitis. *Ophthalmology*, 101, 1267–74.

Stanbury, R.M., Graham, E.M., and Murray, P.I. (1995) Sarcoidosis. *International Ophthalmology Clinics*, 35, 123–37.

Wakefield, D., Montanaro, A., and McCluskey, P. (1991). Acute anterior uveitis and HLA B27. *Survey of Ophthalmology*, 36, 223–32.

Woolf, M.D., Lichter, P., and Ragsdale, C.G. (1987). Prognostic factors in uveitis of juvenile rheumatoid arthritis. *Ophthalmology*, 94, 1242–8.

Zaidman, G.W. and Coles, R.S. (1981). Peripheral uveitis and ulcerative colitis. *Annals of Ophthalmology*, 13, 73–6.

2.8.8 Principles of clinical management of uveitis

C.S. Ng and A. Ralph Rosenthal

The objective in managing patients with uveitis is to alleviate discomfort and to prevent the disruption of ocular structure and function. Decisions in formulating a therapeutic regime are based upon the diagnosis and natural history of the condition, its severity, and the presence of complications. General therapeutic principles for uveitis will be considered in this chapter, and specific treatment measures for individual uveitic entities are discussed in their respective sections.

Medications

Damage from uveitis arises as a consequence of the inflammatory response in the eye. In cases where no obvious infective agents are identifiable, the disease may represent an autoimmune reaction to ocular tissue. Therapeutic agents used in uveitis are therefore aimed at suppressing the inflammatory and immune responses.

Corticosteroids

Mechanisms of action

Corticosteroids are effective anti-inflammatory and immunosuppressive agents and have been regarded as the mainstay of therapy for uveitis since their introduction into ophthalmic use in the 1950s. The mode of action of corticosteroids has not been completely elucidated, but broadly, they affect the production and activities of chemical mediators involved in inflammation, as well as the distribution, concentration, and function of peripheral leucocytes.

More specifically, the synthesis of inflammatory mediators such as prostaglandins and leukotrienes from phospholipids is suppressed due to the inhibition of phospholipase A_2 by corticosteroids. The vasoconstrictive effect of corticosteroids decreases the attendant vascular permeability and minimizes the leakage of fluid, proteins, and inflammatory cells into the affected areas.

Lymphocyte, monocyte, eosinophil, and basophil counts are decreased due to their movement away from the vasculature back into lymphoid tissues, whereas the circulating neutrophil count is elevated due to an increased influx from bone marrow. Corticosteroids, however, have an inhibitory effect on neutrophilic chemotaxis, thereby reducing its migration to inflamed tissue. The rate of lymphocyte proliferation is also suppressed. The net effect is therefore a decrease in leucocyte concentration in the target tissues.

Cell membranes of mast cells and basophils are stabilized by corticosteroids, thus inhibiting their degranulation and the concomitant release of inflammatory mediators like histamines and kinins. Intracellular lysosomal membranes are likewise stabilized resulting in an inhibition of neutrophil degranulation. As a result, the immunocompetence of monocytes and macrophages is compromised, which may lead to an increased susceptibility to infections in patients treated with corticosteroids.

Corticosteroid therapy
Corticosteroids may be administered topically, by periocular injection, orally, or parenterally.

Topical therapy
Topical therapy is the most common means of corticosteroid administration and carries fewer systemic side-effects than periocular injections and systemic therapy. The choice has to be made between the various drugs, concentrations, and base vehicles.

Topically administered corticosteroids enter the eye via the cornea. The lipophilic corneal epithelium and hydrophilic stroma facilitate ocular penetration by preparations that are biphasic in solubility, like dexamethasone alcohol and prednisolone acetate suspensions, rather than hydrophilic ones, such as betamethasone and prednisolone phosphate. In uveitis, where a high drug concentration in the aqueous is important, the use of the former preparations is therefore preferred.

Application of higher concentration corticosteroid preparations result in higher intraocular concentration. The anti-inflammatory effect of prednisolone acetate thus increases in line with its concentration from 0.125 to 1 per cent (although when the concentration is further increased to 2 per cent there is no discernible corresponding augmentation of this anti-inflammatory effect). The intraocular concentration of corticosteroid can be further titrated by adjusting the frequency of instillation.

Ointments yield a more prolonged release of corticosteroids although peak concentrations in the eye are less compared with drops, and are therefore often used mainly as night-time preparations.

Topical corticosteroids are extremely effective in the treatment of anterior uveitis and may also be useful in the management of intermediate uveitis. In posterior uveitides, however,

Table 1 Systemic side-effects of steroids

Endocrine
Cushingoid state
Adrenal suppression
Growth retardation in children
Amenorrhoea
Impotence

Cardiovascular
Hypertension

Central nervous system
Psychosis
Benign intracranial hypertension
Increased appetite

Gastrointestinal
Peptic ulceration
Pancreatitis
Silent intestinal perforation

Healing
Impaired wound healing
Subcutaneous tissue atrophy

Immunological
Immunosuppression

Integumentary
Hirsutism
Panniculitis

Metabolic
Impaired glucose tolerance
Sodium and water retention
Hypokalaemic alkalosis
Hyperosmolar non-ketotic coma
Hyperlipidaemia

Musculoskeletal
Aseptic necrosis of bone
Myopathy
Osteoporosis

although there is some evidence that topically applied corticosteroids can gain access to the posterior pole via the suprachoroidal circulation, they are usually of little therapeutic value.

Periocular injections
Periocular corticosteroids may be delivered through subconjunctival or anterior subtenon injections for anterior segment inflammation, and as posterior subtenon or peribulbar injections for posterior inflammation. They provide a means of administering a large bolus of a drug to the eye whilst minimizing systemic side-effects and also allow the delivery of a depot for a more sustained release of corticosteroid. The duration of action of the various preparations is different: short-acting preparations like betamethasone and dexamethasone are effective for about a day, whilst long-acting corticosteroids such as triamcinolone and methylprednisolone are effective for up to 2 weeks.

Periocular corticosteroid injections are useful adjuncts to topical corticosteroids in severe anterior uveitis. Short-acting preparations are usually given in these instances to avoid potential side-effects. If periocular corticosteroids are used for posterior uveitis or macular oedema, long-acting depot preparations are preferred to minimize the need for repeated injections.

Systemic corticosteroids
There are various preparations of systemic corticosteroids suitable for ophthalmic use including prednisolone, prednisone, methylprednisolone, triamcinolone, betamethasone, and dexamethasone. They are all short-acting corticosteroids, with a biological half-life of between 1 and 3 days. They can be given orally or intravenously.

Side-effects
Corticosteroid therapy can have systemic and ocular side-effects. Systemic side-effects are listed in Table 1 and are more

common with systemic therapy than with periocular injections. Topical treatment carries the least risk of systemic side-effects although systemic absorption can be high enough to cause adrenal suppression in prolonged usage (1 ml of prednisolone acetate 1 per cent contains 10 mg of prednisolone) and punctal occlusion is advisable to minimize systemic absorption.

Ocular complications of topical and periocular corticosteroid therapy include elevated intraocular pressure, cataracts, and a predisposition to infections, especially by herpes simplex virus and fungi. Transient mydriasis and ptosis may occur but will resolve upon cessation of therapy. Complications from periocular corticosteroids may arise as a consequence of the injection as well as from the drug itself. Retrobulbar and subconjunctival haemorrhages, globe perforation, intraocular injection of the drug, optic nerve injury, conjunctival scarring, and subdermal fat atrophy are all potential problems related to periocular injections.

Other immunosuppressive agents

Cytotoxic drugs

Alkylating agents

Alkylating agents interfere with DNA synthesis by inducing intrachain and interchain cross-linking of the DNA molecule during transcription and cell replication which leads to the formation of defective DNA molecules and death of affected cells. They are extremely cytotoxic to lymphoid cells of both B and T classes especially during the clonal proliferative phase of the immune response. Only cyclophosphamide and chlorambucil are in regular use in ophthalmic practice.

Cyclophosphamide This drug is particularly effective in patients with uveitis secondary to polyarteritis nodosa, Wegener's granulomatosis, and rheumatoid arthritis. It has also been used in the treatment of other forms of uveitis unresponsive to conventional therapy.

Cyclophosphamide has a serum half-life of 7 h, and this can be prolonged by allopurinol. It is given at 1–2 mg/kg/day orally. If a rapid response is required, intravenous administration is an alternative. Pulsed intravenous therapy every 3 to 4 weeks is useful in patients who develop haemorrhagic cystitis from daily oral therapy.

Bone marrow depression is a major complication of therapy with cyclophosphamide and blood counts should be monitored regularly in patients treated with it. Some patients may develop haemorrhagic cystitis with cyclophosphamide. This is due to the effect on the bladder mucosa of acrolein, a metabolite of the drug. Patients should be encouraged to drink copious amounts of fluids during treatment to minimize the risk of developing this complication. Mesna is a compound that reacts with acrolein to neutralize its toxicity and can be prescribed for patients known to develop haemorrhagic cystitis with cyclophosphamide. Ocular problems associated with cyclophosphamide therapy include dry eyes, transient blurring of vision, and ocular hypertension. The mechanisms for these effects are uncertain. Other complications include gastrointestinal disturbances, sterility, neoplasms, interstitial pulmonary fibrosis, liver damage, and alopecia.

Chlorambucil Chlorambucil has a major role in the management of patients with Behçet's disease. It has also been used with some success in other uveitic entities including sympathetic ophthalmitis and juvenile chronic arthritis.

Chlorambucil is initially given at 2 mg/day, and this dose can be increased gradually if necessary up to 18 mg/day until a beneficial effect is achieved. Above 10 mg/day, however, the risks of adverse effects increase rapidly.

Complications from chlorambucil are similar to that of cyclophosphamide, with bone marrow suppression as the major problem. Gonadal dysfunction can occur as well as secondary malignancies.

Antimetabolites

Antimetabolites are competitive inhibitors of normal metabolites in DNA synthesis. They are toxic to immunocompetent cells through their interference with purine metabolism and suppress the induction phase of the immune response. Examples of antimetabolites used in ocular inflammatory diseases include azathioprine, mercaptopurine (both antipurines), and methotrexate (an antifolate drug).

Methotrexate Methotrexate has been used in pars planitis, sympathetic ophthalmitis, and juvenile chronic arthritis. Its toxicity limits its use, although coadministration of folinic acid reduces potential complications. Side-effects include bone marrow suppression, gastrointestinal bleeding, pneumonitis, hepatotoxicity, and nephrotoxicity. Ocular symptoms of photophobia and epiphora occur in a quarter of treated patients.

Azathioprine Azathioprine is effective in uveitis related to systemic lupus erythematosus, Behçet's disease, Vogt–Koyanagi–Harada syndrome, idiopathic retinal vasculitis, pars planitis, and sarcoidosis. It is particularly useful as a corticosteroid-sparing agent. Azathioprine carries the least risk of complications amongst the cytotoxic immunosuppressives, and is therefore particularly useful in patients requiring long-term therapy. It is given at 1 to 2.5 mg/kg/day, 25 per cent less if given with allopurinol, which decreases its degradation. Bone marrow suppression, alopecia, and gastrointestinal symptoms are potential side-effects.

Cyclosporin

Cyclosporin, a fungal metabolite with powerful immunosuppressive activity, reversibly inhibits the response of T lymphocytes, in particular, T-helper cells, to antigenic stimulation. It has a role in the management of various forms of posterior uveitides, including sympathetic ophthalmitis, Vogt–Koyanagi–Harada syndrome, and Behçet's disease. The inflammatory activity can usually be adequately controlled in patients receiving a dose of 10 mg/kg/day of cyclosporin alone, but there is an unacceptable risk of irreversible renal failure at this dosage. Owing to this nephrotoxicity, cyclosporin is usually given as a corticosteroid-sparing agent, at a dose of 5 to 7 mg/kg/day. The dosage may be further reduced by inhibiting cyclosporin catabolism by adding ketoconazole. When cyclosporin therapy is withdrawn, an increase in the inflammatory activity is often seen, and the corticosteroid dosage may have to be increased in anticipation, or another immunosuppressive may have to be added. Other complications include hypertension, malaise, gum hypertrophy, gastrointestinal symptoms, hirsutism, and hepato-toxicity.

Rapamycin and tacrolimus have similar mechanisms of action to cyclosporin, and their use in uveitis patients is currently being evaluated.

Miscellaneous immunosuppressives

Colchicine
Colchicine disrupts the function of granulocytes and other motile cells by affecting their fibrillar microtubules and inhibits mitosis through its action on mitotic spindles. It is effective in patients with Behçet's disease, on its own and in combination with other immunosuppressants such as azathioprine. The dosage is 0.5 mg, three times a day. This drug may cause gastrointestinal symptoms, rashes, alopecia, and nephrotoxicity. Prolonged usage can lead to peripheral neuritis, bone marrow suppression, sterility, and alopecia.

Bromocriptine
Prolactin is a competitive inhibitor of cyclosporin through its binding on receptors on T lymphocytes. Bromocriptine, a dopamine agonist which inhibits prolactin secretion, is therefore useful as a supplement to cyclosporin therapy and is useful in patients with refractory iridocyclitis and Behçet's disease. It is given at a dose of 2.5 mg, three to four times a day. Side-effects include gastrointestinal disturbances, headache, confusion, retroperitoneal fibrosis, and dry eyes. Hypotensive reactions may occur during the first few days of therapy.

Miscellaneous therapeutic options

Non-steroidal anti-inflammatory agents
Non-steroidal anti-inflammatory agents act by inhibiting prostaglandin production through the suppression of the cyclo-oxygenase pathway. Their anti-inflammatory effects are not as potent as those of corticosteroids, but they have fewer and less severe side-effects and are sometimes useful as a supplement to corticosteroid therapy. They are effective against episcleritis and scleritis. The use of topical non-steroidal anti-inflammatory agents such as diclofenac in the management of uveitis is still being evaluated.

Interferon
This has been used in the management of severe Behçet's disease. Side-effects includes malaise, myelosuppression, and hepatotoxicity. Cardiovascular disturbances like hypertension, hypotension, and arrythmias have been noted in some patients. In addition, discontinuation of therapy may provoke a relapse of the inflammation. The efficacy of interferon therapy in uveitis remains unproven.

Table 2 Topical mydriatics used in uveitis and their durations of action

Drug	Maximal mydriatic effect (min)	Recovery
Phenylephrine	20	6 h
Tropicamide	40	6 h
Cyclopentolate	60	1 day
Homatropine	60	3 days
Hyoscine	30	7 days
Atropine	40	14 days

Plasmapheresis
The removal of circulating antibodies has been used in the management of patients with collagen vascular diseases but levels of autoantibodies often return rapidly to pretreatment titres. It may, however, be useful if combined with other immunosuppressive therapy. In ophthalmology, patients with Behçet's disease and sympathetic ophthalmitis have been successfully treated with this form of therapy.

Cycloplegics
Cycloplegics prevent the development of posterior synechiae, and if used early in the course of the episode, can break these adhesions. They also relieve the discomfort caused by iris and ciliary body spasms in uveitic patients. Antimuscarinic drugs, for example atropine, homatropine, and cyclopentolate, as well as sympathomimetics such as phenylephrine, are used for this purpose. The duration of action and potency of individual mydriatics vary. Table 2 lists the commonly used mydriatics and their duration of action. Local allergic responses are not uncommon with these preparations and psychotropic effects may occur especially in young children, particularly with atropine and cyclopentolate. Cholinergic effects like dry mouth, flushing, cardiac arrythmias, constipation, and difficulty with micturition may also occur. Adverse effects of phenylephrine include cardiac arrythmias and hypertension.

Treatment of anterior uveitis
Anterior uveitis is usually treated with topical corticosteroids. The severity of the inflammation influences the choice of corticosteroid preparation prescribed and the frequency of instillation. The latter can range from a drop every 30 min in very severe anterior uveitis to 1 drop a week to prevent flare-ups in stable chronic conditions. In general, however, it is important to control and eliminate the inflammation as soon as possible in the initial stages of acute iridocyclitis with a potent corticosteroid, like prednisolone acetate 1 per cent, instilled frequently, for example 1 or 2 hourly, rather than to commence therapy with a weak corticosteroid preparation instilled less often, and subsequently to increase the dosage if the inflammation remains uncontrolled. In very severe disease, subconjunctival injection of short-acting corticosteroids, such as 2 mg of

betamethasone, can be effective in controlling the anterior chamber inflammatory activity. Systemic corticosteroids are rarely needed in the management of uncomplicated anterior uveitis, but may be required in intractable bouts of human leucocyte antigen (HLA) 27 related acute anterior uveitis.

As the uveitis settles, the frequency of instillation can be tapered off, usually over the course of a few weeks. Patients with chronic anterior uveitis who are prone to recrudescence following repeated attempts at cessation of therapy need to be maintained on topical corticosteroids indefinitely.

A topical mydriatic drug, preferably 1 per cent atropine is also prescribed in the active phase of the disease in order to prevent posterior synechia formation and for symptomatic relief. Mydriatics can be withdrawn as the inflammation subsides. Where posterior synechiae have formed, it may be possible to induce their lysis in the acute phase by the intensive use of topical mydriatics, for example atropine, phenylephrine, and tropicamide eye-drops every 10 min for an hour. For refractory cases, a subconjunctival injection of 0.5 ml of Mydriacaine (a mixture of adrenaline, procaine, and atropine) can be effective. In established posterior synechiae with fibrosis, it may not be possible, even with these measures, to break the adhesions.

Treatment of posterior uveitis

Active treatment in patients with posterior uveitis should only be prescribed in cases where clear indications are present. Important factors which must be taken into account in decisions regarding systemic therapy for posterior uveitis include the natural history of the condition being treated, the presence of sight-threatening complications, as well as the severity and the laterality of the inflammation. For example, patients with mild vitritis in intermediate uveitis, do not need treatment as the condition carries a good visual prognosis. Conversely, patients with Behçet's disease often have a poor visual outcome and require a more aggressive approach, with the initiation of systemic immunosuppressive therapy early in the course of the disease. If the patient's vision is significantly affected by complications of inflammation, such as cystoid macular oedema, treatment may have to be initiated. The threshold for commencing therapy is likewise lower when uveitis occurs in the fellow eye of an irreversibly damaged eye, or if there is bilateral disease.

Periocular corticosteroids, for example an orbital floor injection of methylprednisolone, are useful in the management of unilateral disease and avoid the systemic side-effects of oral steroid therapy. Patients who fail to respond after a reasonable period of time after periocular corticosteroids (4–6 weeks) require systemic corticosteroids. The initial course should be of a dose sufficient to suppress the inflammatory process (for example prednisolone 60 mg for a week, then 40 mg for 3–4 weeks); maintenance treatment is then tailored in accordance with the response of the disease and continued until the pathological process resolves. Therapy can be discontinued directly if treatment is given for less than 2 weeks, but needs to be tapered gradually in cases where the treatment programme is

longer. Although most patients can be weaned off corticosteroids, some patients may require a small maintenance dose indefinitely if cessation of treatment leads to a rapid recurrence of the inflammation. Pulsed intravenous methylprednisolone therapy (for example 1 g given over an hour three times a week in the first week, then 500 mg pulses per week for 3 weeks, 250 mg pulses for 2 weeks, then a maintenence of 125 mg pulses weekly) can be used as an alternative to steroid tablets, with less long-term side-effects, but may carry life-threatening complications.

In patients with sight-threatening reversible uveitis that is inadequately controlled with an acceptable dosage of corticosteroids, other immunosuppressive drugs such as cytotoxic agents and cyclosporin may have to be employed. Patients with Behçet's disease, idiopathic retinal vasculitis, and sympathetic ophthalmitis often fall into this category. These drugs are contraindicated for uveitides of infectious origin. Table 3 summarizes the classification, dosage, major indications, and side-effects of non-steroidal immunosuppressive drugs in use in uveitis treatment. If tolerated, a high dose of systemic corticosteroids should also be given together with an immunosuppressive agent for the initial 4 to 6 weeks while awaiting the effects of these drugs to be established. Once the inflammation is controlled, it may be possible to decrease the dosage gradually, and maintain the patient on a minimal amount of drugs necessary to keep the inflammation at bay. Treatment with a particular drug is discontinued if there is no discernible improvement in the condition or when unacceptable side-effects occur.

Before initiating systemic therapy for uveitis, patients should be made aware of the potential side-effects of the treatment (including that of systemic corticosteroids) as well as the likely outcome of therapy, and should be actively involved in the decision over whether or not treatment should be initiated. Patients on systemic immunosuppresive agents should be managed in collaboration with a doctor who is familiar with their use throughout the course of the therapy.

Significant associated anterior uveitis may need treatment with topical corticosteroids and mydriatics. Retinal neovascularization secondary to retinal ischaemia in some forms of uveitides often resolves following adequate control of the inflammatory process, but if not, retinal photocoagulation may be necessary.

Cataract surgery in uveitis patients

Cataracts can develop as a complication of chronic glaucoma or secondary to corticosteroid therapy (especially with systemic rather than topical therapy, prolonged usage, as well as higher dosage). Surgery for cataracts can be performed if necessary when the uveitis is well controlled. The risks of complications following cataract surgery depends upon the type and severity of the attendant uveitis. These risks as well as the presence of pre-existing complications of uveitis such as chronic cystoid macular oedema should be taken into consideration before undertaking cataract surgery. Intensive perioperative corticosteroid therapy starting 24 to 48 h prior to surgery is prescribed to minimize the risks of severe flare-ups and cystoid macular

Table 3 Summary of major non-steroidal immunosuppressive drugs used in uveitis treatment

Class	Drug	Route and dosage	Major indications	Major side-effects
Alkylating agent	Cyclophosphamide	Oral or intravenous; 1–2 mg/kg/day	Polyarteritis nodosa, Wegener's granulomatosis	Bone marrow suppression, haemorrhagic cystitis, secondary neoplasms
Alkylating agent	Chlorambucil	Oral; 2 mg/day	Behçet's disease, systemic lupus erythematosus	Marrow suppression, sterility, secondary neoplasms
Antifolate	Methotrexate	Oral, intravenous, intramuscular; 10–25 mg/m^2 every 1–4 weeks	Sympathetic ophthalmia	Marrow suppression, hepatotoxicity, gastrointestinal bleeding
Antipurine	Azathioprine	Oral; 1–2.5 mg/kg/day	Behçet's disease, sympathetic ophthalmia	Marrow suppression, hepatotoxicity
Antibiotic	Cyclosporin	Oral; 5–7 mg/kg/day	Behçet's disease, sympathetic ophthalmia	Nephrotoxicity, hypertension
—	Colchicine	500 μg three times daily (with azathioprine)	Behçet's disease	Peripheral neuritis, sterility, nephrotoxicity, marrow suppression

oedema. Intraocular lens insertion, especially in-the-bag lens implantation following capsulorhexis (avoiding ciliary body irritation), is well tolerated in patients with Fuchs' heterochromic iridocyclitis and inactive non-granulomatous uveitis. Encouraging results have also been reported following cataract surgery with intraocular lens implantation in patients with inactive intermediate uveitis, chronic iridocyclitis, and sarcoidosis-related uveitis. A surface-modified (heparin-coated) lens engenders a less intense inflammatory response and is a safer alternative in uveitis patients. Lens implants are poorly tolerated and should be avoided in patients with uveitis associated with juvenile chronic arthritis and chronic iridocyclitis in which scarring is a significant feature. Phakoemulsification induces less surgical trauma when compared with manual cataract expression and may be the preferred technique for cataract surgery in uveitis patients. The role of vitrectomy in combination with cataract surgery is controversial, but may have a place in patients with significant chronic vitritis or chronic macular oedema.

Glaucoma in uveitis patients

Intraocular pressure should be monitored regularly during the course of the disease and treatment. Although the intraocular pressure may be low during the earlier stages of uveitis due to the associated ciliary body dysfunction, there may be a rebound elevation of the pressure due to aqueous hypersecretion as the ciliary body recovers. The intraocular pressure may also be elevated secondary to anterior or posterior synechiae, blockage of the trabecular meshwork with cellular or fibrinous debris, trabeculitis, rubeosis iridis, or corticosteroid therapy in susceptible individuals.

Corticosteroid-induced glaucoma is an open angle type glaucoma, occurring more commonly with topical and periocular than with systemic administration of corticosteroids. Three different levels of responses of intraocular pressure to topical corticosteroids are noted in the general population: after 6

weeks of topical corticosteroid treatment, a marked rise in intraocular pressure (over 31 mmHg) occurred in about 5 per cent of subjects, 35 per cent experienced a rise to between 22 and 31 mmHg, while the remainder did not exhibit any rise in their intraocular pressure. Withdrawal of corticosteroids is followed in most cases by a reduction of intraocular pressure to a normal level, although rarely the high pressure may persist due to damage to the trabecular meshwork. In a clinical setting, a rise in intraocular pressure in steroid-responsive patients, which can be abrupt and severe (especially in patients who have had periocular corticosteroid injection, and in particular with long-acting preparations), typically occurs after 4 to 6 weeks of topical therapy and is often associated with a marked reduction of anterior chamber inflammatory activity. Reducing the amount of corticosteroids instilled or switching to preparations like fluorometholone and clobetasone, which have less potential to induce glaucoma, can lead to a lowering of the intraocular pressure for patients with mild uveitis. A distinction needs to be made between corticosteroid-induced glaucoma and the other forms of uveitis-related glaucomas, many of which, by contrast, are accompanied by increased inflammatory activity and an intensive course of topical steroids is often effective in lowering the pressure. A balance needs to be struck between the benefits of corticosteroid therapy and the ability of the treated eye to tolerate the increased pressure.

Topical or systemic ocular antihypertensives (except pilocarpine, which can compromise the blood–eye barrier, promoting further inflammation) are often effective in controlling the intraocular pressure in patients with active uveitis who fail to respond to corticosteroid therapy alone. The role of prostaglandin analogues in uveitic glaucoma is as yet uncertain. Argon laser trabeculoplasty, however, may induce further intraocular inflammation and should therefore be avoided. In refractory cases, trabeculectomy, with or without antimetabolites, may be necessary in cases where the optic nerve head is damaged from the elevated intraocular pressure. Seton surgery can be considered for patients where previous glaucoma surgery has failed. A course of systemic corticosteroids starting 24 to 48 h prior to surgery should be given together with intensive topical corticosteroid therapy and atropine for maximal control of the anticipated inflammation following surgical intervention. In patients with end-stage disease, cyclodestructive procedures can be employed to control the intraocular pressure.

Conclusion

The management of uveitis relies on the suppression of the inflammatory and immune responses and the treatment of the complications arising from these responses. Current therapeutic options have led to significant improvements in the outcome of many conditions that have previously carried devastating visual prognoses. However, these non-specific immunosuppressive agents carry substantial risks to patient health, bearing in mind that most of these patients are otherwise well. Future developments in the field of pharmacology and immunology may yield therapeutic options that are more specific and less harmful than those currently available.

Further reading

Borgioli, M., Coster, D.J., Fan, R.F.T., et al. (1991). Effect of heparin surface modification of polymethylmethacrylate intraocular lenses on signs of postoperative inflammation after extracapsular cataract extraction. Ophthalmology, 99, 1248–55.

Dick, A. (1994). The treatment of chronic uveitic macular oedema: is immunosuppression enough? British Journal of Ophthalmology, 78, 1–2.

Forrester, J.V. (1992). Uveitis. In Recent Advances in Ophthalmology 8, (ed. S.I. Davidson and B. Jay), pp. 107–27. Churchill Livingstone, Edinburgh.

Foster, C.S., Fong, L.P., and Singh, G. (1989). Cataract surgery and intraocular lens implantation in patients with uveitis. Ophthalmology, 96, 281–7.

Hakin, K.N., Pearson, R.V., and Lightman, S.L. (1992). Sympathetic ophthalmia: visual results with modern immunosuppressive therapy. Eye, 6, 453–5.

Helm, C.J. and Holland, G.N. (1995). The effects of posterior subtenon injection of triamcinolone acetonide in patients with intermediate uveitis. American Journal of Ophthalmology, 120, 55–64.

Hemady, R., Tauber, J., and Foster, C.S. (1991). Immunosuppressive drugs in immune and inflammatory ocular disease. Survey of Ophthalmology, 35, 369–85.

Hill, R.A., Nguyen, Q.H., Baerveldt, G., et al. (1993). Trabeculectomy and Molteno implantation for glaucomas associated with uveitis. Ophthalmology, 100, 903–8.

Hooper, P.L., Rao, N.A., and Smith, R.E. (1990). Cataract extraction in uveitis patients. Survey of Ophthalmology, 35, 120–44.

Howe, L.J., Stanford, M.R., Edelsten, C., et al. (1994). The efficacy of systemic corticosteroids in sight-threatening retinal vasculitis. Eye, 8, 443–7.

Ishioka, M., Ohno, S., Nakamura, S., et al. (1994). FK506 treatment of noninfectious uveitis. American Journal of Ophthalmology, 118, 723–9.

Lightman, S. (1991). Use of steroids and immunosuppressive drugs in the management of posterior uveitis. Eye, 5, 294–8.

McGhee, C.N.J. (1992). Pharmacokinetics of ophthalmic corticosteroids. British Journal of Ophthalmology, 76, 681–4.

Martin, D.F., DeBarge, L.R., Nussenblatt, R.B., et al. (1995). Synergistic effect of rapamycin and cyclosporin A in the treatment of experimental autoimmune uveoretinitis. Journal of Immunology, 154, 922–7.

Melmon, K.L., Morrelli, H.F., Hoffman, B.B., et al. (1992). Clinical pharmacology: basic principles in therapeutics, 3rd edn. McGraw-Hill, New York

Moorthy, R.S., Mermoud, A., Baerveldt, G., et al. Glaucoma associated with uveitis. Survey of Ophthalmology, 41, 361–94.

Nussenblatt, R.B. and Palestine, A.G. (1986). Cyclosporine: immunology, pharmacology and therapeutic uses. Survey of Ophthalmology, 31, 159–69.

Shah, S.S., Lowder C.Y., Schmitt M.A., et al. (1992). Low-dose methotrexate therapy for ocular inflammatory disease. Ophthalmology, 99, 1419–23.

Sherwood, R.D. and Rosenthal, A.R. (1991). Cataract surgery in Fuchs' heterochromic iridocyclitis. British Journal of Ophthalmology, 76, 238–40.

Smith, R.E., and Nozik, R.A. (1989). Uveitis: a clinical approach to diagnosis and management, 2nd edn. Williams & Wilkins, Baltimore.

Wakefield, D., McCluskey, P., and Penny, R. (1986). Intravenous pulse methylprednisolone therapy in severe inflammatory eye disease. Archives of Ophthalmology, 104, 847–51.

2.9 Medical retina

2.9.1 Applied anatomy and physiology of the retina

P. Jefferies

Embryology

The eye originates as an outpouching of the prosencephalon at 3 weeks gestation. A double-walled optic cup forms during the fourth week of gestation, the outer wall is the precursor of the retinal pigment epithelium and the inner wall is the precursor of the neural retina. The space between the two walls is the plane of separation in a retinal detachment, and is clinically referred to as the subretinal space.

Retinal pigment epithelium and Bruch's membrane

Retinal pigment epithelium

The retinal pigment epithelium is a monolayer of cells extending from the optic disc to the ora serrata. It lies between the photoreceptor outer segments and Bruch's membrane (Fig. 1).

The basal layer of the retinal pigment epithelium cell membrane, which is infolded to increase its surface area, sits on the cell basement membrane next to Bruch's membrane. The many mitochondria near the base of the retinal pigment epithelium cell reflect the high metabolic activity associated with metabolic transport across the basal membrane. All the nutrients for the highly metabolic photoreceptor outer segments must be transported across the pigment epithelial cell. Adjacent retinal pigment epithelium cells are joined near their apices by tight junctions (zonula occludens and zonula adherens) and form the blood–retinal barrier of the pigment epithelium (see below). There is a constant water flow from the vitreous to the choroid mediated by 'pump' mechanisms, such as the bicarbonate pump, on the cell membrane of the retinal pigment epithelium. Clinically, a focal breakdown in the 'pump' is thought to occur in central serous retinopathy. The 'pump' mechanisms also help to keep the retina flat against the pigment epithelium and remove subretinal fluid following closure of a retinal break in

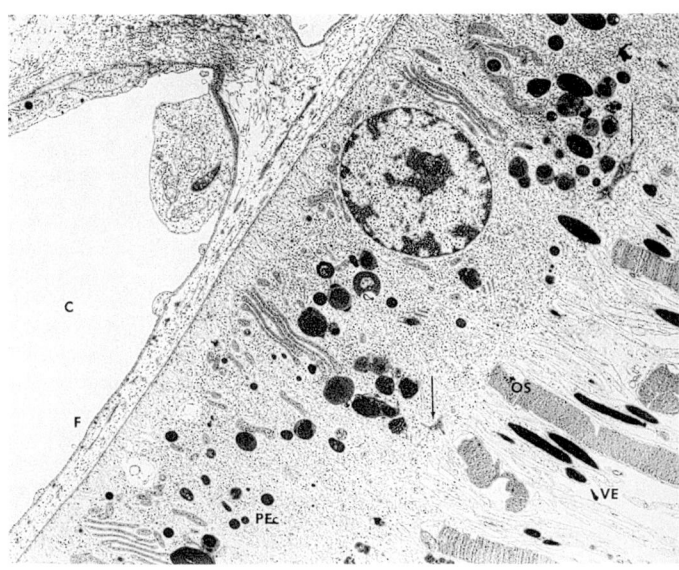

Fig. 1 Pigment epithelium (PE) of rhesus monkey. Outer segment (OS) choroidal capillary (C) with fenestrated wall (F). Arrows indicate tight junctions/terminal bars. 4250× magnification. (Reprinted with permission from Hart 1992.)

retinal detachment surgery. The apices of the retinal pigment epithelium have villi that project up and around the tips of the outer segments but no firm adhesion is formed. The apical region of the cell contains melanosomes (melanin-containing organelles) which absorb scattered light and argon laser light in a photothermal reaction.

The retinal pigment epithelium cell is phagocytic, ingesting fragments of photoreceptor outer segments (Fig. 2). The photoreceptors constantly make new discs and shed fragments of outer segment containing old discs. This shedding of outer segments follows a diurnal pattern, occurring at dawn in rods and at dusk in cones. The fragments phagocytosed by the retinal pigment epithelium cell are digested by lysosomes and the digested material is partially recycled. The residual material accumulates in the retinal pigment epithelium cell as lipofuscin granules, or is deposited in Bruch's membrane as drusen.

The retinal pigment epithelium also plays a key role in the recycling of the vitamin A chromophores of the visual pigments. The four visual pigments are the vitamin A chromophore associated with four different proteins. Electromagnetic radiation in the visible range interacts with visual pigment in the outer segment of the photoreceptor, converting the 11-*cis*-retinaldehyde to all-*trans*-retinaldehyde which is then released

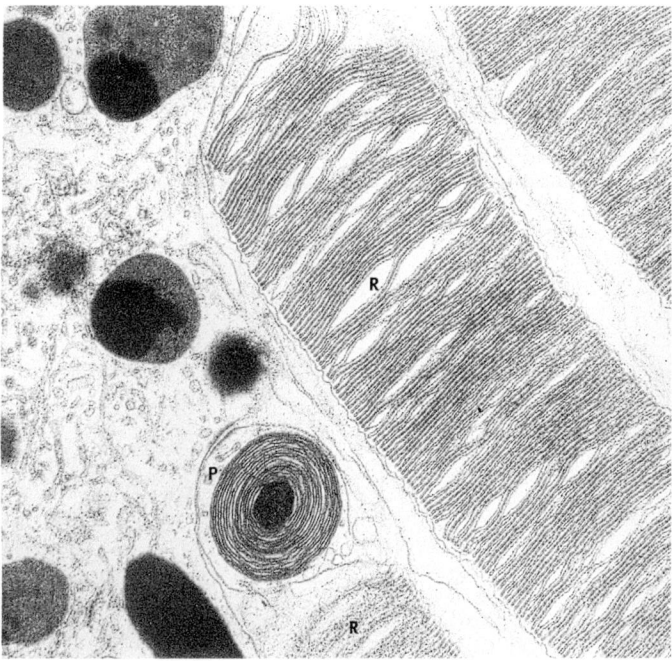

Fig. 2 Rod outer segments (R) abutting on to pigment epithelium of rhesus monkey. Note phagosome (P) forming at rod tip. 29 000× magnification. (Reprinted with permission from Hart 1992.)

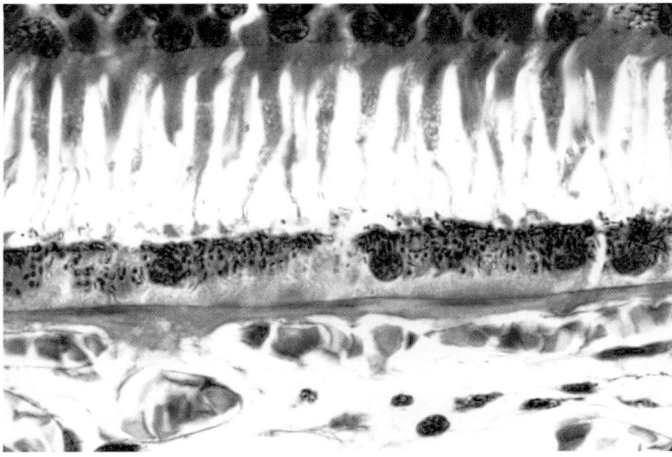

Fig. 3 Clinically normal, 72-year-old male. Early basal laminar deposit (stains blue) developing over a thickened Bruch's membrane. Picro-Mallory stain. 1000× magnification. (Courtesy of Dr John Sarks.)

from the protein component of the visual pigment. The all-*trans*-retinaldehyde is converted to all-*trans*-retinol which is transported to the retinal pigment epithelium by a carrier protein. Reisomerization occurs in the retinal pigment epithelium and 11-*cis*-retinaldehyde is transported back to the photoreceptor.

Bruch's membrane

Bruch's membrane is a condensation of choroidal connective tissue between the choriocapillaris and the pigment epithelium. This connective tissue is a sandwich of three layers: two layers of collagen with a central elastic layer. Bruch's membrane is continuous with the rest of the choroidal connective tissue via tissue pegs between the capillary cells in the lace-like choriocapillaris network. The elasticity of the membrane can be seen clinically following a tear in the retinal pigment epithelium, where the torn edges retract and curl up.

Ageing changes

With increasing age, the retinal pigment epithelium accumulates intracellular residual bodies or lipofuscin granules. The pigment epithelial cells overlying drusen become thinner and depigmented, while cells between drusen become thicker and hyperplastic. Pigment change seen clinically is histologically due to pigment migration into the neural retina and into the subretinal space.

Bruch's membrane becomes thickened and fragmented in an irregular fashion with degeneration of the collagen and elastic tissue. Basal laminar deposit, abnormal collagen material accumulating between the pigment epithelial cell and its basement

membrane, may be a histological marker for the transition from ageing changes to macular degeneration (Fig. 3).

Drusen are commonly seen clinically in the elderly population. Histologically, they consist of deposits of extracellular material that accumulate under the basement membrane of the retinal pigment epithelium, in the inner collagenous layer of Bruch's membrane. Clinically, there are three main types of drusen:

1. Hard drusen are discrete lesions, usually less than 64 μm. Histologically, they are deposits of granular material, including abnormal collagen in discrete nodules.

2. Soft drusen have poorly defined edges and are mostly larger than 64 μm. Histologically, they are like small serous detachments of the pigment epithelial cell and its basement membrane from an abnormal Bruch's membrane.

3. Cuticular drusen are not easily seen biomicroscopically but are clearly seen on fluorescein angiography as a 'starry sky' fluorescent picture. Histologically, they are nodular thickenings of the basement membrane of the pigment epithelium and a diffuse thickening of the inner layers of Bruch's membrane.

Neural retina

There are four types of neural cell in the neural retina: the photoreceptors that detect light, the interconnecting cells that process and relay the information to the ganglion cells, whose axons exit the eye at the optic nerve, and, finally, the retinal glial cells which are mainly Müller cells.

The neural retina is a transparent, 0.4-mm thick sheet of tissue adjacent to the retinal pigment epithelium, and organized into distinct layers on cross-sectional light microscopy (Fig. 4).

1. The outer segments of the photoreceptor cell form the first layer adjacent to the retinal pigment epithe-

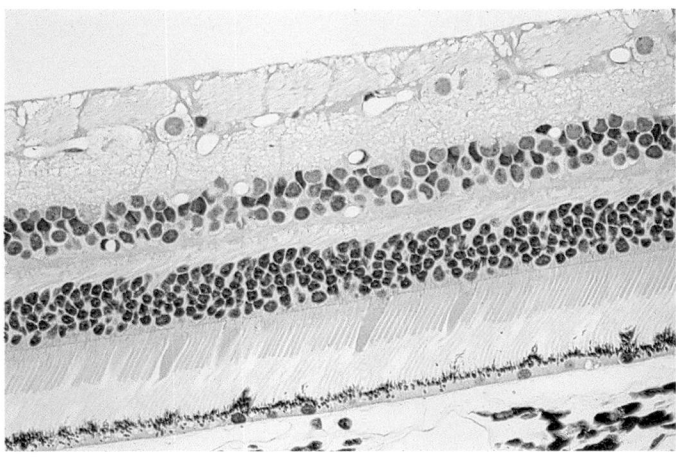

Fig. 4 Rhesus monkey retina. The retinal layers are clearly seen. Haematoxylin and eosin, 400× magnification.

lium. They are embedded in an interphotoreceptor gel of acid mucopolysaccharides and their apices are intimately surrounded by processes of the retinal pigment epithelium. The outer segments of both types of photoreceptor (cones and rods) contain many discs which have the visual pigments within the disc membranes. The discs are arranged in stacks and most are not connected to the cell membrane (see Fig. 2).

2. The inner segments of the photoreceptor cell are connected to the outer segments by a small ciliary stalk. There are two distinct types of inner segment, the larger and the smaller inner segments of the cones and rods, respectively. The apex of the inner segment nearest the outer segment is packed with mitochondria in an area known as the ellipsoid.

3. The outer nuclear layer is comprised of the cell nuclei of the photoreceptors.

4. The outer plexiform layer is mainly comprised of the axons of the photoreceptors. This layer is greatly thickened in the macular area where it is termed Henle's fibre layer.

5. The next nuclear layer, the inner nuclear layer, contains the cell bodies of the bipolar, horizontal, and amacrine cells (interconnecting cells) and of the Mueller cells.

6. The inner plexiform layer is then seen with axons of the interconnecting cells connecting to each other and to the ganglion cells.

7. The nuclei of the ganglion cells form the third nuclear layer and are in a single layer except for the macular region.

8. Finally, the axons of the ganglion cells form the nerve fibre layer as they travel to the optic nerve to exit the eye. Between the nerve fibre layer and the vitreous is a basement membrane of the Müller cells called the internal limiting membrane.

Phototransduction

Photoreceptors are able to detect visible light and to respond with a change in the electrical potential of the cell by a process called phototransduction. In the dark, the photoreceptor cell has sodium entering the outer segment via cyclic guanosine monophosphate dependent sodium channels. The sodium passes to the inner segment via the ciliary stalk where it is actively removed, the cell expending large amounts of energy to pump sodium out of the inner segment. This demanding process accounts for the accumulation of mitochondria in the ellipsoid and about 50 per cent of the oxygen requirement of the retina in the dark.

Visible light activates the visual pigments (see above) that lie in the membrane of the discs in the outer segment. The activated visual pigment activates transducin, another disc membrane protein, which in turn activates phosphodiesterase. The activated phosphodiesterase reduces the levels of cellular cyclic guanosine monophosphate and this causes the sodium channels in the outer segment to close, preventing sodium from entering the cell. This in turn causes the transmembrane cell potential difference to change transiently and the cell to hyperpolarize.

Macula

The retina has a specialized cone-rich area temporal to the optic disc called the macula. This circular area is about 5.5 mm in diameter, with a central depression called the fovea 1.5 mm diameter. The very centre of the fovea is called the foveola (0.35 mm diameter). The foveola is within a 0.5 mm diameter foveal avascular zone. The macula is also referred to as the macula lutea (yellow spot) because of the xanthophyll pigment found here which makes the area look yellow on anatomical gross inspection.

Histologically, the macula is thickened in the perifoveal areas and is at its thinnest at the fovea (Fig. 5). It is densely packed

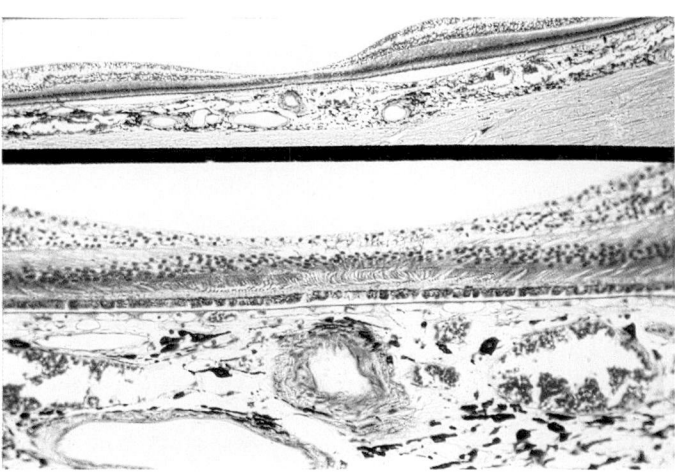

Fig. 5 Normal human macula of 42-year-old male. Picro-Mallory stain, top 45×, bottom 150× magnification. (Reprinted from Sarks 1976, with permission.)

with photoreceptors which are mainly cones, the foveola consisting exclusively of cones. The outer plexiform layer is thickened, with radially running axons, called Henle fibres, from the densely packed photoreceptors at the fovea to their radially displaced interconnecting cells. This is an area of loose tissue that can allow accumulation of fluid and exudates in a radial pattern along the fibres, clinically seen as a macular star. The ganglion cell layer is more than one cell body thick, but ganglion cells are absent from the foveola, which consists solely of photoreceptors.

Physiologically, the macula is a specialized area of maximal spatial, temporal, and colour discrimination at photopic light levels, due to its high concentration of cone photoreceptors.

Visual acuity

Visual acuity is a subjective threshold of the spatial resolving power of the visual system. This is the commonest test of visual function used in ophthalmic practice, usually tested as a Snellen acuity. Images of objects in the environment are formed on the retina. If the images are sharply focused on the retina, the resolving power is limited by the size and spacing of the photoreceptors. These are anatomically spaced at two per minute of arc at the fovea; that is, the anatomical limit of resolving power is half a minute of arc. This corresponds to a 6/3 Snellen acuity.

Optimal visual acuity depends on several factors:

- fully corrected refractive errors
- foveal fixation
- photopic light levels (rod-mediated scotopic acuity is only about 8 minutes of arc)
- high contrast
- no opacities in the media (i.e. cataract).

The 6/6 letters (such as the letter E) on the Snellen chart have the individual limbs and spaces 1 minute of arc in size, and the letters are 5 minutes of arc in total size. To identify the 6/6 letters at 6 m, the minimum angle of resolution of the eye needs to be 1 minute of arc. The minimum angle of resolution difference between two lines of Snellen acuity is not always linear.

Colour vision

The perception of colour is a complex subjective visual experience that is possible because there are three different cone types. This is the anatomical basis of the trichromatic theory of colour vision, where any colour can be matched by a mixture of three primary colours. The three cone types have overlapping spectral sensitivities, but each has a different peak sensitivity: 420 nm blue cones, 530 nm green cones, and 560 nm red cones. The different cone peak spectral sensitivities are possible because a different protein component combines with the vitamin A chromophore for the three cone visual pigment types.

The genes for the visual pigments are on three different chromosomes: rhodopsin (rods) on chromosome 3, blue cones on chromosome 7, and red and green cones on the X chromosome.

In Caucasians, 8 per cent of males and 0.5 per cent of females have an inherited bilateral red/green colour vision defect, with confusion of colours from red to green. A lack of red cone or lack of green cone function is due to a deletion of a gene or a hybrid gene formation for the visual pigments on the X chromosome. Screening and detection of inherited red/green defects can be easily done with colour plates such as the Ishihara pseudoisochromatic plates.

Acquired colour vision defects are usually blue/yellow defects, with confusion of colours from blue to yellow, that tend to involve only one eye or involve the two eyes asymmetrically. The blue/yellow defects are not detected with the Ishihara plates. The Farnsworth panel D15 test is not as sensitive as the Ishihara at detecting the red/green defects, but is a good screening test to detect blue/yellow defects. It is an easier test to use than the more complex Farnsworth–Munsell 100-hue test.

Blood supply

Inner retinal circulation

The ophthalmic artery branches to form the central retinal artery which enters the eye at the optic disc. The inner retina is supplied by end arteries. The central retinal artery divides into upper and lower branches which supply the upper and lower halves of the retina. In about 20 per cent of eyes, part of the macular area is supplied by a cilioretinal artery which is a direct branch of the ciliary arteries. Retinal veins drain into a central retinal vein at the optic disc.

The retinal arteries and veins travel in the nerve fibre layer and frequently cross each other at arteriovenous crossings. There are two types of arteriovenous crossing: (a) artery over vein, with the vein passing under the artery, which accounts for 67 per cent of crossings; and (b) vein over artery, with the vein passing on top of the artery. Anatomically, the two crossings are different. At artery over vein crossings, the vein abruptly deviates to pass under the artery, and a focal compression of the vein cross-sectional area may occur (Fig. 6). Vein deviation and focal narrowing are not seen at vein over artery crossings (Fig. 7). These anatomical differences may explain why virtually all branch retinal vein occlusions occur at artery over vein crossings.

Capillaries in the retinal circulation are in two layers in the outer retina but may be in up to four layers in the macular area. There is a capillary-free zone of 0.5 mm diameter at the fovea (Fig. 8). The capillaries are about 5 μm in diameter and consist of a single endothelial cell lining joined together with tight junctions and surrounded by a basement membrane and a pericyte cell. The function of the pericyte cell is unknown but they are lost in diabetic eye disease.

Outer retinal circulation

Three posterior ciliary arteries, also branches of the ophthalmic artery, divide into up to 20 short posterior ciliary arteries and

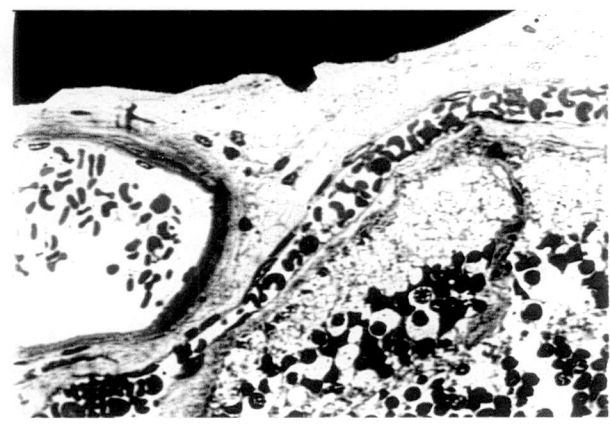

Fig. 6 Human arteriovenous crossing, artery over vein type. The vein abruptly changes direction as it passes beneath the artery. Toluidine blue, 400× magnification. (Reprinted with permission from Jefferies 1993.)

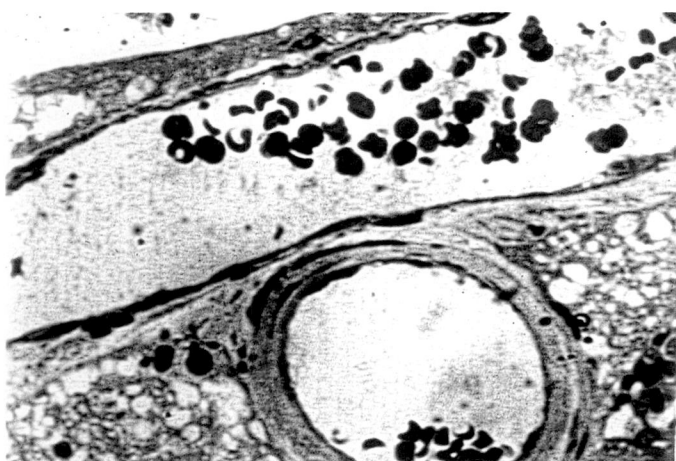

Fig. 7 Human arteriovenous crossing. Longitucinal section of the vein in a vein over artery crossing with no deviation of the ve n as it passes over the artery. Toluidine blue, 400× magnification. (Reprinted with permission from Jefferies 1993.)

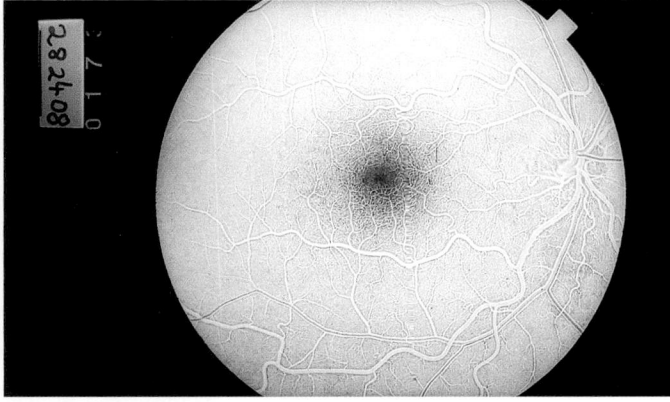

Fig. 8 Right eye fluorescein angiogram of the macula showing the retinal circulation and the well-defined retinal capillaries and foveal avascular zone.

pierce the sclera to form the choroidal arteries. Arterial anastomoses between choroidal vessels enable a good collateral blood supply, and clinically, outer retinal ischaemia from an occluded choroidal artery is rare. The choroiocapillaris is a lace-like sheet of interconnecting capillaries that are supplied in a lobular pattern by the choroidal arterioles. These capillaries are larger than retinal capillaries, and have thin walls which have fenestrations with only a thin membrane between the lumen and the extravascular space. The outer retina is avascular. Oxygen and other metabolic requirements from the choriocapillaris have to travel across Bruch's membrane and the pigment epithelium to reach the photoreceptor outer segments (see Fig. 1).

Ocular blood flow

The ocular blood flow is defined as the perfusion pressure divided by the vascular resistance. The perfusion pressure in the eye is the arterial pressure minus the intraocular pressure. The venous pressure of the central retinal vein is the same as the intraocular pressure. A spontaneous venous pulsation at the disc is seen when the intraocular pressure increases transiently with each arterial pulse, causing the central retinal vein to collapse at the optic nerve head.

The blood flow in the choroid is very high (about 2000 ml/min per 100 g) and acts as a heat sink to protect the eye against thermal damage. This high flow maintains a high oxygen tension and aids diffusion of oxygen to the photoreceptor outer segments. Approximately 65 per cent of the total oxygen demand of the retina is supplied by the choroid to the highly metabolically active retinal pigment epithelium and the outersegments of the photoreceptors. Despite the high oxygen consumption the choroidal arteriovenous oxygen difference is only about 5 per cent.

In contrast, the retinal circulation has a small flow rate (less than 10 per cent of the choroid), and the oxygen extraction is high, with a retinal arteriovenous oxygen difference of about 40 per cent.

Autoregulation of blood flow

Autoregulation of blood flow is a process whereby the blood flow is maintained despite changes in perfusion pressure by altering the vascular resistance. The retinal blood flow is autoregulated and flow rates are maintained over large variations in blood pressure or intraocular pressure. In contrast, there is no autoregulation in the choroid, and the blood flow is reduced with increasing intraocular pressure. The normally very low extraction of oxygen from the choroid can be increased without compromising the supply of oxygen and nutrients, despite significant reductions in choroidal blood flow.

Blood–retinal barrier

The retina has a dual blood supply, both needing a blood barrier to control the permeability of proteins and water-soluble substances to prevent retinal oedema and interference with neurotransmission. A breakdown in the barrier function is clinically seen in diabetic maculopathy or retinal venous occlusive disease. The permeability is controlled in the retinal circulation by the capillary endothelium and the tight junctions (zonula occludens) between these cells, as with the cerebral capillaries in the blood–brain barrier. The choriocapillaris has very permeable capillaries and the barrier to permeability is at the retinal pigment epithelium and the tight junctions between these cells.

The barriers are freely permeable to oxygen and carbon dioxide, but prevent movement of all proteins, glucose, and amino acids. The movement of these substances requires specific carrier-mediated transport systems on the cell membrane of the retinal endothelial and retinal pigment epithelial cells.

Further reading

Anderson, R.E. (1983). *Biochemistry of the eye*, pp. 164–264. American Academy of Ophthalmology, San Francisco.

Fine, B.S. and Yanoff, M. (1972). *Ocular histology: a text and atlas*, Chapter 6. Harper & Row, New York.

Hart, W.M. (1992). *Adler's physiology of the eye*, 9th edn. Mosby Year Book, St Louis.

Jefferies, (1993). An anatomical study of retinal arteriovenous crossings and their role in the pathogenesis of branch retinal vein occlusions. *Australia and New Zealand Journal of Ophthalmology*, 21, 213–17.

Sarks, S.H. (1976). Ageing and degeneration in the macular region: a clinico-pathological study. *British Journal of Ophthalmology*, 60, 324–41.

2.9.2 Diabetic retinopathy

George Turner

The threat of visual disability associated with diabetes mellitus contributes significantly to the burden endured by patients with this common metabolic disorder. Between 1 and 2 per cent of the population of the United Kingdom are diabetic and many develop sight-threatening complications. As young diabetics move into adulthood, many develop diabetic retinopathy, the complications of which are the most prevalent risk factor for visual morbidity in the working population. Older diabetics are also commonly affected by visual problems, often after shorter duration of known diabetes. Although much has been achieved in the detection and management of these complications, and improved metabolic control is of proven efficacy in preventing the evolution of diabetic retinopathy, the extent of visual loss in this population continues to be higher than is acceptable to patients and their carers.

I am grateful to Professor M. Boulton, Department of Cellular Biology, University of Manchester for assistance with the manuscript, Steven Aldington, Department of Diabetic Retinopathy, Royal Postgraduate Medical School for assistance with the illustrations, and Professor David McLeod, Department of Clinical Ophthalmology, University of Manchester for encouragement.

Even in the most advanced health-care systems in the world, diabetic retinopathy regularly leads to blindness, much of which could be ameliorated and a proportion of which is preventable. That it is within the power of national governments and health departments to create conditions to reduce the level of diabetic morbidity was officially recognized in October 1989 in the St Vincent's declaration by the World Health Organization and the International Diabetes Association. Among a number of recommendations made was a commitment to reduce new blindness due to diabetes by a third within 5 years.

As serious sight-threatening complications can for a time be present before any reduction in vision or other visual symptoms occur, comprehensive screening programmes for sight-threatening diabetic eye disease should exist, filtering patients towards eye departments which provide timely access to skilled care.

Epidemiology

Blindness is at least 20 times more common in diabetics than in non-diabetics, with diabetic retinopathy being the commonest cause of blind registration in the working population. The duration of diabetes is the most strongly correlated risk factor to the development of diabetic retinopathy though incidence and prevalence vary with age at diagnosis. Prevalence data from a population-based study conducted by Klein and colleagues in southern Wisconsin demonstrates that where diabetes is diagnosed at less than 30 years, the prevalence of any diabetic retinopathy is very low but increases to greater than 95 per cent after 15 years duration of the disease. Visual impairment is also strongly associated with duration of disease with up to 20 per cent experiencing visual loss after 30 years of metabolic disease, of whom at least 10 per cent are legally blind. In contrast, if the onset of diabetes is after 30 years of age the prevalence of any retinopathy approaches 20 per cent at the outset but rises more slowly to 60 per cent at 15 years duration. The overall rate of sight-threatening retinopathy is lower in the older group, but the prevalence of visual disability is greater due to their overall greater number. These differences may be explained, in part, by the predominance of insulin-dependent diabetes in the younger age group whose disease is metabolically more labile and difficult to control. Diabetes may remain undiagnosed for a significant period in the older non-insulin-dependent diabetic who is thus more likely to have retinopathy at the outset. The prevalence of blindness due to diabetic retinopathy is estimated to be approximately 5 per cent, with an annual incidence of new cases of sight-threatening retinopathy in the region of 1.2 per cent in the United Kingdom. The relationship between poor metabolic control of the diabetes and the development and severity of retinopathy has proved elusive until recently. There is now conclusive evidence that the development and progression of all long-term complications of insulin-dependent diabetes can be reduced by as tight control of the metabolic disorder as can be achieved, without unacceptable episodes of hypoglycaemia. Improved control in non-insulin-dependent diabetes may also have similar benefits.

Pathogenesis

Abnormalities in the retinal capillary bed are the earliest lesions in the development of diabetic retinopathy and current perceptions of the pathogenesis emphasize the role of local microvascular disease, in particular through glucose toxicity to the capillary endothelial cell. Initially the capillary basement membrane thickens, associated with loss of mural pericytes, followed by capillary dilatation, capillary closure, and the formation of microaneurysms. The pathogenesis of microangiopathy is poorly understood but involves in addition to basement membrane thickening, non-enzymatic glycosylation of proteins in the capillary wall, possible increased free radical activity, increased flux through the polyol (sorbitol) pathway, and haemostatic abnormalities. Hyperglycaemia is central and causally related to these abnormalities which together lead to breakdown of the inner retinal barrier. Reduced barrier function leads to retinal oedema and exudation and capillary non-perfusion and shut down gives rise to tissue ischaemia. Inner retinal ischaemia leads to the development of preretinal neovasularization or 'new blood vessel' formation, the most serious and blinding complication of the microangiopathy. Preretinal new vessel growth is initiated by breakdown of the capillary basement membrane, migration of endothelial cells into the break, proliferation of endothelial cells proximal to the migrating tip, with eventual anastomosis of adjacent new vessels allowing blood flow. The vessels are fragile, however, and easily bleed resulting in vitreous haemorrhage and visual loss. The new vessels generally originate from the superficial veins and extend into the vitreous cortex, which acts as a scaffold. An abnormally firm attachment develops between the neovascular complex and the vitreous at each point producing a fulcrum for retinal tractional displacement or detachment and further haemorrhage. A pre-existent posterior vitreous separation from the retina prevents this abnormal relationship developing between the vitreous and retina and is associated with 'abortive' neovascular outgrowth from the surface of the retina with failure to develop into typical neovascular membranes. Preretinal new vessels are fragile and prone to haemorrhage and leak plasma factors. The latter act as chemoattractants for other retinal cell types including glial cells, fibroblast-like cells, retinal pigment epithelial cells, and inflammatory cells, promoting the growth of fibrous elements within the neovascular complex.

The contractile nature of many of these cell types culminates in the latter stages of proliferative retinopathy being associated with significant tractional forces being applied to the retina in an anteroposterior plane (anteroposterior traction) and across the retinal surface (tangential traction) leading to the development of traction retinal detachment. Tractional forces, in addition to producing a mechanical displacement of the retina, may result in retinal tear or hole formation, leading to rhegmatogenous detachment combined with traction detachment.

The elaboration of a diffusible angiogenic factor from ischaemic retina has long been suspected as a principle factor in the evolution of new vessels. Laboratory research has identified a number of potential angiogenic factors whose regulatory activity is complex and interdependent and include vascular endothelial growth factor, insulin-like growth factor-1, fibroblast growth factor, transforming growth factor-β, platelet-derived growth factor, and epidermal growth factor. Vascular endothelial growth factor, in particular, appears to be of primary importance in the retinal neovascular response, having been shown to directly induce preretinal neovasularization when administered directly into the vitreous in rabbits, a response which can be inhibited by neutralizing antibodies or soluble chimeric receptor proteins. Increased vitreous levels of vascular endothelial growth factor can be measured in response to retinal hypoxia in both humans and other animals, vascular endothelial growth factor messenger RNA expression is increased in ischaemic retina of both monkeys and rabbits, and is measured in increased concentration in the human vitreous in proliferative diabetic retinopathy.

Clinical features

Microaneurysms (Fig. 1)

The earliest clinically visible lesions are microaneurysms, as the initial capillary changes are generally not detectable by conventional ophthalmoscopy. Microaneurysms are localized capillary dilations, which are commonly saccular but may be fusiform, appearing clinically as small red dots often in clusters, though they may occur in isolation.

They are visible ophthalmoscopically or photographically when larger than 30 μm, but vary between 12 to 100 μm so many are only detectable by fluorescein angiography.

Intraretinal haemorrhage

Intraretinal haemorrhages may be 'blot or dot' shaped (see Fig. 1) or 'flame shaped' (Fig. 2) depending on the retinal level at which they lie. The capillary network in the posterior retina is found in two layers, a superficial plexus in the nerve fibre layer and a deeper plexus in the inner nuclear layer. Haemorrhage in the nerve fibre layer tends to be flame shaped, following the orientation of the ganglion cell axons, lying parallel to the surface of the retina. In the inner nuclear layer, haemor-

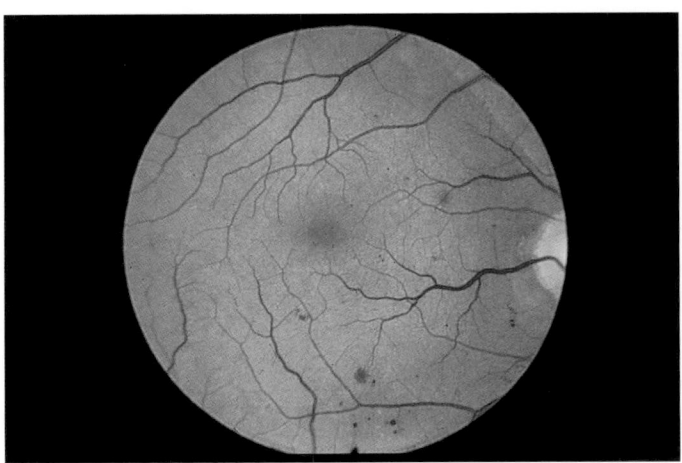

Fig. 1 Microaneurysms and blot haemorrhages.

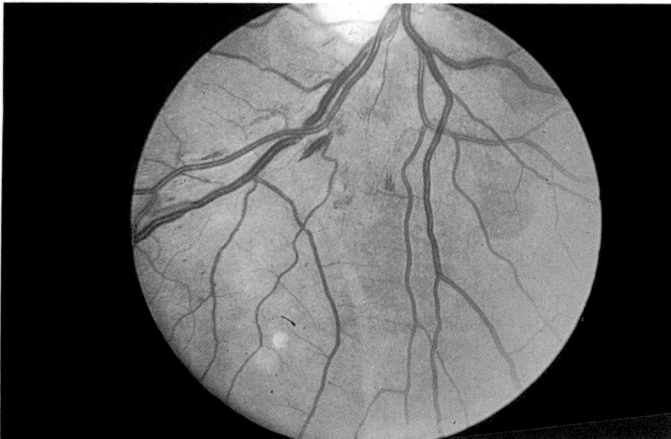

Fig. 2 Flame-shaped haemorrhage.

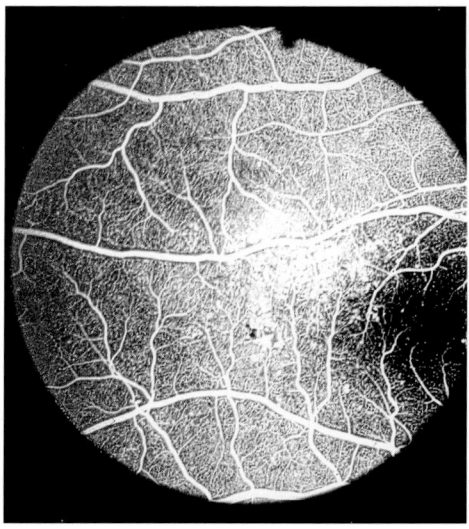

Fig. 4 Circinate exudate with localized leakage on fluorescein angiography.

rhage from the deep capillary plexus is aligned perpendicular to the retinal surface, and is therefore viewed end on, appearing dot or blot shaped. These latter may be difficult to differentiate from microaneurysms clinically, but can be easily distinguished by fluorescein angiography, the microaneurysms 'lighting up' and hyperfluorescing the haemorrhages appearing dark due to masking of the fluorescent dye.

Multiple blot haemorrhages occur when the retina is significantly ischaemic, characteristic of a preproliferative state. This should alert the observer to the underlying ischaemia and the likely development of preretinal neovascularization.

Hard exudates (Figs 3, 4)

Hard exudates are yellow–white intraretinal deposits that can vary from small barely detectable specks initially, evolving to form circinate rings and eventually large confluent plaques. They are composed of extracellular lipid, amorphous extracellular fluid, and macrophages and are found principally in the macula at the level of Henle's layer. Often they can be seen forming a ring or 'circinate' pattern around a cluster of micro-

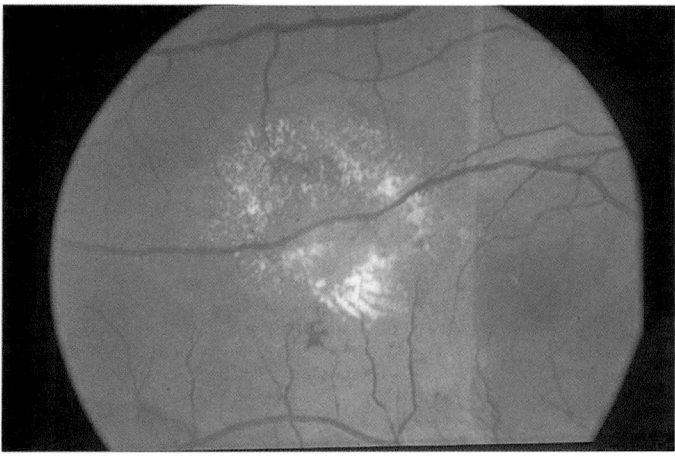

Fig. 3 Circinate exudate with localized leakage on fluorescein angiography.

aneurysms or capillary abnormalities. They arise from leakage of serum from abnormal retinal capillaries with breakdown of the inner retinal barrier, and are thus associated with coexistent retinal oedema. The extracellular lipids coalesce into large smooth-surfaced deposits, which displace the adjacent cells. When they extend into the centre of the macula at the fovea, vision is severely affected.

Cotton-wool spots (Fig. 5)

Cotton-wool spots are seen as greyish-white patches of discoloration in the nerve fibre layer. They result from local ischaemia giving rise to an interruption both orthograde and retrograde axoplasmic flow, seen microscopically as distended stumps of ganglion cell axons in the retinal nerve fibre layer. They are not retinal infarcts as is often stated. They are therefore only seen in the posterior retina where the nerve fibre layer is sufficiently thick, and there is sufficient bulk of axoplasmic flow. Cotton-wool spots are common, but in the majority of patients there are only a few present at any one time. Multiple cotton-wool spots (six to 10 simultaneously in one eye) indicate generalized retinal ischaemia and the likelihood of the development of preretinal neovascularization.

Venous abnormalities (see Fig. 5)

Venous dilation, beading, and duplication occur usually in proportion to the degree of retinal ischaemia. Venous dilation is seen relatively early in the evolution of diabetic retinopathy; beading is a particularly useful sign of generalized retinal ischaemia. Branch venous occlusion is common, but differs from that observed in systemic hypertension in that it is not necessarily associated with occlusion at arteriovenous crossing points. Arteriolar calibre irregularity and sheathing are common in the posterior retina associated with peripheral arteriolar occlusion peripherally and may occur in diabetics in the absence of systemic hypertension.

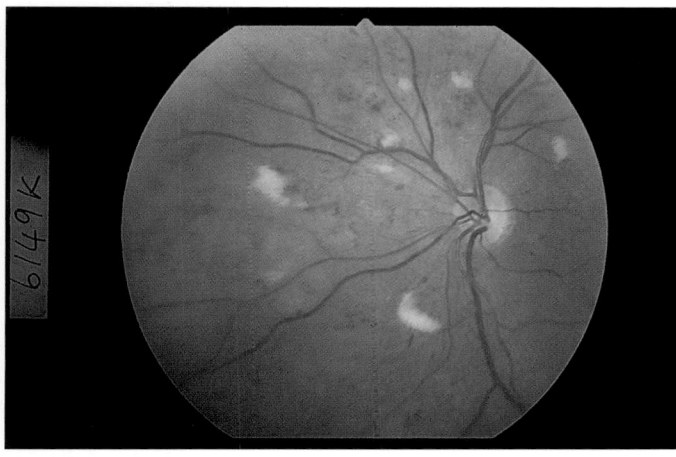

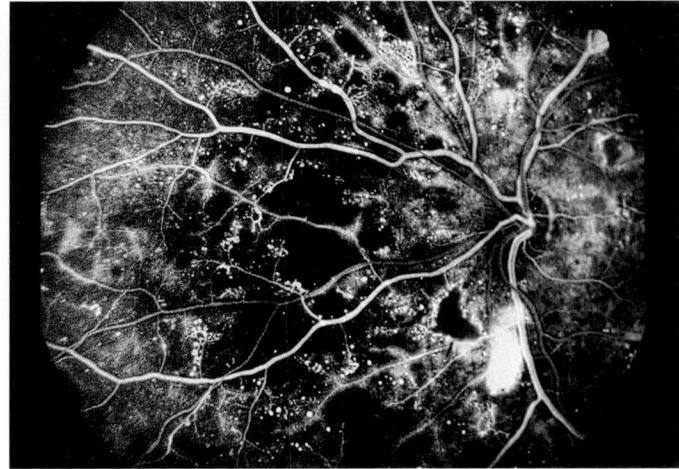

Figs. 5 and 6 Generalized retinal ischaemic picture with multiple blot haemorrhages, cotton-wool spots, and intraretinal microvascular abnormalities. Capillary non-perfusion demonstrated on fluorescein angiography. Note leakage from early new vessels (by courtesy of Mr B. Leatherbarrow).

Intraretinal microvascular abnormalities (Fig. 6)

Intraretinal microvascular abnormalities are ophthalmoscopically visible areas of capillary dilation and tortuosity, capillary shunts, and intraretinal new vessels. They occur adjacent to and within areas of capillary non-perfusion and form in response to generalized retinal ischaemia, and are thus associated with a high risk of preretinal neovascularization.

Extraretinal neovascularization (Figs 7–10)

As the retina becomes progressively more ischaemic new blood vessels may arise either from the optic disc or from the retinal periphery. These vessels usually originate from the major veins, initially as fine delicate tufts either on the surface of the disc or originating from the vessels in the major arcades. As they grow they often form a precapillary network which extends over the surface of the adjacent retina. Where the vitreous remains attached they form abnormal adhesions between the

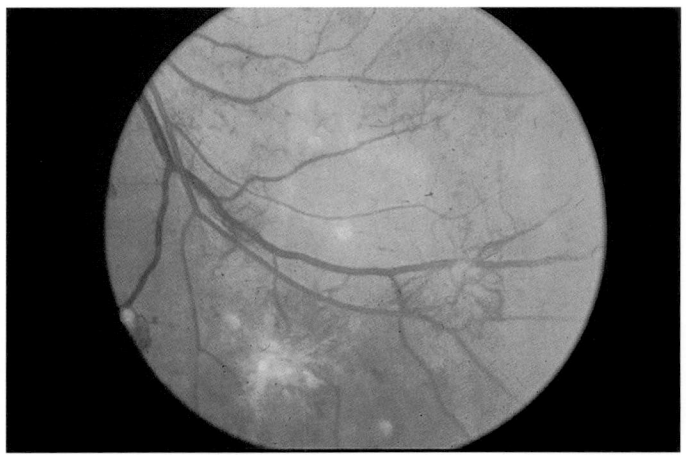

Fig. 8 Peripheral new vessels and fibrosis.

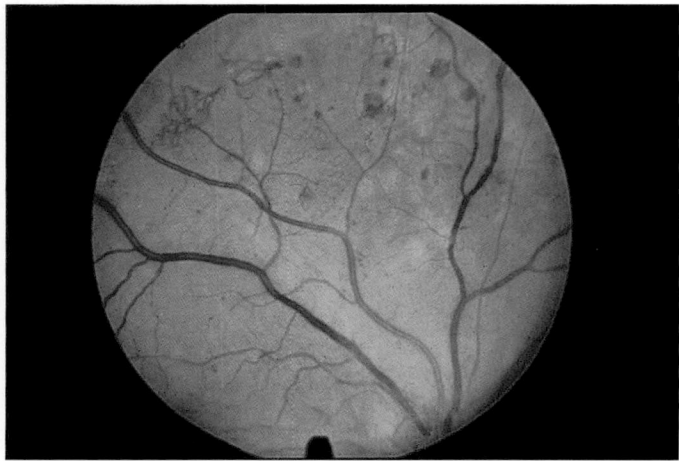

Fig. 7 Fine peripheral new vessels (by courtesy of Mr S. Aldington).

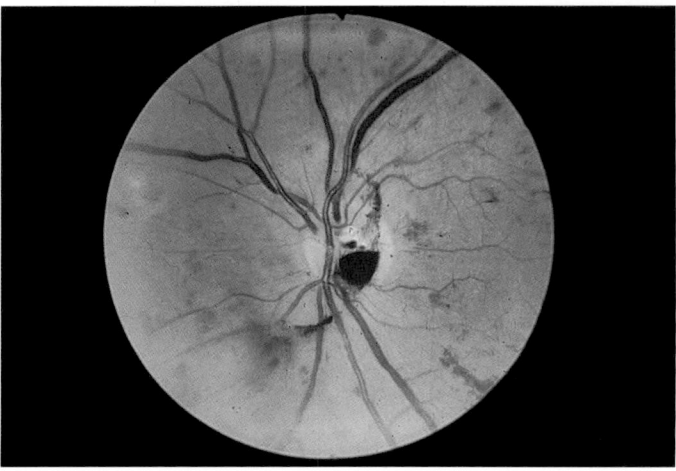

Fig. 9 Disc new vessels, limited haemorrhage (by courtesy of Mr S. Aldington).

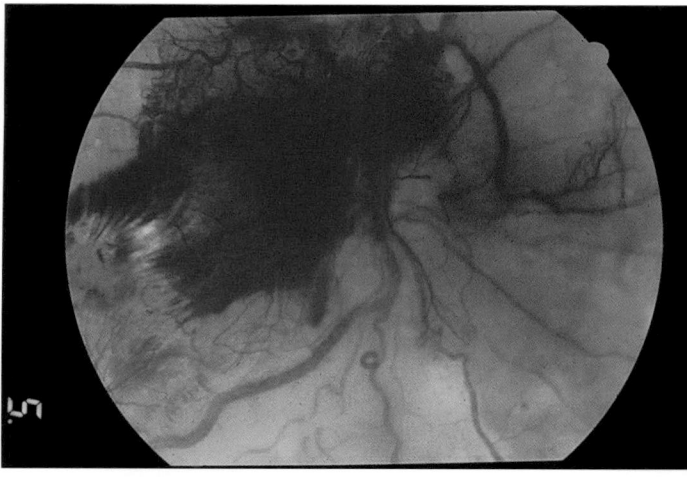

Fig. 10 Disc new vessels, severe preretinal haemorrhage.

Table 1 Classification of diabetic retinopathy

Background retinopathy
Minimal
Moderate
Preproliferative – Severe
　　　　　　　　Very severe

Maculopathy (background retinopathy involving the macula)
Exudative (focal)
Diffuse
Ischaemic
Mixed

Proliferative retinopathy
New vessels on the disc or within 1 disc diameter
New vessels elsewhere in the retina (more than 1 disc diameter from the disc)

vitreous and the vessels themselves, which can give rise to haemorrhage as the vitreous separates. As the vessels mature connective tissue or fibrosis develops, resulting in more firm attachments allowing the vitreous to exert traction which may give rise to retinal traction and consequent retinal detachment. Where vitreous detachment predates the appearances of retinal neovascularization the neovascular process is interrupted, leaving aborted stumps, demonstrating that new vessels require the vitreous scaffold on which to proliferate. Disc new vessels (see Figs 9, 10) and new vessels elsewhere (see Figs 7, 8) are fragile and bleed easily. When the vitreous it detached only locally in the vicinity of a new vessel, blood may accumulate between the retina and the vitreous adopting a characteristic boat-shaped appearance or subhyaloid haemorrhage. Vitreous haemorrhage usually gives rise to profound loss of vision initially as only a small volume of haemorrhage dissolved in the vitreous is sufficient to obscure the retina (see Fig. 11).

Classification
See Table 1.

Background retinopathy

Mild and moderate non-proliferative retinopathy
These include the following.

1. Microaneurysms.

2. Intraretinal haemorrhages: mild to moderate in fewer than four quadrants.

3. Hard exudates.

4. Macular oedema.

5. Foveal avascular zone abnormalities.

Background diabetic retinopathy, also described as non-proliferative diabetic retinopathy, is so called because the lesions lie within the retina and always predate the development of proliferative disease. Initially background diabetic retinopathy consists of microaneurysms only, progressing to microaneurysms with small haemorrhages (dots and blots from the deep capillary plexus), and flame-shaped splinter haemorrhages (in the nerve fibre layer, often associated with hypertension). Hard exudate and retinal oedema are seen as part of the spectrum of background diabetic retinopathy, but where they becomes related to the fovea or centre of the macula, a 'maculopathy' (see below) is identified, principally to highlight the sight-threatening nature of these changes in the macula.

The occasional cotton-wool spot and mild venous dilation with enlargement of foveal avascular zone (bound by the perifoveal capillary net) is consistent with mild or moderate background retinopathy. These changes, however, herald the beginnings of ischaemic change within the retina.

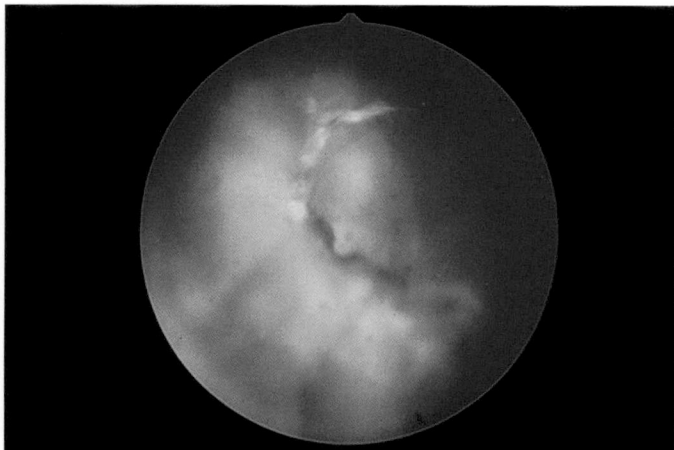

Fig. 11 Diffuse vitreous haemorrhage obscuring view of the retina.

Severe and very severe

With increasing ischaemia, cotton-wool spots become more prevalent and venous changes progress. Variations in vessel calibre develop in the major retinal veins described as beading, which along with venous loops and reduplication are an important indicator of retinal ischaemia.

Severe background retinopathy consists of multiple cotton-wool spots, venous beading, multiple dot and blot haemorrhages, and intraretinal microvascular abnormalities (see Fig. 6). As the ischaemic changes progress, but frank neovascularization has yet to develop on either the optic disc or in the retinal periphery, the retinopathy is classified as very severe, recognizing the high risk of new vessel development.

Maculopathy (Figs 12, 13)

Maculopathy is diagnosed when retinal oedema and hard exudate, with or without ischaemia, is present within 500 μm

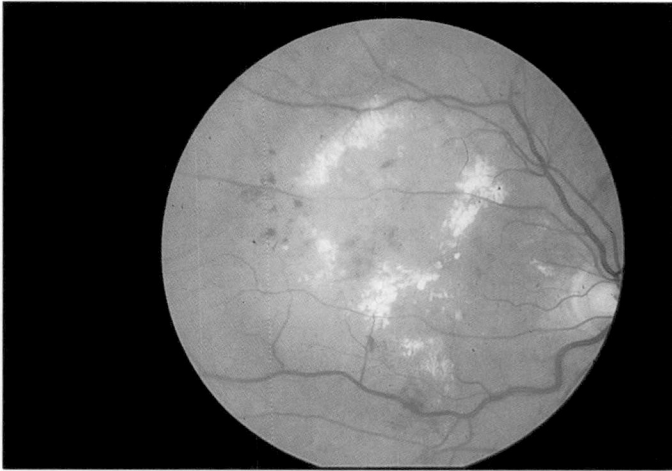

Fig. 12 Right macula. Oedema and hard exudate from leaking microaneurysms and capillaries.

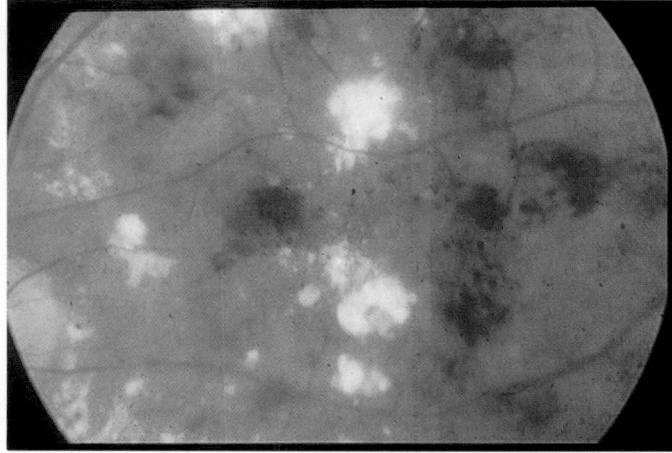

Fig. 13 Left macula. Multiple haemorrhages in addition to exudates indicate ischaemia.

of the centre of the fovea, and is considered to pose a threat to central acuity. Maculopathy is generally further classified into focal, diffuse, and ischaemic types, though this classification overlaps considerably and in many instances a mixed type is identified. Nonetheless it is useful to subdivide types, as there are implications for management and prognosis.

Visual loss in diabetic maculopathy is the result of macular oedema and/or ischaemia. Macular oedema may be detected clinically by observation of retinal thickening on binocular stereoscopic slit lamp examination. Fluorescein angiography may reveal leakage of vessels and pooling in the late stage but is particularly useful in identifying the degree of capillary non-perfusion or ischaemia that is also affecting the macula.

Clinical types of maculopathy

Focal maculopathy (Fig. 14)

The macula develops focal areas of oedema centred on microaneurysms and abnormal leaking capillaries often with complete or incomplete rings of exudate at the margins of the oedema, often referred to as circinate exudates. Exudate tends to gravitate towards the fovea. Oedema results from leakage from the abnormal capillaries with breakdown of the inner retinal barrier, in association with disordered pigment epithelial function. When healthy, the pigment epithelium pumps fluid from the retinal interstitial space towards the choroid, and reduced movement of tissue fluid out of the retina may contribute to the pathogenesis of retinal oedema.

Diffuse maculopathy (Fig. 15)

There is generalized leakage from dilated capillaries, and the entire macula may become oedematous. Severe cystoid spaces may appear similar to those seen in non-diabetic cystoid oedema, often without significant exudation. This type of maculopathy is more often associated with acute systemic abnormalities such as significant systemic hypertension and renal failure with albuminuria and may improve with correction of the underlying medical problem.

Ischaemic maculopathy (see Fig. 13)

Capillary non-perfusion results in foveal ischaemia and is usually associated with blot haemorrhages and venous dilation. Fluorescein angiography will demonstrate the true extent of the ischaemia, often with more extensive capillary closure than clinically apparent.

Mixed maculopathy

There is often no clear distinction between types of maculopathy, as capillary microangiopathy is generalized, with some areas of the macula more affected by oedema associated with localized areas of ischaemia; in such a case the maculopathy would be described as mixed type. It is helpful to decide clinically if a maculopathy is of a predominately focal, diffuse, or ischaemic type, as the method and expected response to laser treatment tend to vary with type.

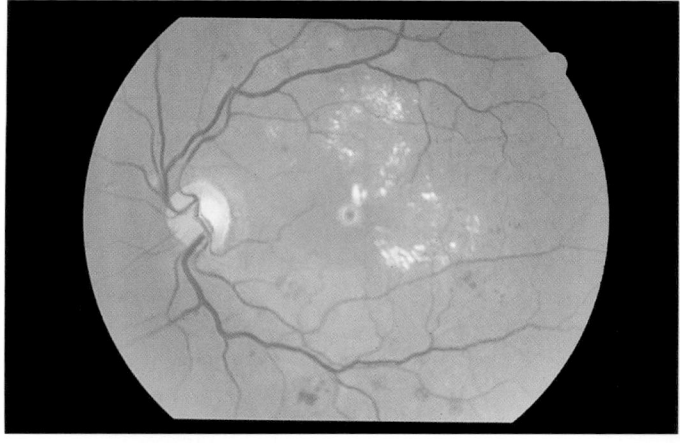

(a)

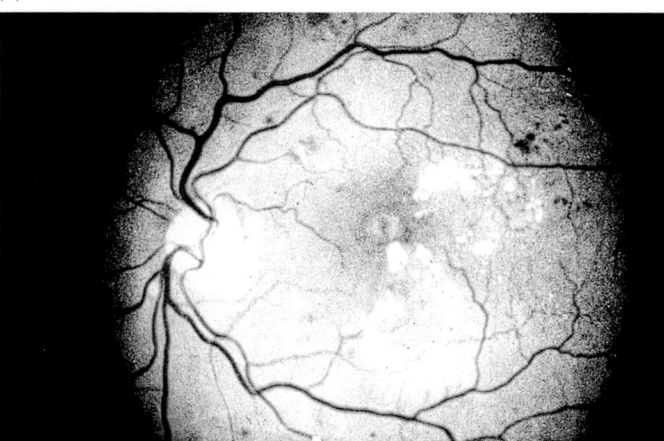

(b)

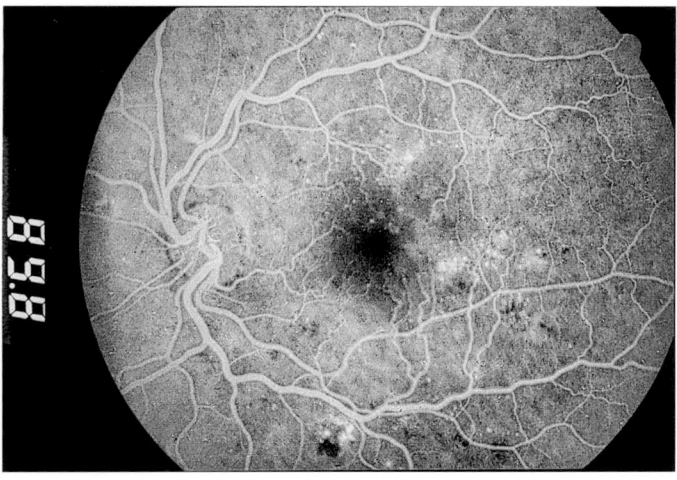

(c)

Fig. 14 Left focal maculopathy (a) colour, (b) red-free, and (c) fluorescein.

Proliferative diabetic retinopathy (see Figs 6–11)

Proliferative diabetic retinopathy usually appears late in the disease. Most importantly severe sight-threatening retinopathy can occur at a time when visual acuity is unaffected. Prior to the development of vitreous haemorrhage or traction retinal

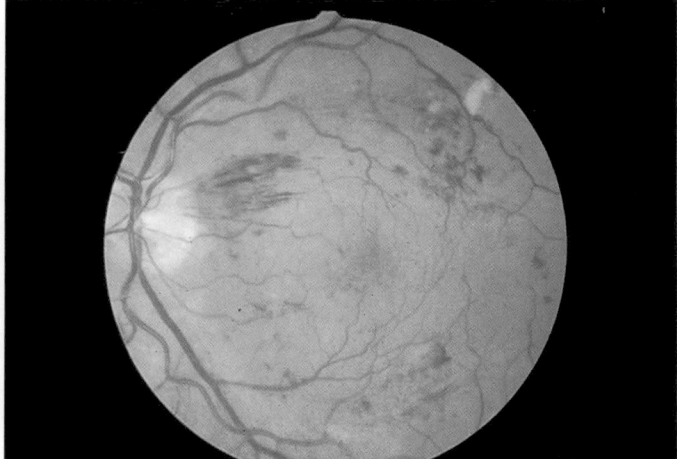

Fig. 15 Diffuse maculopathy.

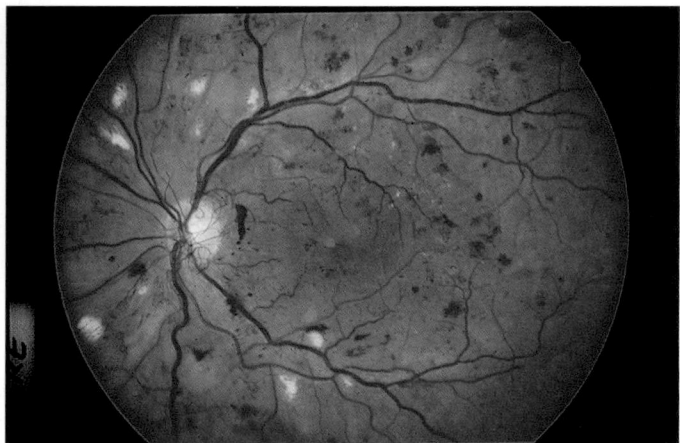

Fig. 16 Disc new vessels with widespread retinal ischaemia.

detachment involving the centre of the macula, visual acuity may be normal. The likelihood of vitreous haemorrhage increases with severity of new vessels and their proximity to the optic disc (Fig. 16). In the control eyes of the large treatment studies carried out in the 1970s, 25 per cent of control eye were blind with disc new vessels within 24 months, increasing to 50 per cent at 4 years. As fibrovascular complexes develop, traction retinal detachment may result. At the outset, fine folds in the inner limiting lamina and inner layers of retina radiate from an 'epicentre' or multiple epicentres of contraction. With continuing contraction of the epiretinal tissue, tangential or traction parallel to the surface of the retina is exerted. The exaggerated attachments of vitreous to retina serve to maintain the attachment of the posterior hyaloid at the posterior pole and when posterior vitreous detachment proceeds more anteriorly this gives rise to an anteroposterior traction band between the vitreous base anteriorly and the vitreoretinal adhesions at the posterior pole. A bridging fibroglial membrane may develop anterior to the macula spanning between the fibrovascular attachments along the superior and inferior major vascular arcades, giving rise to a 'tabletop' detachment of the macula.

Normally traction detachment is initially localized and progresses usually only very slowly. The macula is rarely involved initially and therefore vision is unaffected. Retinal detachment may extend much more rapidly should the traction produce a localized retinal hole allowing fluid from the retrohyaloid space to gain access to the subretinal space, and thereby creating a rhegmatogenous component to the detachment.

Risk factors for the development of diabetic retinopathy

The most significant risk factor in the evolution of diabetic retinopathy is the duration of the metabolic disease itself. There is now conclusive evidence that tight metabolic control of diabetes can reduce the onset of retinopathy. Other factors associated with progression include pregnancy, hypertension, puberty, renal disease, and hyperlipidaemia. Pregnant diabetics with established retinopathy in particular should be screened regularly during pregnancy, as retinopathy can advance very rapidly in a small proportion of patients. Predictive factors include poor prepregnancy control of diabetes, too rapid tightening of control during the prepregnancy period, and the development of complications during pregnancy such as pre-eclampsia and fluid imbalance.

Screening

Diabetic retinopathy is an important public health problem that has a presymptomatic stage detectable in the at-risk population, and for which there is a recognized treatment that is generally available in ophthalmic units throughout the United Kingdom. Diabetic retinopathy therefore fulfils the criteria for a disease for which screening is effective. Screening may be by ophthalmoscopy, either by optometrists or doctors, or by standard or non-mydriatic fundus photography. Each method has its advantages and drawbacks with comparable rates of sensitivity and specificity though ophthalmoscopy should be conducted through dilated pupils and by a trained observer. Fundus photography is equally effective, but more expensive than ophthalmoscopy. It has the advantage of producing permanent objective records acquired by technical personnel, allowing the images to be assessed later by a specialist. Ideally, screening for eye disease including diabetic retinopathy should be done by a dedicated ophthalmologist and more specialists should be specifically trained for this purpose. It is recommended that the organization of screening be primarily the responsibility of the doctor in charge of the diabetic patient. Close collaboration with the nearest ophthalmic department, adequately equipped for further assessment and laser treatment, is required. Many units have developed training and certification programmes for local optometrists to carry out screening. There should be established channels for rapid referral of patients with sight-threatening lesions.

Patients should be screened on an annual basis following the onset of background retinopathy. At diagnosis in young insulin-dependent diabetics, if there is no evidence of retinopathy, further screening can be deferred for at least 3 years. Screening frequency should be increased if there are high-risk associations, such as pregnancy, renal failure, or poorly controlled hypertension. With rapid advancement in technology, newer methods of screening may become available including digital photography and computerized methods of detection and assessment.

Treatment

The treatment of diabetic retinopathy by photocoagulation is of proven efficacy both for proliferative diabetic retinopathy and for maculopathy. A laser is used to produce a retinal burn normally applied through a dilated pupil using a contact lens or an indirect ophthalmoscope, and occasionally externally through the sclera. Transpupillary laser is delivered at the slit lamp using a wide-angle contact lens for panretinal photocoagulation for new vessels, and a narrower angled more magnifying lens such as a Goldmann contact lens for macula treatment. Any wavelength of laser that produces a pigment epithelial and retinal burn can be utilized. Despite many theoretical considerations there is no evidence that one laser wavelength is more efficacious than another. Lasers that operate within the visual spectrum tend to be taken up more easily and are less uncomfortable. Useful wavelengths for retinal photocoagulation vary from blue at 488 nm, green at 532 nm, yellow at 577 nm, red at 640 nm, and infrared at 810 nm. It is recommended that the blue wavelength (488 nm), in the argon laser is avoided particularly in the macular area, due to the presence of the xanthophyll pigment, which absorbs energy at the blue end of the spectrum which may lead to a greater and undesirable degree of inner retinal damage. Yellow laser (577 nm) has the advantage of ability to coagulate red lesions directly, though the principal uptake of energy for all laser types is absorption in the pigment epithelium where the majority of the tissue reaction is induced, but photoreceptors usually receive thermal collateral damage overlying the burn (Fig. 17).

Management of new vessels on the disc and new vessels elsewhere

The rationale of treatment is to produce sufficient retinal photocoagulation scars to induce regression of new vessels. In general this involves producing a panretinal covering of retinal burns in a non-confluent pattern avoiding the macula. Treatment usually comprises between 1000 and 2000 burns of between 200 and 500 μm spot size (Fig. 18). The spot size varies considerably with the type of contact lens applied, a larger burn being achieved by a wide-angled contact lens. Spot size varies with indirect application. The endpoint for each burn is a grey–white lesion on the pigment epithelium (Fig. 19) with the laser power starting at approximately 200 mW, increasing incrementally until the desired burn intensity is achieved. The amount of energy required depends on the degree of pigment present in the pigment epithelium (more power for a pale fundus) and is influenced by retinal thickness

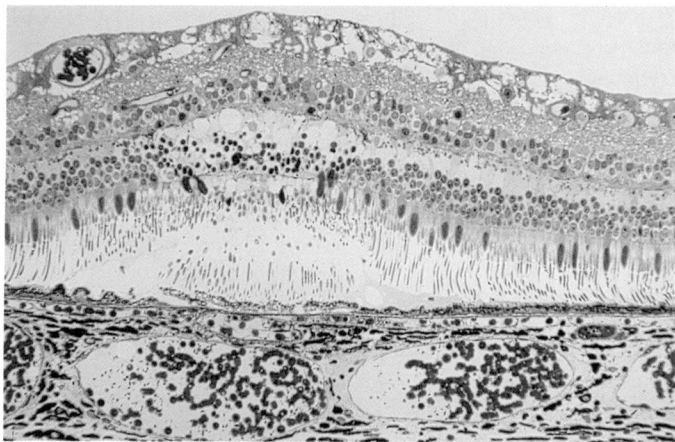

Fig. 17 Histological section of retinal burn with photoreceptor damage (by courtesy of Professor D. McLeod).

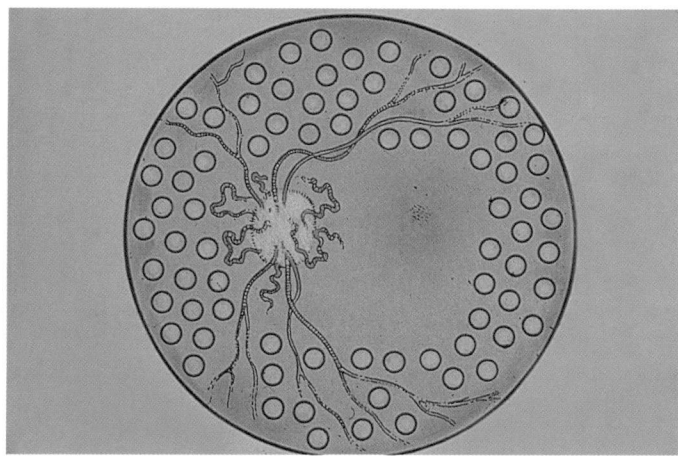

Fig. 18 Schematic representation of laser burns in panretinal photocoagulation.

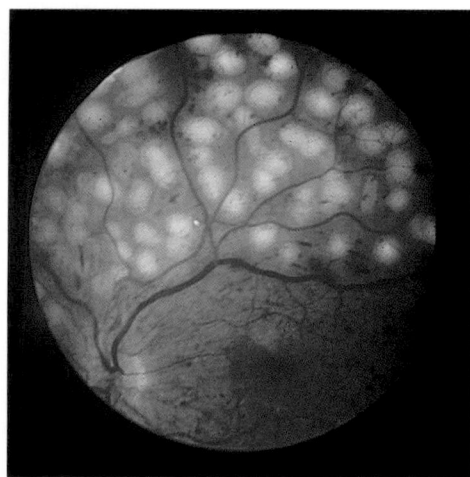

Fig. 19 Acute retinal burns immediately after panretinal photocoagulation.

and oedema. Treatment is usually delivered in two sessions with the inferior half of the retina being treated initially, as the upper retina usually remains more accessible to treatment should a vitreous haemorrhage occur between treatments. The precise number of burns will be dependent on the response to treatment, which should be monitored generally at monthly intervals. In certain circumstances where there is very florid neovascularization, particularly in young poorly controlled diabetics and in pregnancy, treatment may need to be delivered more intensively with the entire panretinal ablation being delivered in a single session.

Management of peripheral new vessels is generally by panretinal photocoagulation (Fig. 20). Where new vessels elsewhere are not fully responding they may be treated directly and closed down by application of the laser around the source of the new vessels elsewhere. Where new vessels elsewhere are associated with fibrous tissue (see Fig. 8) and traction, local laser therapy to the fibrovascular tissue should be avoided, as this may be associated with increasing traction. Laser treatment should be directed away from areas of gliosis to avoid these complications.

Photocoagulation is carried out at sufficient intensity to induce regression of new vessels. This varies between individuals in general requiring titration against the extent of retinal ischaemia. A proportion of patients fail to respond to laser photocoagulation frequently due to inadequate amounts of photocoagulation, often associated with poor patient compliance, due to the uncomfortable nature of the treatment and the often associated temporary reduction in vision. Though the retina has been completely covered outside of the macular area retreatment of treated areas may be performed. This is usually associated with constriction of the visual field. Patients may then find that they are unable to fulfil the DVLC criteria for holding a driving licence. Non-response may also be associated with forward new vessels, held at a distance from the retinal surface by vitreous attachment. An endpoint should be recognized when further photocoagulation is unlikely to induce regression in such vessels. Should they be associated with vitreous haemorrhage then vitrectomy may be used as an effective form of management.

Rubeosis iridis

Rubeosis iridis describes neovascularization of the anterior segment and in particular at the anterior chamber angle and associated development of robotic glaucoma. Rubeosis iridis is often associated with advanced proliferative diabetic retinopathy, though rubeosis in diabetes is often not as aggressive as that associated with ischaemic retinal vein occlusion. A panretinal photocoagulation is urgently required, however, and in the presence of vitreous haemorrhage a vitrectomy and endolaser should be carried out promptly. Glaucoma associated with rubeosis should be treated once the neovascularization is no longer progressing by either an enhanced drainage procedure, drainage tube, or cycloablation. Blind eyes with rubeotic glaucoma should be kept pain-free and topical steroids with atropine may be all that is necessary.

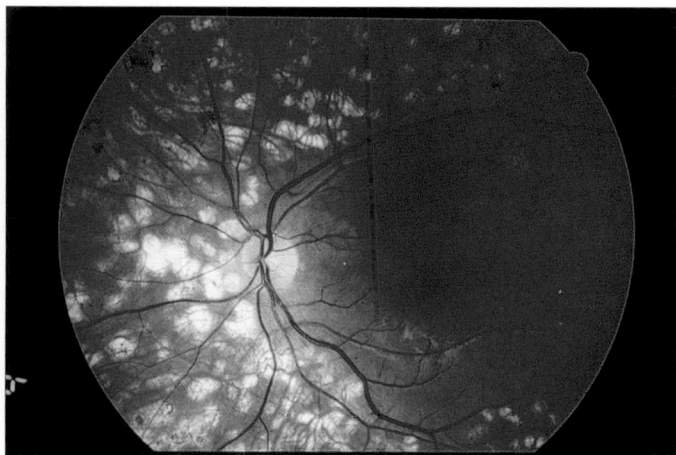

Fig. 20 Pattern of retinal scars after successful panretinal photocoagulation.

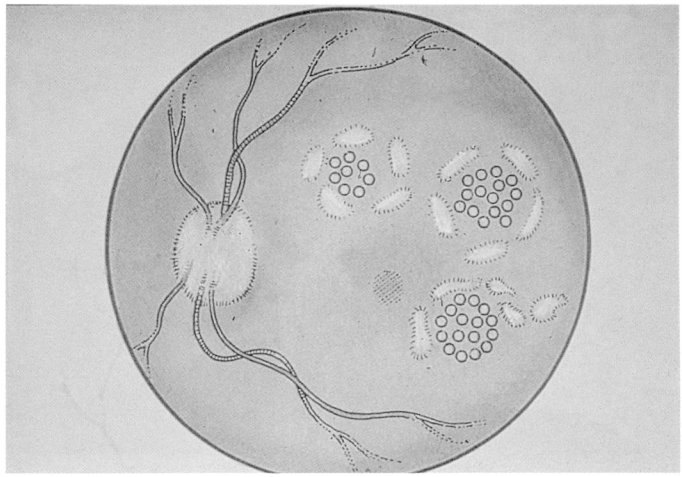

Fig. 21 Schematic representation of focal laser photocoagulation.

Complications of panretinal laser treatment

Pain

The intensity of pain experienced in panretinal photocoagulation varies between individuals, and is influenced by factors such as the power required to achieve an adequate retinal burn, laser wavelength, retinal location, and intensity of previous treatment. There is more likelihood of pain the higher the power, the longer wavelength (diode or krypton lasers), and along the horizontal meridian temporally and nasally. Pain is also more likely following frequent retreatment.

Retrobulbar anaesthesia is desirable where there is significant discomfort, and many operators use this almost routinely if extensive treatment is to be delivered.

Worsening macular oedema

Panretinal photocoagulation is associated with exacerbation of exudative maculopathy and oedema. Usually this is temporary but it is recommended that maculopathy is treated if possible, with oedema resolved, prior to embarking on panretinal photocoagulation if the clinical situation allows.

Pupillary abnormalities

These may arise from direct application of the laser beam and uptake in the pupil pigment epithelium by direct application. In addition treatment along the temporal and nasal horizontal meridian may damage the long posterior ciliary nerves giving rise to pupillary dysfunction.

Macula burn

Very occasionally damage to the fovea results from an inadvertent macula burn. It is important that at all times the laser operator is aware of the anatomical location in the retina to which the laser is being delivered. Loss of orientation is more likely

to occur with the Goldmann three-mirror system than the wide-angle lenses or indirect laser.

Choroidal detachment

Choroidal detachment is not uncommon following anterior panretinal photocoagulation, especially with the indirect laser. Often this is of little significance, but occasionally the induced shallowing of the anterior chamber can precipitate an acute angle closure episode of glaucoma. The acute pressure rise may give rise to limited macular perfusion during the acute episode, especially if there was a coexistent ischaemic maculopathy.

Visual field defects

Visual field defects occur in field areas corresponding to areas of capillary non-perfusion. In addition panretinal photocoagulation gives rise to increasing field defects particularly where applied in the posterior retina and where heavy confluent application is necessary.

Some authorities have attempted to reduce visual field loss induced by photocoagulation by concentrating photocoagulation in the mid-periphery to avoid this complication, but very often the amount of photocoagulation required to control the neovascular process make this approach impractical. Non-confluent treatment reduces the impact of laser photocoagulation on the visual field.

Management of diabetic maculopathy (Figs 14(a)(b)(c) and 21–25)

Clinical trials in the United Kingdom and the United States have demonstrated the efficacy of photocoagulation in the reduction of visual morbidity associated with maculopathy.

Neither of these studies, however, differentiated between the previously described types of retinopathy but treatment protocols have generally employed focal, modified grid, or grid

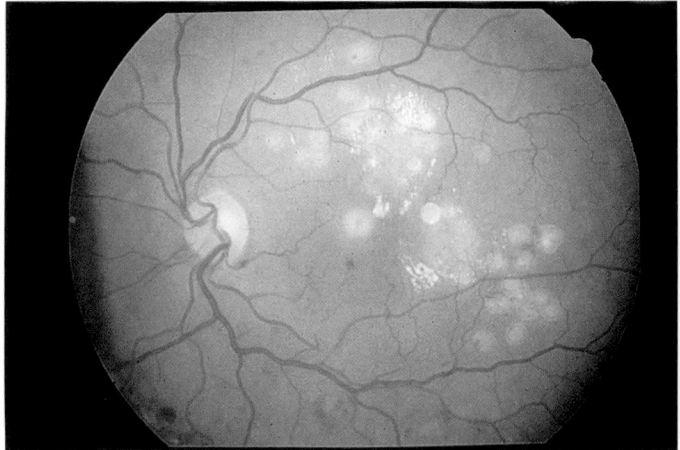

Fig. 22 Immediately postfocal photocoagulation.

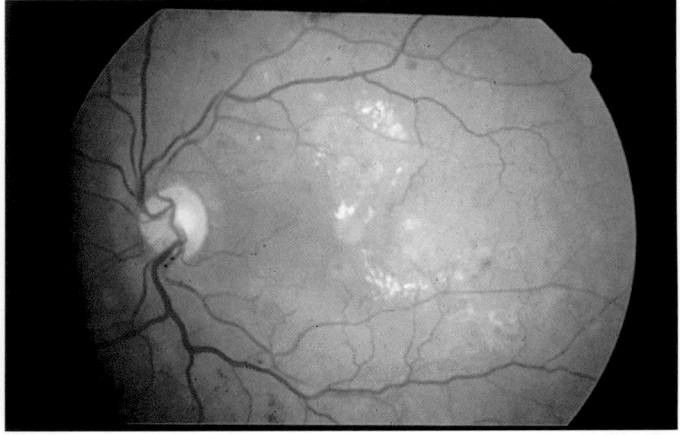

(a)

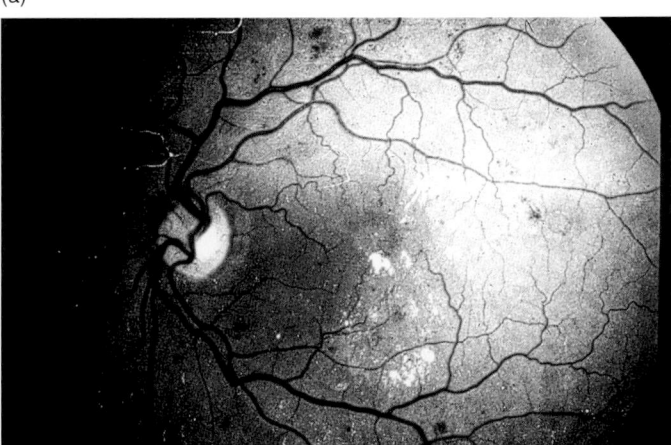

(b)

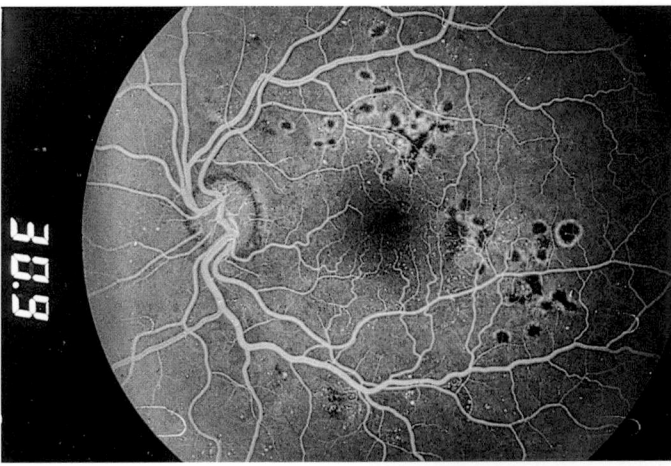

(c)

Fig. 23 Four months postlaser treatment. Resorbing exudate on (a) colour, (b) red-free, and (c) reduced angiographic leak.

photocoagulation. The Early Treatment of Diabetic Retinopathy study demonstrated that photocoagulation of clinically significant diabetic macular oedema reduced visual loss by one half, the diagnosis being based on clinical examination regardless of visual acuity and not dependent on angiographic findings. Thus where retinal oedema is shown to exist within 500 micron of the macula assessed either by a Goldmann contact lens or a hand-held 78- or 90-dioptre lens, photocoagulation can reduce the risk of visual deterioration in 50 per cent of patients.

Treatment strategy is directed initially to focal leakage and secondarily to diffuse leakage. All points of focal leakage, that is microaneurysms located between 500 μm and 2 disc diameters, are treated directly using a 50 to 100 μm spot size of 0.1 s duration. Lesions between 300 and 500 μm from the centre of the fovea are also treated if the perifoveal avascular zone can be preserved. Grid treatment is also applied to areas of oedema consisting of burns of 50 to 200 μm spot size of lighter intensity then required for panretinal photocoagulation, placed one burn width apart at 0.1 s duration. These burns are applied to areas of diffuse leakage or capillary non-perfusion and can be placed within the papillomacula bundle but outside a radius of 500 micron from the edge of the optic disc and not within 500 μm of the centre of the macula. Initial treatment is repeated at 4 months if there is still persistent oedema. Optimal management depends on detection and treatment by photocoagulation of oedema before the fovea is involved. Where the vision is reduced due to macular ischaemia photocoagulation is ineffective, though it should be recognized that many cases of diabetic maculopathy involve coexisting macular oedema, and ischaemia should not necessarily preclude treatment of the oedema.

It is essential when embarking on macula treatment that the exact location of the fovea is identified and that the intensity of the burns particularly between 200 and 500 μm are not excessively intense. There is no specific advantage to a particular wavelength though blue light should be avoided for the reasons previously described. Treatment is commonly carried out using the green component of the argon laser (515 nm).

Maculopathy can recur after treatment and additional treatment may be necessary 4 months after the initial treatment if there is residual thickening of the macula retina involving the margins of the foveal avascular zone. If there is persistent oedema or the visual acuity is deteriorating, fluorescein angiography may be helpful in identifying areas of continuing leakage

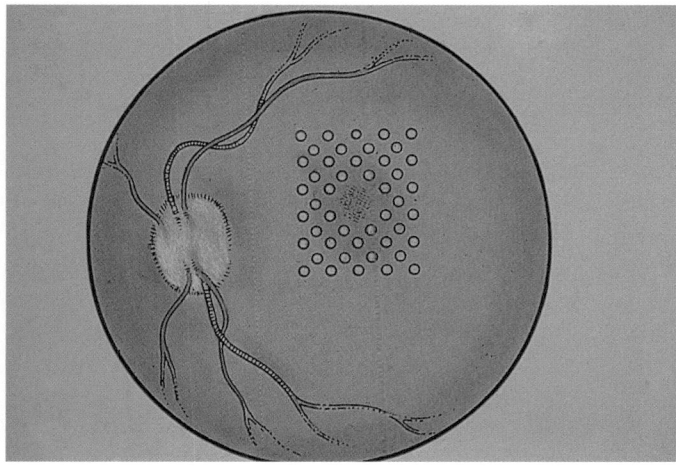

Fig. 24 Schematic representation of grid laser treatment.

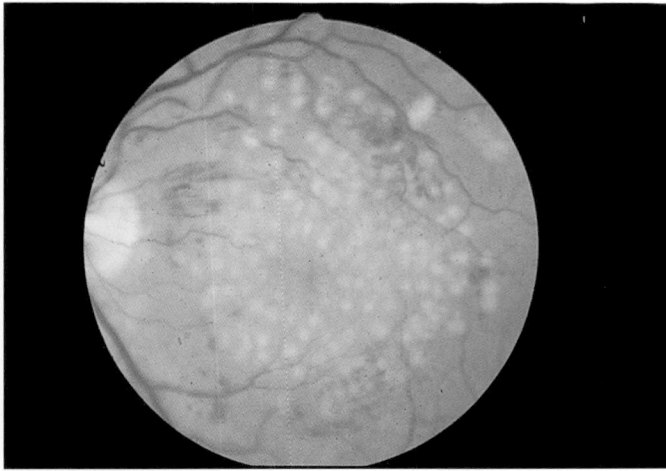

Fig. 25 Immediately postgrid laser treatment.

which can be retreated. Exudates may take much longer to absorb and in a dry-treated macular specks of residual exudate may persist indefinitely.

Cataract and surgery for cataract in diabetes

Cataract is a common complication in diabetes with a prevalence of 10 per cent of diabetics either with cataracts or who have had cataract surgery. It is estimated that up to 15 per cent of cataract surgery is performed on diabetics. Cataracts may interfere with accurate screening for diabetic retinopathy, and surgery is indicated if lens opacity prevents an adequate examination of the fundus or produces excessive scatter of light during laser therapy. The main indications for surgery are identical to those for non-diabetic patients. Standard surgical treatment is applicable by phacoemulsification or by extracapsular extraction. Special considerations include the fashioning of a wider anterior capsulorhexis and scrupulous cleaning of

lens epithelial cells from the underside of the capsulorhexis rim to prevent opacification and difficulty with subsequent laser treatment. In proliferative disease where cataract prevents application of laser, indirect panretinal photocoagulation can be applied intraoperatively and most beneficially prior to intraocular lens implantation. Surgical results are poorer in those eyes with active proliferative retinopathy often being associated with a severe uveitis with fibrinous response. Where rubeosis iridis is present this may be exacerbated by cataract surgery, and maculopathy may worsen. Capsular thickening is more common in diabetics and neovascularization of the anterior segment may increase following yttrium–aluminium–garnet capsulotomy. Vision outcome is often related to the state of the retinopathy and particularly the macula and major complications relate to the progression of retinopathy.

Driving, visual acuity, and visual fields

Retinal ischaemia and photocoagulation may produce visual field defects. All diabetic patients undergoing laser treatment should be aware of this potential complication prior to consenting for treatment. Eligibility can be assessed following treatment using a visual field test such the Estermann programme on automated perimeter.

Conclusion

The prevention, detection, management, and understanding of diabetic retinopathy pose continuing challenges for patients and health-care professionals, and there is still much to be achieved. If patients, who have developed sight-threatening complications are identified, have timely access to treatment facilities, and treatment is applied appropriately, a significant proportion of diabetes-associated visual disability can be ameliorated and avoided. Providing an affordable comprehensive solution to this major public health problem remains a challenge rather than a reality for many health-care systems worldwide.

Further reading

British Multicentre Study Group (1984). Photocoagulation for proliferative diabetic retinopathy: a randomised controlled trial using the xenon arc. *Diabetologia*, **26**, 109.

Diabetes Control and Complications Trial Research Group (1993). The effect of intensive treatment of diabetes on the development and progression of long-term complications in insulin-dependent diabetes mellitus. *New England Journal of Medicine*, **329**, 977–86.

Diabetic Retinopathy Study Research Group (1978). Photocoagulation treatment of proliferative diabetic retinopathy. *Ophthalmology*, **85**, 82–106.

Diabetic Retinopathy Vitrectomy Study Research Group (1983). Early vitrectomy for severe proliferative diabetic retinopathy in eyes with useful vision: results of a randomised trial. Diabetic Vitrectomy Study Report 3. *Ophthalmology*, **95**, 1307.

Diabetic Retinopathy Vitrectomy Study Research Group (1990). Early vitrectomy for severe vitreous haemorrhage in diabetic retinopathy. Four years results of a randomised trial. DRVS report No 5. *Archives of Ophthalmology*, **108**, 958–64.

Early Treatment Diabetic Retinopathy Study Research Group (1985). Photocoagulation for diabetic macular oedema. *Archives of Ophthalmology*, **103**, 1796–806.

Hamilton, P., *et al.* (1996). *Management of diabetic retinopathy.* BMJ Publishing, London.

Olk, and Lee, (1993). *Diabetic retinopathy: practical considerations.* Lippincott, New York.

St Vincent Joint Task Force for Diabetes (1994). *Report of the Visual Impairment Subgroup.* British Diabetic Association/Department of Health, London.

2.9.3 Age-related macular degeneration

Sharon Fekrat, Neil M. Bressler, and S. Bressler

Introduction

In Western countries, age-related macular degeneration is the principal cause of severe loss of central vision among adults aged 65 years or more. It can be classified into non-neovascular and neovascular forms. The non-neovascular form is characterized by macular drusen, abnormalities of the retinal pigment epithelium (including focal hyperpigmentation, non-geographic atrophy, and geographic atrophy), or both. The neovascular form may be accompanied by any or all of the features characteristic of the non-neovascular form, but its hallmark is the presence of choroidal neovascularization and related manifestations, including detachment of retinal pigment epithelium and subretinal fibrovascular and fibroglial (disciform) scars.

Epidemiology

Prevalence

The prevalence of age-related macular degeneration has been examined in several population-based studies with similar, but slightly varying, definitions and terminology. The Framingham Eye Study examined two-thirds of the surviving patients from the original Framingham Heart Study. Ophthalmological examinations were made on 2631 patients, 52 to 85 years old, over a 2-year period. Age-related macular degeneration was defined as visual acuity of 20/30 or less in association with one or more of the following: macular or perimacular drusen, pigment alterations (not secondary to another cause), elevation of retinal pigment epithelium, or circinate exudates. Based on these criteria, age-related macular degeneration was present in at least one eye of 5.7 per cent of the participants. Its prevalence increased with participants' age, being 1.2 per cent in those of 65 years or less, 6.4 per cent in those aged 65 to

Supported in part by the Heed Ophthalmic Fellowship Foundation (SF)

74 years, and 19.7 per cent in those of 75 years and more. Non-neovascular was 15 times more prevalent than neovascular age-related macular degeneration in this population.

The National Health and Nutrition Examination Survey examined 3056 participants, aged 45 to 64 years, over a 3-year period. Age-related macular degeneration was defined by visual acuity of 20/25 or less and the presence of drusen, disciform scarring, lipid, subretinal blood, or loss of the macular reflex with pigmentary disturbance. Disease prevalence varied with age and race. In Caucasian females or males of 45 to 64 years, the prevalence was 2.3 per cent, but increased to 7 per cent for females and 9.6 per cent for males of 65 to 75 years. African-American females and males of 45 to 64 years had a prevalence of 2.4 and 3.8 per cent, respectively, which increased to 11.4 per cent for females and 9.3 per cent for males of 65 to 75 years.

The Chesapeake Bay Watermen Study examined 777 men to determine the prevalence of individual characteristics of age-related macular degeneration. The prevalence of large, confluent, or soft drusen ranged from 4 to 6 per cent among the 50- to 59-year-olds; this was doubled among participants aged 60 to 69 and doubled again for those aged 70 to 79 years. Non-geographic was more common than geographic atrophy in each age group. The prevalence of neovascular age-related macular degeneration was 0.5 per cent among the total population studied.

The Beaver Dam Eye Study examined 4926 adult residents of Beaver Dam, Wisconsin, to determine the prevalence of specific fundus characteristics associated with age-related macular degeneration in this predominantly Caucasian population. Age-related maculopathy was defined as soft drusen, focal hyperpigmentation of retinal pigment epithelium, atrophy of retinal pigment epithelium, or evidence of choroidal neovascularization. Early age-related maculopathy was defined as the presence of any type of drusen except the hard, with degeneration of retinal pigment epithelium or increased retinal pigment in the macula. Late age-related maculopathy was defined as the presence of clinical signs of neovascular age-related macular degeneration or geographic atrophy. Visual acuity was not a criterion for disease classification. One or more drusen were present in 95.5 per cent of participants aged 43 to 84 years. The prevalence of age-related maculopathy increased with age in this population. The youngest group studied, those 43 to 54 years old, had a prevalence of 8.5 per cent, whereas the oldest group, those 75 years and older, had a prevalence of 37 per cent.

The Rotterdam Study examined 6251 participants over the age of 55 years residing in The Netherlands; the prevalence of atrophic or neovascular age-related macular degeneration was 1.7 per cent. Again, prevalence increased with age. In that study, atrophic age-related macular degeneration was defined as an area of well-demarcated atrophy of retinal pigment epithelium with visible choroidal vessels. Neovascular age-related macular degeneration was defined as serous or haemorrhagic detachment of retinal pigment epithelium, or subretinal neovascular membrane, or subretinal haemorrhage, or periretinal fibrous scar.

Although these population-based studies differ slightly in

their definitions and terminology, each found that the prevalence of age-related macular degeneration increased with age and that the non-neovascular form is more prevalent than the neovascular.

Incidence

Information on the incidence of individual features of age-related macular degeneration is provided by a follow-up study of the Chesapeake Bay watermen (see above), but the findings are limited by the relatively small, homogeneous population studied. In the follow-up study, 483 of the originial 777 participants underwent repeat ophthalmic examinations. At the initial examination, 412 participants age 30 years or more did not have large (> 63 μm) drusen; however, 5 years later, 8 per cent of these individuals had developed large drusen. The incidence of large drusen was age-related, increasing from 5 per cent among participants aged 30 to 39 years to 17 per cent in those 60 to 69 years old. Disappearance of drusen also was noted over time. Furthermore, increasing numbers of small drusen at the initial examination increased the risk of having developed larger drusen at the follow-up examination. Three per cent of the group without focal hyperpigmentation of retinal pigment epithelium initially developed this specific feature within the 5-year follow-up. The incidence of neovascular age-related macular degeneration was somewhat low, with only 1 of 474 participants developing choroidal neovascularization or disciform scarring during the follow-up.

Additional incidence data from a larger population are provided by a follow-up study from the Beaver Dam Eye Study (see above). Among the 3611 individuals who participated in the 5-year follow-up examination, the 5-year incidence of early age-related maculopathy (defined above) was about 8 per cent, whereas that of late age-related maculopathy (0.9 per cent) varied with age from 0 per cent in individuals of less than 55 years of age to almost 6 per cent for those of 75 years or more at baseline. These older participants were three and twelve times more likely to develop early and late age-related maculopathy, respectively, than those less than 55 years old. Women of 75 years or more were about eight times more likely to develop late age-related maculopathy than men in this age group. The risk of developing late age-related maculopathy was associated with the presence of soft drusen, confluent drusen, and focal hyperpigmentation of retinal pigment epithelium.

Risk factors

Numerous ocular, systemic, and personal risk factors have been reported to be associated with age-related macular degeneration without reference to whether the degeneration was non-neovascular or neovascular (Table 1). More recent studies have evaluated risk factors with reference to whether the specific form was non-neovascular (Table 2) or neovascular (Table 3).

Risk factors for age-related macular degeneration that cannot be modified include increasing age, positive family history, and race (for neovascular age-related macular degeneration). The observation that few African-Americans participated in the Macular Photocoagulation Study of neovascular age-related

Table 1 Risk factors for age-related macular degeneration (non-neovascular or neovascular)

Arteriosclerosis
Cerebrovascular disease
Left ventricular hypertrophy
Infrequent dietary intake of vitamins A and C
Reduced vital capacity or prior lung infection
Age
Decreased hand-grip strength
Hyperopia
Lower educational level
Short stature

Table 2 Risk factors for non-neovascular age-related macular degeneration

Positive family history
Positive smoking history
Higher calorie intake
Greater recent exposure to blue light and visible light (associated with geographic atrophy)
Higher plasma vitamin A
Light iris colour
High intake of saturated fat and cholesterol

Table 3 Risk factors for neovascular age-related macular degeneration

Diastolic blood pressure greater than 95 mmHg
Antihypertensive medication usage
Higher plasma vitamin A
Lower serum carotenoids
Lower serum antioxidant index
Light iris colour
Positive smoking history
Higher caloric intake
Elevated serum cholesterol
Lower serum cholesterol
Greater elastotic degeneration in sun-protected dermis
Greater exposure to blue light and visible light (associated with disciform scarring)
Positive family history
Increased beer consumption
Greater body mass index (kg/m²)

macular degeneration, when coupled with the findings of other studies, perpetuates the clinical impression that the neovascular form may be less prevalent among African-Americans than Caucasians. The Baltimore Eye Survey examined 2913 Caucasians and 2395 African-Americans aged 40 years or more, and determined that all blindness associated with age-related macular degeneration in this population was found only among the Caucasian participants. The Barbados Eye Study examined 3444 blacks residing in Barbados; the mean age of participants was 56 years and neovascular age-related macular degeneration was found in only 0.6 per cent of this group.

The identification of modifiable risk factors associated with age-related macular degeneration could provide insights for future studies on prevention and intervention. Multiple epidemiological studies have suggested a positive association between age-related macular degeneration and cigarette smoking. Epidemiological studies have been inconsistent in citing an association between hypertension and age-related macular degeneration, higher serum cholesterol, the presence of cardiovascular disease, or other risk factors for cardiovascular disease. The positive association of cigarette smoking, hypertension, cardiovascular disease, or other risk factors for cardiovascular disease with age-related macular degeneration does not necessarily indicate a causal relation, but it does provide yet another reason to try to minimize these habits and conditions. Epidemiological data are also inconsistent in finding an association between exposure to ultraviolet or visible light and age-related macular degeneration, as well as between specific serum concentrations of vitamins and micronutrients or dietary histories of the consumption of foods with various amounts of micronutrients. The use of sunglasses poses little, if any, risk to the patient and may reduce the risk of cataract; therefore, their use need not be discouraged. Until the results of clinical trials, such as the Age-Related Eye Disease Study, demonstrate that micronutrients are beneficial and clarify the potential risk of long-term toxicity, micronutrient supplementation probably should not be recommended to treat age-related eye disease (see below).

Clinical and angiographic features

Non-neovascular age-related macular degeneration

Drusen

Originating from the German word *drüse*, meaning gland, drusen are small, multiple, variably sized and shaped, yellow-white deposits at the level of the retinal pigment epithelium.

Small, hard drusen

Hard drusen are small, generally 63 μm or less in diameter, and typically have well-defined borders (Fig. 1). During fluorescein angiography, hard drusen may behave like transmission defects of the retinal pigment epithelium. In the early transit phase, thinning and depigmentation of the retinal pigment epithelium overlying the druse can lead to enhanced transmission of background choroidal fluorescence. Late in the angiogram, hard drusen fade as the background choroidal fluorescence normally fades. The histopathological equivalent of hard drusen may be lipidized retinal pigment epithelium cells or a focal collection of hyaline material in the inner and outer collagenous zones of Bruch's membrane.

Hard drusen are ubiquitous, noted in nearly 90 per cent of all age groups studied over the age of 30 years. For this reason, hard drusen are not considered sufficient to diagnose age-related macular degeneration. At present, there is no evidence that a few hard drusen increase the risk that an eye will develop

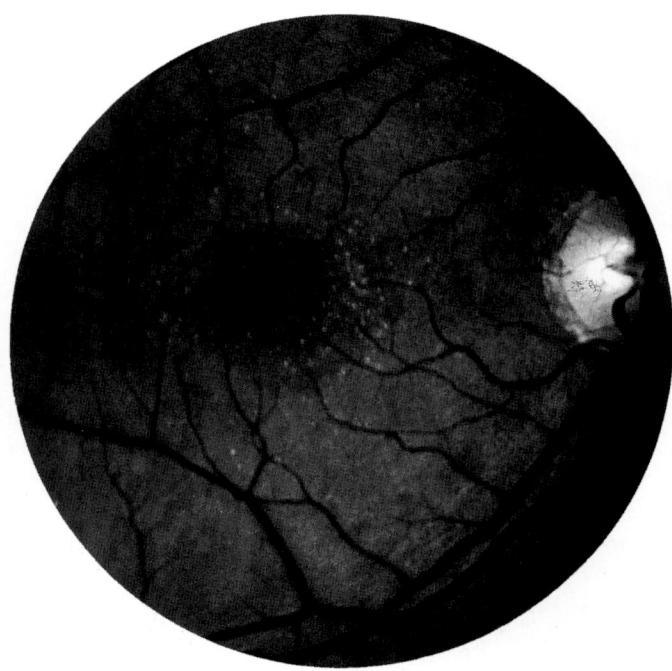

Fig. 1 Hard drusen: small, round, discrete, yellowish-white deposits are present in the posterior pole. (Printed with permission from the American Medical Association: Bressler *et al.* 1988.)

choroidal neovascularization, although increasing numbers of small, hard drusen may identify an eye at increased risk for developing large, soft drusen.

Large, soft drusen

Soft drusen are often large, measuring more than 63 μm in diameter, and have poorly demarcated borders (Fig. 2(a)). Soft drusen may merge with one another. During the transit phase of fluorescein angiography, soft drusen hyperfluoresce whenever there is hypopigmentation of the retinal pigment epithelium overlying them allowing increased visualization of background choroidal fluorescence. Alternatively, some soft drusen hyperfluoresce because material within Bruch's membrane stains with the dye or a cleft within the membrane allows pooling of the dye. Some soft drusen remain hyperfluorescent even in the late phase of the study. Histopathologically, soft drusen correspond either to diffuse thickening of the inner aspect of Bruch's membrane with hypopigmentation of overlying retinal pigment epithelium or to amorphous material located between the detached, thickened inner aspect and the remainder of Bruch's membrane (Fig. 2(b)).

Soft drusen are age-related and, in some patients, they represent a significant risk factor for the development of choroidal neovascularization. Soft drusen are considered an early feature of age-related macular degeneration.

Reticular pseudodrusen

Reticular pseudodrusen appear ophthalmoscopically as yellow, interlacing patterns of linear deposits at the level of the retinal pigment epithelium that are 125 to 250 μm wide and may be

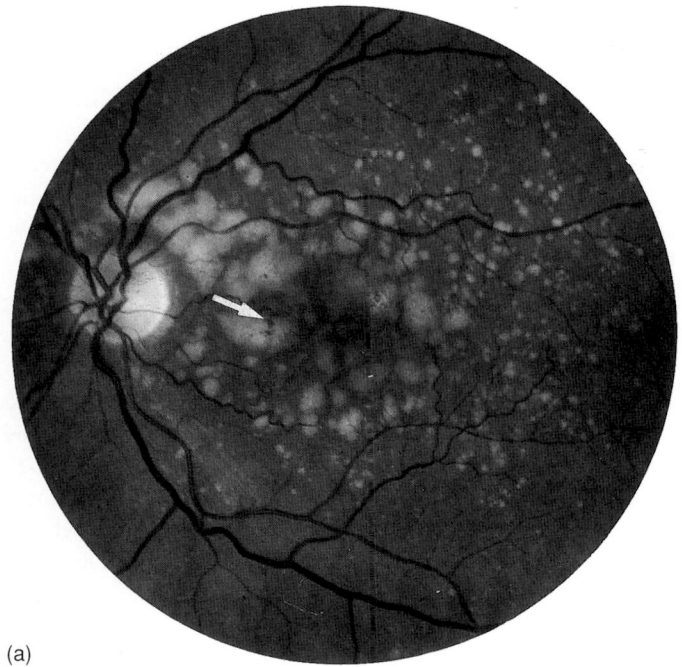

(a)

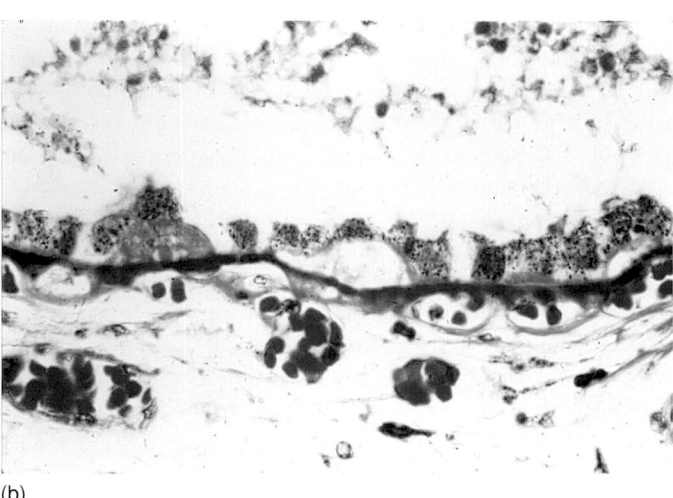

(b)

Fig. 2 (a) Soft drusen: these are larger than hard drusen and have poorly demarcated borders. Focal hyperpigmentation (arrow), corresponding to hyperplasia of retinal pigment epithelium at the level of the outer retina, may be associated. (Printed with permission from the American Medical Association: Bressler *et al.* 1988). (b) Histopathologically, there is either diffuse thickening of the inner aspect of Bruch's membrane with hypopigmentation of overlying retinal pigment epithelium or amorphous material between the detached, thickened inner aspect and the remainder of Bruch's membrane.

relatively flat, soft drusen. They are most prominent in the superotemporal macula but can continue circumferentially around the posterior pole (Fig. 3). Reticular pseudodrusen may not differ from typical soft drusen except for their prominent location in the superotemporal macular. Their lack of obvious hyperfluorescence during fluorescein angiography may be because of little depigmentation of the retinal pigment epithelium overlying the drusen material.

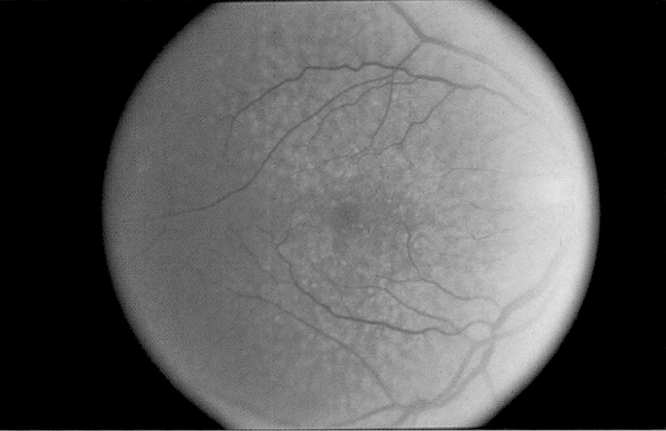

Fig. 3 Reticular pseudodrusen appear ophthalmoscopically as a yellow, interlacing pattern of linear deposits at the level of the retinal pigment epithelium.

Abnormalities of the retinal pigment epithelium

Focal hyperpigmentation
Focal hyperpigmentation is characterized by areas of increased pigmentation at the level of the outer retina (Fig. 2a) and corresponds to hyperplasia of retinal pigment epithelium. During the transit phase of fluorescein angiography, areas of focal hyperpigmentation of retinal pigment epithelium block choroidal fluorescence. Areas of hyperpigmentation seen clinically in eyes with non-neovascular age-related macular degeneration correlate histopathologically with areas of intraretinal pigment migration to the level of the photoreceptor nuclei. Eyes with hyperpigmentation do not necessarily harbour choroidal neovascularization, but have been associated with an increased risk of subsequently developing choroidal neovascularization.

Non-geographic atrophy
Non-geographic atrophy of the retinal pigment epithelium is seen clinically as an area of stippled, punctate depigmentation or hypopigmentation without increased visibility of the underlying choroidal vasculature (Fig. 4). In the affected area, the overlying retina may appear thinned. During the early phase of fluorescein angiography, non-geographic atrophy appears as a flat area of stippled hyperfluorescence. These hyperfluorescent areas may fade in the later phase of the study. Clinicopathological correlation shows mottled regions of relative depigmentation or hypopigmentation of the retinal pigment epithelium interspersed with clumps of hyperpigmentation overlying a diffusely thickened inner aspect of Bruch's membrane. Non-geographic atrophy in the fellow eye may identify patients at an increased risk of developing recurrent choroidal neovascularization after prior successful laser photocoagulation.

Geographic atrophy
Geographic atrophy appears as one or more sharply demarcated areas of depigmentation or hypopigmentation of the retinal pigment epithelium, usually with increased visibility of underlying choroidal vessels and associated thinning of the overlying retina

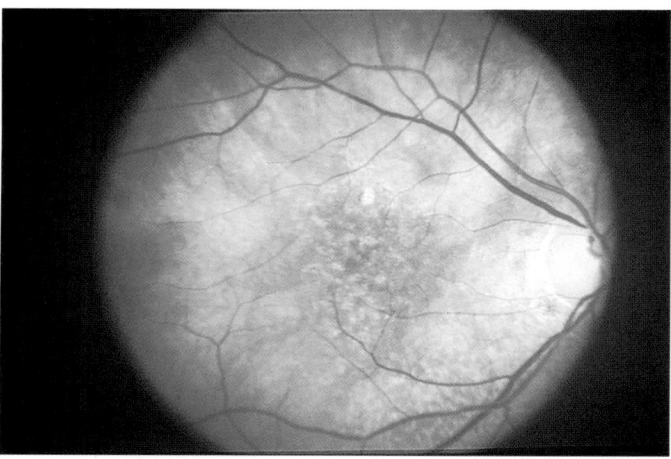

Fig. 4 Non-geographic atrophy of the retinal pigment epithelium is seen clinically as an area of depigmentation or hypopigmentation without increased visibility of the underlying choroidal vasculature.

(Fig. 5). Large, confluent drusen or small areas of reticulated hyper- and depigmentation may precede the development of geographic atrophy at a specific site. As soft drusen atrophy, glistening yellow specks may develop within them, representing calcification within drusen. With time, emerging areas of geographic atrophy coalesce into larger areas that extend more or less contiguously in a horseshoe pattern around the fovea. The geographic atrophy eventually surrounds and slowly progresses to engulf the foveal centre.

Fluorescein angiography demonstrates early, uniform hyperfluorescence throughout the area of geographic atrophy. The increased transmission of choroidal fluorescence may be due to hypopigmentation, depigmentation, attenuation, or absence of the retinal pigment epithelium. Later in the angiogram, the atrophic areas stain with fluorescein due to increased visibility of the normal staining of choroidal and scleral tissues. Histopathological examination of various stages of geographic

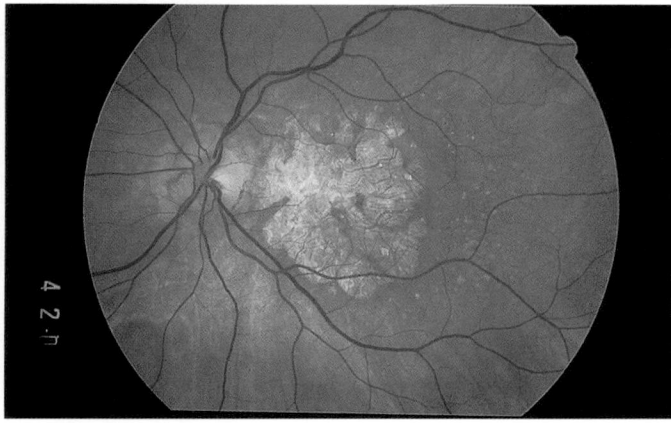

Fig. 5 Geographic atrophy appears as one or more sharply demarcated areas of depigmentation or hypopigmentation of the retinal pigment epithelium, usually with increased visibility of underlying choroidal vessels. A small remnant of remaining retinal tissue within the fovea has not yet been affected in this eye.

atrophy demonstrates the replacement of soft drusen with fibrous tissue or dystrophic calcification. With time, the overlying retinal pigment epithelium completely atrophies and exposes the underlying choroidal vasculature. The choriocapillaris may be sclerosed, with thickening of the intercapillary septa. As the retinal pigment epithelium atrophies, the overlying photoreceptors are secondarily lost, although it is often difficult to predict accurately the acuity from the anatomical configuration of the geographic atrophy.

Neovascular age-related macular degeneration

Neovascular age-related macular degeneration is characterized by the presence of choroidal neovascularization, which occurs when new capillaries grow from the choriocapillaris through Bruch's membrane and proliferate under the retinal pigment epithelium. The capillaries may eventually grow through the epithelium and proliferate in the subretinal space. The choroidal neovascularization itself is usually not visible ophthalmoscopically unless there is atrophy of the overlying retinal pigment epithelium. Rather, the neovascularization leads to multiple clinical signs suggesting its presence, such as subretinal haemorrhage, intraretinal or subretinal lipid or fluid, or serous detachment of the retinal pigment epithelium. Eventually the process leads to the development of subretinal fibrosis (disciform scar), with destruction of macular photoreceptors.

Choroidal neovascularization should be suspected in any patient with non-neovascular manifestations of age-related macular degeneration and a new history of metamorphopsia, a scotoma, or any sudden, non-specific change in visual acuity. A stereoscopic fluorescein angiogram should be obtained promptly to determine whether choroidal neovascularization is present, and if so, to determine if treatment is indicated. Visual acuity and the angiographic features of the choroidal neovascularization should be evaluated to determine if laser photocoagulation of the lesion should be considered.

Classic choroidal neovascularization

Classic choroidal neovascularization is present when the early phase of a fluorescein angiogram demonstrates a bright and fairly well-demarcated source of hyperfluorescence (Fig. 6(a)) that progressively leads to dye leakage and, often, to pooling within the subretinal space (Fig. 6(b)). A lacy capillary network may sometimes be visualized during the early phase of the angiogram, but this is not as common as in eyes with choroidal neovascularization from other causes such as the ocular histoplasmosis syndrome.

Occult choroidal neovascularization

Occult choroidal neovascularization may be recognized by one of two features, or a combination of both features, which have been termed fibrovascular pigment epithelial detachment and late leakage of an undetermined source. The identification of occult choroidal neovascularization is facilitated by a detailed review of stereoscopic frames from the entire fluorescein angiographic sequence.

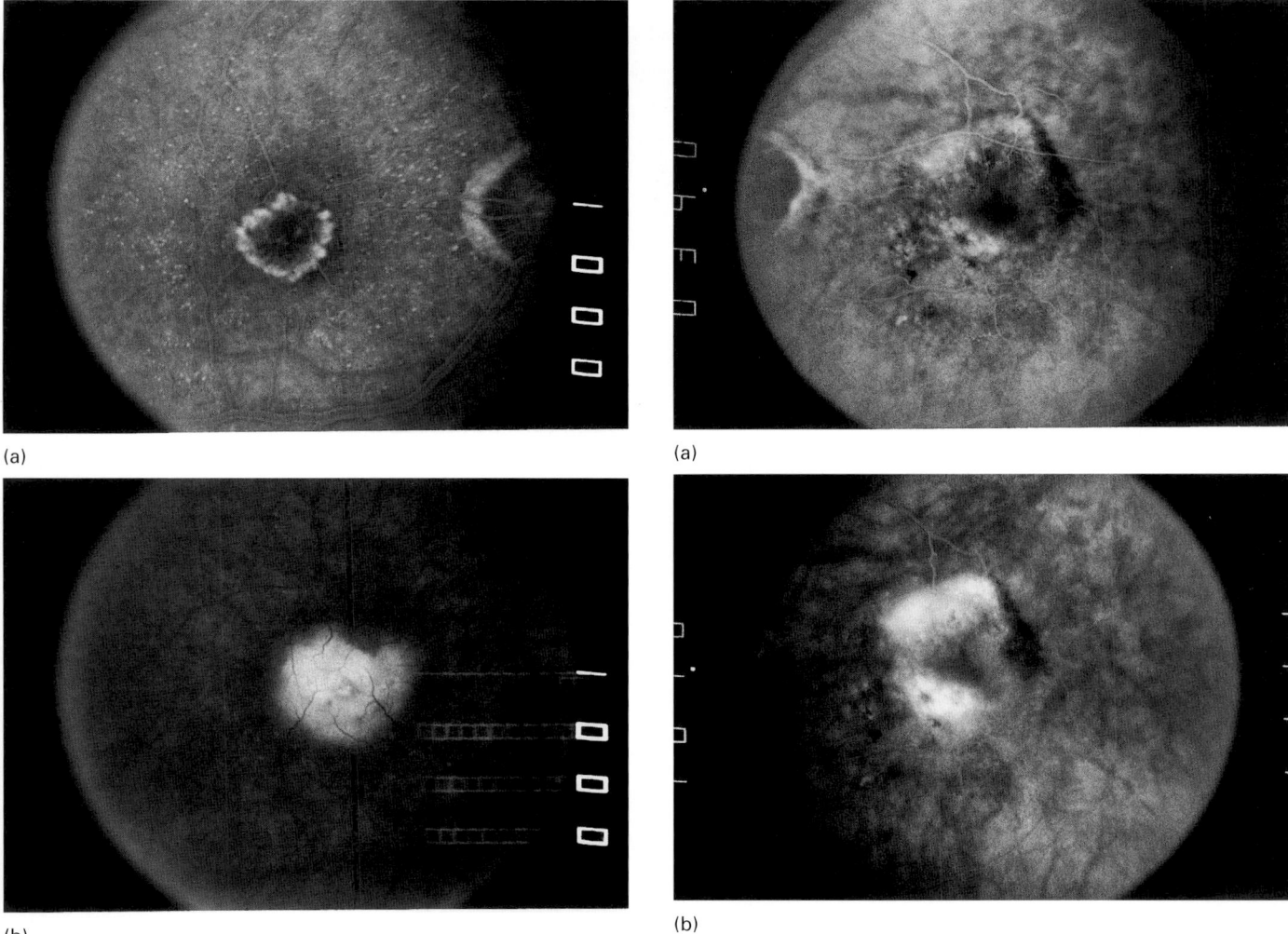

(a)

(b)

(a)

(b)

Fig. 6 (a) Fluorescein angiogram of classic choroidal neovascularization, early phase. A bright and fairly well-demarcated source of hyperfluorescence may suggest the presence of classic choroidal neovascularization. (b) Fluorescein angiogram of classic choroidal neovascularization, late phase. In the late-phase frames, fluorescein leakage, and often pooling within the subretinal space, from an earlier bright and fairly well-demarcated source of hyperfluorescence suggest the presence of classic choroidal neovascularization. (Printed with permission from the American Medical Association: Macular Photocoagulation Study Group, 1991.)

Fig. 7 (a,b) Fluorescein angiogram of occult choroidal neovascularization. An area of speckled hyperfluorescence, with poorly demarcated boundaries, becomes evident within an area of irregularly elevated retinal pigment epithelium 1 to 2 min after dye injection, consistent with a pattern of fibrovascular pigment epithelial detachment.

Fibrovascular pigment epithelial detachment

A stereoscopic fluorescein angiogram is helpful in detecting the irregular elevation of the retinal pigment epithelium that characterizes a fibrovascular pigment epithelial detachment. One to two minutes after the fluorescein injection, an area of speckled hyperfluorescence becomes evident within the irregularly elevated retinal pigment epithelium (Fig. 7). In comparison to classic choroidal neovascularization, this area of stippled hyperfluorescence becomes apparent later during the transit phase, does not appear as bright or as homogeneous, and may have boundaries that are either well- or poorly demarcated. These lesions stain with fluorescein or show leakage into the overlying subretinal space during the latest phases of the angiogram. Histopathologically, a fibrovascular pigment epithelial detach-

ment corresponds to choroidal neovascularization with interspersed fibrocellular tissue, which may account for the multifocal, punctate areas of blocked fluorescence observed angiographically. The irregular elevation of retinal pigment epithelium may be due to the fibrovascular tissue within Bruch's membrane, although fibrocellular or fibrovascular tissue also may be seen in the subretinal space between the photoreceptors and the retinal pigment epithelium.

Late leakage of an undetermined source

Late fluorescein leakage of an undetermined source is identified as an area of late, fuzzy hyperfluorescence that cannot be attributed to any focal sources of classic choroidal neovascularization or a fibrovascular pigment epithelial detachment in the early or middle phase of the angiogram (Fig. 8). This type of occult choroidal neovascularization always has poorly demarcated boundaries and often is appreciated by 5 to 10 min after dye

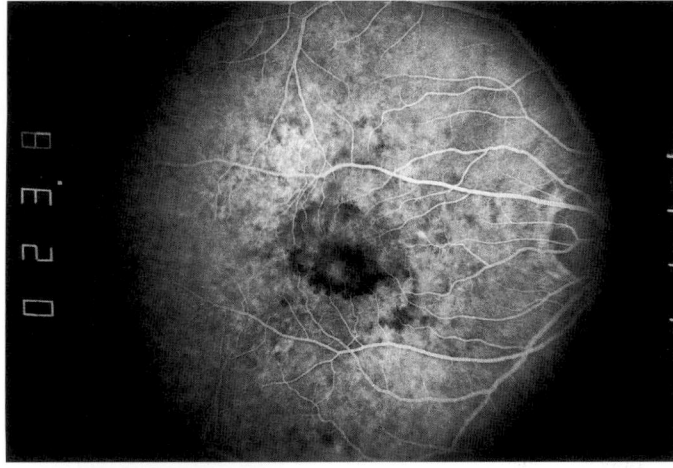

(a)

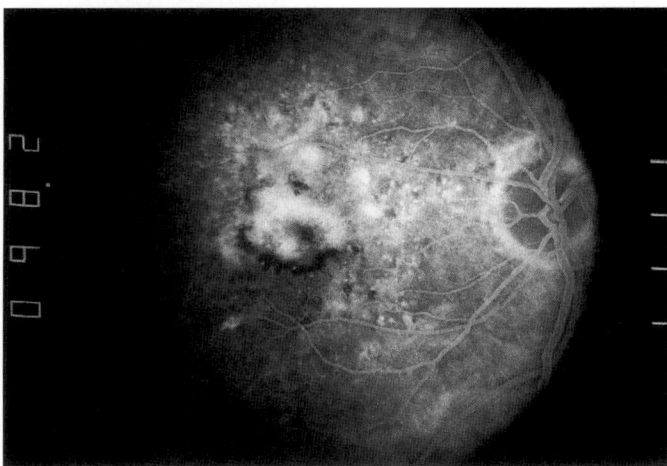

(b)

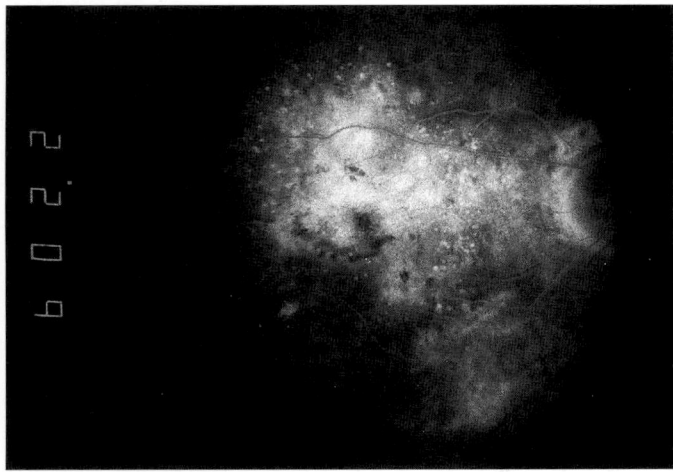

(c)

Fig. 8 Occult choroidal neovascularization represented by a pattern of late fluorescein leakage of an undetermined source. In the mid-phase of the angiogram (b), pinpoint areas of speckled hyperfluorescence and larger areas of hyperfluorescence, with collection of dye leakage in the overlying subretinal space in the later phase (c), are present. The late leakage (c) cannot be attributed to any focal sources of classic choroidal neovascularization or fibrovascular pigment epithelial detachment in the early (a) or middle phase (b) of the angiogram. (Printed with permission from the American Medical Association: Macular Photocoagulation Study Group, 1991).

injection. Histopathologically, late leakage corresponds to choroidal neovascularization.

Features of choroidal neovascularization boundaries

The boundaries of choroidal neovascularization may be either well or poorly demarcated. The term 'well demarcated' should not be used synonymously with classic choroidal neovascularization, and the term 'poorly demarcated' should not be used synonymously with occult choroidal neovascularization, since the boundaries of the angiographic pattern of both classic and occult choroidal neovascularization (fibrovascular pigment epithelial detachment) may be well demarcated. When the boundaries of the lesion of choroidal neovascularization are well demarcated, its location may be described as extra-, juxta-, or subfoveal. When the posterior boundary of the lesion is at least 200 μm from the foveal centre, it is considered extrafoveal. If its posterior boundary lies between 1 and 199 μm from the foveal centre, the choroidal neovascularization is classified as juxtafoveal. Subfoveal choroidal neovascularization underlies the geometric centre of the foveal avascular zone.

Angiographic features obscuring boundaries

Three features that commonly interfere with defining the angiographic boundaries of choroidal neovascularization (classic and occult) include blocked fluorescence presumably due to fibrous tissue or hyperpigmentation or both, blocked fluorescence due to thick blood adjacent to the neovascularization, and hyperfluorescence due to a serous pigment epithelial detachment. When these features are contiguous with areas of choroidal neovascularization, they are considered components of the lesion as they may harbour neovascularization beneath them. Accordingly, these areas are taken into account when considering the size of the lesion that might receive laser photocoagulation.

Blocked fluorescence is identified in stereoscopic frames of the middle and late fluorescein angiogram. Thick blood may be present in the subretinal or subretinal pigment epithelial space and also is identified as dense blockage of choroidal fluorescence throughout the angiogram. A serous pigment epithelial detachment demonstrates early, uniform bright hyperfluorescence on fluorescein angiography, with a smooth contour to the elevated retinal pigment epithelium. Serous pigment epithelial detachments usually have minimal to no leakage into the overlying subretinal space.

Other angiographic features associated with choroidal neovascularization

Feeder vessels

Feeder vessels are of choroidal origin and supply an area of choroidal neovascularization that leaks in the later phases of an angiogram (Fig. 9). Visible during the transit phase, feeder vessels may be seen in previously untreated eyes where choroidal neovascularization peripheral to the feeder may be connected by the vessels to more central choroidal neovascularization that is beginning to form a disciform scar. Feeder vessels may also extend from an area of laser treatment, across the edge

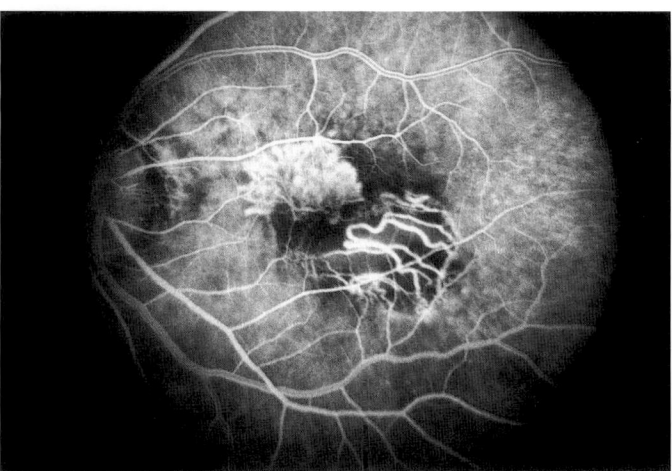

Fig. 9 Feeder vessel, visible during the transit phase, is of choroidal origin. It extends from an area of previous laser treatment to adjacent recurrent choroidal neovascularization. (Printed with permission from the American Medical Association: Macular Photocoagulation Study Group, 1991.)

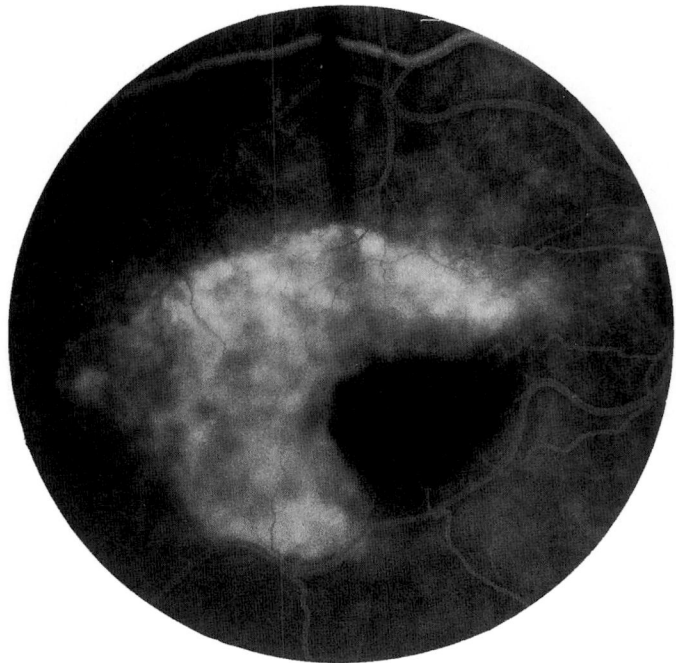

(a)

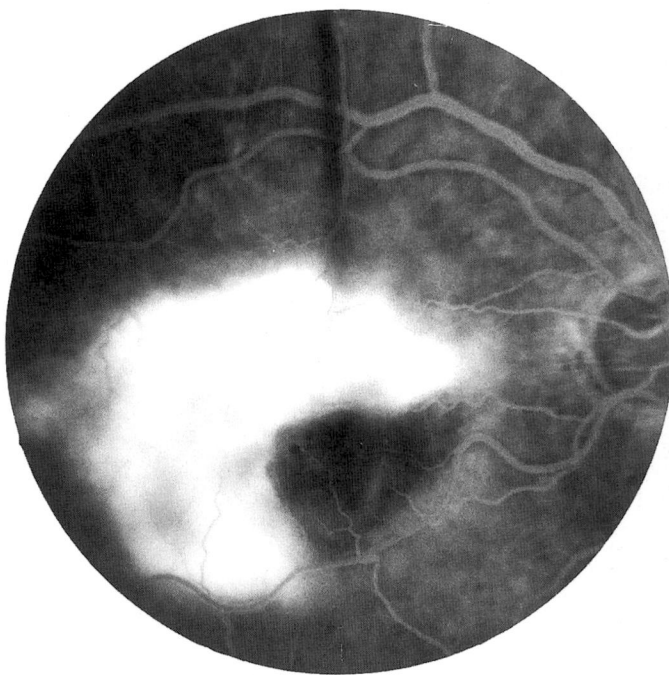

(b)

Fig. 10 Fluorescein angiogram of a tear of the retinal pigment epithelium. An early transit frame (a) demonstrates sharp, well-demarcated hyperfluorescence with continued intense staining in a later frame (b) with minimal dye leakage. The redundant, folded, torn retinal pigment epithelium blocks fluorescence.

of the treated area, to an area of recurrent choroidal neovascularization.

Loculated fluid

Loculated fluid is an angiographic finding that may accompany choroidal neovascularization and needs to be differentiated from the choroidal neovascularization itself to avoid confusion when defining the extent of the lesion. Loculated fluid may be found in the late phase of an angiogram as an area of well-demarcated, bright hyperfluorescence. However, it is pooling of dye into a compartmentalized space anterior to choroidal neovascularization leakage. Sometimes loculated fluid may collect in a typical cystoid pattern. Loculated fluid may obscure the underlying choroidal neovascularization and its boundary should not necessarily be interpreted as the boundary of the lesion, which must be defined in an earlier phase of the study whenever this feature is present.

Retinal pigment epithelial tear

A tear of the retinal pigment epithelium (Fig. 10) may occur spontaneously in eyes with neovascular age-related macular degeneration, a serous pigment epithelial detachment, or as a complication of laser photocoagulation of choroidal neovascularization. Since the retinal pigment epithelium is absent within the tear and cannot provide a barrier to the free movement of fluid, an overlying neurosensory detachment may be present. However, a secondary neurosensory detachment may be absent if the osmotic pressure of the choroid is higher than that of the subretinal space, allowing sufficient fluid absorption despite the absence of retinal pigment epithelium. The prognosis for vision in an eye with a tear in the retinal pigment epithelium is variable, but when accompanied by choroidal neovascularization it is usually poor.

During fluorescein angiography, early, intense, uniform, and well-demarcated hyperfluorescence occurs within the torn area as dye within the choriocapillaris stains the choroidal and

scleral tissues. The scrolled-up retinal pigment epithelium on one side of the tear is seen as a ridge of blocked fluorescence. In the frames of the later phase, the torn area stains with fluorescein, with dye leakage into the subretinal space in those eyes with an overlying neurosensory detachment.

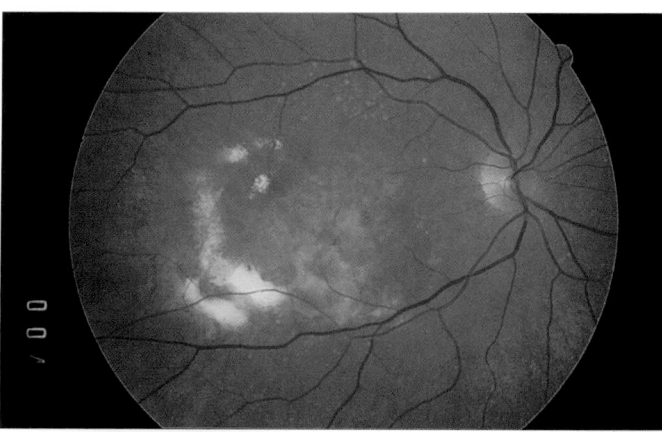

Fig. 11 Disciform scar: fibrous tissue accompanies the ingrowth of neovascular tissue, eventually leading to the development of subretinal fibrosis termed a disciform scar.

Subretinal haemorrhage

Choroidal neovascularization is often accompanied by subretinal haemorrhage along its perimeter. In some cases the haemorrhage may be extensive, and it may obscure much of the choroidal neovascularization and directly underlie the foveal centre. Visual outcome is variable in these eyes; a few improve and the majority deteriorate. A clinical trial to evaluate the surgical removal of extensive subretinal haemorrhages should include an adequate sample size with randomization between surgery and observation to determine the potential long-term benefits.

Aspirin use has not been shown to affect visual outcome in eyes with neovascular age-related macular degeneration. The presence of choroidal neovascularization with haemorrhage has not been proved to be an indication for stopping systemic medications that affect the clotting cascade or platelet function if such medications were medically indicated in a particular patient. Although some patients with subretinal haemorrhages may be using medications that alter haemostasis, such medications are commonly prescribed and their use may be coincidental.

Vitreous haemorrhage

Any bleeding from choroidal neovascularization may potentially extend into the vitreous cavity. If vitreous haemorrhage obscures visualization of fundus detail, B-scan ultrasonography may exclude the presence of a coexisting retinal tear or detachment, or of choroidal melanoma. If no tumour or peripheral vitreoretinal pathology are identified and the fellow eye has evidence of age-related macular degeneration, then choroidal neovascularization as the source of the vitreous haemorrhage becomes a realistic possibility. The vitreous haemorrhage will clear spontaneously in a majority of these eyes, but a pars plana vitrectomy may restore peripheral vision in cases that prove not to clear.

Disciform scar

Fibrous tissue accompanies the ingrowth of neovascular tissue, eventually leading to the development of a disciform scar (Fig. 11). Disciform scars represent a continuum between choroidal neovascularization, choroidal neovascularization with visible scar, and mature scar. In a mature scar, fibrovascular tissue replaces the choriocapillaris–basement membrane–retinal pigment epithelium–photoreceptor layers, resulting in a permanent scotoma. The ophthalmoscopic appearance of the disciform process varies depending on the extent of associated proliferation or atrophy of retinal pigment epithelium, the degree of fibrous tissue proliferation, the amount of coexistent leaking choroidal neovascularization, and the presence or absence of a chorioretinal anastomosis.

The disciform process may occur eccentric to the posterior pole. Eccentric disciforms may be large, irregularly shaped, and accompanied by significant retinal or vitreous haemorrhage. B-scan ultrasonography may be necessary to rule out a malignancy and support the diagnosis of an eccentric disciform in some of these cases.

Indocyanine-green videoangiography

Indocyanine-green videoangiography absorbs and emits fluorescence in the near-infrared wavelengths of light. Infrared light can theoretically penetrate haemorrhage, xanthophyll, melanin, and turbid fluid better than the visible light used in fluorescein angiography. These properties make indocyanine-green angiography an attractive alternative in evaluating eyes with choroidal neovascularization, pigment epithelial detachment, and subretinal haemorrhage. Preliminary work has been done with indocyanine green to evaluate occult choroidal neovascularization and guide laser management in selected cases. However, randomized trials that have demonstrated a significant benefit of laser treatment for choroidal neovascularization have used fluorescein angiography to define the extent of the lesion for photocoagulation. Indocyanine-green angiography has not yet been used to guide laser treatment of choroidal neovascularization in any randomized trials. There is no reason to assume that defining a lesion with indocyanine green and applying a treatment shown to be of value based on fluorescein angiographic features will yield outcomes that are any better or worse than basing the lesion definition on fluorescein angiography. When and if data become available showing that patients treated on the basis of features demonstrated by indocyanine green have better outcomes than untreated patients or those treated on the basis of fluorescein angiographic features, then indocyanine green may be reliably integrated into patient care for age-related macular degeneration. Until that time, indocyanine green-guided treatment of choroidal neovascularization should probably be done within trials designed to determine if it affects vision outcome in patients with neovascular age-related macular degeneration.

Differential diagnosis

Macular or perimacular alterations in the pigmentation of retinal pigment epithelium may be attributed to a variety of ocular conditions other than non-neovascular age-related macular degeneration (Table 4). Basal laminar drusen present as innumerable, small, uniformly sized, discretely round, slightly raised, subretinal lesions seen best with fluorescein angiography

Table 4 Differential diagnosis of non-neovascular age-related macular degeneration

Basal laminar (cuticular) drusen
Dominant drusen in young patients
Pattern dystrophy of the retinal pigment epithelium:
   Adult vitelliform dystrophy
   Adult-onset foveomacular pigment epithelial dystrophy
Bull's eye maculopathy

in middle-aged patients. Pattern dystrophy of the retinal pigment epithelium presents as a reticulated pattern of pigmentation, usually symmetrical between the two eyes, and often in the absence of more typical soft drusen. These dystrophies may show a yellowish deposition at the level of the outer retina, often overlying a central area of greenish hyperpigmentation, and are occasionally surrounded by a petalloid pattern of hyperpigmentation more obvious on fluorescein angiography. Age of onset, symptoms, detailed medical history, visual acuity, fluorescein angiography, and examination of family members may be helpful in establishing a specific diagnosis.

Choroidal neovascularization may be attributed to many ocular conditions other than age-related macular degeneration (Table 5). A thorough history and associated ophthalmoscopic findings will provide clues to the aetiological diagnosis. The presence of peripapillary and peripheral, focal atrophic areas of the retinal pigment epithelium will confirm the diagnosis of the ocular histoplasmosis syndrome. A highly myopic refractive error or an elongated axial length in an eye without large, soft drusen will suggest the diagnosis of pathological myopia as the cause of the choroidal neovascularization. In the presence of large, soft drusen or abnormalities of retinal pigment epithelium in a patient over the age of 50 years, however, choroidal neovascularization is most probably due to age-related macular degeneration.

Subretinal blood may develop in the absence of choroidal neovascularization in cases of retinal macroaneurysm, a lacquer

Table 5 Differential diagnosis of neovascular age-related macular degeneration

Ocular histoplasmosis syndrome
Angioid streaks
Pathological myopia
Optic-disc drusen
Choroidal rupture
Idiopathic
Other inflammatory diseases (e.g. multifocal choroiditis, serpiginous choroidopathy)
Macular neurosensory detachments may be associated with central serous chorioretinopathy, choroidal tumours, or choirdal inflammatory processes
Subretinal haemorrhage may be associated with retinal macroaneurysm, posterior vitreous detachment, lacquer cracks, choroidal tumours, retinal venous occlusive disease
Pseudovitelliform detachments with basal laminar drusen

crack in pathological myopia, tramautic choroidal rupture, posterior vitreous detachment, choroidal tumours, or occasionally retinal vascular occlusive disease. Subretinal fluid also may occur in the absence of choroidal neovascularization, for example, in eyes with central serous chorioretinopathy, choroidal inflammatory conditions, or choroidal tumours.

Natural history

Drusen

Limited data are available on the natural course of non-neovascular age-related macular degeneration in patients with bilateral evidence of the disease but no choroidal neovascularization. Small retrospective studies of patients with non-neovascular age-related macular degeneration limited to evidence of bilateral drusen at baseline suggest that 8.5 to 18 per cent will lose vision to the level of 20/200 or worse, in at least one eye, when followed for an average period of 4 to 5 years. Almost all loss of vision in these patients is due to the development of choroidal neovascularization. This conclusion may not necessarily be applicable to the total population of people who have non-neovascular age-related macular degeneration, since the studies quoted are retrospective reviews of patients who presented to tertiary referral centres. In a prospective study of 126 patients with non-neovascular age-related macular degeneration defined as bilateral drusen at baseline, 56 were available for the 3-year follow-up examination. Among these 56 patients, the 3-year cumulative incidence of the development of a neovascular lesion, defined as any occult or 'manifest' choroidal neovascularization or pigment epithelial detachment, was 13 per cent. The cumulative incidence increased to 18 per cent at 3 years in the subgroup of individuals who were 65 years or older. The Age-Related Eye Disease Study, a multicentre national trial in the United States, is prospectively following over 3000 individuals with non-neovascular age-related macular degeneration. Within the next decade, more precise information on its natural history should be available in this large group of patients.

The Macular Photocoagulation Study Group has reported that the fellow or non-study eyes of patients with age-related macular degeneration with neovascular age-related macular degeneration in the study eye but no evidence of neovascular maculopathy in the fellow eye at baseline are unlikely to develop loss of vision during 5 years of follow-up unless choroidal neovascularization has developed. Fellow eyes without neovascular maculopathy at baseline and at the 5-year follow-up visit suffered an average loss of vision of 0.4 lines, whereas eyes that developed choroidal neovascularization during follow-up developed an average loss of 8 lines of vision. Rates of progression to neovascular maculopathy in the second eye have varied from 3 to 7 per cent per year. In the Macular Photocoagulation Study Group argon–age-related macular degeneration trial, in which data were collected in a prospective fashion and few data were lost during the follow-up period, 28 per cent of these fellow eyes developed choroidal neovascularization over 5 years, at a fairly steady pace of 6 per cent per year.

Specific fundus features of non-neovascular age-related macular degeneration can be evaluated in the fellow eyes of patients with unilateral neovascular maculopathy to predict the rate of progression to neovascular disease in the second eye. The risk of developing choroidal neovascularization in a fellow eye that has small drusen and no large drusen or focal hyperpigmentation may be as low as 10 per cent over 5 years; whereas fellow eyes with either large drusen or focal hyperpigmentation within 1500 μm of the foveal centre may have up to a 30 per cent risk of developing choroidal neovascularization. These risk factors appear to be additive, as those with both large drusen and focal hyperpigmentation have at least a 58 per cent risk of developing choroidal neovascularization within 5 years.

Geographic atrophy

Geographic atrophy usually begins outside the foveal centre, as demonstrated in one study of 208 patients. One way geographic atrophy may progress is to involve areas initially affected by incipient or non-geographic atrophy. These areas are characterized by regions of diffuse, stippled hyperpigmentation and hypopigmentation of retinal pigment epithelium. Alternately, geographic atrophy can progress by resorption of confluent patches of soft drusen. The precise rate at which geographic atrophy progresses, as well as the rate at which significant scotomas form and compromise visual function, remain under investigation. Eyes with geographic atrophy may still be at risk of developing choroidal neovascularization, especially when noted in the fellow eye of a patient whose first eye has choroidal neovascularization.

If a subretinal haemorrhage develops in an eye with geographic atrophy, it does not necessarily imply the presence of choroidal neovascularization. These haemorrhages may represent the rupture of normal choriocapillaries, as described in eyes with pathological myopia. In one study, eight patients with geographic atrophy developed small subretinal haemorrhages that spontaneously cleared over a mean follow-up period of 15 months without developing clinical evidence of choroidal neovascularization.

Choroidal neovascularization

In the Macular Photocoagulation Study, the study eyes that were assigned randomly to observation provide a wealth of information on the course of choroidal neovascularization. Among the untreated eyes with extrafoveal choroidal neovascularization, mean visual acuity was 20/200 at the 5-year examination, with 62 per cent experiencing at least a 6-line fall in their visual acuity since presentation. Among untreated eyes with juxtafoveal choroidal neovascularization, the median visual acuity was 20/250 at the 5-year examination, with 61 per cent losing 6 lines or more of acuity from their baseline level. Among untreated eyes with new subfoveal choroidal neovascularization (no prior laser treatment), the median visual acuity was 20/500 at the 4-year examination and 47 per cent of these

eyes lost 6 lines or more from their baseline level of visual acuity. Among untreated eyes with recurrent subfoveal choroidal neovascularization, the mean visual acuity was 20/320 at the 3-year examination and 36 per cent of these eyes lost 6 lines or more from their baseline level of visual acuity.

The Macular Photocoagulation Study Group's subfoveal studies were restricted to eyes with relatively small lesions that had evidence of classic choroidal neovascularization and well-demarcated boundaries. The natural history of choroidal neovascular lesions with poorly demarcated boundaries and either occult choroidal neovascularization alone or classic and occult choroidal neovascularization in combination was retrospectively reviewed in a study of 84 eyes. Eighty-nine per cent of these lesions initially involved the foveal centre, and the average initial visual acuity was 20/80. After an average follow-up of 28 months, the mean visual acuity had fallen to 20/250. Two-thirds of these lesions progressed to disciform scarring during follow-up, while one-third continued to demonstrate occult choroidal neovascularization without associated scarring at the final examination. Severe loss of vision ($\geq$ 6 lines) developed in 53 per cent of eyes with disciform scarring and in only 21 per cent of those with persistent occult disease ($p < 0.006$). In another retrospective review of 82 untreated eyes with occult choroidal neovascularization only, the mean initial visual acuity was 20/40, and 32 per cent of lesions involved the foveal centre initially. After a mean follow-up of 34 months, the mean visual acuity had decreased to 20/70. Eleven per cent progressed to disciform scarring, and 40 per cent developed severe visual loss. A more recent prospective study demonstrated that 25 per cent of untreated eyes with occult choroidal neovascularization only (no classic choroidal neovascularization) had not lost any vision 3 years after presentation. However, 41 per cent had lost over 3 lines of vision by 12 months after entry into the study: 40 per cent of these eyes had developed classic choroidal neovascularization by 3 months and a further 30 per cent by 12 months. Eyes with asymptomatic occult choroidal neovascularization only and excellent vision, however, may not have the same natural history as those in that study by the Macular Photocoagulation Study Group since their study's eyes were symptomatic and had decreased visual acuity at presentation. In another recent prospective study, 38 per cent of untreated eyes with poorly demarcated, subfoveal, occult choroidal neovascularization and no classic choroidal neovascularization had severe loss of visual acuity by 24 months.

Management

Non-neovascular age-related macular degeneration

The management of non-neovascular age-related macular degeneration was reviewed recently (see Bressler, 1995 in Further Reading). There are at present no means of preventing the development or progression of this form of age-related macular degeneration. Patients with this form should be educated about the potential risk of progression to neovascular disease. Each patient should be taught to monitor their central acuity regularly in a monocular fashion. New symptoms of metamorphopsia, scotoma, or other changes in acuity should be brought to their ophthalmologist's attention promptly. Repeat examination to look for choroidal neovascularization will often be needed under these circumstances. A low-vision evaluation may be required in patients with geographic atrophy or extensive, foveal, non-geographic atrophy.

Oral micronutrient supplementation

As outlined above, the long-term ocular and systemic effects of oral micronutrient supplementation are currently unknown, although multiple epidemiological studies have reported lower rates of age-related macular degeneration in individuals with higher serum concentrations or dietary intake of a variety of antioxidants. One small, prospective, randomized, controlled trial with no more than 24 months of follow-up suggested that oral zinc supplementation may delay loss of vision in patients with non-neovascular age-related macular degeneration. In fact, in the Eye Disease Case-Control Study, a higher serum zinc was found in patients with neovascular age-related macular degeneration than in controls. Long-term evaluation was not done in the small trial mentioned above, and, consequently, the existence and magnitude of long-term benefits or side-effects from zinc remain unknown. Confirmation of the preliminary findings from the zinc trial in a larger number of patients followed for an extended period of time is being sought in the Age-Related Eye Disease Study, which is prospectively following patients with varying degrees of non-neovascular age-related macular degeneration, with random assignment to micronutrient therapy consisting of antioxidants alone, zinc alone, both nutrients, or placebo. (Effects on age-related lens changes also are under investigation in this study.) A clearer understanding of long-term benefits for vision and morphology as well as of the potential toxicity of these agents should become available through this endeavour. The Physicians' Health Study and the Women's Health Study are two other trials evaluating systemic effects of antioxidant vitamins, and these trials should provide supporting information on the role of vitamin supplementation in age-related macular degeneration.

Prophylactic laser

Macular laser photocoagulation appears to promote the resolution of large, soft drusen. Gass first observed the disappearance of drusen in areas near laser scars in 1973. In a pilot study of 20 eyes with confluent soft drusen, argon green-laser treatment of each soft druse in the temporal macula led to the disappearance of both treated and untreated drusen in all 20 eyes at a mean of 2 and 10 months, respectively. The mechanism by which drusen disappear in these photocoagulated eyes remains unknown. Several multicentre trials are currently seeking to evaluate the effectiveness of macular laser in eyes with soft drusen in preventing the subsequent development of choroidal neovascularization and loss of vision. Strategies under investigation include limited scatter treatment of the macula or focal treatment directed specifically at soft drusen. Potential complications, such as the development of geographic atrophy or iatrogenic induction of choroidal neovascularization, will be monitored in these prospective trials.

Neovascular age-related macular degeneration

Laser photocoagulation

Several randomized clinical trials have demonstrated the effectiveness of laser photocoagulation in treating choroidal neovascularization that meets specific criteria, whether extrafoveal or subfoveal in location (Table 6).

Indications and treatment benefit

Extrafoveal choroidal neovascularization A well-demarcated lesion of extrafoveal choroidal neovascularization, consisting of classic choroidal neovascularization with or without a component of occult choroidal neovascularization, is a candidate for laser treatment. Intense and confluent photocoagulation should cover the lesion and extend 100 µm beyond the boundaries of all its components.

In the Macular Photocoagulation Study Group's argon–age-related macular degeneration trial, 64 per cent of the untreated eyes developed severe visual loss 5 years after entry compared to 46 per cent of the treated eyes (RR = 1.5, p = 0.001). Untreated eyes lost, on average, two additional lines of vision as compared to treated eyes (p = 0.01). Five years after entry, the mean visual acuity was 20/200 in the untreated group and 20/125 in the treated group (p = 0.002). Recurrent choroidal neovascularization had occurred in 54 per cent of treated eyes by 5 years. Those eyes that developed recurrences had a worse mean visual outcome (20/250) at the 5-year examination than those that did not (20/50). Seventy-five per cent of the recurrences occurred within the first post-treatment year.

Juxtafoveal choroidal neovascularization A well-demarcated lesion of juxtafoveal choroidal neovascularization, consisting of classic choroidal neovascularization with or without a component of occult choroidal neovascularization, is a candidate for laser treatment. Intense and confluent treatment should cover all lesion components. Treatment along the foveal edge should extend only up to the perimeter of the lesion, attempting to avoid extension through the foveal centre. If the posterior boundary of the choroidal neovascularization is more than 100 µm from that centre, and there is contiguous blood on the foveal side, then treatment should extend 100 µm into the blood and not beyond it. On the non-foveal side of the lesion, photocoagulation should extend 100 µm beyond the perimeter of the lesion.

In the Macular Photocoagulation Study Group's krypton–age-related macular degeneration study, 61 per cent of untreated eyes had developed severe visual loss 5 years after entry compared to 52 per cent of treated eyes (RR = 1.2, p = 0.04). The untreated eyes had lost, on average, 1.2 lines more of visual acuity than the treated eyes at the 5-year examination. The median 5-year visual acuity was 20/250 in untreated and 20/200 in treated eyes (p = 0.02).

The estimated 5-year rate of persistent or recurrent chor-

Table 6 Laser management of choroidal neovascularization (CNV)

Entity	Lesion location and angiographic characteristics	Laser technique	Post-treatment visual acuity	Untreated visual acuity	Persistence and/or recurrence frequency and outcome
Extrafoveal CNV[1]	Posterior edge of classic CNV (and blockage by pigment or blood, if present) 200–2500 μm from foveal centre	Cover CNV, contiguous blockage and 100 μm beyond	At 5 years: 46 per cent ≥ 6-line loss Mean: 20/125	At 5 years: 64 per cent ≥ 6-line loss Mean: 20/200	Treated eyes at 5 years: REC: 54 per cent ≥6 line loss: 78 per cent with REC 17 per cent without REC
Juxtafoveal CNV[2]	Posterior edge of classic CNV 1–199 μm from foveal centre or Posterior edge of classic CNV >199 μm from foveal centre with blockage by pigment or blood <200 μm from foveal centre	*Non-foveal side*: Cover CNV, contiguous blockage, and 100 μm beyond *Foveal side*: Cover CNV, if CNV > 100 μm from foveal centre and contiguous blood is present, also cover contiguous blood up to 100 μm beyond CNV	At 5 years: 49 per cent ≥ 6-line loss Mean: 20/200	At 5 years: 58 per cent ≥ 6-line loss Mean: 20/250	Treated eyes at 4 years: PER: 58 per cent REC: 76 per cent ≥ 6-line loss: 58 per cent with PER 69 per cent with REC 16 per cent without PER/REC
New subfoveal CNV[3,4] (≤3.5 MPS DA)	CNV under foveal centre	Cover CNV, blockage, and 100 μm beyond	At 4 years: 22 per cent ≥ 6-line loss Mean: 20/320	At 4 years: 47 per cent ≥ 6-line loss Mean: 20/500	Treated eyes at 3 years: PER: 13 per cent REC: 35 per cent ≥ 6-line loss: 36 per cent with PER 19 per cent with REC 27 per cent without PER/REC
Recurrent subfoveal CNV[4,5] (≤6.0 MPS DA)	Recurrent CNV under foveal centre	Cover CNV, blockage, and 100 μm beyond[6]	At 3 years: 12 per cent ≥ 6-line loss Mean: 20/250	At 3 years: 36 per cent ≥ 6-line loss Mean: 20/320	Treated eyes at 2 years: PER: 13 per cent REC: 35 per cent ≥6-line loss: 10 per cent with PER 13 per cent with REC 10 per cent without PER/REC

REC, recurrence; PER, persistence.
Data after Bressler (1993).
[1]Macular Photocoagulation Study Group (MPS) (1982); MPS (1986); MPS (1991b).
[2]MPS (1990a); MPS (1990b).
[3]MPS (1991a); MPS (1991c); MPS (1993b); MPS (1994b); MPS (1994d).
[4]At least some CNV must be classic; CNV (either classic or occult) must underlie the foveal centre; any occult CNV (fibrovascular pigment epithelial detachment) must have well-demarcated boundaries; features that could obscure boundaries of CNV (such as blood or elevated blocked fluorescence) must be smaller in area other than CNV.
[5]MPS (1991a); MPS (1991d); MPS (1993d); MPS (1994d).
[6]At interface between recurrence and prior laser, extend treatment spots 300 μm into prior laser scar; cover feeder vessels 100 μm beyond lateral border and 300 μm radially beyond base (origin) of feeder vessel.

oidal neovascularization among the treated eyes in that study was 78 per cent. Treated eyes that developed recurrent choroidal neovascularization had a worse mean visual outcome (20/250) than treated eyes that escaped this complication (20/80) ($p < 0.001$). Recurrent disease can emerge at any time after treatment, but the majority of events develop in the first year.

Subfoveal choroidal neovascularization The Macular Photocoagulation Study Group's new subfoveal trial evaluated laser treatment for subfoveal lesions in eyes that had not received prior photocoagulation. Eligible eyes had choroidal neovascularization underlying the foveal centre with well-demarcated boundaries of all lesion components. Lesions measuring 3.5 or fewer Macular Photocoagulation Study disc areas

(**DA**) in total size had a component of classic choroidal neovascularization, and had choroidal neovascularization as their main component. All patients were 50 or more years old and had baseline visual acuity of between 20/40 and 20/320. All components of the lesion received intense and confluent photocoagulation. Treatment extended 100 μm beyond the perimeter of the lesion, except in the case of thick, contiguous blood, where treatment fully covered the blood but did not extend beyond it.

Laser photocoagulation has not been shown to be beneficial for new, well-demarcated subfoveal lesions of more than 3.5 DA total size, lesions with poorly demarcated boundaries, or those with occult but no classic choroidal neovascularization. Subgroup analysis within the subfoveal trials suggests that the treatment benefit diminishes with larger lesions entered into the study.

When deciding which eyes will benefit from subfoveal laser treatment, the angiographic criteria for eligibility used in the Macular Photocoagulation Study Group trial should be used in assessment since subgroup analysis demonstrated no significant treatment benefit among eyes inadvertently enrolled in the trial that did not meet those criteria. For example, study eyes with poorly demarcated lesions or with occult but no classic choroidal neovascularization did not do better with treatment than similar untreated eyes. Thus laser photocoagulation should usually be considered only for eyes with new, subfoveal choroidal neovascularization that meet the Group's eligibility criteria.

Most subfoveal lesions with a contiguous, serous pigment epithelial detachment do not meet those eligibility criteria, not because of the presence of the serous detachment but for one or more of the following reasons. There is an associated component of choroidal neovascularization with poorly demarcated boundaries; no classic choroidal neovascularization is present; the serous pigment epithelial detachment rather than choroidal neovascularization is under the foveal centre; or the area of the serous detachment is larger than the area of choroidal neovascularization. Most eyes with ophthalmoscopic evidence of subretinal scarring do not meet the eligibility criteria, not because of the presence of the scarring but because no component of classic choroidal neovascularization is present, the lesion is more than 3.5 DA, or it has poorly demarcated boundaries.

In the Macular Photocoagulation Study Group's new subfoveal trial, 47 per cent of untreated eyes had severe loss of vision compared to 22 per cent of treated eyes 4 years after entry ($p = 0.002$). Mean acuity 4 years after entry was 20/500 among untreated eyes and 20/320 among treated eyes. The median speed for reading letters of approximately 20/1500 in size was only 13 words/min in untreated eyes compared to 22 words/min in treated eyes at the 4-year examination ($p = 0.01$). The median contrast threshold needed to discern letters of approximately 20/750 size was 28 per cent in untreated eyes compared to 14 per cent in treated eyes ($p = 0.004$).

The patient's initial visual acuity and the initial size of the new lesion of choroidal neovascularization influenced the magnitude of the treatment benefit and resulted in the categoriz-

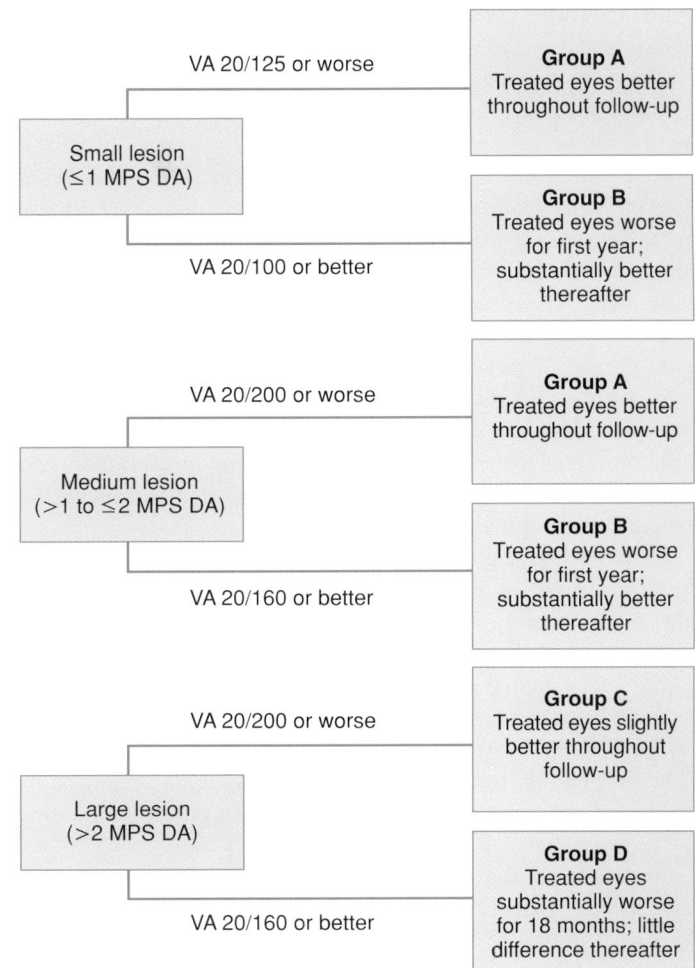

Fig. 12 Schematic aid for determining the pattern of visual loss in eyes with new subfoveal choroidal neovascularization. MPS indicates Macular Photocoagulation Study; DA, disc area; and VA, visual acuity. (Printed with permission of the American Medical Association: Macular Photocoagulation Study Group, 1994.)

ation of eyes into four groups (Fig. 12). Eyes with small or medium-sized lesions (<2 DA) that had poorer levels of visual acuity at presentation had visual loss corresponding to a pattern A in which the treated rather than the untreated eyes always had a lower risk of severe loss. Eyes with initially larger lesions (≥ 2 DA) and better visual acuity (> 20/200) had visual loss corresponding to a pattern D in which the risk of severe loss was worse in treated than untreated eyes for the first 18 months after the initial examination, with little difference thereafter between treated and untreated. Frequent follow-up examinations of eyes in group D may identify the few that develop further loss of visual acuity to 20/200 or worse before the lesion acquires poorly demarcated boundaries or exceeds 3.5 DA. If this occurs, then these eyes may be reclassified into pattern C, in which treated eyes have a slightly smaller risk of severe visual loss. Small and medium-sized lesions with better levels of acuity had visual loss corresponding to pattern B, with a greater risk of severe loss with treatment until 1 year after presentation, when untreated eyes had a significantly greater risk for severe visual loss thereafter (Fig. 12).

For poorly demarcated lesions that include a component of classic choroidal neovascularization, confluent laser treatment to the classic lesion only does not appear to more beneficial than observation, even though without treatment, significant loss of visual acuity will probably develop within several years of follow-up. In eyes with both classic and occult choroidal neovascularization in which only the classic lesion is photocoagulated, there was no significant difference in visual outcome between treated eyes and untreated eyes ($p = 0.66$), with similar rates of severe visual loss at 3 years ($p = 0.90$). Treated eyes with occult, but no classic, choroidal neovascularization were less likely to develop severe visual loss (odds ratio 1.5) than untreated eyes, but the broad confidence interval (0.5, 4.8) suggests that the number of eyes was too small to determine whether these differences were significant.

Perifoveal laser photocoagulation of subfoveal choroidal neovascularization has been attempted to minimize destruction of the foveal centre. One hundred and sixty eyes with either poorly or well-demarcated subfoveal choroidal neovascularization were assigned randomly to observation or confluent laser treatment to the periphery of the choroidal lesion in a doughnut shape, sparing the central 400 μm of the foveal avascular zone. The criteria for inclusion included angiographic evidence of subfoveal choroidal neovascularization, with or without serous pigment epithelial detachment, extending by more than 200 μm from the foveal centre but less than 2.5 disc diameters wide and without detectable fibrous tissue. Visual acuity was maintained or improved in 20 per cent of 59 untreated eyes compared to 41 per cent of 68 treated eyes ($p = 0.04$) over a mean follow-up of 26 months. This technique has not been directly compared with confluent subfoveal treatment.

Subfoveal recurrent choroidal neovascularization   The Macular Photocoagulation Study Group's trial on subfoveal, recurrent choroidal neovascularization evaluated eyes with recurrent subfoveal lesions that had developed after initial photocoagulation of extrafoveal or juxtafoveal choroidal neovascularization. To be eligible for this study, the choroidal lesion had to have recurrent neovascularization beneath the fovea (or within 150 μm of the foveal centre if the previous laser treatment had resulted in extension of depigmented retinal pigment epithelium into that centre). The only other eligibility criterion that differed from the trial discussed above on new subfoveal choroidal neovascularization was the maximum size of the lesion. The previous area of photocoagulation plus the new area to be treated had to be less than or equal to 6 DA. Moreover, some part of the retina within 1 disc diameters of the foveal centre had to remain uninvolved by previous photocoagulation and any treatment subsequently applied to the recurrent choroidal neovascularization was according to the protocol described next.

Treatment of recurrent subfoveal choroidal neovascularization was to extend 100 μm beyond all lesional boundaries, except in the case of thick blood. Treatment covered such blood but was not required to extend beyond it. At the junction of

the area of prior laser treatment and the recurrent lesion, treatment was to extend 300 μm into the previously treated area. If a feeder vessel was present, treatment was to be applied directly to it, extend 100 μm beyond its lateral borders, and 300 μm radially beyond its origin.

Treatment of recurrent subfoveal choroidal neovascularization was shown to be beneficial in relation to the natural course of these lesions. Thirty-six per cent of untreated eyes with the recurrent neovascularization had severe visual loss compared to 12 per cent of treated eyes at 3 years ($p = 0.009$). Mean acuity 3 years after entry was 20/320 in untreated eyes compared to 20/250 in treated eyes. In this Macular Photocoagulation Study Group's trial, the treatment benefit was not influenced by the size of the lesion or baseline level of visual acuity, unlike the treatment benefits for new subfoveal lesions, which varied depending on the initial size of the lesion and the initial visual acuity. Median reading speed was only 15 words/minute in untreated eyes compared to 35 words/minute in treated eyes ($p = 0.02$). The median contrast threshold was 20 per cent in untreated eyes compared to 14 per cent in treated eyes ($p = 0.04$).

Preoperative preparation

Several issues should be discussed with, and understood by, the patient as part of the informed consent that precedes laser treatment. The natural history of their disease should be reviewed. The patient should understand that the goal of treatment is to decrease the risk of further severe loss of vision beyond what has already developed rather than to improve visual acuity. The patient must realize that treatment will create a permanent and absolute scotoma that will usually be worse than the pretreatment vision, but that the possible loss of vision with laser treatment will probably be less than that which would occur within the next 3 to 18 months without treatment. The patient should be prepared for additional recurrent choroidal neovascularization, particularly within the first 1 to 2 years after treatment, that may be amenable to further laser photocoagulation. The likelihood of developing neovascular disease in the fellow eye, if this event has not yet occurred, and the possible need for a low-vision evaluation (see below), should also be addressed.

For laser treatment, a fluorescein angiogram of less than 96 h old is usually recommended to delineate accurately the boundaries of the lesion to which treatment should be applied. Growth of choroidal neovascularization is generally unpredictable, and the availability of a recent angiogram may reduce the chance that the boundaries have enlarged significantly since the study was performed. Treatment is facilitated by projecting the angiogram within viewing distance of the treating ophthalmologist to serve as a precise guide to where photocoagulation should be applied. Periodic comparison of the retinal vascular landmarks in the fundus to the angiogram should assist in adequate coverage and minimize treatment of uninvolved retina.

A retro- or peribulbar injection of anaesthetic is optional. However, it may dampen eye movement that may potentially interfere with either adequate photocoagulation of the entire

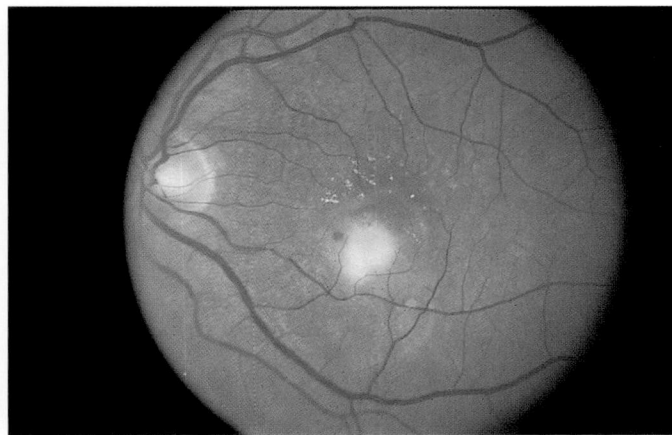

Fig. 13 Treatment intensity standard. Treatment protocol specified a uniform, white burn at least as intense as the treatment standard. (Printed with permission from the American Medical Association: Macular Photocoagulation Study Group, 1989.)

neovascular complex or inadvertent treatment of uninvolved retina. However, the anaesthetic does not prevent head or body movements that also may arise unexpectedly and interfere with accuracy of photocoagulation.

Treatment measures

Suggested measures for obtaining the desired endpoint of a uniform and white laser burn at the level of the outer retina (Fig. 13) include a spot size of 200 μm at a duration of 0.2 to 0.5 s. Avoiding smaller spot sizes and shorter durations reduces the risk of intraoperative choroidal haemorrhage when trying to produce a relatively white burn. Treatment begins by placing contiguous laser burns to outline the choroidal neovascularization. This approach decreases the likelihood that subsequent bleeding will lead to incomplete treatment by obscuring the perimeter of the lesion. The interior of the lesion is then photocoagulated, sometimes broadening the size of the spot to 500 μm. Treatment intensity may vary between different areas of the lesion depending on the presence of haemorrhage and atrophy of retinal pigment epithelium; thus, the surgeon may need to modulate the laser power during the treatment to maintain the desired white intensity of photocoagulation.

Wavelength selection

Limited research studies have been done to determine if there is a clinical advantage in using a particular laser wavelength to photocoagulate choroidal neovascularization. However, on empirical grounds, argon blue-green laser is the least favoured wavelength for macular pathology since macular xanthophyll pigment will absorb the blue rays and cause direct damage to the inner retina. Dye yellow laser (577 nm wavelength) theoretically affords several advantages for treating choroidal neovascularization. This wavelength is absorbed by melanin within the retinal pigment epithelium enveloping the lesion and by haemoglobin within the choroidal neovascularization, it readily traverses the aged nuclear sclerotic lens with minimal dispersion of the laser beam, and it spares the outer retina since it is

poorly absorbed by macular xanthophyll. However, the outcome of treatment with this wavelength has not been compared with that for other wavelengths in randomized clinical trials.

In the Macular Photocoagulation Study Group's new and recurrent subfoveal trials, patients assigned to laser treatment were also assigned randomly to either argon-green or krypton-red laser photocoagulation. In the new subfoveal study, eyes treated with krypton red lost, on average, 0.6 lines more of acuity than eyes treated with argon green ($p = 0.20$). However, the patients treated with krypton red were older and had larger lesions of choroidal neovascularization than those treated with argon green, two baseline features known to be associated with a poor visual outcome. Multivariate analysis demonstrated that the additional loss of vision suffered in the krypton-red group was only 0.06 lines or a difference of one letter. The argon green-treated eyes also performed slightly better than krypton red-treated eyes in their reading speed and contrast-sensitivity threshold, although these differences also were not statistically significant. In the Group's recurrent subfoveal trial, multivariate analysis showed a mean decrease in acuity of an additional 0.2 lines in eyes treated with krypton red compared to argon green ($p = 0.86$). In addition, eyes treated with krypton red read, on average, 16 words/min slower ($p = 0.02$) than eyes treated with argon green. The red-treated eyes also required 1.4 times more contrast to read 20/1500-sized letters ($p = 0.05$). Neither of these studies has identified a major clinically or statistically significant difference between red and green wavelengths in managing these cases.

Laser-related complications

Ocular complications may arise during and after laser photocoagulation. 'Overtreatment' occurs when laser treatment extends beyond the area of pathology and may be associated with unnecessary loss of visual function. 'Undertreatment' occurs when coverage of the choroidal neovascularization lesion is inadequate in extent or intensity, or both, predisposing the eye to an increased risk of persistent disease and subsequent loss of vision.

Other infrequently encountered complications include perforation of Bruch's membrane, intraoperative haemorrhage, rips in the retinal pigment epithelium, the formation of holes in the retina, and full-thickness burns with wrinkling of the inner retina. Intraoperative haemorrhage may be sub- or intra-retinal, and may obscure lesional landmarks and prevent laser uptake at the level of the choroidal neovascularization. Manual pressure on the fundus contact lens and treatment over the haemorrhage during the event often stops the active bleeding. Laser may be applied directly to the bleeding site to coagulate the source while exerting this increased pressure.

Post-laser management

A post-treatment photograph can be obtained immediately after treatment. The adequacy of lesion coverage can be assessed by comparing the area of the laser lesion with that of the choroidal neovascularization lesion from the pretreatment angiogram using an overlay technique. If undertreatment is recognized, additional laser treatment may be done promptly to decrease the risk of persistent choroidal neovascularization.

Follow-up visits are suggested at 2 to 4 weeks, 6 to 8 weeks, 3 to 4 months, 6 to 9 months, 12 months, and then twice yearly through the second or third post-treatment year to search for recurrent disease. In the follow-up examination one should consider including measurement of the best corrected visual acuity, biomicroscopic examination of the fundus, and fluorescein angiography during the first post-treatment year. Clinical examination without fluorescein angiography may allow some treatable recurrent disease to go undetected. In one prospective study, contact-lens biomicroscopy without fluorescein angiography had a sensitivity of 59 per cent for detection of recurrent disease (using fluorescein angiography as the standard for detecting recurrent choroidal neovascularization). Of the cases in which a definite recurrence was detected on angiography but not by clinical examination alone, the majority were amenable to laser treatment. Thus, angiography is suggested as part of the routine follow-up examination to maximize detection of all treatable recurrent disease.

Persistent choroidal neovascularization If leakage of fluorescein is present along the periphery of the laser scar within 6 weeks of treatment, the term 'persistent' is used to describe the choroidal neovascularization that is present. Some features associated with an increased risk of developing persistent choroidal neovascularization include failure to recognize preoperatively and treat the entire extent of the original neovascularization, and inadequate intensity of photocoagulation.

Recurrent choroidal neovascularization Recurrent choroidal neovascularization is the term used to describe any angiographic leakage present at the perimeter of the laser lesion at visits beyond the first 6 weeks postoperatively. The term 'recurrence' could also be used whenever there is leakage at the periphery of a laser scar if previous studies unequivocally demonstrated the absence of leakage, even if within 6 weeks of treatment. In one series the rate of recurrence after photocoagulation in patients with age-related macular degeneration ranged between approximately 50 and 80 per cent within 3 years of treatment. The majority of recurrences present within the first post-treatment year.

Specific patterns on post-treatment angiograms may suggest that recurrent choroidal neovascularization could develop; these patterns include focal staining along the edge of the laser lesion, new speckled hyperfluorescence beyond the margins of the laser treatment, and blocked fluorescence not from new subretinal haemorrhage. Eyes with these features should be monitored carefully for possible progression to definitive evidence of choroidal neovascularization. New subretinal haemorrhage noted at follow-up after laser photocoagulation often, but not always, identifies an eye that has developed recurrent choroidal neovascularization.

Surgical intervention

An important limitation of macular laser photocoagulation is the concurrent destruction of overlying retinal tissue, especially when a choroidal neovascularization lesion is subfoveal. Although laser treatment of subfoveal lesions results in less loss of vision than occurs in the natural course of the process, patients can anticipate a loss of visual acuity at the time of treatment. Surgical removal of choroidal neovascularization lesions has the potential to preserve overlying retinal tissue; therefore, vision may potentially be unaffected by this intervention, or possibly improved in certain cases. In additon, the surgical removal of choroidal neovascularization is possible in lesions with poorly demarcated boundaries or those obscured by significant haemorrhage; it may therefore provide a treatment for this group of lesions in which the laser has been unsuccessful.

In 1988, the surgical removal of subfoveal choroidal neovascularization was pioneered by de Juan and Machemer. The next decade saw the surgical technique refined and encouraging short-term results have been reported. However, cases reported to have stable or improved visual acuity postoperatively have had short (generally 6 months or less) or incomplete follow-up, lack of concurrent controls for comparison, and nonstandardized methods for assessing visual outcome. Comparisons have been drawn with published cases of laser-treated or untreated eyes and are subject to the difficulties often encountered when reviewing data reported by different investigators, including a lack of standardization of patient selection, surgical technique, visual-acuity measurement, or follow-up schedules.

Results from these preliminary series of cases have prompted the organization of multicentre, prospective, randomized clinical trials to compare the long-term outcome for vision in patients undergoing submacular surgery with that produced by the conventional management of age-related macular degeneration with new or recurrent subfoveal or haemorrhagic choroidal neovascularization, or of subfoveal choroidal neovascularization due to the ocular histoplasmosis syndrome or idiopathic causes. The Submacular Surgery Trials' pilot study is investigating the feasibility of a full-scale, properly designed evaluation of this form of treatment. If the pilot study confirms that such clinical trials are indicated, then a full-scale randomized trial may be started to provide information that will assist ophthalmologists in deciding whether to recommend surgery for selected cases of choroidal neovascularization.

Future horizons

Current investigations are in various stages of evaluating safety or efficacy to determine if pharmacological intervention can prevent or stabilize choroidal neovascularization. Pharmacological intervention could provide an option for treatment that might not destroy the overlying retinal tissue as much as with photocoagulation. Preliminary analysis of the results from a multicentre, double-blind, randomized clinical trial to determine the minimal effective dose for the stabilization or improvement of visual acuity and the tolerability of interferon-$\alpha_{2\alpha}$ in patients with age-related macular degeneration and subfoveal choroidal neovascularization suggests that the interferon offers no treatment benefit compared to placebo 1 year after entry into the study and may be associated with significant systemic toxicity. Pilot studies of ionizing radiation are also in progress to determine if this treatment can promote the involution of choroidal neovascularization. However, these studies were not randomized clinical trials; therefore, the potential merits of this therapy as compared to the natural history have not, as yet, been elucidated. Photodynamic therapy is also under investigation to determine if this might stabilize visual acuity, compared to conventional management, because of its potential to stop neovascular growth selectively without significant destruction of the overlying retina.

Low vision assistance

Once central vision has been permanently damaged in both eyes, due either to geographic atrophy, disciform scar, or laser photocoagulation, a low vision evaluation should be considered. The low vision specialist may prescribe spectacles and various magnifying aids to facilitate daily tasks such as writing, typing, reading, sedentary distance viewing, and distance spotting. The examination often employs glare-free, high-intensity lighting and large trial lenses to promote eccentric fixation. A variety of magnification levels are available, some of which have an illumination source. Combinations of aids may be best for a patient's individual visual needs. A low vision consultation should also include informing the patient of support groups, community resources, and products for people with visual disabilities such as large-print books or books on audiotape.

Aids for reading include reading glasses, hand-held lenses, stand magnifiers, and electronic devices. Reading glasses provide fairly large fields of view but shorter working distances because of the high-powered lenses required. The working distance may be lengthened by using telescopic reading glasses, but they provide a smaller field of view and shorter depth of focus than simple reading glasses. Hand-held magnifiers are helpful for simple, quick tasks at arm's length. A stand magnifier is a mounted lens that maintains a consistent focused image of a printed page when positioned so that its focal point correlates to that of the patient's near correction. This device is better suited for a weak or tremulous patient or one who requires longer working distances and/or prefers an incorporated illumination source. Electronic magnifiers, such as a closed-circuit television, provide greater magnification than optical devices. Closed-circuit television permits binocular viewing at a practical reading distance, but its cost and lack of easy portability limit its widespread use.

Distance-viewing devices include opera and binocular field-glasses. Light-weight telescopes may be hand-held or mounted in spectacles. These devices limit peripheral vision, however, and distort distances, so their use is confined to sedentary distance viewing and spotting. The Low Vision Enhancement System is a relatively expensive, battery-powered, binocular, head-mounted video display system that provides 3× to 10× magnification for distance viewing and up to 25× for near viewing.

Most patients with low vision from age-related macular degeneration should be offered a low vision evaluation and training in the use of low vision devices; however, patient motivation and the size and location of the scotoma influence the success of these aids. Patients should be informed that aids are meant to enhance magnification or lighting for their remaining vision, but are not a means of treating or curing their ophthalmological disease.

Further reading

Arnold, J. J., Sarks, S. H., Killingsworth, M. C., and Sarks, J. P. (1995). Reticular pseudodrusen: a risk factor in age-related maculopathy. *Retina*, **15**, 183–91.

Avery, R. L., Fekrat, S., Hawkins, B. S., and Bressler, N. M. (1996). Natural history of subfoveal subretinal hemorrhage in age-related macular degeneration. *Retina*, **16**, 183–9 .

Bennett, S. R., Folk, J. C., Blodi, C. F., and Klugman, M. (1990). Factors prognostic of visual outcome in patients with subretinal hemorrhage. *American Journal of Ophthalmology*, **109**, 33–7.

Berger, A. S. and Kaplan, H. J. (1992). Clinical experience with the surgical removal of subfoveal neovascular membranes. *Ophthalmology*, **99**, 969–76.

Bergink, G. J., Deutman, A. F., Van Den Broek, J. E. C. M., Van Daal, W. A. J., and Van Der Maazen, R. M. W. (1995). Radiation therapy for age-related subfoveal choroidal neovascular membranes: a pilot study. *Documenta Ophthalmologica*, **90**, 67–74.

Bird, A. C. *et al.* (1995). An international classification and grading system for age-related maculopathy and age-related macular degeneration: the international ARM epidemiologic study group. *Survey of Ophthalmology*, **39**, 367–74.

Bischoff, P. M. and Flower, R. W. (1985). Ten years experience with choroidal angiography using indocyanine green dye: a new routine examination or an epilogue? *Documenta Ophthalmologica*, **60**, 235–91.

Blumenkranz, M. S., Russell, S. R., Robey, M. G., Kott-Blumenkranz, R., and Penneys, N. (1986). Risk factors in age-related maculopathy complicated by choroidal neovascularization. *Ophthalmology*, **93**, 552–8.

Bressler, N. M. (1995). Natural history of subfoveal subretinal hemorrhage in age-related macular degeneration: an example of a case with good visual outcome. *Wilmer Retina Update*, **1**, 3–9.

Bressler, N. M. (1995). Submacular surgery: are randomized trials necessary? *Archives of Ophthalmology*, **113**, 1557–60.

Bressler, N. M. and Bressler, S. B. (1995). Preventative ophthalmology. Age-related macular degeneration. *Ophthalmology*, **102**, 1206–11.

Bressler, N. M. and Bressler, S. B. (1996). Indocyanine green angiography: can it help preserve the vision of our patients? *Archives of Ophthalmology*, **114**, 747–9.

Bressler, N. M., Frost, L. A., Bressler, S. B., Murphy, R. P., and Fine, S. L. (1988). Natural course of poorly defined choroidal neovascularization associated with macular degeneration. *Archives of Ophthalmology*, **106**, 1537–42.

Bressler, N. M., Bressler, S. B., West, S. K., Fine, S. L., and Taylor, H. R. (1989). The grading and prevalence of macular degeneration in Chesapeake Bay watermen. *Archives of Ophthalmology*, **107**, 847–52.

Bressler, N. M., Finklestein, D., Sunness, J. S., Maguire, A. M., and Yarian, D. (1990). Retinal pigment epithelial tears through the fovea with preservation of good visual acuity. *Archives of Ophthalmology*, **108**, 1694–7.

Bressler, N. M., Bressler, S. B., Alexander, J., Javornik, N., Fine, S. L., and Murphy, R. P. (1991). Loculated fluid: a previously undescribed fluorescein angiographic finding in choroidal neovascularization associated with macular degeneration. Macular photocoagulation study reading center. *Archives of Ophthalmology*, **109**, 211–15.

Bressler, N. M., Silva, J. C., Bressler, S. B., Fine, S. L., and Green, W. R. (1994). Clinicopathologic correlation of drusen and retinal pigment epithelial abnormalities in age-related macular degeneration. *Retina*, **14**, 130–42.

Bressler, N. M. *et al.* (1995). Five-year incidence and disappearance of drusen and retinal pigment epithelial abnormalities: Waterman Study. *Archives of Ophthalmology*, **113**, 301–8.

Bressler, N. M. *et al.* (1996). Macular scatter ('grid') laser treatment of poorly demarcated subfoveal choroidal neovascularization in age-related macular degeneration: results of a randomized, prospective pilot trial. *Archives of Ophthalmology*, **114**, 1456–64.

Bressler, S. B. (1993). Does wavelength matter when photocoagulating eyes with macular degeneration of diabetic retinopathy? *Archives of Ophthalmology*, **111**, 177–80.

Bressler, S. B., Maguire, M. G., Bressler, N. M., Fine, S. L., and the Macular Photocoagulation Study Group (1990). Relationship of drusen and abnormalities of the retinal pigment epithelium to the prognosis of neovascular macular degeneration. *Archives of Ophthalmology*, **108**, 1442–7.

Bressler, S. B., Silva, J. C., Bressler, N. M., Alexander, J., and Green, W. R. (1992). Clinicopathologic correlation of occult choroidal neovascularization in age-related macular degeneration. *Archives of Ophthalmology*, **110**, 827–32.

Bressler, S. B. *et al.* (1995). Laser to drusen trial: an assessment of short term safety within a randomized, prospective, controlled clinical trial. *Investigative Ophthalmology and Visual Science*, **36**, S225.

Buring, J. E. and Hennekens, C. H. (1992). The Women's Health Study: summary of the study design. *Journal of Myocardial Ischemia*, **4**, 27–9.

Chakravarthy, U., Houston, R. F., and Archer, D. B. (1993). Treatment of age-related subfoveal neovascular membranes by teletherapy: a pilot study. *British Journal of Ophthalmology*, **77**, 265–73.

Chamberlin, J. A. *et al.* (1989). The use of fundus photographs and fluorescein angiograms in the identification and treatment of choroidal neovascularization in the Macular Photocoagulation Study. *Ophthalmology*, **96**, 1526–34.

Chandra, S. R., Gragoudas, E. S., Friedman, E., Van Buskirk, E. M., and Klein, M. L. (1974). Natural history of disciform degeneration of the macula. *American Journal of Ophthalmology*, **78**, 579–82.

Chang, B., Yannuzzi, L. A., Ladas, I., Guyer, D. R., Slakter, J. S., and Sorenson, J. A. (1995). Choroidal neovascularization in second eyes of patients with unilateral exudative age-related macular degeneration. *Ophthalmology*, **102**, 1380–6.

Christen, W. G. *et al.* (1992). A prospective study of cigarette smoking and risk of cataract in men. *Journal of the American Medical Association*, **268**, 989–93.

Chumbley, L. C. (1977). Impressions of eye diseases among Rhodesian blacks in Mashonaland. *South African Medical Journal*, **52**, 316–18.

Coffey, A. J. H. and Brownstein, S. (1986). The prevalence of macular drusen in postmortem eyes. *American Journal of Ophthalmology*, **102**, 164–71.

Coscas, G., Soubrane, G., Ramahefasolo, C., and Fardeau, C. (1991). Perifoveal laser treatment for subfoveal choroidal new vessels in age-related macular degeneration: results of a randomized clinical trial. *Archives of Ophthalmology*, **109**, 1258–65.

Cruickshanks, K. J., Klein, R., and Klein, B. E. K. (1993). Sunlight and age-related macular degeneration: the Beaver Dam Eye Study. *Archives of Ophthalmology*, **111**, 514–18.

Custis, P. H., Bressler, S. B., and Bressler, N. M. (1993). Laser management of subfoveal choroidal neovascularization in age-related macular degeneration. *Current Opinion in Ophthalmology*, **4**, 7–18.

de Juan, E. Jr. and Machemer, R. (1991). Vitreous surgery for hemorrhagic and fibrous complications of age-related macular degeneration. *American Journal of Ophthalmology*, **105**, 25–9.

Duvall, J., and Tso, M. O. M. (1985). Cellular mechanisms of resolution of drusen after laser coagulation: an experimental study. *Archives of Ophthalmology*, **103**, 694–703.

Dyer, D. S., Brant, A. M., Schachat, A. P., Bressler, S. B., and Bressler, N. M. (1995). Angiographic features and outcome of questionable recurrent choroidal neovascularization. *American Journal of Ophthalmology*, **120**, 497–505.

El Baba, F., Green, W. R., Fleischmann, J., Finkelstein, D., and de la Cruz, Z. C. (1986). Clinicopathologic correlation of lipidization and detachment of the retinal pigment epithelium. *American Journal of Ophthalmology*, **101**, 576–83.

Eye Disease Case-Control Study Group (1992). Risk factors for neovascular age-related macular degeneration. *Archives of Ophthalmology*, **110**, 1701–8.

Eye Disease Case-Control Study Group (1993). Antioxidant status and neovascular age-related macular degeneration. *Archives of Ophthalmology*, **111**, 104–9.

Fekrat, S. and Bressler, S. B. (1996). Are antioxidants or other supplements protective for age-related macular degeneration? *Current Opinion in Ophthalmology*, **7**, 65–72.

Figueroa, M. S., Regueras, A., and Bertrand, J. (1994). Laser photocoagulation to treat macular soft drusen in age-related macular degeneration. *Retina*, **14**, 391–6.

Frennesson, I. C. and Nilsson, S. E. G. (1995). Effects of argon (green) laser treatment of soft drusen in early age-related maculopathy: a 6 month prospective study. *British Journal of Ophthalmology*, **79**, 905–9.

Gass, J. D. M. (1984). Pathogenesis of tears of the retinal pigment epithelium. *British Journal of Ophthalmology*, **68**, 514–19.

Goldberg, J., Flowerdew, G., Smith, E., Brody, J. A., and Tso, M. O. (1988). Factors associated with age-related macular degeneration. An analysis of data from the first National Health and Nutrition Examination Survey. *American Journal of Epidemiology*, **128**, 700–10.

Green, W. R. (1991). Clinicopathologic studies of treated choroidal neovascular membranes: a review and report of two cases. *Retina*, **11**, 328–56.

Green, W. R., and Wilson, D.J. (1986). Choroidal neovascularization. *Ophthalmology*, **93**, 1169–76.

Green, W. R., McDonnell, P. H., and Yeo, J. H. (1985). Pathologic features of senile macular degeneration. *Ophthalmology*, **92**, 615–27.

Gregor, Z. and Joffe, L. (1978). Senile macular changes in the black African. *British Journal of Ophthalmology*, **62**, 547–50.

Gregor, Z., Bird, A. C., and Chisholm, I. H. (1977). Senile disciform macular degeneration in the second eye. *British Journal of Ophthalmology*, **61**, 141–7.

Guyer, D. R., Puliafito, C. A., Mones, J. M., Friedman, E., Chang, W., and Verdooner, S. R. (1992). Digital indocyanine green videoangiography in chorioretinal disorders. *Ophthalmology*, **99**, 287–91.

Guyer, D. R., Yannuzzi, L. A., Slakter, J. S., Sorenson, J. A., Hope-Ross, M., and Orlock, D. R. (1994). Digital indocyanine green videoangiography of occult choroidal neovascularization. *Ophthalmology*, **101**, 1727–37.

Holz, F. G. *et al.* (1994). Bilateral macular drusen in age-related macular degeneration. Prognosis and risk factors. *Ophthalmology*, **101**, 1522–8.

Hyman, L. G., Lilienfeld, A. M., Ferris, F. L., and Fine, S. L. (1983). Senile macular degeneration: a case-control study. *American Journal of Epidemiology*, **118**, 213–27.

Hyman, L., He, O., Grimson, R., Oden, N., Schachat, A. P., and Leske, M. C. (1992). Risk factors for age-related maculopathy. *Investigative Ophthalmology and Visual Science*, **33** (Suppl.), 801.

Jampol, L. M. and Tielsch, J. (1992). Race, macular degeneration, and the Macular Photocoagulation Study. *Archives of Ophthalmology*, **110**, 1699–700.

Klein, B. E. and Klein, R. (1982). Cataracts and macular degeneration in older Americans. *Archives of Ophthalmology*, **100**, 571–3.

Klein, M. L. (1991). Macular degeneration: is aspirin a risk for progressive disease? (Questions and answers). *Journal of the American Medical Association*, **266**, 2279.

Klein, R., Davis, M. D., Magli, Y. L., Segal, P., Klein, B. E., and Hubbard, L. (1991). The Wisconsin age-related maculopathy grading system. *Ophthalmology*, **98**, 1128–34.

Klein, R., Klein, B. E., and Linton, K. L. P. (1992). Prevalence of age-related maculopathy: the Beaver Dam Eye Study. *Ophthalmology*, **99**, 933–43.

Klein, R., Klein, B. E. K., and Franke, T. (1993). The relationship of cardiovascular disease and its risk factors to age-related maculopathy: the Beaver Dam Eye Study. *Ophthalmology*, **100**, 406–14.

Klein, R., Rowland, M. L., and Harris, M. I. (1995). Racial/ethnic differences in age-related maculopathy: third national health and nutrition examination survey. *Ophthalmology*, **102**, 371–81.

Klein, R., Klein, B. E. K., Jenson, S. C., and Meuer, S. M. (1996). The 5-year incidence of age-related maculopathy in the Beaver Dam Eye Study. *Investigative Ophthalmology and Visual Science*, **37**, S412.

Lambert, H. M., Capone, A., Jr, Aaberg, T. M., Sternberg, P., Jr, and Lopez, P. F. (1992). Surgical excision of subfoveal neovascular membranes in age-related macular degeneration. *American Journal of Ophthalmology*, **113**, 257–62.

Leibowitz, H. M. *et al.* (1980). The Framingham Eye Study Monograph: an ophthalmological and epidemiological study of cataract, glaucoma, diabetic retinopathy, macular degeneration, and visual acuity in a general population of 2631 adults, 1973–1975. *Survey of Ophthalmology*, **24** (Suppl.), 335–610.

Lim, J. I., Sternberg, P., Jr, Capone, A., Jr, Aaberg, T. M., Sr, and Gilman, J. P. (1995). Selective use of indocyanine green angiography for occult choroidal neovascularization. *American Journal of Ophthalmology*, **120**, 75–82.

Macular Photocoagulation Study Group (1982). Argon laser photocoagulation for senile macular degeneration: results of a randomized clinical trial. *Archives of Ophthalmology*, **100**, 912–18.

Macular Photocoagulation Study Group (1986). Recurrent choroidal neovascularization after argon laser photocoagulation for neovascular maculopathy. *Archives of Ophthalmology*, **104**, 503–12.

Macular Photocoagulation Study Group (1989). Persistent and recurrent neovascularization after krypton laser photocoagulation for neovascular lesions of ocular histoplasmosis. *Archives of Ophthalmology*, 107, 344–52.

Macular Photocoagulation Study Group (1990*a*). Persistent and recurrent neovascularization after krypton laser photocoagulation for neovascular lesions of age-related macular degeneration. *Archives of Ophthalmology*, 108, 825–31.

Macular Photocoagulation Study Group (1990*b*). Krypton laser photocoagulation for neovascular lesions of age-related macular degeneration: results of a randomized trial. *Archives of Ophthalmology*, 108, 816–24.

Macular Photocoagulation Study Group (1991*a*). Subfoveal neovascular lesions in age-related macular degeneration: guidelines for evaluation and treatment in the Macular Photocoagulation Study. *Archives of Ophthalmology*, 109, 1242–57.

Macular Photocoagulation Study Group (1991*b*). Argon laser photocoagulation for neovascular maculopathy: five-year results from randomized clinical trials. *Archives of Ophthalmology*, 109, 1109–14.

Macular Photocoagulation Study Group (1991*c*). Laser photocoagulation of subfoveal neovascular lesions in age-related macular degeneration: results of a randomized clinical trial. *Archives of Ophthalmology*, 109, 1220–31.

Macular Photocoagulation Study Group (1991*d*). Laser photocoagulation of subfoveal recurrent neovascular lesions in age-related macular degeneration: results of a randomized clinical trial. *Archives of Ophthalmology*, 109, 1232–41.

Macular Photocoagulation Study Group (1993*a*). Five-year follow-up of fellow eyes of patients with age-related macular degeneration and unilateral extrafoveal choroidal neovascularization. *Archives of Ophthalmology*, 111, 1189–99.

Macular Photocoagulation Study Group (1993*b*). Laser photocoagulation of subfoveal neovascular lesions of age-related macular degeneration: updated findings from two clinical trials. *Archives of Ophthalmology*, 111, 1200–9.

Macular Photocoagulation Study Group (1994*a*). Laser photocoagulation for juxtafoveal choroidal neovascularization: five-year results from randomized clinical trials. *Archives of Ophthalmology*, 112, 500–9.

Macular Photocoagulation Study Group (1994*b*). Visual outcome after laser photocoagulation for subfoveal choroidal neovascularization secondary to age-related macular degeneration: the influence of initial lesion size and initial visual acuity. *Archives of Ophthalmology*, 112, 480–8.

Macular Photocoagulation Study Group (1994*c*). Evaluation of argon green vs krypton red laser for photocoagulation of subfoveal choroidal neovascularization in the Macular Photocoagulation Study. *Archives of Ophthalmology*, 112, 1176–84.

Macular Photocoagulation Study Group (1994*d*). Persistent and recurrent neovascularization after laser photocoagulation for subfoveal choroidal neovascularization of age-related macular degeneration. *Archives of Ophthalmology*, 112, 489–99.

Macular Photocoagulation Study Group (1995). The influence of treatment extent on the visual acuity of eyes treated with krypton laser for juxtafoveal choroidal neovascularization. *Archives of Ophthalmology*, 113, 190–4.

Macular Photocoagulation Study Group (1996). Occult choroidal neovascularization: influence on visual outcome in patients with age-related macular degeneration. *Archives of Ophthalmology*, 114, 400–12.

Mares-Perlman, J. A., Brady, W. E., Klein, R., VandenLangenberg, G. M., Klein, B. E. K., and Palta, M. (1995). Dietary fat and age-related maculopathy. *Archives of Ophthalmology*, 113, 743–8.

Mares-Perlman, J. A. *et al.* (1995). Serum antioxidants and age-related macular degeneration in a population-based case-control study. *Archives of Ophthalmology*, 113, 1518–23.

Marshall, J. and Bird, A. C. (1979). A comparative histopathological study of argon and krypton laser irradiations of the human retina. *British Journal of Ophthalmology*, 63, 457–668.

Nasrallah, F., Jalkh, A. E., Trempe, C. L., McMeel, J. W., and Schepens, C.L. (1989). Subretinal hemorrhage in atrophic age-related macular degeneration. *American Journal of Ophthalmology*, 107, 38–41.

Newsome, D. A., Swartz, M., Leone, N. C., Elston, R. C., and Miller, E. (1988). Oral zinc in macular degeneration. *Archives of Ophthalmology*, 106, 192–8.

Pieramici, D. J., Bressler, N. M., Bressler, S. B., and Schachat, A. P. (1994). Choroidal neovascularization in black patients. *Archives of Ophthalmology*, 112, 1043–6.

Ritter, L. L., Klein, R., Klein, B. E. K., Mares-Perlman, J. A., and Jensen, S. C. (1995). Alcohol use and age-related maculopathy in the Beaver Dam Eye Study. *American Journal of Ophthalmology*, 120, 190–6.

Roy, M. and Kaiser-Kupfer, M. (1990). Second eye involvement in age-related macular degeneration: a four-year prospective study. *Eye*, 4, 813–18.

Sarks, S. H. and Sarks, J. P. (1994). Age-related macular degeneration: atrophic form. In *Retina* (ed. S. J. Ryan), pp. 1071–102. Mosby, St. Louis.

Sarks, J. P., Sarks, S. H., and Killingsworth, M. C. (1988). Evolution of geographic atrophy of the retinal pigment epithelium. *Eye*, 2, 552–77.

Schachat, A. P., Hyman, L., Leske, C., Connell, A. M. S., Wu, S. Y., and Barbados Eye Study Group. (1995). Features of age-related macular degeneration in a black population. *Archives of Ophthalmology*, 113, 728–35.

Sigelman, J. (1991). Foveal drusen resorption one year after perifoveal laser photocoagulation. *Ophthalmology*, 98, 1379–83.

Slakter, J. S., Yannuzzi, L. A., Sorenson, J. A., Guyer, D. R., Ho, A. C., and Orlock, D. A. (1994). A pilot study of indocyanine green videoangiography-guided laser photocoagultion of occult choroidal neovascularization in age-related macular degeneration. *Archives of Ophthalmology*, 112, 465–72.

Small, M. L., Green, W. R., Alpar, J. J., and Drewry, R. E. (1976). Senile macular degeneration: clinicopathologic correlation of two cases with neovascularization beneath the retinal pigment epithelium. *Archives of Ophthalmology*, 94, 601–7.

Smiddy, W. E. and Fine, S. L. (1984). Prognosis of patients with bilateral macular drusen. *Ophthalmology*, 91, 271–7.

Sommer, A. *et al.* (1991). Racial differences in the cause-specific prevalence of blindness in East Baltimore. *New England Journal of Medicine*, 325, 1412–17.

Sorenson, J. A., Yannuzzi, L. A., Slakter, J. S., Guyer, D. R., Ho, A. C., and Orlock, D. A. (1994). A pilot study of digital indocyanine green videoangiography for recurrent occult choroidal neovascularization in age-related macular degeneration. *Archives of Ophthalmology*, 112, 473–9.

Soubrane, G., Coscas, G., Francais, C., and Koenig, F. (1990). Occult subretinal new vessels in age-related macular degeneration. Natural history and early laser treatment. *Ophthalmology*, 97, 649–57.

Strahlman, E. R., Fine, S. L., and Hillis, A. (1983). The second eye of patients with senile macular degeneration. *Archives of Ophthalmology*, 101, 1191–3.

Sykes, S. O., Bressler, N. M., Maguire, M. G., Schachat, A. P., and Bressler, S. B. (1994). Detecting recurrent choroidal neovascularization: comparison of clinical examination with and without fluorescein angiography. *Archives of Ophthalmology*, 112, 1561–6.

Taylor, H. R., West, S., Munoz, B., Rosenthal, F. S., Bressler, S. B., and Bressler, N. M. (1992). The long-term effects of visible light on the eye. *Archives of Ophthalmology*, 110, 99–104.

Thomas, M. A. and Kaplan, H. J. (1991). Surgical removal of subfoveal neovascularization in the presumed ocular histoplamosis syndrome. *American Journal of Ophthalmology*, 111, 1–7.

Thomas, M. A., Grand, G. M., Williams, D. F., Lee, C. M., Pesin, S. R., and Lowe, M. A. (1992). Surgical management of subfoveal choroidal neovascularization. *Ophthalmology*, 99, 952–68.

Thomas, M. A., Dickinson, J. D., Melberg, N. S., Ibanez, H. E., and Dhaliwal, R. S. (1994). Visual results after surgical removal of subfoveal choroidal neovascular membranes. *Ophthalmology*, 101, 1384–96.

Valmaggia, C., Bischoff, P., and Ries, G. (1995). Low dose radiation on the subfoveal neovascular membranes (SNVM) in age-related macular degeneration. *Klinische Monatsblatter Fur Augenheilkunde*, 206, 343–6.

Vander, J. F., Morgan, C. M., and Schatz, H. (1989). Growth rate of subretinal neovascularization in age-related macular degeneration. *Ophthalmology*, 96, 1422–9.

Vingerling, J. R. *et al.* (1995). The prevalence of age-related maculopathy in the Rotterdam study. *Ophthalmology*, 102, 205–10.

West, S. K. *et al.* (1989). Exposure to sunlight and other risk factors for age-related macular degeneration. *Archives of Ophthalmology*, 107, 875–9.

Wetzig, P. C. (1988). Treatment of drusen-related aging macular degeneration by photocoagulation. *Transactions of the American Ophthalmological Society*, 86, 276–90.

Yannuzzi, L. A., Slakter, J. S., Sorenson, J. A., Guyer, D. R., and Orlock, D. A. (1992). Digital indocyanine green videoangiography and choroidal neovascularization. *Retina*, 12, 191–223.

2.9.4 Vascular occlusive disease of the retina

Rodney H.B. Grey

Arterial occlusion

The retina is supplied by arterial blood from branches of the ophthalmic artery. The inner layers of the neuroretina, that is those layers between the outer plexiform layer and the nerve fibre layer, are supplied by the central retinal artery. This system is one of endarteries and, therefore, occlusion of either the central retinal artery or one of its branches will lead to ischaemia of the territory supplied. There is no anastomotic circulation peripherally to alleviate the affects of anoxia. The photoreceptors and retinal pigment epithelium are supplied by multiple short ciliary arteries which arise via the ophthalmic artery near the apex of the orbit. The short ciliary arteries penetrate the sclera in a circle around the optic nerve supplying both the circle of Zinn around the optic nerve head and also branching into multiple choroidal arteries supplying the highly vascular choriocapillaris. On account of the lobular nature of the choriocapillaris with anastomotic channels between lobules obstruction of a choroidal arteriole rarely produces infarction of the outer retinal layers.

Central retinal artery occlusion

Obstruction of the central retinal artery may occur as a result of thickening of the vessel wall from atheromatous disease or an arteritic process, or alternatively by impaction of an embolus. Vessel wall disease normally occurs at, or posterior to, the lamina cribrosa whereas emboli lodge at the bifurcation of the central retinal artery into upper and lower branches anterior to the lamina cribrosa. The majority of patients suffering arterial obstruction are elderly and frequently have other manifestations of arteriosclerotic disease or systemic hypertension. Younger patients demonstrating arterial occlusion should be thoroughly investigated for a vasculitic process or for sources of emboli arising from the heart or major vessels.

Clinical features

Patients suffering central retinal artery occlusion are aware of sudden painless profound loss of vision in one eye. They frequently describe a curtain moving across the vision over a period of a few minutes, ultimately finishing with bare perception of light.

Clinical examination demonstrates an afferent pupil defect at the outset. Within a few hours the retina shows a greyish pallor of the posterior retina with sparing of the central fovea, giving the appearance of a cherry red spot. The pallor results from of axonal swelling of the nerve fibre layer of the retina. The pallor is, therefore, clinically obvious where the nerve fibre layer is

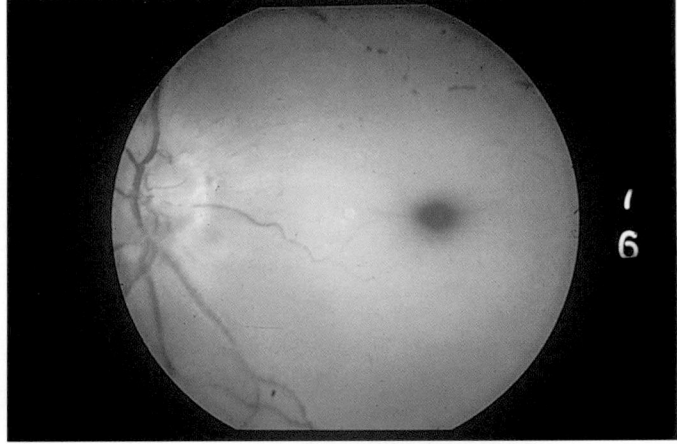

(a)

(b)

Fig. 1 (a) Central retinal artery occlusion. Note the peripapillary tissue whitening from blocked retrograde axoplasmic transport. (b) Angiogram of (a) showing absent retinal vessel filling, normal choroidal filling, and hyperfluorescence of the optic disc supplied from the ciliary circulation.

thickest between the temporal vascular arcades (Fig. 1). The fovea is devoid of ganglion cell axons and normal choroidal coloration is seen in contrast to the surrounding pale retina. The circulation within the retinal arterioles is slowed and the blood column frequently breaks into small nearly stationary segments (cattle trucking). Examination of the optic nerve head may reveal a cholesterol or platelet embolus at the bifurcation of the central retinal artery.

Within hours of occlusion taking place the cell bodies of the bipolar and ganglion cells show cytoplasmic swelling and the nuclei undergo pyknosis. Orthograde cytoplasmic transport of axonal organelles ceases but retrograde transport in the distal portion of the ganglion cell axons continues temporarily. This frequently leads to deposition of organelles passing into the neuroretina from the optic nerve causing a white infiltration in the peripapillary nerve fibre layer of the retina (Fig. 1(a)).

Within a few weeks there is complete atrophy of the inner layers of the neuroretina with loss of the bipolar cells, ganglion cells, and their neuronal connections. Retinal pallor subsides and the optic disc becomes atrophic. It is unusual for recovery of vision to take place, but sometimes, if treatment can be administered quickly or if the obstruction is not total, treatment may allow restoration of useful function (see below).

Investigation

It is essential to investigate for a possible source of emboli and also to exclude any arteritic process, particularly giant cell arteritis. In general the younger the patient, the more likely a non-atheromatous cause may be found.

Duplex ultrasound scanning of the carotid arteries in the neck should be performed to identify atheromatous plaques at the carotid bifurcation. If plaques and carotid stenosis is revealed the opinion of a vascular surgeon should be sought in order to reduce the likelihood of further retinal embolization or cerebrovascular embolization. Carotid obstruction of 75 per cent or greater has been found to respond well to endarterectomy with increased survival, decreased rate of stroke, and abolition of further episodes of visual symptoms.

Plasma erythrocyte sedimentation rate or viscosity should be measured, particularly in patients over the age of 60 years. In patients in whom giant cell arteritis is suspected temporal artery biopsy is advisable in order to confirm the diagnosis. If confirmed or if the clinical suspicion is strongly in favour of giant cell arteritis high dose systemic steroids should be administered without delay in order to prevent occlusion in the fellow eye.

Diabetes mellitus should be excluded and more unusual causes of central retinal artery occlusion should be considered, particularly in patients who are less than 60 years of age. These include cardiac valvular disease or atrial myxoma, collagen vascular diseases such as polyarthritis nodosa, systemic coagulopathies, and also taking oral contraceptive pills.

Fluorescein angiography is rarely required to establish the diagnosis. If performed, the dye enters the retinal circulation after considerable delay and in the acute state shortly after occlusion may fail to pass completely into the arterial circulation (Fig. 1(b)). Background choroidal fluorescence is normal and the optic disc stains brightly.

Treatment

After the passage of a few hours it is unusual for treatment of central retinal artery occlusion to lead to visual improvement because of irreversible neuronal degeneration. If a patient is fortunate to present quickly and is observed to have a retinal embolus attempts to move the embolus further into the vascular bed should be attempted to try and restore at least part of the retinal arterial flow. A number of therapeutic techniques have been employed, but often with disappointing results. However, occasional successes are witnessed and patients should be given the benefit of the doubt. Most treatments centre around reducing the ocular pressure to encourage the embolus to become dislodged at the bifurcation of upper and lower divisions. Paracentesis of the anterior chamber to reduce the ocular pressure sharply has many advocates. Alternatively massage of the eye for a period of 15 min or administration of intravenous acetazolamide can also be tried. Rebreathing in a paper bag can be done easily to try to cause vascular dilatation

from hypercarbia. A further treatment of acute occlusion which has been advocated is breathing high oxygen and high carbon dioxide concentrations. High oxygen leads to increasing oxygen saturation in the retina, particularly via the choroidal circulation. High carbon dioxide concentration acts as a vasodilator of the retinal circulation and may allow improved retinal perfusion.

Approximately 5 per cent of central retinal artery occlusions may later develop neovascularization arising either in the fundus or on the iris. Panretinal photocoagulation is then required to regress new vessel formation.

Patients with suspected emboli from the carotid arteries may also be given anticoagulation for future prophylaxis. Aspirin administration has been demonstrated to reduce further morbidity from embolization. Patients with giant cell arteritis should have prednisolone orally. Initially this is given in high doses (80–100 mg/day) and is reduced every few days in line with the reduction of erythrocyte sedimentation rate. Low dose maintenance of steroid usage is normally required for at least 2 years.

Branch retinal artery obstruction

Embolization may result in obstruction of peripheral retinal arterioles by lodging at vessel bifurcations. The smaller the embolus the further down the vascular tree the site of impaction will occur and, therefore, the smaller the visual disturbance. Tiny emboli are often asymptomatic and may be discovered on routine ophthalmoscopy. The majority of emboli are seen in the territory of either the upper or lower temporal arterioles but nasal vessels may also be involved. The appearance of the emboli depend on their constituents and may be composed of cholesterol (Hollenhorst plaque) or platelets. Rarely a branch arterial obstruction may occur when an arteriole lies close to a focus of retinal infection, for example septic embolus. The vessel wall becomes infiltrated and the lumen constricted.

Pallor of the affected sector is observed beyond the embolus similar to that seen in central retinal artery occlusion (Fig. 2). The visual field shows an arcuate scotoma concurring with the affected territory of infarction. Unlike central retinal artery occlusion visual acuity is often normal with the fovea maintaining perfusion from the unaffected area of retinal circulation. Small emboli in the finer branches may produce no sign of infarction and may be observed in patients having brief loss of vision from transient ischaemic attacks. Patients exhibiting emboli should undergo a cardiovascular examination including duplex scanning of the carotid arteries. They should be treated with low dose aspirin daily. Systemic hypertension and cardiac abnormalities should be treated appropriately.

After 2 or 3 weeks the white appearance of the swollen retina resolves leaving a quadrantic atrophy and pallor of the optic disc. The field defect is usually permanent.

Cilioretinal artery occlusion

Cilioretinal arteries have been described in up to 20 per cent of normal individuals. They are derived from the choroidal

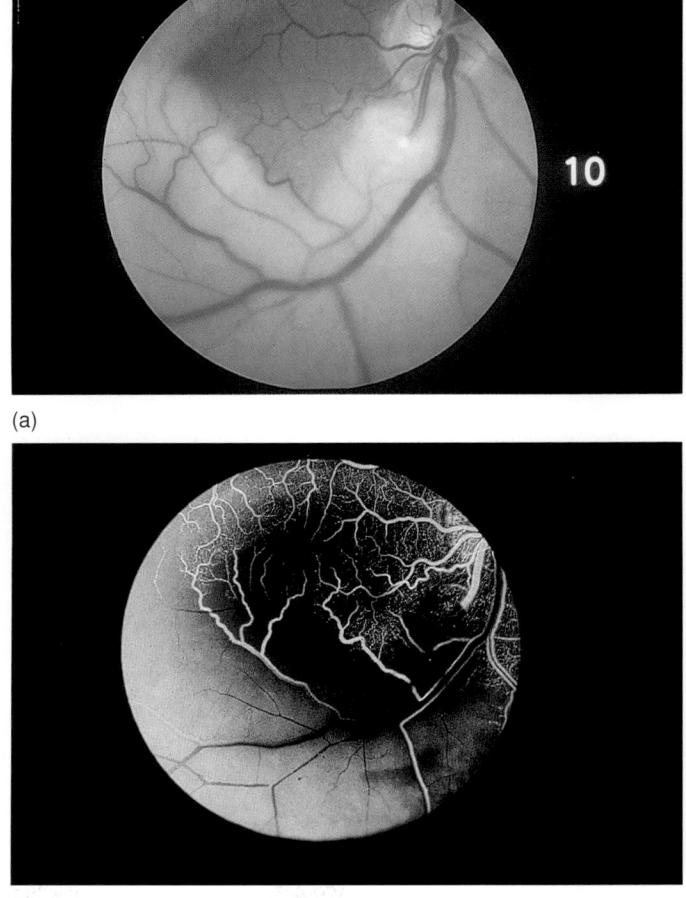

(a)

(b)

Fig. 2 (a) Cholesterol embolus of inferotemporal arteriole. (b) Angiogram of (a) with absent circulation beyond the embolus and showing laminar filling of the veins from adjacent perfused retina.

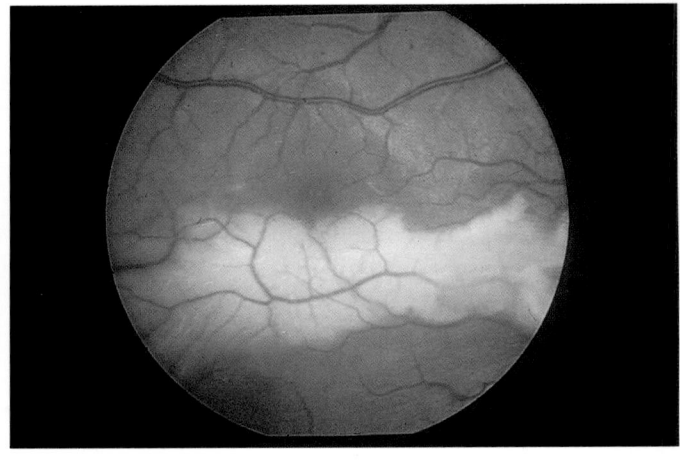

(a)

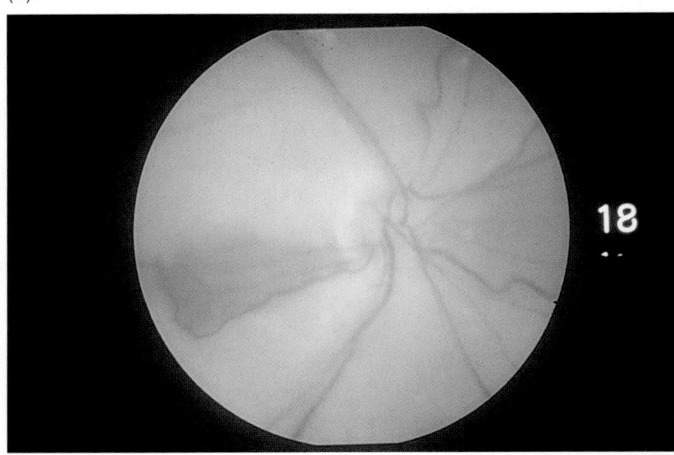

(b)

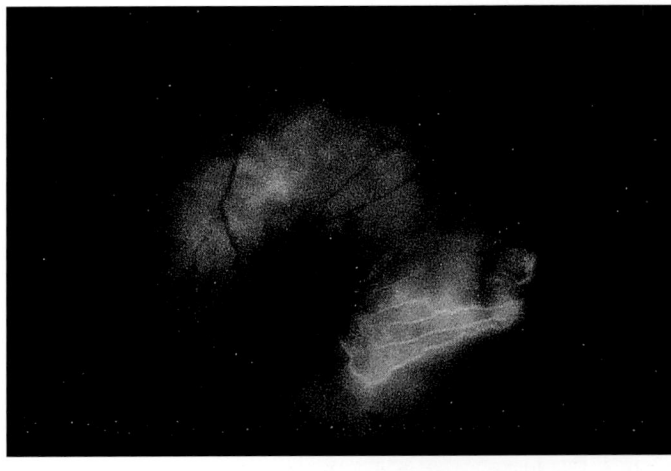

(c)

Fig. 3 (a) Cilioretinal artery occlusion with blocked orthograde axoplasmic transport particularly near the disc at the lower border of the infarcted territory. (b) Obstructed central retinal artery with cilioretinal sparing. (c) Angiogram of (b) showing continued perfusion of the area supplied by the cilioretinal artery.

circulation, emerge at the optic disc, and supply a variable territory of the inner retina. Most commonly cilioretinal arteries are found on the temporal side of the disc, frequently supplying a part of the macula. Less commonly nasal cilioretinal arteries are found.

Predisposing conditions leading to cilioretinal artery obstruction are similar to those for central retinal artery occlusion, namely arteriosclerosis and hypertension but it is rarely associated with emboli. Clinical presentation of cilioretinal artery occlusion is similar to branch retinal artery occlusion. An area of the visual field is lost and patients notice a rapid painless loss of part of their sight over a few minutes.

Fundoscopy at the acute stage of occlusion reveals an area of retinal pallor which is in stark contrast to the surrounding normal retina (Fig. 3). There are accompanying obstructions of axoplasmic transport giving white cotton-wool spots in the nerve fibre layer.

Cilioretinal artery obstruction also may be found with central retinal vein occlusion. The reason for this is not well understood but it is possible that the lower perfusion pressure of the choroidal circulation compared with the retinal circulation, may

allow more profound vascular stasis when the central retinal vein is obstructed (Fig. 4).

Depending on the precise area of supply by the affected cilioretinal artery the loss of vision may be relatively minor or

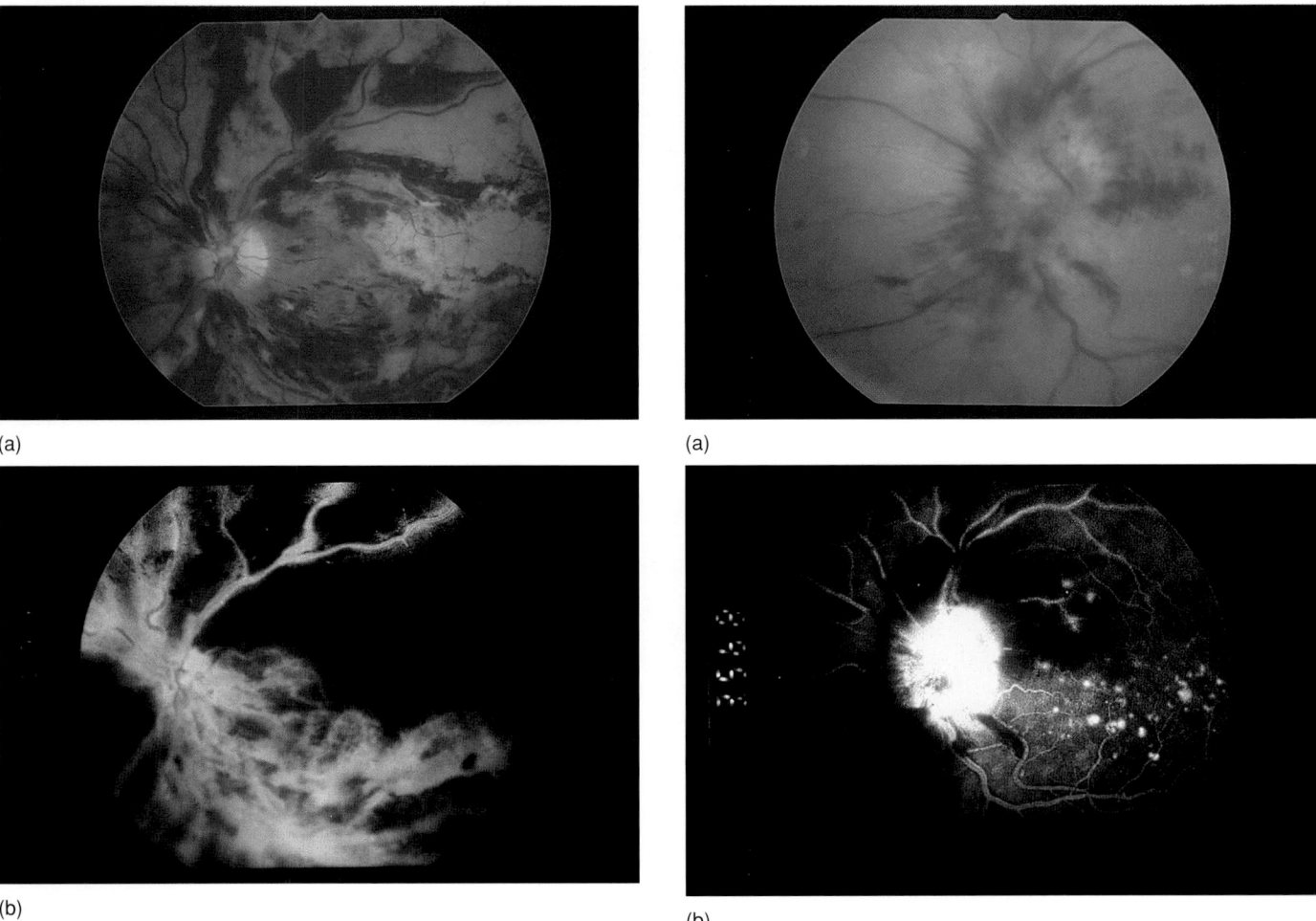

(a)

(b)

Fig. 4 (a, b) Central retinal vein occlusion with associated closure of the arterial circulation above the macula. Note the area superotemporal to the fovea with increased pallor of the retina and considerably fewer retinal haemorrhages.

(a)

(b)

Fig. 5 (a) Anterior ischaemic optic neuropathy with marked disc swelling and peripapillary haemorrhages. (b) Angiogram of (a) with hyperfluorescence of the disc, masking of the fluorescein by the haemorrhages, and normal retinal vessel filling. There are incidental macular drusen showing uptake of fluorescein dye.

may involve a large area of the macula. Recovery of function in the affected territory is uncommon.

Investigation and treatment is similar to retinal branch artery occlusion.

Anterior ischaemic optic neuropathy

Arterial occlusions of the retinal circulation should be differentiated from the sudden loss of vision occurring as a result of ischaemia from the ciliary circulation supplying the circle of Zinn in the optic nerve head (anterior ischaemic optic neuropathy).

Symptomatically patients experience symptoms similar to retinal artery obstruction, namely sudden painless loss of vision in part or all of the visual field of one eye. The area of field loss depends on the extent of the ischaemia of the optic nerve head. Field charting may show an arcuate defect radiating from the blind spot, quadrantic, hemianopic, or complete loss.

On fundoscopy the optic disc appears swollen in contrast to retinal artery occlusion. The peripheral retina is usually normal but obstructed orthograde axoplasmic flow shows as infiltration of the disc head (Fig. 5). The causes are similar to retinal arter-

ial occlusion although embolism is rarely involved. Giant cell arteritis must be excluded in the elderly.

Venous occlusion

Central retinal vein occlusion

Central retinal vein occlusion is the second most common vascular cause of serious visual loss after diabetes. Obstruction of venous outflow at the level of the laminar cribrosa leads to the typical fundus appearance of central retinal vein occlusion. Histology of affected eyes has demonstrated obstruction of the vessel lumen by thrombus in the majority of instances but this is not invariably the case. In some histological specimens the venous lumen appears patent.

Predisposing factors for central venous occlusion have been implicated, namely pre-existing essential hypertension, diabetes, arteriosclerosis, hypercoagulability states, and raised ocular pressure. Central vein occlusion normally occurs in the older population and such underlying systemic disease is common in this age group. A true association between cardio-vascular disease and central vein occlusion has been difficult to identify. A well-established predisposing factor is raised intra-ocular pressure. Patients presenting with central vein occlusion should always have the ocular pressure of both eyes measured because the affected eye may temporarily have a period of hypotension following the occlusion. The predisposing ocular hypertension may, therefore, be missed if the tension in the fellow eye is not measured.

It is well recognized that central vein occlusion has a strong tendency to occur overnight while the patient is asleep. It has been suggested that in susceptible individuals the normal pos-tural ocular pressure adjustment within the eye may not occur with the result that the venous circulation is embarrassed by back pressure in the supine position.

Other systemic disorders associated with central retinal vein occlusions are hyperviscosity syndromes such as multiple myel-oma or polycythaemia, and there is increased risk in younger women taking the contraceptive pill.

Clinical features

Central vein occlusion presents with painless uniocular loss of vision. The degree of visual disturbance is variable depending on the severity of the causative obstruction. Some patients pre-sent with reasonable visual acuity better than 6/18 but the majority of affected eyes have an acuity of 6/24 or less and many are worse than 6/60.

Typically the fundus appearance is one of scattered retinal haemorrhages throughout the retina. Venous congestion and tortuosity with swelling of the optic disc is seen and in addition there may be scattered cotton-wool spots if there is capillary closure (Figs 6 and 7). Depending on the degree of retinal isch-aemia a relative afferent pupil defect may be observed and in some cases this may be the best available method of assessing a risk of later neovascular glaucoma if angiography cannot be performed (see below). Intraocular pressure is frequently found to be elevated and some patients have pre-existing symptoms and signs of primary open angle glaucoma or ocular hyperten-sion.

In the acute stage macular oedema is almost invariably pre-sent, although this can resolve spontaneously in less seriously affected cases during the succeeding weeks or months. Over a period of many months the retinal haemorrhages absorb and retinal venous calibre returns to normal. Enlargement of venous collaterals on the optic disc can be observed in the late stage of venous occlusion from redirection of retinal blood flow into the choroidal circulation (opticociliary shunts). If profound retinal ischaemia has occurred the optic disc becomes pale. In long-standing cases after some years there may be little abnormal to see in the fundus except a slight pigmentary irregularity at the macula and reduced visual acuity.

Variations from the usual clinical presentation are sometimes encountered. Mild cases of central retinal vein occlusion some-times show only a few peripheral retinal haemorrhages and the picture can be confused with venous stasis retinopathy from reduced arterial perfusion secondary to low ophthalmic artery pressure. Careful investigation with carotid ultrasound scan-

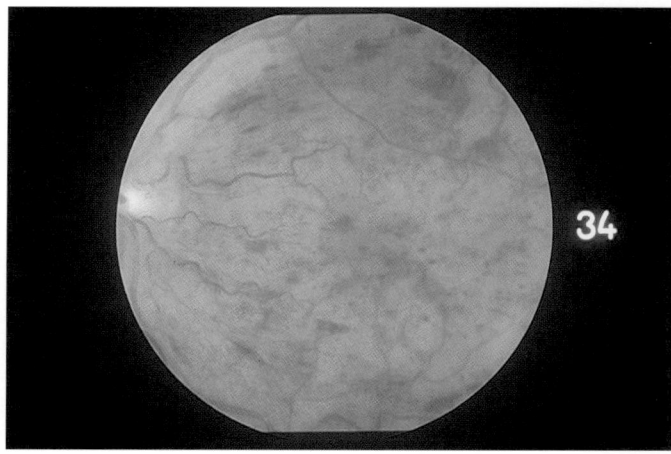

(a)

(b)

Fig. 6 (a) Central retinal vein occlusion. (b) Angiogram of (a) showing complete capillary survival but considerable dilatation and dye exudation through the vessel walls.

ning and ophthalmodynamometry will differentiate between these two conditions; venous stasis retinopathy shows retinal arterial collapse with low external pressure applied to the eye unlike the normal pressure encountered with vein occlusion. A further variation is the presence of a cilioretinal artery occlusion in conjunction with central vein occlusion. In rare cases a branch retinal arterial obstruction can occur.

Between 5 and 10 per cent of cases sustaining central retinal vein occlusion are only mildly affected when they initially pre-sent. However, during the following few weeks a second occlus-ive episode can occur which almost invariably leads to profound retinal ischaemia and further serious loss of vision. Such double occlusions are particularly prone to neovascular glaucoma.

Investigation

Haematological evaluation to exclude underlying predisposing causes of occlusion should be considered in all cases. Blood pressure, plasma glucose, and plasma viscosity should be meas-ured. In younger patients causes of vasculitis should be sought such as lupus erythematosis and conditions causing hypercoag-ulability like multiple myeloma and polycythaemia should be excluded.

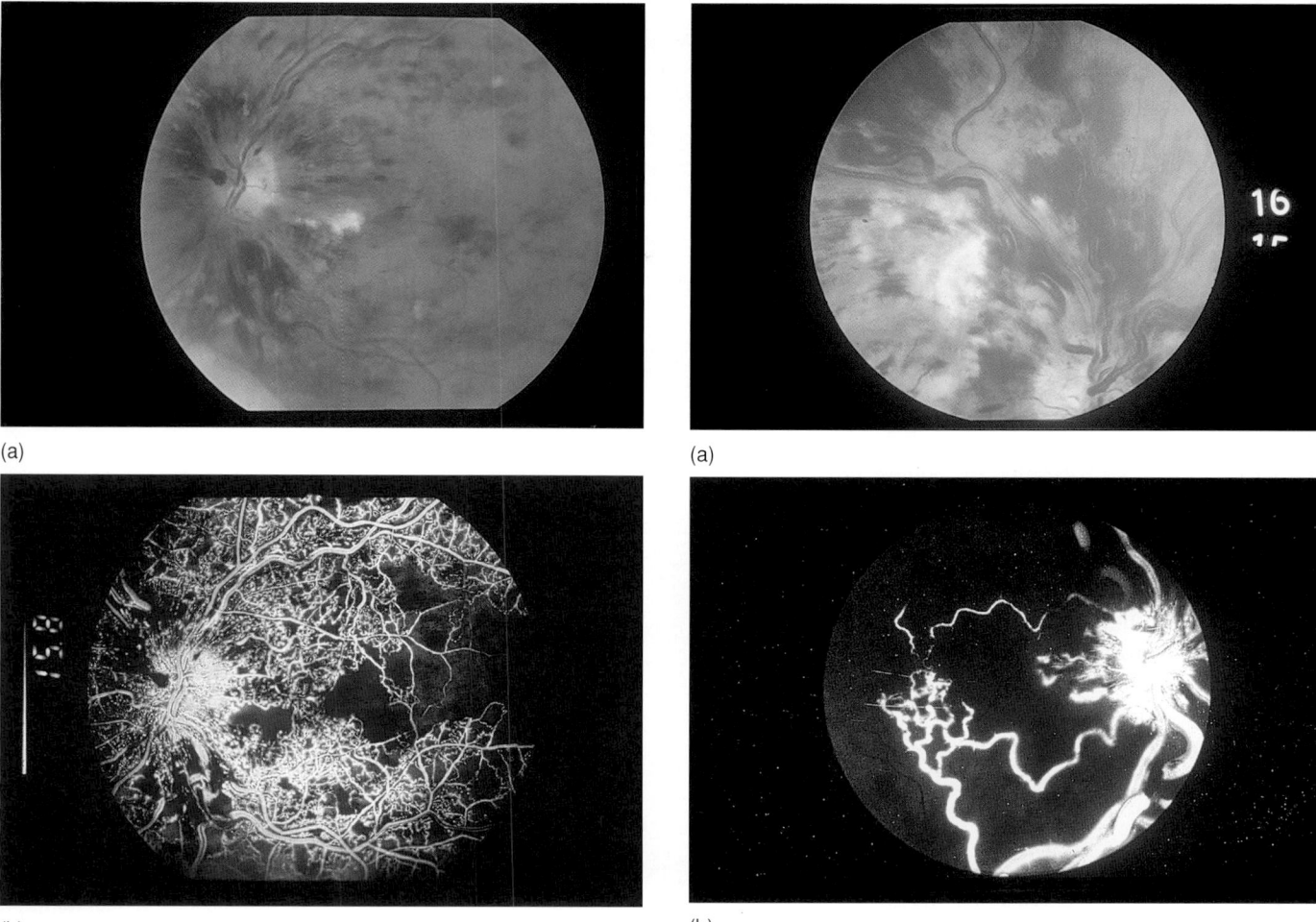

(a)

(b)

(a)

(b)

Fig. 7 (a) Central retinal vein occlusion with a few cotton-wool spots. (b) Angiogram of (a) showing marked capillary dilatation with tortuosity and also areas of closure temporal to the macula.

Fig. 8 (a) Central retinal vein occlusion with diffuse sheet haemorrhages, venous tortuosity, and cotton-wool spots. (b) Angiogram of (a) demonstrating complete capillary loss. Note that assessment of capillary loss is possible even with the presence of multiple haemorrhages.

Fluorescein angiography should be undertaken in all patients with central retinal vein occlusion provided the patient is systemically well enough to tolerate the procedure. This may not be the case in the extreme elderly patient and reliance may have to be placed on the relative afferent pupil defect to assess retinal ischaemia.

Fluorescein angiography has demonstrated that central retinal vein occlusion divides into those cases with good capillary survival, which accounts for approximately two-thirds of cases, and those showing variable degrees of retinal capillary closure (Figs 6–8). With increasing areas of capillary closure the risk of neovascular glaucoma increases. Severe retinal ischaemia should be treated by panretinal photocoagulation (see below). The visual prognosis in cases showing extensive capillary closure is much worse than the non-ischaemia type.

When capillary closure does not occur the capillary bed in acute cases shows dilatation with tortuosity and fluorescein leakage in the later stages of the angiogram. Chronic macular oedema is the usual cause of persistently reduced acuity in long-standing non-ischaemic retinal vein occlusion. It is important to establish soon after the occlusion the degree of

retinal capillary leakage or ischaemia, as this has a direct bearing on the later management of the patient. Although haemorrhages may mask some parts of the angiogram and make interpretation more difficult it is usually possible at an early stage following central vein occlusion to assess the degree of ischaemia in spite of haemorrhages.

Electrophysiology has been shown to be useful in assessing retinal vein obstruction, with particular regard to identifying extensive ischaemia. The electroretinogram frequently shows a reduced B wave and also a reduced B to A wave ratio. The electro-oculogram demonstrates a reduced light rise when compared with the fellow eye in those eyes showing ischaemia.

Treatment

Treatment of patients with central retinal vein occlusion depends upon the degree of capillary disturbance. Those patients showing macular oedema should be followed for signs of diminishing visual acuity. Although the risk of developing neovascular glaucoma does not arise acuity may gradually be reduced, particularly if cystoid spaces develop at the fovea.

When deteriorating visual acuity is observed between 6 and 12 months postocclusion grid photocoagulation can be considered for the persistent oedema. The results of such grid treatment are frequently disappointing but some patients have resolution of oedema with concomitant stabilization or improvement of visual acuity.

An alternative laser treatment by creating a retinochoroidal anastomosis in the peripheral retina has been tried for cases of non-ischaemic persistent macular oedema. For some patients the technique seems to work satisfactorily but serious complications have been reported, such as vitreous haemorrhage and vasoproliferation.

Ischaemic central venous occlusion may need peripheral panretinal photocoagulation, depending upon the degree of retinal capillary closure. Extensive closure carries more than an 80 per cent risk of iris neovascularization and should have prophylactic panretinal laser treatment. Intermediate degrees of ischaemia carry an approximate 25 per cent risk of iris new vessels and can, therefore, be observed monthly for the first 6 months. If early new vessels are observed on the iris, prophylactic photocoagulation should be administered without delay.

Optic disc neovascularization is uncommon in cases of central retinal vein occlusion but has been well described, particularly in patients having received previous photocoagulation to prevent iris new vessels. If disc new vessels are observed panretinal laser treatment should be given.

Patients with underlying systemic disease should be referred for management of their condition and women taking the contraceptive pill should be advised to discontinue it and use alternative methods of contraception. Anticoagulants have not been shown to have any long-term benefit in the management of central retinal vein occlusion but trials have been reported demonstrating benefit from haemodilution.

Neovascular glaucoma

Extensive hypotoxia of the neuroretina may be followed by subsequent endothelial cell proliferation, mainly from the retinal vessels. This fibrovascular growth is stimulated by the production of polypeptide neovascular factors from the poorly perfused retina. Secondary glaucoma resulting from iris neovascularization and growth of fibrovascular tissue over the trabecular meshwork is a well-recognized complication of central retinal vein occlusion, in common with other retinal vascular diseases inducing extensive ischaemia. The development of neovascular glaucoma occurs approximately 3 months from the time of venous obstruction, hence the term '90-day glaucoma' previously applied to this condition. The likelihood of neovascular glaucoma is related to the area of retinal vascular ischaemia and those who have total capillary loss have an 80 per cent risk of developing intractable painful glaucoma. Prophylactic retinal ablation should be given in such cases to regress the new vessels if possible. If laser treatment fails, peripheral retinal cryotherapy can be tried.

Careful observation of patients with recent onset ischaemic central vein occlusion should be undertaken on a monthly basis initially with particular regard to the development of fine iris new vessels. If these are observed panretinal photocoagulation is required in an attempt to prevent the later onset of full blown neovascular glaucoma. Once neovascular glaucoma is established further treatment is of little avail and mydriatics and steroid drops are the mainstay of keeping the affected eye comfortable. Enucleation is occasionally required.

Retinal branch vein occlusion

Tributaries of the retinal venous system may become occluded at the site of arteriovenous crossings. Retinal arterioles and venules share a common adventitial sheath at the point of crossing and conditions which cause thickening of the arteriolar wall may lead to embarrassment of the venous return and ultimately to occlusion. Most commonly vein occlusions occur where the arteriole lies superficial to the vein and the majority occur in the upper temporal quadrant. However, any area of the venous circulation may be involved, either centrally or peripherally. As with other vascular occlusions it is mainly the older population who are at risk, particularly those with essential hypertension. Medial hypertrophy of the arterioles in hypertension cause arteriovenous nipping and a tendency to subsequent occlusion. In many cases retinal branch vein occlusion occurs in the absence of any underlying systemic abnormality. Branch vein occlusions may occur just anterior to the lamina cribrosa causing a hemispheric vein occlusion. More commonly the upper or lower temporal arcade may be involved but the nasal retina, retinal periphery, or small macular tributaries, may be occluded.

Clinical features

The symptoms and signs of branch vein occlusion depend upon the site and area of retina involved. Small peripheral vein occlusions tend to be asymptomatic but when macular function is disturbed patients are aware of sudden onset of painless blurring of acuity.

In the acute stage the retina is oedematous with scattered haemorrhages and sometimes cotton-wool spots are seen (Fig. 9). In time the haemorrhages absorb but lipid exudate may be deposited as a result of chronic vascular leakage.

With long-standing vascular occlusions the exudates and oedema absorb and leave attenuated sheathed vessels in the affected territory. Macular oedema may persist for many months or years with consequent gradual deterioration of central acuity.

The natural history of retinal branch vein occlusions is encouraging in many cases. Fifty per cent of patients showing macular oedema initially will return to, or maintain, 6/12 vision or better, with resolution of the oedema.

Investigation

Fluorescein angiography is useful in branch vein occlusions in which a quadrant or more of the venous system is occluded. In cases of quadrantic occlusions or more it is important to establish whether the retinal capillary circulation has been occluded with consequent retinal ischaemia (Fig. 10). In those cases showing good capillary survival observation for persistent macular oedema is all that is required. Those patients with considerable ischaemia have a risk of developing vasoprolifer-

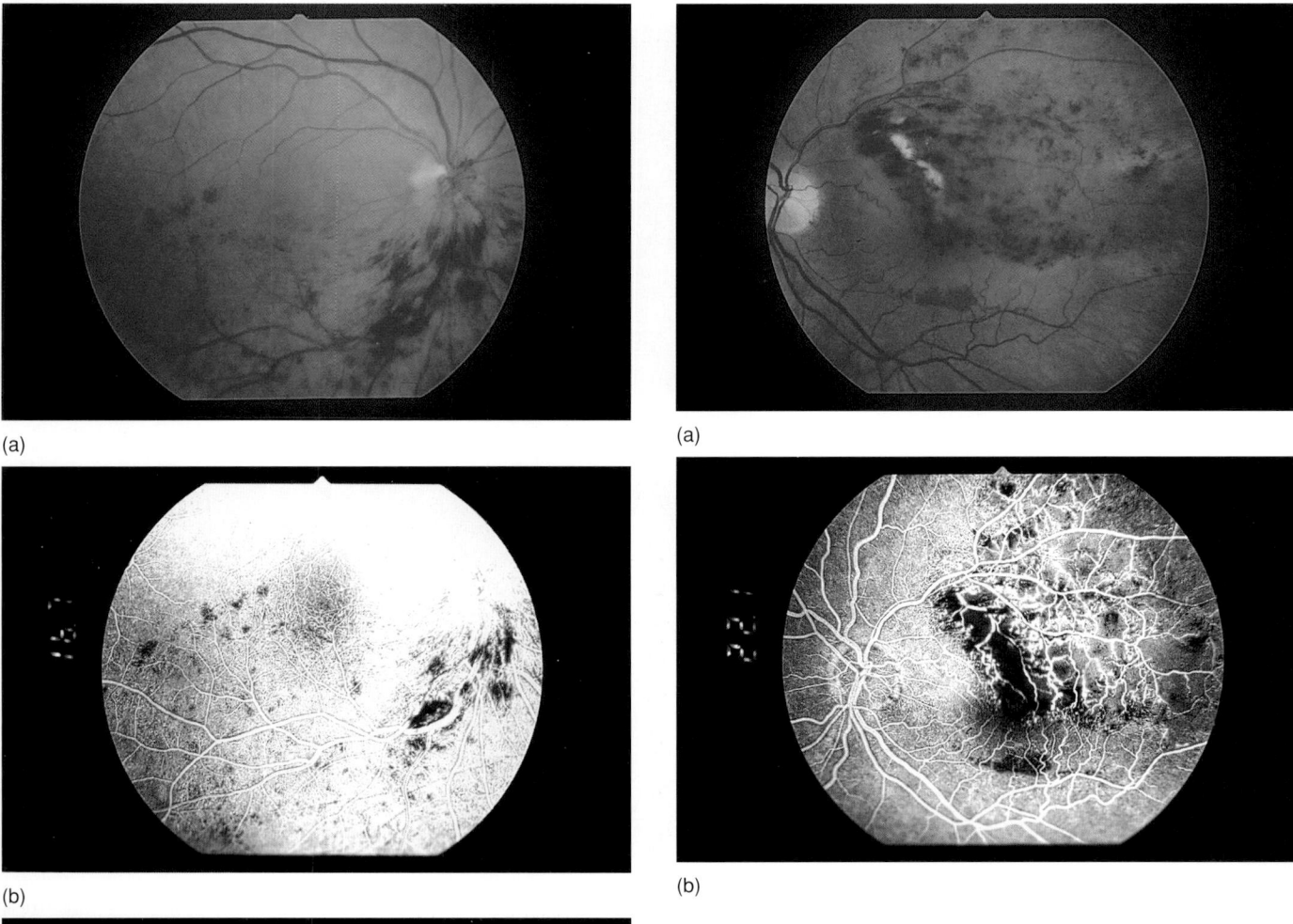

(a)

(b)

(c)

Fig. 9 (a) Acute branch retinal vein occlusion in the lower half of the retina. (b) Angiogram of (a) showing good capillary survival but considerable dilatation, especially below the fovea. (c) Diffuse leakage and macular oedema from damaged capillary tight junctions.

(a)

(b)

Fig. 10 (a) Upper temporal retinal branch vein occlusion at an arteriovenous crossing site one disc diameter from the disc edge. (b) Angiogram of (a) with considerable retinal capillary closure in the territory drained by the venous tributary.

ation on the optic disc or from the peripheral retinal circulation between 1 and 3 years after occlusion. Patients showing marked ischaemia must be followed 6 or 9 monthly until the risk of neovascularization has receded, that is 3 years or so. Unlike central retinal vein occlusion iris neovascularization is rare and neovascular glaucoma does not occur. It is, therefore, advant-

ageous to wait 3 months or more prior to carrying out fluorescein angiography so that the angiogram is not obscured by retinal haemorrhage and more detail can be assessed. Small macular branch vein occlusions do not usually require angiography either to establish the diagnosis or to assess macular oedema, which is apparent on slit lamp biomicroscopy. However, sometimes angiography can be helpful in macular branch vein occlusions following unsuccessful laser treatment in order to delineate those areas continuing to leak and needing further photocoagulation. Complications of retinal branch vein occlusion are persistent macular oedema and retinal neovascularization with subsequent vitreous haemorrhage.

Treatment

Patients showing macular oedema should be followed on a regular basis and if visual acuity is worse than 6/18 after 12 months or if visual acuity is demonstrated to be deteriorating during the first year of follow-up laser photocoagulation should be undertaken. Focal treatment to the areas of capillary leakage should be used initially but if this is unsuccessful grid treatment in the leaking territory should be tried.

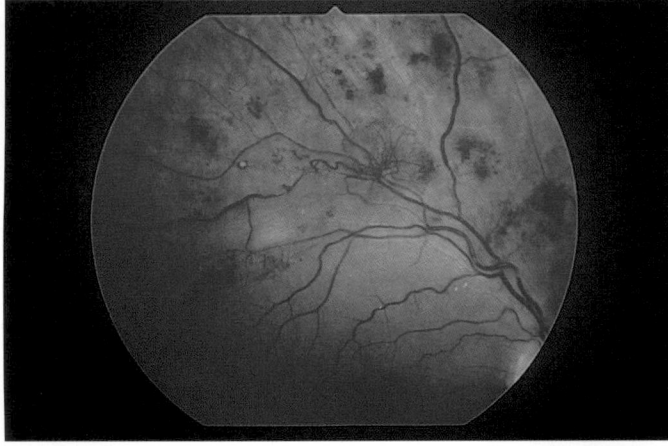

(a)

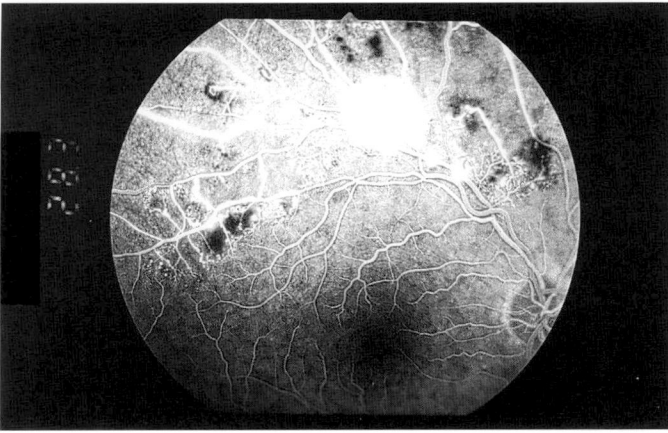

(b)

Fig. 11 (a) Long-standing upper temporal vein occlusion with a frond of forward new vessels. (b) Angiogram of (a) demonstrating intense fluorescein leakage from the new vessel complex. Note the point of origin of the new vessels lying at the margin of the hypoxic and normally perfused retina.

Patients with 25 per cent or more of the retina showing ischaemia are at risk of developing neovascularization from the disc or retinal periphery (Fig. 11). Such neovascularization requires panretinal photocoagulation in the ischaemic territory involved by the vein occlusion to reverse the proliferative process and reduce the risk of vitroeus haemorrhage. Sometimes peripheral branch vein occlusions remain undetected until vitreous haemorrhage supersedes from forward new vessels.

Although the incidence of vitreous haemorrhage is reduced by laser treatment once proliferative retinopathy is established a proportion of patients may still suffer vitreous haemorrhage. If this fails to clear in reasonable time a vitrectomy may be indicated. Often macular function in such cases remains remarkably good unless previously compromised by chronic macular oedema or unless the foveal capillaries have been occluded.

Further reading

Arterial occlusion

Appen, R.E., Wray, S.H., and Cogan, D.G. (1975). Central retinal artery occlusion. *American Journal of Ophthalmology*, **79**, 374–81.

Augsburger, J.J. and Magargal, L.E. (1980). Visual prognosis following treatment of central retinal artery obstruction. *British Journal of Ophthalmology*, **64**, 913–17.

Baghdassarian, S.A., Crawford, J.B., and Rathburn, J.E. (1970). Calcific emboli of the retinal and ciliary arteries. *American Journal of Ophthalmology*, **69**, 372–5.

Brown, G.C. and Shields, J.A. (1979). Cilioretinal arteries and retinal artery obstruction. *Archives of Ophthalmology*, **97**, 84–92.

Brown, G.C., Magargal, L.E., and Sergott, R. (1986). Acute obstruction of the retinal and choroidal circulations. *Ophthalmology*, **93**, 1373–82.

Ealing, E.M., Sanders, M.D., and Miller, S.J.H. (1974). Ischaemic papillopathy. *British Journal of Ophthalmology*, **58**, 990–1008.

Ffytche, T.J. (1974). A rationalisation of treatment of central retinal artery occlusion. *Transactions of the Ophthalmology Society UK*, **94**, 468–79.

McLeod, D. and Ring, C.P. (1976). Cilioretinal infarction after retinal vein occlusion. *British Journal of Ophthalmology*, **60**, 419–27.

McLeod, D., Marshall, J., Kohner, E.M., and Bird, A.C. (1977). The role of exoplasmic transport in the pathogenesis of retinal cotton wool spots. *British Journal of Ophthalmology*, **61**, 177–91.

Manschott, W.A. and Lee, W.R. (1985). Development of retinal neovascularisation in vascular occlusive disease. *Transactions of the Ophthalmology Society UK*, **104**, 880–6.

Yannof, M. and Fine, B.S. (1996). *Ocular pathology*, (4th edn), pp. 365–72. Mosby-Wolfe.

Venous occlusion

Branch Retinal Vein Occlusion Study Group (1984). Argon laser photocoagulation for macular oedema in branch retinal vein occlusion. *American Journal of Ophthalmology*, **98**, 271–82.

Branch Retinal Vein Occlusion Study Group (1986). Argon laser scatter photocoagulation for prevention of neovascularisation and vitreous haemorrhage in branch vein occlusion. *Archives of Ophthalmology*, **104**, 34–41.

Clemett, R.S., Kohner, E.M., and Hamilton, A.M. (1973). The visual prognosis in retinal branch vein occlusion. *Transactions of the Ophthalmology Society UK*, **93**, 523–35.

Eye Disease Case–Control Study Group (1996). Risk factors for central retinal vein occlusion. *Archives of Ophthalmology*, **114**, 545–54.

Grey, R.H.B. and Bloom, P.A. (1991). Retinal ischaemia and afferent pupil defects in central retinal vein occlusion. *European Journal of Ophthalmology*, **1**, 85–8.

Hayreh, S.S. (1983). Classification of central retinal vein occlusion. *Ophthalmology*, **90**, 458–74.

Hayreh, S.S., Rogas, P., Podhajsky, P., Montague, P., and Woolson, R.F. (1983). Ocular neovascularisation with retinal vein occlusion. *Ophthalmology*, **90**, 488–506.

Kearns, T.P. (1983). Differential diagnosis of central retinal vein obstruction. *Ophthalmology*, **90**, 475–80.

Kohner, E.M., Laatikainen, L., and Oughton, J. (1983). The management of central retinal vein occlusion. *Ophthalmology*, **90**, 484–7.

Laatikainen, L. and Kohner, E.M. (1976). Fluorescein angiography and its prognostic significance in central retinal vein occlusion. *British Journal of Ophthalmology*, **60**, 411–17.

Laatikainen, L., Kohner, E.M., Khoury, D., and Blach, R.K. (1977). Panretinal photocoagulation in central retinal vein occlusion. *British Journal of Ophthalmology*, **61**, 741–53.

Magargal, L.E., Donoso, L.A., and Sanborn, G.E. (1982). Retinal ischaemia and risk of neovascularisation following central retinal vein occlusion. *Ophthalmology*, **89**, 1241–5.

Ring, C.P., Pearson, T.C., Sanders, M.D., Wether, S.E.Y., and Mein, G. (1976). Viscosity and retinal vein thrombosis. *British Journal of Ophthalmology*, **60**, 397–410.

Sabates, R., Hirose, T., and McMeel, J.W. (1983). Electroretinography in the prognosis and classification of central retinal vein occlusion. *Archives of Ophthalmology*, **101**, 232–5.

Shilling, J.S. and Kohner, E.M. (1976). New vessel formation in retinal branch vein occlusion. *British Journal of Ophthalmology*, **60**, 810–15.

2.9.5 Hereditary pigmentary retinal and macular dystrophies

Kevin Gregory-Evans and Alan C. Bird

Definitions

Retinal dystrophies comprise a number of conditions in which atrophy of mature retinal tissue (retinal pigment epithelium and neurosensory retina) occurs as a consequence of a genetically determined defect. These conditions are distinguished from dysplasias in which an embryonic abnormality results from failure of maturation, and degenerations where deterioration of mature tissue is secondary to an acquired influence such as trauma, toxic agent, vascular disease, or inflammation. These distinctions are important clinically. The term dystrophy implies that visual disability will progress, and that the disease may also develop in relatives of the patient.

Prevalence

No comprehensive statistics on the prevalence of retinal dystrophies exist. However, in two Royal National Institute for the Blind surveys, 24 per cent of adults reported genetic causes for their blindness. The parents of 23 per cent of British children blind or partially sighted, reported 'heredity' or 'parents incompatible' as a cause for their visual deficit. Studies in Europe, Australia and the United States have suggested that as much as 50 per cent of blindness in children in the developed world is genetically determined.

More precise information exists concerning retinitis pigmentosa which affects approximately 1.5 million people worldwide with 100 000 sufferers in Europe, and a similar number in the United States. Prevalence figures from developed countries report figures of approximately 1 in 5000 with the highest figure (1 in 1878) in the Navajo Indians.

Molecular genetics

Great advances have been made in our understanding of the genetic basis of retinal dystrophies. Molecular genetic linkage analysis has been especially important in the localization of a number of genes causing retinal dystrophy (Table 1). Heterogeneity identified by linkage analysis indicates that many genes expressed in the retina will be causally related to retinal dystrophies with the promise of establishing a detailed understanding of these conditions at a molecular level.

To date, three retinal genes have been shown to be particularly important. *Rhodopsin*, a gene encoding rod photopigment, has been associated with dominant and recessive retinitis pigmentosa and congenital stationary night-blindness (Fig. 1(a)). *Peripherin/RDS* encodes a structural protein found in the outer segment membranes of both rod and cone photoreceptors. In

humans, *peripherin/RDS* mutations give rise to a variety of dominant phenotypes including retinitis pigmentosa, central areolar choroidal dystrophy, adult viteliform macular dystrophy, and macular, cone–rod, and pattern dystrophies (Figs 1(b and c)). Virtually all *peripherin/RDS*-associated phenotypes show evidence of widespread cone and rod dysfunction on detailed investigation indicating generalized photoreceptor dysfunction. Mutations in *TIMP3* have recently been associated with Sorsby's fundus dystrophy a phenotype with many similarities to age-related macular degeneration (Fig. 1(d) and see below). The TIMP3 protein (tissue inhibitor of metalloproteinase-3) plays an important role in the regulation of matrix metalloproteinases, enzymes involved in the synthesis and degradation of extracellular matrix.

Clinical assessment and classification

Most retinal dystrophies can be identified from a brief history, detailed clinical examination, and a few investigations. A family survey will often help in cases with minimal symptoms or nonspecific signs, and is invaluable in establishing the mode of inheritance. Night-blindness is usually, not invariably the first reported symptom in peripheral retinal dystrophies with peripheral field loss usually indicating advanced disease. A preference for subdued illumination when reading may indicate a macular or cone dystrophy. Visual acuity and colour vision testing are important and formal visual field assessment mandatory in drivers of motor vehicles. An adequate fundus examination requires indirect ophthalmoscopy and posterior pole biomicroscopy with a 90- or 78-dioptre lens. Bilateral symmetrical disease is usual.

Electrophysiological assessment is an important clinical investigation. Qualitative and quantitative information can be obtained from electroretinography and electro-oculography. Ancillary information can be obtained from dark-adapted static perimetry, dark adaptometry, fluorescein angiography, and autofluorescence imaging using the scanning laser ophthalmoscope.

Classification may be based on clinical signs, characterization of functional deficit, or mode of inheritance. An arbitrary differentiation into those dystrophies that principally affect the peripheral retina and those that principally affect the posterior pole or macula will be used here. This distinction is the most useful clinically since it can be made by simple clinical assessment, and it helps to predict the nature and progression of visual loss.

Dystrophies principally affecting the peripheral retina

Retinitis pigmentosa

Retinitis pigmentosa identifies a group of disorders that are associated with night-blindness (nyctalopia) and constricted peripheral field as early manifestations. Major differences are found in the age of onset of symptoms, the nature of visual

Table 1 Chromosomal localizations and genes implicated in retinal dystrophies

Chromosome	Gene	Inheritance	Retinal dystrophy
1p21–p13		AR	Stargardt's disease
1q13–q32.1		AR	Retinitis pigmentosa
1q32–q41		AR	Usher's syndrome (type II)
3p11–p13		AR	Bardet–Biedl syndrome
3q21	Rhodopsin	AD	Retinitis pigmentosa
3q21	Rhodopsin	AR	Retinitis pigmentosa
3q21–q25		AR	Usher's syndrome (type III)
4p16.3	PDEB	AR	Retinitis pigmentosa
5q13–q14		AD	Wagner's syndrome
5q13–q14		AD	Erosive vitreoretinopathy
6p12	Peripherin/RDS	AD	Retinitis pigmentosa
6p12	Peripherin/RDS	AD	Macular dystrophy
6p12	Peripherin/RDS	AD	Central areolar choroidal dystrophy
6p12	Peripherin/RDS	AD	Adult vitelliform macular dystrophy
6p12	Peripherin/RDS	AD	Pattern dystrophy
6q11–q15		AD	Stargardt's disease
6q16		AD	North Carolina macular dystrophy
6q16		AD	Progressive bifocal chorioretinal atrophy
6q26–q26		AD	Cone dystrophy
7p15–p21		AD	Cystoid macular oedema
7p14		AD	Retinitis pigmentosa
7q		AD	Retinitis pigmentosa
8cen		AD	Retinitis pigmentosa
8q24		AD	Atypical vitelliform macular dystrophy
10q26	OAT	AR	Gyrate atrophy
11p15		AD	Helicoid peripapillary chorioretinal dystrophy
11p13–p15		AR	Usher's syndrome (type 1c)
11q13		AD	Exudative vitreoretinopathy
11q13		AD	Inflammatory vitreoretinopathy
11q13		AD	Best's disease
11q13		AR	Bardet–Biedl syndrome
11q13	ROM1	AR	Retinitis pigmentosa
11q13.5	Myosin VIIA	AR	Usher's syndrome (type Ib)
12q13.1–13.3	COL2A1	AD	Stickler's syndrome
13q34		AD	Stargardt's disease
14q32		AR	Usher's syndrome (type Ia)
16q13–q22		AR	Bardet-Biedl syndrome
17p12–p13		AD	Cone dystrophy
17p13.1		AD	Retinitis pigmentosa
17q		AD	Retinitis pigmentosa
17q11		—	Cone–rod dystrophy
18q21		—	Cone–rod dystrophy
19q13.3		AD	Cone–rod dystrophy
19q13.4		AD	Retinitis pigmentosa
22q13–qter	TIMP3	AD	Sorsby's fundus dystrophy
Xp22		XL	Retinoschisis
Xp21.3		XL	Retinitis pigmentosa (RP6)
Xp21		XL	Retinitis pigmentosa (RP3)
Xp21.1–11.3		XL	Cone dystrophy
Xp11		XL	Exudative vitreoretinopathy
Xp11.3–p11.2		XL	Retinitis pigmentosa (RP2)
Xp11–q11		XL	Åland eye disease
Xq21	GGT	XL	Choroideraemia
Xq28		XL	Cone dystrophy

AD, autosomal dominant; AR, autosomal recessive; XL, X-linked inheritance.

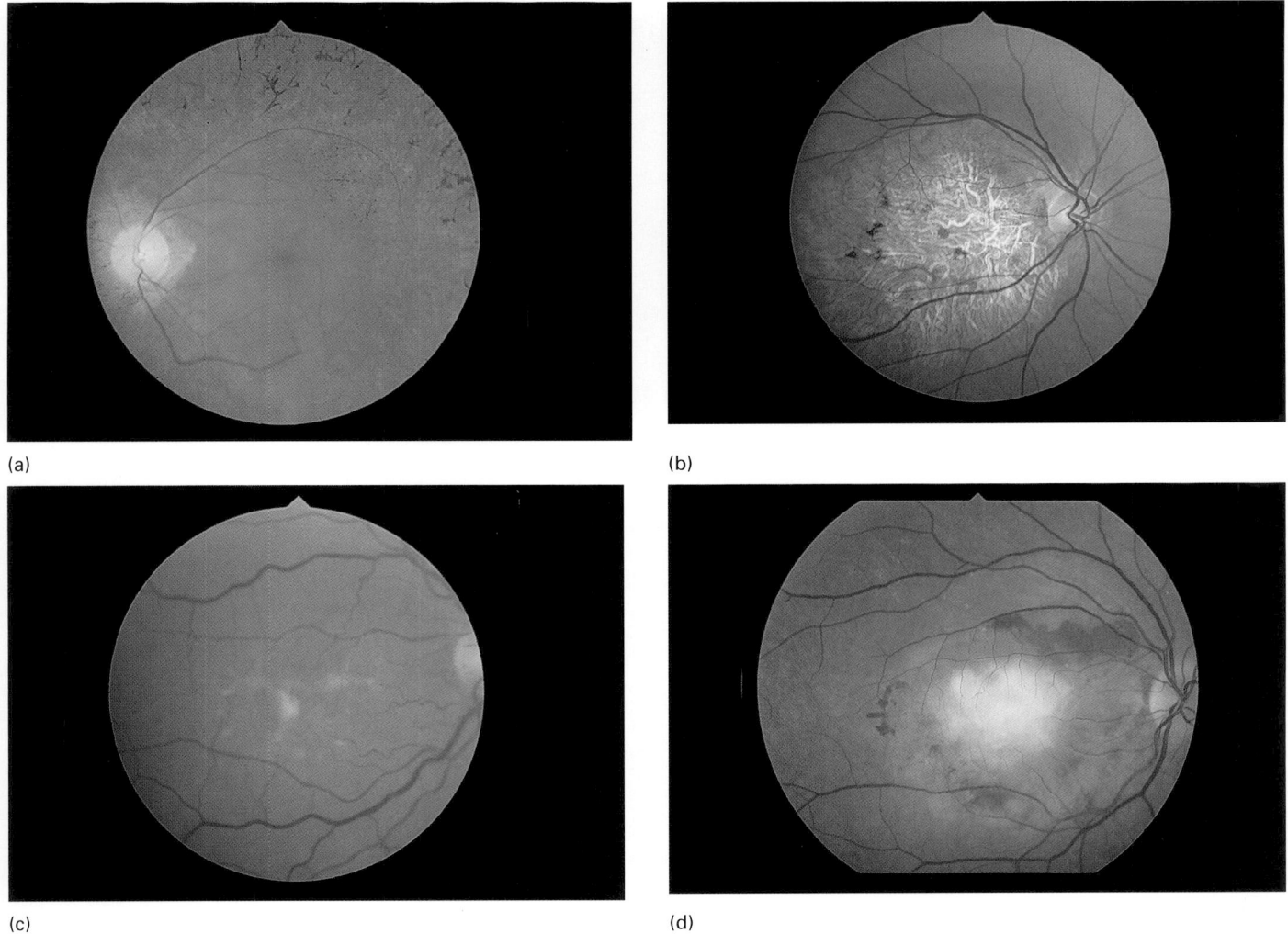

(a)

(b)

(c)

(d)

Fig. 1 Retinal dystrophies associated with specific genetic mutations. (a) Retinitis pigmentosa (*rhodopsin, lys296glu*), (b) macular dystrophy (*peripherin/RDS, arg172tyr*), (c) pattern dystrophy (*peripherin/RDS, tyr140ins*), (d) Sorsby's fundus dystrophy (*TIMP3, ser181cys*).

loss, and speed of progression between the different disorders within this group. Abnormal, bilateral, symmetrical 'bone spicule-like' intraretinal pigmentation is seen which can later develop into extensive chorioretinal atrophy with attenuation of retinal vasculature and secondary optic atrophy. In these later stages, central acuity is often diminished. Other commonly associated ocular features include cystoid macular oedema, myopia, and cataract.

Genetics

Autosomal dominant, autosomal recessive, and X-linked inheritance exist. In 15 to 50 per cent of cases no inheritance pattern is clearly identified (simplex retinitis pigmentosa). If information of an extensive pedigree is not available, severity of disease may be used as a guide to inheritance, for example early onset severe disease is a consistent finding in X-linked disease and common with recessive inheritance, whereas sectorial or altitudinal disease is usually inherited as a dominant trait. Diverse genetic heterogeneity exists. As well as specific mutations of the *rhodopsin* and *peripherin/RDS*, autosomal recessive disease

has been associated with mutations of the gene encoding the β-subunit of phosphodiesterase. Six loci containing dominant retinitis pigmentosa genes and at least two for X-linked disease are known.

Clinical features

Dominant disease may be subclassified into type I and II. The former is characterized as 'diffuse' in that widespread loss of rod function is associated with relative preservation of cone function at some stage of the disease. The latter is characterized by 'regional' distribution of disease with loss of both rod and cone function in some areas but near normal function in others. Although the particular type of disease exhibited is usually consistent within a family, this subclassification does not identify the mutant gene in that both type I and II are seen associated with different rhodopsin mutations. A common feature of dominant disease is variable expressivity in which severity at a particular chronological age varies within a single family. This attribute is a particular feature of the phenotype associated with the 7p14 locus, and is seen in its more extreme form in families linked to the 19q13 locus where members carrying the disease-associated haplotype may either be severely affected or symptomless with effectively normal electrophysiological and psychophysical responses (bimodal expressivity).

Systemic associations

Retinitis pigmentosa, especially in its recessive form, is found in a number of syndromes including Usher's syndrome type I and III (severe, mild, or progressive sensorineural deafness), Bardet–Biedl syndrome (obesity, polydactyly, hypogonadism), Refsum's syndrome (phytanic acid storage disease with peripheral neuropathy and cerebellar ataxia), and abetalipoproteinemia.

Choroideraemia

Choroideraemia is an uncommon X-linked condition due to mutations of the gene encoding a component of RAB geronylgeronyl transferase, a protein involved in intracellular trafficking.

In affected males, symptoms and electrophysiological responses are similar to those seen in retinitis pigmentosa. Differentiation is based on clinical examination and angiography which shows loss of the retinal pigment epithelium and granular subretinal deposits within the first decade of life. By the third decade, characteristic centripetal spread of scalloped areas of retinal pigment epithelium and choroidal atrophy occurs. Abnormal pigmentation of the retinal pigment epithelium starting in the midperiphery is almost invariable in heterozygous females who are virtually symptomless until late in life. Little inter- or intrafamilial variation in phenotypic expression has been reported. Choroideraemia with mental retardation and deafness is associated with microdeletions of the Xq21 region.

Gyrate atrophy

This autosomal recessive condition is due to reduced activity of ornithine aminotransferase, a mitochondrial matrix enzyme. Enzyme activity can be used as the basis for diagnosis. Hyperornithinaemia is an invariable finding thought to be a secondary manifestation not directly pathogenic.

Patients present with nyctalopia within the first decade that progresses to loss of peripheral field and then diminished visual acuity. High myopia is evident in approximately 90 per cent of cases. Sharply demarcated, scalloped areas of chorioretinal atrophy are seen extending from the periphery as early as the second decade. These become confluent and affect the macula with severe visual acuity loss by the fifth decade of life. Occasionally crystalline deposits are seen between atrophic patches. Non-ocular associations include abnormal electroencephalographic responses, type 2 skeletal muscle abnormalities, and alopecia.

Dystrophies principally affecting the macula

These may be subclassified into those that exclusively affect the posterior pole, those that to a lesser extent affect the peripheral retina, and finally those that involve non-retinal tissues. The first two categories will be considered here.

Primary macular dystrophies

In this group, bilateral visual loss within the first two decades of life is usual, with symmetric macular pigmentary (bull's eye) abnormalities. Peripheral colour discrimination is unaffected and flash electroretinographic responses are often normal. Many different disorders exist within this group which are as yet incompletely characterized except on the basis of the mode of inheritance.

North Carolina macular dystrophy is an uncommon, early onset, non-progressive, autosomal dominant macular dystrophy. It is completely penetrant but is variably expressive. Disorders previously described as dominant progressive foveal dystrophy, central aerolar pigment and choroidal degeneration, and central areolar pigment epithelial dystrophy form part of the spectrum of North Carolina macular dystrophy. Affected individuals may be asymptomatic or have a dense central scotoma. In the most mildly affected individuals there are numerous macular drusen (stage 1) which may be confluent (stage 2). In stage 3 disease there is marked atrophy of the retinal pigment epithelium and choriocapillaris. Visual prognosis of stage 1 and 2 is good unless complicated by choroidal neovascularization. Even with large atrophic macular lesions the visual acuity may be remarkably good. Electrophysiological and colour vision assessments are normal.

Generalized choroidoretinal dystrophies with macular involvement

X-linked juvenile retinoschisis

This condition usually presents in childhood with mild loss of central vision. Foveal schisis which does not leak on fluorescein angiography, is seen in affected males. Peripheral retinal abnormalities including schisis, retinal vascular closure, and pigmentary retinopathy are said to occur in 50 per cent of cases. The flash electroretinography has a negative waveform with a-wave greater than b-wave amplitude. This and histological studies suggest that Mueller cells are the site of the primary defect. Carrier females show no ophthalmoscopic or electroretinographic abnormalities but may have evidence of reduced rod–cone interaction on psychophysical testing.

A dominantly inherited form of retinoschisis has been reported. Affected patients had peripheral retinoschisis and pigment epithelial atrophy with some showing typical macular schisis. Most had normal electroretinographic responses. Foveal schisis may also be seen in autosomal recessive Goldmann–Favre disease. Severe nyctalopia, peripheral pigmentary retinopathy, and extinguished electroretinographic responses help differentiate this disorder from other causes of retinoschisis.

Dominant cystoid macular dystrophy

This rare condition is characterized by early loss of acuity and macular oedema with leakage evident on fluorescein angiography. Other early findings include hyperopia and blue–yellow colour vision deficit. Later there may be macular atrophy and peripheral pigment deposition. Electro-oculographic responses are abnormal in older patients indicating panretinal disease.

Progressive cone/cone–rod dystrophies

Cone and cone–rod dystrophies may be inherited as autosomal dominant, recessive, or X-linked disorders (Table 1). They are a heterogeneous group characterized by early loss of visual acuity and colour vision with electrophysiological and psychophysical evidence of widespread cone dysfunction. A bull's eye maculopathy is often present. Mild rod dysfunction is often evident in the later stages which is progressive in cases of cone–rod dystrophy.

Best's disease

Best's disease is dominantly inherited with a variable expression. Half those with the abnormal gene have normal or near normal fundi and good vision. Classically, a round or oval yellow (viteliform) deposit is seen under the macula. With time this material gradually resorbs leaving a large area of atrophy often with submacular fibrosis. Choroidal neovascularization is associated with a poor prognosis. There is histological and electrophysiological evidence of widespread abnormality of the retinal pigment epithelium. The electro-oculogram shows lack of light-induced rise of ocular potential with the abnormal gene and serves to identify the distribution of the gene within a family. Identification of dominant inheritance may depend upon demonstration of an abnormal electro-oculogram in a parent of the propositus.

A dominantly inherited adult viteliform dystrophy has been reported. Affected patients have a small subfoveal lesion similar to those seen in Best's disease with normal electro-oculographic responses. Adult viteliform macular dystrophy usually presents after the third decade of life with minimal loss of visual acuity, and is compatible with retention of good vision throughout life. A yellow focal subretinal deposit is seen at each fovea. Although superficially similar to Best's disease, patients present later, the foveal lesion is smaller and non-progressive, and electro-oculographic responses are normal. A mutation in *peripherin/RDS* has been demonstrated in this condition.

Stargardt's disease

Autosomal recessive Stargardt's disease comprises several disorders characterized by visual loss and macular atrophy presenting in late childhood. They are characterized by white flecks at the level of the retinal pigment epithelium which in some are widespread with little macular atrophy. The term fundus flavimaculatus is used to describe this appearance but it is evident that the two terms represent variations in expression of the same recessive disorder. Characteristically a 'dark choroid' is seen on fluorescein angiography which is thought to be due to widespread lipofuscin accumulation in the retinal pigment epithelium. Recessive Stargardt's disease may be genetically homogeneous in that all affected-family studies have shown linkage to the same chromosomal region.

There have been reports of dominantly inherited retinal dystrophies similar to Stargardt's disease. The 'dark choroid' characteristic of recessive disease was not seen. Also, mutations of mitochondrial DNA at nucleotide position 15257 have been associated with a retinal dystrophy similar to Stargardt's disease.

Benign concentric annular dystrophy

This is a particularly mild dominantly inherited condition. A ring of pigment epithelial atrophy surrounding the macula at about 12°, is evident in the young with little if any reduction of visual acuity. Later mild nyctalopia and a peripheral pigmentary retinopathy may be seen.

Dominant drusen

Dominantly inherited drusen phenotypes are characterized by the appearance of drusen deposits at the posterior pole prior to the sixth decade of life. The term represents a group of conditions, for example Doyne's honeycomb retinal dystrophy (in which peridiscal drusen are pathognomonic) and malattia leventinese (associated with basal lamina drusen). Patients may be asymptomatic despite quite striking macular changes. Visual loss is related to atrophy or subretinal neovascularization.

Pattern dystrophies of the retinal pigment epithelium

The pattern dystrophies are characterized by mild loss of acuity with yellow or pigmented subretinal deposits in various configurations. Electroretinography is usually normal although the electro-oculogram may show reduction of light-induced rise. They are usually classified by the pattern of the pigment epithelial abnormality, for example butterfly-shaped dystrophy and macroreticular (spider) dystrophy. Different patterns may be seen within the same family so it is not clear how many distinct nosological entities exist within this group of conditions. The *peripherin/RDS* gene has been implicated in some families.

Sorsby's fundus dystrophy

Sorsby's fundus dystrophy is an uncommon dominant disorder characterized by slow recovery from bright light in the third decade and loss of central vision from macular atrophy or choroidal neovascularization in the fourth or fifth decade. The earliest features are a rod threshold elevation and a tritan colour vision defect. Widespread bilateral deposition of yellow material beneath the retinal pigment epithelium, accumulation of drusen, and slow choroidal filling on fluorescein angiography at the macula are the earliest ophthalmoscopic features.

Progressive bifocal chorioretinal atrophy

This is an extremely rare progressive autosomal dominant condition in which a large oval area of chorioretinal–retinal atrophy can be seen to extend from the optic disc to temporal to the macula within the first few weeks of life. Later a similar area of atrophy develops on the nasal side of the disc with a peripheral pigmentary retinopathy. Most patients are myopic with manifest nystagmus.

Helicoid peripapillary chorioretinal dystrophy

Most individuals with this rare autosomal dominant condition originate from Iceland. Younger patients are often asymptomatic with slowly progressive 'wings' of chorioretinal atrophy extending from the optic nerve head. Nyctalopia is not a feature but as atrophy extends to the macular, visual acuity is lost. Most affected individuals are myopic.

Clinical management

Ophthalmic genetic counselling requires on the part of the practitioner a detailed knowledge of the consequences of different phenotypes, modes of inheritance and molecular genetics. The knowledge passed to patients and their families has profound effects on their futures, and is best undertaken in a unit in collaboration with a low visual aid facility, an obstetric department, a molecular genetic laboratory, and representatives of support groups such as the Retinitis Pigmentosa Society.

Three broad areas need to be addressed: refined diagnosis, therapeutic options, and an assessment of risk to subsequent children. Accurate clinical diagnosis—for example, distinguishing between retinitis pigmentosa, and cone–rod and cone dystrophies—will have a substantial bearing on the form and age of onset of symptoms, as well as the rate of disease progression. Molecular genetic linkage analysis and gene mutation screening can help to establish a precise diagnosis in many cases. Such techniques can be employed before a phenotype is clinically evident, for example in prenatal diagnosis.

That no treatment regimen has been proven to cure retinal dystrophies should be established early with the patient while at the same time reporting that some therapeutic options are available. Specific treatments exist for abetalipoproteinaemia (vitamin A and E supplements), Refsum's disease (dietary restriction of phytanate compounds such as those in dairy products and meat), and gyrate atrophy (pyridoxine supplements, restriction of dietary arginine). Retinitis pigmentosa patients often develop cataracts which are well worth treating surgically when significant. Cystoid macular oedema is also a common complication. Of the therapeutic options available, treatment with carbonic anhydrase inhibitors (acetazolamide) has been found to be the most beneficial. However, systemic side-effects often limit effectiveness.

Dietary supplements of vitamin A have been suggested as a means of limiting the progression of retinitis pigmentosa, although this is not universally accepted; it is also contraindicated in pregnancy. Megadoses (50 000 IU/day) have also been shown to eliminate night-blindness in early cases of Sorsby's fundus dystrophy, but the effect is short lived. The effectiveness of vitamin A supplements has yet to be proven in follow-up studies and potential side-effects (including teratogenicity) of high dose regimens may limit their use in normal clinical practice.

Assessing the risk to future generations is based on determining the manner of inheritance in the family. A detailed family pedigree is required, accurately documenting relationships between affected family members and any consanguineous unions. An autosomal dominant trait would imply a 50 per cent risk to the offspring. Autosomal recessive inheritance implies a 25 per cent risk to each sibling. An affected individual with an autosomal recessive condition has a small risk of having an affected offspring depending on the frequency of the carrier state in the population. If there is a tradition of consanguinity within the family, there is a much greater risk. Classically, X-linked traits are only symptomatic in affected males who cannot transmit the abnormal gene to their sons. However, all daughters will be carriers (obligate heterozygotes). A common problem is the assessment of risk to offspring in simplex cases where there is no family history of disease. Generally speaking this is less than 5 per cent unless the proposed union is consanguineous or the phenotype is classically dominant or X-linked. Superimposed upon this are a number of phenomena such as variable expressivity, anticipation, meiotic drive, and digenic inheritance which should be taken into account when predicting risk. This also complicates the prediction of disease severity in affected children. The prevalence of such influences in ophthalmic disease is unknown.

Further reading

Bird, A.C. (1995) Retinal photoreceptor dystrophies. Edward Jackson Memorial Lecture. *American Journal of Ophthalmology*, **118**, 543–62.

Evans, K., Gregory, C.Y., Fryer, A., *et al.* (1995). The role of molecular genetics in the prenatal diagnosis of retinal dystrophies. *Eye*, **9**, 24–8.

International Standardization Committee (1989). Standard for clinical electroretinography. *Archives of Ophthalmology*, **107**, 816–19.

Jacobson, S., Cideciyan, A.V., Regunath, G., *et al.* (1995). Night-blindness in Sorsby's fundus dystrophy reversed by vitamin A. *Nature Genetics*, **11**, 27–32.

Newsome, D.A. (ed.) (1988). *Retinal dystrophies and degenerations*. Raven Press.

Weleber, R.G. (1994). Retinitis pigmentosa and allied disorders. In *Retina* (ed. S.J. Ryan), pp. 335–466. Mosby.

Wright, A.F. and Jay, B. (ed.) (1994). *Molecular genetics of inherited eye disorders*. Harwood Academic.

2.10 Glaucoma

2.10.1 Anatomy and physiology in glaucoma

2.10.1.1 Anatomy and physiology of the anterior chamber angle

George L. Spaeth and Robert Ritch

The anterior chamber, the 'front room' of the eye, has several characteristics that make it truly remarkable. In order to allow the eye to function as an effective visual organ, the contents of the anterior chamber cannot impede or distort the transmission of light. Furthermore, so that the eye may function well from an optical point of view the eye must be sufficiently firm to permit the primary refracting surface, the cornea, to be an excellent optical device. But the eye, obviously, is composed of living tissues that must be nourished. The pressure within the eye, then, cannot be so high that it interferes with adequate flow of blood, especially to the oxygen-sensitive neurotissues of the retina and optic nerve. Additionally, though somewhat as an aside, the extremely effective barrier that exists in the blood–aqueous barrier in the normal eye prevents many of the immunologically evoked responses of the other tissues in the body. One consequence of this is of extreme importance for all those with anatomically narrow anterior chamber angles due at least partially to an increased pressure in the posterior as opposed to the anterior chamber; specifically, the hole that can be created in the iris to equalize the pressure between the anterior and the posterior chambers does not, in the normal eye, heal. Because of this lack of healing, millions of people throughout the world can, as a result of a relatively simple surgical operation, be prevented for their entire remaining lives from developing a blinding condition.

The anterior chamber angle is a small area of great importance to the eye, as it contains the mechanism that is largely responsible for regulating the outflow of aqueous humour from the eye, a function critical to maintaining proper pressure within the globe of the eye.

This chapter reviews the anatomy of the anterior chamber angle, discusses in detail the method of examination of the anterior chamber angle, and considers several systems of describing the anterior chamber angle (grading).

Embryology of the anterior chamber angle

The angle recess begins to deepen during the third month of gestation. At 4 months, the anterior surface of the iris and corneal endothelium have come in contact to define the angle. Just anterior to this junction, a nest of mesenchymal cells is destined to develop into the trabecular meshwork. Cells in the apex of the angle begin to differentiate into ciliary muscle fibres. By the fifth month, the chamber has become rounded and is lined by an unbroken, but attenuated layer of endothelial cells. The iris root consists of stroma, vascular channels, and the pigmented and non-pigmented ciliary epithelia. The iris root and ciliary body, initially located at the level of the future mid-trabecular meshwork, begin to move posteriorly relative to the meshwork, while the ciliary body moves posteriorly relative to the iris, probably due to a differential growth rate of these tissues. A continuous layer of corneal endothelial cells line the angle recess until about 7 months of gestation. In the final trimester, this cell layer develops fenestrations to expose the underlying trabecular meshwork to the anterior chamber. At birth, the apex of the angle has progressed posterior to Schlemm's canal and is at the level of the scleral spur. In early childhood, the angle opens to the anterior ciliary body face.

Anatomical considerations

The normal anterior chamber is bounded anteriorly by the corneal endothelium, laterally by the structures of the anterior chamber angle, and posteriorly by the anterior surface of the lens and iris (Fig. 1). The area where the peripheral cornea meets the iris or ciliary body forms an acute angle designated as the anterior chamber angle. The width of the anterior chamber angle is related to the depth of the anterior chamber; in general, the deeper the anterior chamber the wider the anterior chamber angle. However, a variety of other factors, some normal and some pathological, also affect the width of the anterior chamber angle. These include the inherited anatomy of the anterior chamber angle, the degree of relative pupillary block, and pathological conditions such as the iridocorneal endothelial syndromes, neovascularization, ciliary body swelling, and inflammation.

The anterior chamber angle extends from the variably bulbous termination of Descemet's membrane at Schwalbe's line, posteriorly to the trabecular meshwork and the scleral spur. In some individuals this continues posteriorly so that the inner

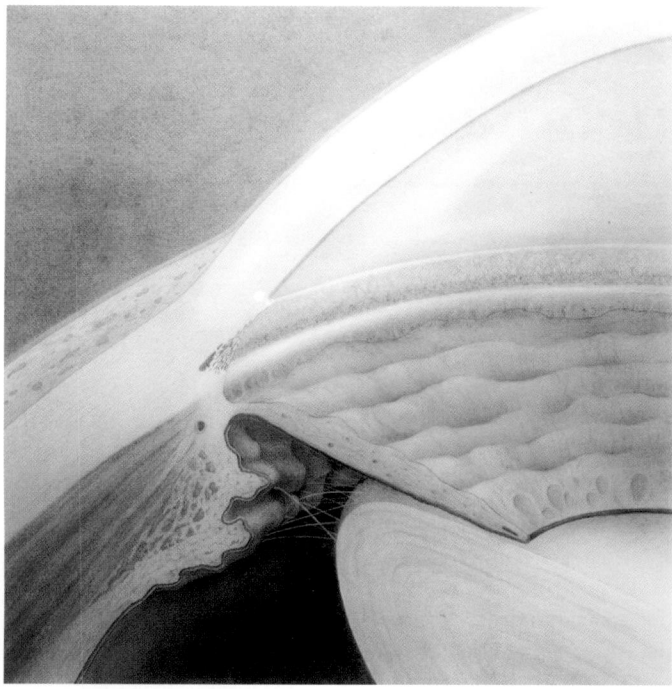

Fig. 1 The anterior chamber angle. The ciliary body is easily visible just anterior to the iris. This tissue varies in colour from individual to individual, sometimes being grey (as it is here) or varying shades of brown. The shiny white scleral spur is easily seen as a thin, well-defined line just anterior to the ciliary body. In younger individuals and those with brown eyes iris processes frequently extend over the posterior portion of the scleral spur. The trabecular meshwork has a different consistency from the scleral spur, being velvety and having depth. The pigmentation of the posterior trabecular meshwork (here around 2+/4+) at the 12 o'clock position of the eye is not related to the colour of the iris; at the 6 o'clock position the amount of pigment in the trabecular meshwork is directly related to the colour of the iris. In the pigment dispersion syndrome the amount of pigment in the 6 and the 12 o'clock positions of the eyes tends to be about the same, whereas in the exfoliation syndrome the pigment is concentrated inferiorly and anterior to Schwalbe's line, which is the junction between the angle tissues and the endothelial surface of the cornea, and which is clearly seen here.

surface of the anterior portion of the ciliary body is also part of the angle, whereas in others the posterior aspect of the angle, the anterior surface of the iris, normally inserts immediately posterior to the scleral spur. The vertical and horizontal diameters of the anterior chamber are normally between 11 and 12.5 mm. The depth of the normal anterior chamber varies considerably, depending upon the age, race, sex, and refractive error of the individual. The volume of the anterior chamber varies markedly, but averages around 0.25 cm³. The anterior chamber is deepest in the most central position and shallowest toward the periphery. Both the anterior and the posterior boundaries of the anterior chamber are variably curved. The dome of the cornea varies relatively little in the normal, but the posterior surface of the angle may be anteriorly convex, flat, or posteriorly concave. It is largely because of this variable feature of the posterior surface that there are discrepancies between the depth of the anterior chamber and the width of the anterior chamber angle.

There are considerable differences between the anatomy of the anterior chamber angle in different species. The angle of

the primate differs considerably from the gonioscopic appearance of the anterior chamber angle in other species. The angles of cats and dogs have a large number of iris processes which extend in a meridional direction, but otherwise are relatively similar to those of primates. In contrast, the anterior chamber angles of pigs, sheep, and cattle appear to have a narrower recess, with prominent, fine, comb-like iris processes and a band of pigmented horizontal streaks limited anteriorly by a grey circumcorneal pigment ring. In the pigmented rabbit the ciliary board of the iris appears separated from the cornea by a dark brown band that consists of small conical or cylindrical fibres of the same colour as the iris. These fibres attach the iris membrane to the inner part of the cornea, giving the angle a more closed appearance than in the other species.

In the normal human, the anterior chamber angle becomes shallower with increasing age. This is partially related to gradual shallowing of the anterior chamber depth. This decreases from an average depth essentially of around 3.5 mm at age 15 years to less than 3.0 mm by the age of 50 years, and gradual continuing narrowing after that. In contrast, the anterior chamber depth increases from the time of birth up until around the age of 20 years.

The normal angle width is roughly 40°. In pupillary block, plateau iris, or other conditions producing angle closure, the angle inlet narrows. Two factors are important in angle parameters, width and occludability. The iris contour is important, as is the position of iris insertion on the anterior ciliary face (Fig. 2). The width of the angle may be irregular or variable, again depending on the contour of the anterior iris surface. Ishikawa *et al.* have defined the angle recess area and developed software to measure it. The dimensions and configuration of the angle may change dramatically with pupillary dilation.

The distance of the iris insertion from the base of the scleral spur may be variable and in some cases suggestive of pathology (Fig. 3(a,b)) . Eyes with pigment dispersion syndrome have a posterior iris insertion, more so than age-, sex-, and refraction-matched myopes. In these eyes, the iris is also characteristically concave, related to reverse pupillary block (Fig. 3(c)). Eyes with angle closure glaucoma often have what appears to be an anterior iris insertion at the base of the scleral spur (see Fig. 3(d)). This may be a result of a gradually progressing synechial closure of the farthest angle recess over a period of years before the angle closure becomes evident (creeping angle closure). Still other eyes appear to have the iris insertion arising from the anterior ciliary processes. In eyes with plateau iris, the insertion site may be variable, and angle closure is caused by large or anteriorly situated ciliary processes holding the iris up against the trabecular meshwork (Fig. 3(e)).

The depth of the anterior chamber has not been extensively studied in different races, but there does not appear to be a significant difference between Caucasian and black Africans, whereas the anterior chamber of the Innuit is shallower.

The anterior chamber depth is greater in males than in females.

The anterior chamber depth and volume decrease with the

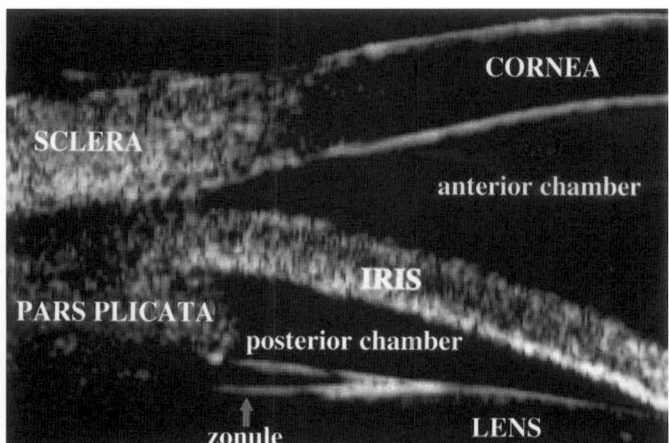

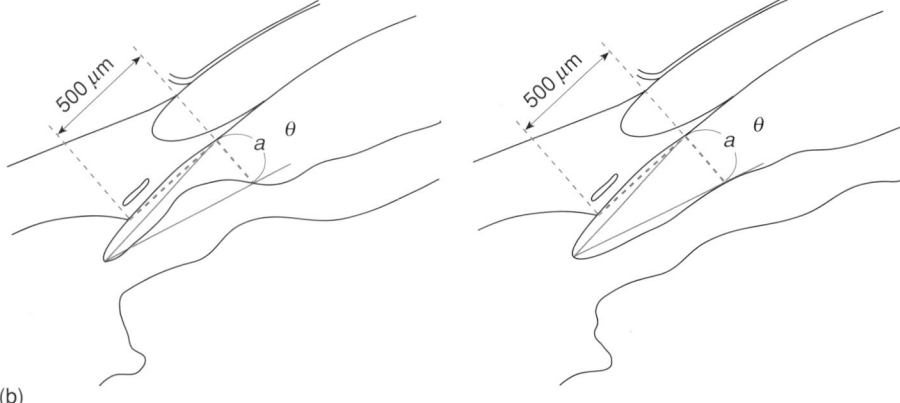

Fig. 2 (a) A normal open angle as seen with ultrasound biomicroscopy. (b) Line drawings showing width and angularity of the angle. At the level of Schwalbe's line the width (a) and angle (θ) are the same, but the angle recesses differ due to differences in the more peripheral portions of the iris. (By courtesy of Hiroshi Ishikawa.)

degree of hyperopia and increase with myopia, the changes being prominent in some individuals.

The anterior chamber angle width also varies with age, race, and refractive error. As discussed below, the width of the angle is affected markedly by the peripheral curvature of the iris, and this varies markedly with age (Tables 1 and 2). The average width of the angle is around 35 to 40° in the young adult but narrows to 20° by the age of 70 years and to less than 10° by the age of 85. The peripheral configuration of the iris tends to be increasingly convex in an anterior chamber, with increasing hyperopia and age. The light blue iris also tends to bow anteriorly more markedly than does the brown iris, and other factors also influence the contour of the iris.

The anatomy of the anterior chamber angle is also affected by race, the site of iris insertion varying considerably in this regard. The angle width tends to be greatest, that is the distance between the posterior extent of the trabecular meshwork and the point at which the iris is adherent to the inner wall of the eye, in Caucasians, less in black Africans, and still less in Far Eastern Asians.

The area through which the aqueous exits is the trabecular meshwork, and as such it is this portion of the anterior chamber angle which is of greatest interest. This meshwork has a trabeculated and reticular appearance and is composed of fibrocellular sheets. It is in the shape of a prismatic band, the apex terminating anteriorly in the deep lamellae of the cornea, and

the base being connected with the scleral spur. Between the trabecular sheet lining the anterior chamber, and Schlemm's canal, which represents the 'internal' extent of the trabecular meshwork is a meshwork of beams covered with endothelial cells.

The corneoscleral trabeculae are connected posteriorly to the anteromedial border of the scleral spur. Anteriorly, these sheets gradually merge with the corneal lamellae. The collagen fibrils of the core are continuous with the fibrils of the internal corneal lamellae, and this portion of the trabecular meshwork does not appear to allow aqueous humour to filter through it.

The 'uveal' trabeculae are connected posteriorly with the circular and radial ciliary muscle fibres, and in a different portion, the meridional ciliary muscle fibres. The number of uveal trabecular sheets varies from two to five, some of which extend anteriorly almost as far as Schwalbe's line. It is this portion of the trabecular meshwork which allows the exodus of aqueous humour and in which are deposited pigment granules, and other particles such as blood cells and exfoliated material.

The scleral spur is a hard, fibrous projection from the inner aspect of the sclera. Its base borders Schlemm's canal. The longitudinal portion of the ciliary muscle inserts into the posterior surface of the scleral spur. Composed of collagen and elastic tissue, the scleral spur gradually merges with the sclera. Contraction of the ciliary muscle pulls the scleral spur poster-

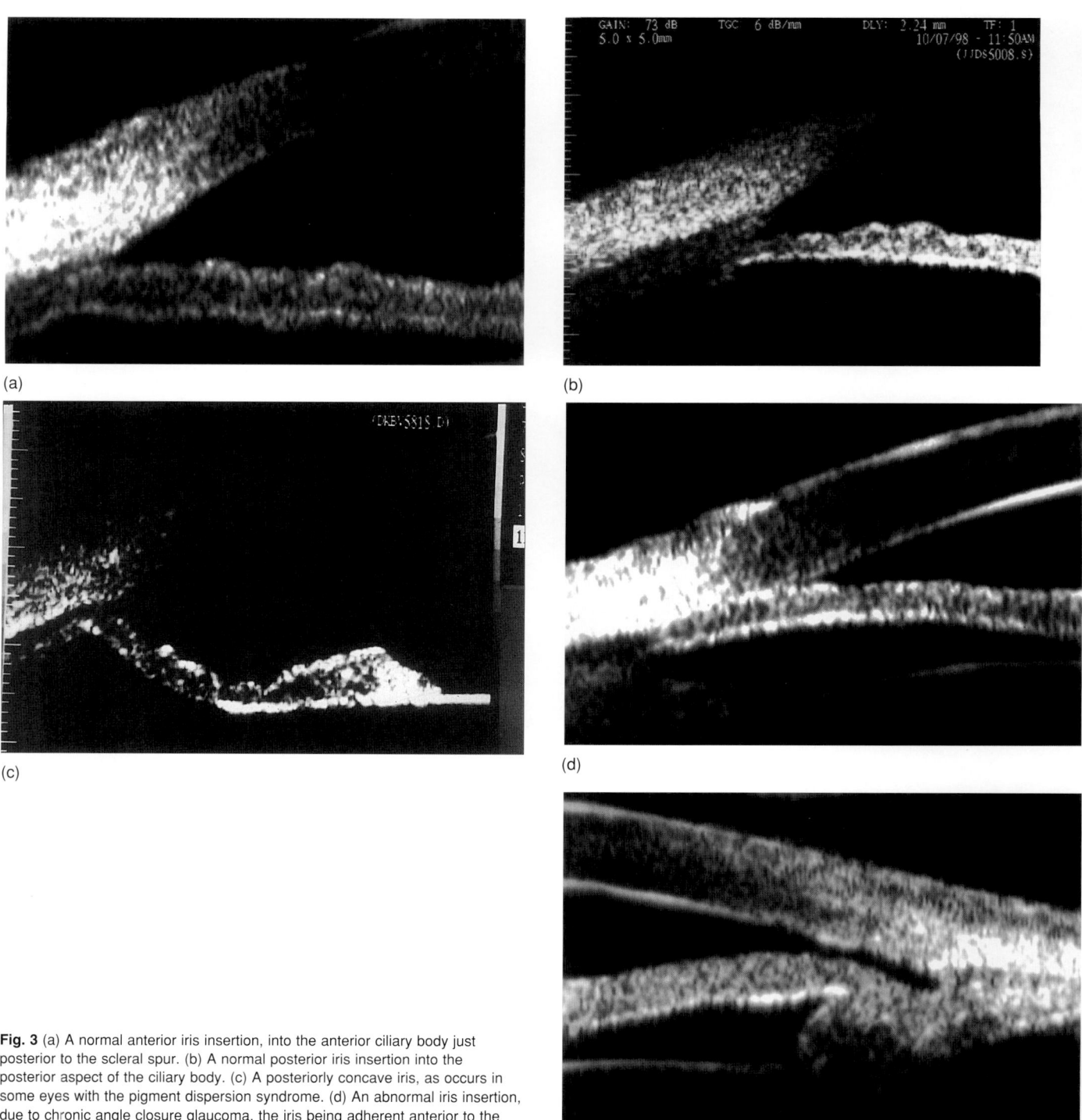

Fig. 3 (a) A normal anterior iris insertion, into the anterior ciliary body just posterior to the scleral spur. (b) A normal posterior iris insertion into the posterior aspect of the ciliary body. (c) A posteriorly concave iris, as occurs in some eyes with the pigment dispersion syndrome. (d) An abnormal iris insertion, due to chronic angle closure glaucoma, the iris being adherent anterior to the trabecular meshwork. (e) A plateau iris, with an extremely narrow recess depth, but a normal angular approach to the recess.

iorly, changing the width of the trabecular spaces and helping maintain patency of Schlemm's canal.

Iris

The iris forms the most anterior portion of the uveal tract and separates the anterior and posterior chambers. By dilating and constricting, it regulates the size of the pupil and the amount of light entering the eye. Increasing evidence suggests that the iris is also an important source of growth factors and other regulatory molecules which influence the cellular activities of the structures of the anterior segment.

The iris is about 12 mm in diameter and normally angles forward from the root, so that the centre of the iris resting on the lens surface is about 0.5 mm more anterior than the root. It is thickest at the collarette. The anterior surface of the iris is in contact with the aqueous humour of the anterior chamber. Under normal circumstances, the posterior iris peripheral to its

Table 1 Various factors affecting anterior chamber depth

Age
Infant	Moderately shallow
Adult	Deep
Elderly	Shallower

Race
All races similar (except Innuit)

Sex
Male deeper than female

Refractive error
Myope	Deepest
Emmetrope	Average
Hyperope	Shallowest

Inheritance
Narrow angle is inherited autosomal dominant fashion

area of contact with the lens is in contact with aqueous humour in the posterior chamber. Abnormally extensive iridolenticular contact and iridozonular contact are present in pigment dispersion syndrome. In pupillary block, the opposite is true; iridolenticular contact is often minimal and increases after laser iridotomy (Fig. 4).

Posterior chamber

The posterior chamber is bounded anteriorly by the iris, laterally by the ciliary body, and posteriorly by the lens. Peripheral to the lens, the posterior border consists of the anterior vitreous face. The zonules pass through the posterior chamber. The volume of the posterior chamber is approximately $0.06\ cm^3$, but it appears larger or smaller in some eyes, particularly those with plateau iris syndrome and pigment dispersion syndrome. The positions of ciliary body and iris appear to be major determinants in the size of the posterior chamber. In eyes with pupillary block, when blinking is inhibited, or with miotic agents, its volume increases because of forward bowing of the iris, and in eyes with reverse pupillary block (pigment

Table 2 Various factors affect the configuration of the anterior chamber angle

Age (years)	0–20	20–50	50–80	80+
Width (degree)	30	35	25	15
Bowing anteriorly peripherally	Slight to none	None	Mild	Moderate
Peripheral insertion				
q*	Uncommon	Uncommon	Rare	Rare
r*	Usual	Usual	Usual	Common
s*	Very rare	Rare	Rare	Infrequent
PTM+ pigment	1	1–2	2	2+
Visibility of Schwalbe's line	Easy	Moderately easy	Harder	Hardest
Race	*Caucasian*	*Black African*	*Asian*	*Eskimos*
Site of iris insertion	Most posterior (D or G)	Usually at scleral spur (C)	At posterior edge of PTM+	At posterior edge of PTM+
Pigmentation of PTM+				
at 12 o'clock	Not related to race			
at 6 o'cclock	1	2+	1–2+	?
Width (degree)	30	30	30	20
Refractive error	*Myope*	*Emmetrope*	*Hyperope*	
Peripheral curvature	q or r	r	r with iris bowing	
Iris insertion	D or E	D	D	
Iris colour	*Brown*	*Hazel*	*Blue*	
PTM+ pigment at 12 o'clock	No effect on PTM+ pigment			
Iris insertion	C	D	D	
Genetics	Autosomal dominant inheritance patterns of angle configuration			
Miotics	Long-term use makes angle shallower: acute deeper, or shallower			
Many pathological factors				

*See text under Gonioscopic grading of the iridocorneal angle for definitions of q, r, and s.
PTM, posterior trabecular meshwork.

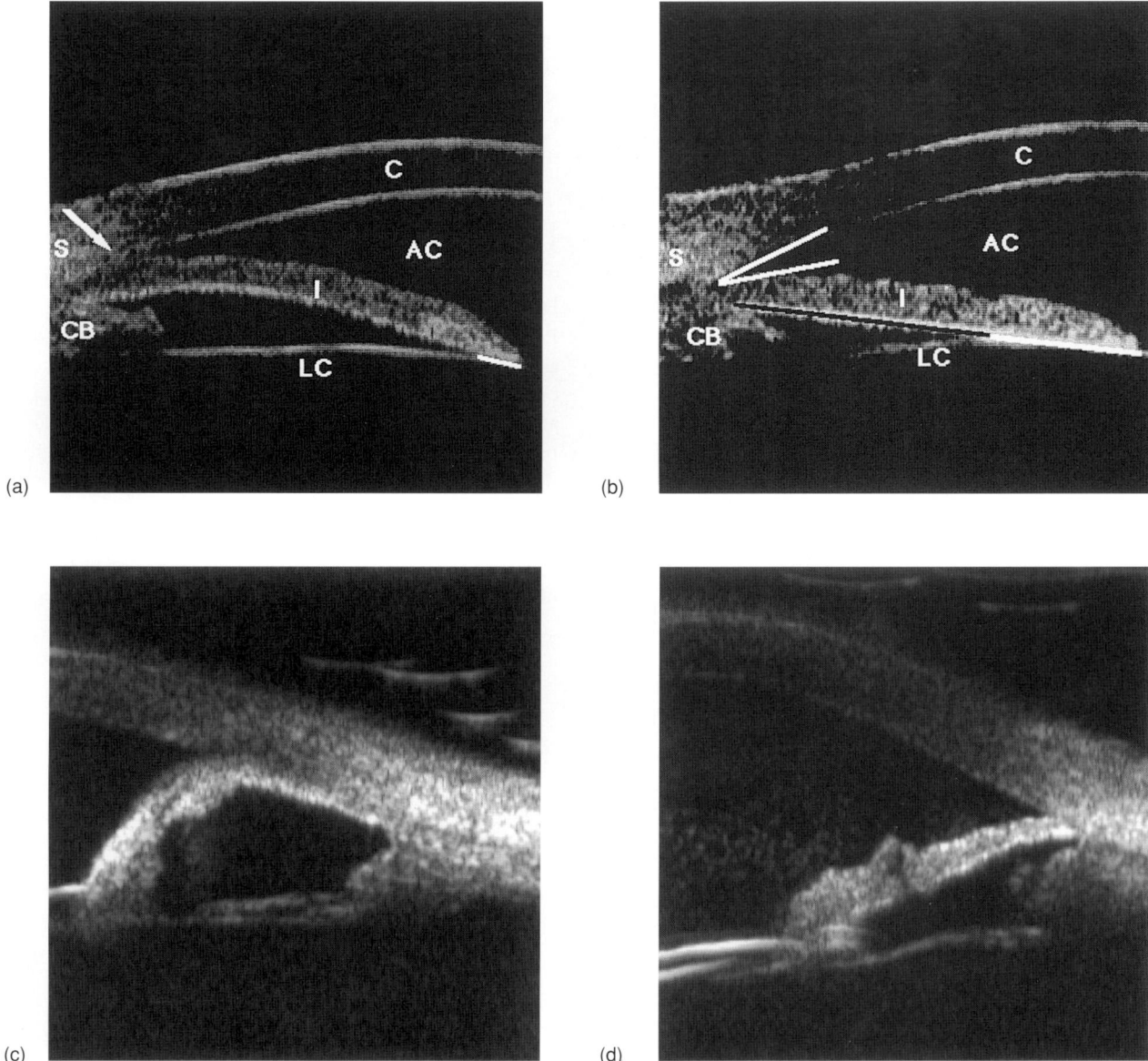

Fig. 4 (a) Iris configuration before (a) and after (b) laser iridotomy. The narrow anterior chamber angle recess becomes deeper as the anterior iris bow is eliminated by lessening the relative pupillary block. C = cornea; I = iris; S = sclera; AC = anterior chamber; CB = ciliary body; LC = lens capsule. (Reprinted with permission from Cariona *et al.* 1996.) (c) Shows angle closure in association with pupillary block. (d) Following peripheral iridotomy, the angle deepens markedly.

dispersion syndrome) or during active accommodation, its volume decreases. The posterior chamber also varies in size depending on the size of the pupil. Aqueous humour enters the posterior chamber from the ciliary body and flows towards and through the pupil into the anterior chamber.

Ciliary body

The ciliary body forms the portion of the uveal tract between the iris and choroid (Fig. 1). It is highly vascular and consists of the ciliary muscle, which functions in accommodation and regulation of trabecular outflow facility, and the ciliary epithelium, which functions in aqueous humour production. The outermost longitudinal fibres of the ciliary muscle insert into the corneoscleral trabecular meshwork and scleral spur. Contraction of the ciliary muscle increases aqueous humour outflow facility by increasing tension on the meshwork. Because the ciliary muscle fibres are only loosely adherent to the sclera, a potential supraciliary space exists which can expand when filled with blood or serous fluid (Fig. 5).

The ciliary processes form the pars plicata which, along with the more posterior pars plana, constitute the lateral wall of the posterior chamber (Fig. 1). The 70 or so major ciliary processes are approximately 2 mm long, 0.5 mm wide, and 1 mm high. Their anterior borders arise from the iris root and are separated from the posterior iris by the ciliary sulcus.

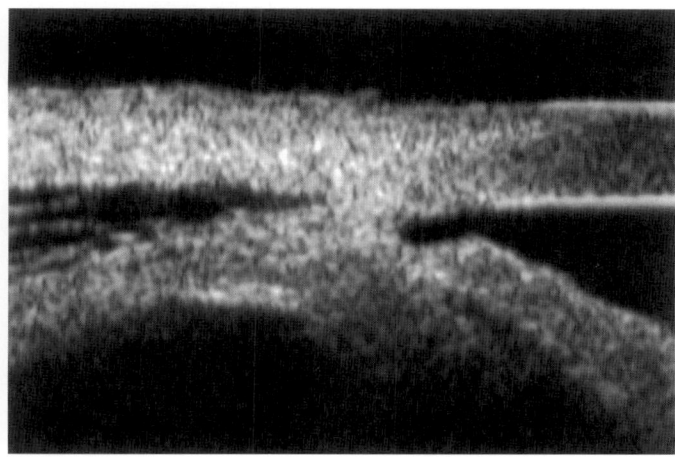

Fig. 5 Ultrasound biomicroscopy showing fluid in the supraciliary space.

Smaller, minor ciliary processes commonly lie between the major processes and do not project as far into the posterior chamber.

The zonular bundles originate primarily from between the inner, non-pigmented epithelial cells of the pars plana and their basement membrane, while some arise from between the ciliary processes. These sweep anteriorly, fuse variably with the anterior vitreous and pars plicata basement membrane, and straddle the equator of the lens, inserting into the lens capsule. When the ciliary muscle contracts, reduced tension on the zonules produces a forward shift of the lens–iris diaphragm and allows the lens curvature to increase during accommodation. Recently, this classic teaching has been challenged.

Examination of the anterior chamber angle

The angle of the anterior chamber is not directly visible due to the anterior extent of the opaque edge of the sclera. In order to visualize the angle, it is necessary to see 'underneath' this ledge and to neutralize the problems associated with the change in refractive index that render ineffective the use of instruments such as an ophthalmoscope. Credit for the initial examination of the anterior chamber angle is usually given to Trantas of Constantinople, who in 1898 described a method of observing the eye by depressing the outside of the globe. In 1900 he reported the angle appearance in a patient with keratoglobus. Saltzman of Vienna, 1913, developed the first contact lens to visualize the angle directly, a method later modified by Koeppe in Germany, Troncoso in New York, and Barkan in San Francisco.

In 1927 Thorburn of Sweden described the difference between wide and narrow anterior chamber angles and introduced a method of photography of the anterior chamber angle. It was not until 1938, however, that Goldmann introduced the concept and the technique of indirect gonioscopy using a mirror within a contact lens to visualize the angle. Prior to that time, identification had been provided by the use of a hand-held microscope, a method well described and developed by Troncoso.

But the ability to examine the angle with the biomicroscope slit lamp allowed both greater convenience and better visual definition of the structure of the anterior chamber angle. The development of a lens with a curvature more similar to that of the cornea and a smaller area of contact allowed performance of gonioscopy without a viscous solution to bond the cornea to the lens. This method of gonioscopy, using a Zeiss four-mirror contact lens, was used by Forbes to deepen the anterior chamber peripherally, allowing differentiation between peripheral anterior synechias and mere contact of the iris to the internal lining of the globe.

The use of the Zeiss four-mirror lens allowed gonioscopy to be performed quickly and conveniently, without the need to use a solution that blurred the patient's and the doctor's vision following the performance of gonioscopy. This method is the most suitable for current clinical practice.

In 1940, Gradle conceptualized the concept of developing quantitative gonioscopy, but was unable to accomplish his goal. Shibata introduced an image-processing technique to attempt a better quantitative measurement of the anterior chamber angle, but this important ability has not yet been accomplished practically. Unlike ophthalmoscopy which, following its introduction in 1850, rapidly became a standard part of the ophthalmic examination, gonioscopy was practised mainly by specialists, and even today is still not a routine part of the ophthalmic examination. Indeed, in a recent determination by the American Academy of Ophthalmology of what constitutes a 'comprehensive ophthalmic examination', gonioscopy was not included. This probably reflects a poor general understanding of the nature of the anterior chamber angle in health and disease, the need to use a specialized instrument that has little applicability in other parts of the examination, and a spuriously apparent lack of practical information derived from performing gonioscopy.

Barkan was a strong advocate for gonioscopy in clinical practice, but until the introduction of the Zeiss four-mirror gonioscopy the methodology was cumbersome and the results often seem to be of little use. The development of argon laser trabeculoplasty, and the effectiveness of neodymium–yttrium-aluminium-garnet (Nd–YAG) laser peripheral iridotomy in the treatment of narrow anterior chamber angles brought a clinical applicability to the technique of gonioscopy which has greatly increased the interest in examining and understanding the anterior chamber angle. A truly quantitative method is still awaited, but should be forthcoming in the near future. A good start has been made by Congdon, who has utilized a reticule in association with slit-lamp indirect gonioscopy to measure the angle depth.

Gonioscopic evaluation

The following description applies to gonioscopy with the indirect method using a gonioscopic lens capable of being used for indentation gonioscopy (Zeiss, Iwata, Posner) (Fig. 6). The descriptions deal primarily with the average situation, and the marked variability of appearance that occurs even in normal subjects must be recalled. One of the many specific differences, for example, is the distance from the posterior edge of the scleral spur to Schwalbe's line, which tends to be around 600 micra, but in myopic eyes or those with congenital glaucoma it is usually larger, whereas in hyperopic or nanophthalmic eyes it tends to be less.

It is also essential that the examiner recall that every examination system introduces certain artefacts. The anterior chamber angle when examined with a Koeppe lens will be deeper than when examined with a Goldmann-type lens at the slit lamp, because in the former situation the patient is supine. Different angularities of the mirror used with Goldmann-type indirect ophthalmoscopy give apparent differences in the configuration of the angle. These are not real differences, however, and can be appreciated by moving the lens or having the patient move his or her eye so that the actual configuration of the angle is considered. The angle can be deformed during the examination technique, as when a small gonioprism indents the cornea, deepening the anterior chamber recess, or the edge of a larger lens compresses one quadrant of the sclera, making the angle appear shallower than it actually is. The lens most likely to introduce errors is the four-mirror type lens, and it must be used with the awareness of this propensity.

The anterior segment should be examined with a biomicroscope prior to placing the lens used for gonioscopy. The cornea is observed and the following questions answered: Is the epithelium intact? Is the tear film normal? Will the epithelium tolerate prolonged use of a contact lens? Is there an arcus, is it regular, and will it interfere with placement of the laser burns? Is the corneal stroma clear and of normal thickness? Are there endothelial changes? How close is the corneal endothelium to the anterior surface of the iris? Is the anterior chamber depth uniform? Are posterior synechias present? What is the condition of the lens? If aphakic, where is the anterior vitreous face and any capsular or inflammatory membranes? If pseudophakic, what is the position of the lens, especially in reference to the pupil margin, secondary membranes, vitreous, and corneal endothelium?

Once the gonioscopy lens is in place, the angle is also examined systematically (Fig. 7). View starts at the pupil margin and sweeps over the iris surface to the iris root. If blood vessels are seen at the pupil margin, neovascularization of the iris is present. Any blood vessels on the iris surface are also noted. The iris is normally almost flat, but with increasing age becomes more bowed anteriorly. Marked anterior convexity of the iris, so-called iris bombe, is not normal and is usually a sign that there is interference with the flow of aqueous humour from the posterior to the anterior chamber.

The iris root in the normal eye should be easily seen as it merges with the ciliary body. At that point the colour changes, as does the texture of the tissue. The ciliary body may be brown or grey, but it is almost invariably different in appearance from the iris. The rugal folds of the iris are not present on the ciliary body. If the anterior chamber angle is deep and peripheral

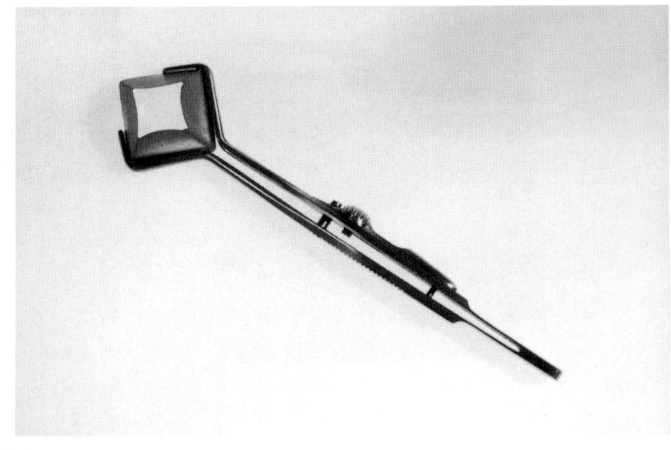

(a)

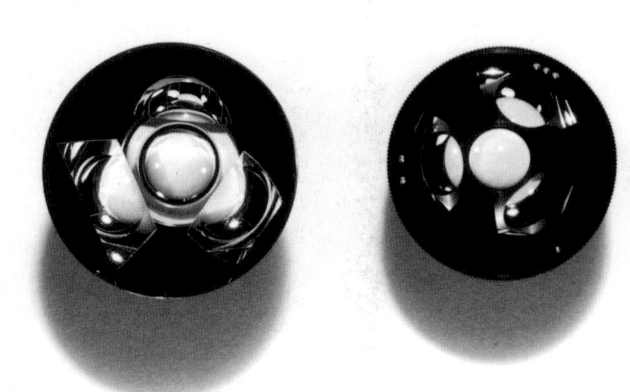

(b)

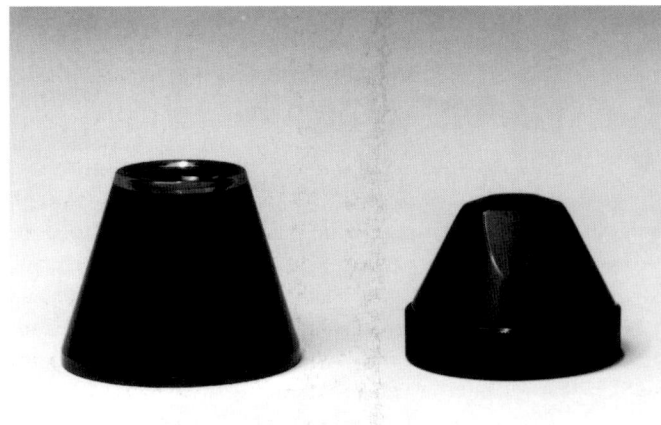

(c)

Fig. 6 (a) The Zeiss four-mirror gonioscopic lens on an Unger handle. This lens permits rapid evaluation of the anterior chamber angle without the need to use an optical bonding solution such as methylcellulose. As it is glass, it is easily cleaned without becoming scratched. The curvature of the lens surface is similar to that of the cornea. This lens is excellent for routine clinical use, including indentation gonioscopy. (b) The standard for indirect gonioscopic evaluation is the Goldmann lens, initially made with one mirror, but now most often used with three mirrors at slightly different angles to permit examination of the anterior chamber angle as well as the peripheral retina. The posterior pole can be viewed well through the central portion of the lens. (c) The Iwata lens has a smaller area of contact with the cornea and a surface which is less curved. This permits optical bonding between the lens and the cornea without the need to use a viscous solution such as methylcellulose. It also permits indentation gonioscopy as described in the text.

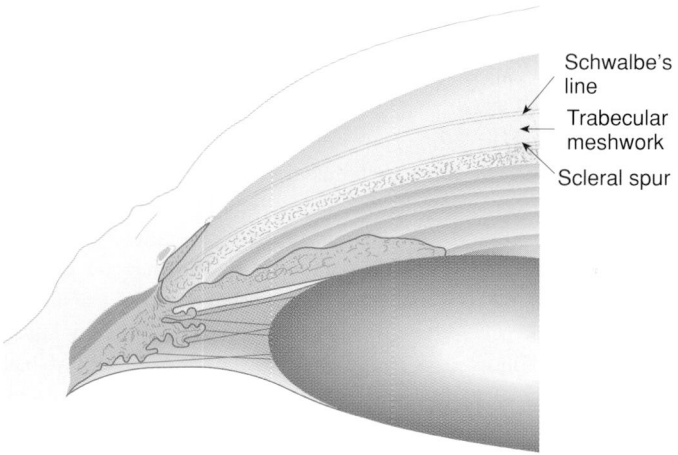

Schwalbe's line

Trabecular meshwork

Scleral spur

Fig. 7 A typical, blue-eyed anterior chamber angle. The appearance of the normal anterior chamber angle varies markedly depending upon age, race, iris colour, and refractive error. The angle shown here is made up of one relatively curved surface (the cornea), and one relatively flat surface (the iris), but in many cases the iris is concave posteriorly or convex anteriorly. Nestled in the depths of the angle recess is the posterior trabecular meshwork, which is often best recognized, especially when it is lacking in pigment, by noting that it does not share the solidity of Schwalbe's line, which protrudes slightly into the anterior chamber and scleral spur, which is flush with the surface; in contrast it is possible to see into the posterior trabecular meshwork.

anterior synechias are visible, it is probable that they are of an inflammatory nature, rather than the type of adhesion associated with primary angle closure glaucoma. Unless such synechias extend anterior to the posterior trabecular meshwork, they usually do not have any effect on aqueous dynamics. Thus, the noting of such adhesions is important to permit arriving at a correct diagnosis, but they usually do not play a role in determining the level of intraocular pressure. These tend to be more prominent inferiorly than superiorly, in contrast to the adhesions seen with primary angle closure, which are invariably more frequent in the superior part of the chamber angle.

If the ciliary body cannot be seen because of anterior bowing of the iris, indentation gonioscopy should be employed to force the iris posteriorly, and to permit the best obtainable view of the angle recess.

Once the ciliary body is identified, the nature and extent of the iris processes are noted. These are, normally, prominent in younger persons and those with brown eyes; they decrease with increasing age. Furthermore, they should normally not extend anterior to the posterior trabecular meshwork. They may be sufficiently dense that they obscure the scleral spur in some cases, making certain identification of landmarks difficult. In such instances, it is best to look more anteriorly, obtaining a sure landmark from Schwalbe's line, and then return the gaze to the area of the ciliary body, using the identified Schwalbe's line as a new guidepost.

The scleral spur is usually shiny white and is most easily identified at the 12 o'clock position of the eye, where it is least likely to be covered with adventitious pigment. It should be at least 200 micra anterior to the insertion of the iris; if it is less than this, the observer should suspect the presence of peripheral anterior synechias. This distance will vary from eye to eye, and in one eye from area to area; at the position where the felt fissure closes, usually inferonasally or inferotemporally, the insertion of the iris is often more anterior; the observer should not be misled into mistaking this for a synechia. Iris processes usually can be identified as individual strands, even where they are matted on top of each other. As such they contrast with peripheral anterior synechias, which resemble tiny volcanoes, some with the apex still in place, and others with the top having been 'blown off', leaving the truncated shape of a mesa. Thus, it is usually possible to distinguish iris processes from peripheral anterior synechias even when they are limited to the depths of the angle recess.

Large or small blood vessels, often quite tortuous, can often be seen running in a meridional direction in the depths of the angle, especially in the blue-eyed individual; these are normal. However, blood vessels that extend anteriorly over the scleral spur, no matter how tiny, are not normal, and are a sure sign of developing neovascular glaucoma.

Trabecular meshwork

The trabecular meshwork is most easily identified at the 12 o'clock position, since the viewer is not confused by the pigment that so characteristically collects in a puddle inferiorly, or by the pigment granules that so typically paint Schwalbe's line at the 6 o'clock position. The trabecular meshwork, unlike scleral spur or Schwalbe's line, has a soft velvety texture, due to the fact that it is a sieve rather than a surface. When the slit lamp is meticulously focused and the gonioscopy lens properly used, the viewer will note this characteristic velvety appearance of the trabecular meshwork, its most unique attribute and one that allows almost sure identification even in the absence of pigmentation. The tissue actually has *depth*, and with careful focus one can see into the depths of the posterior trabecular meshwork. This is not true for Schwalbe's line or the scleral spur, which are solid, translucent structures, or ciliary body, which is a solid, opaque structure. Because the trabecular meshwork may or may not have pigment, the nature of the angle will not always be properly appreciated unless the viewer learns to identify trabecular meshwork in the absence of pigment; clearly, the surgeon will not be able to place laser burns with appropriate accuracy if the trabecular meshwork is not properly recognized.

When pigment is present, it often collects most densely in the posterior position of the posterior trabecular meshwork, presumably because it is the posterior trabecular meshwork through which the aqueous flows to the underlying canal of Schlemm. In some cases, the entire trabecular meshwork is pigmented. This finding is seen most typically in the exfoliation syndrome, in which condition there is always marked pigmentation of the angle. The pigmentation of the posterior trabecular meshwork seen in the pigment dispersion syndrome is usually more sharply delineated than the pigmentation in the exfoliation syndrome; furthermore, in the pigmentation dispersion syndrome the 6 and 12 o'clock positions usually appear similar to each other, whereas in the exfoliation syndrome the pigment is more prominent inferiorly than superiorly. In fact, correct identification of the posterior trabecular meshwork at the 6 o'clock position of the angle may be difficult in the exfoliation syndrome because the pigment may spread over the entire angle recess, obscuring the usual landmarks. Of help in such cases is recognition of Schwalbe's line, which, in patients with exfoliation syndrome, is invariably coated with pigment granules. The coating is in the form of a wavy, scalloped line, usually extending from about 4 to 8 o'clock and densest at 6 o'clock; the granules deposit on the surface, anterior to Schwalbe's line. The pigment in the pigment dispersion syndrome tends to be brown and in the exfoliation syndrome blacker, and, in addition, is not denser inferiorly than superiorly, unlike the exfoliation syndrome. There is usually a decreased amount of pigmentation in the posterior trabecular meshwork at the 3 and 5 o'clock positions. It is almost pathognomonic of the exfoliation syndrome.

Inflammatory conditions also result in deposition of pigment in the inferior angle, but in such cases the pigment is usually located in the depths of the recess, overlying the pocket formed by the junction of the iris and the inner wall of the globe.

Schwalbe's line

Schwalbe's line, the termination of Descemet's membrane, marks the anterior limit of the angle. Identification of this boundary can be made by noting the apex of the wedge formed by the anterior and posterior aspects of the corneal parallelepiped of the well-focused slit lamp beam; this is not an easy method, however, and is not recommended. It is performed as follows. The corneal endothelial surface follows a perfectly smooth curve that merges at Schwalbe's line with the less steeply curved arc of the internal surface of the trabecular meshwork. Just at Schwalbe's line the inner surface is usually extruded, producing a bump on the endothelial surface. At the 6 o'clock position, this bump collects pigment granules, so that an irregular line of dotted pigment develops directly on Schwalbe's line. This pigmentation is not usually visible in the young individual, but becomes increasingly apparent with age. The presence of this sign, and the normally deeper recess of the inferior angle, are the reasons that most observers choose to start their gonioscopic evaluation with the mirror at 12 o'clock, viewing the 6 o'clock position. However, correct identification of the posterior trabecular meshwork is the most important objective of gonioscopy, and this is most easily accomplished at the 12 o'clock position, where pigment debris is least confusing.

One satisfactory gonioscopic technique is to start with the view at 6 o'clock (that is, with the mirror at 12 o'clock), sweep the gaze up from the pupil margin to the angle recess, estimating the angular depth of the anterior chamber, identifying tentatively the point of iris insertion, characterizing the anterior convexity of the iris, trying to note the velvety posterior trabecular meshwork, and settling the gaze on what seems to be Schwalbe's line, noting whether or not Sampaolesi's pigment line is present. A system of describing the configurational changes is described in the following paragraphs. Then, with

the eye focused on Schwalbe's line, the gonioscopy lens is rotated clockwise so that the view goes from 6 to 12 o'clock, never losing sight of what is believed to be Schwalbe's line. It is important to stress that the observer does not take his other eyes from the slit lamp, but follows what is believed to be Schwalbe's line in the mirror as the lens is rotated. As the mirror turns, the pigment on Schwalbe's line should become less and less visible until it has disappeared completely, usually around the 9 o'clock position. Here the gaze may be shifted posteriorly to what is believed to be the posterior trabecular meshwork. Its velvety texture is identified, and this new landmark is then followed as the mirror is rotated. If the PTM has been correctly identified, the amount of pigmentation present will be quite similar in all areas, with the exception of the 3 and 9 o'clock positions, at which points there is usually slightly less pigment.

Indentation gonioscopy

To visualize the angle of patients with narrow anterior chamber angles, indentation gonioscopy must be performed. An appropriate lens is used. The edge of the angle is first determined with the lens held very lightly so that no indentation is occurring. The view at that point should be crystal clear. Pressure is then directed against the cornea with the lens, pushing directly into the orbit. As this is done, striae will develop in the cornea, obscuring the view partially. Aqueous humour is displaced from the central to the peripheral portion of the anterior chamber, and this displaced aqueous will push the peripheral portion of the iris posteriorly in areas where it is not either adherent or lying on a non-compressible surface. Therefore, the iris position will not change where it is in contact with the internal surface of the globe, and it will not change where it is on the anterior surface of the lens. Between the lens and the site of iris insertion, however, the iris is usually not supportive, and when the pressure in the anterior chamber is higher than that in the posterior chamber, the iris is bowed posteriorly. The angle is evaluated in its 'indented' state and then pressure on the gonioscopy lens is released, allowing the displaced aqueous to return to its former position. At this point, the posteriorly bowed iris should then move anteriorly to its pre-indented position (Fig. 8).

Gonioscopic grading of the iridocorneal angle

The advent of gonioscopy and differentiation of angle closure glaucoma from open angle glaucoma in the 1950s required the development of a grading system to describe the anatomical configuration of the angle seen gonioscopically. The first of these, defined by Scheie, consisted of a simple description of the angle width as seen gonioscopically. Grade 0 represented a wide open angle and grade 5 the narrowest. Shaffer devised a similar system with a grade 0 angle being closed and a grade 4 angle the widest. This grading method has proven the most widely accepted one over the years. The Scheie system uses the most posterior angle structure that can be seen, while the

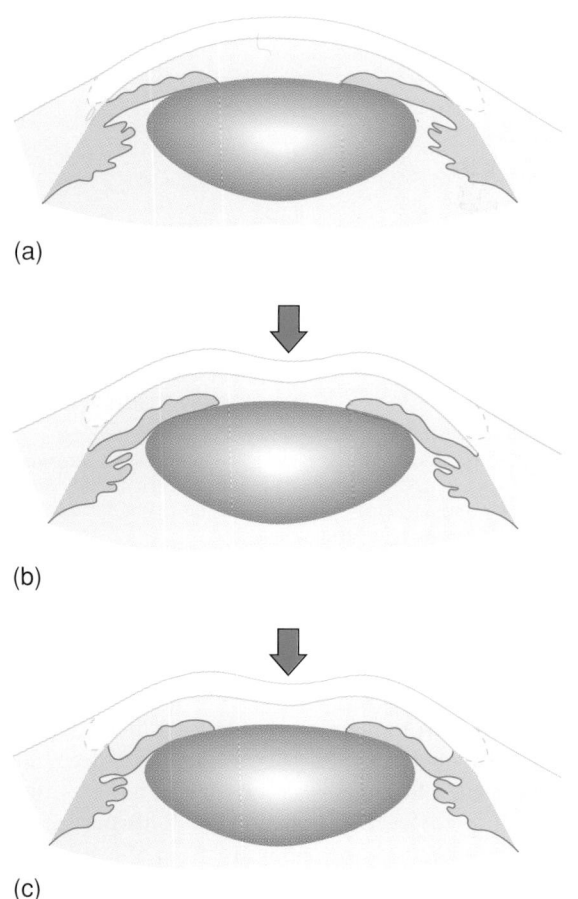

(a)

(b)

(c)

Fig. 8 (a) Before indentation gonioscopy. (b) Pressure is directed against the cornea with the lens, pushing directly into the orbit (c) Aqueous humour is displaced from the central to the peripheral portion of the anterior chamber, and this displaced aqueous pushes the peripheral portion of the iris posteriorly in areas where it is not either adherent or lying on a non-compressible surface.

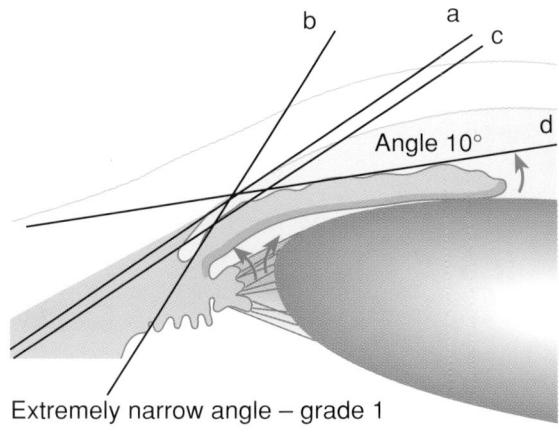

Extremely narrow angle – grade 1

Fig. 9 The most widely used gonioscopic grading system is that devised by Shaffer. The grade of the angle is related to the angularity of the approach to the angle recess, a 40° approach being graded 4, a 30° approach 3, a 20° approach 2, a 10° approach 1, and a closed angle 0. This has the benefit of simplicity and is easily learned. However, as is shown in the illustration here, it does not take account the peripheral curvature of the iris. The figure shows an iris that is bowed forward convexly. This angle is described in the discussion on the Shaffer system as a 'grade 1' angle. However, due to the curvature the angularity could actually be described in a variety of different ways.

Shaffer system is based on an estimate of the angularity of the approach to the angle, a grade 4 angle representing a 40° approach, grade 3 a 30° approach, grade 2 a 20° approach, grade 1 a 10° approach, and grade 0 a closed angle. This Shaffer system is simple and is probably the grading system that has been most widely used. However, the periphery of the angle is frequently curved, so that such a grading system may be misleading (Fig. 9). Scheie's system does not describe the actual nature of the angle, but varies depending upon the optical artefacts of the gonioscopic technique. The method that will be described in most detail here recognizes that to describe the configuration of the angle properly requires at least three different considerations: firstly, the position at which the iris is actually connected to the internal surface of the cornea or angle recess; secondly, the space between the anterior surface of the iris and the posterior surface of the cornea (the angle described by Schaffer); and thirdly, the peripheral curvature of the iris, which can be bowed anteriorly, be flat, or be bowed posteriorly, with varying degrees of suddenness of bowing.

Figure 7 shows the gonioscopic appearance of the anterior chamber in an average eye. Again, it should be stressed that this appearance will vary markedly depending upon eye colour, race, refractive error, and other factors.

The point of contact between the iris and the inner wall of the globe is noted (Fig. 10). In the majority of Caucasian eyes the iris is adherent to the ciliary body, preventing visualization of the structures anterior to that juncture. If this point of adherence cannot be seen because of iris bowing, the angle is indented so that the site of actual insertion can be determined with certainty. Figure 10 shows the general scheme of grading this characteristic of the angle. When the iris is adherent anterior to Schwalbe's line, the angle is graded as an 'A' (Fig. 11). This is always a pathological condition. An angle is designated 'B' when the iris is adherent to the trabecular meshwork so that Schwalbe's line is visible but the scleral spur is not, even with indentation (Fig. 12). A 'C' angle describes the angle in which the trabecular meshwork is totally visible, and in addition Schwalbe's line can be seen (Fig. 13). When the

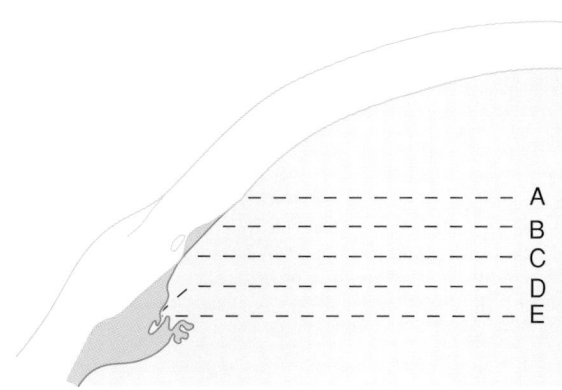

Fig. 10 Schematic drawing of the variability of iris insertion.

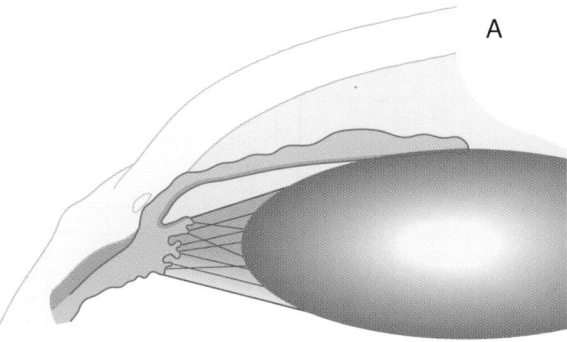

Fig. 11 The iris is adherent to the cornea and to Schwalbe's line, which is always a pathological condition and is not in the range of normal variability. Most typically, this type of angle is seen in patients with neovascular membranes or following various types of trauma. This angle is designated as 'A'.

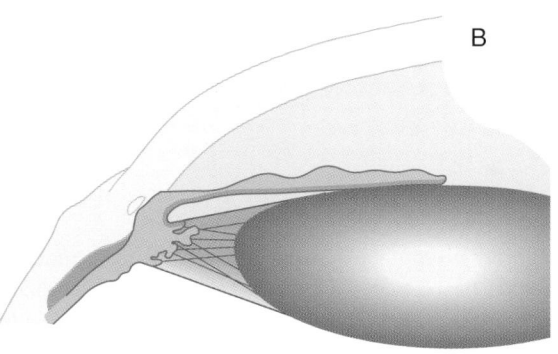

Fig. 12 The iris is adherent to the trabecular meshwork, behind Schwalbe's line. This is always a pathological condition and is frequently seen in patients who have chronic angle closure glaucoma.

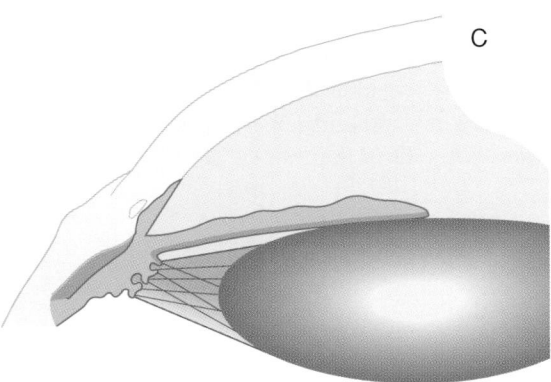

Fig. 13 A 'C' configuration angle in which the iris is adherent just posterior to the scleral spur which is, therefore, visible. This type of angle is normal in patients who have brown irides, especially when they are young. Thus a 'C' angle can be normal. However, a 'C' angle would be unusual in patients with blue irides or those who are older than 20 years of age. 'C' angles are common in black people and Asians, and rare in Caucasians.

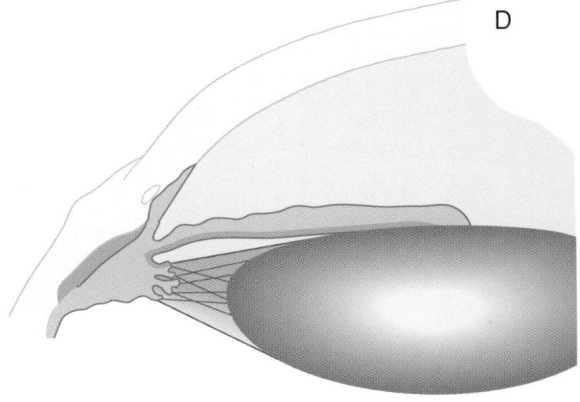

Fig. 14 The iris inserts into the anterior ciliary body. This is the commonest configuration of the anterior chamber angle in Caucasians. In black Africans or the Asian patient, this angle may also be normal, but is less common. This is designated as 'D', standing for 'deep' angle.

ciliary body is also visible, the angle is termed 'D' (Fig. 14), and when a millimetre or more of ciliary body is visible, the angle is designated as 'E' (Fig. 15). The letters themselves can be of some help in remembering that for which they stand: A is anterior, B is behind (Schwalbe's line), D is deep, and E is extremely deep. The angle is also graded in terms of the width of approach to the recess (Figs 16, 17). This measurement is made approximately 3 mm centrally from the iris root, just anterior to Schwalbe's line, and represents an estimate of the anterior chamber depth. This angularity is relatively easily estimated with a thin beam on the slit lamp. It is important to keep the angle of the beam at approximately 30°. The accuracy of this estimate has been validated by ultrasound biomicroscopy.

The curvature of the peripheral iris must be described (Fig. 18). The iris is designated as an 's' when there is a sudden anterior convexity, bending the iris sharply to a flat central iris. This is the appearance described as 'plateau iris' (Fig. 19).

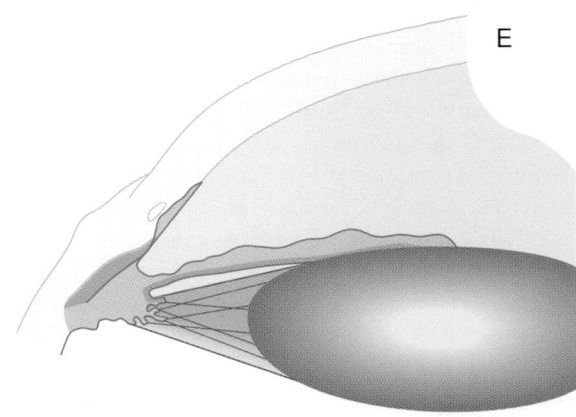

Fig. 15 Where the iris inserts in the ciliary body one millimetre or more posterior to the scleral spur, the angle is designated as an 'E' for 'extremely' deep. This appearance is typical of myopes. Where it occurs in a brown-eyed patient, a black African, or an Asian, it must be distinguished from the pathology associated with a cyclodialysis or angle recession.

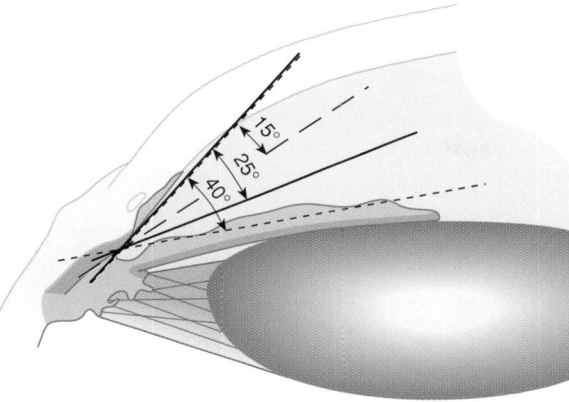

Fig. 16 The approach to the angle recess is estimated in angular degrees at Schwalbe's line.

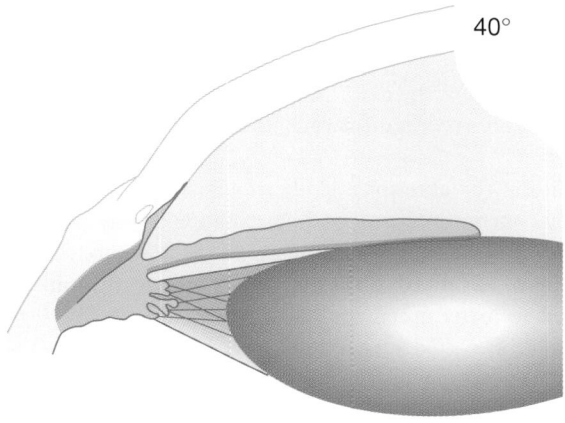

Fig. 17 A 40° approach to the anterior chamber angle is characteristic of the young and the myope.

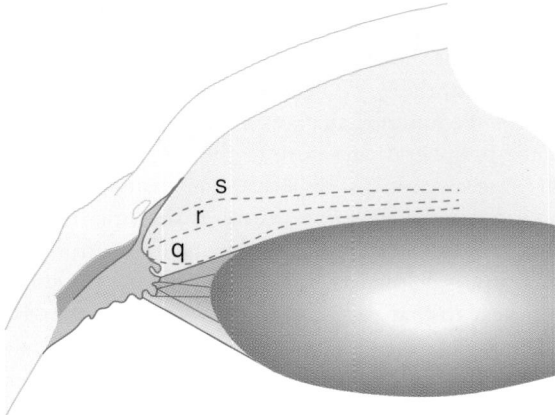

Fig. 18 q', 'r', and 's'. The peripheral configuration of the iris must be considered in evaluating the configuration of the anterior chamber angle. This may bow anteriorly in a gradual fashion, it may bow in a sudden fashion, where the curve of the periphery is not continued in the more central portion of the iris, or the bow may be more posterior in a concave fashion. This is notated with lower case q, r, or s.

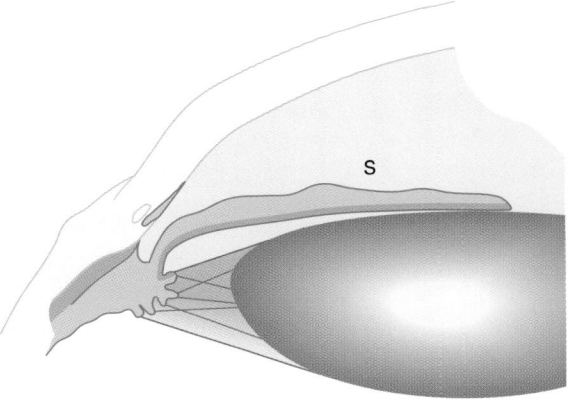

Fig. 19 A plateau iris occurs rarely, and is not a normal iris appearance. It needs to be differentiated from the peripheral configuration, in which there is a more consistent convexity to the iris without the discontinuity shown here. In the plateau iris (designated 's' for 'sudden', 'steep') the most central portion of the iris has no curvature.

Where the iris has no sudden change in curvature, but rather a flat or gradual bow, it is designated as an 'r' or a regular or rounded curve (Fig. 20). Where the peripheral iris bows posteriorly so that it is concave peripherally it is called a 'q' iris (Fig. 21). This is not a common appearance, and q refers to 'queer' or 'quixotic'.

The grading system that has been described at this point attempts to describe the angle configuration validly, that is, as the angle actually is, not simply as it 'appears'. When the angle is so narrow that indentation is required, valid description of the angle demands a notation that indicates the appearance of the angle, and how that appearance can be misleading. The angle illustrated in Fig. 22 would be described as follows: 'This anterior chamber angle is associated with an anterior chamber of relatively normal depth. The approach to the angle is normal. There is a steep, sudden anterior convexity of the iris limited to the extreme iris periphery, following which the iris has an unbowed anterior surface. This anterior peripheral convexity of the iris blocks the view of the deeper portions of the angle recess. However, when the peripheral of the portion

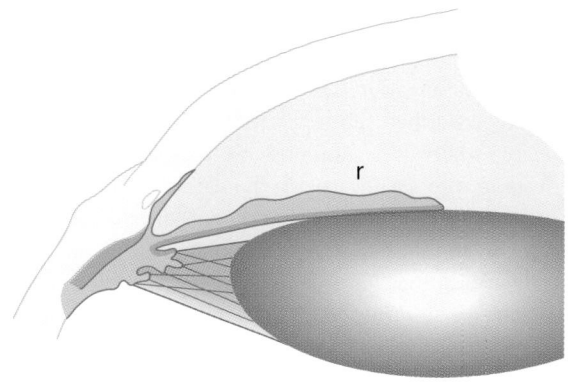

Fig. 20 In most normal angles there is a flat or mild anterior rounded curve of the peripheral iris that continues all the way towards the pupillary margin. This regular appearance is designated 'r'.

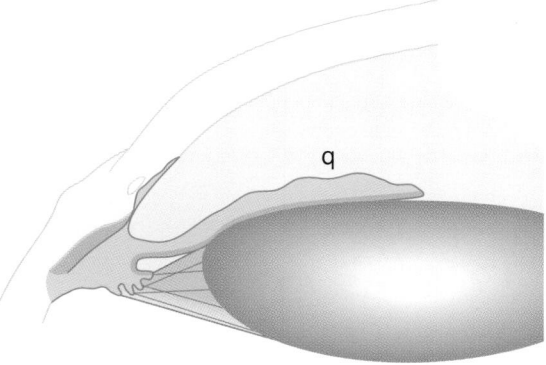

Fig. 21 In some myopes, the peripheral iris bows posteriorly as shown here. This is a rather clear appearance, and is designated 'q'. This is also seen in pathological conditions in association with a dislocated lens and aphakia.

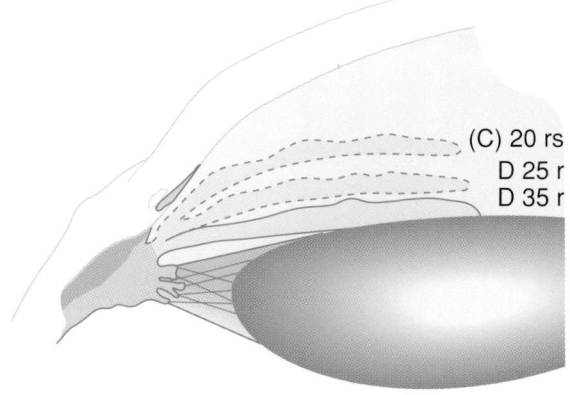

Fig. 23 Three various angled configurations, all with the same iris insertion, but with different degrees of iris bowing and angularity of approach. The angle is described by first listing the site of iris insertion with a capital letter, then the angular approach, and lastly the peripheral curvature. Thus, using these three descriptors, one can describe the entire configuration of the anterior chamber angle.

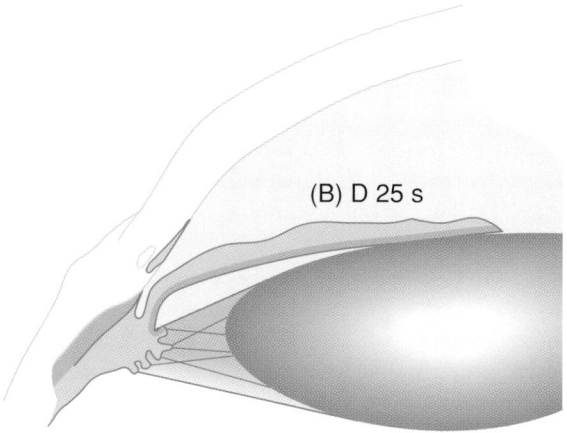

Fig. 22 When it is not possible to visualize the anterior chamber angle without indentation, the site of iris insertion may be mistaken. In the angle shown here, the view into the anterior chamber angle would be limited by the anterior bowing of the iris, due to an 's' (plateau iris configuration). The approach to the angle is average depth (25°) and the actual site of iris insertion (the anterior ciliary or 'd') is normal. However, because the view is limited to the posterior trabecular meshwork in an unindented state, the angle is designated as a (B)D25s.

different parts of the eye. The configuration of the angle should be separately recorded for each area in which the configuration differs.

Grading the anterior chamber angle should also provide an estimate of the intensity of pigmentation of the posterior trabecular meshwork. This can be graded as none, mild, moderate, marked, or advanced, or in the numerical system similar to that utilized in many other grading systems, specifically, 0 = none, 1 = mild, 2 = moderate, 3 = marked, 4 = advanced (Fig. 24). The pigmentation of the posterior trabecular meshwork must be graded at the 12 o'clock position. The amount of pigment inferiorly should also be noted. The notation of the angle that is recorded in the chart is performed as follows. The site of the iris insertion is recorded first as a capital letter. If it is impossible to see the actual site of insertion, then the most posterior structure visible is indicated in parentheses, following which the actual site of insertion as determined by indentation gonioscopy is indicated in a capital letter without parentheses. Next, the angularity of the approach to the recess in degree is indicated, measuring the angle between the posterior surface of the cornea and the anterior surface of the iris at Schwalbe's line. Then, the peripheral curvature of the iris is indicated as q, r, or s, in lower case letters. Finally, the intensity of pigmentation of the posterior trabecular meshwork is shown as 0 to 4+ (Fig. 24). Where the characteristics of the angle vary from quadrant to quadrant it is helpful to draw a circle and use the appropriate notation next to that part of the circle that corresponds to the angle being described. Thus, an anterior chamber angle in which the most anterior structure visible without indentation gonioscopy at the 12 o'clock position was the scleral spur, and in which the actual iris insertion was into the ciliary body, which had an angular approach of 20° with a regular curvature and moderate pigmentation of the posterior trabecular meshwork, but in which at the 6 o'clock position inferiorly the angle was deeper so that it was possible to see that the iris inserted

is displaced by forcing the aqueous humour posteriorly, the actual site of the iris insertion can be seen; this is at the anterior portion of the ciliary body. No pathological adhesions are present.'

This same description can be recorded by using the grading system described above with one important addition. Specifically, where it is not possible to see the actual site of iris insertion, the structure of the angle that is able to be visualized in the unindented state is noted, and recorded with a parenthesis around the letter. The parenthesis indicates that this is an appearance, and not an actuality. The actual site of iris insertion, in this case the anterior ciliary body or D, is indicated following the parenthesis. Figure 23 illustrates three slightly different configurations and how they would be notated.

The consideration of the anterior chamber angle varies in

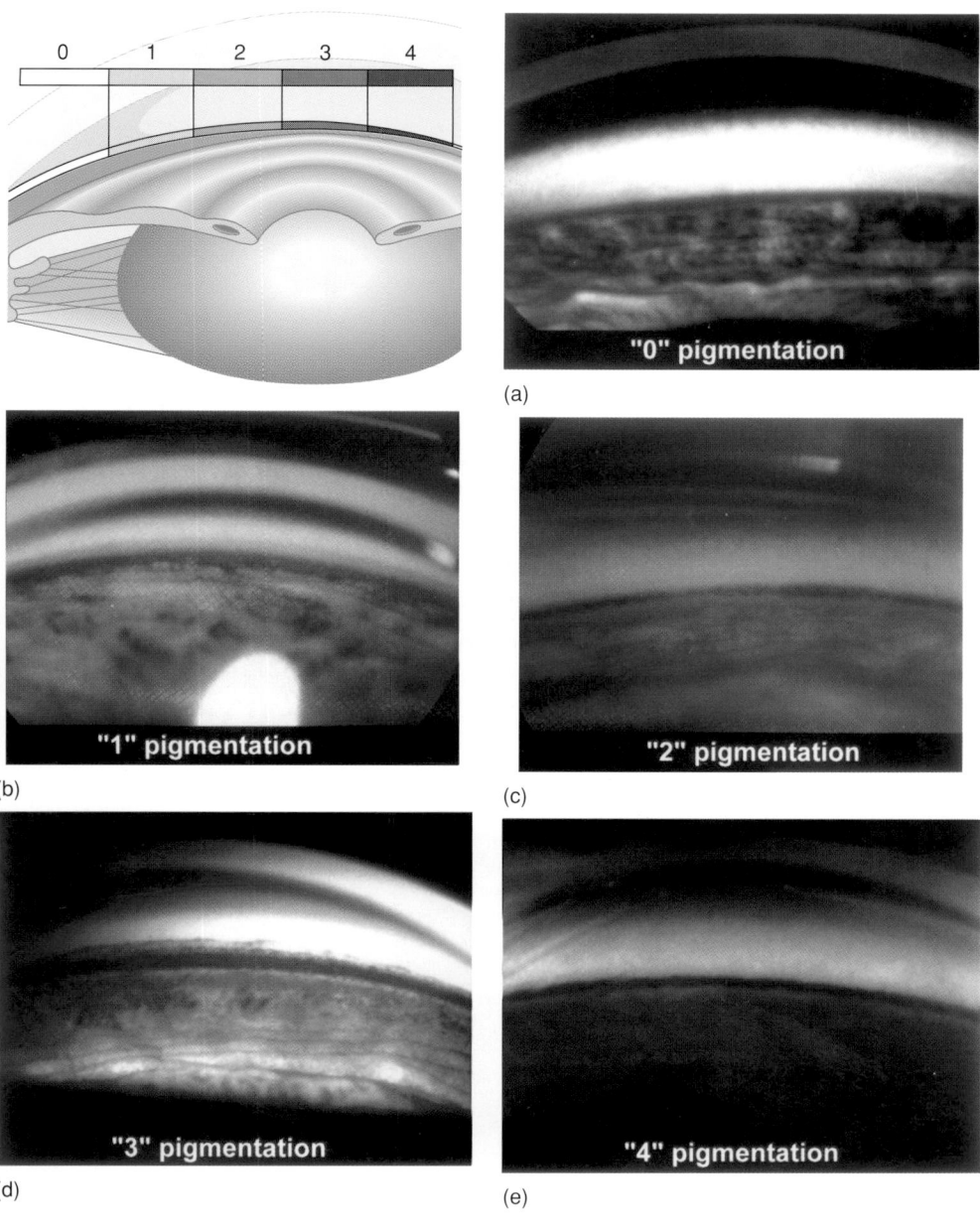

"0" pigmentation

(a)

"1" pigmentation

(b)

"2" pigmentation

(c)

"3" pigmentation

(d)

"4" pigmentation

(e)

Fig. 24 Four different intensities of pigmentation in the posterior trabecular meshwork. (a) There is a wide ciliary body band, but no pigmentation in the trabecular meshwork. (b) The ciliary body band is brown and just anterior to it is a very lightly pigmented trabecular meshwork. (c) The pigmentation is more marked, varying from 1+ to 2+. This is a frequent appearance in normal individuals. In this slide, the 6 o'clock position of the eye is to the left, the 12 o'clock position to the right, and the 9 o'clock position in the middle of the illustration. Typically there is less pigment in the posterior trabecular meshwork at the 3 and 9 o'clock positions. (d) There is intense pigmentation in the posterior trabecular meshwork and moderate pigment anterior to the trabecular meshwork on Schwalbe's line. The 6 o'clock position is to the left, which is where pigment on Schwalbe's line is likely to accumulate. (e) There is extremely dense pigmentation of the posterior trabecular meshwork without pigmentation anterior to this. This appearance is typical of the angle at the 12 o'clock position. This extent of pigmentation is not a normal finding. The schematic drawing illustrates the method of grading pigmentation in the posterior trabecular meshwork based on pigment intensity. This is done at the 12 o'clock position.

into the anterior ciliary body without using indentation gonioscopy, and in which there was a regular curvature and more marked pigmentation of the posterior trabecular meshwork would be notated by drawing a circle at the top of which one would write (C)D20r 2+ posterior trabecular meshwork, and at the bottom of which one would write D30r 3+ posterior trabecular meshwork.

Variations of normal

It should be stressed that the configuration of the angle changes. The dimensions of the anterior chamber have a diurnal variation and so likewise does the anterior chamber angle itself, varying with time and other changing circumstances.

Some of the changes in the anterior chamber angle related to age, race, and iris colour have already been mentioned. In the normal eye the depth of the anterior chamber is usually similar in all quadrants. In eyes with primary angle closure glaucoma (relative pupillary block type of angle closure) the angle is usually narrowest just inferior to the 12 o'clock position and deepest at the 6 o'clock position. When the angle is narrow in association with the exfoliation syndrome, it tends to be narrowest at the 6 o'clock position and deepest superiorly.

The pigmentation that occurs in association with the pigment dispersion syndrome is usually brown and concentrated within the posterior trabecular meshwork. There is as much pigmentation at the 12 o'clock position as at the 6 o'clock position. The colour of the iris does not affect the intensity of pigmentation of the posterior trabecular meshwork at 12 o'clock, but in brown-eyed individuals there may be increased pigment inferiorly, the pigment usually being on the surface of

Schwalbe's line, trabecular meshwork, and the ciliary body. In the exfoliation syndrome, the pigmentation of the inferior angle is much denser than that superiorly and tends to be black.

Further reading

Alsbirk, P.H. (1986). Limbal and axial chamber depth variations. *Acta Ophthalmologica*, **64**, 593–600.

Anderson, D.R. (1981). The development of the trabecular meshwork and its abnormality in primary infantile glaucoma. *Transactions of the American Ophthalmology Society*, **79**, 458.

Barkan, O. (1936). New operation for chronic glaucoma: restoration of physiological function by opening Schlemm's canal under direct magnified vision. *American Journal of Ophthalmology*, **19**, 951.

Barkan, O. (1938). Glaucoma: classification, causes, and surgical control. Results of micro-gonioscopic research. *American Journal of Ophthalmology*, **21**, 1099–117.

Barkan, O., Boyle, S.F., and Maisler, S. (1936). On the genesis of glaucoma. An improved method based on slit lamp microscopy of the angle of the anterior chamber. *American Journal of Ophthalmology*, **19**, 209–15.

Barkhoff, E.R. and Kaizik, O. (1969). Vergleichende gonioskopische und tonographische Untersuchungen verschiedener Altersklassen. *Klinische Monatsblatter für Augenheilkunde*, **155**, 518–25.

Berliner, M. (1943). *Biomicroscopy of the eye*, Vol. I, p. 262. Paul B. Hoeber/Harper, New York.

Busacca, A. (1964). *Biomicroscopie et histopathologie de l'oeil*, Vol. II, p. 736. Schweizer Druck & Verlagshaus, Zurich.

Campbell, D.G. (1979). A comparison of diagnostic techniques in angle-closure glaucoma. *American Journal of Ophthalmology*, **88**, 197–204.

Caprioli, J., Spaeth, G.L., and Wilson, R.P. (1986). Anterior chamber depth in open angle glaucoma. *British Journal of Ophthalmology*, **70**, 831–6.

Caronia, R.M., Liebmann, J.M., Stegman, Z., Sokol, J., and Ritch, R. (1996). Iris–lens contact increases following laser iridotomy for pupillary block angle-closure. *American Journal of Ophthalmology*, **122**, 53–7.

Delmarcelle, Y. and Luyckx-Bacus, J. (1970). Influence de la cataracte senile sur l'epaisseur du cristallin et la profondeur de la chambre anterieure. *Bulletin de la Societe Belge d'Ophthalmologie*, **155**, 465–73.

Fontana, S.T. and Brubaker, R.F. (1980). Volume and depth of the anterior chamber in the normal aging human eye. *Archives of Ophthalmology*, **98**, 1803–8.

Forbes, M. (1966). Gonioscopy with corneal indentation. A method for distinguishing between appositional closure and synechial closure. *Archives of Ophthalmology*, **76**, 488–92.

Gandham, S., Spaeth, G.L., Baez, K.A., Smith, M., Katz, L.J., Orengo, S., and Bond, J.B. (1992). Diurnal variation of anterior chamber depth and angle. *Investigative Ophthalmology and Visual Science*, **33** (suppl.), 732 Abstr.

Goldmann, H. (1938). Zur Tecknik der Spaltlampenmikroskopie. *Ophthalmologica*, **96**, 90.

Gradle, H.S. and Sugar, H.S. (1940). Concerning the chamber angle. III. Clinical method of goniometry. *American Journal of Ophthalmology*, **23**, 1135.

Hansson, H.A. and Jerndal, T. (1971). Scanning electron microscopic studies on the development of the irido-corneal angle in human eyes. *Investigative Ophthalmology*, **10**, 252.

Henkind, P. (1964). Angle vessels in normal eyes. A gonioscopic evaluation and anatomic correlation. *British Journal of Ophthalmology*, **48**, 551–7.

Ishikawa, H., *et al.* (1996). A new method of quantifying the anterior chamber angle with ultrasound biomicroscopy. *Investigative Ophthalmology and Visual Science*, **37** (suppl), S820.

Karickhoff, J.R. (1993). Reverse pupillary block in pigmentary glaucoma: follow up and new developments. *Ophthalmic Surgery*, **24**, 562–3.

Knisely, T.L., *et al.* (1991). Production of latent transforming growth factor-beta and other inhibitory factors by cultured murine iris and ciliary body cells. *Current Eye Research*, **8**, 761–71.

Koeppe, L. (1919–1920). Die mikroskopie des lebenden Kammerwinkels intramuscular fokalen Lichte der Gullstrandschen Nernstspaltlampe. *Archiv für Ophthalmologie*, **101**, 48, 238.

Kupfer, C., Datiles, M., and Kaiser-Kupfer, M. (1982). Development of the anterior chamber of the eye: embryology and clinical implications. In *Basic aspects of glaucoma research*, (ed. E. Lütjen-Drecoll). Schattauer Verlag, Stuttgart.

Lichter, P.R. (1969). Iris processes in 340 eyes. *American Journal of Ophthalmology*, **68**, 872–6.

Liebmann, J.M., *et al.* (1995). Prevention of blinking alters iris configuration in pigment dispersion syndrome and in normal eyes. *Ophthalmology*, **102**, 446–55.

Liebmann, J.M., Sokol, J., and Ritch, R. (1996). Management of chronic hypotony following glaucoma filtration surgery. *Journal of Glaucoma*, **5**, 210–20.

Lowe, R.F. (1964). Primary creeping angle-closure glaucoma. *British Journal of Ophthalmology*, **48**, 544.

Mapstone, R. and Clark, C.V. (1985). Diurnal variation in the dimensions of anterior chamber. *Archives of Ophthalmology*, **103**, 1485–6.

Morrison, J.C. and Freddo, T.F. (1996). Anatomy, microcirculation, and ultrastructure of the ciliary body. In *The glaucomas*, (ed. R. Ritch, M.B. Shields, and T. Krupin), (2nd edn), pp. 125–38. Mosby, St Louis.

Oh, Y.G., Minelli, S., Spaeth, G.L., *et al.* (1994). The anterior chamber angle is different in different racial groups. *Eye*, **8**, 104–8.

Olurin, O. (1977). Anterior chamber depths of Nigerians. *Annals of Ophthalmology*, **9**, 315–26.

Plouet, J. and Gospodarowicz, D. (1990). Iris-derived melanocytes contain a growth factor that resembles basic fibroblast growth factor. *Experimental Eye Research*, **51**, 519.

Potash, S.D., Tello, C., Liebmann, J., *et al.* (1994). Ultrasound biomicroscopy in pigment dispersion syndrome. *Ophthalmology*, **101**, 332–9.

Raeder, J.G. (1923). Untersuchungen uber die Lage und Dicke der Linse intramuscular menschlichen Auge bei physiologischen und pathologischen Zustanden, nach einer neuen Methode gemessen. Klinische Beobachtungen und Messungen der Vorderkammertiefe bei primaren und sekundaren Glaukomen. *Archives of Ophthalmology*, **44**, 112.

Raviola, G. (1971). The fine structure of the ciliary zonule and ciliary epithelium: with special regard to the organization and insertion of the zonular fibrils. *Investigative Ophthalmology and Visual Science*, **10**, 851.

Ritch, R., Liebmann, J., and Stegman, Z. (1995). Mapstone's hypothesis confirmed. *British Journal of Ophthalmology*, **79**, 300.

Salzmann, M. (1914). Die Ophthalmoskopie der kammerbucht. *Zeitschrift für Augenheilkunde*, **31**, 1.

Scheie, H.G. (1957). Width and pigmentation of the angle of the anterior chamber: a system of grading by gonioscopy. *Archives of Ophthalmology*, **58**, 510.

Shaffer, R.N. (1960). Gonioscopy, ophthalmoscopy, and perimetry. *Transactions of the American Academy of Ophthalmology and Otolaryngology*, **64**, 112.

Shibata, T., Kazuyuki, S., Sakamoto, Y., *et al.* (1990). Quantitative chamber angle measurement utilizing image-processing techniques. *Ophthalmic Research*, **22**, 81–4.

Smelser, G.K. and Ozanics, V. (1971). The development of the trabecular meshwork in primate eyes. *American Journal of Ophthalmology*, **71**, 366.

Sokol, J., *et al.* (1996). Location of the iris insertion in pigment dispersion syndrome. *Ophthalmology*, **103**, 289–93.

Spaeth, G.L. (1971). The normal development of the human anterior chamber angle: a new system of descriptive grading. *Transactions of the Ophthalmology Society UK*, **91**, 709–39.

Spaeth, G.L., Araujo, S., and Azuara, A. (1995). Comparison of the configuration of the human anterior chamber angle, as determined by the Spaeth gonioscopic grading system and ultrasound biomicroscopy. *Transactions of the American Academy of Ophthalmological Society*, **93**, 377.

Stegman, Z.X., *et al.* (1996). Reduced trabecular meshwork height in juvenile primary open-angle glaucoma. *Archives of Ophthalmology*, **114**, 660–3.

Streeten, B.W. (1982). Zonular apparatus. In *Biomedical foundations of ophthalmology*, (ed. T.D. Duane and E.A. Jaeger). Harper & Row, Philadelphia.

Thorburn, T. (1932). A gonioscopic study of anterior peripheral synechia in primary glaucoma (thesis). *Acta Ophthalmologica*, **10**, 112.

Tiedeman, J.S. (1991). A physical analysis of the factors that determine the contour of the iris. *American Journal of Ophthalmology*, **111**, 338–43.

Trantas, A. (1907). Ophthalmoscopie de la region ciliaire et retrociliaire. *Archives d'ophtalmologie*, **27**, 581.

Tripathi, R.C. and Tripathi, B.J. (1982). Functional anatomy of the anterior chamber of the angle. In *Biomedical foundations of ophthalmology*, Vol. 1 (ed. T.D. Duane and E.A. Jaeger). Harper & Row, Hagerstown.

Tripathi, B.J., Tripathi, R.C., and Wisdom, J.E. (1996). Embryology of the anterior segment of the human eye. In *The glaucomas*, pp. 3–38, (ed. R. Ritch, M.B. Shields, T. Krupin, and J.E. Wisdom). Mosby, St Louis.

Uribe Troncoso, M. (1921). *Gonioscopy with the electric ophthalmoscope*. New York Academy of Medicine.

Uribe Troncoso, M. (1942). Microanatomy of the eye with the slit lamp microscope. II. Comparative anatomy of the ciliary body, zonula, and related structures in mammalia. *American Journal of Ophthalmology*, **25**, 1.

Uribe Troncoso, M. and Castroviejo, R. (1936). Microanatomy of the eye with slit lamp microscope: I. Comparative anatomy of the angle of the anterior chamber in living and sectioned eyes of mammalia. *American Journal of Ophthalmology*, **19**, 371, 481, 583.

Van Buskirk, E.M. (1981). Clinical implications of iridocorneal angle development. *Ophthalmology*, **88**, 361.

Weekers, R., Delmarcelle, Y., Collignon, J., and Luyckx, J. (1973). Mesure optique de la profondeur de la chambre anterieure applications cliniques. *Documenta Ophthalmologica*, **34**, 413–34.

Measuring the depth of the anterior chamber

Chandler, P.A. and Grant, W.M. (1965). *Lectures on glaucoma*, pp. 54–107. Lea & Febiger, Philadelphia.

Cloakes, R.L., Lloyd-Jones, D., and Hitchings. R.A. (1979). Anterior chamber volume—its measurement and clinical application. *Transactions of the Ophthalmology Society UK*, **99**, 78–81.

Cohen, J.S. and Tilton, T. (1988). Technique for slit lamp comparison of anterior chamber depth. *Ophthalmic Surgery*, **19**, 58–60.

Dellaporta, A. (1975). Historical notes on gonioscopy. *Survey of Ophthalmology*, **20**, 137–49.

Dimitrakos, S.A. (1982). Comparaison de trois methodes pour la mesure de la profondeur de la chambre anterieure. *Klinische Monatsblatter für Augenheilkunde*, **180**, 417–19.

Douthwaite, W.A. and Spence, D. (1986). Slit-lamp measurement of the anterior chamber depth. *British Journal of Ophthalmology*, **70**, 205–8.

Hitchings, R.A., Romano, J., and Clark, P. (1984). Measurements of axial and peripheral anterior chamber depth: accuracy of a photographic method. *British Journal of Ophthalmology*, **68**, 212–14.

Jacobs, I.H. (1979). Anterior chamber depth measurement using the slit-lamp microscope. *American Journal of Ophthalmology*, **88**, 236–8.

Pavlin, C.J., *et al.* (1992). Ultrasound biomicroscopy of anterior segment structures in normal and glaucomatous eyes. *American Journal of Ophthalmology*, **113**, 1381.

Pavlin, C.J., *et al.* (1991). Clinical use of ultrasound biomicroscopy. *Ophthalmology*, **98**, 287.

Pavlin, C.J., Ritch, R., and Foster, F.S. (1992). Ultrasound biomicroscopy in plateau iris syndrome. *American Journal of Ophthalmology*, **113**, 390–5.

Pavlin, C.J., *et al.* (1994). Ultrasound biomicroscopic features of pigmentary glaucoma. *Canadian Journal of Ophthalmology*, **29**, 187.

Richards, D.W., Russell, S.R., and Anderson, D.R. (1988). A method for improved biometry of the anterior chamber with a Scheimpflug technique. *Investigative Ophthalmology and Visual Science*, **29**, 1826–35.

Shibata, T., Kazuyuki, S., Sakamoto, Y., *et al.* (1990). Quantitative chamber angle measurement utilizing image-processing techniques. *Ophthalmic Research*, **22**, 81–4.

Smith, R.J.H. (1979). A new method of estimating the depth of the anterior chamber. *British Journal of Ophthalmology*, **63**, 215–20.

van Herick, W., Shaffer, R.N., and Schwartz, A. (1969). Estimation of width of angle of anterior chamber. Incidence and significance of the narrow angle. *American Journal of Ophthalmology*, **68**, 626–33.

The field of gonioscopy

Alward, W.L.N. (1994). *Color atlas of gonioscopy*. Mosby, London.

Berliner, M. (1943). *Biomicroscopy of the eye*, Vol. I, p. 262. Paul B. Hoeber/ Harper, New York.

Busacca, A. (1945). *Elements de gonioscopie: normale, pathologique et experimentale*. Tipografia Rossolillo, Sao Paulo, Brazil.

Dellaporta, A. (1975). Historical notes on gonioscopy. *Survey of Ophthalmology*, **20**, 137–49.

Donaldson, D. (1973). *Atlas of external diseases of the eye*, Vol. IV. *Anterior chamber, iris, and ciliary body*. Mosby, St Louis.

Francois, J. (1948). *La gonioscopie*. Fonteyn, Louvain.

Gorin, G. and Posner, A. (1961). *Split-lamp gonioscopy*. Williams & Wilkins, Baltimore.

Palmberg, P. (1996). Gonioscopy. In *The glaucomas*, (2nd edn), (ed. R. Ritch, M.B. Shields, and T. Krupin), pp. 455–71. Mosby, St Louis.

Tripathi, R.C. and Tripathi, B.J. (1982). Functional anatomy of the anterior chamber angle. In *Biomedical foundations of ophthalmology*, Vol. I, pp. 1–188. Harper & Row, Philadelphia.

Uribe Troncoso, M. (1921). *Gonioscopy with the electric ophthalmoscope*. New York Academy of Medicine.

Uribe Troncoso, M. (1942). Microanatomy of the eye with the slit lamp microscope. II. Comparative anatomy of the ciliary body, zonula, and related structures in mammalia. *American Journal of Ophthalmology*, **25**, 1.

Uribe Troncoso, M. and Castroviejo, R. (1936). Microanatomy of the eye with slit lamp microscope: I. Comparative anatomy of the angle of the anterior chamber in living and sectioned eyes of mammalia. *American Journal of Ophthalmology*, **19**, 371, 481, 583.

Vogt, A. (1930). *Lehrbuch und Atlas der Spaltlampenmikroskopie des Lebende Auges*. Verlag von Julius Springer, Berlin.

2.10.1.2 **Aqueous humour dynamics**

Theodore Krupin

Intraocular pressure reflects a balance between the rate of aqueous humour formation by the ciliary body and the rate of fluid exit from the eye via the trabecular meshwork and the uveoscleral pathways. Dynamic processes contributing to the maintenance of intraocular pressure include the following.

1. Aqueous humour formation or flow (F). Each ciliary process consists of a loose connective tissue containing a central vascular core covered by a bilayered epithelium. Active transport by the ciliary epithelium is the main mechanism for the entry of fluid into the posterior chamber, which is measured in μl/min. Ultrafiltration (dialysis in the presence of hydrostatic pressure) is only a minor mechanism for aqueous humour formation when the normal blood–aqueous barrier is intact.

2. Aqueous humour outflow. Aqueous humour exits the anterior chamber via two routes at the anterior chamber angle. Pressure-sensitive flow (C), measured as μl/min/mmHg, occurs through the trabecular meshwork, where the fluid enters Schlemm's canal and drains into episcleral veins. Pressure-insensitive flow (U), the so-called uveoscleral outflow, measured in μl/min, occurs across the anterior face of the ciliary body with subsequent aqueous flow through the sclera

into orbital tissue or absorption into uveal blood vessels. Trabecular outflow constitutes the major portion of aqueous humour outflow. Uveoscleral outflow may account for a greater than normal percentage of outflow in glaucomatous eyes with decreased trabecular outflow. It may also be the route by which topically applied drugs, after penetrating the cornea and entering the anterior chamber, reach the ciliary body to affect aqueous production. In addition, approximately 5 to 10 per cent of aqueous exits the anterior chamber by exchange across the iris.

3. Episcleral venous pressure (P_v). Flow of aqueous humour into the recipient episcleral veins is directly dependent upon the pressure in these vessels. For each mmHg change in episcleral venous pressure, there is an associated change of approximately 1 mmHg in intraocular pressure.

Under normal steady-state conditions the hydraulics of aqueous humour dynamics may be reasonably approximated for clinical purposes by

$$\text{flow}_{in} = \text{flow}_{out} = C(\text{intraocular pressure} - P_v) + U.$$

Typical values for these parameters in the normal human eye are as follows:

$$\text{flow}_{in} = \text{flow}_{out} = 2.5 \ \mu l/min$$

$$C = 0.3 \ \mu l/min/mmHg$$

$$\text{intraocular pressure} = 16 \ mmHg$$

$$P_v = 9 \ mmHg$$

$$U = 0.4 \ \mu l/min$$

so that

$$2.5 = 0.3(16 - 9) + 0.4$$

In glaucoma, increased intraocular pressure is usually related to reduced trabecular outflow facility. An increased rate of aqueous humour formation is rarely, if ever, the aetiology for the increased pressure in glaucoma. However, pharmacological reduction of intraocular pressure decreasing the normal rate of aqueous formation is a mainstay of treatment for glaucoma. In addition, the importance of aqueous production to the level of intraocular pressure (and to the therapy of glaucoma) is underscored by a diurnal fluctuation in the rate of aqueous formation: the highest rate being usually in the morning and decreasing during the day to reach a low point (approximately a 50 per cent decrease) during sleep.

Aqueous humour

Aqueous fulfills a number of important functions within the anterior segment.

1. The constant flow of aqueous helps to inflate the globe and maintain an adequate intraocular pressure which is necessary for the structural integrity and normal optical functioning of the eye.

2. Aqueous serves a metabolic function for avascular anterior segment tissues including the cornea, lens, and trabecular meshwork. Substrates (e.g. glucose, oxygen, and amino acids) are supplied to these tissues while metabolic wastes (e.g. lactic acid, pyruvic acid, and carbon dioxide) are carried away.

3. Aqueous humour in many species, including humans, contains a high concentration of ascorbate, which may affect catecholamine storage in the iris, serve as an antioxidant, regulate the sol-gel balance of glycosaminoglycans in the trabecular meshwork, serve to partially absorb cataractogenic ultraviolet radiation, or act as a superoxide radical scavenging agent.

4. Aqueous humour facilitates cellular and humoural immune responses under adverse conditions, such as inflammation and infection.

The composition of aqueous humour depends upon the nature of its production, on the metabolic interchanges that occur during its flow through the posterior and anterior chambers (diffusional and metabolic alterations occur as ionic and solute exchanges take place across the vitreous, lens, cornea, and iris), and its rate of outflow. In fact, insights into aqueous production were first gained by comparing the concentration of substances in the aqueous humour and in plasma. The complex make-up of aqueous suggests that it is not a simple ultrafiltrate of plasma.

A number of observations suggest the presence of functional barriers in the anterior segment to the movement of substances from the plasma to the aqueous humour. For example, the concentration of proteins in the anterior chamber (approximately 25 mg/dl) is markedly lower than plasma levels (approximately 6 g/dl). Physiologically the blood–aqueous barrier has been recognized to be located at a site other than the walls of blood vessels, since albumin and other proteins exit the vessels of the ciliary body at a faster rate than they enter the anterior chamber. Horseradish peroxidase, a tracer which readily exits the ciliary process vessels, is blocked by the junctions at the apical portions of the non-pigmented ciliary epithelial cells. The blood–aqueous barrier consists of tight junctions (zonulae occludentes) that appear as fused bands encircling the apical ends of the lateral plasma membranes of the non-pigmented ciliary epithelial cells, sealing adjacent cell membranes. Structurally, the barrier consists of a series of fibrillar networks that form discontinuous ridges. This organization could effectively block the passage of large molecules while still allowing a flux of ions and low molecular weight solutes through channels within the junction.

Formation of aqueous humour

Aqueous formation results from net fluid movement across the epithelial layers of the ciliary processes. There are approximately 70 processes which are radiating villiform ridges projecting into the posterior chamber. Each process is composed of blood vessels embedded in a loose connective tissue with a double layer of epithelial cells lining the surface. The apices of the two epithelial layers face each other, with the basolateral membrane of the outer pigmented cells facing the stroma and the basolateral membrane of the inner non-pigmented epithelial cells facing the posterior chamber. These anatomical relationships result embryologically from invagination of the optic vesicle to form the optic cup. The ciliary body stroma is separated from the pigmented epithelium by the forward continuation of Bruch's membrane, while the non-pigmented epithelium is separated from the posterior chamber by an internal limiting membrane that is continuous with that of the retina. The two epithelial layers are connected by gap junctions and desmosomes. The entire group of processes can be thought of as an everted gland.

Fluid transport across the ciliary epithelium can occur by three basic mechanisms.

1. Diffusion, the passive movement of solutes, especially lipid soluble substances, across cell membranes in response to a concentration gradient

2. Ultrafiltration (dialysis under pressure), the passive movement of water and water-soluble substances across the cell membrane in response to a non-enzymatic process regulated by both the differential hydrostatic pressure in the blood and the osmotic pressure of the ciliary body

3. Secretion, the active, energy-dependent movement of solutes across the cell membrane.

As for all epithelia, transfer can proceed both between the cells (paracellular route) and through the cells (transcellular route) as a direct or indirect result of differences in hydrostatic or osmotic pressure across the tissue. The concentration of many elements of the aqueous humour differ from those of plasma (see above) more than would be expected on the basis of the Gibbs–Donnan equilibrium, indicating that aqueous humour is not a simple dialysate of plasma. While the relative contributions of ultrafiltration and secretion in aqueous humour formation has been controversial, a number of observations which are presented below do not support ultrafiltration as a major mechanism for aqueous humour production. These observations indicate that active, rather than passive, forces are more important to aqueous humour formation.

Ultrafiltration

As much as 70 per cent of aqueous humour formation occurs by the passive movement of water and water-soluble substances from the plasma into the posterior chamber in response to a differential hydrostatic pressure in the blood and the osmotic pressure of the ciliary body. The theoretical considerations for the importance of ultrafiltration depend on the presence of 'leaky' junctional complexes on the channel between ciliary epithelial cells which would allow the possibility of pressure-dependent flow through the channel. The possible importance

of ultrafiltration was based on Cole's reported low value of short-circuit current in the isolated iris–ciliary body preparation and on high measurements of hydraulic conductivity of ciliary processes *in vitro*.

The proportional role of ultrafiltration and secretion in the formation of aqueous humour is important in understanding the effect of a drug on the rate of aqueous humour production. However, a number of observations do not support ultrafiltration as a major mechanism for aqueous humour production.

1. Bill (Bill 1973) demonstrated that experimentally induced variations in systemic blood pressure result in only small changes in aqueous humour formation.

2. Biochemical observations support secretion as the primary mechanism of aqueous production (i.e. the low concentration of non-ionized freely diffusible urea in aqueous humour, the effect of aqueous outflow on steady-state solute concentrations, the rates of entry and turnover of radioactive tracers into the aqueous, and the higher concentration of ascorbate in the posterior rather than in the anterior chamber or the plasma).

3. Metabolic poisons and cardiotonic-steroid inhibitors of the sodium pump (e.g. ouabain), reduce the *in vivo* rate of aqueous formation by 70 to 80 per cent.

4. The necessary pressure within in the ciliary capillaries in order for the proposed rate of ultrafiltration to occur has been postulated to be 49 to 57 mmHg. This value is higher than measured values (25 to 33 mmHg). In fact, Bill (Bill 1973) has indicated that the hydrostatic and oncotic forces across the ciliary epithelium favour reabsorption of aqueous humour into the ciliary process rather than ultrafiltration.

5. Studies in the rabbit and monkey report low values for hydraulic conductivity and osmotic fluid permeability across the iris–ciliary body. These studies suggest that the previously reported values may be too high by a factor of 18 times.

These observations indicate that active, rather than passive, forces are more important to aqueous humour formation. The product of secretion by the ciliary epithelium consists of two processes: (a) ultrafiltration of the plasma from the capillaries of the ciliary processes into the extracellular space (stroma) of the ciliary processes; and (b) the transport of a modified form of this extracellular fluid across the two layers of the ciliary epithelium. However, even though ultrafiltration is of little importance for the normal formation of aqueous humour, it may affect movement of fluid across the ciliary epithelium when there is damage to the blood–aqueous barrier (e.g. inflammation, intraocular surgery, ciliodestructive surgery).

Secretion

Aqueous humour formation is now recognized to result from solute transfer from the ciliary process stroma to the posterior chamber, creating an osmotic pressure difference across the ciliary epithelial layers. Water movement follows passively along its chemical gradient. The bilayered structure makes it more difficult to study secretory processes in the ciliary epithelium than in other epithelia. Although the specific roles of the non-pigmented and pigmented layers are not yet established, it is now clear that the two layers function as a syncytium. Gap junctions provide the structural basis for intercellular communication both within each epithelial layer and between the two layers. Functional intercommunication within the ciliary epithelium was first demonstrated by intracellular electrical recording and histological analysis by Green et al. (Green et al. 1985), and has since been supported by electrophysiological studies, electron probe X-ray microanalysis, and scanning confocal microscopy demonstrating spread of the fluorescent dye Lucifer yellow between the two epithelial layers. Exchange of dye has also been observed with isolated pigmented and non-pigmented ciliary epithelial cells. The biochemistry of transport processes across the ciliary epithelium has been studied using *in vivo* and *in vitro* techniques.

In vivo techniques

As discussed above, differences in the composition of aqueous and the plasma indicate that aqueous humour is not a simple dialysate of plasma. However, current techniques for measurement of ion movement between aqueous and plasma are not suitable for human studies. Measurements of ion concentrations in the posterior chamber have not been performed in humans.

The biochemistry of aqueous formation has been studied in animals by measuring the transfer rate of ionic species (e.g. Na^+, Cl^-, HCO_3^-) from plasma to aqueous in the anterior and/or posterior chamber. Turnover of ^{24}Na in the posterior and anterior chambers, aqueous humour flow, and intraocular pressure all decrease following systemic hypothermia by cold water immersion. A temperature-related reduction in metabolic and enzymatic processes resulting in decreased sodium transport and aqueous secretion is suggested by these results. Cole (Cole 1960) measured the effects of two metabolic inhibitors, dinitrophenol and fluoracetamide, by blocking the drainage angle with silicone, collecting aqueous continuously through an anterior chamber cannula, and measuring the flow with a calibrated measuring capillary. Both inhibitors caused approximately a 33 per cent reduction of aqueous flow and influx of Na^+, Cl^-, and K^+.

The effects of specific metabolic inhibitors which reduce transcellular but not paracellular routes (e.g. inhibition of the Na,K-exchange pump with ouabain and studies with carbonic anhydrase inhibitors) have provided important biochemical information on the accession rate of radioactive ionic species, and the formation of aqueous humour. The similarity of results in various animal models support basic patterns of aqueous humour formation which appear to be a fundamental element of vertebrate physiology.

In vitro studies

Study of the intact ciliary epithelium in the excised iris–ciliary body has formed the basis for an understanding of aqueous humour formation, free from the complexities of uncontrolled variations in ciliary blood flow and outflow dynamics of the aqueous humour. Cole (Cole 1961a) was the first to apply the short-circuiting approach used by Ussing and Zerahn (Ussing and Zerhan 1951) to study transport across the ciliary epithelium. Preparations from a broad spectrum of species have been investigated. Given the structural complexities of the iris–ciliary body, a number of alternative preparations have also been developed, including the isolated ciliary epithelium, separated non-pigmented and pigmented cell layer, primary cultures of non-pigmented and pigmented ciliary epithelial cells, cultures and immortalization of both types of cell lines.

Short-circuit current

When the iris–ciliary body is mounted between the two halves of a chamber and bathed with identical Tyrode's solution on its two surfaces, a spontaneous potential difference (V_{ba}, aqueous with respect to blood surface) is observed. The magnitude and even the sign of this difference in electrical potential were initially uncertain. Experimental inconsistencies have been ascribed partly to the use of different experimental animals and different bathing solutions. The aqueous side was initially reported to be positive for the isolated iris–ciliary body of the rabbit and ox. However, subsequent studies demonstrated that the sign and magnitude of V_{ba} and the short-circuit current across the isolated iris–ciliary body of the rabbit are dependent on the bicarbonate concentration. Many of the early studies used nominally bicarbonate-free solutions, so that bubbling with or without CO_2 produced undefined concentrations of bicarbonate. In the presence of bicarbonate, the aqueous surface is negative relative to the contralateral surface of the preparation. The polarity is reversed when HCO_3^- is omitted from the solutions bathing the rabbit preparation. The aqueous has been established to be negative for the bicarbonate-bathed iris–ciliary body of the rabbit, cat, dog, toad, and human preparations. Thus, all isolated preparations of vertebrate ciliary epithelia studied with bicarbonate-containing solutions display a negative value for V_{ba}. Ionic dependence of the short-circuit current indicates that the major ions transported by the ciliary epithelium are Na^+, K^+, Cl^-, and HCO_3^-. In addition, the short-circuit current has been most productively used to monitor hormonal and pharmacological effects and to identify the sidedness (aqueous or stromal) of the actions. Biochemical uncoupling agents (e.g. 2,4-dinitrophenol), inhibitors of citrate cycle metabolism, and anoxia reduce the short-circuit current. A number of drugs reduce transepithelial measurements across the isolated iris–ciliary body including ouabain (an inhibitor of Na,K-activated adenosine triphosphatase), carbonic anhydrase inhibitors, adrenergic agonists, and halogenated inhalation anaesthetic agents.

Intracellular analysis and membrane transport

Many biophysical and biochemical techniques have been applied to identify the basic transport processes responsible for aqueous humour formation. These include intracellular electrical recording, and radioactive and spectroscopic measurements during and after ion substitutions and application of inhibitors. In addition, patch clamping, as well as the development of molecular strategies, have enormously facilitated identification of the membrane transporters in the ciliary epithelium. Details of these techniques are reviewed by Krupin and Civan (Krupin and Civan 1996).

Measurements of the intracellular potential (V_m) have been conducted by impaling both intact tissues and isolated cells with ion-insensitive micropipettes. In the intact rabbit ciliary epithelium bathed with bicarbonate-containing solution, measurements of V_m display a unimodal distribution with a mean of -68.2 ± 0.4 mV. Intracellular pH (pH_i) and intracellular Ca^{2+} [$(a_{Ca})_c$] activity have been measured fluorometrically in both the iris–ciliary body and isolated ciliary epithelial cells. In the presence of CO_2 and bicarbonate, pH_i has been reported to be 7.1 ± 0.1. The baseline level of $(a_{Ca})_c$ has been reported to be 140 ± 10 nmol/litre.

The volume of ciliary epithelial cells in culture has been measured by a variety of techniques. Either swelling or shrinking of the cells triggers regulatory transport mechanisms acting to restore cell volume to its baseline level. Investigators have taken advantage of these phenomena to identify membrane transport processes and the regulatory cascades modifying them.

Development of patch clamping, as well as molecular strategies, have enormously facilitated identification of the membrane transporters. The techniques of molecular biology are only now being applied to the ciliary epithelium. Patch clamping permits observation of ion channel transitions among the closed and one or more open states and characterization of the kinetics, selectivity, and current–voltage relationship of a single channel. This technique can also be conducted after excising the membrane patch with the external surface oriented towards the bath ('outside-out patch') or with the cytoplasmic surface directed towards the bath ('inside-out patch'). This approach provides an opportunity to control the solutions on both surfaces of the membrane and the membrane potential. By excluding cytoplasmic factors (other than those adhering to the membrane surface), the excised-patch mode facilitates study of second-messenger cascades in isolation.

Basic components of ion transport

Several basic transport proteins have been described in the plasma membranes of the ciliary epithelial cells: the Na,K-exchange pump, symports (producing cotransport of different ions in the same direction), antiports (producing countertransport of ions in opposite directions), and ion channels. In the next section, these elements will be considered to formulate a current heuristic model of aqueous humour formation (Fig. 1).

Na,K-exchange pump

The Na,K-exchange pump is the fundamental basis for the asymmetry in ionic composition across the plasma membranes of almost all vertebrate cells. With time, extracellular Na^+ tends to leak into, and intracellular K^+ to leak out of, the cell. The pump counteracts these leak processes by driving Na^+ outwards and accumulating K^+ in the cell. This basic pump–leak hypothesis has been a central tenet of cellular physiology for four decades.

The functional cycle of the pump is thought to be well described by the Post–Albers model, which postulates two different conformational states of the enzyme. In the E1 state (facing the cytoplasmic surface), the pump displays a low affinity for K^+ and a high affinity for Na^+. In the E2 state (facing the external surface), these relative affinities are reversed. With physiological concentrations of Na^+, K^+, Mg^{2+}, and adenosine triphosphate, the forward cycling of the pump is strongly favoured, extruding three Na^+ and accumulating two K^+ at the expense of 1 adenosine triphosphate. Thus, each physiological cycle of the pump transfers one net positive charge from the inside to the outside of the cell, resulting in net current flow. Under non-physiological conditions, the stoichiometry and mode of operation of the pump can be altered, and adenosine triphosphate can even be generated by forcing the pump to run in the reverse sense.

Symports and antiports

Of the multiple symports and antiports presented in Fig. 1, the $Na^+/K^+/2Cl^-$ exchanger of the pigmented epithelial cells is likely most important in the formation of the aqueous humour. Evidence has been presented that a furosemide- and bumetanide-blockable $Na^+/K^+/2Cl^-$ symport is found in the ciliary epithelium. The symport probably provides the major route of entry of Na^+, K^+, and Cl^- from the stroma into the pigmented ciliary epithelial cells. These ions can then diffuse through gap junctions into the non-pigmented cells, from which they are extruded into the aqueous humour.

The $2Na^+$/ascorbate$^-$ symport is also clearly involved in transepithelial secretion. By coupling to the favourable electrochemical gradient driving Na^+ into the cell, this phloretin-inhibitable cotransport permits intracellular ascorbate to accumulate in the ciliary epithelium. Isolated pigmented cells have been found to increase the intracellular ascorbate level some 20-fold over that of the external medium. This concentration gradient provides the driving force for the ascorbate to exit into the aqueous humour by sodium-independent facilitated diffusion. The coupling of ascorbate to Na^+ transport not only provides the energy needed for secretion of ascorbate into the aqueous humour against a concentration gradient, but also enhances transepithelial Na^+ movement (albeit to a small degree).

The role of the many other symports and antiports incorporated in Fig. 1 in aqueous humour formation is as yet unclear. These mechanisms may be primarily involved in maintaining the homeostasis of the intracellular milieu, particularly volume, pH, and intracellular Ca^{2+} activity. For example, Na^+/H^+ antiports are found not only in the ciliary epithelial cells, but seem to be ubiquitous. Multiple isoforms of the Na^+/H^+ antiport have been sequenced. Intracellular pH is also likely regulated by HCO_3^- entry through Na^+-dependent and Na^+-independent HCO_3^-/Cl^- antiports and through a $Na^+/2HCO_3^-$ symport.

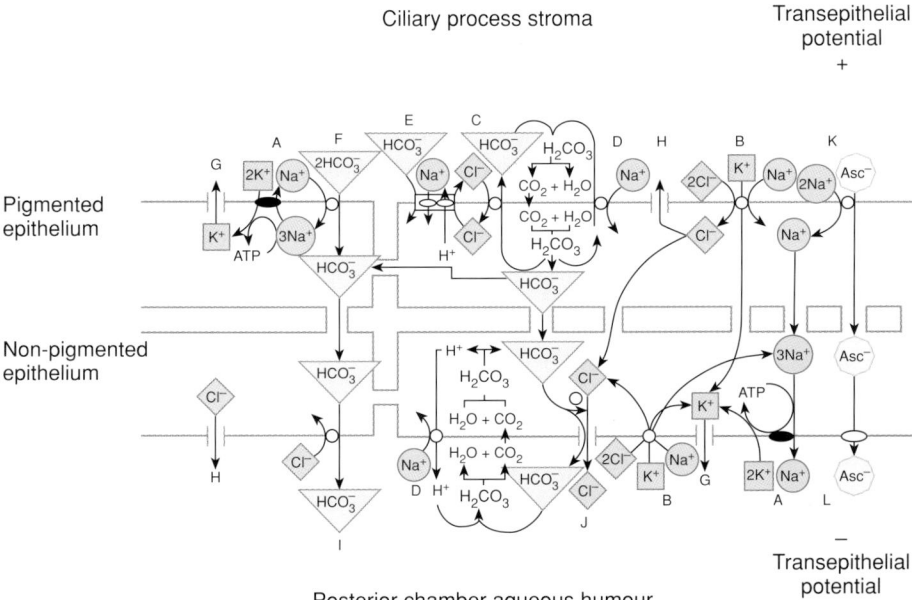

Fig. 1 Diagram presenting many of the transport components likely present in the plasma membranes of the pigmented and non-pigmented ciliary epithelial cells. Because of electrical coupling among the pigmented and non-pigmented cells through gap junctions, the epithelium functions as a syncytium. Tight intercellular junctions are present only between the non-pigmented cells, so that only this layer presents a complete barrier to transepithelial movement of solutes and water. Na^+,K^+-pumps (A) are shown on the basolateral membranes of both the pigmented and non-pigmented epithelial cells. The pigmented cells contain a $Na^+/K^+/2Cl^-$ symport (B), an electroneutral, Na^+-independent HCO_3^-/Cl^- antiport (C) coupled to the Na^+/H^+ antiport (D), an Na^+-dependent HCO_3^-/Cl^- antiport (E), an Na^+/H^+ antiport (D), and a negative $Na^+/2HCO_3^-$ symport (F). These processes will affect Cl^-/Na^+-coupled transport, which in addition to the Na^+,K^+-exchange pumps function to maintain the Cl^- electrochemical gradient. K^+ channels (G) are present on the pigmented and non-pigmented ciliary epithelial cells with channels on the non-pigmented layer most likely providing the major access route of K^+ into the aqueous humour. Cl^- channels (H) are present on both cell layers. The non-pigmented cells contain Na^+/H^+ antiport (D), an $Na^+/K^+/2Cl^-$ symport (B), HCO_3^-/Cl^- antiport (I), and an anion channel which passes both Cl^- and HCO_3^- (J). Also displayed are the $2Na^+$/ascorbate symport (K) subserving ascorbate uptake from the stroma and the transporter which translocates ascorbate across the aqueous-side membrane (L).

Ion channels

As in the case of symports and antiports, ion channels serve a dual function for epithelial cells, performing housekeeping chores for the cells themselves (particularly in terms of regulation of volume and membrane potential) and participating in transepithelial ion movement. Like other cells, the ciliary epithelial cells display calcium- and voltage-activated outwardly-rectifying K^+ channels, inwardly-rectifying K^+ channels, Cl^- channels, Ca^{2+} channels, Na^+ channels, and cation-non-selective channels. The kinetics, rectifying properties, selectivity, and pharmacological characteristics of these ciliary epithelial channels are reviewed in detail elsewhere. However, Fig. 1 presents one view of how some of these channels may be involved in forming aqueous humour.

The membrane potential of both the pigmented and non-pigmented cells in culture is reduced upon applying the K^+-channel blocker Ba^{2+}. Application of Ba^{2+} to the surface of the intact iris–ciliary body produces a much larger change in transepithelial potential when applied from the aqueous than from the stromal surface. This suggests that the basolateral membrane of the non-pigmented cells has a higher density of

K^+ channels than does the contraluminal membrane of the pigmented cells. Like other cells, the ciliary epithelial cells display a number of different K^+ channels. The full physiological importance of so rich a heterogeneity of K^+ channels is not clear, but a major function of such channels is clearly to regulate the membrane potential. As with other vertebrate cells, intracellular K^+ is accumulated by the operation of the Na,K-exchange pump and symports. Thus, the non-pigmented cells are poised to release K^+ down its electrochemical gradient into the aqueous humour.

An analogous condition holds for the chloride ion. Through the operation of symports and antiports, Cl^- is also accumulated within the ciliary epithelial cells against an electrochemical gradient. As noted above, the $Na^+/K^+/2Cl^-$ exchanger of the pigmented cells is likely to be the most important of these mechanisms in accumulating Cl^- in the cell against its electrochemical gradient. Cl^- channels have been detected at the aqueous surface of the intact rabbit ciliary epithelium, but their density is low under baseline conditions. The Cl^- conductance is also much lower than the K^+ conductance of non-pigmented cells under baseline conditions in culture. As in the case for K^+, the non-pigmented cells are poised to release Cl⁻ into the aqueous humour in response to signals upregulating the activity of the Cl⁻ channels.

Model of aqueous humour formation

Figure 1 presents most of the transport components thought to be present in the ciliary epithelium. A simplification is presented in Fig. 2 to emphasize those elements likely critical in secreting aqueous humour.

In the presence of CO_2/bicarbonate, the isolated ciliary epithelium generates a spontaneous transepithelial potential, the aqueous surface negative to the stromal surface. That small potential provides an electrical driving force for the predominant extracellular cation (Na^+) to be secreted into the aqueous humour. That same transepithelial voltage tends to favour reabsorption of Cl⁻ from the aqueous humour back into the blood. In the absence of a substantial difference in Cl⁻ concentration between the aqueous and blood phases in most species, it is unlikely that much net Cl⁻ is secreted through the paracellular pathway. There are a number of possible transport mechanisms which might extrude Cl⁻ into the aqueous humour. However, the concentration gradients driving the HCO_3^-/Cl⁻ antiports favour uptake (not release) of Cl⁻ from the aqueous into the cell.

It is possible that an electroneutral K^+/Cl⁻ symport might drive Cl⁻ into the aqueous humour. This symport is involved in the regulatory volume response activated by anisosmotic swelling of some cells. Like other vertebrate cells, non-pigmented cells display a period of secondary spontaneous shrinkage in response to an initial period of anisosmotic swelling, either of the intact epithelium or of cultured preparations. This regulatory response is termed the regulatory volume decrease. Studies of the regulatory volume decrease involving ion substitutions and inhibitors have clearly demonstrated that the regulatory volume decrease of the non-pigmented ciliary epithelial cells must largely reflect the release of K^+ and Cl⁻ through parallel K^+ and Cl⁻ channels. Given the responses to blockers of the K^+ channels (e.g. Ba^{2+} and quinidine) and Cl⁻ channels (e.g. NPPB, DIDS, and niflumic acid), it is implausible that the K^+/Cl⁻ symport contributes significantly to Cl⁻ transport into the aqueous humour. Cl⁻ is largely secreted through Cl⁻ channels at the aqueous surface of the non-pigmented cells. K^+ is secreted through parallel K^+ channels at the same surface. Na^+ is extruded into the aqueous humour, both by the Na,K-exchange pump of the non-pigmented cells and by paracellular movement in response to the transepithelial electrical driving force.

This model is fully consonant with the formulation of Frizzell et al. (Frizzell et al. 1979) which has served as the basic working model for secretory epithelia over the past 15 years. Aqueous humour formation is based on the transfer of solutes from the plasma, with water passively following (see Figs 1, 2). Most of this solute transfer occurs by passage through, rather than between, the cells. The exception to this rule is that positive ions, especially the major extracellular cation Na^+, also cross through the paracellular pathway in response to the small electrical gradient across the ciliary epithelium. It is likely that a Na^+/K^+/$2Cl^-$ symport is important in loading the pigmented ciliary epithelial cells with these ions. The pigmented and non-pigmented ciliary epithelial cells are interconnected with gap junctions, permitting Na^+, K^+, and Cl⁻ to diffuse to the aqueous surface of the non-pigmented ciliary epithelial cells. At this membrane, Na^+ is extruded by the Na,K-exchange pump, while K^+ and Cl⁻ are released down their electrochemical gradients through ion-selective channels. The low density or open probability of the Cl⁻ channels under baseline conditions indicates that Cl⁻ secretion at the aqueous surface of the non-pigmented cells may be an important rate-limiting factor in aqueous humour formation.

Pressure-dependent outflow

Aqueous humour leaves the anterior chamber by passive bulk flow via the following pathways at the anterior chamber angle.

1. The trabecular or conventional route: through the trabecular meshwork, across the inner wall of Schlemm's canal, and then into collector channels, aqueous veins, and the general venous circulation.

2. The posterior, unconventional, or uveoscleral route: across the iris root and the anterior face of the ciliary muscle, through the connective tissue between muscle bundles, into the suprachoroidal space, and then out through the sclera.

In monkeys, the trabecular route accounts for approximately half of the total drainage of aqueous humour, the uveoscleral pathway draining the remainder. In the normal human eye, the importance of the uveoscleral pathway has not been well

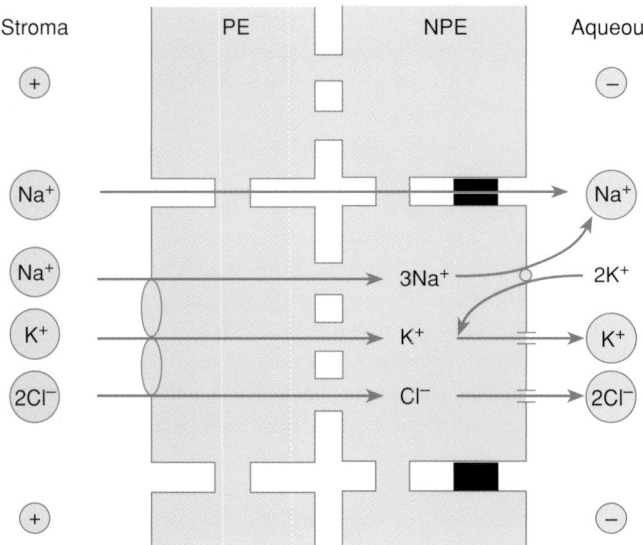

Fig. 2 Simplified form of Fig. 1 emphasizing the transport components thought critical in the formation of aqueous humour. For clarity, the ascorbate pathway has been omitted. Tight intercellular junctions are shown as dark boxes between the non-pigmented cells (NPE). Gap junctions are represented as shaded areas between the pigmented cells (PE), the PE and NPE, and the NPE cells.

quantitated. In the eyes of middle-aged or elderly people with posterior segment tumours, this pathway accounts for 5 to 20 per cent of total aqueous humour drainage, but may comprise one-third of the total drainage in younger individuals. There is relatively little uveoscleral drainage of aqueous humour in cats or rabbits. Other potential routes of aqueous humour egress include reabsorption of nascent fluid by the ciliary processes themselves, and flow posteriorly across the vitreoretinal interface. There is little net water movement across the iris vasculature.

Fluid mechanics

The chamber angle tissues offer a certain normal resistance to fluid outflow. In the glaucomatous eye, this resistance is unusually high, causing an elevated pressure. Although the proportionate distribution of this resistance within the chamber angle tissues is unsettled, the general consensus is that most of the resistance lies across and within the trabecular meshwork, perhaps in the cribriform region adjacent to the inner wall of Schlemm's canal.

Flow from the anterior chamber across the trabecular meshwork into Schlemm's canal is pressure dependent, but drainage via the uveoscleral pathway is virtually independent of pressure at intraocular pressure levels greater than 7 to 10 mmHg in the uninflamed eye. Although the actual drainage rates (μl/min) via the trabecular and uveoscleral routes in the monkey may be approximately equal, the measured facility of uveoscleral outflow is only about 0.01 to 0.02 μl/min/mmHg. Thus, uveoscleral facility constitutes at most only about 5 per cent of total facility.

The ultrafiltration component of aqueous humour formation is pressure-sensitive, decreasing with increasing intraocular pressure. This phenomenon is quantifiable and is termed pseudofacility, because a pressure-induced decrease in inflow will resemble an increase in outflow facility when tonography and constant pressure perfusion are used without special modification to measure outflow facility.

Direct measurements of aqueous humour formation in monkeys by isotope dilution at different intraocular pressures suggest that pseudofacility is approximately 0.02 μl/min/mmHg and thus amounting to no more than 5 to 10 per cent of total facility. This seems consistent with the predominant role of active aqueous humour secretion, which is rather unaffected by intraocular pressure within the near-physiological range, as opposed to passive ultrafiltration in the entry of newly formed aqueous humour into the posterior chamber. In situations in which the blood–aqueous humour barrier is disrupted, such as inflammation, ultrafiltration may become more pronounced and pseudofacility thus increases. This blunts the tendency for intraocular pressure to increase under such conditions.

Trabecular outflow is not completely independent of intraocular pressure or episcleral venous pressure. In human and monkey eyes, there is a decline of 1 to 2 per cent per mmHg increase in pressure, perhaps from compression of the trabecular meshwork or Schlemm's canal. Trabecular outflow increases with increasing episcleral venous pressure, presumably from inflation of Schlemm's canal and opening of collapsed segments. Intraocular pressure also increases with increasing episcleral venous pressure, but slightly less than mmHg for mmHg.

Measurement of trabecular outflow and outflow facility

Tonography affords a non-invasive means of estimating total outflow facility, which under normal circumstances reflects primarily trabecular outflow. The basic principle involves an estimation from the rate at which the intraocular pressure decreases when a known weight is applied to the eye. The method may be used in living humans and, with less reliability and more assumptions, in live animals. By combining tonography with measurement of P_v and/or aqueous flow, contamination of the tonographic facility estimate by pseudofacility and uveoscleral outflow can be minimized. However, in situations where the blood–aqueous barrier has been substantially compromised or uveoscleral outflow has become substantially pressure dependent, such contamination may remain significant.

More precise measurement of total outflow may be made invasively in live animal eyes or in enucleated postmortem animal and human eyes by various anterior chamber perfusion techniques. The chamber may be perfused at a constant flow rate, the resulting intraocular pressure reflecting total outflow. Alternatively, a constant pressure may be maintained, the flow rate then reflecting total outflow. Either technique may be run at two sequential levels (i.e. two-level constant rate, two-level constant pressure perfusion). In both instances, the difference between flow rates divided by the difference between the pressures defines outflow. The two-level constant pressure method has been preferred during the past two decades. Although less subject to various artefacts than tonography, these methods are still contaminated by uveoscleral facility and, in living animal eyes, by pseudofacility. By incorporating radioactive tracers, typically radioiodinated albumin, into the perfusate, it is possible to measure only trabecular outflow and outflow facility from living monkey eyes. Since outflow via Schlemm's canal and the trabecular route enters the systemic circulation immediately, one determines the radioactivity in arterial or venous blood and, by concurrently measuring the radioactivity in the anterior chamber and the distribution space for albumin in the body, determine the volume of fluid which has entered the circulation from the anterior chamber. Dividing this volume by the elapsed time gives the rate of trabecular outflow, and if measurements are performed successively at two different pressures, dividing the difference between the flow rates by the pressure difference gives a value for trabecular facility. This measurement is generally free of aqueous production (endogenous production is free of radioactivity) and uveoscleral outflow (labelled fluid leaving via this pathway requires several hours to enter the general circulation).

Fluid movement across the inner wall of Schlemm's canal

There has been considerable debate as to the route and mechanism by which aqueous passes from the trabecular to the luminal side of the endothelium of the inner wall of Schlemm's canal. For the past few decades, it has been widely held that most of the fluid transfer occurs via a pressure-dependent system of transcellular channels, rather than via intercellular pathways. These transcellular channels begin as invaginations on the trabecular (basal) side of the inner wall endothelial cell and progressively enlarge concurrent with the thinning of the cytoplasm on the luminal (apical) aspect of the cell. Eventually, the giant vacuole thus formed opens to the canal lumen, forming a through-and-through channel, with a pore opening to both sides (albeit not necessarily simultaneously). This is a dynamic intraocular pressure-dependent process which is probably not energy dependent. Transcellular channels and pores can also occur without the formation of giant vacuoles. Micropinocytosis and paracellular pathways have been thought to contribute very little to fluid movement across the inner wall. Recently, the paracellular pathway has received renewed attention, and some investigators feel that its role may have been underestimated.

Particulate sieving probably occurs in the juxtacanalicular region of the meshwork, where the flow pathways narrow progressively as the inner wall is approached from the meshwork side. This system may act as a one-way valve, permitting fluid and particulate matter to exit the anterior chamber into Schlemm's canal while preventing reflux. However, it probably provides no more than 10 to 25 per cent of the overall resistance to aqueous humour outflow. Most investigators believe that the majority of the resistance resides in the juxtacanalicular region of the meshwork. However, some feel that the continuous layer of trabecular cells comprising aqueous channels terminating in cul-de-sacs proximal to the juxtacanalicular region provides substantial resistance to flow.

Fluid movement through the entire conventional pathway obey all the laws of passive bulk flow. However, the synthetic, phagocytic, contractile, and other properties of the biologically active endothelial cells are undoubtedly crucial to the normal functioning of the system, and its response to hormones, autacoids, and drugs. The earlier concept of the trabecular meshwork/Schlemm's canal as an inert 'sieve' is clearly erroneous. Rather, this is a biologically active tissue that mediates and modulates a passive physical process. Innervation to portions of the anterior chamber angle has been known for some time, and the finding of a rich and varied peptidergic innervation has received special attention recently, but the functional roles remain unclear.

Cholinergic mechanisms

In primates the iris root inserts into the ciliary muscle and the uveal meshwork just posterior to the scleral spur; the ciliary muscle inserts at the scleral spur and the posterior inner aspect of the trabecular meshwork. These two contractile, cholinergically innervated structures effect resistance to aqueous humour outflow. Voluntary accommodation and cholinergic agonists (topical, intracameral, or systemically administered) decrease outflow resistance, whereas ganglionic blocking agents and cholinergic antagonists increase resistance. These findings suggest that iris sphincter and ciliary muscle contraction physically alter meshwork configuration so as to decrease resistance, whereas muscle relaxation deforms it so as to increase resistance. The monkey model of total iris removal and ciliary muscle disinsertion confirms that the acute resistance-decreasing action of pilocarpine is mediated entirely by drug-induced ciliary muscle contraction, with no direct pharmacological effect on the meshwork itself. In this preparation, the ciliary muscle retains its normal morphology and its contractility in response to pilocarpine, and the meshwork exhibits essentially its normal light and electron microscopic appearance. However, there is virtually no acute resistance response to either intravenous or intracameral pilocarpine, and no response to topical pilocarpine. Light and electron microscopic studies of the trabecular meshwork and Schlemm's canal demonstrate pilocarpine-induced alterations in the size and shape of the intertrabecular spaces and in various characteristics, including vacuolization, of the inner canal wall endothelium.

Outflow resistance and meshwork biology

In the primate eye, approximately 75 per cent of the resistance to aqueous humour outflow resides in the tissues between the anterior chamber and the lumen of Schlemm's canal. A small percentage of this resistance, perhaps 10 to 25 per cent, resides in the inner wall of Schlemm's canal. Most investigators believe that the primary resistance site is in the cribriform portion of the meshwork—the outermost part of the meshwork consisting of several layers of endothelial cells embedded in a ground substance composed of a wide variety of macromolecules, including hyaluronic acid, other glycosaminoglycans, collagen, fibronectin, and other glycoproteins.

The endothelial cells of the meshwork have phagocytic capabilities. It has been proposed that the meshwork is in effect a self-cleaning filter and that in most of the open angle glaucomas, the phagocytic function is deficient or at least inadequate to cope with the amount of material present. In eyes with chronic open angle glaucoma, there appears to be deposition of an as yet only partially characterized electron-dense material in the cribriform region, although the influence of the confounding variables of age, trabecular cell loss and prior medical therapy needs further assessment. Pigmentary and exfoliation glaucoma may also be examples of glaucoma caused by deposition of specific materials clogging or damaging the meshwork.

Pharmacological manipulation

Aqueous humour outflow via the conventional drainage pathway is a physical process that can be altered pharmacologically. Several classes of pharmacological agents unequivocally alter aqueous humour outflow in the primate: cholinomimetics, catecholamines, cytochalasins, chelators, α-chymotrypsin, and ethacrynic acid to name some. Some of these compounds (e.g. cytochalasins, chelators, ethacrynic acid) produce structural alterations in the chamber angle that would seem to account for their effects on outflow. Other agents may affect outflow secondarily, such as pilocarpine-induced ciliary muscle contraction. However, the complete sequence of physical events by which a drug alters aqueous humour outflow are unknown. Narrowing or collapse of Schlemm's canal may decrease outflow facility. Ciliary muscle tendons connect directly with the cribriform meshwork and inner canal wall in such a way that muscle contraction might spread the cribriform meshwork and widen the canal, whereas muscle relaxation might tend to collapse them. Such studies begin to address the real issues but do not explain conclusively the physics behind the physiology. Even with agents such as cytochalasins, which have a presumably specific subcellular action (interference with actin filament formation, and a clearly disruptive effect on the structural integrity of the outflow pathways, the precise pathophysiological sequence of events is unclear.

Further reading

Alvarado, J.A. and Murphy, C.G. (1992). Outflow obstruction in pigmentary and primary open angle glaucoma. *Archives of Ophthalmology*, **110**, 1769–78.

Alvarado, J., Murphy, C., and Juster R. (1984). Trabecular meshwork cellularity in primary open-angle glaucoma and nonglaucomatous normals. *Ophthalmology*, **91**, 564–79.

Bárány, E.H. (1978). The influence of extraocular venous pressure on outflow facility in *Cercopithecus ethiops* and *Macaca fascicularis*. *Investigative Ophthalmology and Visual Science*, **17**, 711–17.

Bárány, E. and Langham, M.E. (1955). On the origin of the ascorbic acid in the aqueous humuor of guinea pigs and rabbits. *Acta Physiologica Scandanavica*, **34**, 99–115.

Barros, F., Lipez-Briones, L.G., Coca-Prados, M., *et al.* (1991). Detection and characterization of Ca²⁺-activated K⁺ channels in transformed cells of human non-pigmented ciliary epithelium. *Current Eye Research*, **10**, 731–8.

Becker, B. (1961). The effect of hypothermia on aqueous humor dynamics. III. Turnover of ascorbate and sodium. *American Journal of Ophthalmology*, **51**, 1032–9.

Bill, A. (1966). Conventional and uveo-scleral drainage of aqueous humor in the cynomolgus monkey (*Macaca irus*) at normal and high intraocular pressures. *Experimental Eye Research*, **5**, 45–54.

Bill, A. (1968). Capillary permeability to and extravascular dynamics of myoglobin, albumin, and gammaglobulin in the uvea. *Acta Physiologica Scandanavica*, **73**, 204–19.

Bill, A. (1973). The role of ciliary body blood flow and ultrafiltration in aqueous humor formation. *Experimental Eye Research*, **16**, 287–96.

Bill, A. (1975a). Blood circulation and fluid dynamics in the eye. *Physiology Review*, **55**, 383–417.

Bill, A. (1975b). The drainage of aqueous humor (editorial). *Investigative Ophthalmology*, **14**, 1–3.

Bill, A. and Phillips, C.I. (1971). Uveoscleral drainage of aqueous humor in human eyes. *Experimental Eye Research*, **12**, 275–81.

Bill, A. and Svedbergh, B. (1972). Scanning electron microscopic studies of the trabecular meshwork and the canal of Schlemm—an attempt to localize the main resistance to outflow of aqueous humour in man. *Acta Ophthalmologica*, **50**, 295–320.

Bill, A., Lütjen-Drecoll, E., and Svedbergh, B. (1980). Effects of intracameral Na₂ EDTA and EGTA on aqueous outflow routes in the monkey eye. *Investigative Ophthalmology and Visual Science*, **19**, 492–504.

Butler, G.A.D., Chen, M., Stegman, Z., *et al.* (1992). Separation of the rabbit ciliary body epithelium cell layers in viable form and identification of distinct mechanisms of bicarbonate transport. *Investigative Ophthalmology and Visual Science*, **33**(suppl.), 1109.

Candia, O.A., Shi, X.P., and Chu, T.C. (1991). Ascorbate-stimulated active Na⁺ transport in rabbit ciliary epithelium. *Current Eye Research*, **10**, 197–203.

Caprioli, J. (1992). The ciliary epithelium and aqueous humor. In *Adler's physiology of the eye: clinical application*, (ed. W.M. Hart). Mosby, St Louis.

Carré, D.A., Tang, C.-S.R., Krupin, T., *et al.* (1992). Effect of bicarbonate on intracellular potential of rabbit ciliary epithelium. *Current Eye Research*, **11**, 609–24.

Carré, D.A., Anguita, J., Coca-Prados, M., *et al.* (1996). Cell-attached patch clamping of intact rabbit ciliary epithelium. *Current Eye Research*, **15**, 193–201.

Chu, T.C., Candia, O.A., and Iiuzka, S. (1986). Effects of forskolin, prostaglandin F₂ₐ, and Ba⁺⁺ on short-circuit of the isolated rabbit iris–ciliary body. *Current Eye Research*, **5**, 511–16.

Chu, T.C., Candia, O.A., and Podos, S.M. (1987). Electrical parameters of the isolated monkey ciliary epithelium and effects of pharmacological agents. *Investigative Ophthalmology and Visual Science*, **28**, 1644–8.

Civan, M.M., Bowler, J.M., Zellhuber-McMillan, S., *et al.* (1991). Microanalysis of rabbit ciliary epithelium. *Investigative Ophthalmology and Visual Science*, **32** (suppl.), 978.

Civan, M.M., Peterson-Yantorno, K., Coca-Prados, M., *et al.* (1992). Regulatory volume decrease by cultured nonpigmented ciliary epithelial cells. *Experimental Eye Research*, **54**, 181–91.

Civan, M.M., Coca-Prados, M., and Peterson-Yantorno, K. (1994). Pathways signaling the regulatory volume decrease of cultured nonpigmented ciliary epithelial cells. *Investigative Ophthalmology and Visual Science*, **35**, 2876–86.

Civan, M.M., Coca-Prados, M., and Peterson-Yantorno, K. (1996). Regulatory volume increase of cultured non-pigmented ciliary epithelial cells. *Experimental Eye Research*, **62**, 627–40.

Coca-Prados, M. and Kondo, K. (1985). Separation of bovine pigmented ciliary epithelial cells by density gradient and further characterization in culture. *Experimental Eye Research*, **40**, 731–9.

Cole, D.F. (1960). Effects of some metabolic inhibitors upon the formation of the aqueous humour in rabbits. *British Journal of Ophthalmology*, **44**, 739–50.

Cole, D.F. (1961a). Electrical potential across the isolated ciliary body observed *in vitro*. *British Journal of Ophthalmology*, **45**, 641–53.

Cole, D.F. (1961b). Electrochemical changes associated with the formation of the aqueous humour. *British Journal of Ophthalmology*, **45**, 202–17.

Crook, R.B., Lui, G.M., and Polansky, J.R. (1992). Thrombin stimulates inositol phosphates formation, intracellular calcium levels and DNA synthesis in cultured human non-pigmented ciliary epithelial cells. *Experimental Eye Research*, **55**, 785–95.

Delamere, N.A. and Williams, R.N. (1987). A comparative study on the uptake of ascorbic acid by the iris–ciliary body of the rabbit, guinea pig and rat. *Comparative Biochemistry and Physiology*, **88**, 847–9.

Edelman, J.L., Sachs, G., and Adorante, J.S. (1994). Ion transport asymmetry and functional coupling in bovine pigmented and nonpigmented ciliary epithelial cells. *American Journal of Physiology*, **266**, C1210–21.

Epstein, D.L. and Rohen, J.W. (1991). Morphology of the trabecular meshwork and inner wall endothelium after cationized ferritin perfusion in the monkey eye. *Investigative Ophthalmology and Visual Science*, **32**, 160–71.

Erickson-Lamy, K., Schroeder, A., and Epstein, D.L. (1992). Ethacrynic acid induces reversible shape and cytoskeletal changes in cultured cells. *Investigative Ophthalmology and Visual Science*, **33**, 2631–40.

Farahbakhsh, N.A. and Fain, G.L. (1988). Volume regulation of non-pigmented cells from ciliary epithelium. *Investigative Ophthalmology and Visual Science*, **28**, 934–44.

Farahbakhsh, N.A. and Cilluffo, M.C. (1994). Synergistic effect of adrenergic and muscarinic receptor activation on [Ca²⁺]ᵢ in rabbit ciliary body epithelium. *Journal of Physiology London*, **477**, 215–21.

Frizzell, R.A., Field, M., and Schultz, S.G. (1979). Sodium-coupled chloride transport by epithelial tissues. *American Journal of Physiology*, **236**, F1–8.

Glynn, I.M. (1993). Annual review prize lecture: all hands to the sodium pump. *Journal of Physiology London*, **462**, 1–30.

Gooch, A.J., Morgan, J., and Jacob, T.J.C. (1992). Adrenergic stimulation of bovine non-pigmented ciliary epithelial cells raises cAMP but has no effect on K⁺ or Cl⁻ currents. *Current Eye Research*, **11**, 1019–29.

Grant, W.M. (1963). Experimental aqueous perfusion in enucleated human eyes. *Archives of Ophthalmology*, **69**, 783–801.

Green, K. and Pederson, J.E. (1972). Contribution of secretion and filtration to aqueous humor formation. *American Journal of Physiology*, **222**, 1218–26.

Green, K., Bountra, C., Georgiou, P., *et al.* (1985). An electrophysiologic study of rabbit ciliary epithelium. *Investigative Ophthalmology and Visual Science*, **26**, 371–81.

Grierson, I. and Johnson, N.F. (1981). The post-mortem vacuoles of Schlemm's canal. *Albrecht von Graefes Archiv für Klinische und Experimentelle Ophthalmologie*, **215**, 249–64.

Grierson, I. and Lee, W.R. (1973). Erythrocyte phagocytosis in the human trabecular meshwork. *British Journal of Ophthalmology*, **57**, 400–15.

Helbig, H., Korbmacher, C., and Wiederholt, M. (1987). K^+-conductance and electrogenic Na^+/K^+ transport of cultured bovine pigmented ciliary epithelium. *Journal of Membrane Biology*, **99**, 173–86.

Helbig, H., Korbmacher, C., Berweck, S., *et al.* (1988). Kinetic properties of Na^+/H^+ exchange in cultured pigmented ciliary epithelial cells. *Pflügers Archiv*, **412**, 80–5.

Helbig, H., Korbmacher, C., Wohlfarth, J., *et al.* (1989a). Effect of acetylcholine on membrane potential of cultured human nonpigmented ciliary epithelial cells. *Investigative Ophthalmology and Visual Science*, **30**, 890–6.

Helbig, H., Korbmacher, C., Wohlfarth, J., *et al.* (1989b). Electrogenic Na^+-ascorbate cotransport in cultured bovine pigmented ciliary epithelial cells. *American Journal of Physiology*, **256**, C44–9.

Helbig, H., Korbmacher, C., Stumpff, F., *et al.* (1989c). Role of HCO_3^- in regulation of cytoplasmic pH in ciliary epithelial cells. *American Journal of Physiology (Cell Physiology)*, **257**, C696–705.

Holmberg, A. and Bárány, E.H. (1966). The effect of pilocarpine on the endothelium forming the inner wall of Schlemm's canal: an electron microscopic study in the monkey *Cercopithecus aethiops*. *Investigative Ophthalmology*, **5**, 53–8.

Jacob, T.J.C. (1991a). Identification of a low-threshold T-type calcium channel in bovine ciliary epithelial cells. *American Journal of Physiology*, **261**, C808–13.

Jacob, T.J.C. (1991b). Two outward K^+ currents in bovine pigmented ciliary epithelial cells; $I_{K(Ca)}$ and $I_{K(V)}$. *American Journal of Physiology (Cell Physiology)*, **261**, C1055–62.

Jacob, T.J.C. and Civan, M.M. (1996). Role of ion channels in aqueous humor formation. *American Journal of Physiology (Cell Physiology)*, **271**, C703–20.

Kaufman, P.L. and Bárány, E.H. (1976a). Loss of acute pilocarpine effect on outflow facility following surgical disinsertion and retrodisplacement of the ciliary muscle from the scleral spur in the cynomolgus monkey. *Investigative Ophthalmology and Visual Science*, **15**, 793–807.

Kaufman, P.L. and Bárány, E.H. (1976b). Residual pilocarpine effects on outflow facility after ciliary muscle disinsertion in the cynomolgus monkey. *Investigative Ophthalmology and Visual Science*, **15**, 558–61.

Kaufman, P.L. and Bárány, E.H. (1977). Cytochalasin B reversibly increases outflow facility in the eye of the cynomolgus monkey. *Investigative Ophthalmology and Visual Science*, **16**, 47–53.

Kaufman, P.L. and Crawford, K. (1989). Aqueous humor dynamics: how PGF2α lowers intraocular pressure. *Progress in Clinical Biology Research*, **312**, 387–416.

Kaufman, P.L., Bill, A., and Bárány, E.H. (1977). Formation and drainage of aqueous humor following total iris removal and ciliary muscle disinsertion in the cynomolgus monkey. *Investigative Ophthalmology and Visual Science*, **16**, 226–9.

Kishida, K., Miwa, Y., and Iwata, C. (1986). 2-Substituted 1,3,4-thiadiazole-5-sulfonamides as carbonic anhydrase inhibitors. Their effects on the transepithelial potential difference of the isolated rabbit ciliary body and on the intraocular pressure of the living rabbit eye. *Experimental Eye Research*, **43**, 981–95.

Krupin, T. and Civan, M.M. (1996). Physiologic basis of aqueous humor formation. In *The glaucomas*, (ed. R. Ritch, M.B. Shields, and T. Krupin). Mosby-Year Book, St Louis.

Krupin, T., Reinach, P.S., Candia, O.A., *et al.* (1984). Transepithelial electrical measurements on the isolated rabbit iris–ciliary body. *Experimental Eye Research*, **38**, 115–23.

Krupin, T., Wax, M.B., Carré, D.A., *et al.* (1991). Effects of adrenergic agents on transepithelial electrical measurements across the isolated iris–ciliary body. *Experimental Eye Research*, **53**, 709–16.

Lütjen-Drecoll, E., Kaufman, P.L., and Bárány, E.H. (1977). Light and electron microscopy of the anterior chamber angle structures following surgical disinsertion of the ciliary muscle in the cynomolgus monkey. *Investigative Ophthalmology and Visual Science*, **16**, 218–25.

Lütjen-Drecoll, E., Futa, R., and Rohen, J.W. (1981). Ultrahistochemical stud-

ies on tangential sections of the trabecular meshwork in normal and glaucomatous eyes. *Investigative Ophthalmology and Visual Science*, **21**, 563–73.

Mitchell, C.H, and Jacob, T.J.C. (1994). Two maxi-conductance channel types in bovine pigmented ciliary epithelial cells. *Investigative Ophthalmology and Visual Science*, **35** (suppl.), 1455.

Moses, R.A., Grodzki, W.J. Jr, Etheridge, E.L., *et al.* (1981). Schlemm's canal: the effect of intraocular pressure. *Investigative Ophthalmology and Visual Science*, **20**, 61–8.

Oh, J., Krupin, T., Tang, L.-Q, *et al.* (1994). Dye coupling of rabbit ciliary epithelial cells *in vitro*. *Investigative Ophthalmology and Visual Science*, **35**, 2509–14.

Pederson, J.E. (1982). Fluid permeability of monkey ciliary epithelium *in vivo*. *Investigative Ophthalmology and Visual Science*, **23**, 176–80.

Pederson, J.E. and Green, K. (1973). Aqueous humor dynamics: experimental studies. *Experimental Eye Research*, **15**, 277–97.

Raviola, G. (1974). Effects of paracentesis on the blood–aqueous barrier: an electron microscope study on *Macaca mulatta* using horseradish peroxidase as a tracer. *Investigative Ophthalmology*, **13**, 828–58.

Raviola, G. and Raviola, E. (1978). Intercellular junctions in the ciliary epithelium. *Investigative Ophthalmology and Visual Science*, **17**, 958–81.

Reiss, G.R., Lee, D.A., Topper, J.E., *et al.* (1984). Aqueous humor flow during sleep. *Investigative Ophthalmology and Visual Science*, **25**, 776–8.

Rohen, J.W., Futa, R., and Lütjen-Drecoll, E. (1981). The fine structure of the cribriform meshwork in normal and glaucomatous eyes as seen in tangential sections. *Investigative Ophthalmology and Visual Science*, **21**, 574–85.

Sears, M.L., Yamada, E., Cummins, D., *et al.* (1991). The isolated ciliary bilayer is useful for studies of aqueous humor formation. *Transactions of the American Ophthalmology Society*, **89**, 131–52.

Stelling, J.W. and Jacob, T.M.C. (1992). The inward rectifier K^- current underlies oscillatory membrane potential behaviour in bovine pigmented ciliary epithelial cells. *Journal of Physiology London*, **458**, 439–56.

Tang, L.Q., Krupin, T., Milner, M., *et al.* (1991). Halogenated inhalation anesthetic agents decrease transepithelial electrical measurements across the isolated iris–ciliary body. *Investigative Ophthalmology and Visual Science*, **32**, 1912–15.

Toris, C.B. and Pederson, J.E. (1985). Effect of intraocular pressure on uveoscleral outflow following cyclodialysis in the monkey eye. *Investigative Ophthalmology and Visual Science*, **26**, 1745–9.

Tripathi, R.C. (1977). The functional morphology of the outflow systems of ocular and cerebrospinal fluids. *Experimental Eye Research*, **25** (suppl.), 65–116.

Ussing, H.H. and Zerahn, K. (1951). Active transport of sodium as the source of electric current in the short-circuited isolated frog skin. *Acta Physiologica Scandanavica*, **23**, 110–27.

Watanabe, T. and Saito, Y. (1978). Characteristics of ion transport across the isolated ciliary epithelium of the toad as studied by electrical measurements. *Experimental Eye Research*, **27**, 215–26.

Wiederholt, M. and Zadunaisky, J.A. (1986). Membrane potentials and intracellular chloride activity in the ciliary body of the shark. *Pflügers Archiv*, **407**, S112–15.

Wiederholt, M., Flügel, C., Lütjen-Drecoll, E., *et al.* (1989). Mechanically stripped pigmented and non-pigmented epithelium of the shark ciliary body: morphology and transepithelial electrical properties. *Experimental Eye Research*, **49**, 1031–43.

Wiederholt, M., Helbig, H., and Korbmacher, C. (1991). Ion transport across the ciliary epithelium: lessons from cultured cell and proposed role of the carbonic anhydrase. In *Carbonic anhydrase*, (ed. F. Botré, G. Gross, and B.T. Storey). VCH Verlagsgesellschaft, Weinheim, Germany.

Wolosin, J.M., Bonanno, J.A., Hanzel, D., *et al.* (1991). Bicarbonate transport mechanisms in rabbit ciliary body epithelium. *Experimental Eye Research*, **52**, 397–407.

Yantorno, R.E., Coca-Prados, M., Krupin, T., *et al.* (1989). Volume regulation of cultured, transformed, nonpigmented cells from human ciliary body. *Experimental Eye Research*, **49**, 423–37.

Yantorno, R.E., Carré, D.A., Coca-Prados, M., *et al.* (1992). Whole-cell patch clamping of ciliary epithelial cells during anisosmotic swelling. *American Journal of Physiology*, **262**, C501–9.

2.10.2 Anatomy and circulation of the anterior optic nerve

George A. Cioffi

The anterior optic nerve has been examined and its vasculature detailed by a variety of observers. Despite this intensive scrutiny, the exact anatomy of the optic nerve microvasculature has remained a point of controversy. This chapter details the basic anatomy of the anterior optic nerve and its microcirculation.

General anatomy of the anterior optic nerve

The anterior optic nerve extends from the superficial retinal surface of the optic disc to the retrobulbar space where the nerve exits the globe. The anterior optic nerve is composed of the axonal elements of the retinal ganglion cells, neural glial tissue, blood vessels, and connective tissue. Each optic nerve contains approximately 1.2 million axons. At the superficial retinal level of the optic nerve, axons of the retinal nerve fibre layer comprise approximately 90 per cent of the nerve tissue volume. The ganglion cell bodies are located in the innermost nuclear layer of the retina away from the nerve head. Single axons arise from each retinal ganglion cell and are grouped into fibre bundles to compose the nerve fibre layer of the retina. At the optic nerve head, the axons of the retinal nerve fibre layer turn to exit the eye. Axons from the nasal retina travel directly to the nerve and enter along the nasal margin of the optic disc. Axons within the papillomacular bundle transit directly from the macula to the temporal margin of the optic disc. Fibres of the temporal retina arch around the foveal area to enter the superior and inferior poles of the temporal optic nerve.

The anterior portion of the optic nerve may be divided into four regions: the superficial nerve fibre layer, the prelaminar region, the laminar region, and the retrolaminar region (Fig. 1). The superficial nerve fibre layer is the portion of the optic nerve anterior to an imaginary plane extending across the optic nerve from the peripapillary Bruch's membrane, and is primarily composed of axons extending from the retinal ganglion cells. Immediately posterior to the superficial nerve fibre layer is the prelaminar region, which lies adjacent to the peripapillary choroid. The prelaminar region is distinguished by hypercellular glial septae with minimal connective tissue. The laminar region is characterized by a gradual transition from glial columns to dense connective tissue plates. The laminar cribrosa is continuous with the peripapillary sclera but is fenestrated, allowing transit of the neural fibres. Each plate of laminar tissue has approximately 300 to 600 perforations. The laminar plates are composed of fibroblasts, collagen, ground substance, glycos-

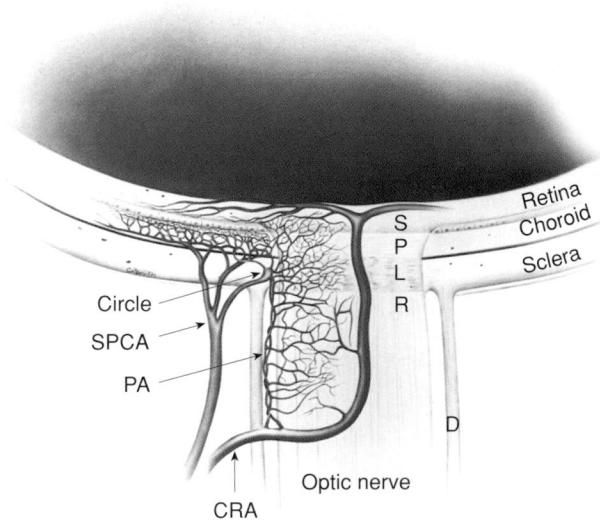

Fig. 1 Arterial supply of the anterior optic nerve. The anterior optic nerve (ON) is divided into four regions: the superficial nerve fibre layer (S), the prelaminar region (P), the laminar region (L), and the retrolaminar region (R). The anterior optic nerve is principally supplied by the short posterior ciliary arteries (SPCA), with some contribution from the central retinal artery (CRA). Circle of Zinn-Haller (circle), pial arteries (PA), dura mater (D). (Modified from Cioffi and Van Buskirk 1995.)

aminoglycans, and basement membranes. Posterior to the laminar region is the retrolaminar region, which is marked by the beginning of the meningeal sheaths, myelinated axons, and delicate connective tissue septae. The myelin sheaths enlarge the optic nerve to approximately 3 mm as it exits the globe.

The neural glial cells of the anterior optic nerve are primarily astrocytes, while in the retrobulbar optic nerve, oligodendrocytes and microglia are more prevalent. An astrocytic network surrounds the fascicles of the nerve axons and is continuous from the retinal edge, posteriorly to the laminar cribrosa and the retrobulbar optic nerve.

General vasculature of the orbit

The orbital contents receive their vascular supply from several arteries, including the ophthalmic artery, the meningolacrimal artery (a branch from the middle meningeal artery), and palpebral arteries which branch from the facial artery. The middle meningeal artery and the facial artery belong to the external carotid arterial system. The ophthalmic artery provides most of the blood supply to the eye and is the first branch of the internal carotid artery, arising as the internal carotid artery turns to pierce the dura and emerge from the cavernous sinus. The vascular supply to the intraorbital optic nerve, retina, and choroid arises predominantly from the ophthalmic arterial circulation via the posterior ciliary arteries, the central retinal artery, and the pial vascular network along the optic nerve (see Fig. 1). The ophthalmic artery exits the intracranial cavity through the optic canal and, in most individuals, lies inferolateral to the optic nerve. The ophthalmic artery has several intraorbital collateral vessels from the external carotid artery system, the most significant of which are the lacrimal and the ethmoidal anastomoses. The ocular branches of the ophthalmic artery are the central retinal artery and one to five posterior ciliary arterial trunks. These trunks branch into the main posterior ciliary arteries. Most individuals have two to three posterior ciliary trunks which supply the medial and lateral posterior ciliary arteries. Each main posterior ciliary artery further divides into several short posterior ciliary arteries, just before or after entering the sclera (see Fig. 1). In addition, a medial and the lateral long posterior ciliary arteries arise from the ciliary trunks, travel anteriorly along the outside of the globe, before penetrating the sclera at the horizontal meridian of the globe. The long posterior ciliary arteries supply the iris, ciliary body, and the anterior region of the choroid.

The short posterior ciliary arteries course anteriorly after branching from the main posterior ciliary arteries and pierce the sclera immediately adjacent to the optic nerve, predominantly in the nasal and temporal region. Occasionally, short posterior ciliary arteries may have extrascleral anastomosis. The short posterior ciliary arteries supply the posterior choroid, as well as the majority of the anterior optic nerve. The size and shape of the area of the choroid and optic nerve supplied by each short posterior ciliary artery is variable among subjects and even between the eyes of a single individual. Some short posterior ciliary arteries course, without branching, through the sclera directly into the choroid; others divide within the sclera to provide branches to both the choroid and the anterior optic nerve. Often the medial and lateral short posterior ciliary arteries anastomose and form an elliptical circle around the optic nerve, the arterial circle of Zinn-Haller. Branches derived from the circle of Zinn-Haller include recurrent pial branches, choroidal branches, and branches penetrating the optic nerve. This arterial circle is usually intrascleral, but occasionally an incomplete extrascleral arterial network is present. Human intravascular corrosion castings have demonstrated that the anastomoses between the lateral and medial short posterior ciliary arteries form a complete elliptical circle around the optic nerve in 77 per cent of the eyes, but that 43 per cent of these eyes have narrowed segments along the interarterial anastomoses.

The venous drainage of the orbit generally does not follow the arterial supply. The orbital veins, in common with those of the head and neck, contain no valves. The largest of the orbital veins is the superior ophthalmic vein, which accommodates the majority of the orbital venous effluent. The venous drainage of the retina and the anterior optic nerve is almost exclusively via the central retinal vein and its tributaries, which subsequently empties into the superior ophthalmic vein (Fig. 2). The choroid is drained through the vortex venous system which empties into the superior and inferior ophthalmic veins. It is often difficult to identify an inferior ophthalmic vein independent from the superior ophthalmic vein. Numerous anastomoses are generally present between the superior and inferior ophthalmic veins. Both vessels drain into the cavernous sinus. However,

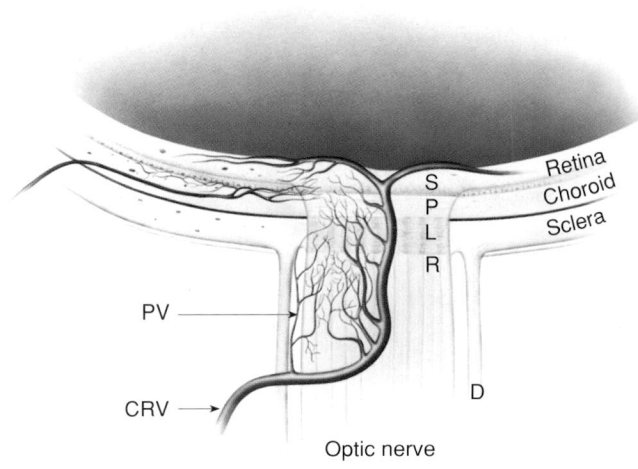

Fig.2 Venous drainage of the anterior optic nerve. The vasculature of the anterior optic nerve (ON) is drained almost exclusively via the central retinal vein (CRV). Superficial nerve fibre layer (S), the prelaminar region (P), the laminar region (L), and the retrolaminar region (R), pial veins (PV), dura mater (D). (Modified from Cioffi and Van Buskirk 1995.)

the inferior ophthalmic vein occasionally drains into the pterygoid plexus through the inferior orbital tissue.

Microvasculature of the anterior optic nerve

The vasculature of the anterior optic nerve varies depending on the region (see Fig. 1). The superficial nerve fibre layer is supplied principally from the arterioles in the adjacent retina. Most of these vessels are capillaries originating in the peripapillary nerve fibre layer. These vessels, as with all capillary beds within the optic nerve, are not fenestrated and the tight junctions between their endothelial cells constitute the blood–ocular barrier. The temporal nerve fibre layer may have an additional arterial contribution from the cilioretinal artery. No direct choroidal contribution is observed in the superficial nerve fibre layer region.

The prelaminar region receives its arterial supply via direct branches of the short posterior ciliary arteries and via vessels originating from the arterial circle of Haller. As detailed above, the posterior ciliary arterial system provides input to both the choroid and the arterial circle of Haller. The origin of the blood supply to the prelaminar region of the anterior optic nerve has evoked controversy. Studies have suggested the presence of a choroidal arterial contribution to the prelaminar and laminar anterior optic nerve. Indeed, fluorescein angiography demonstrates the appearance of fluorescein in these deeper regions of the anterior optic nerve concomitantly with the filling of the choroidal vasculature. This suggests that both the anterior optic nerve and the choroid share a common arterial input. However, further investigations have demonstrated minimal anatomical vascular connections between the peripapillary choroid and anterior optic nerve. Branches from the short posterior ciliary arteries may actually course through the choroid and supply the prelaminar region. These vessels do not actually arise from the choroid, but merely transit through, to directly supply the optic nerve. The direct arterial supply to the prelaminar region arising from the choroidal vasculature is minimal. Therefore, the simultaneous filling of the optic nerve vasculature and the peripapillary choroid with fluorescein angiography appears to be related to their common posterior ciliary arterial supply.

The arterial supply to the laminar region is similar to the supply of the prelaminar region. The short posterior ciliary arteries, either directly or via the arterial circle of Haller, provide the principal arterial input to the laminar region of the optic nerve. As in the prelaminar region, the peripapillary choroid may contribute occasional small arterioles to the laminar region. The precapillary vessels perforate the outer aspect of the lamina cribrosa before branching into an intraseptal capillary network. Most of the blood supply to the retrolaminar portion of the optic nerve occurs through numerous perforating vessels from the pia mater. These pial vessels obtain their supply either directly from the ophthalmic artery or indirectly from recurrent branches from the posterior ciliary arteries. The central retinal artery contributes occasional small branches within the retrolaminar optic nerve. The central retinal artery may also provide small branches to the retrobulbar optic nerve. Some investigators have described 'central optic nerve artery equivalents', which are pial-derived longitudinal arterioles in the retrolaminar nerve.

The rich capillary beds of the peripapillary retina, the anterior optic nerve, and the retrobulbar optic nerve are anatomically confluent and form a continuous vascular network along the anterior optic nerve. These capillary interconnections unite the microvasculature along the length of the anterior optic nerve. There is a subtle transition in the organization of the capillaries between the prelaminar and laminar regions. The capillaries of the prelaminar region are complex and randomly arranged, while the capillaries of the laminar region conform to the pattern of the connective tissue septae which compose the supportive architecture of the lamina cribrosa. The presence of this longitudinal anastomosis of capillaries might be viewed as a protective mechanism against regional ischaemic insult, but the functional importance of these potential collaterals is not known. Flow resistance may be so high in these fine capillaries that it limits potential collateral flow.

The venous drainage of the anterior optic nerve is almost exclusively via the central retinal vein (see Fig. 2). In the nerve fibre layer, blood is drained by small veins that converge and empty, ultimately, into the central retinal vein. In the prelaminar, laminar and retrolaminar regions, venous drainage also occurs via the central retinal vein or centripetal tributaries to the central retinal vein. Occasionally, small venules connecting the optic nerve and the peripapillary choroid can be identified, mainly within the prelaminar region. In the peripheral aspects of the laminar and retrolaminar regions, some optic nerve venous drainage occurs via pial veins, but these pial veins ulti-

mately drain into the central retinal vein as it exits the optic nerve.

Further reading

Anderson, D.R. and Braverman, S. (1976). Re-evaluation of the optic disc vasculature. *American Journal of Ophthalmology*, **82**, 165–74.

Cioffi, G.A. and Van Buskirk, E.M. (1994). Microvasculature of the anterior optic nerve. *Survey of Ophthalmology*, **38** (suppl), S107–17.

Cioffi, G.A. and Van Buskirk, E.M. (1995). Vasculature of the anterior optic nerve and peripapillary choroid. In *The glaucomas*, (2nd edn) (ed. R. Ritch, M.B. Shields, and T. Krupin), pp. 177–88. Mosby, St Louis.

Harris, A., Shoemaker, J.A., and Cioffi, G.A. (1998). Assessment of human ocular hemodynamics. *Survey of Ophthalmology*, in press.

Hayreh, S.S. (1978). Structure and blood supply of the optic nerve. In *Glaucoma: conceptions of a disease: pathogenesis, diagnosis, therapy* (ed. K. Heilman and K.T. Richardson), pp. 78–96. George Thieme, Stuttgart.

Hayreh, S.S. (1989). Blood supply of the optic nerve head in health and disease. In *Ocular blood flow in glaucoma: means, methods and measurements* (ed. G.N. Lambrou and E.L. Greve), pp. 3–48. Kugler and Ghedini, Amsterdam; Berkeley.

Lieberman, M.F., Maumenee, A.E., and Green, W.R. (1976). Histologic studies of the vasculature of the anterior optic nerve. *American Journal of Ophthalmology*, **82**, 405–23.

Olver, J.M., Spalton, D.J., and McCartney A.C.E. (1990). Microvascular study of the retrolaminar optic nerve in man: the possible significance in anterior ischemic optic neuropathy. *Eye*, **4** (part 1), 7–24.

Onda, E., Cioffi, G.A., Bacon, D.R., and Van Buskirk, E.M. (1995). Microvasculature of the human optic nerve. *American Journal of Ophthalmology*, 92–102.

Orgul, S. and Cioffi, M.D. (1996). Embryology, anatomy, and histology of the optic nerve vasculature. *Journal of Glaucoma*, **5**, 285–94.

Orgul, S., Meyer, P., and Cioffi, G.A. (1995). Physiology of blood flow regulation and mechanisms involved in optic nerve perfusion. *Journal of Glaucoma*, **4**, 427–43.

Quigley, H.A. and Addicks, E.M. (1981). Regional differences in the structure of the lamina cribrosa and their reaction to glaucomatous nerve damage. *Archives of Ophthalmology*, **99**, 137-43.

Quigley, H.A. and Green, W.R. (1979). The histology of human glaucoma cupping and optic nerve damage: clinicopathologic correlation in 21 eyes. *Ophthalmology*, **86**, 1803–30.

Varma, R. and Minckler, D.S. (1995). Anatomy and pathophysiology of the retina and optic nerve. In *The glaucomas*, (2nd edn) (ed. R. Ritch, M.B. Shields, and T. Krupin), pp. 139–76. Mosby, St Louis.

2.10.3 Glaucoma definition and classification

Robert N. Weinreb and Alfonso Anton-Lopez

Definition

Glaucoma is a progressive optic neuropathy with characteristic structural changes in the optic nerve head and functional changes in the visual field. It has diverse aetiologies, including

Table 1 Structural characteristics of glaucomatous optic neuropathy

Specific	Suspicious	Non-specific
Progressive excavation of cup	Large optic cup (C/D ≥ 0.7)	Peripapillary atrophy
Progressive local retinal nerve fibre layer change in superior and/or interior arcuate bundles	Asymmetry of C/D (difference > 0.2)	Exposed lamina cribosa
Notching/localized thinning of the rim	Vertical C/D > horizontal C/D (vertical ovalization)	Nasal displacement of vessels
Development of an acquired pit	Splinter haemorrhage Retinal nerve fibre layer defects (localized and/or diffuse) Regional pallor	Baring of circumlinear vessels

C/D, cup to disc ratio.

those which are idiopathic. Previously, the causative role of high intraocular pressure was emphasized widely. More recently, it has been recognized that intraocular pressure is merely a risk factor, albeit an important one. Hence, glaucomatous optic neuropathy can be defined as a final common pathway for a group of conditions which share common biological properties and clinical characteristics.

Biological definition

According to our current understanding, glaucomatous optic neuropathy results from specific pathophysiological changes in retinal ganglion cell axons, also known as optic nerve fibres. Although our knowledge about what damages axons and specifically how they are injured in glaucoma is still incomplete, there are some biological properties which most likely are shared by all forms of glaucoma. These changes are the consequence of a multifaceted and complex biological process which has not been elucidated fully.

Characteristic morphological and physiological changes in the glaucomatous optic nerve are thought to originate at the level of the lamina cribrosa. There is compression and posterior displacement of this lamina and selective loss of retinal ganglion cells. Physiological studies in cats and monkeys with experimentally induced ocular hypertension have demonstrated blockade of both orthograde and retrograde transport in retinal ganglion cells at the lamina cribrosa. In monkey eyes with experimentally induced ocular hypertension and a glaucoma-like condition, there are intra-axonal collections of vesicles and mitochondria, and disorganization of microtubules and neurofilaments adjacent to the level of the posterior lamina cribrosa. In postmortem human eyes with primary open angle glaucoma, similar ultrastructural changes in optic nerve fibres have been observed which are consistent with the experimental change in these monkeys.

Whether glaucomatous optic neuropathy can result from only an intraocular pressure which is sufficiently high is not known. In some cases, it is likely that an impaired microcirculation either separately or in combination with intraocular

pressure, or some other pathophysiological mechanism, may also contribute. Regardless of the cause, a cascade of specific events—compression and posterior displacement of the lamina cribrosa, retinal ganglion cell axonal transport disruption at the lamina cribrosa, and subsequent selective degeneration of the optic nerve fibres—leads to glaucomatous optic nerve damage. This cascade is what appears to distinguish glaucomatous optic neuropathy from other optic neuropathies at the cellular level.

These events may have diverse consequences for retinal ganglion cell physiology and may lead to cell death. For example, there is evidence that axonal transport stasis may block the delivery to the cell body of the retinal ganglion cell of essential target-derived (from lateral geniculate body) neurotrophic growth factors. This may damage the cell, either directly or indirectly, and cause cell death by apoptosis. An enhanced understanding of the cellular and molecular events which occur during the pathological process which culminates in glaucomatous optic neuropathy will most certainly evolve over the next

Table 2 Visual field changes in glaucomatous optic nueropathy

Specific	Non-specific
Arcuate scotoma (cluster of three or more adjacent defects of ≥ 5dB or two adjacent defects > 10 dB within paracentral arcuate region)	Generalized loss of sensitivity
Nasal step	Blind spot enlargement
Central and/or temporal island	Visual field indexes (MD, PSD, CPSD, SF) outside of 95% values of age-matched normals
Glaucoma hemifield test outside of 95% values of age-matched normals	

CPSD, corrected pattern standard deviation; MD, mean deviation; PSD, pattern standard deviation; SF, short-term fluctuation.

decade, and will provide a more definitive biological basis for defining glaucoma.

Clinical definition

From a clinical perspective, glaucoma is a progressive optic neuropathy with characteristic structural damage and a specific type of visual field loss.

Structural changes

With retinal ganglion cell death and nerve fibre loss in glaucoma, particular structural changes in the appearance of the optic nerve head and retinal nerve fibre layer are observed. The optic nerve head becomes progressively excavated and there is concomitant loss of the retinal nerve fibre layer in local and/or diffuse patterns. Although progressive excavation is the charac-

---

Table 3 Classification of glaucoma based on aetiology and pathogenic mechanism

Primary glaucomas

Open angle
Childhood glaucoma (first two decades of life)
Adult (primary open angle glaucoma)

Closed angle glaucoma
With pupillary block
   acute
   subacute
   chronic
Without pupillary block (plateau iris)

Combined mechanism glaucoma

Secondary glaucomas

Childhood
Secondary or associated with ocular abnormalities
   Anterior segment dysgeneses (Axenfeld's anomaly, Rieger's syndrome, Peters' anomaly)
   sclerocornea
   microcoria
   microcornea
   microphthalmos
   megalocornea
   cornea plana
   congenital corneal staphyloma
   aniridia (AD)
   lens anomalies (dislocation, microspherophakia)
   angle closure glaucoma secondary to posterior segment lesions (retinoblastoma, retrolental fibroplasia, persistent hyperplastic primary vitreous)
   trauma
   corticosteroid-induced glaucoma
   iritis
   following surgery for congenital cataract (early onset angle closure glaucoma, late developing open angle glaucoma)
Associated with systemic abnormalities
   chromosomal disorders (Down's syndrome or trisomy 21, Patau's syndrome or trisomy D, Edward's syndrome or trisomy 18, Turner's syndrome (XO/XX))
   others (Sturge–Weber syndrome, neurofibromatosis (AD), Marfan's syndrome (AD), homocystinuria (AR), Weill–Marchesani syndrome, Lowe's syndrome (oculocerebral syndrome, X-linked recessive), Stickler's syndrome (hereditary progressive arthro-ophthalmopathy, AR), Zellweger's syndrome (cerebrohepatorenal syndrome, AR), Hallermann–Streiff syndrome (dysencephalic mandibulo-oculofacial syndrome), Rubinstein–Taybi syndrome (broad-thumb syndrome), oculodentodigital dysplasia (AD), Prader–Willi syndrome, Cockayne's syndrome (AR), maternal rubella syndrome, fetal alcohol syndrome and other rare syndromes and associations (e.g. mucopolysaccharidoses))

Adult
Pigmentary
Exfoliative
Inflammatory
(a) open angle glaucoma
   • iridocyclitis (acute anterior, associated to immune systemic arthropathies, pars planitis, glaucomatocyclitic crisis, Fuchs' heterochromic iridocyclitis)
   • choroiditis and retinitis (Vogt–Koyanagi–Harada syndrome, sympathetic ophthalmia, cytomegalovirus retinitis, toxocariasis)
   • keratitis (herpes simplex, herpes zoster)
   • scleritis
(b) angle closure glaucoma
   • pupillary block
   • peripheral anterior syneciae
Steroid-induced
Traumatic
(a) Open angle glaucoma
   • early onset (direct injury, hyphaemia)
   • late onset (angle recession glaucoma)
(b) Closed angle glaucoma
   • posterior and/or anterior synechiae
Lens-induced
(a) open angle glaucoma
   • phacolytic
   • lens particle
   • phacoanaphylaxis
(b) closed angle glaucoma
   • phacomorphic
   • microspherophakia
Following ocular surgery
(a) Glaucoma
   • aqueous misdirection (also may be spontaneous)
   • choroidal hemorrhage
(b) Cataract
   • open angle (aphakic glaucoma, epithelial ingrowth)
   • closed angle (anterior/posterior synechiae, pupillary block (vitreous)
(c) Vitreoretinal
   • scleral buckling
   • vitrectomy (silicone oil)
(d) Penetrating keratoplasty
(e) Panretinal photocoagulation
Elevated episcleral venous pressure
   carotid–venous fistula
   superior vena cava syndrome
   Sturge–Weber syndrome
Neovascular
Intraocular tumours
Ghost cell glaucoma (also following trauma)

AD, autosomal dominant; AR, autosomal recessive.

teristic change noted in the glaucomatous optic nerve head, other changes may be suspicious including asymmetric cup to disc ratio, notching, vertical ovalization of the cup, splinter haemorrhage, and regional pallor. Progressive retinal nerve fibre layer changes can be observed concomitantly with changes in the optic nerve head (Table 1). Lack of a practical clinical means for objectively and quantitatively studying the optic nerve head and retinal nerve fibre layer has impeded more definitive classification. Occasionally non-glaucomatous optic neuropathies are diagnosed incorrectly as glaucomatous. Unlike other optic neuropathies, the glaucomatous optic nerve head is excavated and the excavation typically exceeds the extent of pallor.

Functional changes

Glaucoma affects several aspects of visual function. The best known functional consequence of glaucoma is the progressive deterioration of visual field which usually begins in the midperiphery, often in the superior field, and may progress in a centripetal manner to a central or temporal island of vision or even to light perception. These localized characteristic visual field defects (Table 2) correspond topographically to retinal nerve fibre loss. Other functional changes in glaucoma include loss of colour sensitivity, especially for short-wavelength (blue) light. Testing for loss of sensitivity of blue light with short wavelength automated perimetry has been demonstrated to be more sensitive for diagnosing and monitoring glaucomatous field loss than standard achromatic perimetry. Furthermore, it is the only diagnostic test to be validated in longitudinal and multicentred investigations. Loss of other visual functions including spatial resolution, motion detection, and temporal contrast sensitivity have also been noted in glaucoma. Although many of these changes have been observed to occur years before abnormalities in standard perimetry are noted, these tests have not been widely used in clinical practice. Ongoing studies should help to define specific characteristics of glaucomatous visual function loss.

Classification

Glaucoma has been classified in numerous ways. These include those based on age of onset (childhood versus adult) and aetiology (primary versus secondary). Some are based on the status of the trabecular meshwork, the major outflow pathway, including the configuration of anterior chamber angle (open versus closed angle) or the specific site of outflow blockade (internal versus external). Others consider the appearance of the optic nerve head (e.g. focal, diffuse, acquired pit, or senile sclerosis). Still others are related to the underlying pathophysiological mechanism (intraocular pressure-dependent versus intraocular pressure-independent) or intraocular pressure (high tension versus normal tension). These latter classification schemes have been vigorously debated in an attempt to discern whether glaucoma is related to a mechanical and/or vascular problem.

During the 1990s, the inheritance pattern of some types of glaucoma has been established and the locus for the responsible gene has been identified. Several pedigrees of an autosomal

dominant inherited juvenile glaucoma have been reported and analysis has shown significant linkage to loci q21–q31 of chromosome 1. This is a different disease-causing mutation than the one associated with the Rieger's syndrome locus on q25 of chromosome 4 which is also inherited with an autosomal dominant pattern. Autosomal dominant posterior polymorphous dystrophy, which leads to glaucoma in 40 per cent of affected individuals, has been linked with the long arm of chromosome 20. Based on these pioneering molecular genetic studies, it may be reasonable to classify some glaucomas in a group according to their mendelian inheritance as autosomal dominant, autosomal recessive, or X-linked recessive. The inheritance of primary open angle glaucoma is more complex; it may be autosomal recessive, perhaps polygenic and probably multifactorial. The latter could be included with other glaucomas, such as primary angle closure glaucoma and primary congenital glaucoma, in another group of polygenic and multifactorial inherited glaucomas. A third group of glaucomas could include those without apparent genetic influence (e.g. traumatic, postsurgical, inflammatory, lens-induced, and neovascular glaucoma). In the future, perhaps a molecular genetic approach to glaucoma diagnosis will allow a better understanding and more satisfying classification of glaucomas.

Given our current stage of knowledge, it appears that no single classification scheme is comprehensive. Table 3 provides a classification based on aetiology and pathogenic mechanism. Primary glaucomas are considered as those without any known underlying aetiology. In contrast, each secondary glaucoma has a known underlying aetiology. Open angle refers to the visible trabecular meshwork which can be observed throughout 360°. In this case, outflow resistance is increased largely within the trabecular meshwork, but proximal to the Schlemm's canal. In closed angle glaucoma, the trabecular meshwork cannot be fully visualized and is obstructed, most often by the iris. Combined mechanism glaucoma includes those eyes in which the outflow resistance is increased both within the trabecular meshwork and proximal to it.

Further reading

Baez, K.A., McNaught, A.I., Dowler, J.G., Poinoosawmy, D., Fitzke, F.W., and Hitchings, R.A. (1995). Motion detection threshold and field progression in normal tension glaucoma. *British Journal of Ophthalmology*, **79**, 125–8.

Fechtner, R.D. and Weinreb, R.N. (1994). Mechanisms of optic nerve damage in primary open angle glaucoma. *Survey of Ophthalmology*, **39**, 23–42.

Heon, E., Mathers, W.D., Alward, W.L., *et al.* (1995). Linkage of posterior polymorphous corneal dystrophy to 20q11. *Human Molecular Genetics*, **4**, 485–8.

Johnson, C.A., Adams, A.J., Casson, E.J., and Brandt, J.D. (1993a). Blue-on-yellow perimetry can predict the development of glaucomatous visual field loss. *Archives of Ophthalmology*, **111**, 645–50.

Johnson, C.A., Adams, A.J., Casson, E.J., and Brandt, J.D. (1993b). Progression of early glaucomatous visual field loss as detected by blue-on-yellow and standard white-on-white automated perimetry. *Archives of Ophthalmology*, **111**, 651–6.

Johnson, A.T., Drack, A.V., Kwitek, A.E., Cannon, R.L., Stone, E.M., and Alward, W.L. (1993c). Clinical features and linkage analysis of a family with autosomal dominant juvenile glaucoma. *Ophthalmology*, **100**, 524–9.

Lachenmayr, B.J., Drance, S.M., Chauhan, B.C., House, P.H., and Lalani, S.

(1991). Diffuse and localized glaucomatous field loss in light-sense, flicker and resolution perimetry. *Graefe's Archives of Clinical and Experimental Ophthalmology*, **229**, 267–73.

Lampert, P.W., Vogel, M.H., and Zimmerman, L.E. (1968). Pathology of the optic nerve in experimental acute glaucoma. *Investigative Ophthalmology*, **7**, 199–213.

Martinez, G.A., Sample, P.A., and Weinreb, R.N. (1995). Comparison of high-pass resolution perimetry and standard automated perimetry in glaucoma. *American Journal of Ophthalmology*, **119**, 195–201.

Minckler, D.S., Bunt, A.H., and Johanson, G.W. (1977). Orthograde and retrograde axoplasmic transport during acute ocular hypertension in the monkey. *Investigative Ophthalmology*, **16**, 426–41.

Minckler, D.S., Bunt, A.H., and Klock, I.B. (1978). Radiographic and cyto-chemical ultrastructural studies of axoplasmic transport in the monkey optic nerve head. *Investigative Ophthalmology*, **17**, 33–50.

Murray, J.C., Bennett, S.R., Kwitek, A.E., *et al.* (1992). Linkage of Rieger syndrome to the region of the epidermal growth factor gene on chromosome 4. *Nature Genetics*, **2**, 46–9.

Netland, P.A., Wiggs, J.L., and Dreyer, E.B. (1993). Inheritance of glaucoma and genetic counseling of glaucoma patients. *International Ophthalmology Clinics*, **33**, 101–20.

Pearson, H.E. and Stoffler, D.J. (1992). Retinal ganglion cell degeneration following loss of postsynaptic target neurons in the dorsal lateral geniculate nucleus of the adult cat. *Experimental Neurology*, **116**, 163–71.

Pearson, H.E. and Thompson, T.P. (1993). Atrophy and degeneration of ganglion cells in central retina following loss of postsynaptic target neurons in the dorsal lateral geniculate nucleus of the adult cat. *Experimental Neurology*, **119**, 113–19.

Quigley, H.A. and Anderson, D.R. (1976). The dynamics and location of axonal transport blockade by acute intraocular pressure elevation in primate optic nerve. *Investigative Ophthalmology*, **15**, 606–16.

Quigley, H.A. and Green, W.R. (1979). The histology of human glaucoma cupping and optic nerve damage: clinicopathologic correlation in 21 eyes. *Ophthalmology*, **86**, 1803–30.

Radius, R.L. and Bade, B. (1981). Pressure-induced optic nerve axonal transport interruption in cat eyes. *Archives of Ophthalmology*, **99**, 2163–5.

Ruben, S.T., Hitchings, R.A., Fitzke, F., and Arden, G.B. (1994). Electrophysiology and psychophysics in ocular hypertension and glaucoma: evidence for different pathomechanisms in early glaucoma. *Eye*, **8**, 516–20.

Sample, P.A. and Weinreb, R.N. (1990). Color perimetry for assessment of primary open-angle glaucoma. *Investigative Ophthalmology and Visual Science*, **31**, 1869–75.

Sample, P.A. and Weinreb, R.N. (1992). Progressive color visual field loss in glaucoma. *Investigative Ophthalmology and Visual Science*, **33**, 2068–71.

Sample, P.A., Weinreb, R.N., and Boyton, R.M. (1986). Acquired dyschromatopsia in glaucoma. *Survey of Ophthalmology*, **31**, 54–64.

Sample, P.A., Ahn, D.S., Lee, P.C., and Weinreb, R.N. (1992). High-pass resolution perimetry in eyes with ocular hypertension and primary open-angle glaucoma. *American Journal of Ophthalmology*, **113**, 309–16.

Sample, P.A., Taylor, J.D., Martinez, G.A., Lusky, M., and Weinreb, R.N. (1993). Short-wavelength color visual fields in glaucoma suspects at risk. *American Journal of Ophthalmology*, **115**, 225–33.

Sheffield, V.C., Stone, E.M., Alward, W.L., *et al.* (1993). Genetic linkage of familial open angle glaucoma to chromosome 1q21–q31. *Nature Genetics*, **4**, 47–50.

Silverman, S.E., Trick, G.L., and Hart, W.M. Jr (1990). Motion perception is abnormal in primary open-angle glaucoma and ocular hypertension. *Investigative Ophthalmology and Visual Science*, **31**, 722–9.

Thoenen, H. (1991). The changing scene of neurotrophic factors. *Trends in Neuroscience*, **14**, 165–70.

Tyler, C.W. (1991). Specific deficits of flicker sensitivity in glaucoma and ocular hypertension. *Investigative Ophthalmology and Visual Science*, **32**, 2552–60.

Tyler, C.W., Hardage, L., and Stamper, R.L. (1994). The temporal visiogram in ocular hypertension and its progression to glaucoma. *Glaucoma*, **3**, S65–S72.

Vrabek, F. (1976). Glaucomatous cupping of the human optic disk; a neuro-histologic study. *Graefe's Archives of Clinical and Experimental Ophthalmology*, **198**, 223–34.

Wiggs, J.L., Haines, J.L., Paglinauan, C., Fine, A., Sporn, C., and Lou, D. (1994). Genetic linkage of autosomal dominant juvenile glaucoma to 1q21–q31 in three affected pedigrees. *Genomics*, **21**, 299–303.

2.10.4 Epidemiology and risk factors for primary open angle glaucoma

James M. Tielsch

Primary open angle glaucoma is a group of disorders characterized by optic nerve damage resulting in peripheral visual field loss which can progress to involve the fovea and central vision. In recent years, there has been a dramatic increase in the number and sophistication of studies on the epidemiology of this disease. Significant problems related primarily to the definition of primary open angle glaucoma have been resolved and population-based studies have provided estimates of prevalence and limited assessment of potential risk factors.

Research on the epidemiology of primary open angle glaucoma are directly related to our knowledge of the pathophysiological mechanism by which damage occurs in primary open angle glaucoma. This process is the subject of much debate with two major hypotheses proposed to account for the observed damage to the optic nerve. The first hypothesis suggests that reductions in vascular perfusion of the optic nerve and nerve fibre layer is the primary mechanism of damage and the second hypothesis centres on mechanical damage occurring at the level of the lamina cribrosa. In both hypotheses, damage to the optic nerve is thought to be mediated through a combination of inherent susceptibility of the optic nerve head and elevation in the intraocular pressure beyond the tolerance of a susceptible eye. It is likely that both mechanisms act to produce damage and that the relative importance of one mechanism over the other may depend on a variety of factors, including the level of the intraocular pressure. Whatever mechanism plays the leading role in producing glaucomatous optic nerve damage, there is little good information about what initiates this process or about the subgroups of the population who are at high risk for the onset of such damage.

Methodological issues

To review the epidemiology of primary open angle glaucoma, a solid understanding of the evolution of diagnostic methods and definitions used for this disorder is necessary. It is accepted widely now that primary open angle glaucoma is fundamentally an optic neuropathy with the defining clinical sign being damage to the axons of retinal ganglion cells. This damage may be evidenced clinically by any combination of abnormalities in the visual field, excavation of the optic nerve, or thinning of the nerve fibre layer.

Issues regarding the definition of primary open angle glaucoma have been at the heart of our confusion about its epidemiology. For many years, the definition of glaucoma was synonymous with elevated intraocular pressure. Early studies often included groups of cases dominated by patients who had elevated intraocular pressure only and neither optic nerve excavation nor visual field loss. This confusion was reinforced by a statistical classification of the distribution of intraocular pressure that mistakenly equated infrequency with abnormality. In response to this problem, two different conditions are now described, glaucoma and ocular hypertension, separating those with optic nerve damage from those with only statistically defined elevated intraocular pressure.

There remain, however, differences in the definitions used for glaucoma. Differences exist in the criteria for glaucomatous optic nerve damage, the techniques used to measure such damage, who is qualified to make such assessments, and whether elevated intraocular pressure is a necessary component of the disease definition. Dilated examinations of the optic nerve head are critical to making full use of the dimensional clues to the status of the optic nerve. Despite the safety of pupillary dilation (risk of dilating a potentially occludable angle using appropriate screening criteria is less than 3/1000), few non-ophthalmologists are able to adequately examine the optic nerve for signs of glaucomatous optic nerve damage. The confusing role of elevated intraocular pressure in the definition of primary open angle glaucoma, has resulted in the categorization of primary open angle glaucoma into classical primary open angle glaucoma, which has elevated intraocular pressure as well as optic nerve damage, and low tension glaucoma, which has intraocular pressure in the 'normal' range, but damage to the optic nerve. While a number of investigators have claimed to demonstrate differences in the clinical presentation of low tension glaucoma as compared with classical primary open angle glaucoma, a growing body of evidence suggests that most cases are part of the expected distribution of primary open angle glaucoma. Nevertheless, it is likely that there is heterogeneity in the aetiology of primary open angle glaucoma in both the classical form as well as those with 'normal' intraocular pressure. A critically important issue regarding the definition of primary open angle glaucoma for epidemiological studies, is the realization that objective structural criteria such as cup to disc ratio or other characteristics of the optic nerve are poorly sensitive to detecting glaucomatous optic nerve damage. Examination of the visual field is necessary, as up to one-third of cases will be missed when using structural criteria alone or in combination with an intraocular pressure criterion.

Prevalence and incidence

A significant number of recent studies have provided solid data on the prevalence of primary open angle glaucoma in the United States, Europe, and the Caribbean. Estimates of prevalence range from 0.42 per cent among Caucasians in Wales to over 14 per cent among black people on St Lucia. Two main factors account for the observed variation in rates (excluding sampling error), racial composition of the study population, and the definition of primary open angle glaucoma used. Persons of African descent have higher rates than Caucasians. Among Caucasians, studies that uniformly conducted visual field testing and did not require elevated intraocular pressure as a criterion for diagnosis suggest that the prevalence is between 1.5 and 2.0 per cent for those 40 years or older (Table 1).

While good data on the prevalence of glaucoma are now available, adequate information on the incidence of primary open angle glaucoma is not. Statistical models which utilize assumptions about the relationship of age-specific cross-sectional prevalence and general population survival rates as well as longitudinal studies which were not population-based have been used to estimate incidence for a variety of populations, primarily white residents of the United States. The longitudinal studies indicate that, even in study populations enriched with subjects who are considered high risk for the development of primary open angle glaucoma, the incidence of new cases is quite low, in the range of 1 in 1000 to 1 in 100 per year. Statistical modelling of incidence indicate that rates are even lower for Caucasians from the general population, ranging from 0.08 per 1000 per year for those in their early forties to 1.46 per 1000 per year for persons in their eighties. Direct estimates of incidence will be available over the next few years from longitudinal studies currently underway in a variety of locations.

The functional consequences associated with primary open angle glaucoma are not well understood but thought to be limited except in far advanced disease that involves visual field loss within 10 or 20° of fixation. Recently, a variety of patient-oriented measures of visual functional status have been developed and applied to patients undergoing cataract extraction. Whether such instruments will be useful for a disease like primary open angle glaucoma, where central vision is generally spared until the latest stage, is not clear, but changes in these instruments will likely be needed in order to detect functional loss associated with peripheral vision deficits. Efforts are currently underway to develop and test such instruments.

Information on the magnitude of the most severe form of visual functional impairment associated with primary open angle glaucoma, blindness, is limited. Most data come from blindness registries which are usually incomplete in their ascertainment of blind persons. The Model Reporting Area Study, which last reported results from 1970, used data from 16 states in the United States that agreed to a common reporting format and criteria for the definition of blindness. Standardization of diagnostic criteria for defining the cause of blindness was not possible, however, nor was there any direct information about the proportion of blind persons ascertained by the registration system. Despite these problems, the Model Reporting Area Study remains a heavily used source of data on the cause-specific rates of blindness in the United States. In 1970, glaucoma was the third leading cause of blindness (after cataract and

Table 1 Prevalence of open angle glaucoma

Location	Age range	Prevalence	Racial composition
Europe			
Wales, 1966	40–75 years	0.42%	White Welsh
Dalby, Sweden, 1981	55–69 years	0.86%	White Swedish
Iceland, 1986	≥50 years	1.91%	White Icelandic
Sweden, 1982	≥50 years	1.4%	White Swedish
Rotterdam, The Netherlands, 1994	≥55 years	1.1%	White Dutch
Ireland, 1993	≥50 years	1.9%	White Irish
United States			
Framingham, USA, 1980	52–85 years	2.1%	White Americans
Baltimore, USA, 1991	≥40 years	1.7%	White Americans
		5.6%	Black Americans
Beaver Dam, Wisconsin, U.S.A., 1992	43–84 years	2.1%	White Americans
Caribbean			
Jamaica, 1969	≥35 years	1.4%	Black Jamaicans
St Lucia, 1989	≥30 years	8.8%	Black St Lucians
		–14.7%	
Barbados, 1994	40–84 years	7.0%	Black Barbadians

age-related macular degeneration) with a prevalence of 16.2 per 100 000 and an incidence of new blindness registrations of 1.5 per 100 000 per year. Data from other population-based sources suggest that these figures are seriously underestimated. The Baltimore Eye Survey estimated the prevalence of glaucomatous blindness at 1.7 per 1000 in a population with equal numbers of black people and Caucasians, of which more than 75 per cent was due to primary open angle glaucoma. The Rotterdam Study found a similar rate of approximately 1 per 1000 among a white population.

Worldwide estimates of the prevalence of glaucomatous blindness are particularly difficult, since adequate information is missing from large parts of the world. The World Health Organization used available prevalence data and population models to estimate that there are 13.5 million persons 40 years or older affected with primary open angle glaucoma, of whom 3 million are blind.

Another perspective on the size of the glaucoma problem is economic. While cost-of-illness studies often suffer from lack of adequate data and can vary widely depending on the structure of the health-care delivery system, reasonable assumptions can be used to develop a more comprehensive picture of the impact of disease on society than prevalence alone can provide. Such efforts divide total costs into those associated with the direct medical care of persons with illness (direct costs), indirect costs such as lost wages, and income transfer. One estimate suggested that, in 1991, the estimate of total direct costs for glaucoma in the United States was approximately $1.6 billion.

This estimate reflects the costs of treating one-half the total number of persons with glaucoma as only 50 per cent of those who have primary open angle glaucoma have been diagnosed. Treating the additional 50 per cent of cases would more than double this estimate, since costly efforts would be required to identify the undiagnosed group. Another $1.1 billion was paid by the United States government to support individuals blind from glaucoma, and indirect costs were estimated very conservatively at over $235 million.

Risk factors

Age

An increased prevalence of primary open angle glaucoma with older age has been found in every population-based study (Fig. 1). The magnitude of this association is large, with prevalence rates between four and 10 times higher in the oldest age groups as compared with persons in their forties. Similarly, the 13-year incidence of glaucomatous visual field defects rose from 0.7 per cent among those less than 40 years of age at baseline to 4.8 per cent among those 60 years or older at baseline in the Collaborative Glaucoma Study. Statistical projections for Caucasian populations show a rise from 0.08 to 1.46 per 1000 per year with increasing age. The linear age-prevalence curve for black people suggests that age may not be associated with incidence of new disease in this ethnic group.

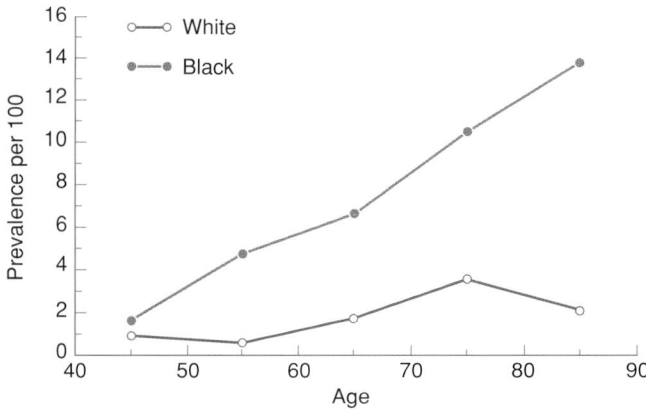

Fig. 1 Prevalence of primary open angle glaucoma in Caucasians and black people. (Based on data from the Baltimore Eye Survey.)

Table 2 Association of intraocular pressure and primary open angle glaucoma

Intraocular Pressure, mmHg	Prevalence (%)	Relative Prevalence
<= 15	0.65	1.0
16–18	1.31	2.0
19–21	1.82	2.8
22–29	8.30	12.8
>= 30	25.5	39.3

Data taken from Sommer *et al.* (1991).

Studies that directly estimate incidence in different racial groups are needed to address this issue.

Gender

Data on the relationship of gender to the prevalence of primary open angle glaucoma are inconsistent. The Framingham and Barbados Eye Studies found that men had a significantly higher prevalence of primary open angle glaucoma than women; the opposite was found in Sweden; and no association was found in Wales, Baltimore, Beaver Dam, or the Collaborative Glaucoma Study. Thus, gender is unlikely to be a major risk factor for primary open angle glaucoma.

Race

Racial differences in the prevalence and severity of primary open angle glaucoma are an important facet of the epidemiology of this disease. Persons of west African ancestry, including black populations in the Caribbean and the United States, have a significantly higher prevalence of primary open angle glaucoma than do Caucasians. The evidence for this excess risk in black people comes from a wide variety of sources including clinic-based studies in which black people comprise a higher proportion of glaucoma clinic attendees than among general eye clinic populations. Black people also have glaucoma surgery at higher rates than Caucasians, and, among those who participate in glaucoma screening programmes, black people are more likely to be diagnosed with glaucoma. Prevalence surveys conducted in primarily black populations have shown higher rates of glaucoma than those using similar methods in Caucasian populations. Black people in Jamaica had a rate three times higher than that found among Caucasians in Wales. More recent studies in St Lucia and Barbados have found extremely high rates, 7 to 16 per cent among those 40 or older, among the black populations of these islands. The only direct comparison of prevalence between black people and Caucasians from the same population comes from the Baltimore Eye Survey which found an age-adjusted 4.3-fold excess prevalence of primary open angle glaucoma in black people as compared with their Caucasian neighbours.

Primary open angle glaucoma also may be a more severe disease among black people. They have a younger age of onset, more advanced disease at the time of first diagnosis, and are more often refractory to medical therapy. Whether these differences reflect a more rapid progression of disease or a combination of higher age-specific incidence and poor access to eye care services is not known. A number of clinical trials and longitudinal studies of primary open angle glaucoma among black people and Caucasians are currently underway and should provide the information required to determine if progression and treatment efficacy are modified by race.

The explanation for the observed excess prevalence among black people is not well understood, but is likely related to an underlying predisposition to this disease. The associations of other conditions such as sickle cell disease, systemic hypertension, and diabetes with black race have led to hypotheses that the racial variation in primary open angle glaucoma risk may be a function of this excess co-morbidity. However, the available data do not support this idea. These factors act independently, if at all, on the risk of primary open angle glaucoma.

Intraocular pressure

The association between intraocular pressure and primary open angle glaucoma is strong and consistent even when elevated intraocular pressure is excluded as a criterion for the diagnosis of primary open angle glaucoma. There is an exponential increase in prevalence with increasing intraocular pressure (Table 2). Additional convincing evidence for an aetiological role for increased intraocular pressure in the development of primary open angle glaucoma comes from studies which show asymmetric optic nerve damage in persons with corresponding asymmetric elevations in intraocular pressure, and from studies that demonstrate a reduction in the risk of optic nerve damage among high-risk populations in whom the intraocular pressure was lowered. Despite this very strong association, even at levels of intraocular pressure considered dangerously high, a significant proportion of persons will never be affected. In addition, there is a significant overlap of intraocular pressure distributions between those with and without primary open angle glaucoma such that a large proportion of primary open angle glaucoma cases have intraocular pressure well within the 'normal' range. The sensitivity of the classical cut-off for intraocular pressure of greater than 21 mmHg is less than 50 per cent, and there is no level at which a reasonable balance of sensitivity and specificity is achieved. The implications of these results for the use of tonometry in glaucoma screening are well known; this approach is now generally discouraged.

Optic disc parameters

Discussion of the association of optic nerve head characteristics with primary open angle glaucoma is confused by their use both to identify population groups with an elevated risk for glaucomatous optic nerve damage and as criteria for the definition of disease. These parameters include the cup to disc ratio, the narrowest neuroretinal rim width, rim area, cup volume, and a variety of others. Many of these descriptors are now based on sophisticated three-dimensional imaging of the optic nerve head. Because these parameters are often used to define primary open angle glaucoma or determine whether or not progression has occurred, they are not risk factors in a traditional aetiological sense, but actual markers of damage. Despite the direct measurement of optic nerve status implied by these parameters, their ability to classify people accurately into diseased and non-diseased states is poor. Similar to the problems with tonometry, there is no cut-off point in the distributions of cup to disc ratio, neural rim width, cup volume, rim area, or disc area that achieves adequate balance in terms of sensitivity and specificity making their use in screening problematic.

The thickness and integrity of the nerve fibre layer as determined by clinical or photographic fundus examination is a more direct measure of damage to the optic nerve and has been shown to be both sensitive and specific in its ability to classify persons into diseased and non-diseased states. It is also useful for predicting who will develop glaucomatous visual field loss. Significant issues remain, however, regarding the transfer of this technology into the general practice of ophthalmology, let alone population screening.

Recently, sophisticated hardware and software systems using stereo video imaging and scanning laser tomography and polarimetry have been developed to three-dimensionally image the optic nerve head and measure the thickness of the nerve fibre layer. At this point in time, there is limited information on how these various technologies perform both for cross-sectional classification of persons with and without disease and for detection of incidence and progression. These technologies are quite early in their development, especially the software algorithms that can summarize the vast quantities of raw data captured by these systems in a meaningful fashion.

Refractive error

The association of refractive error with primary open angle glaucoma has been controversial. Myopia has been associated with glaucoma in a number of studies with relative odds of primary open angle glaucoma between 2 and 5 when compared with either clinic-based controls or national norms for refractive status. The potential for selection bias when using clinic-based ascertainment for cases is strong for a variable such as myopia because those with poor vision due to their myopia are more likely to seek eye care and have a higher probability of being diagnosed with glaucoma. Despite this potential bias, unpublished data from the Baltimore Eye Survey and a small population-based study from Sicily have demonstrated that myopia is associated with the prevalence of primary open angle glaucoma. Whether this association is aetiological in nature or confounded by some other common factor is not yet understood.

Diabetes

It is well known that complications of diabetes can produce secondary glaucoma, but the association of diabetes with primary open angle glaucoma has been less clear. A number of clinic-based case–control studies have reported odds ratios ranging from 1.6 to 4.7. In these studies, controls were ascertained from similar sources as the cases, but selection bias cannot be ruled out as an explanation for these results. Population-based studies in Framingham, Sweden, Baltimore, and the Collaborative Glaucoma Study have found no association between diabetes and primary open angle glaucoma. In contrast, the Beaver Dam Study found a two-fold excess risk of diabetes in persons with primary open angle glaucoma as compared with controls. This conflict with other population-based studies may be due to methodological differences in the examination protocols for these studies. The lack of a direct clinical assessment by an ophthalmologist in the Beaver Dam Study may have missed retinal complications of diabetes that can produce visual field loss similar in appearance to that of primary open angle glaucoma. The overall weight of evidence from population-based studies suggests that diabetes is unlikely to be a major risk factor for primary open angle glaucoma.

Systemic hypertension

Similarly to diabetes, the association of systemic hypertension with primary open angle glaucoma is controversial. Much of the confusion in the literature is due to reports which have associated intraocular pressure with systemic blood pressure. There is relatively strong evidence for this association even though the magnitude of the correlation may be small. Within many of these same investigations, however, no association was found between primary open angle glaucoma and systemic hypertension. Other case–control studies also have shown no association with primary open angle glaucoma, though one has demonstrated a strong and statistically significant association between untreated systolic hypertension and primary open angle glaucoma.

More recent evidence from the Baltimore and Barbados Eye Surveys suggest that the relationship between primary open angle glaucoma and systemic blood pressure is complex and related to a variety of other haemo- and oculodynamic factors. In the Baltimore data, age modified the effect of systemic hypertension on risk of primary open angle glaucoma. Those below the age of 60 were protected, while those older than 70 showed an elevated prevalence of primary open angle glaucoma if they were hypertensive. Such a pattern would be expected if, early in the course of systemic hypertension, the elevated blood pressure resulted in increased perfusion, while later, after significant microvascular damage had occurred, blood flow to the optic nerve head was reduced. An additional important finding was that perfusion pressure (the difference between blood pressure and intraocular pressure) was significantly associated with the risk of primary open angle glaucoma in a way that might be predicted based on autoregulation of blood flow in the retina and optic nerve head. The prevalence of primary open angle glaucoma remained constant across a wide range of perfusion pressure until below 50 mmHg where the prevalence rose dramatically. There was a six-fold excess prevalence in the lowest versus highest perfusion pressure categories. Because of the cross-sectional nature of these data, the directionality of this association cannot be determined nor do we understand how the duration of low perfusion pressure affects this association.

Another mechanism by which primary open angle glaucoma and haemodynamics may be related is through vascular spasm, which can result in an acute reduction in blood flow to the retinal nerve fibre layer and optic nerve head. This hypothesis is supported by studies demonstrating a positive association of migraine and Raynaud's syndrome with low tension glaucoma. However, the single population-based study which examined this issue found no association between migraine-like headache and primary open angle glaucoma.

Family history of glaucoma

A number of studies have suggested that as much as one-quarter of patients with glaucoma have a positive family history. Epidemiological studies have estimated that a positive family history of glaucoma is associated with between a two- and five-fold excess risk of primary open angle glaucoma. In addition, it is well accepted that a number of ocular parameters associated with primary open angle glaucoma are influenced by heredity. These include cup to disc ratio, disc size, intraocular pressure, and others. Also, certain forms of juvenile glaucoma have been found to have a primary genetic basis. The search for genetic markers associated with primary open angle glaucoma or a common mode of inheritance, however, has not been successful. Reports of strong associations between human leucocyte antigens and glaucoma have not been confirmed. While there is little doubt that familial factors play an important role in the underlying susceptibility to the development of primary open angle glaucoma, methodological limitations of previous studies have made it difficult to study familial associations well. Specifically, since primary open angle glaucoma is strongly age-related, complete family studies that apply uniform criteria for diagnosis and staging are very difficult.

Summary

Epidemiological studies have provided us with accurate measures of the magnitude and severity of the disease burden caused by primary open angle glaucoma in selected populations. The latest investigations which have included visual field measurements on all subjects have demonstrated that previous estimates of the prevalence of this disorder were too low, by as much as 30 to 50 per cent. These studies also have confirmed the significantly elevated risk of primary open angle glaucoma among black people, although the basis for this excess risk remains unclear. Age and intraocular pressure remain the strongest risk factors for primary open angle glaucoma across all populations with exponential increases in the rate of primary open angle glaucoma with increasing age and intraocular pressure. Family history of glaucoma is also a major risk factor for this disease; however, the source of this association has yet to be elucidated. Other risk factors for this disease include myopia and vascular disorders which result in lowered perfusion pressure to the eye. Future research on the epidemiology of primary open angle glaucoma will quantify the incidence of this disorder and evaluate the interaction of heredity and environmental factors in producing excess risk.

Further reading

Armaly, M.F. (1980). Lessons to be learned from the Collaborative Glaucoma Study. *Survey of Ophthalmology*, **25**, 139–44.

Bengtsson, B. (1981). Aspects of the epidemiology of chronic glaucoma. *Acta Ophthalmologica*, **146** (suppl), 4–26.

Dielemans, I., Vingerling, J.R., Wolfs, R.C.W., Hofman, A., Grabbee, D.E., and de Jong, P.T.V.M. (1994). The prevalence of primary open-angle glaucoma in a population-based study in The Netherlands. *Ophthalmology*, **101**, 1851–55.

Eddy, D.M., Sanders, L.E., and Eddy, J.F. (1983). The value of screening for glaucoma with tonometry. *Survey of Ophthalmology*, **28**, 194–205.

Hollows, F.C. and Graham, P.A. (1966). Intraocular pressure, glaucoma and glaucoma suspects in a defined population. *British Journal of Ophthalmology*, **50**, 570–86.

Kahn, H.A. and Milton, R.C. (1980). Alternative definitions of open-angle glaucoma. Effect on prevalence and associations in the Framingham Eye Study. *Archives of Ophthalmology*, **98**, 2172–9.

Klein, B.E.K., Klein, R., Sponsel, W.E., et al. (1992). Prevalence of glaucoma. The Beaver Dam Eye Study. *Ophthalmology*, **99**, 1499–504.

Leske, M.C., Connell, A.M.S., Schachat, R.P., Hyman, L., and the Barbados Eye Study Group (1994). The Barbados Eye Study. Prevalence of open angle glaucoma. *Archives of Ophthalmology*, **112**, 821–9.

Mason, R.P., Kosoko, O., Wilson, M.R., et al. (1989). National survey of the prevalence and risk factors of glaucoma in St Lucia, West Indies. Part I: prevalence findings. *Ophthalmology*, **96**, 1363–8.

Ponte, F., Giuffre, G., Giammanco, R., and Dardononi, G. (1994). Risk factors of ocular hypertension and glaucoma. The Casteldaccia Eye Study. *Documenta Ophthalmologica*, **85**, 203–10.

Sommer, A., Tielsch, J.M., Katz, J., et al. (1991a). Racial differences in the cause-specific prevalence of blindness in east Baltimore. *New England Journal of Medicine*, **325**, 1412–17.

Sommer, A., Tielsch, J.M., Katz, J., et al. (1991b). Relationship between intraocular pressure and primary open angle glaucoma among white and black Americans: the Baltimore Eye Survey. *Archives of Ophthalmology*, **109**, 1090–5.

Thylefors, F. and Negrel, A.-D. (1994). The global impact of glaucoma. *Bulletin of the World Health Organization*, **72**, 323–6.

Tielsch, J.M., Katz, J., Singh, K., et al. (1991a). A population-based evaluation of glaucoma screening: the Baltimore Eye Survey. *American Journal of Epidemiology*, **134**, 1102–10.

Tielsch, J.M., Sommer, A., Katz, J., Royall, R.M., Quigley, H.A., and Javitt, J. (1991b). Racial variations in the prevalence of primary open angle glaucoma: the Baltimore Eye Survey. *Journal of the American Medical Association*, **266**, 369–74.

Tielsch, J.M., Katz, J., Quigley, H.A., Javitt, J.C., and Sommer, A. (1995). Hypertension, perfusion pressure and primary open angle glaucoma: a population-based assessment. *Archives of Ophthalmology*, 113, 216–21.

Uhm, K.B. and Shin, D.H. (1992). Positive family history of glaucoma is a risk factor for increased intraocular pressure rather than glaucomatous optic nerve damage (primary open angle glaucoma vs. OH vs. normal control). *Korean Journal of Ophthalmology*, 6, 100–4.

Van Buskirk, E.M. (1994). Glaucomatous optic neuropathy. *Journal of Glaucoma*, 3, S2–3.

Wallace, J. and Lovell, H.G. (1969). Glaucoma and intraocular pressure in Jamaica. *American Journal of Ophthalmology*, 67, 93–100.

Wilson, M.R., Hertzmark, E., Walker, A.M., Childs-Shaw, K., and Epstein, D.L. (1987). A case–control study of risk factors in open angle glaucoma. *Archives of Ophthalmology*, 105, 1066–71.

2.10.5 Diagnostic and clinical tests in glaucoma

2.10.5.1 Intraocular pressure measurement and optic nerve examination

Wojciech S.S. Karwatowski

Intraocular pressure

A measurement of intraocular pressure which is both accurate and consistent is critical in any ocular examination and in particular in one which concerns itself with the diagnosis and management of glaucoma. Whilst many instruments have been used to facilitate this, the vast majority of intraocular pressure measures are now done by Goldmann applanation tonometry.

Applanation tonometry

Applanation tonometry works by applying a measured force to flatten a known area of the cornea, and deducing from it the intraocular pressure. The Goldmann applanation tonometer is a variable force tonometer which is based on the Imbert–Fick law. This states that the pressure $P = F/A$, where the force (F) is needed to flatten a given area of a sphere (A). However, this applies only to a perfect sphere which is infinitely thin, infinitely elastic, and which is subject to no surface tension forces. These criteria are obviously not applicable in the human eye. The main confounding forces are the tendency for the rigidity of the cornea to push away the tonometer (N) and the second is that the tear film creates a surface tension that pulls the applanating surface towards the cornea (M). Thus the equation becomes

$$P = F/A + M - N.$$

Empirical derivations developed by Goldmann and coworkers which allowed for corneal rigidity, surface tension, and the dif-

ference between internal and external area displacement, showed that an applanator of diameter 3.06 mm produces the appropriate area of indentation on the endothelial side of the cornea. This size was also used as it allowed simple conversion from grams force to millimetres of mercury by multiplying by 10.

Use of the Goldmann tonometer

The Goldmann tonometer consists of a tonometric head which contains a bi-prism. When in contact with the cornea two semi-circles are visible through one of the slit lamp oculars when the tonometer is positioned for intraocular pressure measurement (Fig. 1). The patient is positioned as normal on the slit lamp and the corneal surface is anaesthetized, using a topical anaesthetic. An amount of 0.25 per cent fluorescein solution is instilled into the inferior conjunctival sac. Alternatively, a small paper strip impregnated with fluorescein is used to introduce fluorescein into the tear film.

The tonometric prism and cornea are illuminated with a cobalt blue light from the slit lamp and the tonometer moved forward so that the prism face is in contact with the eye (Fig. 2). The semi-circular pattern is then observed and adjusted using the vertical and horizontal adjustment of the slit lamp so that the two semi-circles appear of equal size.

The applanating force is then adjusted so that the inner edge of the upper and lower semi-circles become aligned. The observer will notice the semi-circular meniscus arcs moving reflecting the ocular pulse. The pressure reading is generally

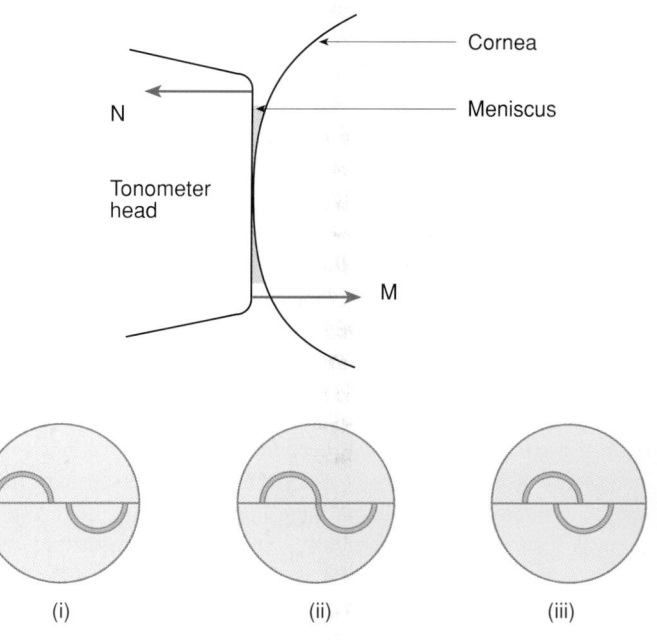

Fig. 1 When the Goldmann applanation tonometer head is pressed against the cornea, it indents it and a fluorescein stained meniscus is seen. The rigidity of the cornea (N) tends to push the tonometer head away from the eye while the surface tension created by the tear film (M) tends to pull the tonometer head towards the eye. The fluorescein stained meniscus is seen through one of the slit lamp oculars (i–iii). The applanating force is increased if the applanating area is too small (i) or decreased if it is too large (iii) to get to the correct endpoint (ii).

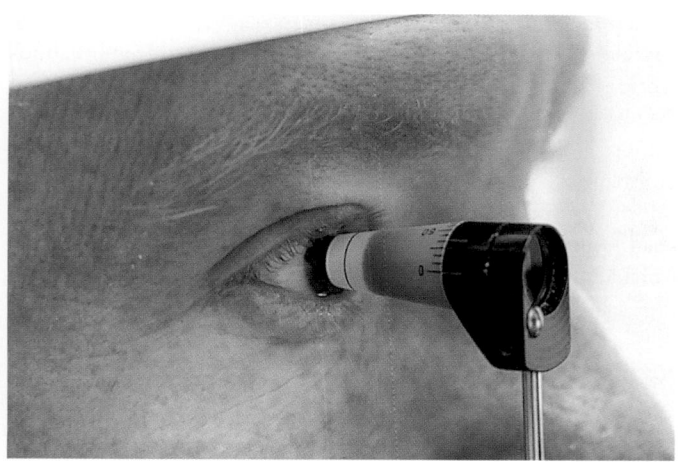

Fig. 2 The Goldmann applanation tonometer head is placed in contact with an anaesthetized eye for intraocular pressure measurement. Note that the tonometer head is centred carefully on the cornea and minimal, if any, force is applied to the eyelid to help achieve an accurate result.

taken as the mean of these movements although some observers use the systolic value as the endpoint.

Care has to be taken to ensure that the tonometer head is adequately sterilized before use. There is concern regarding transmission of the human immunodeficiency virus (HIV) and hepatitis B as well as much more common ocular pathogens such as adenovirus. It is generally recommended that the tonometer should be wiped clean after use. It should then be further sterilized in 0.1 per cent sodium hypochlorite solution for 5 min. The solution should be washed off prior to tonometer use. It has also been suggested that disposable covers for applanation tips can be used as a further precaution when it is considered that the infectious risk is particularly high.

Reliability and accuracy

Allowing for interobserver and interinstrument error, the use of the Goldmann tonometer should give results accurate to +1 or −1 mmHg. However, this depends on removing as many sources of error as possible. The first potential source of error is an inappropriate concentration of fluorescein in the precorneal tear film. An underestimation of the intraocular pressure may occur at too low a concentration, and an overestimate at too high a one.

Refractive error can also influence tonometric results. An increase in corneal curvature by 3 dioptres is capable of increasing the measured pressure by 1 mmHg. Similarly with the mires placed horizontally, intraocular pressure is underestimated by 1 mmHg for every 4 dioptres of with-the-rule astigmatism. To avoid this error the tonometer prism should be rotated so that the axis of least corneal curvature is opposite the red line on the prism holder, alternatively, two readings taken with the mires parallel and at 90° to the axis of astigmatism can be taken. The results are then averaged.

A portable form of the Goldmann tonometer, the Perkins tonometer, is also available.

Mackay–Marg tonometry

In principle the MacKay–Marg tonometer consists of a plunger extending a small distance, 10 μm, beyond the plane of the surrounding probe. When the tonometer is placed against the cornea, the force applied against the plunger increases until the full area of the plunger is flat against the cornea. At this point the force against the plunger is equal to the intraocular pressure and the force necessary to deform the cornea. As the tonometer is advanced further this latter force is transferred from the plunger to the surrounding probe. The tracing showing the forces being used shows a slight dip and thus the intraocular pressure can be calculated from the difference in force from baseline to the dip.

The most recent derivative of the MacKay–Marg principle is the Tonopen. This is a small hand-held device with MacKay–Marg type probe at its tip. With the probe tip covered by a rubber film, a suitably anaesthetized subject's cornea is gently indented a number of times until the device accepts the quality of the MacKay–Marg curve and displays the value for the intraocular pressure with a standard deviation of the average pressure readings measured.

This device has the advantage that it can be used with reasonable confidence on irregular corneas and in difficult situations when it is not possible to use a slit lamp mounted Goldmann tonometer. Although it tends to underestimate high pressures and overestimate low ones there is good correlation in the normal pressure ranges measured with a Goldmann tonometer.

A similar principle to the MacKay–Marg tonometer but rather differently implemented is found in the pneumatonometer. In this case a constant flow of air takes the place of a plunger to measure the intraocular pressure and the force necessary to bend the cornea is transferred to the rest of the pneumatonometer plunger. The instrument provides a constant record of the intraocular pressure and is able to measure effectively the variations between systolic and diastolic intraocular pressures.

Non-contact tonometry

Non-contact tonometry involves a high pressure stream of air flattening the corneal apex. The instrument uses optical means to measure the desired area of flattening and the time of air flow required to produce this is then translated into an intraocular pressure measurement. It is attractive in that it does not require topical anaesthesia and is relatively easy to use. However, due to the extremely short time taken to make an individual reading there can be significant variations between repeat readings and hence possible inaccuracies.

Indentation tonometry

Prior to the development of Goldmann tonometry the Schiotz indentation tonometer was the main form of pressure measurement. The Schiotz tonometer consists of a foot plate and a plunger. The instrument is applied to the surface of an anaesthetized cornea with the subject supine. The extent to which the cornea is indented by the plunger is an indication of intra-ocular pressure. This movement is transmitted via a lever and is read off a scale.

The Schiotz tonometer has been standardized with a given radius of curvature of foot plate and plunger weight. The plunger usually has a weight of 5.5 g but additional weights can be added. The intraocular pressure can then be deduced from the scale reading using a nonagram. The main problem with this tonometer is that the weight of the instrument increases the intraocular pressure depending on the ocular rigidity. Although the nonagrams provided with the instrument allow for this they are averaged. This means that subjects with either high or low ocular rigidity may give false readings. These inaccuracies together with the fact that the patient needs to lie supine has meant that the technique has now been largely superseded by Goldmann tonometry.

Examining the optic disc

The clinical evaluation of the optic discs forms a central part of in the examination of any subject. Whilst there are several new technologically derived methods of documenting the shape and appearance of the optic disc the role of clinical examination is still important. It is therefore necessary for the clinician to master the ability to examine the optic disc using several different techniques.

Direct ophthalmoloscopy

The classical method of the examination is the direct ophthalmoscope. This is the most universally available and portable instrument to examine the optic disc and it provides a direct, magnified, monocular view of the optic disc. The lack of stereoscopic view is the greatest drawback of this technique. Further limitations are the relative smallness of the field of view and their relatively poor image quality that can result from minor opacities in the media and a poorly dilated pupil.

The technique requires that the subject should have pupils that are fully dilated using short-term dilating agents such as tropicamide 1 per cent, phenylephrine 2.5 or 10 per cent, or cyclopentolate 1 per cent. The subject should be seated in a room with subdued lighting and asked to fix on an object straight in front of them at the same height as their head. The examiner's head should approach the subject at the same height with the beam of the ophthalmoloscope angled approximately 15° towards the nasal side. The examiner should ensure that the subject is encouraged to fix straight ahead during this procedure and is encouraged to do so. The focus of the ophthalmoscope should be set to approximately the spherical equivalent of the patient's refractive error with a suitable compensation for the observer's refractive error as well. This should enable a reasonable image to be obtained immediately and further adjustment of the ophthalmoscope's focus can be achieved whilst observing the subject's optic disc or retina. Occasionally, if the observer is highly ametropic they may wish to continue to wear their spectacle correction during the procedure.

The optic disc is observed using an illuminating beam which is ideally smaller than the optic disc. This allows better dynamic imaging and decreases the amount of glare caused by reflections and media opacities. The observation process is usually a dynamic one with small movements of the ophthalmoscope and the observer's head. During this process the optic disc is observed with particular reference to its shape and colour, and the course of the blood vessels. Movement of the ophthalmoscope allows shadows to be created, thus further informing the observer of the topography of the optic nerve head. A combination of these factors allows the observer to construct in their mind an approximation of the three-dimensional shape of the optic nerve head from the two-dimensional observation that has been made. The observations are then recorded by drawing.

Stereobiomicroscopy

One of the most precise methods of examining the optic disc is with stereo biomicroscopy using a slit lamp and a high dioptre plus lens, (usually +90 or +78 dioptres). The lens is held between 1 and 2 cm away from the patient's eye and the slit lamp assembly usually has to be moved backwards from its normal focused position on the anterior segment for an image to be obtained. Once the red reflex is seen, the slit lamp is then moved to allow a focused image of the retina and optic disc. To facilitate accurate imaging of the optic disc the patient can be asked to fixate the non-examined eye slightly temporally. A magnified stereoscopic image of the optic disc can be obtained in this manner. A further advantage is that some degree of media opacity can be overcome by this system.

The main disadvantage of the technique is that the observer has to remember that the image obtained is both upside down and reversed right to left. However, with practice most observers are able to compensate for this phenomenon automatically. A further possible disadvantage is that good pupil dilatation is required for best stereoscopic images although examining lenses are available with small apertures which are specifically designed to overcome this problem.

Recording the image

It is important that the clinician accurately records an interpretation of the appearance of the optic disc gleaned by clinical examination. Although it is well recognized that clinicians assess the appearance of optic nerves differently, it is useful for salient points of an examination to be noted. In particular, drawings of the optic discs are much more useful than approximations of cup to disc ratio. Important features that need to be noted are as follows:

- the shape of the optic disc with particular relevance to the width of the neuroretinal rim

- the depth and dimensions of the cup

- the position of the blood vessels

- the colour of the neuroretinal rim and disc

- the nature of the peripapillary region.

- the presence of optic disc haemorrhages

- any asymmetry between the two optic discs.

Optic disc photography

Photographic records have the clear advantage of providing an objective image of the optic disc. However, a fundus camera is required to produce an image. These cameras usually require a well-dilated pupil and clear media. There are cameras that can be used without mydriasis although there usefulness in optic disc recording is limited. Optic disc pictures are obtained using colour reversal film. Care has to be taken when observing sequential films due to differences in magnification between different fundus cameras and also the colour values of different photographs.

Of potentially more use is stereophotography. Most fundus cameras are able to create pseudostereo pairs by changing the horizontal position of the camera between two photographs thus creating a stereo separation. However, this technique is limited in that the separation may not always be reproducible and the patient's eye may move during the process.

More accurate systems have been devised. An Allen separator can be inserted into the light path of a standard fundus camera producing more reproducible stereo separation although as this still involves sequential photography it does not overcome the problem of eye movement.

A more satisfactory result can be obtained by simultaneous stereo cameras which use a fixed angle image splitting device which allows two images of the optic disc to be made on the same exposure of a 35 mm film frame. This guarantees the reproducibility of stereo separation. The only disadvantage of the system is that the field of view is more limited.

Interpretation of photographic results

The interpretation of the photographic results can be more than subjective. Numerous techniques have been described for standardizing photography and then interpreting it using either planimetry or stereo photogrammetry.

Planimetary involves using stereo photographs and tracing the disc and neuroretinal rim margin usually using digitizing computer-based equipment. The results are then interpreted in a two-dimensional way producing measurement of disc area, cup, and neuroretinal rim areas as well as various dimensional parameters such as cup to disc ratio.

Stereo photogrammetry utilizes stereo photographic pairs and a topographic mapping device to produce a three-dimensional image of the optic disc. This can then be interpreted in three dimensions thus giving value not only for areas but also for cup depth and volume.

Whilst these techniques are capable of producing significant useful information they suffer from several drawbacks. In particular, they require experienced operators to trace optic nerve features manually thus leading to interobserver variations. They also require magnification correction for the patient's refractive error and apparatus used. These techniques have found some role in research but have not enjoyed widespread clinical acceptance.

The desire for standardized numerical data on optic disc morphology has resulted in the development of several different systems which attempt to automatically analyse the three-dimensional nature of the optic nerve head. These are the

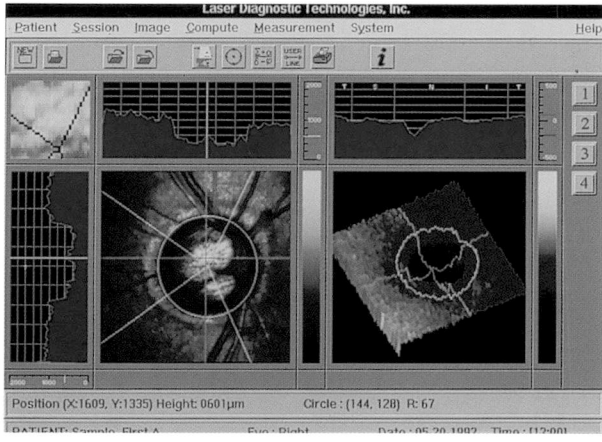

Fig. 3 Computer reconstruction of data produced from a scanning laser ophthalmoscope allows a three-dimensional reconstruction of optic nerve head topgraphy.

Humphrey retinal analyser, the Rodenstock optic nerve head analyser, and the Topcon image analyser. All these technologies rely on photographic techniques and subsequent image disparity analysis of various different forms, with digital image acquisition and computer-aided analysis. However, they all suffer problems from image degradation caused by ocular abnormality, eye movements problems, and require some degree of pupil dilatation. Similarly, they also rely to some degree on operator-dependent choices.

More recently scanning laser ophthalmoscopy has been seen as the emerging technology for optic nerve head analysis. The scanning laser ophthalmoscope relies on the confocal scanning principal in which only the particular plane of scanning is in focus. The scanning laser ophthalmoscope takes a series of 32 digitized images at different focal planes. These images are then computer reconstructed to provide a three-dimensional image of the optic disc (Fig. 3). This image can then be used to investigate the topographic nature of the optic disc. Several manufacturers now make such devices. Images of the optic nerve can be produced through undilated pupils and with some degree of media opacity. However, the images are susceptible to patient eye movement, refractive error, and to some degree to operator experience. The best use of numerical data produced by the system is still to be decided. Various two-dimensional parameters such as cup to disc ratio can be useful in the diagnosis of glaucoma but other more sophisticated analysis using true three-dimensional data such as analysis of the optic disc cup shape show more promise. Whilst initial experience with these instruments is highly encouraging their role in the diagnosis and monitoring of glaucoma still remains to be confirmed.

Nerve fibre layer evaluation

Evaluation of the retinal nerve fibre layer is often useful in detecting early glaucoma. It allows the detection of damage to the nerve fibre layer before it is apparent at the optic disc margin. Whilst the presence of wedge-shaped defects in the nerve fibre layer can often be observed, a more generalized decrease in nerve fibre layer thickness is much more difficult to detect, thus limiting the usefulness of the technique.

The nerve fibre layer is best observed using either the red-free light of the direct ophthalmoscope or of the slit lamp combined with 78- or 90-dioptre lens. The most useful images are often obtained using either the slit function of the direct ophthalmoscope or a fairly narrow slit using the slit lamp. The nerve fibre layer can then be quite clearly observed with the normal distribution of thickened bundles suprotemporally and inferotemporally. Nerve fibre layer defects appear as wedge-shaped darkenings in an overall bright nerve fibre layer bundle.

The main difficulty experienced by most observers is a tendency to overdiagnose the presence of defects. Small slit-like defects in the nerve fibre layer are common and not diagnostic of glaucoma. True defects should be wedge shaped in profile thus reflecting the Purkinje distribution of the nerve fibre bundle. They should also have a width at the optic disc edge greater than the diameter of a first-order arteriole.

Photographic methods using red-free light and black and white film is also useful in detecting nerve fibre layer defects. A good quality wide field image is required as are careful photographic developing techniques to produce a sufficient amount of contrast for the nerve fibre layer defects to be seen.

Quantitative imaging of the nerve fibre layer

Whilst the technique of examining the nerve fibre layer for wedge defects can be extremely useful, particularly in diagnosing early glaucoma, it is clinically difficult to evaluate the nerve fibre in advanced glaucoma and to observe any progressive changes. This difficulty has been addressed to some extent by the development of two further methods of nerve fibre layer assessment.

The nerve fibre analyser relies on the polarizing nature of the nerve fibre layer. Using this phenomenon a computer-aided device can measure the thickness of the nerve fibre layer at different points around the optic nerve. The image produced appears similar to that seen in red-free photography but carries with it quantitative data concerning the thickness of nerve fibre layer. Optical coherence tomography directly measures the thickness of the retina using optical means. Variations in the optical properties of the retina allow the nerve fibre layer thickness to be assessed. These new methods of nerve fibre layer investigation are of considerable interest in that they provide quantitative information but their role in generalized clinical practice is as yet uncertain.

Further reading

Airaksenen, P.J., Tuulonen, A., and Werner, E.B. (1996). Clinical evaluation of the optic disc and retinal fibre layer. In *The glaucomas*, (ed. R. Ritch, M.B. Shields, and T. Krupin). Mosby, St Louis.

Freidenwald, J.S. (1957). Tonometer calibration: an attempt to remove discrepancies found in the 1954 calibration scale for Schiotz tonometers. *Transactions of the American Academy of Ophthalmology and Otolaringology*, **61**, 108.

Jonas, J.B. and Dichtl, A. (1996). Evaluation of the retinal nerve fiber layer. *Survey of Ophthalmology*, **40**, 369.

Whitacre, M.M. and Stein, R. (1993). Sources of error with use of Goldmann-type tonometers. *Survey of Ophthalmology*, **38**, 1.

2.10.5.2 Fields and other visual function tests

William E. Sponsel

Definition and aetiology of glaucomatous visual loss

In glaucoma, discrete bundles of ganglion cell axons cease to transmit visual information to the lateral geniculate body via the optic nerve. Once the outer retina has processed spatial form and motion from photoreceptor stimuli, visual information is transmitted semi-selectively by two broad subclasses of ganglion cell. One class (parvocellular) predominantly transmits information from small retinal receptive fields, and the other (magnocellular) from larger receptive fields. The ganglion cell axons of the magnocellular pathway, which tend to conduct visual input from larger or faster moving stimuli, may appear to be selectively lost early in the glaucomatous disease process.

A proportion of this damage may be transient, but in chronic glaucoma the majority of neural loss is typically irreversible. As the disease proceeds, compromised ganglion cells are ultimately lost, along with their supporting oligodendrogliocytes, producing characteristic cupping of the optic nerve head. In very advanced disease, selective axonal loss may be visualized ophthalmoscopically to correspond with areas of visual field loss (most typically an inferotemporal notch on the nerve corresponding with extensive superior visual field loss perimetrically). Such gross clinicopathological associations are not typically seen, however, in the earlier stages of glaucoma. Minimal disc asymmetry may be associated with substantial visual field asymmetry, or vice versa, in mild to moderate glaucoma. It is thus imperative that the clinician develop the ability to elicit subtle details of clinical relevance from both the ophthalmoscopic and perimetric examination, in order to detect and treat this complex group of diseases appropriately.

Diagnostic issues

Traditionally, glaucoma has been defined as the coexistence of at least two of three clinical signs: characteristic nerve-fibre bundle visual field loss, optic nerve head cupping, and raised intraocular pressure. Pathological definitions for each of these signs vary, but disease prevalence has typically been found to be approximately 2 per cent among individuals of Northern European descent, and around 8 per cent among adults of African heritage.

The inclusion of intraocular pressure as an equally weighted diagnostic parameter alongside visual fields and disc assessment has produced an interesting bias historically, affecting prevalence data, referral criteria, clinical practice patterns, and applied research. Tonometry has always been the easiest of the three diagnostic modalities to execute, followed by optic disc assessment, and visual field testing, in that order. Population screening at the primary care level has thus been based predominantly on pressure testing. This has led to a tendency to evaluate suspects with higher eye pressures, and to perform visual fields only on those with high pressure and visible glaucomatous optic nerve changes. Such practices, along with a presumption that the only therapeutic advantage that can be offered to glaucoma sufferers is pressure reduction, have placed glaucoma diagnosis and all related clinical research in a quagmire from which we are only now emerging. Objective large-scale studies which have taken account of all three traditional diagnostic variables have shown that a majority of individuals with coexisting disc cupping and field loss do not have elevated eye pressure. Moreover, such studies have verified that the vast majority of individuals who do have pressures over 21 mmHg have neither disc nor visual field damage. Thus, while visual field loss and optic nerve change are both quite good indicators of glaucomatous ganglion cell damage, intraocular pressure quite obviously is not.

How can this be, given our knowledge that raised eye pressure is a major risk factor for glaucomatous damage? The key to diagnostic utility for any test is its specificity (that is, its ability to discern normality), since, by definition, diseases of clinical interest are relatively rare among healthy people. A diagnostic test must be applicable to the majority of individuals with the disease in order to be worthwhile, and must incorrectly infer pathology among normal subjects as infrequently as possible. Tonometry has a nearly perfect diagnostic specificity for detecting glaucomatous optic nerve damage once intraocular pressure exceeds 40 mmHg (central retinal diastolic blood pressure), but 98 per cent of glaucomatous eyes never attain such high pressures. As the cut-off pressure level for 'diagnosis' is reduced, the 'true positive' rate (sensitivity) increases linearly but the yield of false positives increases exponentially. Thus, a conservative intraocular pressure cut-off of 24 mmHg, while segregating fewer than half of those in the tested population who have glaucomatous neural damage into the screening failure group, will at the same time inappropriately fail 30 times as many individuals who have no other evidence of disease.

Long-term follow-up studies show that very few of these visually normal ocular hypertensives will ever develop glaucoma. Nevertheless, costly clinical resources have long been devoted to following such individuals, while neglecting the large proportion of the diseased population that such illogical screening practices have missed. 'Normal tension glaucoma' therefore has typically not been seen by the ophthalmologist until sufficient damage has occurred to both the optic nerve and visual field to produce significant visual symptoms, leading to the generalized assumption that glaucoma without high pressure is a peculiar, rapidly progressive, occult process. This does not appear to be the case. Population studies indicate that visual field loss and disc damage associated with normal tension glaucoma is present in early, moderate, and severe forms, following a distribution similar to that seen among higher pressure glaucomas.

Failure to detect mild to moderate normal tension glaucoma (which may account for a majority of extant disease) is an inev-itable consequence of our historic over-reliance on non-specific and non-sensitive detection methods which have effectively excluded such disease from consideration. This realization has prompted North America's largest glaucoma screening organization, Prevent Blindness America, to adopt strict new standards for all future screenings, disallowing the use of tonometry in isolation, and requiring the use of an evaluated and approved visual field test as a component of all adult vision screenings. This new policy has been endorsed by leading glaucoma specialists across the United States.

Glaucoma should ideally be detected and treated long before a diseased individual is consciously aware of visual loss, which usually occurs once sensitivity to light is significantly diminished in corresponding visual retinal zones of both eyes, compromising binocular daylight vision. Success in isolating glaucomatous disease while it remains asymptomatic rests on our ability to perform appropriate visual function tests which are standardized, rapid, and which have good sensitivity and specificity. On these grounds, from today's perspective, the most important contribution to glaucoma diagnosis since the development of ophthalmoscopy has been the introduction of computer-assisted perimetry.

Background to perimetry

Perimetry, as its name implies, involves measuring peripheral vision. All forms of perimetry attempt to create a contour map of light sensitivity over a defined portion of the field of vision, which corresponds inversely in space with an associated area of the retina. Visual fields are typically tested one eye at a time, using illuminated stimuli on a darker background. Stimulus luminosity, size, duration, and degree of contrast with the background are all important determinants of minimal perimetric light perception, or threshold, for a given location within the visual field. In healthy eyes, light sensitivity is greatest centrally, and decreases logarithmically in all directions towards the visual periphery. The ora serrata and optic nerve intraocularly, and the nose, brow, and eyelids extraocularly, define absolute margins to the visual field (Fig. 1), which may therefore extend to almost 90° temporally, but only 60° nasally and superiorly, in normal subjects. A scotoma is an area of visual field with decreased sensitivity within these limits. The universal scotoma or 'physiological blind spot', corresponding to the optic nerve head, is approximately 10° in diameter, centred approximately 15° temporal to the centre of vision.

While ideally testing visual integrity within the above-defined anatomical bounds, perimetry is in fact a complex subjective test of the oculocerebromotor systems. Like all psychophysical tests, perimetry is subject to the compliance and awareness of both the subject and the technician carrying out testing. A learning effect exists, so performance on automated perimetry typically improves even in normal subjects over the first three sets of visual fields tested in each eye. Physiological factors, particularly pharmacologically induced differences in pupil diameter, or time allowed for dark adaptation, may produce substantial variations in visual field response for the same individual under otherwise identical testing conditions. Vari-

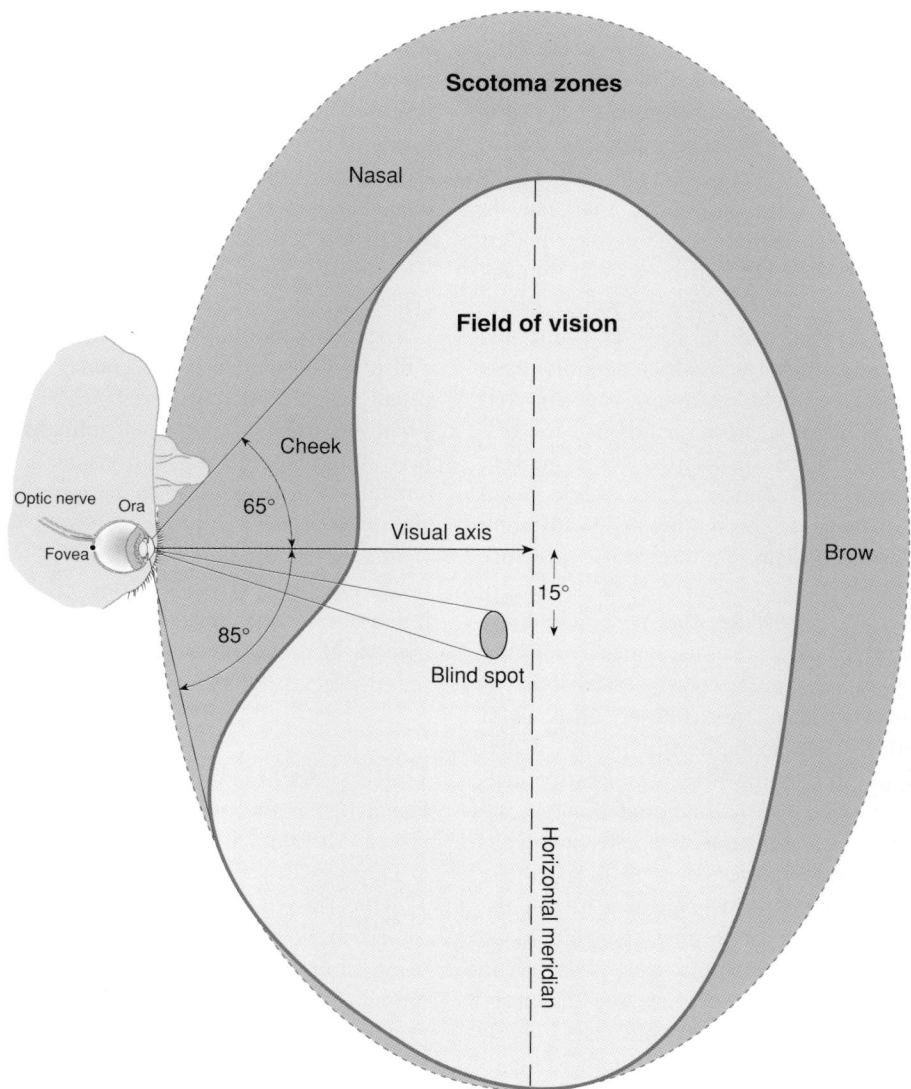

Fig. 1 Field of vision of the right eye, face forward, looking down at a desktop with the left eye covered. Note the relationship of the physiological blind spot to the visual axis, consistent with the 15° nasal displacement of the optic nerve from the fovea. The potentially round (in this case, obliquely oval owing to the angle of view) outer limit of vision is only realized temporally, since anatomical facial features produce peripheral scotomas in all other directions.

ations in room lighting may produce a similar confounding effect. Eyelid closure (rapid blinking or sustained fatigue) or ptosis may diminish the visual field in a manner unrelated to the glaucomatous disease process, producing confusing artefacts on the perimetric trace. Poor refraction, tearing, corneal disease, cataract, and vitreous opacities may also absorb or scatter light, producing potentially confusing visual field changes. Retinal scars, coloboma, and retinal degenerative disease may also mimic glaucomatous visual field defects. Optic nerve head drusen and ischaemic optic neuropathy can produce segmental ganglion cell axon lesions indistinguishable from those seen in glaucoma. Careful and thorough clinical examination is thus critical to proper interpretation of visual fields.

Normal eye movements (microsaccades) or major deviations of the eye or head may destroy the relationship between retina and peripheral field being mapped at any time during visual field testing. The combination of microsaccades and so-called 'angioscotomas' (blood vessels, most commonly adjacent to the optic nerve, which absorb light before it reaches peripapillary photoreceptors) ensure that the blind spot which is mapped perimetrically appears more irregular in shape than the corresponding optic nerve head (Fig. 2). Loss of central fixation during testing can result in a lower than expected sensitivity in one area while producing an area of greater sensitivity than is actually present elsewhere in the visual field.

The following are thus prerequisites to good perimetry.

1. Ensure that the individual carrying out perimetric testing is familiar with the method and goals of testing

2. Ensure that best corrected refraction is in place, with minimal room light and no variable external (especially window) light

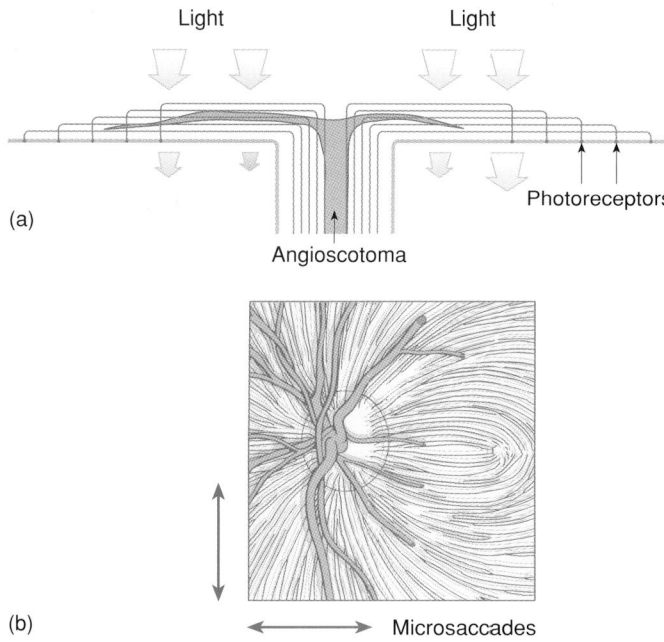

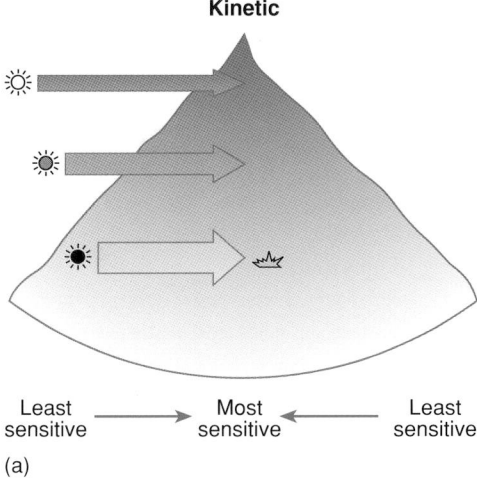

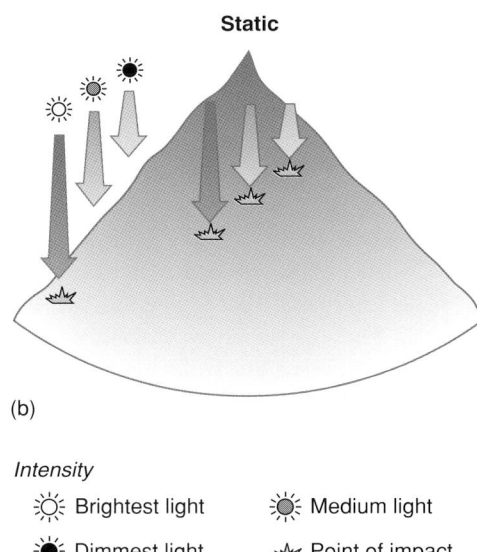

Fig. 2 There are two reasons why light sensitivity near the optic nerve (i.e. adjacent to the physiological blind spot) appears to be highly variable in normal eyes. (a) Branches of the central retinal vein and artery, which are highly concentrated near the disc, actually filter and scatter light before it can reach normal photoreceptors, producing an 'angioscotoma'. (b) Small rotary excursions of the eye (microsaccades) are inevitable during testing in normal subjects, effectively moving the disc and hence the blind spot around despite apparently excellent fixation. Thus, even though neural loss is frequently concentrated near the optic nerve in glaucoma patients, the diagnostic specificity of classic 'baring the blind spot' as an early finding is surprisingly low.

3. Optimize patient awareness and compliance by explaining the goals of testing and proper response technique

4. Establish appropriate neutral, stable head position to minimize brow and ptosis artefacts and discourage head movement

5. Document pupil diameter carefully, and encourage good fixation during testing.

Continuity of testing conditions between visits is essential for meaningful assessment of visual field change over time. Patients receiving miotic eye-drops provide an important clinical logistic challenge, since pupils of 2.5 mm diameter or less tend to produce artefactual visual field constriction, and depression of light sensitivity centrally. Miotic patients should be dilated sufficiently on each occasion before undergoing perimetry, with the knowledge that variations in pupil diameter and accommodation which accompany pharmacological mydriasis can produce variable visual field responses. Conversely, for most non-miosed patients undergoing clinical assessment, pharmacological dilation (for stereo disc assessment or photography) can be deferred until after perimetry has been performed, since the quality and reproducibility of non-dilated fields may actually exceed those of dilated fields

Fig. 3 There are two ways to map three-dimensional visual fields, which both quantify the varying light sensitivity of the eye in a fixed viewing area. (a) Light stimuli of various fixed intensities are brought into the field of vision from many directions, all of which are perpendicular to the direction of gaze. The circumlinear contour lines connecting points of equivalent light sensitivity so obtained are called 'isopters' (iso, same; pter, wing). Because the targets presented radially actually move, the technique is known as 'kinetic perimetry'. (b) Light stimuli at predefined fixed locations can be flashed briefly. Bright lights will be seen through the entire field in normal eyes, but very dim lights will only be seen near the more sensitive central macular zone. Because the stimuli do not move, this technique is known as 'static perimetry'.

for such individuals. This practice has the added advantage of balancing demand for the perimeter throughout the clinical session in a busy glaucoma clinic, avoiding a late afternoon 'perimetry bottleneck'.

Kinetic versus static perimetry

The field of vision can be quantified either by providing stimuli of variable size or intensity in a moving (kinetic) (Fig. 3(a)) or fixed (static) (Fig. 3(b)) manner. The present discussion is intended to clarify the current role of each method.

Kinetic perimetry

Kinetic perimetry, is largely limited to the manually operated hemispheric Goldmann bowl perimeter, although recently several companies (Humphrey, Kowa, and Optikon) have introduced automated kinetic perimeters modelled after the Goldmann perimeter. This device has been a mainstay of glaucoma and neuro-ophthalmology clinics for over 50 years, and in many regards still retains its role as the gold standard for perimetric testing. The Goldmann 30-cm radius bowl has a background luminance of 10 cd/m^2. A recording sheet with a centripetal array of reference circles and radii for mapping the field is affixed behind the bowl, and the perimetrist moves an external light projector in correspondence with sweeping or fixed movements of a hand-held wand over the recording sheet. The subject, seated in an erect posture with chin and forehead secured on moveable rests, views the bowl with the tested eye positioned at the bowl's diametric centre, the fellow eye patched. The brightness of the projected stimulus can be modulated with grey A filters (designated by subscript Arabic numerals 3, 2, and 1, in order of increasing absorption). Modulated intensities relative to the unshielded projection light are 3.15 per cent for filter 1; 10 per cent for filter 2; 31.5 per cent for filter 3; and 100 per cent (i.e. no modulation) for 4. An additional set of auxiliary B (a, 40 per cent; b, 50 per cent; c, 63 per cent; d, 80 per cent; and e, 100 per cent intensity) filters may also be interposed, producing further light attenuation, if desired. These extra filters are rarely used, and the small letter e as a suffix to the Goldmann luminance setting confirms that the supplemental filters have not been employed. Stimulus size can also be adjusted on a base-4 scale using Roman numerals, where II equals a 1 mm^2 round object on the bowl face; size III is a 4 mm^2 object; size IV 16 mm^2; and size V 64 mm^2. Smaller stimuli are size 0, 1/16 mm^2; and size I, 1/4 mm^2. Hence, using a maximal luminance of 318 cd/m^2 against a 10 cd/m^2 background, the Goldmann perimeter allows testing of a luminance range from 10 000 asb (the brightness of a full moon on a clear night) to the least visible stimulus of 0.008 asb, a 10^6 range.

The Goldmann perimeter is particularly useful in monitoring visual field loss in patients with very advanced glaucoma, since testing of severely diminished visual fields with static perimetry can be inordinately time-consuming. Kinetic Goldmann perimetry takes little longer for such individuals than do normal fields. Kinetic fields are also valuable for following patients who have problems complying with automated testing. Well-performed kinetic visual field testing is usually less erratic than static testing, giving a reliable indication of visual field stability or progression. Kinetic fields are, however, typically less useful in detecting early disease than are static fields, and consistency depends on having the same well-trained and highly motivated perimetrist perform each field on a given patient. Failure to employ the same testing parameters on successive visits is a frequent confounding problem which greatly diminishes the utility of a patient's perimetric record, even where a continuity of skilled technical assistance is available. Erratic organization of paper perimetric traces in the clinical record may further restrict the clinician's ability to interpret visual field changes.

In Goldmann kinetic perimetry, a contour map of the hill of vision is produced by bringing stimuli in from beyond the field of vision towards the centre of vision along each of 24 15° radii (see Fig. 2). The stimulus should be moved inward at a rate of only 2° per second, and should be introduced along different radii in a random, unpredictable pattern to encourage central fixation. The subject responds by pressing a buzzer when the light is seen, at which point the examiner should turn off the stimulus, mark the perimetry trace sheet with a recognizable symbol corresponding to the test stimulus in use, and reposition the wand. Brighter, larger stimuli (i.e. V$_4$e) define the outer extremity (the 'coastline' of the island of vision in the sea of blindness), producing the largest isopter. Smaller, dimmer stimuli (i.e. I$_2$e) are typically not perceived until the light has advanced to within 30° of fixation, and are small and dim enough to be used to map the blind spot and other pericentral scotomas. Each isopter should be clearly labelled (not merely colour coded) in order to facilitate interpretation of visual fields which might be photocopied or faxed between clinical centres. A complete glaucoma field would typically include I$_1$e, I$_2$e, I$_3$e, I$_4$e, and III$_4$e (or V$_4$e) isopters.

Absolute or relative scotomas within each isopter are systematically sought by presenting static stimuli of greater luminance within the confines of each mapped isopter. Glaucomatous defects are characterized by two important geographic characteristics: (a) they respect the horizontal meridian; and (b) they follow an arcuate pattern. This is because the 1.2 million ganglion cell axons comprising the optic nerve are segregated along the horizontal raphe into superior and inferior major bundles which do not intermingle, and which arch into the optic nerve. The most commonly seen nerve fibre bundle defects in glaucoma (Fig. 4) include the Bjerrum scotoma, Seidel scotoma, nasal step, baring of the blind spot, and generalized depression (concentric loss).

Static perimetry

Static perimetry involves the generation of non-moving stimuli at preordained locations throughout the visual field. Static testing forms the basis for most computed perimetry, and is now by far the most widely employed method for glaucoma detection and monitoring. Static perimetry does not necessarily require computerization, and may, for example be performed manually on the Goldmann perimeter. One such technique involves the mapping of a single static profile along a predetermined meridian to assess the proximity of a severe visual field defect to the fovea. Various static test charts exist which lend themselves well to detecting moderate to severe glaucoma, particularly the Damato campimeter, which has recently been adopted by screening organizations throughout the world. Another manual method, the venerable Bjerrum screen, remains particularly useful for the rapid detection of factitious visual field loss. Early non-automated static perimeters are also occasionally seen in modern clinics and continue to have their advocates, but all are destined to be replaced by computer-assisted automated devices.

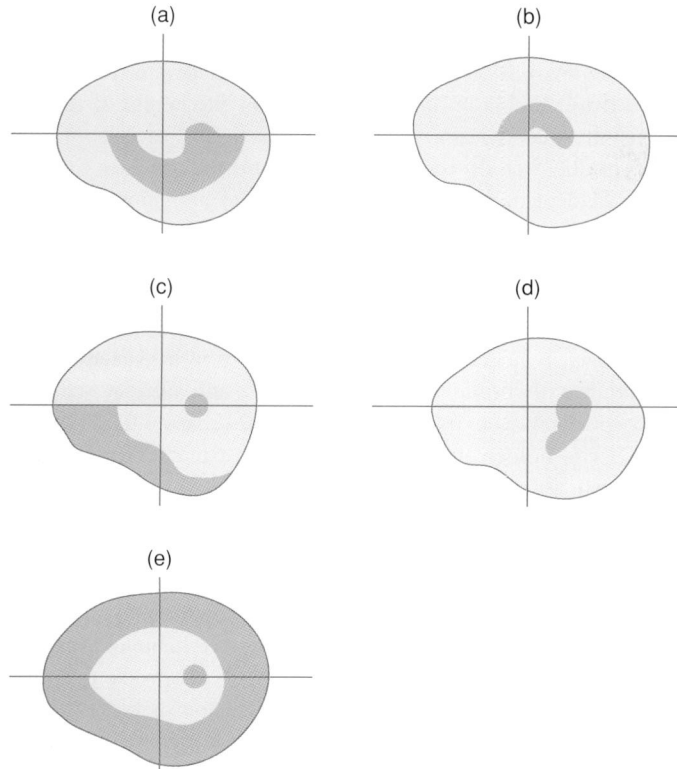

Fig. 4 Classical glaucomatous field loss patterns as seen on right-eye Goldmann kinetic perimetric testing. Configurations of common nerve-fibre layer visual field defects (scotomata). (a) Bjerrum scotoma, (b) Seidel scotoma, (c) nasal step, (d) baring of the blind spot, and (e) generalized depression (concentric loss).

A complete review of the wide array of computer-assisted static perimetry instruments currently available is beyond the scope of this chapter, but an understanding of their general principles and differences is important. Each static perimeter incorporates testing strategies which exploit one of each of the following dichotomous characteristics: (a) projection versus fixed stimulus; (b) bowl versus flat screen; (c) single versus multiple stimulus; (d) central versus oculokinetic fixation; (e) external stimulus versus transpupillary (direct fundus) presentation; (f) full threshold versus suprathreshold testing; and (g) conventional versus complex stimuli.

The most popular composite is a projection bowl, single conventional stimulus, centrally fixating, full thresholding perimeter, like the Humphrey field analyser, Octopus, Dicon, Kowa, Optikon, or Topcon. These machines each have unique software features, but only the first three have incorporated an extensive normative database against which to compare presumptive pathological fields. The Humphrey has rapidly become the predominant instrument in clinics across North America, and has gained prominence elsewhere throughout the world. A greater diversity of instruments is seen throughout Europe, with the Octopus retaining a significant market share.

While many testing computer programs are offered, the more standard tests in widespread use assess the central 24 or 30° using a 6° square grid. Full threshold testing can be carried

out across the entire Goldmann luminance range, usually using a stimulus size equivalent to that of the Goldmann III (i.e. 4 mm^2). Light attenuation is measured in increments related to the brightest Goldmann stimulus (10 000 asb) by an ascending logarithmic (decibel) scale, from 0 (i.e. no attenuation; 10 000 asb) to 40 dB (10 000-fold attenuation, or 1 asb). Thus, 10 dB equals 10-fold attenuation (i.e. 1000 asb), 20 dB equals 100-fold attenuation (i.e. 100 asb), and 30 dB equals 1000-fold attenuation (i.e. 10 asb). A typical normal central 30° visual field would reveal central (foveolar) threshold values less than 40 dB, pericentral thresholds around 30 dB, and peripheral thresholds around 20 dB.

Early glaucomatous fields commonly show (a) asymmetry between the threshold values in corresponding locations of the upper and lower hemifield of each eye; and (b) clustered zones of threshold depression wherein two or more contiguous stimuli are depressed 5 dB or more relative to surrounding values. Statistical software features such as the Humphrey StatPac, Octosoft/Octosmart, or Dicon Field View assist the clinician in the assessment of subtle visual field changes, providing a range of indices which quantify the patient's compliance with testing, intrinsic variation, and the statistical significance of focal and global changes in the visual field. Grey scale plots allow visualization of threshold variation and permit rapid assessments of change over time in a highly organized format.

Fundamentals of automated perimetry

The principles of good perimetry described above are just as critical to success in automated perimetry as with the more labour-intensive traditional manual techniques. Computed perimeters will carry out testing to completion regardless of the attentiveness of the technician or patient, and printed output is produced every time. The clinician should be keenly aware of this fact, and must have the ability to identify tell-tale signs of poor testing compliance and make appropriate mental adjustments in interpreting suboptimal fields, preferably remedying such deficiencies immediately wherever possible by ordering repeat fields. Classic faults alluded to earlier include poor fixation, excessive miosis, and poor refraction. Fixation is commonly monitored using the Heijl/Krakau method, in which light stimuli are periodically presented within the previously mapped physiological blind-spot zone. If the subject does not see the light, fixation is presumed to have been properly maintained. This method works well provided there is adequate initial mapping of the blind spot, good maintenance of head position throughout testing, and, most importantly, a comparatively normal peripapillary visual field. Fixation losses are displayed as a fraction on the perimetric data sheet, indicating the number of times the blind spot was seen over the number of times it was presented. Beware that any patient with advanced field damage may produce a very low fixation loss numerator, suggestive of good compliance, because most of their field is a blind spot, and they are thus unlikely to hit the response button during blind spot monitoring regardless of their direction of gaze.

Another typical error is referred to as the false positive response, a conditioned Pavlovian tendency to hit the response button when no light or light too dim to be seen in a specific region based on previous testing is presented. Such responses upset calculations of focal variation in light sensitivity, and contribute to the variability quotient known as short-term fluctuation. Conversely, a false negative response is deemed to have occurred when a previously mapped visual locus is retested and found to have a significantly lower threshold (i.e. require much brighter stimulus illumination) than on initial testing. False negative responses, which also contribute to short-term fluctuation, may actually arise as part of the pathological process of glaucoma as a consequence of neural fatigue, but may also reflect inattention or lid interference. Fixation loss and false positive responses are thus the two best indicators of compliance in most glaucomatous fields.

Some subjects try to 'outwit' the test, or may respond to intraretinal phosphene flashes. Their Pavlovian button pushing tendency may produce fields with ridiculously high threshold values in all zones. Conversely, other patients may fail to appreciate the need to respond to relatively dim peripheral stimuli as well as apparently brighter central stimuli, producing an artefactually very small concentric field. Such individuals, who at first glance may be presumed to have grossly advanced glaucomatous field loss or even retinitis pigmentosa, can be quickly re-evaluated by simple confrontation testing and are often found to have quite normal peripheral vision! Aphakic spectacles or high-plus hyperopic correction produce a prismatic effect which can also generate artefactually constricted concentric fields. The presence of a horizontal demarcation line in the superior field is usually evidence of ptosis or fatigue, and can be rectified by repeating the visual field test with the brow taped to the forehead. Dense ring scotomas which fall inside areas of apparently normal peripheral vision are frequently the result of a malpositioned lens holder.

Quantifying visual field loss

As discussed above, visual field depression in glaucoma reflects the segmental loss of ganglion cell axons, which project separate arcuate bundles into the optic nerve from the superior and inferior hemiretina. Static visual fields will reflect the same gross pathological features seen on kinetic perimetry, although it should be borne in mind that the diameter of the field being tested statically is usually much smaller. Once severe field loss has occurred, it is useful to decrease the field size even further, from the standard 24 or 30° radius 6° grid, to one of 10° on a 1° matrix. Such tests, like the Humphrey 10-2, have largely supplanted meridional Goldmann testing for patients at risk of losing foveolar function (splitting fixation). Unfortunately, at first glance the round grey scale plot of a 10° field with dense concentric loss looks remarkably similar to that of a 30° field, since the peripheral graticule lines demarcating field size are largely obliterated by the black pericentral scotoma. Testing strategies, including stimulus size, field diameter, plus important reliability indices, date, pupil diameter, and patient identification and age, are usually displayed at the top of the computer print-out, and can be obscured beneath the metal binders of a thick hospital or clinic chart. Since these data are vital, the clinician must be willing to remove fields from such records and organize them in a manner which facilitates logical interpretation.

Glaucomatous field loss is characterized two ways. Global (or diffuse) loss is uniform depression of the height of the hill of vision, reflected as concentric contraction of each isopter on a kinetic field or decrease of numeric threshold values across a static field print-out. Focal loss is isolated or regional depression in light sensitivity accompanying segmental axonal damage which can be discriminated from diffuse loss perimetrically (Fig. 5). While both forms of field loss are typically seen in glaucoma, the latter is the more reliable indicator. As stated previously, poor dark adaptation, variations in background illumination, suboptimal refraction, miosis, and nuclear sclerotic or cortical cataracts may all produce diffuse visual field depression. Lens holder artefacts and ptosis can mimic focal loss as discussed above, but these are more readily identifiable and remediable. Dense subcapsular cataracts and macular disease may also produce focal loss, but such geographical areas of visual field depression rarely respect the horizontal meridian and are usually obvious on clinical examination. Thus, focal rather than diffuse loss is usually the more reliable indicator of glaucomatous damage. Poor compliance can produce erratic fields with apparent zones of focal depression or pseudoelevation, but, again these rarely respect the horizontal meridian, and are usually accompanied by high fixation loss or false positive rates, and abnormally high short-term fluctuation.

Before the advent of automated perimetry, characterization of the severity of field loss was largely descriptive, with attempts at quantitation typically based upon the presence or absence of concentric loss, baring of the blind spot, nasal step, arcuate or altitudinal field loss, and so on. Although experienced clinicians could weigh up all these variables quite well in monitoring their own patients, attempts to use such features to produce numeric data which could be monitored in studies of antiglaucoma therapy were largely futile. This relegation of perimetry to the realm of clinical art rather than numeric science contributed to our historic dependence upon pressure in the diagnosis and treatment of glaucoma. Despite great advances in perimetric science, federal drug regulatory agencies are more interested in the ocular hypotensive effects of a proposed new antiglaucoma medication than in its visual protective effects. There is no logical reason for this situation to persist.

Numerical quantitation of field loss is now indeed a science, and much credit is owed the energetic efforts of the International Perimetric Society and its founders. The two standard measures of visual field survival, mean deviation and pattern deviation, are numerical estimates of global and focal field loss, respectively. Mean deviation (see Fig. 5(a)) reflects the overall height of the hill of vision relative to an age-related normal value, and pattern standard deviation (see Fig. 5(b)) the extent of irregularity existing within the hill of vision, regardless of its height. If the contribution of short-term fluctuation is factored out of the pattern standard deviation value, the resultant corrected pattern standard deviation provides an estimate of actual geographic irregularities (i.e. scotomas) within the hill of vision. These four values—mean deviation, pattern standard deviation, short-term fluctuation, and corrected pattern stand-

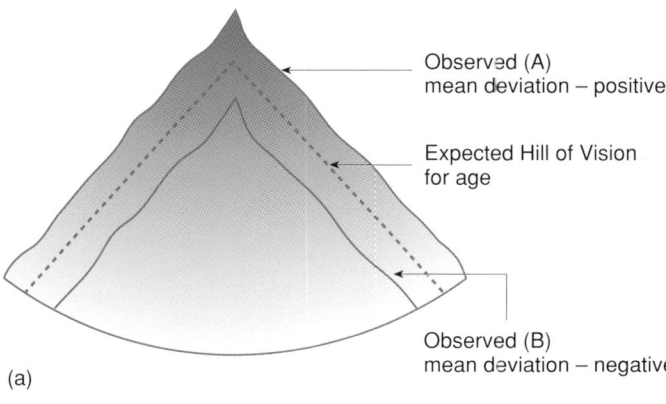

(a)

Observed (A)
mean deviation – positive

Expected Hill of Vision
for age

Observed (B)
mean deviation – negative

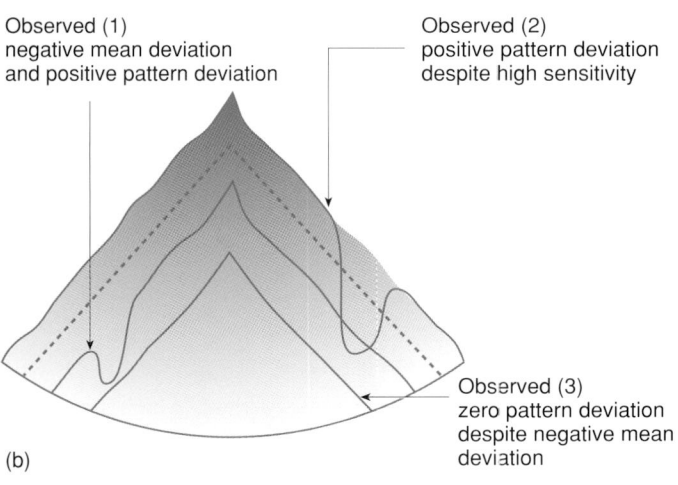

Observed (1)
negative mean deviation
and positive pattern deviation

Observed (2)
positive pattern deviation
despite high sensitivity

Observed (3)
zero pattern deviation
despite negative mean
deviation

(b)

Fig. 5 There are two important concepts in quantifying sensitivity to light, one seeking differences from the age-related normal hill of vision height (mean deviation) and another which looks for unexpected variations in the shape of the hill of vision, regardless of its height (pattern deviation). (a) A cross-section of the expected hill of vision and two others obtained by perimetric testing of two different patients. The higher profile field was from an eye able to see lights dimmer than anticipated across the whole field. Such a result might occur in very healthy subjects, or in individuals who are very dark-adapted, providing a positive mean deviation value. The lower profile might arise in a normal individual with inadequate dark adaptation prior to testing, diffuse cataract or corneal disease, or poor health (including glaucoma, diabetes, or renal disease). Negative mean deviation, without excluding these other causes, is of limited utility in diagnosing glaucoma. (b) A cross-section of the expected hill of vision and three others obtained by perimetric testing of three different patients. The first provides and example of what might occur in a typical glaucomatous eye, overall depression combined with a significant focal defect, which is a cross-section of an arcuate scotoma. This eye would have a negative mean deviation and a positive pattern deviation value. The second has a very high profile, but still exhibits a focal zone of depressed light sensitivity. This eye may well have profound neural loss but the patient would never have known had he not been placed in the dark and asked to respond to very dim lights, since his weakest visual area is still within the normal range. This eye would exhibit positive values for both mean deviation and pattern deviation. The last, like the lower profile in 5(a), is uniformly depressed. Despite having a lower overall sensitivity, this eye exhibits a normal profile, and its pattern deviation is therefore zero.

ard deviation—are known as the global indices, and their progression over time can be monitored graphically for individuals or groups of patients under treatment, facilitating clinical evaluation and objective research.

Numeric and grey-scale plots representing the statistical probability of normality for each specific locus stimulus response are displayed graphically. These are the same two-dimensional arrays of the data from which the global mean deviation and corrected pattern standard deviation values are derived, and can be very helpful in discerning the specific nature of field loss. Thus, widespread depression on the total deviation plot frequently indicates the presence of cataract or other media opacity. A scotoma within the depressed hill of vision, obscured by the cataract on the standard grey-scale plot, may stand out in isolation on the pattern deviation plot. An additional helpful indicator is the glaucoma hemifield test, which compares like zones in the upper and lower fields of the same eye to expose statistically significant altitudinal defects which may be obscured by other features. Ultimately, the clinician must become adroit at scanning the print-out to glean hints from all of these numerical and statistical indicators, but should reserve all assumptions about the field until the actual data, the raw numeric threshold plot, has been reviewed with care. Statistical plots may produce areas of apparent visual depression which are in fact areas of abnormally high retinal light sensitivity, for example. Finally, the fields of both eyes should be assessed side by side, since reproducibility parameters, blind-spot size, mean deviation, and so on are normally highly symmetric, and because neurological disorders are best appreciated on bilateral assessment. Gross differences between eyes at the first perimetric visit are common, and usually reflect a learning effect.

Grading of glaucomatous defects now exploits the utility of global indices as well as classic geographic features of nerve fibre layer damage. The ability to categorize field loss into pathological categories (normal, early, moderate, and severe) can greatly facilitate communication between clinicians, legal documentation, and applied research. One very useful system, proposed by Hodapp, Parrish, and Anderson, is provided in Table 1. This objective grading system has been successfully adapted for use in epidemiological studies, and has been shown to segregate fields into categories in a manner highly concordant with the subjective gradings of glaucoma experts.

Alternative methods of perimetry

As mentioned above in the earlier discussion of static perimetry, computer-assisted instruments each comprise a specific permutation of testing strategies. Most companies produce one or more instruments and programs, with at least one version mirroring the standard Humphrey or Octopus full-thresholding regimen. There are, however, potential advantages of other less conventional strategies that merit brief mention here. Stimuli may be presented directly from light-emitting diode incorporated into the bowl or screen of a perimeter, and many instruments use this approach, including the Henson, Kowa, Optifield, Peristat, and Tomey perimeters. Campimetry, using a flat screen rather than a bowl can decrease the size and expense of a visual field analyser, and such screens are sufficient for testing the central 25 to 30° at the standard working distance. If light-emitting diode stimuli are used, patterns of multiple stimuli can be presented simultaneously. Typically stimuli

Table 1 Humphrey visual field rating criteria

Category	Characteristics

Severe visual field loss	Mean defect worse than −12 dB, or
	On the pattern deviation plot
	  37 or more points depressed at or below 5%, or
	  20 or more points depressed at or below 1%, or
	One or more points in the central 5° at 0 dB, or
	Hemifield point pairs in central 5° at or below 15 dB

Moderate visual field loss	Mean defect between −12 and −6 dB, or
	On the pattern deviation plot
	  18 to 36 points depressed at or below 5%, or
	  10 to 19 points depressed at or below 1%, and
	No points in central 5° at 0 dB, and
	No hemifield pairs in central 5° at or below 15 dB

Early visual field loss	Mean defect greater than −6 dB, and
	On the pattern deviation plot
	  At least three arcuate depressed points, and
	  17 to seven points depressed at or below 5%, and
	  10 or fewer points depressed at or below 1%, and
	No points in the central 5° at 0 dB, and
	No hemifield pairs in central 5° at or below 15 dB

Non-pathological visual field	Defects do not meet early criteria

Adapted from Hodapp *et al.* 1993.

are presented in patterns of two, three, or four, with a maximum of one per quadrant. One such device which has gained favour in Europe and which has been used successfully in major epidemiological studies is the Henson central field analyser. Multiple stimulus perimetry has the advantage of being very rapid, encouraging central fixation, and allowing the use of an audible stimulus prior to each pattern presentation, since there are 16 permutations of response possible which cannot possibly be guessed. Strategies for identifying which stimuli have been seen or missed are various, including a four-button response system in the Marco perimeter, reminiscent of a pinball machine. Such methods present no problem for most patients and can be less tedious than single stimulus perimetry; often patients unable to comply with standard testing perform admirably with these less conventional methods. Flat screen campimetry with a moving fixation target (oculokinetic fixation) allows testing of the entire visual field, and one such device, which uses voice recognition software for recording patient responses, is produced by Dicon.

Fundus-related perimetry has been performed using fundus cameras for over 20 years, and entails directing stimuli at the retina through the pupil, producing a photograph of the posterior pole with isopteric margins demarcated by overexposure spots. Recently, a highly efficient variant of this concept, the Octopus 1-2-3 optometer, was introduced. Eliminating the need for a screen or bowl, this small, portable instrument performs familiar 30° perimetric testing strategies using transpupillary light presentation, employing an automated fixation monitor control system.

Mapping the absolute threshold for each point in the visual field is time-consuming. Short-cut methods which attempt to abbreviate the full-threshold mapping process by decreasing the number of times the threshold is passed before designating each focal threshold value can effectively make field defects disappear (or worsen, depending on conditioned response habits of the patient under testing). A logical and highly effective alternative to abbreviating full-thresholding strategies is suprathreshold perimetry. This method of perimetry has been popular in Europe for over 30 years, having been refined initially in the Friedmann analyser. The 'threshold-related suprathreshold' method takes account of the fact that (a) the slope of the central hill of vision is relatively constant, even among diseased individuals; and (b) average levels of light sensitivity may vary greatly, even among normal individuals. A 'working-threshold' is established by threshold testing a reference series of stimulus locations. This is adjusted across the field, higher centrally and lower peripherally, to establish a normal cone-shaped reference hill appropriate to the individual eye under consideration. Stimuli which are uniformly brighter than the physiologically adjusted working threshold (i.e. which should be readily seen) are then presented all over the field. Points missed at these brighter intensities are retested for confirmation, and then tested again with incrementally brighter lights until seen to quantify defect depth. No field of vision is actually smooth, and suprathreshold techniques identify scotomas of pathological relevance without undertaking the cumbersome task of mapping minor undulations in the otherwise normal hill of vision. Suprathreshold testing can thus dramatically reduce testing time, and tends to produce less noise on the visual field print-out. For screening purposes in particular, this approach has great advantages, the Henson central field analyser having demonstrated a remarkably high sensitivity and specificity for glaucoma detection.

Contrast patterns, flickering, or coloured stimuli can be used as an alternative to single light flashes with standard perimetric testing. Each of these alternative stimuli is intended to elicit putative selective magnocellular neural loss. All of these alternative methods for discriminating selective axonal loss lend themselves to non-perimetric central visual testing techniques.

Other psychophysical methods

Aside from acuity and perimetry, contrast sensitivity is the most widely employed psychophysical test. Static contrast sensitivity tests in the form of wall charts or transilluminated screens are very rapid, and have demonstrated utility for monitoring visual change in glaucoma once the disease has been diagnosed. These methods have a very low diagnostic utility, being little better than tonometry in that regard, because of the very wide range of baseline contrast sensitivity thresholds which exist among individuals with normal vision.

Temporal or flicker sensitivity is determined by adjusting the peak-to-trough luminance of a neutral blank field. At high temporal frequencies, glaucomatous eyes typically require a significantly higher peak-to-trough luminance amplitude for the flickering character of the diffuse light stimulus to be detected. Flicker testing could hold promise as a simple and inexpensive means for early detection of glaucomatous neural damage.

One particularly promising device which incorporates features of standard perimetry, contrast, and flicker testing is the Welch Allyn frequency doubling perimeter. This portable device has been shown to have sensitivity and specificity equal to the most elaborate standard equipment. Zeiss now markets this economic and portable device under contract with its developers.

Variations in colour sensitivity accompany glaucoma, with selective decreases especially prevalent in the Tritan (blue–yellow) axis. Thresholds can be measured perimetrically, and such short-wavelength perimetry with blue stimuli on a yellow background has already demonstrated an ability to detect glaucomatous visual field damage before the same scotomas become evident with standard perimetry. The Tubinger and Humphrey II are both equipped to carry out such testing. Novel computed techniques employing temporally modulated colour contrast patterns in the central visual field have demonstrated very high sensitivity and specificity for glaucoma detection, as well.

Electrophysiological tests

Visual evoked potentials are elicited from the brain by placement of electrodes on the frontal and occipital scalp and mastoid. Checkerboard stimuli are presented at varying temporal frequencies, and both the latency (stimulus–response time) and the amplitude of cortical responses are recorded. Because of the embryological outward twisting of optic radiation geniculate fibres from macular ganglion cell synapses, the visual evoked potential has a high central visual component. While visual evoked potential has a demonstrated utility in detecting demyelinating optic nerve disease, its sensitivity and specificity for glaucoma detection remains uncertain. The visual evoked potential has particular utility in monitoring acute visual function changes which accompany alterations in intraocular pressure or ocular circulation, and unique autoregulatory differences have been demonstrated to exist between glaucomatous and normal individuals in such studies.

Traditional flash electroretinography measures outer retinal activity, and has not been demonstrated to have utility in measuring glaucomatous damage. However, pattern electroretinography, in which a temporally modulated patterned stimulus is provided rather than a flash, is possibly the most sensitive and specific of all diagnostic tests for glaucoma. Studies suggest that low-amplitude (about 1 per cent that of a typical flash electroretinography) pattern electroretinography is a direct measure of ganglion cell integrity. Pattern electroretinography waveforms can be derived for either the transient response (< 10 reversals/s) or the steady-state response, at high temporal frequency. The transient response displays an initial negative deflection at around 35 ms (N35), a positive wave at around 50 ms (P50), and a second negative wave at 95 ms (N95). The steady-state response has only one negative trough and one positive peak, the second negative wave being obliterated by the repetitious waveform. In each instance, the data of greatest value for glaucoma assessment is the amplitude, measured as the trough to peak height. Patients with early and established open angle glaucoma typically exhibit substantial reductions in pattern electroretinography amplitude which are rarely seen in individuals with normal optic nerve function.

The pattern electroretinography procedure can be performed very quickly, since no dark adaptation is required. Testing typically takes 2 to 3 min once electrodes have been placed. Moreover, the test is non-subjective, and no learning curve exists. Interpretation of results is straightforward, and with the most up-to-date instruments Fourier analysis allows specific quantitation of the visual response at every harmonic frequency. Fourier analysis helps eliminate noise and other errors which may arise during smoothing or averaging of responses, and is recommended, since it allows detection of smaller changes and helps eliminate false positive findings.

Basic pattern electroretinography can be performed in most clinics equipped with electroretinography instrumentation. Non-contact lens electrodes (i.e. fibre or foil) should be used, with the reference electrode at the outer canthus, and a ground electrode on the forehead. A black and white reversing checkerboard 10 to 16° wide is presented on a video display unit, with individual checks subtending approximately 40 min of arc. The contrast between black and white squares should be maximal, never less than 80 per cent, with a photopic luminance of white squares greater than 80 cd/m². Typically the transient pattern electroretinography is adequate for separating P50 and N95; steady-state pattern electroretinography recordings may be useful and can be obtained quickly, but should only be undertaken if appropriate instrumentation for proper analysis is available. Reversal rates of 2 to 6/s (1–3 Hz) for transient and 16/s (8 Hz) for steady state are recommended. Each laboratory should establish appropriate age-related normal control values for its own equipment and population, and care should be taken to recalibrate stimuli on a regular basis.

Conclusion

Great strides have been made in recent years towards turning perimetry from an acquired art into a more exact clinical science. Computers and cleverly designed statistical programs have provided the means to quantify field change, and have led to much improved standardization of data between clinics. Numerical visual function indices now allow for clinical trials which can quantify visual survival, which is, after all, the goal of therapy. Further evolution of the available methods for testing the field of vision are inevitable, and clinicians should be acquainted with alternative strategies which may expedite and improve the specificity of testing. Finally, regardless of the technological advances, proper patient management will always require the integration of a thorough ocular examination with a cautious bilateral evaluation of present and past visual fields.

Further reading

Anderson, D. (1992). *Automated static perimetry*. Mosby, St Louis.

Choplin, N.T. and Edwards, R.P. (1995). *Visual field testing*. Slack, New Jersey.

Higgenbotham, E. and Lee, D. (1993). *Clinician's guide to the management of difficult glaucomas*. Medical Economic Books, New Jersey.

Lachenmayr, B.J. and Vivell, P.M.O. (1993). Perimetry and its clinical correlations. Georg Thieme Verlag, Stuttgart.

2.10.6 The natural history of primary open-angle glaucoma

Jeffrey L. Jay

Introduction

It is difficult to study the natural history of primary open-angle glaucoma since the course of the disease is usually modified by treatment, sometimes not fully effective or properly administered. Individual case histories of untreated disease, such as those described below, are occasionally available and suggest wide variation in the rate of progress. They also provide some idea of the connection between disease of the optic nerve and intraocular pressure and other risk factors. There is, however, information now available about the course of ocular hypertension and glaucoma that allows us to propose a working model for the probable course of untreated disease.

Case histories

Case 1

An asymptomatic and healthy 67-year-old woman was found, on routine sight testing, to have a raised intraocular pressure of 32 mmHg, right eye, and 44 mmHg, left eye. The optic discs appeared healthy; cup:disc ratio 0.3 and 0.4 right and left eyes, respectively. Gonioscopy revealed open iridocorneal angles without unusual features. There were no defects in the visual field. Treatment with timolol drops, 0.5 per cent twice daily, reduced the pressure to the low twenties. After 5 months she failed to attend for further follow-up but almost 4 years later sought re-examination because of poor vision. The pressure was then 52 mm, right eye, and 56 mm, left eye, and there was advanced cupping of both optic discs (cup:disc ratio 0.8 right, 1.0 left) The left eye was blind (no perception of light). The right eye maintained good central acuity (6/9 Snellen) but had a tiny central tunnel of residual field that reached out to 5° from fixation in one quadrant only. Thus, in a period of $3\frac{1}{2}$ years, intact visual fields in both eyes had been all but extinguished. Trabeculectomy in each eye reduced the pressures to the range of 9 to 15 mmHg, right eye, and 11 to 19 mmHg, left eye. The last island of field in the right eye remained 7 years later, with only slight further constriction. This case demonstrates that the progress of the loss of visual field in high-pressure glaucoma may be surprisingly rapid and that effective lowering of the pressure will slow the progress.

Case 2

Abnormal cupping of the optic discs, cup:disc ratio 0.75 for each eye, was suspected in a 40-year-old man, but prolonged investigation showed no reduction in sensitivity of the visual field and the maximum intraocular pressure was 20 mmHg. There were no other risk factors for glaucoma. He was in good health and had no family history of glaucoma. CT scan revealed nothing that might have explained the optic-nerve changes. After 1 year of repeated examinations, follow-up without treatment after a further 5 years was recommended, with interim annual review by his optometrist. He was eventually referred again after 14 years and found to have more extensive cupping than before (now the cup:disc ratio = 0.95 right, 0.85 left). There was loss of visual field in the form of relative suppression of the retinal sensitivity in the arcuate areas, typical of primary open-angle glaucoma. Occasionally the untreated intraocular pressure now reached 25 mmHg. There was therefore convincing evidence of progressive glaucomatous optic neuropathy but the pressure was only marginally elevated and he had none of the ocular or systemic vascular features associated with normal-pressure glaucoma. Is this type of disease slower because the pressure is not so high and are factors other than raised intraocular pressure at least partly responsible?

Comment

These two case histories present examples of the extreme ends of the range of the disturbance in intraocular pressure and the optic nerve that is termed primary open-angle glaucoma. Most ophthalmologists will recall similar cases but there is now more objective evidence to confirm that they represent typical variations in the course of untreated disease.

The end and beginning of primary open-angle glaucoma

There is no doubt that primary open-angle glaucoma is often a blinding condition characterized by progressive loss of the visual field and optic-nerve fibres in a recognizable pattern. Scotomas in the arcuate area, with or without a nasal step, progress to extensive peripheral loss, and the last areas to be extinguished are usually small islands of field in the central zone and the temporal periphery. The head of the optic nerve loses axons and appears cupped. Although in most cases the intraocular pressure is high, there are a few exceptions (normal-pressure, low-tension glaucoma) where the pressure is never raised. At or near the end, ischaemic complications such as peripheral retinal haemorrhages and occlusion of central retinal vein may occur. The latter often causes rubeosis (neovascularization) of the iris and secondary angle-closure, which results in a vicious circle of a further rise in pressure, pain, cataract, and distressing corneal oedema.

The earliest stage of the disease is, however, almost impossible to define. Minor abnormalities of intraocular pressure, visual field, or in the appearance of the optic nerve overlap the range of their physiological variance. More precise, modern methods of investigation, such as optic-disc biometry, nerve fibre layer analysis, or computerized perimetry, although more sensitive, have not improved our ability to distinguish the boundary of abnormality from normal variation. They have therefore not provided a method for the diagnosis of the earliest stage of the disease without the need for sequential observation to identify progressive deterioration. The old adage still holds: 'We are unable to detect a criminal by looking at his face. We must have evidence of bad behaviour.'

Progression of ocular hypertension to glaucoma

Raised intraocular pressure without damage to the optic nerve or visual field is termed ocular hypertension. In many cases this state progresses to glaucoma, usually defined as the appearance of defects in the field of vision. There is a transitional phase before the field defects appear, where attenuation of the nerve-fibre population is revealed by changes at the head of the optic nerve such as cupping or haemorrhage. These patients with disc abnormality, with or without detected increases in pressure, are identified as glaucoma suspects. In a recent large-scale population study, increasing age, abnormalities of the optic disc, and the amount of pressure elevation were confirmed as associated with a higher rate of progression to glaucomatous visual-field defects. In other studies the rate of progression

Table 1 Percentage of patients with ocular hypertension who developed glaucoma at mean follow-up of 40 months ($n = 117$)

Intraocular pressure (IOP) (mmHg)	Percentage which developed field defects	Relative risk vs IOP 21–25 mmHg
21–25	2.7	× 1
26–30	12.0	× 4
>30	41.2	× 13

After David *et al.* (1977).

varied considerably (from 6.7 to 30 per cent). This discrepancy may be explained by different periods of follow-up and different patterns of increased pressure in the study populations. For example, the relative risk of developing glaucoma at different pressures in one study is shown in Table 1, and a relative risk approximately × 3 if the pressure is over 26 mmHg has been identified in another. The presence of pseudoexfoliation or optic-disc haemorrhage may increase the risk by factors of ×10 and ×5, respectively.

Ocular hypertension should therefore be considered to be a precursor of glaucoma. Nevertheless, the probability of developing glaucoma is often very low, especially when the pressure is in the low twenties. Only the higher-risk patients are selected for treatment.

Rate of visual-field loss without treatment

Although the experience of individual cases, such as the first patient described above, suggests that progression to blindness in untreated, primary open-angle glaucoma may be surprisingly rapid, it is more difficult to obtain a reliable estimate of the rate of field loss in untreated disease for the whole glaucoma population. A cross-sectional method has been used to estimate the average time taken to progress from the earliest identifiable field loss to the endstage of the disease. The age at diagnosis of patients who presented with mild field loss was compared with the age of those who presented with the field virtually extinguished. The difference in the mean ages at these two points in the disease (Table 2) provides a method for estimat-

Table 2 Statistical analysis of the relation between untreated increases in intraocular pressure (IOP) and the mean interval from early to endstage disease

Untreated IOP at diagnosis (mmHg)	Estimated average interval (years) from early to endstage diseases (SEM)	*p*
21–25	14.4 (2.2)	<0.00001
26–30	6.5 (2.9)	0.029
>30	2.9 (2.1)	0.17

ing the average rate of progression at different pressures before diagnosis and treatment, but it can give no clue to the possible scatter of the population around that average rate. The p-values are shown in the table and statistical significance is reached for the two pressure bands up to 30 mmHg. For pressures over 30 mmHg the interval from early disease to endstage is very short (2.9 years) and does not seem to reach statistical significance. It must be remembered, however, that this indicates that the interval may not be significantly different from zero and emphasizes that there is likely to be very rapid progression when the pressure is very high. These results confirm that the rate of disease is faster at higher pressure. Some eyes show an episodic, curvilinear course of field deterioration with time rather than a linear decay, but these fluctuations are relatively brief and do not invalidate the concept of a gradual, linear decay when a time-scale of several years is considered. The possibly rapid rate of deterioration must be recognized when planning the frequency of repeat examinations in population-screening programmes. Perhaps the maximum interval should be 5 years, as some patients may not have a prolonged phase of relatively mild ocular hypertension but may develop dangerously high pressure near the beginning of their disease.

The rate of field loss in treated disease

Many trials of medical treatment have been unsatisfactory in design or inconclusive in outcome. Often, for reasons of ethics or availability, it is mild forms of the disease that are studied, for example where intraocular pressure is only slightly raised. In these lower pressure ranges the conversion rate from ocular hypertension to glaucoma is, as described above, infrequent, and even when there is already some field reduction, progress may be very slow. It is therefore difficult to construct a trial of therapy with enough patients treated for sufficient time to reach the required power for a valid statistical outcome. Nevertheless, there is now sufficient evidence that treatment to lower intraocular pressure protects the visual field and we should not be misled by the difficulty in demonstrating this benefit in cases that progress only very slowly without treatment. Two studies have estimated the time it might take to progress from the earliest stage of field damage to blindness under conditions of optimal pressure control following drainage surgery. They agree that this interval may be between 30 and 40 years. For patients with similar pressures at diagnosis, that is, greater than 25 mmHg, the expected interval without treatment would be only 3.6 years (Table 3). Not all treatment strategies are as effective as surgery, although medical or laser therapy may be appropriate in lower-risk cases. When medical therapy was compared with drainage surgery (trabeculectomy) as the initial form of treatment, many cases on medical therapy could not be controlled and the slope of the deterioration of the visual field during this unsuccessful trial of medical therapy suggested an interval of about 10 years from an early stage of field loss to blindness. This is better than without treatment but far short

Table 3 Estimated mean interval of progression from early field loss to endstage disease in primary open-angle glaucoma under different conditions

Untreated	3.6 years
During unsatisfactory medical treatment	10 years
After trabeculectomy	38 years

Minimum pressure at diagnosis, 25 mmHg (from Jay and Murdoch, 1993).

of the optimum field protection achieved by successful surgery (Table 3).

The contribution of normal ageing to the course of treated disease

In humans there is gradual reduction in the number of axons in the optic nerve with increasing age. At birth there are between 1.0 and 1.5 million, and several studies indicate a loss of about 5000 per year throughout life. Individual variation is considerable. At a chosen age the number of fibres may show a range twice that of the lower value, and larger discs have more axons but they are less densely packed. Assuming a complement of axons at 60 years of age of 700 000 and a possible loss of up to 40 per cent during a period of ocular hypertension before field defects are detectable by standard tests, it may be that a 60-year-old patient with primary open-angle glaucoma in whom field changes are just appearing has 420 000 axons. If the subsequent decay of these axons can be extended over a 40-year period, which is the estimate for survival of the visual field on optimal treatment, the rate of axon loss will be about 10 000 per annum. Thus, for well-treated glaucoma, the average rate of deterioration in the optic nerve could be only twice that for normal ageing.

Summary

Improved understanding of the of the natural history of this disease emphasizes the value of early diagnosis but allows us to delay treatment until there is a significant threat to vision. We are therefore learning to avoid the disadvantages of unnecessary therapy. At the same time the need for vigorous treatment of high-risk cases is becoming better recognized.

Further reading

Armaly, M. F. *et al.* (1980). Biostatistical analysis of the collaborative glaucoma study. I. Summary report of the risk factors for glaucomatous visual field defects. *Archives of Ophthalmology*, **98**, 2163–71.

Balazsi, A. G., Rootman, J., Drance, S. M., Schulzer, M., and Douglas, G. R. (1984). The effect of age on the nerve fibre population of the human optic nerve. *American Journal of Ophthalmology*, **97**, 760–6.

Crick, R. P. *et al.* (1989). The visual field in chronic simple glaucoma and ocular hypertension: its character, progress, relationship to intraocular pressure and response to treatment. *Eye*, **3**, 536–46.

David, R., Livingston, D. G., and Luntz, M. H. (1977). Ocular hypertension—

a long-term follow up of treated and untreated patients. *British Journal of Ophthalmology*, **61**, 668–74.

Ekstrom, C. (1993). Elevated intraocular pressure and pseudoexfoliation of the lens capsule as risk factors for chronic open angle glaucoma. A population based five year follow up study. *Acta Ophthalmologica*, **71**, 189–95.

Jay, J. L. (1992). Rational choice of therapy in primary open angle glaucoma. *Eye*, **6**, 243–7.

Jay, J. L. and Allen D. (1989). The benefit of early trabeculectomy versus conventional management in primary open angle glaucoma relative to severity of disease. *Eye*, **3**, 528–35.

Jay, J. L. and Murdoch, J. R. (1993). The rate of visual field loss in untreated primary open angle glaucoma. *British Journal of Ophthalmology*, **77**, 176–8.

Johnson, B. M., Miao, M., and Sadun, A. A. (1987). Age related decline of human optic nerve axon population. *Age*, **10**, 5–9.

Jonas, J. B., Müller-Bergh, J. A., Schlötzer-Schrehardt, U-M., and Naumann, G. O. H. (1990). Histomorphometry of the human optic nerve. *Investigative Ophthalmology and Visual Sciences*, **31**, 736–44.

Jonas, J. B., Schmidt, A. M., Müller-Bergh, J. A., Schlötzer-Schrehardt, U-M., and Naumann, G. O. H. (1992). Human optic nerve fibre count and optic disc size. *Investigative Ophthalmology and Visual Sciences*, **30**, 2012–18.

Lundberg, L., Uettreil, K., and Linner, E. (1980). Ocular hypertension. A 20 year follow up at Skvode. *Surveys of Ophthalmology*, **25**, 136–47.

Mikelberg, F. S., Schulzer, M., Drance, S. M., and Lau W. (1986). The rate of progression of scotomas in glaucoma. *American Journal of Ophthalmology*, **101**, 1–6.

Mikelberg, F. S., Drance, S. M., Schulzer, M., Yidegiligne, H. M., and Weiss, M. M. (1989). The normal human optic nerve. *Ophthalmology*, **96**, 1325–8.

Morrison, J. C., Cork, L. C., Dunkelberger, G. R., Brown, A., and Quigley, H. A. (1990). Ageing changes of the rhesus monkey optic nerve. *Investigative Ophthalmology and Visual Sciences*, **31**, 1623–7.

Quigley, H. A., Enger, C., Katz, J., Sommer, A., Scott, R., and Gilbert, D. (1994). Risk factors for the development of glaucomatous visual field loss in ocular hypertension. *Archives of Ophthalmology*, **112**, 644–9.

Rosetti, L., Marchetti, I., Orzales, N., Scorpiglione, N., Torri, V., and Liberate, A. (1993). Randomized clinical trials of medical treatment of glaucoma, are they appropriate to guide clinical practice? *Archives of Ophthalmology*, **111**, 96–103.

Smith, R. J. H. (1986). The enigma of primary open angle glaucoma. *Transactions of the Ophthalmological Societies of the United Kingdom*, **105**, 618–33.

2.10.7 The management of glaucoma (medical, laser) and indications for surgery

Colm O'Brien

Background

Glaucoma is, in public health terms, a common condition which is characterized by a distinctive pattern of optic nerve damage (cupping and pallor) and visual field loss (mid-peripheral arcuate defects). In the majority of patients, these features occur in association with elevated (over 21 mmHg) intraocular pressure, although it can occur in the presence of normal intraocular pressure. Because glaucoma is generally an asymptomatic disease, screening the population for the major risk factors is of critical importance if glaucoma blindness is to be kept to an absolute minimum.

An estimated 30 per cent of all hospital ophthalmic outpatient appointments in the United Kingdom are for glaucoma-related conditions. The challenge to those involved in the care of glaucoma patients involves two separate and distinct issues, namely the philosophical and practical approaches to treatment. The first issue involves having a clear understanding of the natural history and spectrum of the disease, and is the background against which individual patient management is based. The second point not only includes the use of medical, laser, and surgical therapy, but also requires that a clear explanation and likely prognosis be given to each patient emphasizing the likely impact of both the disease and its treatment on the quality of vision and life during the expected lifetime of the patient.

The focus of this chapter is on the commoner types of glaucoma that clinicians face in daily practice, namely primary open angle glaucoma and its related conditions. These include ocular hypertension, low tension glaucoma, and secondary open angle glaucoma entities such as pseudoexfoliation and pigment dispersion glaucoma (angle closure, congenital, and other secondary forms of glaucoma are dealt with elsewhere).

Definitions

In this chapter, the following definitions are used.

1. Primary open angle glaucoma: this is a chronic progressive form of optic neuropathy (cupping and pallor) with an associated pattern of visual field loss, where the intraocular pressure is greater than 21 mmHg, the anterior chamber drainage angle is macroscopically open, and there is no obvious ocular or systemic cause for the elevation in intraocular pressure (other synonyms used are chronic open angle glaucoma or chronic simple glaucoma).

2. Ocular hypertension: raised intraocular pressure (above 21 mmHg), open drainage angle, and normal visual field. The optic disc may be normal or show some cupping.

3. Low tension glaucoma: essentially the same as primary open angle glaucoma except that the intraocular pressure is less than 22 mmHg.

4. Secondary open angle glaucoma: the same features as primary open angle glaucoma, but where there are specific ocular syndromes (such as pseudoexfoliation or pigment dispersion) which play a role in the elevation of the intraocular pressure.

Socioeconomic issues

The prevalence of glaucoma in developed Western countries is approximately 1 per cent of the population over the age of 40 years, and rises with age to 3 per cent of those of 70 years of age and over. Epidemiological surveys indicate that nearly half of those affected with glaucoma in the community are undetected. The prevalence of ocular hypertension is higher at between 5 and 7 per cent of the population over the age of 40 years. Glaucoma in black people is more common, with higher intraocular pressures and more severe damage at presentation, is more difficult to control, and occurs at a younger age than in white Caucasians.

Fifteen per cent of those registered blind or partially sighted in this country suffer from glaucoma, although this figure is considered to seriously underestimate the true number of visually disabled people with glaucoma. Eligibility for registration generally results from gross constriction of the visual field with retention of good central visual acuity. The majority of glaucoma blindness affects individuals over the age of 60 years. Patient support groups with bases in the United Kingdom include the International Glaucoma Association, the Royal National Institute for the Blind, and the Guide Dogs for the Blind Association.

Patients with mild to moderate glaucoma frequently have few symptoms attributable to the disease. However, late in the disease, difficulty with outdoor mobility, glare disability, and a generalized loss of confidence affects patients. The other major social impact of glaucoma relates to driving, where constriction of the visual field might result in the loss of a valid driving licence with significant consequences on independence and mobility.

Disease spectrum

Up until the 1960s all patients with elevated intraocular pressure were incorrectly labelled as glaucoma with the result that many patients were treated unnecessarily (for example pressures in the low 20s without other risk factors, with normal optic discs and visual fields), while others were probably overtreated (for example surgery for ocular hypertension in patients who did not have visual field loss). Numerous epidemiological surveys have shown that for every patient with glaucoma, there are four or five with raised pressure without field loss (this is ocular hypertension). Raised intraocular pressure has been shown to be the most important risk factor for the development of glaucoma. The prevailing concept is that a prolonged period of elevated pressure will result in progressive damage to the axons of the optic nerve with irreversible visual field loss, and the higher the pressure the greater the risk. Consequently, the aim of therapy has focused almost exclusively on lowering the intraocular pressure in an attempt to slow down the rate of attrition of optic nerve fibres. Secondly, this disease model emphasizes the critical nature of early detection at the ocular hypertension stage before irreversible glaucoma damage to the optic nerve, and especially the visual field, occurs. However, long-term follow-up studies show that the conversion rate of ocular hypertension to glaucoma is low at approximately 1 to 2 per cent per year. Other major factors which are associated with an increased risk of getting glaucoma in ocular hypertensive patients include age, myopia, family history of glaucoma, Afro-Caribbean race, and the amount of disc damage (in the absence of field loss) at the time of diagnosis.

Once glaucoma is diagnosed, treatment is aimed at reducing the rate of subsequent visual field loss. Because no trial of treatment versus no treatment has been completed to date, there is no absolute proof that current therapy (aimed at lowering intraocular pressure) is effective. The combination of conventional wisdom, and the clinical experience of glaucoma specialists and indirect evidence on the effectiveness of treatment, all dictate that patients are treated to prevent further loss of vision.

Pathophysiology

Intraocular pressure

This is determined by the balance between aqueous inflow and outflow. Aqueous humour is formed in the ciliary processes by a combination of secretion, ultrafiltration, and diffusion. The normal flow rate is approximately 2.5 µl/min. The formation of aqueous has a diurnal variation, being greater in the morning and falling during the day, and also decreases with age. Aqueous production is not increased in glaucoma.

The outflow of aqueous is mostly via the trabecular meshwork to Schlemm's canal and the venous circulation on the scleral surface. The trabecular meshwork has three layers: the uveal, corneoscleral, and the juxtacanalicular tissue which is the layer closest to Schlemm's canal and the site of greatest resistance to outflow. Aqueous outflow falls with age due to a loss of trabecular meshwork cells and thickening and fusion of trabecular meshwork beams. This process is accelerated and more pronounced in primary open angle glaucoma, and is the cause of the increase in the intraocular pressure.

An alternative outflow pathway is via the uveoscleral route where aqueous flows from the anterior chamber into the ciliary muscle to the supraciliary and suprachoroidal spaces and through the sclera. In the normal eye, this accounts for 20 per cent of aqueous outflow and is a pressure-dependent mechanism.

The pressure in the episcleral venous circulation is generally stable at between 8 and 12 mmHg. An increase in this pressure such as with superior vena caval obstruction, will increase the resistance of aqueous outflow and cause a rise in ocular pressure.

Optic nerve

Approximately 1 million axons from the retinal ganglion cells leave the globe in the optic nerve through a circular/oval canal of 1.8 mm diameter in the sclera. These axons take an arcuate pathway in the retina to reach the optic nerve and are bunched together at the superior and inferior poles of the nerve head. Axons originating close to the optic disc lie in the centre of the nerve head, while axons from the more peripheral parts of the retina occupy the peripheral part of the nerve head.

The axons pass through the lamina cribrosa which is situated at the scleral level. This collagenous fenestrated structure has approximately 10 layers. The fenestrations in the lamina are wider in the vertical poles of the optic nerve head. The horizontal regions of the lamina have more connective tissue and smaller pores. When the intraocular pressure is elevated, the laminae are compressed together and there is backward bowing of the whole lamina. This results in compression of the nerve axons with hold-up of axoplasmic flow, and this represents the mechanical hypothesis of glaucoma damage. A second hypothesis is also proposed whereby ischaemia-induced axonal loss occurs. It is more likely that the pressure–mechanical and vascular–ischaemic theories both occur together to contribute to the pathogenesis of optic nerve damage in glaucoma.

The optic nerve head can be divided into four different anatomical regions. The superficial retinal nerve fibre layer receives its vascular supply from the central retinal artery. The second layer is the prelaminar nerve tissue layer whose blood supply is from branches of the short posterior ciliary artery. The third layer is the laminar layer and again the vascular supply is from the branches of the short posterior ciliary artery. These three layers have a continuous capillary network lined by pericytes and behave like the retinal and central nervous system capillaries, and are capable of autoregulation. The retrolaminar layer lies outside the globe and is supplied by branches from the central retinal artery and meningeal arteries.

Retinal ganglion cells

Broadly speaking there are two different classes of retinal ganglion cell types, the magno and parvo cells. The larger diameter magno cells respond to low contrast stimuli of high temporal frequency and synapse in the magnocellular layer of the lateral geniculate nucleus. The smaller parvo cells respond to colour stimuli and are responsive to high contrast low temporal frequency stimuli. Retinal ganglion cell death in glaucoma can occur by the process of programmed cell death, otherwise known as apoptosis. Raised retinal levels of the excitatory amino acid glutamate may also cause ganglion cell neurotoxicity and cell death in glaucoma.

Genetics of glaucoma

A family history (siblings, parents, and children) of glaucoma is one of the risk factors for developing this disease. The prevalence of primary open angle glaucoma is higher (6 per cent) in first-degree relatives of glaucoma patients than in the general population. A strong familial autosomal dominant inheritance pattern has been observed in the increased intraocular pressure response to topical corticosteroid use. The inheritance of juvenile open angle glaucoma appears to be autosomal dominant with reduced penetrance in several large pedigrees, and a genetic marker has been identified on chromosome 1q. A mutation in the trabecular meshwork, the inducible glucocorticoid response or TIGR gene on chromosome 1q, has been isolated in juvenile glaucoma, and the defect also occurs in 3 per cent of patients with primary open angle glaucoma. No clear pattern of inheritance has been documented in primary open angle glaucoma which appears to be polygenic and multifactorial in nature.

Screening (case detection)

Because the development of irreversible glaucoma damage to the optic nerve and visual field loss is preceded by a period of elevation in intraocular pressure, it is possible to identify those at risk of getting this disease before the raised pressure has caused irreversible damage. The onset of presbyopia ensures that the great majority of people over the age of 40 years attend an optometrist for a sight test, and therefore can be tested for the features of glaucoma. The combined use of tonometry, ophthalmoscopy, and rapid perimetric testing by optometrists significantly increases the diagnostic accuracy of glaucoma referrals to the local hospital eye service. Over 1 million sight tests are performed annually in the United Kingdom and approximately 60 000 are referred for further evaluation of possible glaucoma.

It is somewhat inaccurate to describe the above process as screening as no official national screening programme exists. The current method is more appropriately called opportunistic case detection, the success of which depends on people attending their optometrist regularly and the quality of the ocular examination carried out there. Ideally, the general population should be tested for glaucoma every 4 to 5 years for those between the ages of 40 and 60 years, and every 2 to 3 years thereafter. Individuals with a family history of glaucoma are entitled to a free eyesight test and should be screened more frequently than the general population.

Good clinical practice (evaluation of the patient)

Clinical information

In the United Kingdom, the great majority of patients presenting to the hospital eye service are referred by optometrists via the general practitioner. Few have symptoms suggestive of glaucoma, the majority having visited their optometrist for a change of glasses and found to have features suggestive of glaucoma. Recent evidence indicates that, following assessment, one-third of referrals have glaucoma, a further third require long-term monitoring for ocular hypertension, and one-third are discharged. Accurate diagnosis is a prerequisite for appropriate treatment, and clinically relevant information forms a vital part of patient care.

Careful history taking should include the following.

1. Current ocular symptoms.

2. Past ocular history (inflammation, trauma, the use of topical steroid creams or eye-drops for blepharitis/conjunctivitis).

3. Refractive error (myopia being more common in primary open angle glaucoma; hypermetropic eyes have an increased risk of angle closure glaucoma).

4. Family history of glaucoma (first/second-degree relative, age of onset, and mode of treatment in affected family members).

5. Medical history (systemic vascular disease, diabetes mellitus, respiratory illness especially asthma, vasospastic conditions such as migraine and Raynaud's phenomenon, smoking habits).

6. Medications and allergies: note in particular the use of

systemic β-blockers which lower intraocular pressure; past or present use of corticosteroids in any form (tablets, creams, inhalers, nebulizers) as they may be associated with elevation of intraocular pressure.

Clinical examination skills

1. Best corrected visual acuity; near and distance with spectacle/contact lens correction.

2. Pupil response to light; a relative afferent pupillary defect may be seen with asymmetric disease.

3. Anterior segment examination using slit lamp biomicroscopy. Look for corneal endothelial pigmentation, peripheral and central anterior chamber depth, iris colour configuration and transillumination, pseudoexfoliation material on the pupil margin and anterior lens capsule, heterochromia, and iris neovascularization. Peripheral anterior chamber depth can be assessed by projecting the slit beam at a 60° angle just anterior to the limbus (Van Herick method). If the width of the peripheral anterior chamber (that is the distance between the iris surface and the corneal endothelium) is less than one quarter of the corneal thickness, then the angle is judged to be narrow, and gonioscpopy is indicated. Central anterior chamber depth can be measured with optical devices attached to the slit lamp, and values less then 2 mm indicate a significantly shallow chamber.

Intraocular pressure

Clinical measurement is with the Goldmann contact applanation tonometer. Factors which may influence pressure readings include breath holding, the Valsalva manoeuvre, corneal thickness and scarring, low scleral rigidity, and the 'white coat effect' especially in patients at their first consultation. Because of the diurnal variation, it is often appropriate to get two or three readings at the time of diagnosis (before treatment is started) to include a morning pressure, especially if the initial consultation is in the afternoon. If the intraocular pressure is greater than 21 mmHg then gonioscopy should be performed prior to pupil dilation. In the presence of active corneal infectious disease or scarring, then tonometry with the Tono-pen (a hand-held Mackay–Marg type tonometer) can give reasonably accurate recordings of intraocular pressures.

The mean intraocular pressure in large-scale population studies is 16 mmHg with a standard deviation of 2.5 mmHg. The normal range of pressures is therefore from 11 to 21 mmHg, and values over 21 mmHg are considered as abnormal. If the distribution of pressures had a normal Gaussian pattern, 2.5 per cent of the population would have abnormally high pressures. However, the distribution is non-Gaussian, and is shifted to the right such that between 5 and 7 per cent of the population have pressures greater than 21 mmHg. The normal diurnal range in intraocular pressure is 5 mmHg, while in primary open angle glaucoma it is in the region of 10 to 15 mmHg, with the highest readings in the morning period.

Gonioscopy

Careful examination of the anterior chamber drainage angle is essential when making a diagnosis. Indirect angle assessment at the slit lamp uses a goniolens with a mirror to view the diagonally opposite angle. With the eye in the primary position, the inferior angle is generally wider when the superior angle. If the angle appears narrow or closed, asking the patient to look in the direction of the viewing mirror will improve the clinician's view of the angle structures.

The normal anatomical features, when viewed from anterior to posterior include Schwalbe's line, the trabecular meshwork, scleral spur and the ciliary body. Schwalbe's line can be seen at the junction of two reflected beams of light from the external and internal corneal surfaces. The trabecular meshwork has an anterior non-pigmented and a posterior pigmented surface, and the scleral spur is a pale white stripe immediately anterior to the pigmented ciliary body. Trabecular meshwork pigmentation, if present, is generally best seen in the inferior angle and is increased in heavily pigmented eyes, but most of all in the pseudoexfoliation and pigment dispersion syndromes.

Goniolenses with the same radius of curvature as the cornea and with a smaller diameter than the cornea, such as the Zeiss or Sussmann four-mirror lens, can be used without any coupling fluid. If the trabecular meshwork is not seen in the primary position or the peripheral iris appears in contact with the trabecular meshwork, the clinician can indent the cornea centrally with these lenses to displace aqueous fluid into the angle. If the angle is narrow, this manoeuvre will open the angle to allow visualization of angle structures. However, if the angle is closed due to adhesion (peripheral anterior synechiae) between the iris and trabecular meshwork, then indentation will not open the angle. In general, hypermetropic eyes will have a shallower anterior chamber and narrow angles while myopic eyes will have deeper anterior chambers and open drainage angles. The Goldmann-type goniolens requires a coupling fluid such as methylcellulose, which often results in a loss of corneal clarity after gonioscopy and can limit subsequent fundal examination.

Several classification systems, some of which are somewhat complex and difficult to remember, have been devised to help describe the anatomical features of the angle. Good gonioscopy should include a description of the most posterior angle structure seen in each of the four quadrants (superior, nasal, inferior, and temporal) with the eye in the primary position followed if necessary by indentation or looking towards the relevant mirror if angle closure is suspected. Additional features such as the degree of trabecular meshwork pigmentation, the presence of iris processes (thin strands extending from the peripheral iris to the trabecular meshwork), and the convexity of the peripheral iris should be noted accurately. Estimation of the angle width is helpful, but is a subjective assessment with poor interobserver agreement.

Optic nerve

The optic nerve head is best viewed with either a direct ophthalmoscope to give a monoscopic view or with a slit lamp

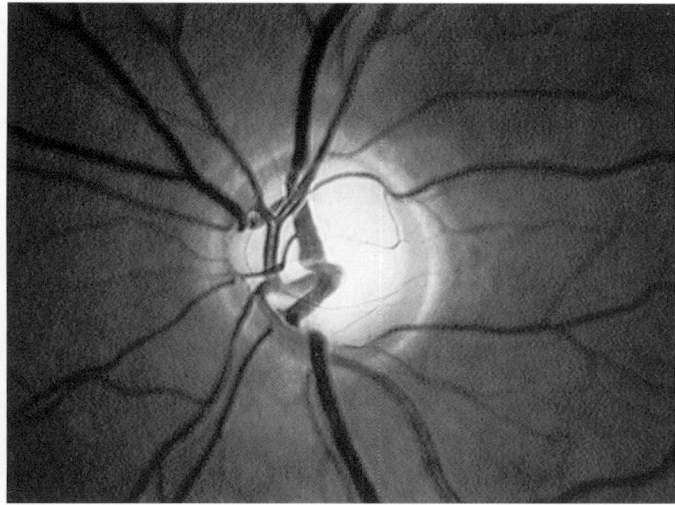

Fig. 1 Diffuse enlargement of the optic cup (loss of the neuroretinal rim) with additional thinning of the rim at the 1 o'clock position (left eye).

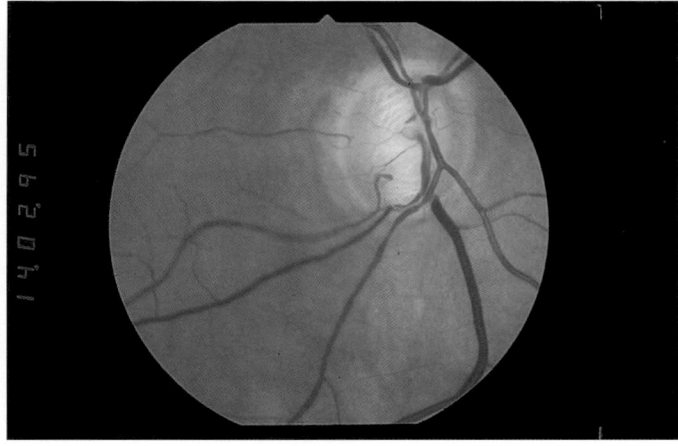

Fig. 2 Localized rim notching at the vertical poles of the optic disc (right eye).

biomicroscope using an indirect lens such as the 60, 78 or 90 dioptre lens, the Hruby lens, or the Goldmann-type contact lens to give a stereoscope three-dimensional view.

There is wide variety in the normal appearance of the optic disc in terms of size, shape, orientation, and colour. The normal disc area is 2.0 mm^2 with a large standard deviation of 0.5 mm^2, with larger discs seen in myopes and smaller discs in hypermetropes. Disc shape is generally circular or oval with the long axis in the vertical meridian. Many myopic optic discs are tilted in either an inferonasal or inferotemporal direction and often accompanied by peripapillary chorioretinal atrophy and hypopigmentation of the corresponding segment of retina. The smaller hypermetropic discs frequently have poorly defined disc margins.

The healthy nerve head has a pink/orange colour due to the presence of healthy neural tissue (neuroretinal rim) surrounding a central pale cup. The size of the physiological cup is determined by the disc size and has a strong genetic inheritance pattern. The appearance of the normal cup may be a small physiological dimple in the centre of the disc, a deep punched-out cup with sharp cup borders and visible lamina cribrosa, or a cup where the nasal border is sharply defined with a sloping temporal cup wall (the edge of which is hard to outline) which extends towards the edge of the disc.

In glaucoma, the size of the neural rim tissue diminishes with a corresponding increase in the cup size (area, depth, and volume) as progressive axonal loss occurs. Generally, this takes the form of concentric enlargement of the cup with diffuse thinning of the rim (Fig. 1) and an increase in disc pallor. This results in nasal shift of the major disc vessels and loss of the temporal rim. With progressive damage, the cup becomes deeper and paler, and the lamina cribrosa pores become visible. Less commonly there will be a focal cup enlargement due to localized rim loss or notching which occurs at the vertical poles of the disc (Fig. 2).

Associated features include the presence of peripapillary

atrophy which generally correlates with the degree of glaucoma damage, and linear flame-shaped haemorrhages on the disc surface in the nerve fibre layer which frequently predate progressive rim and visual field loss.

Retinal nerve fibre layer

In young patients with clear media and dilated pupils it is possible to see the peripapillary nerve fibre layer using red-free light and the slit lamp biomicroscope. This is best seen at the vertical poles of the disc where the nerve fibre bundles are congregated and seen as white striations radiating away from the disc (Fig. 3). In glaucoma the most common change is diffuse atrophy (Fig. 4), although slit-like or wedge-shaped defects which take an arcuate pattern in the nerve fibre layer can also occur.

Clinical assessment of optic disc appearance

All of the above descriptive features of optic nerve damage in glaucoma can be documented in careful drawings of the optic

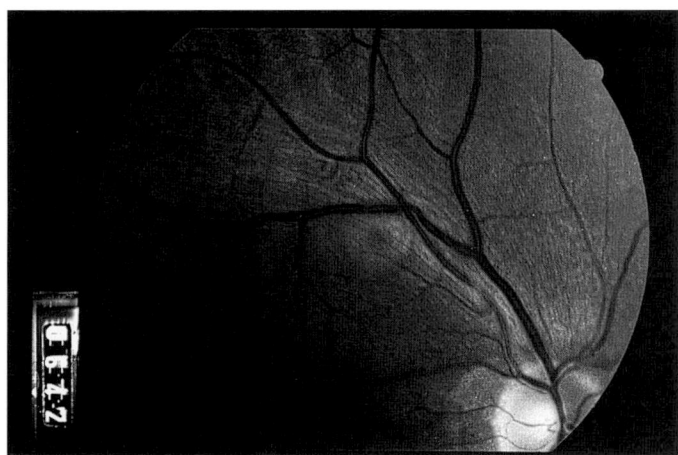

Fig. 3 Red-free photograph showing the retinal nerve fibre layer appearance in a healthy eye (right eye). The bundles of nerve fibres can be seen as striations radiating from the optic disc and are so abundant in places that the retinal vessels are obscured from view.

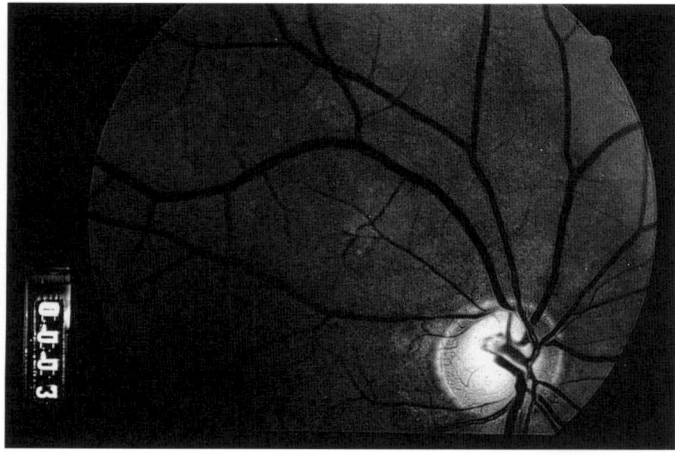

Fig. 4 Diffuse atrophy of the retinal nerve fibre layer in glaucoma (right eye). No striations are seen but the blood vessels are clearly seen.

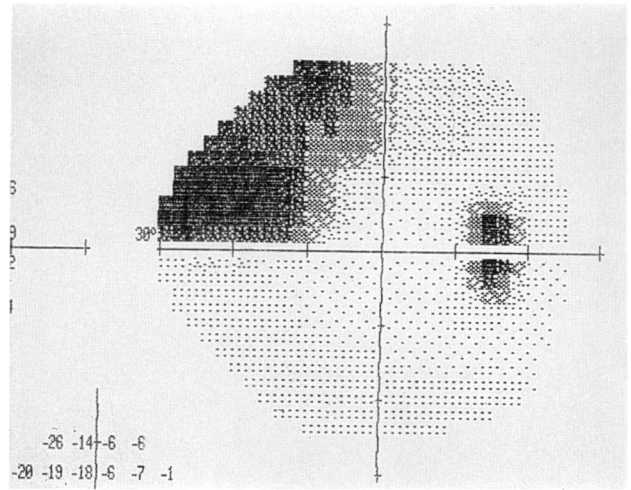

Fig. 5 Grey scale printout of a nasal step (right eye).

nerve, although photography provides a permanent record for future comparisons.

Many clinicians utilize the cup to disc ratio as a summary measure of disc appearance in glaucoma. The ratio expresses the cup size as a fraction of disc size; the greater the ratio, the greater the damage. The usefulness of this term is limited by the poor level of interobserver agreement (even in glaucoma specialists) which curtails the ability to document progressive disc damage. Furthermore, the fact that cup size is to a large extent determined by disc size in normal individuals, implies that it is necessary to know disc area before interpreting the clinical meaning of a given ratio. Consequently, cup to disc ratio is a poor method of describing the overall appearance of optic nerve damage in glaucoma, particularly for long-term follow-up.

Fundus examination

Following pupil dilation, an assessment of the macula and peripheral retina should be carried out looking for non-glaucomatous causes of visual field loss such as chorioretinal scarring and pigmentation, retinoschisis, and long-standing retinal detachment.

Visual field

Traditionally, assessment of optic nerve function in glaucoma is by means of perimetric exploration of the field of vision. Using a moving or static test stimulus, which is usually a white target against a darker background, it is possible to outline the boundary and/or height of the hill of vision. The normal hill of vision shows a progressive increase in retinal sensitivity from the periphery to the centre with the highest sensitivity occurring at the fovea. The technique of threshold perimetry represents the precise measurement of the hill of vision, when the patient is just about capable of detecting the target, while suprathreshold perimetry utilizes a stimulus which is considerably brighter than what the patient should be able to detect.

Glaucoma results in both a localized reduction of sensitivity in the hill of vision (called a scotoma) and, less commonly, a

diffuse depression of the whole hill of vision. The classic patterns of field loss in glaucoma include nasal steps (Fig. 5), arcuate scotomas (Fig. 6), and paracentral defects (Fig. 7). In reality, it is often difficult to discern these classic patterns of field loss. Progression usually takes the form of an increase in the size and depth of existing scotomas, and also the development of new defects in the other hemifield. In advanced stages, the patient is left with a small central island of vision (frequently with good visual acuity) and also a temporal island of vision.

Clinical perimetry of the visual field can be performed with a number of different techniques, the more commonly used methods include automated static and manual kinetic perimetry. Computer-assisted perimeters can measure retinal sensitivity at different locations in the visual field, generating numerical data which can be compared with age-matched normal sensitivity. This form of quantification of neural sensit-

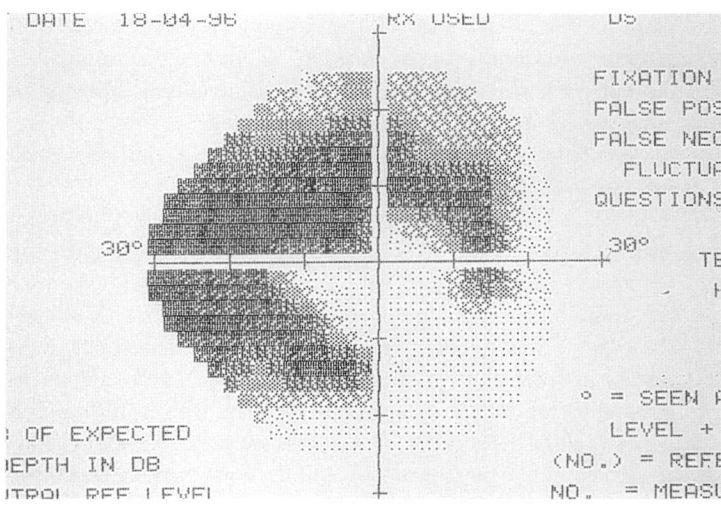

Fig. 6 Superior and inferior nasal loss with superior arcuate scotoma and early inferior arcuate scotoma (right eye).

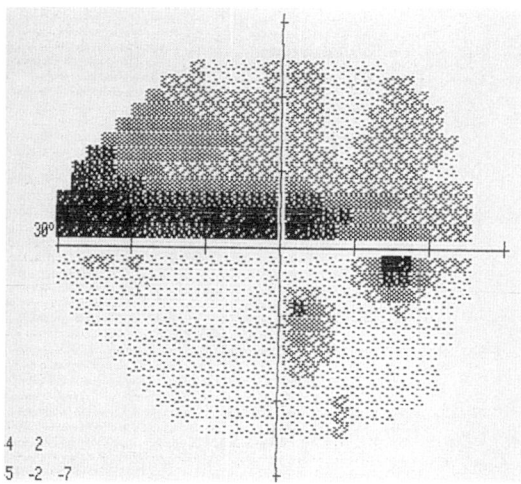

Fig. 7 Superior paracentral scotoma (right eye).

ivity can be used to establish a diagnosis or help monitor the course of the disease during follow-up.

An important aspect in the interpretation of any apparent visual field loss is that it must correspond with the clinical appearance of the optic disc. When a threshold visual field printout shows field loss which is not compatible with the disc appearance, then a repeat test is indicated, possibly with a suprathreshold programme. Further strategies in this situation include the use of a forced-choice method of testing, kinetic perimetry, or, as a last resort, confrontation testing of the hill of vision. Field assessment by the confrontation method (finger counting or the use of red/white targets) plays little or no role in routine glaucoma management, because of the difficulty in detecting the small, localized early field loss which is a characteristic feature of glaucoma. Secondly, monitoring for progressive field loss by the confrontation method is extremely difficult and unreliable for long-term disease.

While automated threshold perimetry has standardized perimetric assessment, not all patients are capable of performing reliable tests. This results from many factors, including the long test duration causing fatigue and loss of concentration, or an inability to understand the nature of the task. Other potential sources of error include patient- and test-related artefact and physiological variation. As a result, many patients are better suited to less demanding tests such as suprathreshold screening or kinetic perimetry.

Clinical investigations

Photography
Colour optic disc photographs taken at the time of the initial examination provide a very useful baseline picture for future comparisons. These can be either mono- or preferably stereoscopic pictures. Retinal nerve fibre layer photographs of good quality can be obtained using a blue- or red-free filter in patients with clear media and dilated pupils, and can be of significant clinical benefit in some ocular hypertensive patients.

Visual function
The goals of visual field assessment by perimetry are firstly to identify any defects in the field of vision, and secondly to monitor any change in an existing defect. It is vitally important to tailor the type of field test to the ability and understanding of each individual patient, and not to have a universal policy of, for example, using a threshold programme for all patients. While threshold tests can detect visual field loss at an earlier stage than suprathreshold evaluation, many elderly patients have great difficulty with the demands of threshold perimetry. It is possible to obtain valuable clinical information from less demanding suprathreshold tests, both for diagnostic purposes and for follow-up. Once a reliable test has been obtained, it is essential during subsequent examination to use the same perimeter and test programme so that a meaningful comparison can be made. Changing from one perimeter to another causes problems with interpretation of results.

Additional tests
The application of computer image analysis techniques to the field of glaucoma may, in the future, provide objective measurements of optic disc and retinal nerve fibre layer topography, thereby providing evidence of abnormality or progression of glaucoma. Techniques currently under evaluation include confocal laser scanning ophthalmoscopy, laser polarimetry, and optical coherence tomography.

In addition to the standard practice of using a white stimulus on a white background (white on white perimetry), a number of alternative tests have been proposed to help identify the earliest signs of retinal ganglion cell dysfunction in glaucoma. These tests include the use of blue on yellow or short wavelength perimetry, flicker perimetry, pattern electroretinography, contrast sensitivity, and scotopic threshold perimetry. The value of these techniques in long-term glaucoma follow-up remains unproven.

Management overview

Making a diagnosis
It is essential that an experienced ophthalmologist is closely involved in the initial decision-making diagnostic and treatment plan. This aspect of care should not be left to a junior or trainee ophthalmologist because mistakes at this stage will lead to problems during follow-up. Combining the clinical history, ocular examination, and appropriate investigations allows the clinician to make an informed and accurate diagnosis. The diagnosis may initially have to be a provisional one because, for example, the patient may be unable to undertake a satisfactory perimetry test. It may be necessary to repeat some aspect of the examination such as applanation tonometry or perimetry to confirm the diagnosis.

While it is important for the clinician to have a general overview of treatment, it is essential to deal with each patient individually. The patient needs to be told of the diagnosis and likely prognosis, whether treatment is indicated, the likely outcome if left untreated, the risks and benefits of treatment, the different forms of treatment, and the one best suited to that patient. An explanation should be given of the irreversible nature of glaucoma damage, the possible effects of the disease and treatment on the patient's quality of life, the fact that treatment and monitoring are long-term, and that treatment is aimed at preventing further loss. If possible an explanatory leaflet should be given to the patient which should include information on the disease, treatment, and patient support groups.

Approach to treatment

Having established the diagnosis, the next step is to determine the severity of the disease which depends on the amount of optic disc damage and visual field loss. The more advanced the disease at presentation then the lower the intraocular pressure needs to be to prevent further visual loss, and this is the basis behind the setting of target pressures to help control the disease. The traditional approach to the treatment of glaucoma is to use topical medications followed possibly by laser trabeculoplasty and finally drainage surgery. This is the principle which underlies the term 'maximum tolerated medical therapy' whereby patients are treated with several topical eye-drops, sometimes systemic medications, and finally laser trabeculoplasty before surgical intervention is indicated. While many patients achieve good glaucoma control using medications alone, the traditional approach to treatment is challenged by two trials which show that patients subjected to a prolonged attempt at medical control fare worse in terms of field survival when compared with patients having early trabeculectomy. Early surgery also achieves better long-term pressure control. The prolonged use of certain topical medications increases the inflammatory conjunctival cell profile and adversely affects the success rate of subsequent drainage surgery.

The treatment protocol for the management of ocular hypertension is not as aggressive as it is for the management of glaucoma. Presenting pressures tend to be lower and trial results show that lowering intraocular pressure by medical means prevents glaucoma damage and loss of visual field. Indeed a large proportion of ocular hypertensive patients probably do not require any therapy, and the decision to treat depends on the level of pressure and the presence of other risk factors.

Currently all treatment is directed towards lowering of intraocular pressure, although future therapies may include neuroprotection and improved perfusion of the optic nerve. Medical therapy needs to be effective at lowering intraocular pressure, well tolerated by the patient with few, if any, side-effects, and to be successful needs to be used regularly by the patient. β-Blockers remain the initial drug of choice, although newer topical agents such as the prostaglandin analogues, carbonic anhydrase inhibitors and the α_2-agonists (all of which are considerably more expensive than β-blockers) may replace β-blockers as first-line agents. Miotics and adrenaline-like drugs, although effective and cheap are possibly regarded as third-line agents. Depending on the presenting level of pressure, initial treatment is with one or two topical drugs followed if necessary by further therapy to control the level of pressure

and stabilize the disease. Patients should be asked directly about specific side-effects at each clinic visit.

Monitoring progression

When treatment has achieved a satisfactory level of pressure, the target pressure, long-term review focuses on regular monitoring of intraocular pressure, the optic disc, and visual field at intervals of 4 to 6 months initially. Disease progression in ocular hypertension results in the development of a field defect, while in glaucoma there will be an increase in the size and depth of existing scotomas.

Progressive loss of the neuroretinal rim or increase in the size of the optic cup can be difficult to detect clinically, but the use of regular photography will help to detect change. Similarly, progressive visual field loss can be difficult to determine because perimetry is a subjective test with short- and long-term fluctuation causing variability in responses, problems with test reliability, and the influence of other factors such as cataract formation and pupil miosis. It is better to study a series of visual field tests for evidence of progression rather than making individual comparisons between the most recent and the baseline field test. A number of statistical methods (for example linear regression analysis) have been used to help identify progressive loss of retinal sensitivity using automated perimeters. If progressive field loss is detected and a change in therapy contemplated (such as filtration surgery) it is imperative to repeat the field test to obtain clear and repeatable evidence that the visual loss is progressing, and that it is glaucomatous in nature. If there is unequivocal evidence of disease progression then additional therapy is needed. This may take the form of a further topical agent, laser trabeculoplasty, or trabeculectomy.

Individual disease management

This section should not be read in isolation and the reader is advised to read the whole chapter to get a better understanding of the disease.

Armed with the above knowledge and information, the clinician is now able to concentrate on the individual circumstances of each patient. For example, a young, well-informed, and motivated patient will have good compliance with medical treatment, while some elderly patients with other medical conditions, will be less motivated and less compliant. In addition, the elderly find threshold perimetry difficult to manage, and as a result produce field results which are frequently unreliable and have artefacts.

Primary open angle glaucoma

This is by far the commonest form of glaucoma in Western populations. As defined above, this condition results in progressive optic nerve damage and visual field loss. Occurring generally in people over the age of 60 years at presentation it is generally bilateral, but asymmetric in terms of the amount of damage. It affects both sexes equally, and is more prevalent in the black population. Associated ocular and systemic features include myopia, retinal venous occlusion, systemic hypertension, and diabetes mellitus. The great majority of patients are initially detected by optometrists during a routine sight test ocular examination. Patients are generally asymptomatic, but on direct questioning, may have difficulty when moving from a bright to a dark room, suffer from glare, bump into objects, and experience difficulty judging steps and kerbs.

Despite the fact that glaucoma has been treated for over 100 years, there is no evidence, in the form of a published clinical trial of treatment versus no treatment of glaucoma that treatment is effective. However, the substantial weight of clinical opinion and judgement warrants that all patients with primary open angle glaucoma should be treated. Treatment takes the form of pressure reduction generally by medical means and possibly laser trabeculoplasty. Patients with uncontrolled disease (intraocular pressure too high with maximum tolerated medical therapy or progressive visual field loss with apparently 'controlled' ocular pressure) require surgery.

While the disease can present with pressures ranging from 22 up to 40 or 50 mmHg, most presenting pressures are in the region of the upper 20s and lower 30s, and consequently require at least two topical medications to achieve satisfactory pressure control. The majority of medically treated patients retain their presenting level of visual function provided they are identified early in the disease, are appropriately treated and monitored, and show good compliance. Once satisfactory pressure control has been achieved, patients should be reviewed every 4 to 6 months initially, and later every 6 to 8 months with regular pressure measurements, optic disc examination, and perimetry once or twice annually.

Because other ocular diseases such as cataract and macular degeneration occur commonly in the same age group, great care is needed to identify the various contributing factors to the level of visual field loss in such patients. Cataract formation generally results in a diffuse depression in the hill of vision, but occasionally a localized lens opacity may produce a scotoma. If cataract surgery is to be undertaken in the glaucoma patient, combining the cataract extraction with a drainage procedure in the form of phacotrabeculectomy, is very successful at visual rehabilitation and at lowering intraocular pressure.

Ocular hypertension

Ocular hypertension is defined here as the presence of elevated intraocular pressures and normal visual fields, with optic discs which may be normal or show some cupping. This common condition, affecting between 5 and 7 per cent of the population over the age of 40 years, constitutes a large proportion of those attending hospital clinics in this country. Only a small proportion of patients with this condition will convert to primary open angle glaucoma, the estimates from long-term studies showing a conversion rate of 1 to 2 per cent per annum. It is important therefore to identify those at risk of converting to glaucoma, so that treatment can be started thereby reducing the risk of progression to glaucoma.

The major risk factors are the level of ocular pressure and the presence of disc cupping. The higher the pressure, the greater the risk, and all patients with pressures of 30 mmHg or more require treatment even in the absence of other risk factors. The available evidence indicates that the risk begins to rise quite significantly if the pressures are consistently greater than 26 mmHg and many clinicians begin treatment at this level of pressure. Likewise having a cup to disc ratio of 0.6 or greater appears to carry an increased risk of subsequently developing glaucoma in the presence of ocular pressures greater than 21 mmHg, and is an indication for treatment. Having the combination of pressure greater than 26 mmHg and a cup to disc ratio of 0.6 or more greatly increases the risk of progression to glaucoma.

Other known risk factors (though possibly not as important as ocular pressure and cupping) to consider include myopia, a family history of glaucoma, Afro-Carribean race, and optic disc haemorrhage. Treatment of ocular hypertension is also indicated if the fellow eye has glaucoma, if it is an only eye situation, or if either eye has suffered a retinal vein occlusion. The presence of systemic diseases such as diabetes mellitus and arterial hypertension which increase the vulnerability of the optic nerve to pressure-induced damage may also be a factor in the decision to treat. Additional findings of a retinal fibre layer defect or an abnormality of some additional test (blue on yellow perimetry, psychophysical or electrodiagnostic assessment) would also be an indication for treatment.

It is important to note that most American glaucoma specialists would label and treat patients with raised pressure and optic disc cupping as glaucoma even in the absence of a visual field defect. In the United Kingdom, these patients would probably be called ocular hypertensives or possibly 'glaucoma suspects', because having elevated pressure and disc damage are the two most important risk factors for the development of irreversible glaucomatous visual field loss.

If treatment is deemed necessary in those with a high risk of developing glaucoma, medical therapy with one or two topical medications will in the majority, bring the ocular pressure to a satisfactory level so that the risk is minimized. Laser trabeculoplasty may be needed, but it is uncommon for ocular hypertensive patients to require drainage surgery because of inadequate pressure control. Once the condition is brought under satisfactory control (a process which may take several clinic visits over a short period), patients should be reviewed every 6 months, perhaps lengthening the time interval between review appointments after 1 or 2 years of monitoring. Likewise, the low-risk untreated patients (pressures less than 26 mmHg with healthy optic discs) need long-term review initially twice a year, but later this may be an annual clinic assessment. Some of these patients (the low-risk and possibly the well-controlled treated ocular hypertensives) may be suitable for a shared-care approach between glaucoma-trained community optometrists and the hospital eye service.

Low tension glaucoma

Also known as normal tension or normal pressure glaucoma, the essential clinical features of this condition are identical to primary open angle glaucoma except that the intraocular pressure level is less than 22 mmHg. Previously regarded as a relatively rare entity, recent prevalence studies show that approximately 25 per cent of all newly diagnosed cases of glaucoma have normal ocular pressure at the time of diagnosis. This apparent increase in prevalence may reflect improved examination skills and greater use of perimetry by optometrists.

Because the eye pressure is normal, a search for other contributing factors shows that vascular risk factors occur commonly in this condition. This search has identified factors which might influence the level of optic nerve perfusion, including cardiovascular (hypertension, angina, peripheral vascular disease) and cerebrovascular disease, systemic hypotension and exaggerated nocturnal dips in systemic blood pressure, and vasospastic disorders such as migraine and Raynaud's phenomenon. Although the pressure is within normal limits (that is less than 22 mmHg), studies on patients with asymmetric disease show that the eye with the higher pressure tends to have greater disc damage and visual field loss.

Although both high and low tension glaucoma result in abnormalities of the optic disc and visual field, there are certain features which tend to occur more commonly in the low pressure variety of glaucoma. Localized or focal rim loss or notching (see Fig. 2), acquired optic disc pits, flame-shaped disc haemorrhages and, peripapillary atrophy are more frequently seen in low tension glaucoma. Visual field defects in low tension glaucoma tend to be deeper and steeper, and occur closer to fixation (Fig. 7) than in primary open angle glaucoma.

It is important to exclude certain ocular and extraocular causes of the field loss. These include optic disc drusen, colobomatous optic discs, tilted discs with hypopigmentation of the inferonasal retina, optic neuropathies, chorioretinal disease, retinoschisis, or long-standing retinal detachment. Compressive lesions of the optic nerve or chiasm can produce visual field loss although it should be possible to differentiate the pattern of the neurological field defect from that of a glaucoma field defect. If the appearance of either the optic disc or the visual field does not equate with glaucoma damage, then further neuro-ophthalmic assessment and investigation is indicated.

At the time of diagnosis, other factors to take into account include a past ocular history of uveitis, trauma, corticosteroid use, or very rarely 'burned-out' pigment dispersion syndrome. Any history of cardiovascular disease, vasoactive medications, and smoking should be documented. It is important to obtain several recordings of intraocular pressure to include a morning reading before confirming the diagnosis. Because the majority of patients have their highest pressure reading in the morning period, an abbreviated form of diurnal phasing (for example from 9 a.m. to 1 p.m.) may suffice when reaching a diagnosis.

Because ocular pressure and vascular perfusion may contribute to optic nerve damage in low tension glaucoma, pressure reduction is probably indicated as this will improve perfusion, particularly if the presenting pressure is at the upper end of the normal range. If the level of ocular pressure is between 10 and 14 mmHg at diagnosis, it is unlikely that pressure *per se* plays a significant role. At this end of the pressure scale, attention should be paid to the vascular risk factors (for example stopping smoking, advising aerobic exercise), and consideration should possibly be given to the use of slow-release systemic calcium antagonists as these may help to improve optic nerve perfusion, provided they do not lower systemic blood pressure and are well tolerated by the patient.

As with primary open angle glaucoma, initial topical therapy is with one of the β-blockers. Combination therapy with a topical carbonic anhydrase inhibitor may help to reduce ocular pressure. When the visual field shows progressive loss, then filtration surgery (possibly with antimetabolites) is needed to achieve a low pressure of between 8 and 12 mmHg. It is important to remember that a large percentage of low tension glaucoma patients remains stable without evidence of progressive field loss.

Secondary open angle glaucoma

Pseudoexfoliation syndrome

Characterized by the deposition of grey–white fibrillar protein material throughout the anterior segment of the eye, the deposits consist of an abnormal mesh of fibrils and filaments consisting of glycoproteins such as fibrillin, elastin, amyloid, and tropoelastin. Initial presentation is frequently unilateral but 40 to 50 per cent of cases subsequently show bilateral involvement. The deposits can be seen on the anterior capsule and zonules of the lens (Figs 8, 9), pupillary margin, drainage angle, and corneal endothelium. Approximately 50 per cent of patients with the pseudoexfoliation syndrome develop open angle glaucoma, which presents with higher intraocular pressure and is more difficult to control that primary open angle glaucoma. It is a common condition in certain countries, particularly in Scandinavia where it is also called glaucoma capsulare. Associated features include pigment release from the iris pigment epithelial layer due to rubbing of the iris against the pseudoexfoliate material on the anterior lens capsule, which gives rise to iris transillumination defects close to the pupil margin. This increase in pigment can be seen on the corneal endothelium and in the trabecular meshwork of the drainage angle, especially in the inferior angle, where an additional line

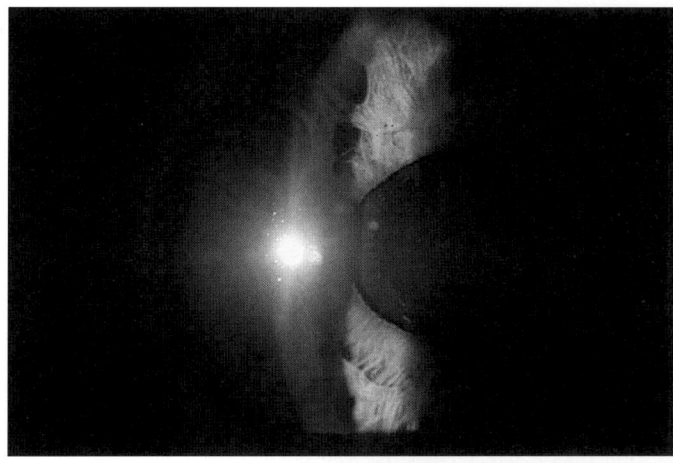

Fig. 8 Pseudoexfoliation material on the peripheral lens capsule. Pupil dilation significantly improves visualization of the pseudoexfoliate material on the capsule.

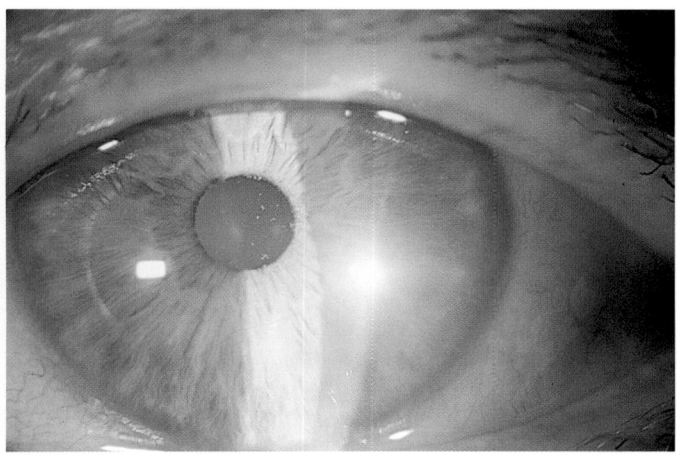

Fig. 9 Dandruff-like deposits of pseudoexfoliation on the pupil margin and central lens capsule.

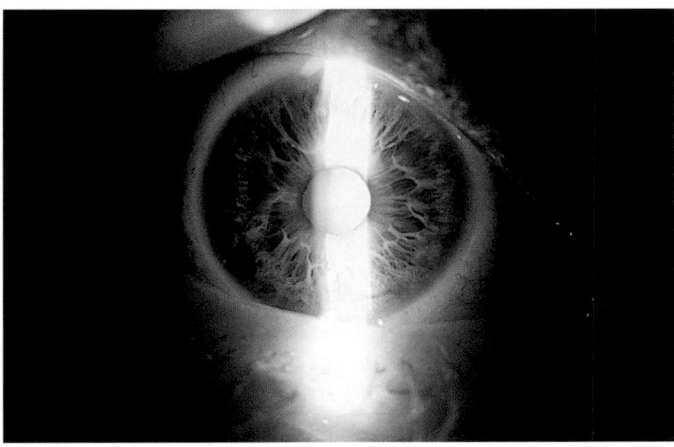

Fig. 10 Slit-like iris transillumination defects in the pigment dispersion syndrome.

of pigment deposition can be seen on or anterior to Schwalbe's line (called Sampolesi's line).

Depending on the level and duration of intraocular pressure, patients can have ocular hypertension or glaucoma. Treatment is similar to the management of these two conditions, although the higher level of pressure in pseudoexfoliative eyes may require several medications to achieve pressure control. Laser trabeculoplasty is generally very effective in this condition because of the increased level of trabecular meshwork pigmentation. Filtration surgery is often required to lower the pressure to a level where progressive field loss is brought under control. Cataract formation is common in the pseudoexfoliation syndrome, and involvement of the lens zonules increases the risk of zonular dehiscence during cataract surgery.

Pigment dispersion syndrome

The features of this condition are the release and deposition of pigment throughout the anterior chamber and peripheral retina due to the rubbing of the iris pigment epithelial layer against the lens zonules, particularly in eyes where there is excessive backward bowing of the mid-peripheral iris.

Typically the patient is a young to middle-aged Caucasian male (male to female ratio of 2–3 to 1) with mild to moderate myopia. Anterior segment examination shows a vertical region of corneal endothelial pigmentation called Krukenberg's spindle, pigment deposits on the lens and the anterior surface of the iris, and mid-peripheral slit-like iris transillumination defects (Fig. 10). Gonioscopy shows an open drainage angle with a dense band of pigmentation throughout the entire 360°, particularly on the posterior trabecular meshwork. Long-term studies indicate that between 20 and 40 per cent of people with this syndrome subsequently develop ocular hypertension or open angle glaucoma.

The mechanism of pigment release is hypothesized to be a form of reverse pupillary block resulting in a higher pressure in the anterior chamber than in the posterior chamber. This causes a backward bowing of the peripheral iris bringing the iris pigment layer into contact with the zonules. This posterior

bowing of the mid-peripheral iris can be relieved by laser iridotomy or miotic therapy.

Treatment of the associated ocular hypertension or glaucoma is similar to the management of primary open angle glaucoma, although the ocular pressure tends to be higher and more difficult to control. Although miotics help to relieve the reverse pupil block, they are poorly tolerated by young myopes. Laser trabeculoplasty is very effective at lowering pressure because of increased trabecular pigmentation although pressure control tends to decline with the passage of time. The success rate of drainage surgery in this condition is similar to that of primary open angle glaucoma. With increasing age, there is a tendency for the amount of pigment released to fall off considerably (termed 'burned-out' pigment dispersion syndrome). Exercise is known to increase pigment dispersion in certain individuals leading to pressure spikes and blurring of vision. In these patients, it may be advisable to use 0.5 per cent pilocarpine or low dose acetazolamide tablets before exercise.

Laser trabeculoplasty

This mode of treatment was first used in glaucoma nearly 20 years ago as an alternative to drainage surgery in poorly controlled disease. Argon and diode laser trabeculoplasty effectively lower intraocular pressure in many patients although its role in the management strategy currently remains unclear. It is generally used when one or two topical medications fail to achieve pressure control, but may have a role to play as a primary form of therapy in some patients. Because it is a surgical procedure with considerable risks and potential complications, it is essential that the doctor performing the treatment has considerable gonioscopy experience.

The standard argon laser protocol is to use a goniolens with a 50 micron spot size, a duration of 0.1 s, and energy levels between 500 and 1000 mW depending on the uptake of laser burns in the trabecular meshwork. The ideal response is to see a mild blanching or a small bubble when the laser is aimed at the anterior border of the pigmented meshwork. Initially, treatment of 180° with 50 laser burns is advised, followed if necessary 6 to 8 weeks later by treatment of the other half of the angle. Retreatment after 360° laser therapy is not indicated.

Before undertaking the procedure, the patient should be told the indication for treatment, what to expect during the procedure, a clear explanation of likely events during the postlaser period, and possible complications. Pretreatment with 250 or 500 mg acetazolamide 30 min before laser therapy helps to prevent post-laser pressure spikes. The intraocular pressure needs to be monitored for 1 to 2 h following treatment and if the pressure spikes to a high level then topical apraclonidine 1 per cent is very effective at rapidly lowering the pressure in this situation. A sustained pressure elevation occurs is a small percentage of patients following laser trabeculoplasty.

Patients should be prescribed topical steroid eye-drops for the mild post-laser uveitis and reviewed 1 week later when the steroids should be stopped. All glaucoma medications should be continued after laser therapy, and the patient should be seen at 6 weeks when, if the intraocular pressure has fallen significantly, consideration should be given to reducing or omitting some of the topical medications. Lowering of intraocular pressure following laser treatment results from an increase in aqueous outflow although the exact mechanism for this remains unclear. Conditions associated with increased angle pigmentation such as the pseudoexfoliation and pigment dispersion syndromes have a better response to argon laser trabeculoplasty than primary open angle glaucoma. The success rate falls with the passage of time, and 40 per cent maintain satisfactory pressure control 2 years after laser trabeculoplasty when performed as a primary therapy without associated medical therapy. The procedure should not be performed in paediatric and other secondary forms of glaucoma associated with closure of the angle due to rubeosis or peripheral anterior synechiae. The latter is a potential complication of laser trabeculoplasty if the laser burns are incorrectly placed or if excessive laser energy is used.

Indications for surgery

In primary and the forms of secondary open angle glaucoma described in this chapter, filtering surgery is generally reserved for patients with poorly controlled intraocular pressure and also for those with apparently well-controlled pressure but progressive glaucomatous damage. Factors influencing the decision to operate include the level of ocular pressure, the severity of optic nerve damage and visual field loss at presentation, and patient compliance with and tolerance of medical treatment.

It is important to establish early in the course of a patient's disease whether the prescribed medical therapy is having the desired effect. It is unwise to have a protracted period of attempted but unsuccessful medical control, and an early decision to operate may be in the patient's best interest.

Drainage surgery is also indicated in medically treated low tension glaucoma patients with progressive visual field loss. Surgical intervention in ocular hypertension is rarely indicated, but if deemed necessary is generally to lower poorly controlled intraocular pressure.

Further reading

Anderson, D.R. (1983). The mechanisms of damage of the optic nerve. In *Glaucoma update*, (ed. G. Kriegelstein and W. Leydhecker), pp. 89–93. Springer-Verlag, Heidelberg.

Caprioli, J. (1990). Automated perimetry in glaucoma. In *Visual fields: examination and interpretation*, (ed. T.J. Walsh), pp. 71–106. American Academy of Ophthalmology, San Francisco.

David, R., Livingston, D.G., and Luntz, M.H. (1977). Ocular hypertension—a long-term follow-up of treated and untreated patients. *British Journal of Ophthalmology*, 61, 668–72.

Drance, S.M. (1997). *Vascular risk factors and neuroprotection in glaucoma—update 1996*. Kugler, Amsterdam.

Fechtner, R. and Weinreb, R.N. (1994). Mechanisms of optic nerve damage in primary open angle glaucoma. *Survey of Ophthalmology*, 39, 23–42.

Flammer, J. (1996). To what extent are vascular risk factors involved in the pathogenesis of glaucoma. In *Ocular blood flows*, (ed. H.J. Kaiser, J. Flammer, and P. Hendrickson), pp. 12–39. Karger, Basel.

Geijssen, H.C. (1991). *Studies on normal pressure glaucoma*. Kugler, Amsterdam.

Grierson, I. (1986). Alterations in the outflow system in chronic simple glaucoma. In: *Glaucoma*, (ed. J.A. McAllister and R.P. Wilson), pp. 1–29. Butterworths, London.

Hitchings, R.A. (1992). Low tension glaucoma—its place in modern glaucoma practice. *British Journal of Ophthalmology*, 76, 494–6.

Hodapp, E., Parrish, R.K., and Anderson, D.R. (1993). *Clinical decisions in glaucoma*. Mosby-Year Book, St Louis.

Mills, R.P. and Weinreb, R.N. (ed.) (1991). *Glaucoma surgical techniques*. American Academy of Ophthalmology, San Francisco.

Quigley, H.A. (1986). Pathophysiology of the optic nerve in glaucoma. In *Glaucoma*, (ed. J.A. McAllister and R.P. Wilson), pp. 30–53. Butterworths, London.

Ritch, R., Shields, M.B., and Krupin, T. (ed.) (1996). *The glaucomas*. Mosby, St Louis.

Schwartz, A.L. (1993). Argon laser trabeculoplasty in glaucoma: what's happening (survey results of American Glaucoma Society members). *Journal of Glaucoma*, 2, 329–35.

Shields, M.B. (1998). *Textbook of glaucoma* (4th edn). Williams & Wilkins, Baltimore.

Sommer, A., Tielsch, J.M., Katz, J., *et al.* (1991). Relationship between intraocular pressure and primary open angle glaucoma among white and black Americans. The Baltimore Eye Survey. *Archives of Ophthalmology*, 109, 1090–5.

Spaeth, G.L. (1994). A new classification of glaucoma including focal glaucoma. *Survey of Ophthalmology*, 38 (suppl), 59–517.

Varma, R. and Spaeth, G.L. (ed.) (1993). *The optic nerve in glaucoma*. Lippincott, Philadelphia.

Yablonski, M.E., Zimmerman, T.J., Kass, M.A., and Becker, B. (1980). Prognostic significance of optic disc cupping in ocular hypertensive patients. *American Journal of Ophthalmology*, 89, 585–90.

2.10.8 Primary angle closure glaucoma

Yoshiaki Kitazawa and Tetsuya Yamamoto

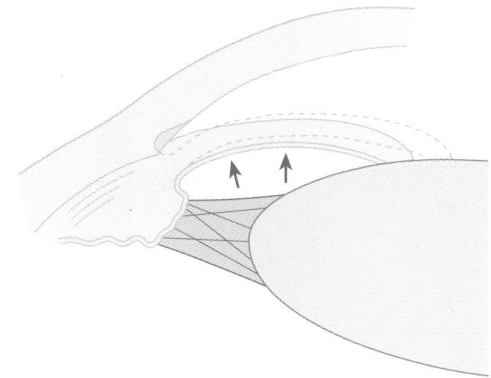

Fig. 1 Relative pupillary block.

Definition and aetiology

Angle closure glaucoma is a type of glaucoma in which the anterior chamber angle is mechanically occluded by the peripheral iris or peripheral anterior synechiae, causing the intraocular pressure to rise. There are two distinct types of the entity: primary angle closure glaucoma and several varieties of secondary angle closure glaucoma. This chapter discusses primary angle closure glaucoma only.

Acute angle closure glaucoma is the oldest recognized type of glaucoma. In fact, the word 'glaucoma' has long been a synonym for all acute glaucomas—mostly acute primary angle closure glaucoma. Hippocrates, speaking of the disease in his *Aphorisms*, characterized it by saying: 'If the pupil becomes sea-coloured, sight is destroyed and blindness of the other eye often follows'. This view continued through the mid-nineteenth century when several chronic types of glaucomas, due to the newly invented ophthalmoscope, were beginning to be recognized as pathological changes in the optic nerve head. In 1622, Banister, an English oculist, theorized for the first time in Europe that the acute condition is associated with high intraocular pressure: 'If one feele the Eye by rubbing upon the Eie-lids, . . . the Eye be growne more solid and hard than naturally it should be'. Since that time, the acute type of primary angle closure glaucoma has gradually come to be widely recognized clinically as a sight-threatening elevation of intraocular pressure in association with some inflammatory changes in the eyeball. However, the chronic type of primary angle closure glaucoma, the aetiology of which is nearly identical to that of the acute type, is much more common.

Mechanisms of angle closure

In primary angle closure glaucoma, the rise in intraocular pressure results from mechanical blockage of the anterior chamber angle by the peripheral iris. The mechanisms of angle blockage or closure in the disease are of two distinct types: the relative pupillary block and the plateau iris types.

Relative pupillary block is by far the more common mechanism (Fig. 1). When the lens is located relatively anterior to the chamber angle, because of a vector force induced by the iris and the lens towards the centre of the eyeball, the aqueous humour in the posterior chamber is more or less prevented from flowing through the pupil into the anterior chamber. Because of the resistance at the pupillary margin, aqueous humour builds up in the posterior chamber, creating a pressure higher than that in the anterior chamber. This pressure differ-

ential exerts a force on the peripheral iris, bending it towards the chamber angle. If the force is strong enough to bring the iris into contact with the angle, the angle begins to close and the intraocular pressure rises. In the early stages, angle closure is reversible; if the relative pupillary block is reduced or eliminated, the angle reopens. At this stage, the condition is referred to as appositional or functional angle closure. However, the closure can become organic with the development of peripheral anterior synechiae, gradually in many chronic cases, or relatively quickly in acute cases. Organic angle closure is permanent unless some of the synechiae can be surgically peeled off.

The other major type of primary angle closure glaucoma is the plateau iris syndrome. Here, when the pupil is dilated, the iris becomes attached to the chamber angle, even when there is no relative pupillary block (Fig. 2). Although pure cases of the syndrome are very rare, the plateau configuration of the iris occurs in about 10 to 15 per cent of eyes with primary angle closure glaucoma in which relative pupillary block is the main cause of closure.

Angle closure is also classified in terms of the site to which the peripheral iris has become attached, that is in the vicinity of Schwalbe's line or at the bottom of the angle recess. A recent ultrasound biomicroscopic study demonstrates that the former type is as common as the latter with respect to the appositional closure (Figs 3 and 4). But in organic angle closure, synechial closures rarely commence near Schwalbe's line; however, in

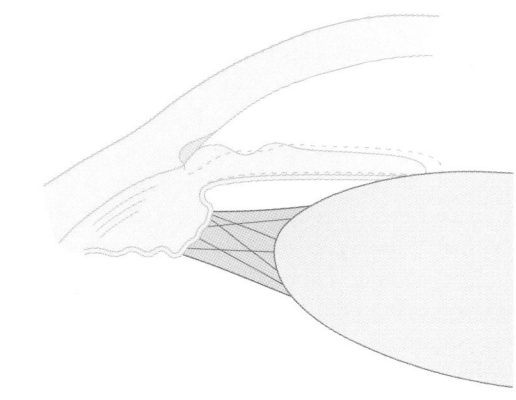

Fig. 2 Plateau iris mechanism.

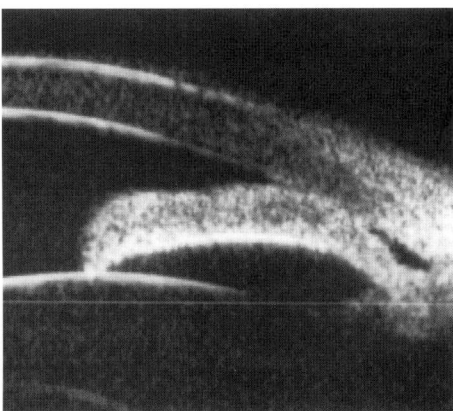

Fig. 3 Angle closure starting in the vicinity of Schwalbe's line (ultrasound biomicroscopic view).

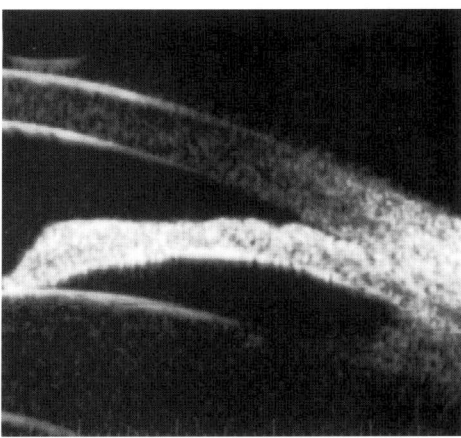

Fig. 4 Angle closure starting from the bottom of the angle recess (ultrasound biomicroscopic view).

width, they vary from small tent-like formations to one that may even cover the entire angle circumference. They tend to occur in the superior quadrant of the chamber angle, probably because the superior angle is physiologically narrower than other parts of it.

Epidemiology

It is well known that the incidence of primary angle closure glaucoma and the prevalence of eyes with a narrow angle vary remarkably among the various ethnic groups. They are highest among the Innuit and lowest among Caucasians and black people, with Asians (including Chinese, Japanese, and so on) somewhere in between. It is estimated that the susceptibility of Innuit women to primary angle closure glaucoma is 40 times higher than it is among Caucasian women. The incidence is estimated to be less than 0.1 per cent in Caucasians, about one-fifth of that of primary open angle glaucoma. A nationwide glaucoma survey conducted in Japan found the incidence to be 0.38 per cent among women aged 40 years or older and 0.21 per cent among men in the same age group. In fact, the

condition usually develops in individuals over 40 years of age, and women are more commonly affected than men. There is also a tendency for it to develop in persons with a positive family history and/or hypermetropia.

Anatomical features

Primary angle closure glaucoma mostly affects eyes with shallow anterior chambers. Thus, affected eyes tend to have distinctive anatomical features: a smaller axial length, a steeper corneal curvature, a shallower anterior chamber, a more thickened lens, and a relatively more anteriorly located lens. Refraction in these eyes is usually hyperopic or emmetropic. As a result of these kinds of morphological variations of the eyeball as a whole, the angle is narrower than in normal eyes. Interestingly, despite the marked differences in the incidence of angle closure among several different ethnic groups, the biometric data are more or less identical. Thus, it is likely that some topological differences in the anatomy of the anterior segment other than these parameters are crucial in the development of angle closure.

Clinical features

Clinical types

Primary angle closure glaucoma is further diagnosed as acute or chronic depending on the presence or absence of the characteristic clinical signs and symptoms of an acute attack. Some investigators prefer to distinguish a third type coming somewhere in between these two, a subacute form in which mild transient symptoms such as headache, eye pain, conjunctival hyperaemia, and halo occur intermittently in otherwise quiet eyes.

Acute primary angle closure glaucoma

Here, because of an acute rise of intraocular pressure, several symptoms and signs appear rapidly. This condition, one of the most important emergency conditions in ophthalmology, is also known as a glaucoma attack. Unless treated immediately, the affected eye may permanently lose sight in a matter of several hours.

Precipitating factors

Several factors that appear to precipitate an acute attack in eyes with a narrow angle have been distinguished. A number of conditions that may induce temporary mydriasis may trigger an attack, including dim light, emotional stress, and medications such as anticholinergics and adrenergics. Thus, mydriatics should be used very cautiously in examining eyes with a narrow angle. Conversely, conditions inducing miosis also sometimes trigger an acute attack. Here, a greater relative pupillary block caused by miosis and anterior displacement of the lens is the suspected mechanism.

Symptoms

Foggy vision, deep eye pain, headache, nausea, and vomiting are common symptoms and they get worse very quickly. Some patients seek non-ophthalmic treatment because of the extraocular symptoms, possibly delaying correct diagnosis and appropriate treatment. The foggy vision mainly results from corneal oedema and circulatory disturbance in the optic disc area. Since the oedematous cornea serves as an optical diffractor, the patient often complains of rainbow-coloured (halo) vision. The eye pain, headache, nausea, and vomiting are caused by irritation of the trigeminal and parasympathetic nerves. Profound sweating, also related to parasympathetic stimulation, is common as well.

Clinical signs

The following clinical findings are very important in the diagnosis of acute primary angle closure glaucoma: highly elevated intraocular pressure, corneal oedema, angle closure, aqueous flare in a shallow anterior chamber, mydriasis, conjunctival hyperaemia, iris atrophy, and glaukomflecken (Fig. 5).

Intraocular pressure usually rises to around 40 to 80 mmHg and even as high as 100 mmHg in a few cases. Spontaneous remission sometimes occurs, with the intraocular pressure decreasing to around 20 mmHg, possibly leading to misdiagnosis.

Corneal oedema, with the accompanying loss of corneal transparency, results from reversible decompensation of corneal endothelium due to the acute rise in intraocular pressure. When the pressure decreases, the pathological corneal condition disappears unless corneal endothelial cells have become irreversibly damaged during an especially long-lasting, severe attack.

Demonstration of angle closure is indispensable to correct diagnosis. But such demonstration is difficult during the attack because of severe corneal oedema and dense aqueous flare. In such cases, gonioscopy should be performed following medical reduction of intraocular pressure with pilocarpine carbonic anhydrase inhibitors and possibly hyperosmotic agents. In these cases, the angle is closed or, at best, slit-like at all areas of the angle circumference. Pressure gonioscopy (i.e. indentation or compression gonioscopy) reveals the presence of peripheral

anterior synechiae in almost all cases. Their extent depends on the duration and severity of the attack.

Determination of a potentially closable, narrow angle in the fellow eye is a key point in correct diagnosis. The anterior chamber is shallow in both eyes in all cases, never exceeding 3 mm. However, it is not as shallow as it is in malignant glaucoma (aqueous misdirection syndrome) or in some eyes with lens dislocation. Aqueous flare, visible upon slit lamp examination, appears as a result of the breakdown of the blood–aqueous barrier, corresponding with the concentration of protein in the anterior chamber. In contrast with secondary glaucoma due to some types of uveitis, mutton fat-like keratic precipitates are not seen.

Due to paralysis of the iris sphincter muscles, the pupil is in a mid-dilated position and the iris loses reactivity to light. In many cases, the pupil is vertically oval.

The conjunctiva is hyperaemic because of congestion of ocular vessels. Unlike in conjunctivitis, ciliary injection is also present.

Iris atrophy and glaukomflecken are positive signs indicating a past attack (Fig. 6). They remain for life. Thus, the occurrence of a past attack can be verified even several decades later. Iris atrophy, sectorial or entirely on the iris surface, results from ischemia of the iris. The atrophic iris also shows depigmentation. Glaukomflecken is a type of cataract that develops following an acute glaucoma attack. White dot-like lens opacities appear in subcapsular areas of the lens and gradually become buried in the anterior cortical zone.

Diagnosis

A diagnosis of acute angle closure glaucoma is established based on clinical signs and symptoms. However, it is difficult to distinguish the condition from several forms of secondary glaucoma, including neovascular glaucoma, secondary angle closure glaucoma due to intumescent cataract, secondary angle closure glaucoma caused by dislocation of the lens, phacolytic glaucoma, Posner–Schlossman syndrome or glaucomatocyclitic

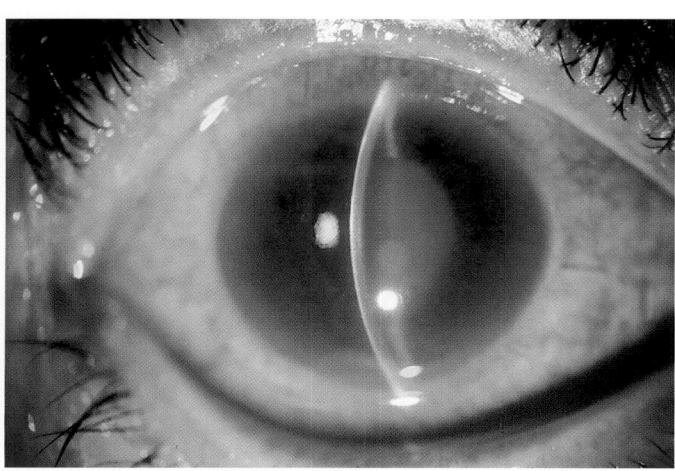

Fig. 5 Acute primary angle closure glaucoma.

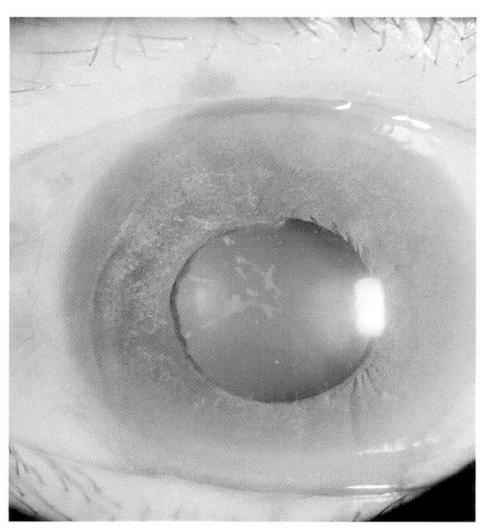

Fig. 6 Glaukomflecken and iris atrophy.

crisis, and secondary glaucoma due to uveitis. In terms of acute onset and severe symptoms, neovascular glaucoma and the three types of lens-related secondary glaucomas are very similar to acute primary angle closure glaucoma. Careful gonioscopy of eyes that have suffered an acute attack as well as of their fellow eyes helps establish the correct diagnosis.

Some clinical findings useful for differential diagnosis are as follows:

- neovascularization in the iris and the angle, a deep anterior chamber, and a history of retinal vascular occlusive diseases such as diabetic retinopathy and central retinal vein occlusion in neovascular glaucoma

- the presence of mature or hypermature cataract with a very shallow anterior chamber in secondary angle closure glaucoma due to intumescent cataract

- anterior chambers of different depths in the same individual in secondary angle closure glaucoma caused by dislocation of the lens

- the presence of mature or hypermature cataract and severe inflammatory reactions in the anterior segment in phacolytic glaucoma

Visual field and optic disc findings are not helpful in diagnosing acute primary angle closure glaucoma.

Prognosis

Visual prognosis of acute primary angle closure glaucoma depends on the status of the optic nerve and the level of intraocular pressure control achieved following the attack. If the attack is successfully treated within a few hours, the prognosis is good; no deterioration will occur in some mild cases. The longer the attack, the more likely it is that the eye will lose sight permanently solely due to the attack. Because of the development of cataract or corneal oedema, some eyes will later require cataract extraction or a corneal transplant.

Chronic primary angle closure glaucoma

In the chronic form of primary angle closure glaucoma, angle closure occurs insidiously. In the beginning, the intraocular pressure stays within normal limits, rising only when functional angle closure occurs over some extent of the angle circumference. With time, the closure becomes organized, and when the organic closure (peripheral anterior synechiae) exceeds a certain area, for example one-third to one-half of the total angle circumference, the intraocular pressure remains higher than 'normal', even when there is no functional closure. The intraocular pressure gradually increases, eventually rising to 50 to 60 mmHg as the extent of the peripheral anterior synechiae broadens. However, because the rise is gradual, affected eyes often seem to adapt, showing no clinical signs of acute attack and no characteristic angle closure symptoms. Some patients complain of mild headache, eye pain, and so on, but the absence of complaints is not unusual.

Except for a shallow anterior chamber and a narrow angle,

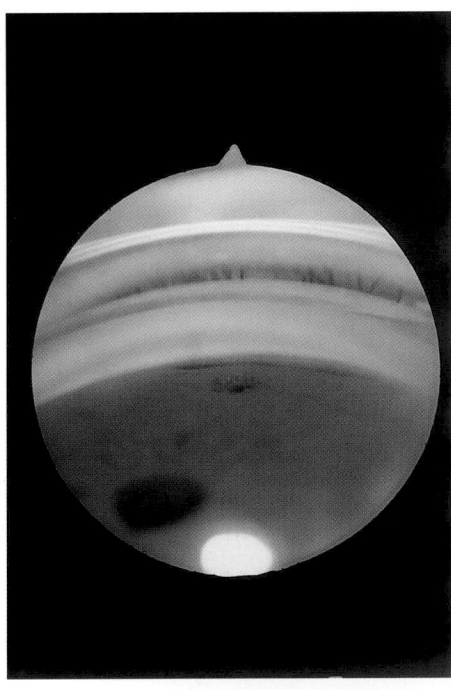

Fig. 7 Gonioscopic view of chronic primary angle closure glaucoma, showing peripheral anterior synechiae.

the clinical findings of chronic primary angle closure glaucoma more closely resemble those of primary open angle glaucoma than those of acute primary angle closure glaucoma. Intraocular pressure is high—around 30 to 60 mmHg—although it fluctuates and is sometimes within normal limits in early cases. The cornea is clear. The anterior chamber is shallow but there is no evidence of aqueous flare. The iris configuration is convex. The angle is narrow: when the intraocular pressure is elevated, the angle is closed or slit-like; when it is normal, the angle is usually Shaffer 1 narrow (Fig. 7). Pressure gonioscopy is indispensable for distinguishing functional closure from organic closure, that is for accurately determining the extent of peripheral anterior synechiae. Direct as opposed to indirect pressure gonioscopy is more suitable for accurate viewing in eyes with a very narrow angle.

Optic disc examination demonstrates essentially the same abnormalities as those seen in primary open angle glaucoma. Accordingly, perimetric abnormalities are also largely the same as those in primary open angle glaucoma.

Diagnosis

The diagnosis of chronic angle closure glaucoma is established by finding evidence of angle closure caused by relative pupillary block or the plateau iris mechanism. Elevation of intraocular pressure and the presence of glaucomatous optic nerve damage are not essential for the diagnosis. Therefore, gonioscopy is especially crucial. If peripheral anterior synechiae are found by pressure gonioscopy in cases with bilateral shallow anterior chamber, and if other conditions known to precipitate peripheral anterior synechiae such as uveitis and lens dislocation can be differentiated, a diagnosis of chronic primary angle closure glaucoma may be established. This is possible even though intraocular pressure is normal and no glaucomatous changes are evident in the optic nerve head or visual field. Provocative tests may also be used.

Differential diagnosis of chronic primary angle closure glaucoma includes primary open angle glaucoma that has developed in narrow-angled eyes, and several forms of secondary angle closure glaucoma. In the former, intraocular pressure remains elevated even though the trabecular meshwork is visible gonioscopically over most of the angle circumference. When both open angle and angle closure mechanisms are present in the same eye, the condition is referred to as combined mechanism glaucoma. However, all single mechanisms of increased intraocular pressure must be ruled out before a double mechanism diagnosis can be entertained. Gonioscopic findings and intraocular pressure information are useful for this purpose. Secondary angle closure glaucomas due to lens dislocation, nanophthalmos, malignant glaucoma, massive lesions in the posterior segment, ciliary body swelling, tumours, and so on, may resemble primary angle closure glaucoma. Careful examination of both eyes, including gonioscopy as well as detailed history taking, are useful in the differential diagnosis.

Prognosis

Intraocular pressure control in chronic primary angle closure glaucoma depends on the extent of peripheral anterior synechiae and of any remaining function of the chamber angle. Generally speaking, if one-third of the angle remains open, medical control of the intraocular pressure at a 20 mmHg level is highly probable. As in primary open angle glaucoma, visual acuity does not deteriorate until the advanced stages in chronic primary angle closure glaucoma. Visual field defects depend on glaucomatous changes in the optic nerve head: if glaucomatous changes are absent or mild, the visual prognosis is good; if they are advanced, visual prognosis is only fair or poor.

Provocative tests

Differentiating simple narrow angle from primary angle closure glaucoma is especially challenging. Several provocative tests as well as pressure gonioscopy have been designed to differentiate between the two. All of these tests exploit the essential character of the disease, namely angle closure with a consequent rise of intraocular pressure. The dark-room provocative test, the mydriatic provocative test, and the prone position provocative test are common. For example, in the prone position test, a suspected patient is kept in a prone position for 60 min and immediately following the provocation, tonometry and gonioscopy are performed. A rise of intraocular pressure of at least 8 mmHg is deemed positive. However, the non-physiological character of all of the provocative tests limits their usefulness; their sensitivity and specificity reportedly range from 48 to 90 per cent at the most. Thus, a positive provocative test may be considered positive evidence of primary angle closure glaucoma, but a negative result does not exclude the presence of

the disease in a particular eye, and further careful follow-up is required to confirm the diagnosis.

Principles of management

Management of acute attack

Medical therapy is used for treating an acute attack, firstly, to reduce the intraocular pressure as quickly as possible to preserve useful vision, and, secondly, to break the pupillary block by mechanically pulling the iris toward the pupillary centre. Immediately after a diagnosis of acute attack is established, intensive measures should be taken.

To reduce the intraocular pressure carbonic anhydrase inhibitors with or without hyperosmotic agents such as mannitol, glycerol, and isosorbide are administered intravenously or orally; topical β-blockers or dorzolamide also may be used. Carbonic anhydrase inhibitors and β-blockers reduce the pressure by suppressing aqueous production. Hyperosmotic agents reduce the intraocular pressure via reduction of vitreous volume by creating an osmotic gradient between blood and intraocular fluid and by removing water from the vitreous. Hyperosmotic agents and carbonic anhydrase inhibitors cannot be administered orally in many cases because of the nausea and vomiting that typically occur during a severe attack.

Pilocarpine, a parasympathomimetic medication, is administered to break pupillary block. The action of pilocarpine is through parasympathomimetic stimulation of the iris sphincter muscle. Dosage should be small enough to avoid any toxic effects: a couple of drops of 1 or 2 per cent pilocarpine are enough to break the pupillary block if the intraocular pressure is reduced. During a severe attack, more intensive instillation is needed. Once the pupillary block is broken, instillation of 1 or 2 per cent pilocarpine four times daily should be continued to avoid reclosure of the angle until the pupillary block is permanently resolved by surgical intervention.

Laser iridotomy

Pupillary block can be resolved by creating a bypass between the anterior and posterior chambers. Laser iridotomy is the preferred method of doing this. Figure 8 shows how the pro-

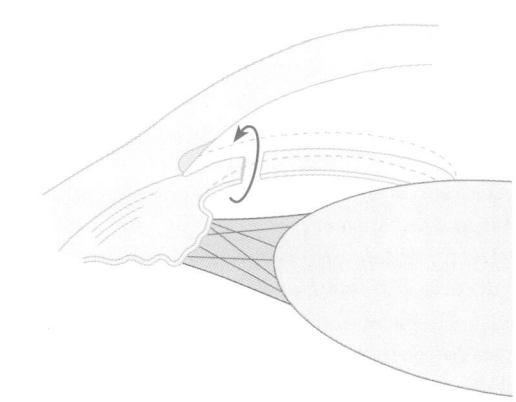

Fig. 8 Mechanism of action of the laser iridotomy.

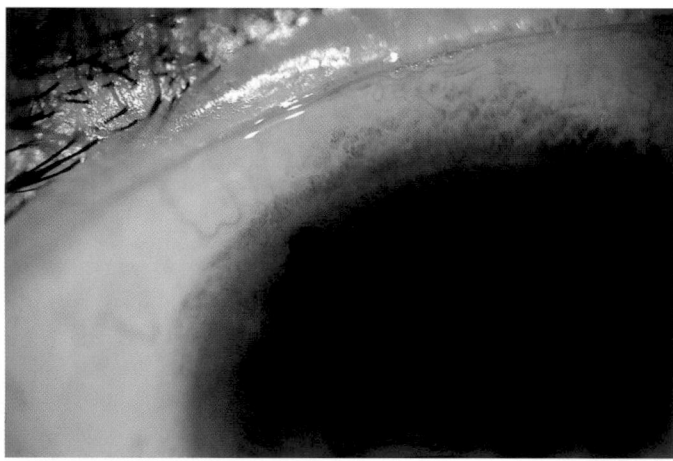

Fig. 9 Argon laser iridotomy.

cedure works to break pupillary block. The two major lasers presently available for the procedure are the argon laser and the neodymium–yttrium–aluminium-garnet (Nd–YAG) laser. The argon laser can create an iridotomy by thermal effect (Fig. 9); the Q-switched Nd–YAG laser by optical breakdown. Laser iridotomy should be performed without delay in all cases of primary angle closure glaucoma once the diagnosis has been established.

The success rate of creating a patent iridotomy in eyes with chronic angle closure glaucoma by either the argon or Nd–YAG laser is almost 100 per cent. With the argon laser, a shot with shorter laser duration and higher energy is preferable for brown or dark irides. However, it is difficult to create a patent iridotomy in some acute cases, especially when corneal oedema and/or dense aqueous flare are present. In such cases, the iridotomy may be delayed for a couple of days as long as the angle has been reopened and the intraocular pressure normalized with medical treatment. Topical corticosteroids are recommended to reduce inflammatory reaction in eyes waiting to undergo the procedure.

Medical therapy

Medical treatment of primary angle closure glaucoma should be restricted to cases involving an acute attack, those for which laser iridotomy is planned, and those with uncontrollable intraocular pressure following iridotomy. Adrenaline and dipivefrin may increase pupillary block and definitely should not be used before laser iridotomy. Intraocular pressure may be controlled medically without laser iridotomy in chronic primary angle closure glaucoma. However, continuing medical treatment without performing laser iridotomy could increase peripheral anterior synechiae formation and, eventually, loss of pressure control.

Therefore, early resolution of pupillary block by laser iridotomy is of the utmost importance. If the intraocular pressure is uncontrollable following laser iridotomy, additional medical treatment should be instituted. In such circumstances, medications should be used as in primary open angle glaucoma.

Other surgical procedures

Another laser procedure, laser gonioplasty, is preferred for some eyes in which laser iridotomy is difficult to perform, especially in those suffering a fulminating attack. In laser gonioplasty, argon laser is delivered evenly to all portions of the peripheral iris to open up the angle by shrinking the peripheral iris. The advantage of laser gonioplasty over laser iridotomy is that it can be performed even in eyes undergoing a severe attack. Since the effect of the gonioplasty may not be permanent, laser iridotomy should be performed in such eyes after the acute inflammatory reaction subsides.

Incisional iridectomy also can be performed, and, in fact, it used to be the first-choice treatment before the introduction of laser iridotomy.

Lens extraction with implantation of a posterior chamber intraocular lens is another method of breaking the pupillary block. Recent advances in cataract surgery, with better surgical outcomes, make this the preferred procedure in eyes with medically controllable primary angle closure glaucoma with moderate to advanced lens opacity.

In eyes in which intraocular pressure is uncontrollable with maximum tolerable medication after a patent iridotomy has been created, glaucoma filtering surgery is indicated. Trabeculectomy, a guarded filtering surgery, should be performed in these circumstances. Primary angle closure glaucoma is a well-known risk factor for the development of several postoperative complications such as malignant glaucoma (aqueous misdirection syndrome) and shallow anterior chamber. Therefore, preventative measures such as preoperative use of hyperosmotic agents and tight closure of the scleral flap should be adopted.

Surgical reconstruction of the chamber angle by releasing peripheral anterior synechiae has been reported. The long-term effectiveness of the procedure (goniosynechialysis) remains to be demonstrated.

Management of the fellow eye

Primary angle closure glaucoma is bilateral. With acute primary angle closure glaucoma, the probability of an acute attack in the non-attack fellow eye within 5 years following an attack in the first eye is estimated to be around 80 per cent if no treatment is given, and about 50 per cent even if pilocarpine is used. Therefore, when one eye suffers an acute attack, it is highly desirable to perform prophylactic laser iridotomy in the fellow eye.

Treatment of plateau iris syndrome

Treatment of plateau iris syndrome (primary angle closure glaucoma caused by plateau iris mechanism) is distinct. Resolving relative pupillary block is useless in treating the plateau iris syndrome, as one might guess from the definition of this rare clinical entity. Laser gonioplasty and pilocarpine are the two preferred treatments. However, even in eyes in which plateau iris syndrome is suspected based on the iris configuration, laser iridotomy is usually performed in order to eliminate the pupillary block component, which is more or less present in most of the cases, and to confirm the diagnosis. If the angle becomes closed following laser iridotomy when the pupil is dilated, the diagnosis of the syndrome is confirmed.

Other related information

Ultrasound biomicroscopy

Ultrasound biomicroscopy, recently developed for investigating the anterior segment of the eye, is particularly useful for estimating relative pupillary block and detecting functional angle closure in eyes with a narrow angle. Using this technique, it has been found that in about two-thirds of eyes with chronic primary angle closure glaucoma the angle closes functionally in dark-room conditions before laser iridotomy is performed. Ultrasound biomicroscopy is also valuable for detecting appositional angle closure and plateau iris configuration. It is a promising tool for the early diagnosis of primary angle closure glaucoma.

Further reading

Cairns, J.E. (ed.) (1986). *Glaucoma*. Grune & Stratton, London.

Epstein, D.L. (1996). *Chandler and Grant's glaucoma*, (4th edn). Williams & Wilkins, Baltimore.

Hoskins, H.D. Jr and Kass, M. (1989). *Becker and Shaffer's diagnosis and therapy of the glaucomas*, 6th edn. Mosby, St Louis.

Ritch, R., Shields, M.B., and Krupin, T. (ed.) (1996). *The glaucomas*, (2nd edn). Mosby, St Louis.

Shields, M.B. (1997). *Textbook of glaucoma*, (4th edn). Williams & Wilkins, Baltimore.

Van Buskirk, E.M. (1986). *Clinical atlas of glaucoma*. Saunders, Philadelphia.

2.10.9 The secondary glaucomas

Simon Ruben and R.A. Hitchings

The secondary glaucomas are a protean group of conditions that cause elevated intraocular pressure and together account for about a third of all cases of glaucoma seen by the ophthalmologist. Unlike primary open angle glaucoma, which is often associated with an intraocular pressure within normal limits, secondary glaucomas can be diagnosed by pressure alone on the assumption that optic nerve damage will ensue if the high pressure remains untreated. Strictly speaking the majority of patients with secondary glaucoma could be considered as having 'secondary ocular hypertension', although if untreated these eyes have a high risk of developing glaucomatous damage (as intraocular pressures are often considerably higher than

Figures 2 to 7, 10, 13, and 14 are reproduced with permission of the Western Eye Hospital Photographic Department. Figures 8 and 16 are reproduced with permission of Wolfe Medical Publications.

normal) and using the term glaucoma for all cases removes the risk of complacency in management. How the patient presents will depend on the underlying aetiology. For example, secondary acute angle closure glaucoma may have similar symptoms and signs to primary angle closure glaucoma, glaucoma associated with uveitis will usually be diagnosed by the ophthalmologist, and secondary open angle glaucoma may be picked up within the community by primary health-care screening.

Classification

Because of the diverse nature of the secondary glaucomas classification is not simple, but commonly two approaches have been made (Table 1): firstly, with respect to the mechanism of the raised pressure, and secondly, by aetiology. The mechanistic approach to classification is important in understanding the pathological processes involved in causing raised intraocular pressure whereas the aetiological classification considers the underlying disorder which would seem to be a more sensible approach for the clinician, as management is often directed as much at treatment of the cause as at the glaucoma.

Glaucomas associated with corneal pathology

Iridocorneal endothelial syndromes

This spectrum of diseases was originally described as three separate entities: Chandler's syndrome, essential iris atrophy, and iris–naevus syndrome of Cogan–Reese, but all have in common an abnormality of the corneal endothelium, the anterior chamber angle, and iris. These conditions typically present in the 20–40-year-old age group with corneal oedema, blurred vision, and pain, and are usually unilateral and more commonly occur in females. The underlying pathology is an endothelial degeneration with the appearance of fine guttata which migrates over the anterior chamber angle, trabecular meshwork, and anterior surface of the iris. Specular microscopy reveals a typical appearance of large irregular endothelial cells with abnormal morphology. The unaffected eye will in contrast show healthy endothelial cells (Fig. 1).

In Chandler's syndrome the predominant features are corneal with marked oedema (even with normal intraocular pressures), but only mild iris atrophy and corectopia. Iris changes are most severe in essential iris atrophy with progressive atrophy, iris holes (causing pseudopolycoria), and marked corectopia. The endothelial membrane tends to contract towards the angle causing pupillary distortion and the formation of full thickness holes. In the Cogan–Reese syndrome there are, in addition to this picture, multiple pigmented nodules over the surface of the iris. These are thought to be protrusions of iris stroma through defects in the endothelial membrane. The majority of patients present with variable features of all these subgroups. Herpes simplex viral DNA has been identified in ocular tissues of patients with iridocorneal endothelial syndrome and has been implicated in its pathogenesis. This inflammatory aetiology may account for the unilateral nature of

Table 1 Classification of secondary glaucoma
(a) According to mechanism

Open angle glaucoma	Pretrabecular (e.g. neovascular or inflammatory membrane)
	Trabecular (e.g. pigment clogging or trabecular trauma)
	Post-trabecular (e.g. raised episcleral venous pressure)
Closed angle glaucoma	Secondary to pupil block (e.g. subluxed lens)
	Secondary to anterior 'pulling' (e.g. formation of PAS, e.g. uveitis)
	Secondary to forward 'pushing' (e.g. cileolenticular block)

PAS, peripheral anterior synechiae.

Table 1 Classification of secondary glaucoma
(b) According to aetiology

Secondary to ocular disease	Cornea (e.g. ICE syndromes)
	Iris (e.g. iris cysts)
	Lens (e.g. lens-induced uveitis)
	Retina (e.g. post-traumatic retinal detachment)
	Raised episcleral venous pressure (e.g. Sturge–Weber)
	Tumours (e.g. iris melanoma) (melanocytic glaucoma)
	Inflammation (e.g. heterochromic cyclitis)
Steroids	Topical
	Systemic
Trauma	Angle recession
Postsurgery	Ciliary block
	Aphakia/pseudophakia
	Retinal surgery
Associated with congenital abnormalities of the eye	Aniridia
	Anterior segment cleavage syndromes
	Chromosomal abnormalities

ICE, iridocorneal endothelial syndrome.

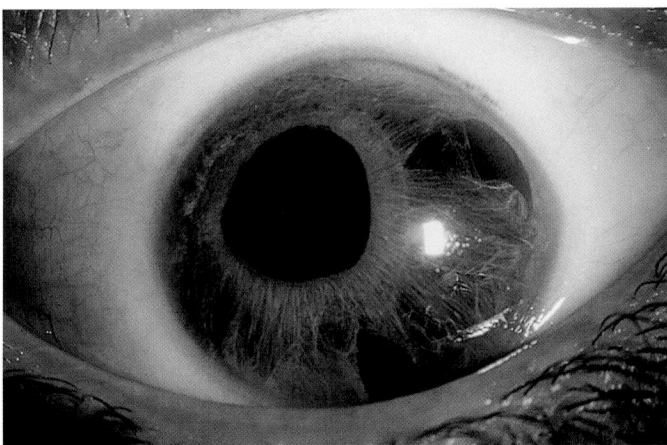

(a)

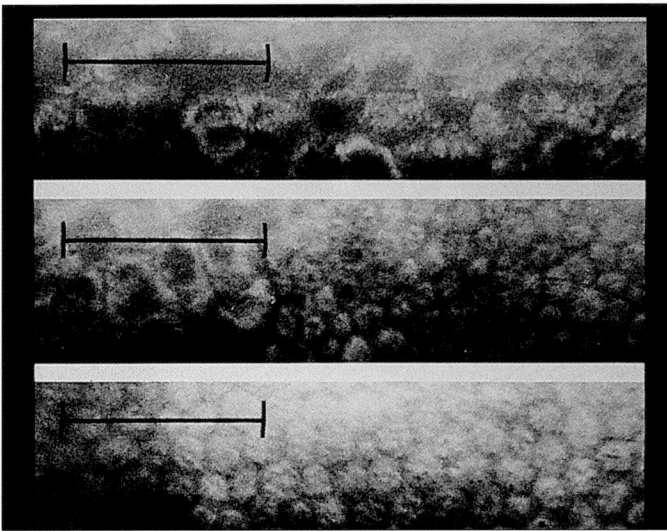

(b)

Fig. 1 Iridocorneal endothelial syndrome. (a) Typical anterior segment appearance showing iris thinning, corectopia, and pseudopolycoria. (b) Upper two sections show typical abnormal large iridocorneal endothelial syndrome cells, with normal appearance of endothelium from the fellow eye (bottom).

antimetabolites in glaucoma filtration surgery may lead to an improvement in intraocular pressure control but the use of these agents in young patients is not without risk as the long-term effects of hypotony and leaking blebs are still not fully realized.

Posterior polymorphous dystrophy

This is a dominantly inherited condition that is bilateral, often progressive, and tends to manifest in childhood. Posterior polymorphous dystrophy usually does not become symptomatic until early adulthood. Slit lamp examination reveals irregular lesions of the posterior cornea involving either a small area or occurring diffusely across the whole surface. Signs and symptoms may show marked asymmetry between the two eyes. Glaucoma occurs in about 15 per cent of eyes. Extensive iridocorneal adhesions may lead to angle closure glaucoma similar in mechanism to the iridocorneal endothelial syndromes.

the condition together with the occasional report of cases where mild iritis was noted at initial presentation.

The glaucoma can often be initially controlled with medical therapy but surgery is often required as the disease progresses. Surgery may fail due to endothelial growth over the fistula making tube surgery or diode laser ablation of the ciliary body necessary. In addition to glaucoma surgery a number of patients will need corneal grafting and cataract surgery. This combination of problems is often difficult to manage with patients having to undergo multiple surgical procedures resulting in a poor long-term visual prognosis. The increasing popularity of

Glaucoma may also occur in the presence of an open angle in association with a 'high' insertion of the iris. Differentiation from iridocorneal endothelial syndrome may be difficult but can be made on the basis of bilateral endothelial lesions in posterior polymorphous dystrophy. Glaucoma, if it occurs is managed in the same manner as for primary open angle glaucoma.

Glaucomas associated with diseases of the iris

Pigmentary glaucoma (pigment dispersion syndrome/glaucoma)

Pigment dispersion typically occurs in young myopic men with blue irides although there are many exceptions to this rule. Melanin pigment is lost from the pigment epithelium of the iris leading to radial slit-shaped defects which can be seen on transillumination. The pigment is deposited on structures within the anterior chamber including lens and zonules, iris, trabecular meshwork, and corneal endothelium (Krukenberg spindle).

The presence of pigment dispersion does not universally lead to glaucoma or even raised intraocular pressure, with only about 10 per cent of patients actually developing glaucoma. Although pigment dispersion glaucoma usually follows a progressive course, a few patients show a decrease in the trabecular pigment with time and iris transillumination defects may even disappear.

The pathophysiology of pigment dispersion is not entirely clear. The disease may occur in two stages. Initially pigment granules may themselves cause clogging of the trabecular meshwork causing transient spikes of intraocular pressure which may not necessarily lead to chronic glaucoma. In addition transient pressure spikes can occur after exercise with increase in pigment release. In the second stage, excessive phagocytosis of pigment leads to migration and/or autolysis of trabecular endothelial cells with trapping of cell debris by the meshwork and sclerosis of the denuded trabecular beams. It is unlikely that pigment itself causes the chronic state as in eyes with chronic pigment dispersion glaucoma only 3.5 per cent of the pigment is found in the juxtacanalicular tissue. On electron microscopy there is no difference from normal subjects in the total number of electrolucent spaces within the juxtacanalicular tissue. Furthermore, pigment dispersion glaucoma is not a condition seen in black people despite the clinical appearance of a pigmented trabecular meshwork.

Mechanism of pigment loss from the iris

It has been noted that the iris transillumination defects often correspond to the position of the zonules and that simple rubbing of the iris against these may lead to dispersion of pigment. There is often an unusual anterior chamber configuration with concave backward bowing of the iris caused by so-called reverse pupil block. This appearance disappears if blinking is withheld and/or a large laser peripheral iridotomy is performed. This change in appearance has been elegantly shown on high definition ultrasound biomicroscopy. The proposed mechanism of reverse pupil block is that small aliquots of aqueous are forced through the pupil into the anterior chamber during blinking, exercise, or accommodation leading to a temporary situation in which the pressure is higher in the anterior chamber than in the posterior chamber leading to the backward bowing of the iris that can sometimes be seen. This would also explain why the pressure is not necessarily high when measured as the rise in pressure due to this mechanism is likely to be transient. Alternatively the backward bowing of the iris may allow for the traumatic release of pigment and physical clogging of the trabecular meshwork. Peripheral iridotomy may prevent the pressure difference between anterior and posterior chambers from occurring. Reverse pupil block would also explain why pigment dispersion syndrome sometimes improves with age for as the lens increases in size it may pull the peripheral iris away from the zonules and relieve the reverse pupil block.

Management of pigment dispersion glaucoma is the same as that for primary open angle glaucoma, although laser trabeculoplasty appears to have a higher than average success rate in these eyes. A number of patients also respond well to miotics although the coincident myopia may make the treatment difficult to tolerate. Ocuserts have a place here with low dose pilocarpine minimizing the side-effects. Alternative treatments such as laser iridotomy need further evaluation with prospective randomized trials.

Iridoschisis

This uncommon bilateral condition usually occurs in the older age group. It is characterized by separation of stromal layers to give a ragged threadbare appearance on slit lamp examination (Fig. 2) . Raised intraocular pressure occurs in about 50 per cent of cases and occasionally the iris strands may touch the corneal endothelium causing localized corneal oedema. Glaucoma may be closed angle due to pupil block or open angle due to blockage of the trabecular meshwork by iris strands or released pigment.

Patients with angle closure can be treated with peripheral

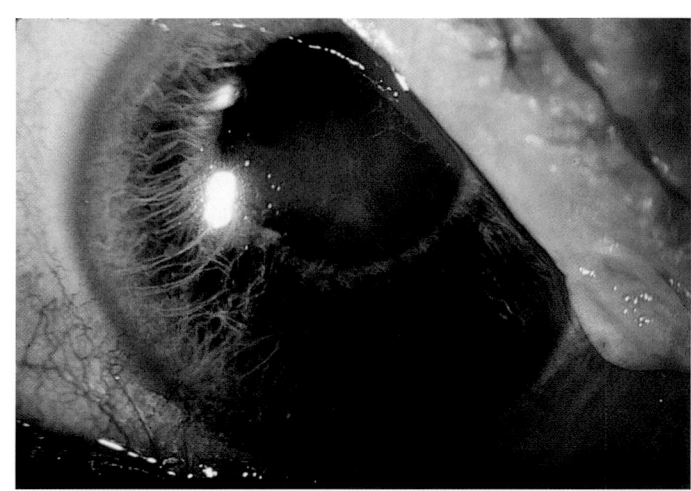

Fig. 2 Iridoschisis. Note moth-eaten appearance of iris stroma.

Table 2 The lens-induced glaucomas

Open angle	Mechanical obstruction of the angle	True exfoliation of the lens capsule
		Pseudo exfoliation of the lens capsule
	Inflammatory	Phacolytic
		Phacoanaphylactic
	Subluxation/dislocation of the lens	Inflammatory
		Associated angle anomaly
Closed angle	Subluxation/dislocation of the lens	Pupil block
		lens
		vitreous
	Secondary angle closure	Phacomorphic

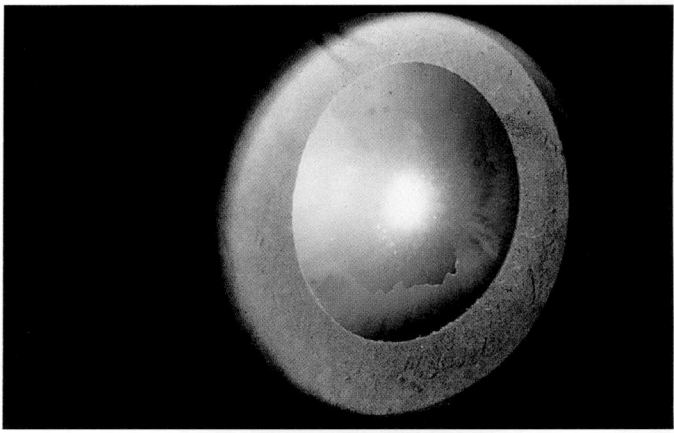

Fig. 3 Typical appearance of pseudoexfoliation of anterior lens. Note the clear ring devoid of exfoliation material thought to represent rubbing by the posterior surface of the iris.

iridotomy whilst the open angle forms are treated as for primary open angle glaucoma.

Glaucoma associated with disease of the lens

Disease of the lens may predispose to glaucoma through a variety of mechanisms (Table 2). The lens may be subluxed due to disease or trauma: there may be deposition of abnormal substances on the surface of the lens as occurs in pseudoexfoliation; in phacomorphic glaucoma the anteroposterior diameter of the lens increases to such an extent that it causes pupil block and may precipitate angle closure; in phacolytic glaucoma there is a leakage of lens protein from a hypermature or mature cataract leading to inflammation and blockage of the trabecular meshwork; and in phacoanaphylactic glaucoma there is a severe inflammatory response due to sensitization to lens protein antigens which may occur in the ipsilateral or contralateral eye following surgery or trauma to the lens.

Pseudoexfoliation syndrome

The term pseudoexfoliation is often used to differentiate this condition from true exfoliation of the anterior lens capsule which occurs in relation to infrared heat damage as occurs typically in glass-blowers' cataract. Although it is thought that the prevalence of pseudoexfoliation is highest in Scandinavian countries epidemiological studies have found the condition to be present in almost all populations. The condition may easily go undetected if it is not specifically looked for. Prevalence increases with age being 10 to 20 times more prevalent in the eighth decade than in the fifth, making pseudoexfoliation a disease of the elderly population.

It is generally accepted that the presence of pseudoexfoliation is a risk factor in the development of glaucoma, but to what extent is difficult to say as the reported prevalence of pseudoexfoliation in patients with glaucoma ranges between 0 and over 90 per cent depending on the population studied.

Conversely, the prevalence of glaucoma in eyes with pseudoexfoliation is far higher than occurs in eyes without it.

The condition may be unilateral or bilateral and patients with uniocular disease may develop it in the other eye after a period of many years. There is no sex predilection for the development of glaucoma in eyes with pseudoexfoliation. Familial occurrence and population genetics have suggested an autosomal dominant mode of inheritance in some populations.

The clinical picture is characterized by the deposition of pseudoexfoliation material in a typical configuration on the anterior surface of the lens, the pupillary margin, and in the anterior chamber angle (Fig. 3). Pseudoexfoliation material has been found in association with many ocular structures including the ciliary body and even the conjunctiva. Pseudoexfoliative fibrillopathy has also been identified in many systemic organs including skin, heart, lung, liver, and gallbladder. The fibrillar material is found to be present in fibrovascular septa adjacent to elastic and oxytalan fibres. In addition there is nearly always pigment deposition in the trabecular meshwork and also on Schwalbe's line (Sampaolisi's line).

The exact biochemical nature and origin of pseudoexfoliation material is not clear and several theories have been suggested. It has been shown to have features of an amyloid-like substance, a proteoglycosaminoglycan, and oxytalan, a microfibrillar constituent of elastic tissue which may be part of its composition. The mechanism by which pseudoexfoliation causes glaucoma is also unclear. It has been proposed that the material simply blocks the trabecular meshwork. This theory is confounded by the not uncommon finding of exfoliation occurring without glaucoma and bilateral glaucoma in patients with uniocular pseudoexfoliation. However, both are common conditions and it is not unlikely that primary open angle glaucoma may occur in an eye with pseudoexfoliation. Iris angiography reveals an abnormal capillary pattern with early breakdown of the blood–aqueous barrier.

The management of patients with pseudoexfoliation is the same as that of primary open angle glaucoma, but they may be more resistant to treatment. However, argon laser trabeculoplasty tends to have a favourable outcome in pseudoexfoliation. Extra care should be exercised when performing cataract surgery in the presence of pseudoexfoliation as the zonules are often weak and there may be localized areas of zonular dehiscence with up to 2 per cent of patients having some degree of lens subluxation. Phacoemulsification can be performed in eyes with pseudoexfoliation but if there is zonular weakness or dehiscence the use of a capsular ring will reduce the risk of vitreous loss. Surgery may also be complicated by bleeding from iris or angle vessels. Lax or dehisced zonules may allow forward movement of the lens predisposing to pupil block and acute angle closure glaucoma.

Phacolytic glaucoma

Leakage of lens protein from a mature or hypermature cataractous lens may cause blockage of the trabecular meshwork by both lens proteins themselves and also by macrophages which have engulfed the lens material.

Patients with phacolytic glaucoma may have an acute onset of very high intraocular pressure with symptoms not unlike those of acute angle closure, including severe conjunctival injection and pain. There is usually a history of gradually diminishing vision due to the underlying cataract, but acuity may drop further with the onset of the acute elevation of intraocular pressure. Clinical examination usually reveals diffuse corneal oedema, marked flare, and macrophages (which are larger than typical leucocytes) in the anterior chamber. There may be small particles of lens material within the anterior chamber and calcium oxalate crystals have also been observed. The anterior chamber is of normal depth and the chamber angle open on gonioscopy which differentiates phacolytic from acute angle closure glaucoma.

The management of phacolytic glaucoma is essentially planned early cataract extraction. Although the high intraocular pressure may be refractory to medical therapy it is worth treating with topical β-blockers/aproclonidine and steroids and also with intravenous, oral, or topical carbonic anhydrase inhibitors. If the intraocular pressure remains high, care must be taken not to suddenly decompress the eye at the time of surgery. Extracapsular extraction is probably the safest method as phacoemulsification of a mature lens in the presence of corneal oedema is not straightforward. Some surgeons still advocate intracapsular extraction in this situation but extracapsular surgery should be safe and technically straightforward using modern methods and instrumentation.

Phacoanaphylaxis

Phacoanaphylaxis is a granulomatous uveitis which may occur following extracapsular cataract surgery either in the ipsilateral eye or in the contralateral eye if there is subsequent cataract surgery or leakage of lens protein from a mature cataract. It may also occur following rupture of the lens capsule either spontaneously or secondary to trauma. The inflammatory response may occur at any time from hours to months following the initial trauma or surgery. On examination there is marked inflammation with keratic and intraocular lens precipitates and hypopyon is common. Residual lens material is always present. Pupillary block glaucoma may occur as a result of anterior and posterior synechiae. Although there may be some response to steroid therapy the uveitis often returns when they are withdrawn. Phacoanaphylaxis does not always cause glaucoma and is often associated with ocular hypotony.

It is important to differentiate this condition from other postoperative inflammations in particular bacterial endophthalmitis. The clinical picture should help in the differential diagnosis but if doubt exists a diagnostic paracentesis may reveal the presence of typical foamy macrophages. Treatment consists of surgical removal of any retained lens particles. If cataract occurs in the other eye intracapsular extraction is the method of choice to prevent the occurrence of an accelerated immune response to lens material due to the presence of previously formed antibodies.

Phacomorphic glaucoma (lens-induced angle closure)

Phacomorphic glaucoma occurs when the crystalline lens becomes too large for the anterior segment causing pupillary block and secondary acute angle closure glaucoma. It may be due to an intumescent lens in a normal anterior segment or due to the normal ageing change in an eye with hypermetropia and/ or short axial length. This is one of the proposed pathomechanisms of acute angle closure glaucoma. As a secondary condition in eyes of normal axial length phacomorphic glaucoma is likely to be seen less often if the trend towards earlier cataract surgery continues.

The patient presents in much the same way as primary acute angle closure glaucoma and it may be difficult to distinguish between the two. However, the fellow eye in phacomorphic glaucoma may have a normal anterior chamber depth and open chamber angle. In primary acute angle closure glaucoma the fellow eye also has a shallow anterior chamber and closeable angle. The cataractous lens of the affected eye will also be obvious once the corneal oedema has cleared sufficiently.

Despite relief of pupil block by medical means and surgical or laser peripheral iridotomy the anterior chamber may remain shallow and the pressure uncontrolled. In such cases lens extraction with or without trabeculectomy is the treatment of choice.

Glaucoma secondary to lens subluxation or dislocation

A lens partly displaced due to incomplete zonular dehiscence and remaining at least in part within the pupillary aperture is said to be subluxed. If there is total loss of zonular support the lens becomes dislocated or luxated. Table 3 shows the major causes of ectopia lentis. Fully or partly dislocated lenses may cause a secondary glaucoma due to a variety of mechanisms.

The most usual cause is pupil block either because of forward movement of the lens or more dramatically by the dislocation of the entire lens into the anterior chamber (Fig. 4) when pupil block occurs due to contact with the posterior surface of the lens. If posterior lens dislocation occurs into the vitreous

Table 3 Causes of ectopia lentis

Congenital	Marfan's syndrome
	Homocystinuria
	Aniridia
	Ehlers–Danlos syndrome
	Weill–Marchesani syndrome
	Crouzon disease
	Sturge–Weber syndrome
	Familial miscrospherophakia
	Sprengel's deformity
	Sulphite oxidase deficiency
	Oxycephaly
Trauma	
Secondary to other ocular disease	Buphthalmos
	High myopia
	Chronic inflammation
	Pseudo exfoliation
	Hypermature cataract
	Congenital syphilis

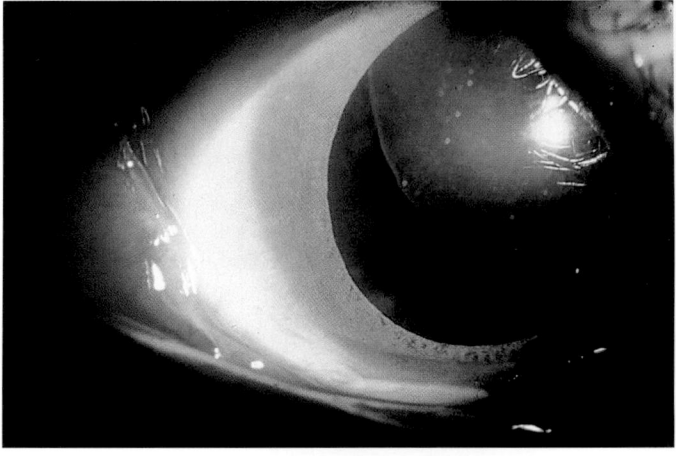

Fig. 5 A patient with Marfan's syndrome showing typical upward subluxation of the lens.

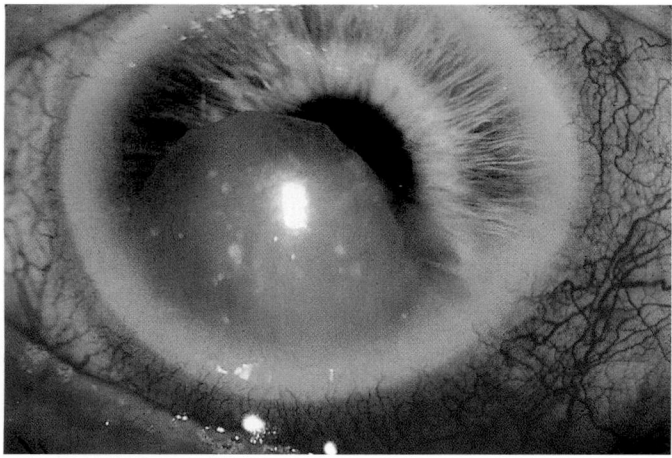

Fig. 4 An anteriorly subluxed lens may induce acute glaucoma due to pupil block by contact with the posterior surface of the lens.

cavity secondary glaucoma is unlikely unless due to phacolytic or inflammatory complications although pupil block may occur due to anterior displacement of a knuckle of vitreous through the pupillary aperture (Fig. 5). In some developmental conditions (e.g. Marfan's syndrome) there may be an associated angle abnormality giving rise to open angle glaucoma unrelated to the lens abnormality.

Management of these cases is difficult. Miotics may induce pupil block either by constricting the pupil around a knuckle of vitreous or by allowing forward displacement of the lens. Conversely, mydriatics may allow the lens to pass completely through the pupil. If a cataractous lens is dislocated into the anterior chamber it should be removed as soon as the intraocular pressure has been reduced by medical means. It may be possible to coax a partially dislocated lens back behind the pupil by use of mydriatics and lying the patient in the supine posi-

tion. Long-term miotic therapy in conjunction with a peripheral iridotomy may keep the lens safely in position. Lenses dislocated into the posterior segment are best left alone, unless there are phacolytic or phacoanaphylactic complications when a pars plana approach is probably the safest way to effect removal.

Glaucoma associated with retinal disorders

Neovascular glaucoma

Neovascular glaucoma epitomizes the philosophy of 'prevention is better than cure'. Once the patient presents with severe iris neovascularization, extremely high intraocular pressure with bullous keratopathy, and profound loss of vision the prognostic outcome is very poor (Fig. 6). The prognosis can be greatly improved if the iris neovascularization is diagnosed at an early stage and the underlying retinal condition treated adequately.

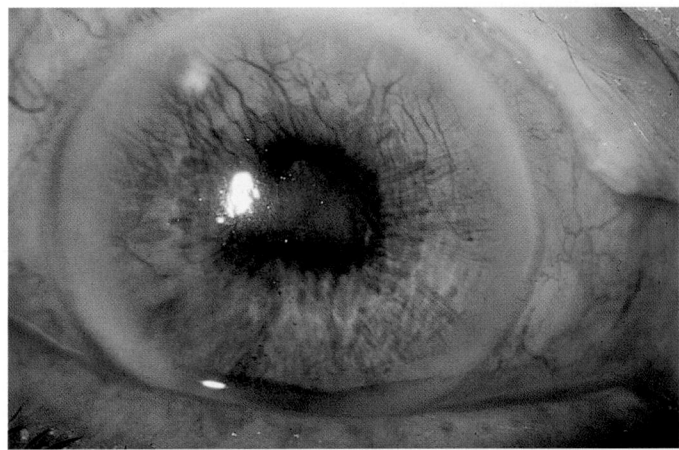

Fig. 6 Advanced neovascularization of the iris. Early intervention and treatment may prevent this late appearance.

Iris neovascularization may be associated with any condition that leads to chronic retinal ischaemia. About one-third of cases are associated with diabetic retinopathy, one-third with central retinal vein occlusion, and one-third with other miscellaneous conditions, of which about 40 have been described including carotid artery disease, retinal and choroidal tumours, sickle cell retinopathy, and long-standing retinal detachment.

Iris neovascularization begins at the pupil margin and often coincidently in the anterior chamber angle. It is important when managing patients with conditions associated with iris neovascularization to make a detailed high magnification examination of the iris before mydriatics are used as early new vessels are easily missed once the pupil is dilated.

The probable pathomechanism involves the release of an angiogenic factor from the ischaemic posterior segment that diffuses through to the aqueous. Because the pupillary margin and angle are the two areas exposed to the highest flow of aqueous this may explain the predisposition of these areas to the early onset of new vessel formation. New vessels are associated with the formation of fibrous tissue membranes on the anterior iris and overlying the trabecular meshwork. In the angle this leads to peripheral anterior synechiae with secondary angle closure and at the pupil margin causes ectropion uveae and may lead to a fixed dilated pupil in the later stages. In the early stages before synechial closure has occurred there may be a secondary open angle glaucoma due to obstruction of the trabecular meshwork by the fibrovascular membrane. Whilst treatment of the underlying condition may cause regression of the new vessels, the fibrous membrane and synechial angle closure are not reversible.

Management can be divided into prophylactic and therapeutic. If the retinal condition is diagnosed before there is evidence of iris neovascularization steps can be taken to prevent its onset. This usually takes the form of panretinal laser ablation in eyes with proliferative diabetic retinopathy or central retinal vein occlusion. About 20 per cent of central retinal vein occlusions will be ischaemic and of these 60 per cent will develop iris neovascularization and 30 per cent glaucoma. The glaucoma can occur within as little as 2 weeks following vein occlusion but more typically occurs within 3 months, hence the term '100-day glaucoma'.

If the patient presents with established glaucoma the initial therapy is medical in order to reduce the pressure enough to allow clearing of the cornea for subsequent retinal laser ablation. If direct laser photocoagulation is not possible because of media opacities trans-scleral cryoablation of the peripheral retina can be undertaken. Trials using diode laser ablation are also underway. In eyes with visual potential in which the optic nerve and retinal blood flow is severely compromised the quicker the intraocular pressure can be normalized, the better the prognosis. This may require conventional filtration procedures in conjunction with antimetabolites, the insertion of a glaucoma tube and plate (e.g. Molteno tube) or the use of cyclodestructive procedures. If there is little visual potential medical treatment is aimed at keeping symptoms of inflammation and bullous keratopathy at a minimum.

Glaucoma associated with other retinal pathology

A wide variety of retinal pathology may be associated with raised intraocular pressure. This includes glaucoma associated with retinal detachment (Schwartz's syndrome), or with neonatal retinal diseases such as retinopathy of prematurity and persistent hyperplastic primary vitreous. There is a high incidence of angle closure glaucoma associated with choroidal effusion in nanophthalmic eyes. This can be treated successfully with laser iridotomy or by performing a posterior sclerostomy or sclerectomy. Surgical decompression of the vortex veins has also been successfully used in the management of exudative retinal detachment/choroidal effusion in nanophthalmic eyes. A posterior sclerostomy performed at the time of cataract or glaucoma surgery is useful prophylaxis against formation of choroidal effusions. An alternative approach in small eyes with angle closure glaucoma due to crowding of the anterior segment structures is to consider clear lens extraction and insertion of a high power intraocular lens.

Glaucoma secondary to raised episcleral venous pressure

The final exit site of the aqueous after it has passed through the trabecular meshwork and Schlemm's canal is via the aqueous veins and into the episcleral venous system. The intraocular pressure is very much dependent upon the episcleral venous pressure and any condition which causes this to be raised will cause a secondary rise in intraocular pressure.

The episcleral venous pressure may be elevated by increased central venous pressure (superior vena cava syndrome), by local orbital pathology (orbital varices, Sturge–Weber syndrome), or by arteriovenous fistulas. The site of the underlying pathology will determine whether the raised episcleral venous pressure is unilateral or bilateral. The typical appearance is of dilated and engorged episcleral veins and there may be chemosis and proptosis. On gonioscopic examination the angle is invariably open and blood may be visible in Schlemm's canal. If the underlying disorder leads to generalized orbital ischaemia there may rarely be associated iris neovascularization.

One of the more common conditions to cause orbital congestion is dysthyroid eye disease, although raised pressure may also occur secondary to tethering of the extraocular muscles with spikes of pressure occurring on up or down gaze. Arteriovenous fistulas may occur between the carotid artery and cavernous sinus and are often traumatic in aetiology, more typically in men, but (especially in elderly females) may occur spontaneously. High flow arterial shunts are associated with proptosis, chemosis, and a bruit heard over the orbit. In contrast low flow shunts between the cavernous sinus and dural vessels may be far less conspicuous and difficult to diagnose in elderly women unless there is a certain degree of suspicion. The clues that may indicate the correct diagnosis are the appearance of arteriolized veins in non-sticky and otherwise uninflamed eyes and often present with a history of 'conjunctivitis'.

The Sturge–Weber syndrome is associated with haemangiomas in the territory of the trigeminal nerve with or without intracranial involvement. Elevated episcleral venous pressure is one of several mechanisms postulated for the secondary glaucoma associated with this syndrome. Others include the presence of an abnormal anterior chamber angle or choroidal haemangiomas. In contrast to arteriovenous fistulas the episclera has a more fleshy pink appearance with less prominent veins.

Management is initially medical. However, medical treatment cannot lower the intraocular pressure below that of the raised episcleral venous pressure. In cases where medical therapy is insufficient it is necessary to resort to conventional fistulizing surgery. High episcleral venous pressure may predispose to choroidal effusions and haemorrhage at the time of or after surgery. For this reason prophylactic posterior sclerostomy at the time of filtering surgery has been advocated. When performing filtration surgery on patients with the Sturge–Weber syndrome an ultrasound b-scan should be done to exclude the presence of large choroidal haemangiomas which may predispose to choroidal effusion and/or haemorrhage. In such cases peroperative precautions such as hypotensive anaesthesia, a tightly sutured scleral flap with releasable sutures, and viscoelastics in the anterior chamber should be employed.

Glaucoma associated with ocular inflammation

Glaucoma may be associated with any inflammatory condition of the ocular coats or uvea. All patients with ocular inflammation should have regular intraocular pressure monitoring throughout their treatment as pressure may not only be associated with the disease itself but also with the steroids used in treatment.

Glaucoma associated with uveitis

Eyes with uveitis may have subnormal intraocular pressure due to inflammation of the secretory epithelium of the ciliary body. About 1 in 5 will have an associated secondary glaucoma which may become manifest by one of three mechanisms.

1. Open angle glaucoma secondary to blockage of the trabecular meshwork by inflammatory cells and debris (Fig. 7). These include white blood cells, macrophages, fibroblasts, and pigment granules. In chronic granulomatous conditions (e.g. sarcoidosis) the angle may be compromised by the presence of granulomas which appear gonioscopically not unlike peripheral anterior synechiae but tend to disappear with adequate steroid therapy. In long-standing disease the trabecular meshwork may become permanently damaged. The inflammatory process may affect the trabecular meshwork itself causing a reduction in the size of the intertrabecular spaces. This trabeculitis is typically seen in acute anterior uveitis associated with herpes simplex and herpes zoster infections. There is also evidence that recurrent unilateral uveitic glauc-

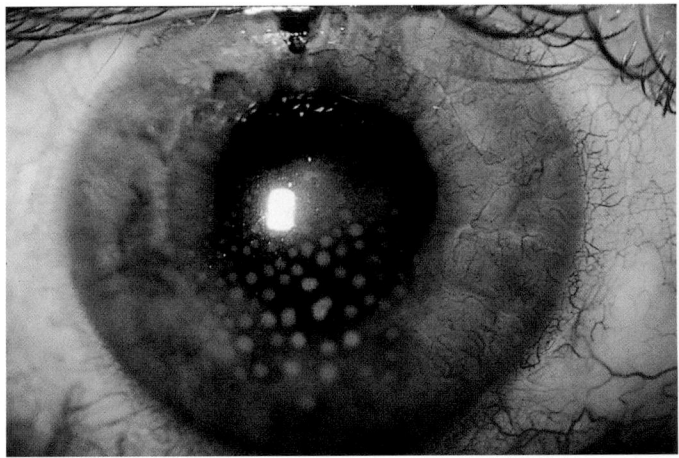
Fig. 7 Granulomatous uveitis. Note large mutton fat keratic precipitates, engorged iris vessels, and iridectomy associated with trabeculectomy. Glaucoma may occur due to a variety of mechanisms (see text).

oma may be due to herpes simplex virus even in the absence of any corneal involvement and herpes virus has been identified in the aqueous of such eyes.

2. Angle closure glaucoma secondary to the formation of 360° posterior synechiae (seclusio pupillae) leading to pupil block with iris bombé. In these eyes the pressure may be extremely high and require early peripheral iridotomy to prevent the formation of peripheral anterior synechiae. Once permanent peripheral anterior synechiae have been established fistulizing surgery may be necessary.

3. Angle closure secondary to the formation of peripheral anterior synechiae. This is a slowly progressive process and is more commonly associated with chronic granulomatous conditions such as tuberculosis and sarcoidosis. Peripheral anterior synechiae in uveitis tend to be irregular and may be in the form of cones and cylinders or tent-like structures. There may be sectors of normal looking open angle interspersed with areas of peripheral anterior synechiae.

Any or all of these mechanisms may be present at any one time and management must be directed both towards the primary inflammatory process and the glaucoma. It is important to try to dilate the pupil as fully as possible from the outset in order to prevent the formation of posterior synechiae. Cycloplegia will also alleviate ciliary spasm and decrease pain and photophobia. Aqueous suppressants (β-blockers, carbonic anhydrase inhibitors) are the medical treatment of choice. Cholinergic agents tend to exacerbate the inflammation and increase ciliary spasm and should therefore be avoided. In refractory cases filtration or drainage tube surgery in conjunction with antimetabolites may be necessary although there is a high failure rate for such surgery, especially if performed in the presence of active inflammation. Cyclodestructive techniques are also an option but carry a real risk of phthisis.

Glaucoma associated with specific inflammatory conditions

Posner–Schlossman syndrome (glaucomatocyclic crisis)

The Posner–Schlossman syndrome is a very characteristic and specific condition that occurs in young adult life and more commonly in males. It was first described by Posner and Schlossman in 1948. It is almost always unilateral and takes the form of recurrent episodes of very high (often 40–80 mmHg) intraocular pressure. The attacks are associated with a very mild anterior chamber inflammatory reaction with only a few white cells and one or two 'sentinel' keratic precipitates in a white eye. Posterior synechiae do not occur. There may be fine corneal oedema and the pupil may be semi-dilated. Gonioscopic examination reveals a normal looking open angle. The symptoms are usually associated with the corneal oedema consisting of slight blurring of vision and haloes around lights. Individual attacks may last from a few hours to a few days and are generally self-limiting. Diagnosis is made on clinical findings and history.

The aetiology of Posner–Schlossman syndrome remains unclear. An allergic reaction associated with prostaglandin release has been suggested but not proven. As with other forms of unilateral uveitic glaucoma the herpes simplex virus has been implicated. Management involves the use of carbonic anhydrase inhibitors and β-blockers to cause remission of the attack. Treatment between attacks is not usually necessary. Steroids are of limited value and are probably best avoided as a high proportion of these patients have been shown to be steroid responders. Although the Posner–Schlossman syndrome *per se* is not thought to lead to chronic glaucoma associated with optic nerve damage there does seem to be a higher than average incidence of primary open angle glaucoma in these patients, presumably secondary to chronic repetitive insults to the trabecular meshwork.

Fuchs' heterochromic cyclitis

Fuchs first described this syndrome consisting of mild anterior uveitis, iris heterochromia, cataract, and occasional glaucoma in 1906. It affects males and females equally and occurs unilaterally in about 90 per cent of cases. It tends to occur in young to middle-aged adults. Patients may have the condition for many years and remain symptom-free until vision is affected by cataract or the condition is noted during a routine eye examination.

The heterochromia is usually manifest by hypochromia of the affected eye and tends to be more obvious in patients of 'mixed' colour. On slit lamp examination the iris appears thin and moth-eaten even in the absence of hypochromia. The anterior chamber angle shows the presence of fine blood vessels which have a tendency to bleed when the anterior chamber is opened, as at the time of cataract surgery, which is said to be pathognomonic of Fuchs' cyclitis.

The cyclitis tends to be chronic and mild with the presence of anterior chamber cells and mild flare. Posterior synechiae are conspicuous by their absence. The keratic precipitates are of medium size, round or stellate in appearance, and tend to cover the whole cornea rather than being confined more inferiorly as in acute anterior uveitis. They are connected by fine filaments and transiently disappear following cataract surgery. There are also opacities in the anterior vitreous which may cause symptoms in the form of floaters and may become more troublesome following cataract surgery.

Cataract takes the form of posterior cortical opacity and is probably related to the long-standing cyclitis. Surgery is seldom complicated and has a good prognosis. However, there is a wide spectrum of disease severity with some cases requiring more involved surgery such as vitreolensectomy. The underlying aetiology is not clear although there is evidence of a vasculitic mechanism which is supported by angiographic evidence.

The cyclitis itself does not usually require treatment with steroids but cataract and glaucoma will require intervention. Glaucoma is the most serious complication of Fuchs' cyclitis. It has an incidence of about 10 per cent in unilateral and 25 per cent in bilateral cases. The exact mechanism is unclear and it tends to resemble primary open angle glaucoma although it may be related to the presence of abnormal vessels in the anterior chamber angle or secondary to chronic inflammation.

Glaucoma associated with scleritis

Glaucoma occurs in up to 12 per cent of eyes with scleritis. In about a third of these the glaucoma will be coincidental primary open angle glaucoma which may be exacerbated by the ocular inflammation or by a steroid response. Secondary open angle glaucoma may arise because of anterior uveitis/trabeculitis or be associated with active limbal scleritis or episcleral vaculitis. Such secondary glaucomas usually respond well to high dose steroid treatment. It is rare to have secondary glaucoma associated with posterior scleritis, although choroidal effusion may lead to secondary angle closure. The presence of angle closure will be suggested by finding asymmetrical anterior chamber depths on clinical examination and can be confirmed by ultrasound if there is no adequate fundal view. Management is aimed at treatment of the underlying inflammation together with antiglaucoma medication as needed. In some cases surgical intervention will be required, but should be performed in an area of uninvolved sclera if possible, and after the inflammation has been brought under control. If there is active inflammation it is advisable to use antimetabolites in conjunction with filtration surgery although care should be taken as mitomycin C itself may cause scleritis.

Glaucoma associated with intraocular tumours

Intraocular tumours may cause glaucoma by a variety of mechanisms. Large posterior tumours may be associated with iris neovascularization due to ischaemia, or may cause forward displacement of the lens–iris diaphragm causing angle closure. Tumour cells may directly block the trabecular meshwork or more anterior tumours may directly infiltrate the trabecular meshwork. The finding of high intraocular pressure as a consequence of an intraocular tumour is inevitably a poor pro-gnostic sign. In adults the commonest tumours are metastases and malignant melanomas but others include lymphoid tumours, neurofibromas, haemangiomas, and adenomas. In children the most important intraocular tumour is retinoblastoma.

It is important to keep in mind the possibility of intraocular tumour especially in any atypical unilateral glaucoma. If visualization of the posterior pole is not possible ultrasound should be performed if there is any doubt about the diagnosis. Glaucoma secondary to tumours may masquerade as uveitis, neovascular glaucoma, or even as unilateral primary open angle glaucoma.

The commonest tumour to present with glaucoma is malignant melanoma. About 20 per cent of eyes with melanomas develop raised intraocular pressure. This may be caused by any of the mechanisms discussed above. Large posterior pole tumours may push the lens–iris diaphragm forwards leading to angle closure. Ciliary body tumours may extend directly into the angle and trabecular meshwork and may spread around the entire circumference producing a ring-shaped melanoma. In the rare melanomalytic glaucoma a melanoma may become necrotic and macrophages laden with digested tumour particles may block the trabecular meshwork in a similar fashion to phacolytic glaucoma.

More uncommon is glaucoma associated with primary cysts of the iris and ciliary body. These are not associated with any systemic abnormality and in some cases may be inherited as an autosomal dominant trait. The cysts may enlarge and cause acute angle closure. Pigmented cysts may be amenable to puncture using argon laser. If angle closure is long standing and peripheral anterior synechiae form, filtration surgery may be necessary.

Glaucoma associated with steroids

Steroid-induced glaucoma is almost always caused by exogenous steroids. These may be applied topically as eye-drops or steroid cream applied to the skin around the eyes and eyelids; orbital floor injections of depot preparations; or applied systemically. On rare occasions it may be related to the overproduction of endogenous corticosteroids in Cushing's syndrome or adrenal hyperplasia.

In cases of exogenous steroid use the intraocular pressure may rise after as little as a week or after many months or years and it is therefore vital that patients on long-term treatment have regular intraocular pressure monitoring.

The clinical picture resembles primary open angle glaucoma with little in the way of symptoms unless the intraocular pressure is high enough to cause corneal oedema. The condition may not become evident until many years after the initial event that caused steroids to be used and may mimic low tension glaucoma. Alternatively, the long-term use of steroids may lead to a permanent rise in intraocular pressure which will masquerade as primary open angle glaucoma. For these reasons the cause can be ascertained only if a thorough history of past ophthalmic and systemic steroid use is taken from the patient. In some cases (for instance uveitic glaucoma) it may be impossible to differentiate steroid-induced glaucoma from that secondary to the underlying condition. On examination there may be associated systemic or ocular signs of steroid use such as posterior subcapsular cataracts if the steroid use has been long standing.

The underlying pathomechanism by which steroids cause glaucoma remains unclear although the raised intraocular pressure is due to a decrease in outflow facility. One theory suggests that steroids cause an accumulation of glycosaminoglycans in the trabecular meshwork by inhibiting their breakdown. Alternatively, steroids may inhibit the phagocytic action of the trabecular endothelial cells leading to a build-up of debris in the meshwork. It has also been postulated that the secondary glaucoma is due to the effect of steroids on prostaglandin synthesis, which is an interesting idea in the light of the current development of prostaglandin derivatives as therapeutic agents for glaucoma.

The management of steroid-induced glaucoma is aimed at decreasing and stopping the steroids. It may not be possible to stop the drug completely in which case the dose should be reduced as far as possible or a weaker steroid substituted. It is important that the management of the condition requiring steroids is not compromised and they should not be decreased purely in an attempt to lower intraocular pressure. Whether the steroid is stopped or not the intraocular pressure may take several weeks to return to normal during which time antiglaucoma medication should be used. If intraocular pressure cannot be controlled medically, filtration surgery may be required.

Glaucoma associated with trauma

The mechanism of raised intraocular pressure following trauma will depend upon the type of damage inflicted on the globe, whether it be blunt trauma, penetrating injury, or damage caused by chemical injury or irradiation.

Blunt ocular trauma may lead to a rise in intraocular pressure as an acute event secondary to hyphaema or inflammation, or may occur much later as a consequence of damage to angle structures. Damage to other structures within the eye may also cause glaucoma as in the case of lens subluxation.

Hyphaema usually occurs at the time of injury due to tearing of structures within the eye, typically between the circular and longitudinal fibres of the ciliary body. The patient will invariably complain of blurred vision due to the blood within the aqueous. The haemorrhage is usually self-limited by the tamponade effect of the subsequent rise in intraocular pressure. The initial high pressure is usually short lived, but in 10 to 30 per cent rebleeding may be a complication after 4 to 5 days as clot lysis occurs. The rise in intraocular pressure is due to a mechanical blockage of the trabecular meshwork by red blood cells and blood clot. Usually conservative management with aqueous suppressants is all that is required until the hyphaema resolves. In the case of a total (eight ball or black ball) hyphaema associated with an intraocular pressure rise unresponsive to medical management surgery (clot evacuation with or without peripheral iridotomy) may be necessary in order to prevent permanent bloodstaining of the cornea (Fig. 8).

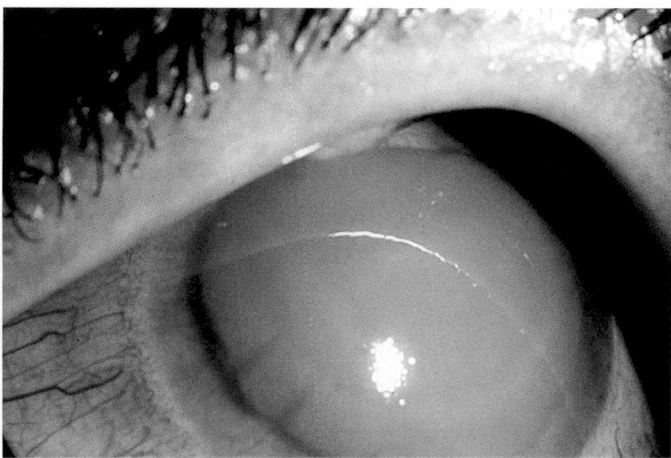

Fig. 8 Traumatic hyphaema associated with raised intraocular pressure may result in permanent bloodstaining of the cornea.

Zonular rupture with subluxation of the lens may cause pupillary block glaucoma with an acute rise in intraocular pressure. Treatment with mydriatics may alleviate the block but it may be necessary to perform iridectomy or lens extraction to prevent long-term problems caused by the formation of peripheral anterior synechiae. Blunt trauma may also be severe enough to cause damage to the lens capsule leading to the formation of cataract and the risk of phacolytic glaucoma.

Blunt trauma may be associated with a marked inflammatory response which may give rise to glaucoma in the same fashion as other inflammatory glaucomas.

Damage to the trabecular meshwork with the formation of scarring can cause marked resistance to outflow in the early post-trauma period, although the condition often resolves spontaneously. Angle recession due to a tear in the ciliary body typically appears as a deepening of the anterior chamber angle with prominence of the scleral spur on gonioscopy (Fig. 9). The diagnosis is facilitated by comparison with the contralateral eye. Scarring may lead to resolution, and the formation of

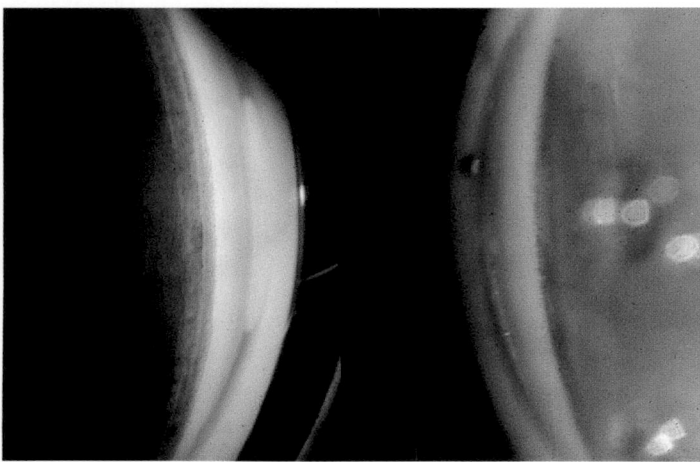

Fig. 9 Gonioscopic view of angle recession.

peripheral anterior synechiae may obscure any underlying damage to the ciliary body. The incidence of glaucoma following traumatic angle recession is in the order of 2 to 10 per cent and occurs with higher frequency if the angle recession involves more than 270°. The associated glaucoma may occur at any time from weeks to many years following the original injury, so that long-term monitoring of intraocular pressure is important. Subsequent ocular hypertension and glaucoma should be managed as for primary open angle glaucoma.

Trauma sufficient to cause complete separation of the ciliary body and/or iris from its attachment to the scleral spur may present with an iridodialysis or cyclodialysis cleft with associated hypotony.

Glaucoma associated with penetrating ocular injury will depend on the extent of the injury and involvement of different ocular structures. There may be damage to the lens, severe inflammation, or peripheral anterior synechiae secondary to prolonged loss of the anterior chamber in addition to all the mechanisms of glaucoma associated with blunt trauma.

Chemical injuries, in particular alkali burns may cause a refractory glaucoma due to structural damage to anterior segment structures and subsequent scarring. A number of mechanisms may be involved including direct damage to the trabecular meshwork, the formation of peripheral anterior synechiae, or posterior synechiae with pupil block. Severe damage to the episcleral venous system may cause a chronic post-trabecular type of glaucoma. Once the acute phase is over, glaucoma filtration or tube surgery may be necessary although in some cases the conjunctiva may be so scarred as to preclude this. In such cases ciliary destruction may be a useful alternative.

Glaucoma following intraocular surgery

Raised intraocular pressure may occur after almost any intraocular surgery. It may occur in the early postoperative period and be either self-limiting or chronic in nature or may occur some time after surgery. It is important to be able to recognize the cause of a postoperative pressure rise as management will depend very much on the underlying mechanism of the glaucoma.

Glaucoma in aphakia and pseudophakia

Acute postoperative rises in intraocular pressure may occur secondary to the use of viscoelastic agents used peroperatively or from blockage of the trabecular meshwork with retained lens matter or inflammatory cells. These types of glaucoma are usually self-limiting and can be treated with topical β-blockers and/or carbonic anhydrase inhibitors together with intensive topical steroids if there is significant inflammatory activity in the anterior chamber. If it is likely that some viscoelastic material remains after surgery the patient should be given a prophylactic dose of acetazolamide or topical β-blocker or apro-clonidine in order to prevent a pressure spike that may occur during the first 24 h postoperatively. This is especially important after phacoemulsification because of the self sealing nature

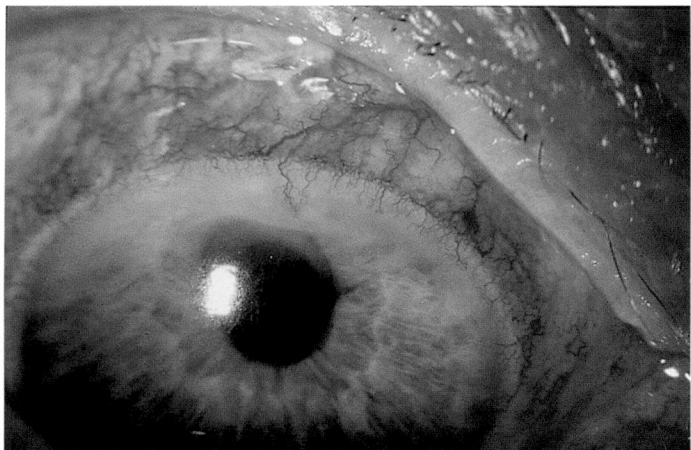

Fig. 10 Downgrowth of epithelium through cataract wound.

of the wound. In cases which do not settle with conservative treatment it may be necessary to wash retained viscoelastic from the anterior chamber.

Chronic glaucoma in aphakia may be related to continuing uveitis or secondary to peripheral anterior synechiae if there has been prolonged shallowing of the anterior chamber during the immediate postoperative period. Shallowing of the anterior chamber may occur due to wound leak, pupillary block, malignant glaucoma, or choroidal detachment or haemorrhage. If there has been vitreous loss during surgery with incarceration of vitreous in the wound glaucoma may occur because of continuing inflammation or because of epithelial ingrowth (Fig. 10). Management of any postoperative glaucoma depends first on recognizing and treating the underlying problem. Chronic glaucoma will require long-term treatment which may be medical or need further laser or surgical intervention.

Malignant glaucoma

The term malignant glaucoma was first coined by von Graefe in 1869 when he noticed that following peripheral iridectomy for angle closure glaucoma a number of eyes developed shallowing of the anterior chamber associated with a rise in intraocular pressure. The term 'malignant' was used as von Graefe noted that once this clinical appearance was recognized the outcome was usually very unfavourable. A variety of other terms have since been introduced including ciliolenticular block, ciliary block, and aqueous misdirection glaucoma in an attempt to describe the condition in terms of the underlying pathomechanism. However, these terms are based largely on hypothetical mechanisms and unlike the term malignant glaucoma do not conjure up the seriousness of the condition. Malignant glaucoma remains a condition with a relatively poor outcome because it can be difficult to recognize early and medical treatment is therefore not instituted early enough or is ineffective. Furthermore, surgical management remains difficult and controversial.

Malignant glaucoma typically occurs following filtration surgery in eyes with chronic angle closure but can occur following cataract surgery, surgical iridectomy, or laser iridotomy. It may occur in phakic, aphakic, or pseudophakic eyes and has even been reported following miotic therapy. The specific mechanism remains unclear but the most popular theory advocates the posterior diversion of aqueous behind or into the vitreous. A number of distinctive anatomical features have been noted in eyes developing malignant glaucoma. There is anterior rotation of the ciliary processes and the tips of the ciliary processes may actually be in contact with the lens. Optically clear areas within the vitreous may be seen clinically or with the aid of ultrasonography.

It is important to recognize the clinical signs of malignant glaucoma early to give the best chance of relieving the attack with medical treatment alone. Malignant glaucoma presents as a shallow anterior chamber with normal or high intraocular pressure in the presence of a patent peripheral iridotomy. Unlike pupil block the iris is not typically bowed forwards, but if the patency of the iridectomy is in doubt a repeat laser iridotomy can be performed to exclude pupil block. Figure 11 shows an algorithm that can be followed if there is a shallowing of the anterior chamber following glaucoma filtration surgery.

Treatment

In the first instance medical management of malignant glaucoma consists of mydriatic/cycloplegic drops, topical β-blockers or apraclonidine, oral carbonic anhydrase inhibitors, and if necessary oral glycerol. This combination shrinks the vitreous, decreases aqueous production and encourages backward displacement of the lens–iris diaphragm. Fifty per cent of cases will be relieved within 5 days. If high pressure continues after this time or if lens–corneal touch occurs surgical intervention should be considered as prolonged shallowing of the anterior chamber will lead to the formation of peripheral anterior synechiae, posterior synechiae, cataract, and damage to the corneal endothelium.

Surgical intervention may require laser or more invasive surgical procedures. Direct argon laser through a peripheral iridectomy may be used in an attempt to shrink the ciliary processes and thus relieve ciliolenticular block to anterior flow of aqueous. Alternatively in aphakic or pseudophakic eyes the neodymium–yttrium aluminium garnet laser may be used to perform posterior capsulotomy/hyaloidotomy. This manoeuvre will only be effective if a direct communication between the vitreous cavity and anterior chamber can be established. In 1968 Chandler described the technique of vitreous aspiration through an 18 gauge needle via a pars plana sclerostomy in conjunction with anterior chamber reformation with air. More recently pars plana vitrectomy with or without lensectomy or extracapsular lens extraction have been reported. In a series of 20 eyes requiring surgical treatment at Moorfields Eye Hospital pars plana vitrectomy was successful in 67 per cent of pseudophakic but only 25 per cent of phakic eyes. Combined cataract surgery and vitrectomy with intact posterior capsule had a success rate of 17 per cent whereas in patients in whom a primary posterior capsulotomy was performed the success

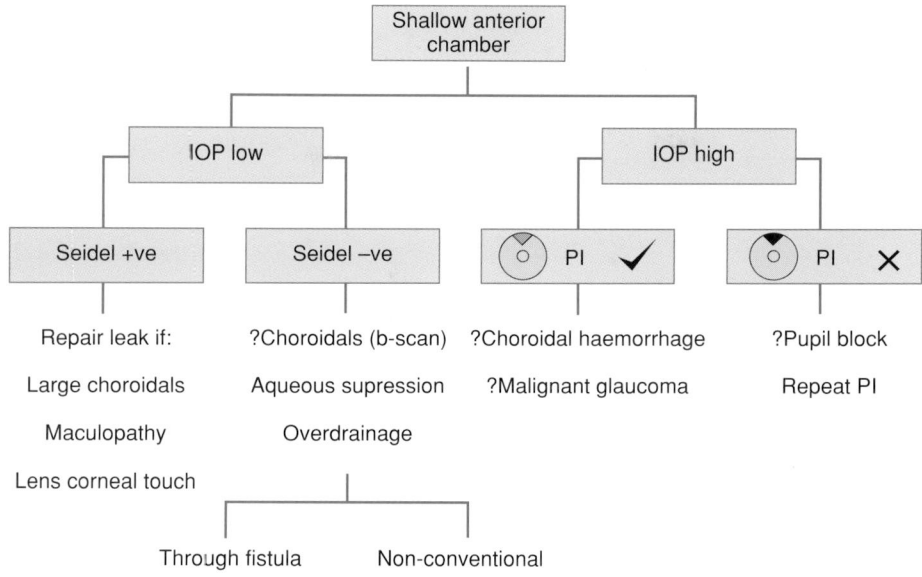

Fig. 11 Algorithm showing management of a shallow anterior chamber following glaucoma filtration surgery

rate was 80 per cent. Combined extracapsular cataract extraction or phacoemulsification together with posterior capsulorrhexis and anterior vitrectomy would seem reasonable in any patient with lens opacity. In the presence of a clear lens treatment is rather more controversial, although clear lens extraction should be considered. The flow chart in Fig. 12 outlines the steps taken in managing malignant glaucoma.

Precautions should be taken to avoid the development of malignant glaucoma at the time of surgery in susceptible eyes. Any eye with chronic angle closure, previous acute angle closure, or short axial length is at high risk. Ultrasound may reveal large or anteriorly rotated ciliary processes. If filtration surgery is being performed the use of viscoelastic in conjunction with extra releasable sutures in the scleral flap to maintain a deep anterior chamber during the early postoperative period should be considered.

Glaucoma following vitreoretinal surgery

High intraocular pressure may occur following vitreoretinal surgery due to several different mechanisms. Ghost cell glaucoma occurs secondary to trabecular obstruction by degenerated erythrocytes. These are spherical, khaki-coloured, and less pliable than normal red blood cells. Ghost cell glaucoma may occur following vitreous haemorrhage from any cause as long as there has been disruption of the anterior hyaloid face allowing the ghost cells entry into the anterior chamber. Typically, it occurs following either incomplete vitrectomy for vitreous haemorrhage or vitreous haemorrhage as a complication of vitrectomy. The pressure rise associated with this type of glaucoma may occur over weeks or months following the initial haemorrhage. Slit lamp examination will reveal the khaki-coloured cells in the anterior chamber and on the corneal endothelium and if present in sufficient numbers there may be a

greenish coloured pseudohypopyon. Once the diagnosis has been made the initial management is medical. If this is insufficient the surgical procedure of choice is irrigation of the anterior chamber. Occasionally vitrectomy is required to remove old blood. However, the condition is invariably self-limiting and does not lead to permanent trabecular damage so that where possible, conservative management is preferable.

Angle-closure glaucoma is a recognized complication of scleral buckling procedures. The underlying mechanism may be related to obstruction to venous outflow through the vortex veins with subsequent swelling of the ciliary body and choroidal detachment. Resolution usually occurs spontaneously over several weeks.

The use of expanding intraocular gases such as sulphur hexafluoride (SF_6) or perfluorocarbons (C_3F_8) may cause an acute postoperative pressure rise and there is a danger of precipitating a central retinal artery occlusion. Such pressure spikes usually occur within the first 24 h of surgery and can be managed medically. In some instances it will be necessary to remove some of the gas.

The use of intraocular silicone oil may be associated with acute or chronic secondary glaucoma occurring at any time from 1 day to many months postoperatively. In a proportion of eyes the pressure elevation will be transient and can be treated with medical treatment alone. In other cases the glaucoma is more persistent and may require removal of the silicone oil, although this does not always lead to resolution. Resistant cases can often be successfully treated with cyclodestructive procedures of the ciliary body. The overall prognosis is poor in eyes which develop glaucoma secondary to silicone oil. The mechanism of the glaucoma may partly be due to physical blockage of the trabecular meshwork by emulsified oil droplets which can be seen in the anterior chamber, but other mechanisms may also play a role.

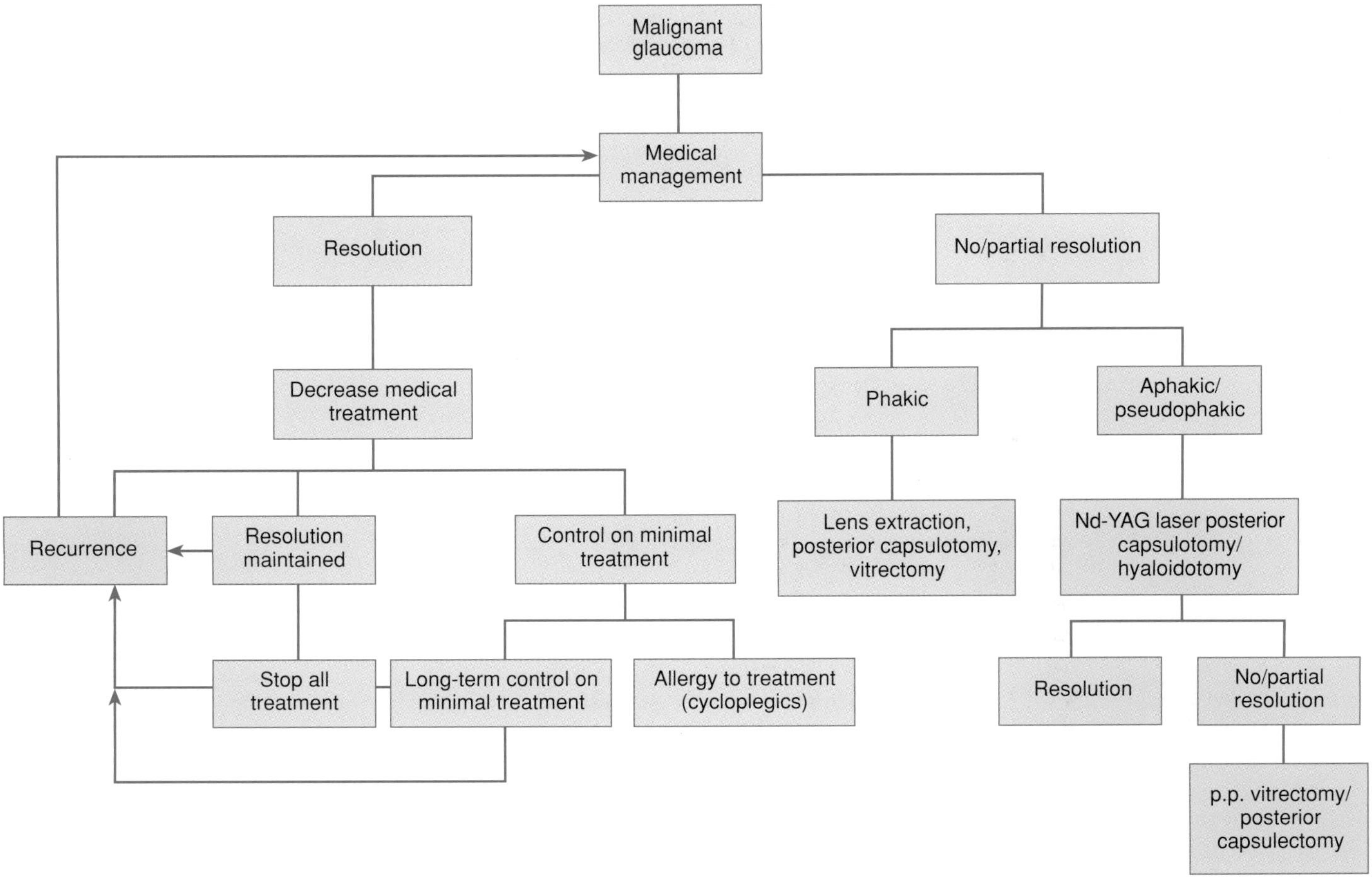

Fig. 12 Algorithm outlining the management of malignant glaucoma (see text for details).

Secondary glaucomas related to congenital abnormalities of the eye

There are an enormous number of congenital conditions which may either be confined to abnormalities of the eye, or may form part of a more complex syndrome, which may be associated with glaucoma. Those affecting predominantly the eye include aniridia and other so-called 'anterior chamber cleavage' syndromes, whereas conditions with other systemic manifestations include many chromosomal syndromes, congenital rubella, and the phakomatoses.

Anirida

This is a rare condition occurring with an incidence of 1 in 60 000. It is characterized by absence of a normal iris and is associated with foveal hypoplasia and poor vision (Fig. 13). The condition is dominantly inherited in about two-thirds of cases. Of the sporadic cases two-thirds are due to a new autosomal dominant gene mutation. In others there is a deletion of the short arm of chromosome 11 (11p13) which is also associated with a high risk of developing Wilms' tumour. This usually develops within the first 2 years of life and during this time it is important that regular renal ultrasound examinations are carried out as the prognosis is good if the tumour is detected at an early stage.

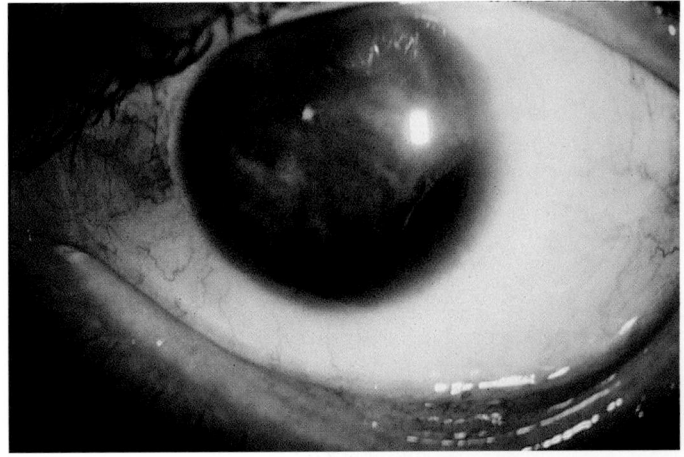

Fig. 13 Aniridia is often associated with cataract.

The abnormality is thought to be associated either with abnormal mesodermal, or more likely, neuroectodermal embryogenesis and development. There is a wide spectrum of abnormality ranging from almost complete absence of the iris to mild iris hypoplasia. Other ocular abnormalities include foveal hypoplasia, optic nerve hypoplasia, nystagmus, microcornea, corneal pannus formation, cataract, microphakia, and lens subluxation.

The glaucoma associated with aniridia may be related to either developmental abnormalities of the anterior chamber angle or from progressive angle closure by apposition of the rudimentary iris stump. Initial management is medical but surgical intervention by trabeculotomy or filtration procedures may be required. Trabeculotomy is the approach of choice. Fistulizing surgery may be followed by marked lens corneal touch if there is shallowing of the anterior chamber. Glaucoma tube surgery may also be required in some cases. Many eyes have coincidental lens subluxation. In such cases trabeculotomy or tube surgery is best approached from the quadrant opposite to the direction of subluxation.

Axenfeld–Rieger syndrome

This is a spectrum of developmental disorders that over the years have been referred to by a variety of eponyms. The term anterior chamber cleavage syndromes is often used but more recent studies have failed to support the theory of incomplete anterior chamber cleavage during embryological development. Mesodermal dysgenesis is another misnomer as the tissues involved are derived from neural crest cells and not from mesodermal tissues as was previously believed. Whatever the underlying mechanism these conditions all have in common a developmental defect of the anterior chamber angle. The term Axenfeld–Rieger syndrome covers the complete spectrum of conditions that can be separately classified as Axenfeld's anomaly, Rieger's anomaly, and Rieger's syndrome. All can be inherited in an autosomal dominant fashion. All usually show bilateral ocular involvement, and occur equally in both sexes.

Posterior embryotoxon (Fig. 14) was the term used by Axenfeld to describe the appearance of an abnormally prominent anteriorly placed Schwalbe's line which can be seen on slit lamp examination as a white band on the posterior cornea just inside the limbus. Posterior embryotoxon occurs in about 15 per cent of normal eyes. In Axenfeld's anomaly posterior embryotoxon is associated with multiple iris processes which are inserted anteriorly into Schwalbe's line. These vary in thickness from thin strands to broad bands. In isolated Axenfeld's anomaly the iris is otherwise normal in appearance. In more severe forms of Axenfeld–Rieger syndrome the iris shows degrees of hypoplasia ranging from mild stromal thinning to the formation of full thickness holes, ectropion uveae, and corectopia causing displacement of the pupil away from the area of iris thinning (Fig. 15).

About 50 per cent of eyes with Axenfeld–Rieger syndrome develop glaucoma. Although the glaucoma may present in infancy it more commonly occurs between the first and third decades of life. Management will depend on the time of presentation, but if surgery becomes necessary trabeculectomy is the operation of choice.

Axenfeld–Rieger syndrome may be associated with other congenital defects including maxillary hypoplasia which causes flattening of the mid-face and typical dental defects (microdontia, hypodontia, and oligodontia). Hypertelorism may also occur and is a prominent feature in some pedigrees.

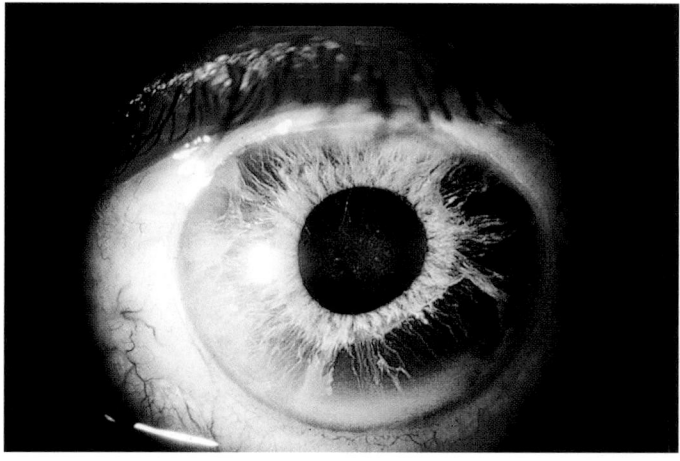

(a)

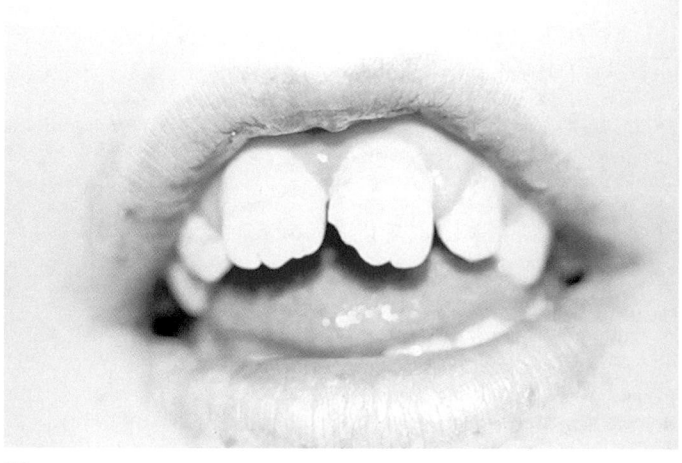

(b)

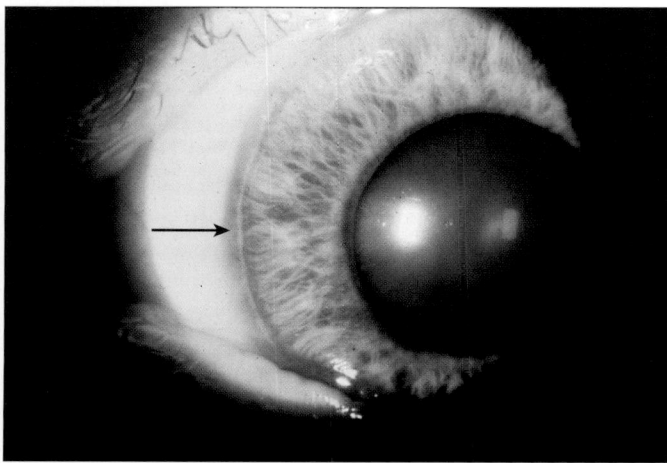

Fig. 14 Posterior embryotoxon (arrow) occurs in up to 15 per cent of normal eyes.

Fig. 15 Axenfeld–Rieger syndrome. (a) Appearance of anterior segment. (b) Oligodontia with typical notched teeth.

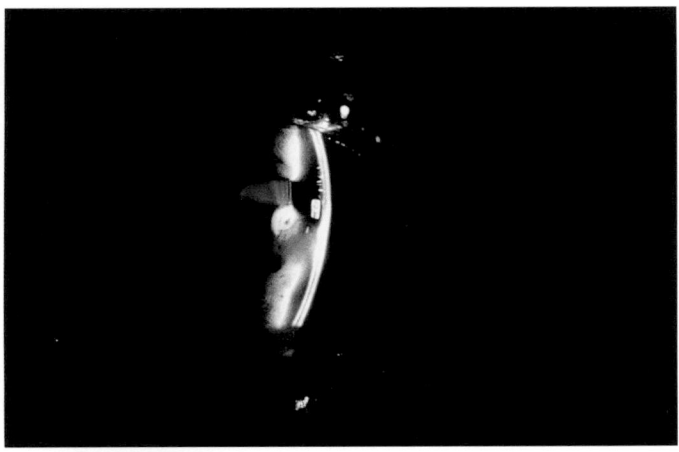

Fig. 16 Peters' anomaly showing adhesions between iris/cornea and cornea.

Peters' anomaly

Peters' anomaly is characterized by a central corneal leucoma associated with thinning of the stroma and a deficiency in Descemet's membrane. There are usually adhesions between the corneal opacity and the central iris (Fig. 16). There is a wide spectrum of disease. The cornea may remain almost totally clear or the opacity may be so great as to totally obscure the anterior chamber. In most cases the anomaly is bilateral. In some cases there is an associated keratolenticular adhesion with lenticular opacity. About two-thirds of cases develop glaucoma. The pathogenesis is not fully understood and many theories have been proposed including intrauterine infection, incomplete separation of lens vesicle from the surface ectoderm, anoxia, or a failure of differentiation of neural crest cells. There is no typical inheritance pattern with some cases appearing to show a recessive pattern of inheritance or autosomal dominant with incomplete penetrance, although the majority of cases occur sporadically. Glaucoma when it occurs is typically difficult to manage, and usually each case has to have strategies planned depending on the site and extent of the lesions.

Further reading

Brown, G.C., Magargal, L.E., Schachat, A., and Shah, H. (1984). Neovascular glaucoma. Etiologic considerations. *Ophthalmology*, **91**, 315–20.

Chan, C. and Okun, E. (1986). The question of ocular tolerance to intravitreal liquid silicone. A long-term analysis. *Ophthalmology*, **93**, 651–60.

Chi, T.S. and Netlan, P.A. (1995). Angle recession glaucoma. *International Ophthalmology Clinics*, **35**, 117–26.

Christensen, G.R. and Records, R.E. (1979). Glaucoma and expulsive hemorrhage mechanisms in the Sturge–Weber syndrome. *Ophthalmology*, **86**, 1360–6.

Ellant, J.P. and Obstbaum, S.A. (1992). Lens-induced glaucoma. *Documentation in Ophthalmology*, **81**, 317–38.

Farrar, S.M. and Shields, M.B. (1993). Current concepts of pigmentary glaucoma. *Survey of Ophthalmology*, **37**, 233–52.

Hayreh, S.S., Rojas, P., Podhajsky, P., Montague, P., and Woolson, R.F. (1983). Ocular neovascularization with retinal vascular occlusion. III. Incidence of ocular neovascularization with retinal vein occlusion. *Ophthalmology*, **90**, 488–506.

Jones, N.P. (1993). Fuchs' heterochromic uveitis: an update. *Survey of Ophthalmology*, **37**, 253–72.

Luntz, M.H. and Rosenblatt, M. (1987). Malignant glaucoma. *Survey of Ophthalmology* **32**, 73–93.

Murphy, C.G., Johnson, M., and Alvarado, J.A. (1992). Juxtacanalicular tissue in pigmentary and primary open angle glaucoma. The hydrodynamic role of pigment and other constituents. *Archives of Ophthalmology*, **110**, 1779–85.

Pasquale, L.R. and Green, W.R. (1993). Exfoliation syndrome: slit lamp biomicroscopy and pathological findings of the anterior segment. *New Trends in Ophthalmology*, **8**, 117–29.

Ritch, R. and Shields, M.B. (1982). *The secondary glaucomas*. Mosby, St Louis.

Ritch, R., Shields, M.B. and Krupin, T. (1989). *The glaucomas*. Mosby, St Louis.

Ritch, R., Steinberger, D., and Liebmann, J.M. (1993). Prevalence of pigment dispersion syndrome in a population undergoing glaucoma screening. *American Journal of Ophthalmology*, **115**, 707–10.

Streeten, B.W., Li, Z.Y., Wallace, R.N., Eagle, R.C. Jr, and Keshgegian, A.A. (1992). Pseudoexfoliative fibrillopathy in visceral organs of a patient with pseudoexfoliation syndrome. *Archives of Ophthalmology*, **110**, 1757–62.

Tello, C., Chi, T., Shepps, G., Liebman, J., and Ritch, R. (1993). Ultrasound biomicroscopy in pseudophakic malignant glaucoma. *Ophthalmology*, **100**, 1330–4.

Traboulsi, E.I. and Maumenee, I.H. (1992). Peters' anomaly and associated congenital malformations. *Archives of Ophthalmology*, **110**, 1739–42.

Urban, R.C. and Dreyer, E.B. (1993). Corticosteroid induced glaucoma. *International Ophthalmology Clinics*, **33**, 135–9.

2.10.10 Genetics of glaucoma

James E. Morgan

Glaucomatous optic neuropathy results in cupping of the optic disc and characteristic arcuate loss of visual field. Raised intraocular pressure is often included in the diagnosis but it is becoming clear that this is not an essential feature since a significant proportion of patients will have intraocular pressures within the normal range. It has been known for many years that various types of glaucoma tended to run in families though the mode of inheritance was complicated. For the most prevalent form, adult onset open angle glaucoma, the risk of a first-degree relative developing the condition can be up to 16 per cent, compared with an overall risk for the population of 2 per cent. Many of the factors that are thought to be implicated in disease pathogenesis, such as intraocular pressure, cup to disc ratio, outflow facility, and susceptibility to steroid-induced ocular hypertension all have heritable components.

Several forces have driven the search for the genetic basis of the disease. Glaucoma encapsulates a wide range of optic disc morphologies and modes of disease progression suggesting a number of pathophysiological processes for which the final common pathway is cupping of the optic disc. Some patients will be very sensitive to moderate increases in intraocular pressure whereas others will not develop any field loss in spite of consistent long-term increase in intraocular pressure. Treatment strategies should, therefore, be tailored to the particular disease subtype suffered by the patient. This approach requires a knowledge of the disease at the molecular level for which an understanding of the disease's genetic basis is invaluable. In conjunction with this, it is important that tests are developed that pinpoint those patients requiring intervention. At present we rely on the detection of visual field or optic nerve damage. Unfortunately, considerable damage may have been done before these changes in the appearance of the optic disc and visual field can be detected using available clinical techniques. If suitable genetic markers can be found patients can be screened for the presence of disease prior to the onset of damage.

In any genetic study it is important to determine the interaction of the environment and genotype in determining the phenotype. In glaucoma, genetic studies have been facilitated by the apparent lack of any clear major environmental influence. Even so, factors such as diet and the degree of exercise can affect the intraocular pressure. Seasonal variation has also been reported to influence the frequency of glaucoma in the population. In the United Kingdom, for example, the risk of development of primary open angle glaucoma was significantly lower for patients born between October and December compared with the rest of the year.

Methods used in molecular genetics

The considerable progress that has been made in recent years in our understanding of the genetic basis of glaucoma is due the development of molecular tools that can identify and localize parts of the genome. Sequencing of the DNA base sequence has been a slow and laborious process in the past. Now it has been automated to a large extent and laboratories can routinely in a single day determine the order of many thousands of base pairs.

DNA markers

Early work on the identification of particular parts of the genome was hampered by the limited availability of suitable markers. For example, early studies of glaucoma inheritance used markers such as the ABO group on chromosome 9 and the HLA system of chromosome 6 that were of little help in pinpointing those chromosomes involved in the disease. Subsequent work has shown that it is unlikely that genes on these chromosomes are involved in the development of disease.

The use of restriction enzymes has revolutionized the development of chromosomal markers. The DNA from subjects in a pedigree is isolated and fragmented using these enzymes that cleave the DNA at particular locations. Because of variation in the base sequence between individuals, the lengths of the resultant fragments will vary, generating so-called restriction fragment length polymorphisms. These segments of DNA are inherited in a mendelian fashion and their course can be plotted through a particular pedigree. These markers are, however, only useful if the individual under study is heterozygous at the marker and disease locus.

Linkage maps can be constructed using these markers that can plot the location of genes on a particular chromosome. The

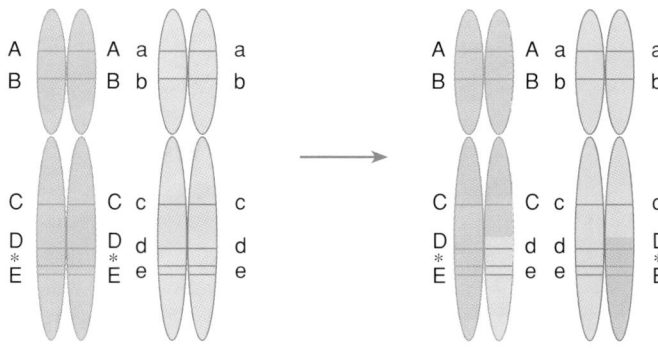

Fig. 1 Crossing over (recombination) can occur between adjacent chromosomes during meiosis. The gene responsible for disease is marked with an asterisk. It is flanked by the markers D and E, lying closer to E. Thus during recombination, the marker E is most likely to stay linked with the disease gene. This is much less likely with the more distant markers A, B, and C. (Redrawn from Alward *et al.*,1996, with permission.)

greater the number of markers, the greater the precision with which genomic locations can be defined. The linkage map of the human chromosome has benefited greatly from the discovery of regions of DNA with variable length repetitions of simple DNA sequences (in particular the sequence adenine-cytosine) that have generated large numbers of microsatellite repeats or short tandem repeat polymorphisms. A linkage map comprising 800 such markers is now available for the human.

The general principle is to find a marker whose allele cosegregates with the allele causing the illness. The closer the marker and the allele, the less likely that they will be separated during meiosis (i.e. become recombinant). The separation of the marker and the allele (or between any locus) can conveniently be expressed in terms of the probability that they will be separated during meiosis (Fig. 1).

In linkage studies the separation of genes and markers on the chromosome is measured in centimorgans, each unit representing a 1 per cent chance of recombination between loci as the chromosome passes from parent to child. In physical terms this is equivalent to approximately 1 million base pairs. This represents a tiny fraction of total human genome which has been estimated to be 3700 cM in length.

If the frequency of recombination is low (less than 5 per cent), loci are said to be linked. If the frequency is over 50 per cent, the loci are unlinked. In humans it is not possible simply to count the frequency of recombination and a statistical method, the maximum likelihood method, is used to express the likelihood that two loci might be linked. This is expressed as the lod score in which the logarithm of the ratio of the odds of linkage is divided by the odds that no linkage has occurred. By convention, a lod score of 3 or greater (representing an odds for linkage of 1000 to 1) is taken as indicating linkage. The criterion is conservative to take account of the low background probability that any two loci might be linked. Linkage is excluded with a lod score of -2 (indicating 100 to 1 odds against linkage).

Using these techniques, there are a number of ways in which linkage analysis can be used.

Candidate gene approach

If there is good evidence that a single gene is key to the development of a disease then linkage analysis can be used to see if the gene strictly cosegregates with the disease phenotype. Once this has been established the relevant gene is then cloned to allow the identification of relevant mutations. This approach has worked well in the identification of mutations in the peripherin-retinal degeneration slow (RDS) gene in retinitis pigmentosa. Attempts to use this technique in glaucoma, looking at a range of candidate genes (such as those for collagen and elastin) that might reasonably be thought to play a role in disease pathogenesis, have not been successful. In many respects this is not surprising. Glaucoma may result from the interaction between a larger number of genes, ranging from those involved in trabecular meshwork structure and metabolism to those affecting the optic nerve head and its vasculature.

Positional cloning

This method has the advantage that it does not require prior knowledge of the disease pathogenesis. The physical location of loci that cosegregate with the disease is calculated using relevant markers. If a genome-wide search is undertaken, the method is time-consuming. However, it can be narrowed if changes in the chromosome can be identified cytogenetically. For example, the identification of translocations and deletions linked to Rieger's syndrome has shown that the gene for this condition lies on the long arm of chromosome 4 (4q25 region). Similar techniques have also been useful in determining the genetic basis of aniridia (chromosome 11, 11p13 region). Once the site of the mutation is known, hypotheses can be constructed with regard to disease pathogenesis. This is the method that has yielded the most results in the search for a genetic basis to glaucoma.

Linkage analysis in complex disease

Existing data on the genetic bias of glaucoma is based on disease inherited in simple mendelian fashion (that is autosomal dominant or recessive) and due to mutation in a single gene. However, it is clear that for the majority of cases of open angle glaucoma the disease phenotype may result from the interaction of several genes. In this respect, association rather than linkage studies will be more useful.

Association studies compare the frequency of a marker in samples of patients and controls. The techniques used in these studies allow for the detection of genes that may have only a small effect in the disease pathogenesis. For theoretical reasons these studies require a much more detailed map of the genome than is currently available with a resolution of 1 to 2 cM. However, given the present speed with which the genome is being investigated such a map will soon be available.

Glaucoma associated with normal anterior segment anatomy

Primary open angle glaucoma is by far the most important type, occurring in over 2 per cent of the population over 65 years of age. The evidence for a genetic component to this disease is compelling. For first-degree relatives of patients with the condition the risk of developing the disease can be up to 16 per cent. Of the average open angle glaucoma population, approximately 70 per cent will have increased intraocular pressure (over 21 mmHg). For the majority of patients, inheritance will be complex and multifactorial, with low penetrance and for these elucidation of the genetic basis is a formidable task. Not surprisingly, the greatest progress has been made with the minority of patients with an autosomal dominant mode of inheritance. These patients usually have an earlier onset of the disease and have been described as having juvenile open angle glaucoma (or juvenile primary open angle glaucoma) to distinguish them as distinct from the more common adult onset of the disease (adult onset primary open angle glaucoma).

Juvenile primary open angle glaucoma

The juvenile form of the disease typically affects individuals in the teenage years though the age range extends from over 3 years to under 35 years. Several large pedigrees of juvenile primary open angle glaucoma in the United States, France, and the United Kingdom have been described. The inheritance is autosomal dominant but with variable penetrance of 80 to 100 per cent at 20 years. Although this form of glaucoma is rare it should be considered in patients under 40 years with high pressures and marked optic nerve cupping (Fig. 2).

Juvenile primary open angle glaucoma is distinct from congenital glaucoma. Patients do not develop buphthalmos and the corneas remain clear with the majority of cases having a normal anterior segment. The intraocular pressure is usually significantly raised (over 40 mmHg, range 30 to 50 mmHg) with a large diurnal fluctuation. The response to medical treatment is usually poor, with most patients requiring filtration surgery. Some distinguishing anterior segment characteristics have been noted. Prominent iris processes have been described that do not seem to correlate with the severity of the intraocular pressure rise. Goniodysgenesis has been described in one Danish pedigree in which affected patients had a high iris insertion and persistent uveal meshwork. In most cases, however, the trabecular meshwork is not significantly abnormal. An association with myopia has also been reported.

A major breakthrough with this condition came from Sheffield et al., studying a large affected family in the Midwest of the United States. Linkage studies with over 90 short tandem repeat polymorphisms localized the gene (called GLC1A) to the long arm of chromosome 1. Subsequent linkage analysis by this and other groups narrowed the affected region to 1q21–q31 (Fig. 3).

In 1997 the gene was isolated and shown to be responsible for the expression of trabecular meshwork induced glucocorticoid response protein. This protein can induce increased intraocular pressure by obstruction of aqueous flow and may be involved in the induction of steroid-induced glaucoma. Three mutations have so far been described, two being amino acid substitutions and one a nonsense mutation (glutamine to stop). The trabecular meshwork induced glucocorticoid response pro-

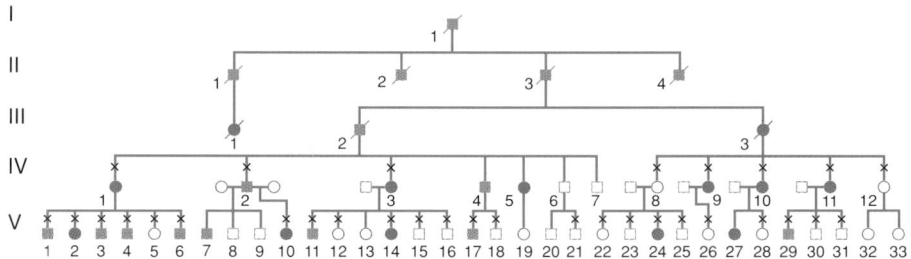

Fig. 2 Pedigree of family with juvenile primary open angle glaucoma. Affected individuals with intraocular pressure over 30 mmHg are represented by solid symbols. Lines drawn through symbols indicate those patients who are deceased. (Redrawn from Sheffield *et al.*, 1993, , with permission.)

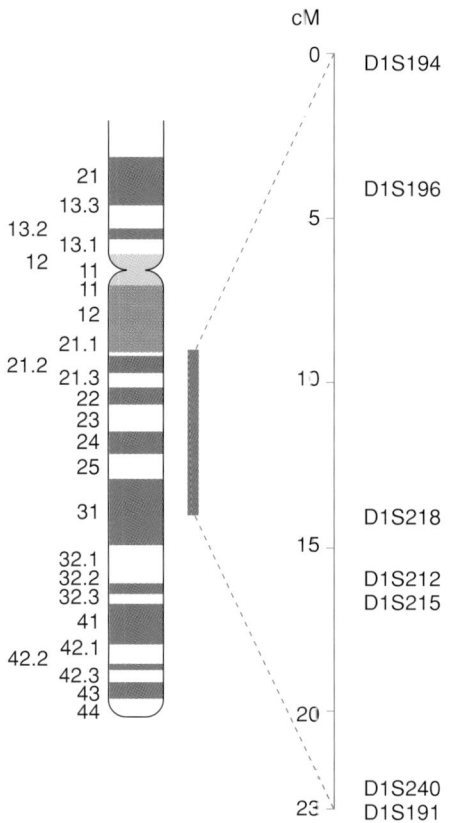

Fig. 3 Chromosome map showing the location of the gene causing juvenile primary open angle glaucoma. (Redrawn from Sheffield *et al.*, 1993, with permission.)

tions may have been missed and that the gene defect may be present in higher frequencies.

Although juvenile primary open angle glaucoma is a relatively rare form of open angle glaucoma, the high prevalence of the disease has led to estimates that mutations in GLC1A may cause glaucoma in 100 000 individuals in the United States. Tests that are based on the detection of mutations in this gene may usefully be incorporated into a screening process.

In view of the phenotypic variation seen in juvenile primary open angle glaucoma and the size of the q21–31 interval, it is likely that other gene interactions can affect the phenotypic expression of mutations in this region. One pair of monozygotic twins has been reported that illustrates this possibility. One twin developed severe glaucoma by 19 years of age whilst the other, although he had moderately increased intraocular pressure (25 and 28 mmHg), had minimal optic nerve degeneration and full visual fields. Whilst additional involved genes may lie on other chromosomes, other candidate genes lie within the q21–31 interval and include: atrial natriuretic peptide receptor, laminin, and adenosine triphosphatase 1B1 and B2. Indeed, receptors for this atrial natriuretic factor have been found on the ciliary body though it remains to be seen how changes in the level of this protein could decrease aqueous outflow. There is also evidence for juvenile primary open angle glaucoma phenotypes that do not show linkage to 1q21–31. These may form a different subset of disease since the patients developed severe optic nerve damage (before 10 years of age) and the intraocular pressure is slightly lower than expected for juvenile primary open angle glaucoma, in the range 25 to 30 mmHg.

Adult onset primary open angle glaucoma

The peak age of onset for this disease is approximately 40 years—at the time when the prevalence of juvenile primary open angle glaucoma is falling off. The genetic basis for this condition is strong but more complicated than for the juvenile onset type. Relatives of an affected member have a 7 to 10 times greater risk of developing the diseases compared with the unrelated and unaffected population with the age-adjusted risk being 4 times greater for those of African origin compared with Caucasians. High concordance has been shown for monozygotic twins and the propensity to develop ocular hypertension fol-

tein gene product is expressed in ciliary body and trabecular though the precise role of the gene in the pathophysiology of glaucoma remains to be elucidated (Fig. 4).

When the trabecular meshwork induced glucocorticoid response protein gene assay was used to screen eight families with chromosome 1q-linked glaucoma, five of the eight showed one of these amino acid mutations. Mutations were found also in 3.9 per cent of unrelated glaucoma patients studied compared with 0.2 per cent of controls. However, since the assay used only a portion of the gene, it is possible that other muta-

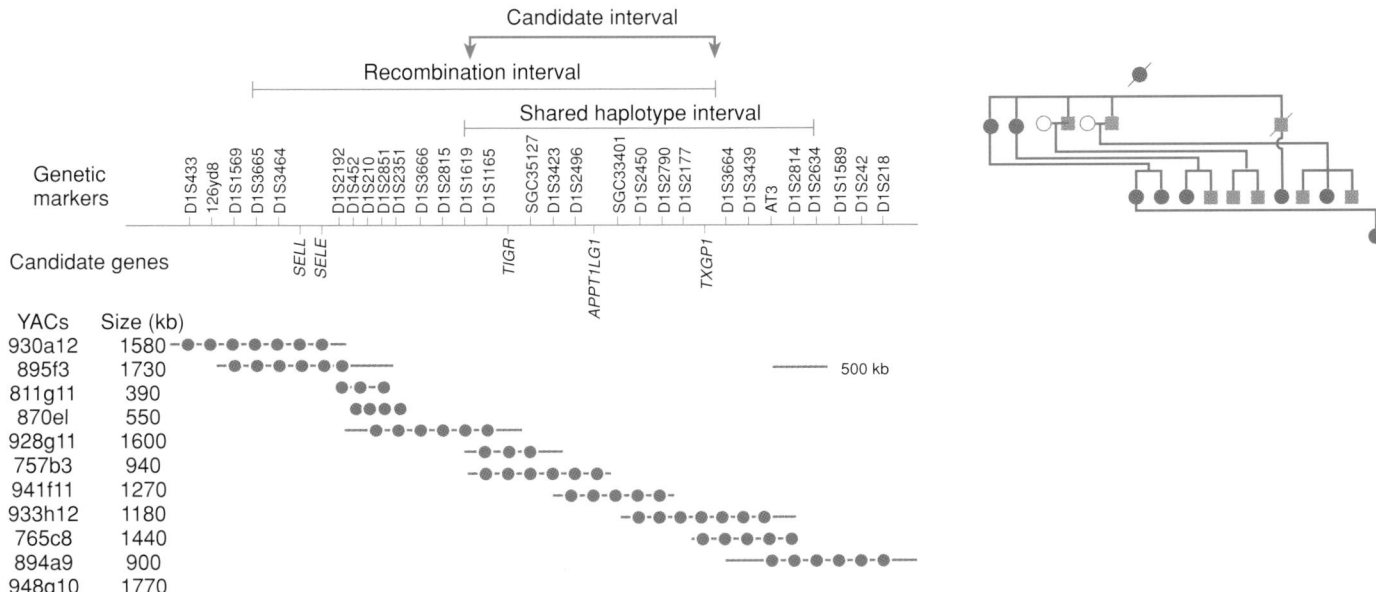

Fig. 4 Pedigree showing segregation of a glycine to valine mutation in a four generation family with adult onset open angle glaucoma. The white symbols indicate spouses who are unaffected. Filled symbols show affected spouses. Below this the various polymorphisms have been aligned so that each gel lane lies directly below the pedigree symbol of the family member supplying the DNA for that lane. Clinically unaffected family members are not shown. (Redrawn from Stone *et al.*, 1997, with permission.)

lowing the administration of topical steroids is closely related to the inheritance of primary open angle glaucoma.

A key question is the relationship of juvenile primary open angle glaucoma to adult onset primary open angle glaucoma and, in particular, whether the latter shows linkage to the site of the gene on chromosome 1. Mutations in the trabecular meshwork induced glucocorticoid response protein gene have been reported in 15 affected members of a family with autosomal dominant adult onset disease. Testing of a consecutively ascertained adult onset primary open angle glaucoma group showed the mutation in 2.9 per cent of patients. This figure could well be higher since only a portion of the gene was used in the analysis and the sensitivity of the detection techniques was less that 100 per cent.

The variable phenotype that can occur with juvenile primary open angle glaucoma can be problematic when attempts are made to define the phenotype for adult onset disease. If the effect of GLC1A is only partially penetrant, then the rate of disease progression may be slowed. Individuals with this phenotype who have been diagnosed as adults may therefore be erroneously classified as adult onset primary open angle glaucoma patients. Analysis of a large French Canadian pedigree illustrates this problem well and supports the idea that there is a continuum of phenotype severity, blurring the distinction between juvenile and adult onset primary open angle glaucoma. For a large French Canadian pedigree of 142 individuals, 36 were classified as juvenile primary open angle glaucoma, four as primary open angle glaucoma, with six having ocular hypertension. All cases showed tight linkage to 1q21–25q (this lies within the 1q21–31 interval). Work on a large French pedigree also showed age-dependent penetrance of the effect of the GLC1A gene. Affected individuals were typical for

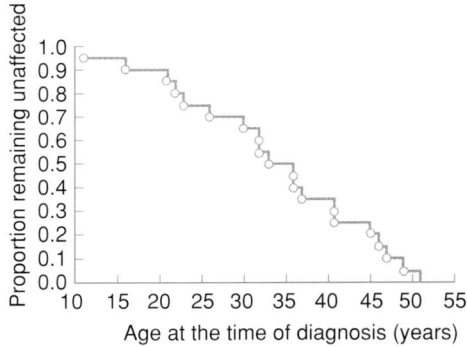

Fig. 5 Age-dependent penetrance of the gene for open angle glaucoma in a large French pedigree. The proportion of subjects remaining unaffected is plotted as a function of age at diagnosis. (Redrawn from Meyer *et al.*, 1996, with permission.)

juvenile primary open angle glaucoma in that the intraocular pressure was poorly controlled medically with filtration surgery being required in 17 of 20 affected individuals. The penetrance of the disease showed a striking variation with age; the cumulative proportion of affected patients was 25 per cent at 23 years, increasing to 75 per cent at 41 years of age (Fig. 5).

Evidence for a distinct form of adult onset primary open angle glaucoma comes from studies of patients in whom the age of onset is significantly greater than for the juvenile form (over 40 years) and the intraocular pressure increase modest (highest intraocular pressure less than 35 mmHg). For a family in the American Midwest with this form of disease, linkage could not be demonstrated to the GLC1A locus (lod score of −3.28).

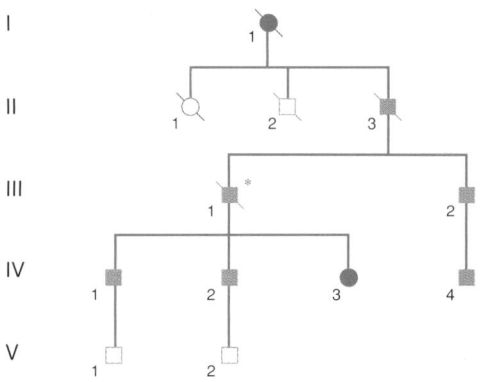

Fig. 6 Optic disc and macula of the right eye of an affected individual showing retinal folds radiating from the optic disc. The location of patients with this phenotype in the pedigree is shown inset. (Redrawn from Bennet *et al.* 1989, with permission.)

It may be more logical therefore to define disease not by age of onset but by the size of the intraocular pressure increase. Two other loci for patients with late onset primary open angle glaucoma are associated with modest increase in intraocular pressure. The GLC1B locus occurs at 2-cen-q13 in patients for whom mean age of onset was 47 years. The intraocular pressure was only slightly elevated, with 50 per cent having intraocular pressure less than 22 mmHg and the remainder having intraocular pressures in the range of 22 to 30 mmHg. Only one patient had an intraocular pressure greater than 30 mmHg. In contrast with juvenile primary open angle glaucoma, more than half the patients showed a good response to medical treatment. Using intraocular pressure as a criterion, some of these patients would be classified as having normal tension glaucoma. However, the affected families comprised patients with high and normal intraocular pressure. The 2-cen-q13 region is large, estimated at 8 to 17 cM, possibly comprising as many as 40 million base pairs. Candidate genes that lie in this region include *RALB* (*ras*-like protein b), *ADRA2B* (α-2b-adrenergic receptor), and *PAX8* (paired box homeotic gene 8). Considerable further refinement of this region is required before any candidate genes can be isolated.

The GLC1C locus has been described on chromosome 3 (3q21–q24) in patients with autosomal dominant glaucoma with a modest increase in intraocular pressure (over 24 mmHg and less than 30 mmHg) with ages at diagnosis in the range of 38 to 80 years. Candidate genes in the 11.1 cM interval for the GLC1C locus include a membrane endopeptidase that is expressed in the trabeculae and has been implicated as involved in the regulation of intraocular pressure.

Low tension glaucoma

An autosomal dominant form of low tension glaucoma has been described. However, the phenotype is atypical in that patients were affected early in life with pronounced cupping seen early in childhood. Two of the six affected patients also had retinal folds radiating from the optic disc that are not part of the normal glaucoma phenotype (diagnosis is usually made in middle age) (Fig. 6).

Histological analysis of the eyes from one deceased patient show cupping of the optic nerve head and extensive loss of retinal ganglion cells typical of glaucoma and did not suggest an alternative pathological mechanism.

Sex-linked glaucoma

Sex-linked glaucoma is very rare. A few pedigrees have been described. Large surveys have failed to show any association with sex for primary open angle glaucoma.

Glaucoma associated with abnormal anterior segment anatomy

Primary congenital glaucoma

Although this condition is rare with an incidence in the West of 1 in 10 000, increasing to 1 in 2000 in the Middle East, it can have a devastating impact on both patient and family. Control of intraocular pressure can be difficult and frequently requires surgical intervention. The inheritance is usually autosomal recessive with most patients being diagnosed at birth, often because of buphthalmos; earlier diagnosis can be facilitated by the presence of diffuse corneal opacification or other symptoms such as photophobia, tearing or blepharospasm. In many cases the anterior segment anatomy is abnormal, sometimes secondary to a membrane lying over the trabecular meshwork that provides a mechanical barrier to aqueous outflow. It is also possible that the drainage angle is defective following abnormal mesodermal cleavage during embryogenesis.

Families with buphthalmos have been analysed that map to 2p21 (GLC3A) and 1p36 (GLC3B). Heritable mutations of the cytochrome P4501B1 gene (CYP1B1) have been described in the affected individuals of five well-characterized families linked to the GLC3A locus. Three types of mutation were found. Two involved a deletion of base pairs and the other the insertion of a single cytosine base. All resulted in frame shift mutations that were not detected in normal subjects. P4501B1 is expressed constitutively in the trabecular meshwork and may be involved in the metabolism of a molecule that is active in development. An arachidonate metabolite of the P450 enzyme has also been implicated in the inhibition of sodium, potassium, and adenosine triphosphatase. This may affect corneal transparency and ciliary body function, explaining in part the corneal opacity and increased intraocular pressure in buphthalmos.

Juvenile glaucoma with iris hypoplasia

Affected individuals have characteristically bilateral slate grey or chocolate brown irides. Inheritance is autosomal dominant with linkage analysis indicating involvement of the 4q25 region. Note that this also corresponds to the region implicated in Rieger's syndrome.

Rieger's syndrome

Rieger's syndrome is inherited in an autosomal dominant manner. Affected eyes show iris hypoplasia, prominent iridotrabecular, processes. and posterior embryotoxon. Glaucoma develops in 60 per cent of patients though its severity does not appear to correlate with the degree of iris pathology. The corneal endothelium may be affected and corneal opacification may be a presenting sign. Cytogenetic abnormalities have been found at chromosomes 6 (inversion) and 13 (deletion). Linkage analysis has most consistently indicated involvement of chromosome 4q25.

Aniridia

Aniridia shows autosomal dominant inheritance. Glaucoma will develop in 6 to 75 per cent of patients with cataract developing in up to 85 per cent. Deletions involving the short arm of chromosome 11 have been demonstrated. The severity of the disease appears to depend on the extent of the deletions. Thus, large deletions are associated with the development of Wilms' tumours, aniridia, genitourinary abnormalities, and mental retardation (WAGR syndrome). Linkage analysis has shown the *PAX6* gene to be involved. This is important in the regulation of the activity of other genes during development. Mutations in this gene would therefore be consistent with abnormal development of the anterior segment; not surprisingly, mutations in this gene have been described in Peters' anomaly in which anterior segment development can be significantly disrupted.

Secondary glaucomas

Glaucoma may also account for part of several ophthalmic syndromes for which the inheritance pattern, is known. These include the following.

Lowe's oculocerebrorenal syndrome (X-linked recessive)

Linkage has been demonstrated to Xq25. The gene at this location is similar to inositol polyphosphate-5-phosphatase suggesting the role of a defect in inositol metabolism in this disease.

Weil-Marchesani (autosomal recessive)

Glaucoma usually results from pupil block and angle closure. Patients have spherophakia sometimes combined with lens subluxation.

Homocystinuria (autosomal recessive)

This results in osteoporosis, arterial venous thrombosis, and mental retardation. Ocular signs include spherophakia, ectopia lentis, myopia, and retinal detachment. Glaucoma can result from pupil block.

Neurofibromatosis (autosomal dominant)

The glaucoma is usually unilateral and associated with an ipsilateral plexiform neuroma.

Pigment dispersion

Several pedigrees have been described that show autosomal dominant inheritance. The glaucoma usually presents in young adulthood. Patients often have a moderate degree of myopia.

Iris pigment is dislodged by rubbing against the lens zonules. Up to 36 per cent of males and 33 per cent of females will develop increased intraocular pressure. Pigment may not be the sole factor that contributes to the rise in intraocular pressure and it is possible that some type of mesodermal dysgenesis may also be occurring to contribute to the increase in intraocular pressure.

Future work

Glaucomatous optic neuropathy is very much defined by changes in the optic nerve and visual field which may be inadequate to differentiate the various subtypes of the disease. In this respect it may be similar to retinitis pigmentosa in which a number of different mutations can give rise to a similar phenotype. Precise characterization of the various phenotypic subtypes of adult onset primary open angle glaucoma will be important in determining the genetic basis of the disease. Although the discovery of the trabecular meshwork induced glucocorticoid response protein gene has been a major step forward, it seems likely that this represents only one pathway to the generation of increased intraocular pressure. For the majority of patients the variable expression of their glaucoma phenotype will result from the interaction of a number of genes. Fortunately, the great advances that have been made in molecular genetics will permit the elucidation of these interactions.

Further reading

Alward, W., *et al.* (1996). Molecular genetics in glaucoma: current status. *Journal of Glaucoma*, **5**, 276–84.

Bennet, S., Alward, W., and Folberg, R. (1989). An autosomal dominant form of low-tension glaucoma. *American Journal of Ophthalmology*, **108**, 203.

Francois, J. (1981). Genetic predisposition to glaucoma. *Developmental Biology*, **3**, 1–45.

Graff, C., Urbak, S., Jerndal, T., and Wadelius, C. (1995). Confirmation of linkage to 1q21–q31 in a Danish autosomal dominant juvenile-onset glaucoma family and evidence of genetic heterogeneity. *Human Genetics*, **96**, 285–9.

Meyer, A., Béchetoille, A., Vallot, F., *et al.* (1996). Age-dependent penetrance and mapping of the locus for juvenile and early onset open angle glaucoma on chromosome 1q (GLC1A) in a French family. *Human Genetics*, **98**, 568.

Morisette, J., Cote, G., Anctil, J.-L., *et al.* (1995). A common gene for juvenile and adult-onset primary open-angle glaucomas, confined on chromosome 1q. *American Journal of Human Genetics*, **56**, 1431–42.

Richards, J., Lichter, P., Hermans, S., *et al.* (1996). Probable exclusion of GLC1A as a candidate glaucoma gene in a family with middle-age onset primary open angle glaucoma. *Ophthalmology*, **103**, 1035–40.

Sheffield, V., Stone, E., Alward, W., *et al.* (1993). Genetic linkage of familial open angle glaucoma to chromosome 1q21–q31. *Nature Genetics*, **4**, 47–50.

Stewart, W. (1995). The effect of lifestyle on the relative risk to develop open-angle glaucoma. *Current Opinion in Ophthalmology*, **6**, 3–9.

Stoilova, D., Child, A., Trifan, O., Pitts Crick, R., and Coakes, R.M.S. (1996). Location of a locus (GLC1B) for adult onset primary open angle glaucoma to the 2cen-q13 region. *Genomics*, **36**, 142–50.

Stone, E., Fingert, J., Alward, W., *et al.* (1997). Identification of a gene that causes primary open angle glaucoma. *Science*, **275**, 668–70.

Wiggs, J., Del Bono, E., Schuman, J., Hutchinson, B., and Walton, D. (1995). Clinical features of five pedigrees genetically linked to the juvenile glaucoma locus on chromosome 1q21–q31. *Ophthalmology*, **102**, 1782–9.

Wirtz, M., Samples, J., Kraemer, P., *et al.* (1997). Mapping a gene for adult-onset primary open angle glaucoma to chromosome 3p. *American Journal of Human Genetics*, **60**, 296–304.

Index

low vision *(continued)*
  patient evaluation 319–21
  sources of data 953–4
  see also visual impairment
Low Vision Enhancement System 595
lubricants, ocular **79–80**
  in facial nerve palsy 884
  see also tear(s), replacements
lumbar puncture 833
lumican
  in corneal stroma 375
  in macular corneal dystrophy 389, 390
lung carcinoma, intraocular metastases 927–8
lupus erythematosus
  cutaneous 754
  systemic, *see* systemic lupus erythematosus
Lyell's syndrome (toxic epidermal necrolysis) 343, 754
Lyme disease *524*, **526–7**
  facial palsy *883*, 884
  intermediate uveitis 539
  optic neuropathy 840
  risk factors 515
  treatment 527
lymphadenopathy, preauricular 334, 336, 407
lymphangioma 1032–3
lymphatics
  eyelids 357
  intraocular absence 3, 509
  orbit 199
lymphocytes 47
  in chronic inflammation 48
  intraocular traffic 518
  in multiple sclerosis 898–9
  see also B lymphocytes; T cells
lymphogranuloma venereum 41
lymphoid hyperplasia
  atypical 371
  benign reactive 371, **931**
  orbit 209–10
lymphoma
  conjunctiva 344–5
  Epstein–Barr virus and 430
  eyelids 371
  lacrimal gland 221–2, 1159
  ocular **550–1**, 735, **931**
    in AIDS/HIV infection 791
    clinical features 550, *550*
  optic nerve infiltration 842
  orbital 209, 218
lymphoproliferative lesions
  conjunctiva 344–5
  lacrimal gland **221–2**
Lynch incision 219, 1162
  superior oblique underaction after 266
lyonization 13
lysinuric protein intolerance *802*, 803
lysosomal disorders 451, *802*, **807–9**, 811
lysosomal enzymes 50
lysosomal phosphotransferase deficiency 451
lysozyme 4, 24–5, 79

M
Macaca cyclops 43
Mackay–Marg based tonometers 115, 653
McLure Reading Text book 1018
McNeill/Goldmann speculum 1174–5, 1177
macroaneurysms, retinal arteriolar, in hypertension 739–40
macrolide antibiotics, ocular side-effects *768*
macrophages 46–7
  in acute inflammation 47–8
  in chronic inflammation 48
  epithelioid 47, 48
  HIV infection 781
  intraocular 3

macrophages *(continued)*
  in multiple sclerosis 899
  in necrosis 50
  in thyroid eye disease 723–4
macrorcticular dystrophy 611
macro-square wave jerks 881
macula 814–15
  age-related degeneration, *see* age-related macular degeneration
  annular reflex, in infants 1030
  burns, nadvertent laser-induced 575
  cherry red spot, *see* cherry red spot
  coloboma 1000–1
  detachment, in diabetic retinopathy 1273, 1274
  development 990
  disorders
    diagnosis 822
    electroretinography 180
    fluorescein angiography 158
  dystrophies 609, **610–12**
    adult vitelliform *608*, 611
    atypical vitelliform *608*
    benign concentric annular 611
    childhood **1054–5**
    dominant cystoid *608*, 610–11
    fluorescein angiography 158
    molecular genetics *608*
    North Carolina *608*, 610
    primary **610**
  hypoplasia 1052
    and congenital cataract 1207
  ischaemia, in diabetic retinopathy 571
  parafoveal zone 814
  perifoveal zone 814–15
  schisis 1053
  serpiginous choroidopathy involving 543
  sparing 818, 823, 824
  zones 814–15
maculae ceruleae 971
maculae occludentes 376
macula lutea 563, 814
macular corneal dystrophy *389*, **389–90**
  clinical features 390
  definition/aetiology 389
  epidemiology 389
  pathophysiology/biochemistry 389–90
  treatment 395
  type I 389–90
  type II 389
macular oedema
  cystoid
    in acute anterior uveitis 520
    after cataract surgery 1203, 1206, 1253
    in Behçet's disease 546, 557
    in birdshot retinochoroidopathy 543
    dominant *608*, 610–11
    fluorescein angiography 155, 156
    in intermediate uveitis 521, 539
    in multifocal choroiditis 540
    in posterior uveitis 522
    in sarcoidosis 547
    sympathomimetic-induced 66
    treatment 75
  diabetic 571, 713–14, 1274
    laser therapy 98, 576
    see also diabetic maculopathy
  fluorescein angiography 158
  panretinal laser photocoagulation exacerbating 575
  post-traumatic 1298
  in retinal vein occlusions 602, 603–4, 605
Macular Photocoagulation Study Group trial 587–8, 589–92, 593
macular star exudates 564, 814
  in optic atrophy 211, 213
maculopathy
  arc welding 743
  diabetic, *see* diabetic maculopathy
Maddox rods 251, 258, 1022
MAGE genes 11

magnesium fluoride 293
magnetic resonance angiography (MRA) 150, 151, 829
  arteriovenous malformations 895
  indications 829
  in orbital disease 204
  in paediatric patients 1029
magnetic resonance imaging (MRI) **148–50**, 827–9
  blood flow studies 830
  contraindications 828, 1281
  contrast media 828
  future developments 150–1
  indications 828–9
  in multiple sclerosis 828, 903
  in orbital disease 204, 218, 828
  in orbital fractures 1281
  in orbital pseudotumour 209
  in paediatric patients 1029
  in papilloedema 833
  in retinoblastoma 920
  in thyroid eye disease 149, 150, 725
  in uveal melanoma 149, 911
  vs computed tomography 828
magnetic resonance spectroscopy 151
  in orbital disease 220
magnification
  in aphakic correction 312–13
  empty 116
  lateral 284
  loupe 103
  slit lamp biomicroscope, *see* slit lamp biomicroscope, magnification
  spectacle, *see* spectacles, magnification
  by spherical reflecting surfaces 282
  telescopes 324
magnifiers
  electronic 595
  hand 321–2, 595
  illuminated 323–4
  stand 322–3, 595
magnocellular system 816, *816*, 819
Mainster lens 119–20
major circle of iris (mci, major arterial circle) 162, 164
  anatomy 502, 503, 507
  development 989
  normal blood flow *163*
  pathological blood flow 167, 173
  to ciliary body 504
major histocompatibility complex (MHC) 7–8, 517
  class I genes 8
  class II genes 8
    knockout mice 43
  see also HLA
major outer membrane protein (MOMP) 42, 43, 44
malar bone, *see* zygomatic bone
malar eminence, flattening 1280, 1284, 1285
malaria *35*
malathion 972
malattia leventinese 611
MALE procedure, in "A" and "V" pattern exotropia 1243
Malherbe, calcifying epithelioma of 370
malignant disease, *see* cancer
malingering, visual evoked potentials in 182
malondialdehyde, in cataract 461
Maltese cross intracellular inclusions 451
mandibular hypoplasia 794, 796
mandibulofacial dysostosis *1039*
mannitol 68, 1103
mannosidosis *802*, 809, 1038
  cataracts 477, 481, 803, 1046
manometry, intraocular pressure measurement 113
map–dot–fingerprint corneal dystrophy 381–3, 448
  clinical features 382–3
  definition and aetiology 381–2

map–dot–fingerprint corneal dystrophy *(continued)*
  pathophysiology and biochemistry 382
Marchesani's syndrome *802*
Marcus Gunn jaw-winking (phenomenon) 359, 821, 886
  inverse 359, 886
  surgical management 1139, 1140
Marfan's syndrome *802*, 810, *1039*
  glaucoma 1081
  lens changes 803
marginal arcades, eyelids 356, 357
marginal bundle of Drualt 992
marginal degeneration, cornea, *see* Terrien's disease
marginal myotomy 1245
marginotomies, orbital 1162
Marin–Amat syndrome 886
Marinesco–Sjögren(–Larssen) syndrome *802*, 1047
Maroteaux–Lamy syndrome 809, *1038*
masking (blinding) 946
"masquerade syndrome" 369
mast cells 47
  in allergic conjunctivitis 5, 340
matching *937*, 944–5
maturation, delayed visual, *see* delayed visual maturation
maxilla 195, 196
  anterior lacrimal crest 195, 1280, 1286
  fractures 798, 799, 1281
    Le Fort II/III 798, 1158
    see also zygomaticomaxillary fractures
  hypoplasia 792, 794, 796
  orbital plate 1279
maxillary sinus 196
Mazzotti reaction 40
Mazzotti test 40
MB-45 antibody 53
measles 979–81
  corneal ulceration 979–80
  immunization 980, 984
  keratoconjunctivitis 979
  prevention of blindness 980
  uveitis (retinitis) *524*, **530**
  virus *29*
  vitamin A deficiency 979
measurement, clinical *933–6*
measurement scales
  interval 933–4
  nominal or classificatory 933
  performance 934–6
  rank ordered or ordinal 933
  ratio 934
  reliability 934
  repeatability 934–5
  sensitivity/responsiveness to change 935–6
  types 933–4
  validity 934
Mectizan, *see* ivermectin
medial canthal incision, in craniofacial anomalies 1128
medial canthal ligament/tendon 197, 355, 356
  congenital anterior displacement 1155–6
  in hypertelorism 1128
  laxity, repair 1138
  traumatic disruption 1158, 1280, 1286
  traumatic loss 1138
medial canthal repair 1145
medial check ligament 196, 232, 233
medial longitudinal fasciculus (MLF) 235, 237
  demyelination 902
  lesions 867, 868, 872
  in oculomotor control 238, 867, 868
  rostral interstitial nucleus (riMLF) 867
    lesions 868, 872
    in vertical gaze control 238, 868
medial ophthalmic vein 199
medial palpebral arteries 198, 356, 357
medial palpebral ligament, *see* medial canthal ligament/tendon

paracentesis *(continued)*
  in trabeculectomy 1217
paracetamol, ocular side-effects *771*
paraesthesia, in migraine 890
parallax angle 239–40
paramedical workers
  in developing countries 981, 983
  see also ophthalmic assistants
parametric statistics 935
Paramyxoviridae 29, *423*
paranasal sinuses
  carcinoma, surgical management 1131
  pain referred from 886
  squamous cell carcinoma 799–800
  surgical approaches 1163
paranasal sinusitis
  lacrimal obstruction 1156
  orbital cellulitis secondary to 206, 207
paraneoplastic diseases
  bilateral diffuse uveal melanocytic
    proliferation 932
  cancer-associated retinopathy 8, 551,
    932
  uveitis 551
paraplegia, in neuromyelitis optica 905
parasitic infections/infestations
    34–41, *35*
  cornea 419–23
  tropical 961–72
  uvea 532–3
  see also specific diseases
parasympathetic nerves
  ciliary body 504
  in Holmes–Adie syndrome 865
  iris/pupil 502, 503, 819
  lacrimal gland 197, 200
  orbit 200
parasympathomimetic drugs
  in glaucoma 65, 1215
  in paediatric patients 1026
paratrigiminal neuralgia (Raeder's
    syndrome) 864, 891
paraxial theory 122
parents
  age, in retinoblastoma 918
  in paediatric glaucoma 1082
  preoperative instructions 1111
  see also family
parietal lobe
  demyelination 902
  lesions 823
  in oculomotor control 868–9
parieto-occipital cortex lesions 860,
    861
Parinaud's oculoglandular syndrome
    338, 529
Parinaud's syndrome, *see* dorsal
    midbrain syndrome
Parkinson's disease 886
  blepharospasm 277
  saccadic disorders 869
parotid lymph nodes 204
paroxetine, ocular side-effects *771*
Parry–Romberg syndrome 537, *760*
pars plana 503, 618
  development 989
pars plicata, *see* uveitis, intermediate
pars plicata 503, 618
  lens zonules 455
partial sight, *see* visual impairment
parvocellular system 816, *816*, 819
Pasteur, Louis 23
Patau's syndrome (trisomy 13) 756–7,
    1045
patch clamping 633
patching, *see* occlusion
Paton's folds 833
pattern dystrophies of retinal
    pigment epithelium 587, *608*, 609,
    611
Paul–Bunnell heterophile antibody
    431
pause cells 867
pavingstone retinal degeneration 1258
PAX gene family 999, 1006

PAX2 gene 999, 1006
PAX6 gene
  in eye development 1036–7
  mutations
    anterior chamber dysgenesis 708,
      758, 1006, 1037
    cataract 1045, 1046
    homozygous 1037
    prenatal diagnosis 1009
    protein (PAX6) 459, 1006
  in retinal development 1002
PDEB mutations 608
PDS II (polydioxanone) sutures 1121,
    1123
"peculiar substance" 384
pediculosis 971–2
Pediculus humanus
  var. *capitis* 971
  var. *corporis* 971
Pelli–Robson low contrast letter chart
    113, 821, 1018
  in cataract 486–7
pellucid marginal corneal
    degeneration 301, *434*
pemphigoid, cicatricial 4–5, **750–3**
  antigen 753
  clinical features 750–2
  conjunctival changes 330, *342–3*, 751
  corneal changes 438, 751, 752
  diagnosis 750, *750*
  entropion 1135, 1136
  pathology 752–3
  treatment/prognosis 753
pemphigus 5, 754
penetrating keratoplasty (PKP)
    1174–81
  in *Acanthamoeba* keratitis 38, 422, *422*
  acute anterior uveitis after 535
  in alkali burns 1177, 1178, 1301
  in aphakic bullous keratopathy 1176
  in bacterial keratitis 417, 1176
  combined with cataract extraction/
    implant (triple procedure) 1176
  complications
    delayed 1180–1
    early postoperative 1179–80
    surgical 1178–9
  computed videokeratography after 137
  in corneal dystrophies 387, 395, 400
  in corneal perforation 1173, **1176–7**
  donor cornea assessment 1170
  donor tissue preparation 1174
  in herpes zoster 430
  indications 1173
  in keratoconus 405
  in peripheral ulcerative keratitis *436*,
    1176
  postoperative management 1179
  in pseudophakic bullous keratopathy
    1176
  repeat 1177–8
  in rheumatoid arthritis 745–6
  special procedures 1175–8
  surgical technique 1174–5, *1175*
  sutures
    management 1180
    placement 1187
    in postgrafting astigmatism 1181,
      1186
  see also corneal transplantation
penicillin 70
  ocular side-effects *768*, *771*
Penicillium 418
pen torch, in paediatric examination
    1012–13, 1023
pentose-phosphate pathway, lens 459
peptidoglycan 24, 26
peracetic acid sterilization 1118
perfluorocarbons
  anaesthetic considerations 1112–13
  causing glaucoma 699
  in epiretinal membrane dissection
    1269
  in retinal detachment repair 1264–5,
    1271, 1276

perfusion pressure, ocular 507, 565
  primary open angle glaucoma and 651
periaqueductal grey 235, 237
peribulbar anaesthesia (block) 1109–
    10
  in choroidal neovascularization 592–3
  in glaucoma surgery 1211–12
  injection technique 1109–10
  local anaesthetic solution 1109
  needles 1109
  oculopression 1108
pericytes, retinal 564
  in diabetes 716, 717, 804
perimeter, Goldmann 185
perimetry **657–66**
  alternative methods 663–6, 675
  automated **185–92**, 661–3
    factors affecting results 188–9,
      657–8, 675
    false negatives 189, 662
    false positives 189, 661–2
    fixation losses 189, 661
    fundamentals 661–2
    graphical display of results 187–8
    greyscales 187, 188
    learning effect 189, 657
    reliability indices 189
    in series 190–2
    statistical analysis 189–90, 662–3
    summary measures 190
  full threshold 186–7
  fundus-related 664
  in glaucoma 674–5
  kinetic 185, 186, 659, **660**
  manual **185**, 186
  multiple stimulus 663–4
  in neuro-ophthalmology 821
  prerequisites for good 658–9
  static 185–7, 659, **660–1**
  suprathreshold 187, 664–5, 675
perineuritis, orbital 208
peri-optic nerve arteriolar
    anastomoses, *see* Haller–Zinn,
    arterial circle of
periorbital fascia 196
periorbital incisions, in craniofacial
    surgery 1128–9
periorbital skeletal abnormalities, *see*
    facial skeletal disorders
periorbital trauma 1280
peripheral arcade, upper lid 356, 357
peripheral cystoid degeneration, retina
    1256–7
peripheral nerve tumours, lacrimal
    gland 224
peripherin/RDS mutations 607, *608*,
    609
  in pattern dystrophies 609, 611
  in retinitis pigmentosa 609, 1057
peritoneal shunt, lumbar, in
    papilloedema 834
periventricular leucomalacia,
    retinopathy of prematurity and 1064
Perkins tonometer 653
  in paediatric patients 1028, 1083
perlecan 377
permethrin 972
peroxisomal disorders *802*, **809**, 811
perseveration, visual 858
persistent hyperplastic primary
    vitreous (PHPV) 992, **1001–2**
  cataract 1048
  clinical features 1014, 1015
  secondary glaucoma 693
  vs toxocariasis 533
pes pedunculi, syndrome of (Weber's)
    236, 876, *876*
Peters' anomaly 702, 1010, *1036*, 1037
  congenital cataract 1045
  genetics 708
  glaucoma 702, 1079–80
  glaucoma surgery 1214
petrolatum 972
petrous tip, apex of 238
P-glycoprotein 922

pH
  bacterial growth and 27
  local anaesthetic solutions 1106, 1107–8
phacoanaphylaxis 481, 690, **691**
phacodonesis 1298, 1299
phacoemulsification **1198–203**
  advantages 1198
  capsulorhexis 1200
  complications 1198, 1203
  disadvantages 1198
  glaucoma complicating 697–8
  hydrodissection 1200
  incisions 1198, 1199–200
  intraocular lenses 1201–2
  irrigation/aspiration of cortical material
    1201
  learning curve 1198
  machines 1198
    aspiration 1199
    infusion 1199
    power 1199
  principles 1198
  surgical technique 1200–1
  in uveitis 558, 1251
  viscoelastic materials 1200
  wound closure 1202–3
phacomatoses **759–67**, 1058–9
  glaucoma 1081
  molecular genetics 765–6
phacometry 122
phacotrabeculectomy, *see*
    trabeculectomy, combined with
    cataract surgery
phaeochromocytoma 763, 1059
phagocytosis 46
  apoptotic cells 51
  by retinal pigment epithelial cells 561
  by trabecular meshwork endothelial
    cells 637
phakinin (CP49) 461
phako-, *see* phaco-
pharmaceutical companies,
    anticataract drugs 489, 497
pharmacology **57–78**
  principles 57–63
pharyngoconjunctival fever 336, 431,
    432
phase separation inhibitors 495
phenoxymethyl-penicillin, ocular
    side-effects *771*
phenylephrine
  in episcleritis 348, 349
  for fundoscopic examination 61
  in paediatric patients 1067, 1091
  preoperative use 1103
  in scleritis 351
  in uveitis 556, *556*
  before cataract surgery 1250
phenylketonuria 802
phenytoin, ocular side-effects *771*
phlebography, orbital 826
phlyctenular disease *434*, 437
pholedrine, in Horner's syndrome 864
phoria, *see* deviation, ocular, latent
phosducin 8
phosphenes 858
phosphodiesterase 563, 1057
phosphoinositol cycle, lens 461
phospholipase A_2 76, 78
phosphorus-32 (^{32}P) uptake test, uveal
    melanoma 911
photic stimulation
  electrodiagnosis 177
  electro-oculography 177
  electroretinography 179–80
photoablation, laser 95, 99–100, 1189
  clinical applications 100
photoastigmatic refractive
    keratectomy (PARK), corneal
    topography 137
photochemical reactions 95
photochromic tints 293
photocoagulation, laser **96–8**
  in choroidal neovascularization 98,
    589–94, *590*